Disorders
of the
Respiratory Tract
in Children

by 29 Authorities

Edited by

EDWIN L. KENDIG, Jr., M.D., (1911-

Professor of Pediatrics, Medical
College of Virginia; Director of Child
Chest Clinics, Medical College
of Virginia Hospitals, Richmond

W. B. SAUNDERS COMPANY

Philadelphia and London, 1967

W. B. Saunders Company: West Washington Square,
Philadelphia, Pa. 19105

12 Dyott Street
London, W.C.1

DISORDERS OF THE RESPIRATORY TRACT
IN CHILDREN

For

Emily, Randolph and Corbin

Contributors

WILLIAM CURTIS ADAMS, M.D. Associate Professor of Pediatrics, University of Miami School of Medicine. Attending Pediatrician, Variety Children's Hospital, Jackson Memorial Hospital and Doctors Hospital, Miami, Florida.

GAYLE G. ARNOLD, M.D. Assistant Clinical Professor of Pediatrics, Medical College of Virginia, Richmond, Virginia.

MARY ELLEN AVERY, M.D. Eudowood Associate Professor of Pulmonary Diseases of Children, Johns Hopkins Medical School, Baltimore, Maryland.

JAMES W. BROOKS, M.D. Associate Professor of Surgery, Medical College of Virginia. Attending Surgeon, Division of Cardiac and Thoracic Surgery, Medical College of Virginia and McGuire Veterans Administration Hospitals, Richmond, Virginia.

VICTOR CHERNICK, M.D. Assistant Professor of Pediatrics, Johns Hopkins Medical School, Baltimore, Maryland.

AMOS CHRISTIE, M.D. Professor and Chairman, Department of Pediatrics, Vanderbilt University School of Medicine. Pediatrician-in-Chief, Vanderbilt University Hospital, Nashville, Tennessee.

HENRY G. CRAMBLETT, M.D. Professor of Pediatrics, and Professor and Chairman, Department of Medical Microbiology, Ohio State University College of Medicine. Chief of Infectious Diseases Section, Children's Hospital, Columbus, Ohio.

SUSAN C. DEES, M.D. Professor of Pediatrics (Allergy), Duke University School of Medicine. Assistant Pediatrician and Director of Pediatric Allergy, Duke University Medical Center; Consultant in Pediatric Allergy, Watts Hospital, Durham, North Carolina.

CHARLES F. FERGUSON, M.D. Instructor in Otolaryngology, Harvard Medical School. Otolaryngologist, Children's Hospital Medical Center; Consultant, New England and Boston Lying-in Hospitals, Boston, Massachusetts.

VINCENT V. HAMPARIAN, Ph.D. Associate Professor of Pediatrics and Medical Microbiology, Ohio State University College of Medicine, Columbus, Ohio.

G. DOUGLAS HAYDEN, M.D. Clinical Professor, Department of Otolaryngology, Medical College of Virginia, Richmond, Virginia.

DOUGLAS C. HEINER, M.D. Associate Professor of Pediatrics, University of Utah College of Medicine. Associate Physician, University of Utah Medical Center; Consultant, Primary Children's Hospital, Salt Lake City, Utah.

ROBERT H. HIGH, M.D. Chairman, Department of Pediatrics, Henry Ford Hospital, Detroit, Michigan.

WILLIAM A. HOWARD, M.D. Professor and Chairman, Department of Pediatrics, George Washington University Medical School. Chief of Allergy Division, and Senior Attending Physician, Children's Hospital; Consultant in Pediatrics, Walter Reed Army Hospital, Washington, D.C.

EDWIN L. KENDIG, Jr., M.D. Professor of Pediatrics, Medical College of Virginia. Director of Child Chest Clinic, Medical College of Virginia Hospitals, Richmond, Virginia.

v

WILLIAM E. LAUPUS, M.D. Professor
and Chairman, Department of Pediatrics,
Medical College of Virginia. Director of
Pediatrics, Medical College of Virginia
Hospitals, Richmond, Virginia.

ROSA LEE NEMIR, M.D. Professor of
Pediatrics, New York University School of
Medicine. Attending Physician, and Direc-
tor of Children's Chest Clinic, Bellevue
Hospital; Attending Pediatrician, Uni-
versity Hospital, New York University
Medical Center, New York, New York.

ROBERT H. PARROTT, M.D. Professor of
Pediatrics, Georgetown University School
of Medicine. Director, Children's Hospital
and Research Foundation of Children's
Hospital, Washington, D.C.

PETER N. PASTORE, M.D. Professor and
Chairman, Department of Otology, Rhin-
ology, Laryngology, Audiology and Speech,
Medical College of Virginia. Attending
Physician and Consultant, Medical Col-
lege of Virginia Hospitals, Crippled Chil-
dren's Hospital, Richmond Eye, Ear, Nose
and Throat Hospital, Richmond Memorial
Hospital, St. Mary's Hospital and McGuire
Veterans Hospital, Richmond, Virginia.

E. O. R. REYNOLDS, M.B. Lecturer in
Paediatrics, University College Hospital,
London, England.

ARNOLD M. SALZBERG, M.D. Associate
Professor of Surgery, Medical College of
Virginia. Attending Pediatric Surgeon,
Medical College of Virginia Hospitals;
Attending Thoracic Surgeon, Medical
College of Virginia and McGuire Veter-
ans Administration Hospitals, Richmond,
Virginia.

JOHN H. SEABURY, M.D. Professor of
Medicine, Louisiana State University
School of Medicine. Senior Visiting Phy-
sician, and Director of the Lung Station,
Charity Hospital of Louisiana, New Or-
leans, Louisiana.

HARRY SHWACHMAN, M.D. Clinical
Professor of Pediatrics, Harvard Medical
School. Chief of Laboratory of Clinical
Pathology, and Senior Associate in Medi-
cine, Children's Hospital Medical Center,
Boston, Massachusetts.

LEROY SMITH, M.D. Associate Clinical
Professor of Surgery, and Associate Professor of Oral Surgery, Medical College of
Virginia. Director of Plastic Surgery, Crippled Children's Bureau of State of Virginia, Richmond, Virginia.

MARGARET H. D. SMITH, M.D. Pro-
fessor of Pediatrics and Epidemiology,
Tulane University School of Medicine.
Visiting Physician, Charity Hospital of
Louisiana, New Orleans, Louisiana.

MILDRED T. STAHLMAN, M.D. Associate
Professor of Pediatrics, Vanderbilt University School of Medicine. Vanderbilt
Hospital, in charge of Newborn and Premature Nurseries, Nashville, Tennessee.

SAMUEL STONE, M.D. Professor of Clin-
ical Pediatrics, New York University
School of Medicine. Visiting Physician,
Bellevue Hospital; Attending Pediatrician,
University Hospital, New York, New York.

J. A. PETER TURNER, M.D. Assistant
Professor of Pediatrics, Faculty of Medi-
cine, University of Toronto. Physician-in-
Charge of Chest Service, Hospital for Sick
Children, Toronto, Ontario, Canada.

WILLIAM W. WARING, M.D. Professor
of Pediatrics, and Lecturer in Physiology,
Tulane University School of Medicine.
Attending Physician, Charity Hospital of
Louisiana, New Orleans, Louisiana.

Foreword

Physicians who care for children have come to recognize that there is nothing pathognomonic about the lesions noted in the chest roentgenogram of a child. Cavity-like lesions, even with fluid levels, may be pneumatoceles, blebs or cysts, infiltrations may be pyogenic or mycotic, and adenopathy may be malignant or inflammatory. Only when these shadows are interpreted with the knowledge gained by a good history, careful and repeated physical examination, appropriate skin testing and microbiological and pathologic studies and when they are correlated with size, location and extent do they represent our best and most reliable means for an early and accurate diagnosis of chest disease in children.

These facts pinpoint some of the differences between adult and childhood disease, not only of the chest, but in other organ systems as well. In pediatrics we deal not with little men and little women, but with individuals who are in a state of constant growth and development. A shadow of certain size or shape may be normal today, but no longer normal tomorrow. As a matter of fact, it may not even be present in the next phase of respiration. This makes our work frustrating and difficult, but always challenging and interesting. In pediatrics we deal with diseases in which hereditary factors play a large part. Certain results of infection or injury at birth are common. Immunologic immaturity with susceptibility to infection is obvious to the skilled physician. Congenital defects are probably more frequent. Examples of anatomic, physiologic and immunologic differences are a part of our everyday thinking. To

the chest physician hemoptysis in a 35-year-old woman has a certain meaning, but the meaning is entirely different when the patient is a three-year-old with anemia and hepatosplenomegaly.

John Caffey writes learnedly and well as he epitomizes our dilemma and challenge: "The physician needs to know intimately each living patient through whom the racing black light darts, flashes hidden depths to reveal them in a glowing mirage of thin images, each cast delicately in its own halo, but all veiled and blended endlessly."

This statement seems to me to highlight much of our effort, and particularly that of Dr. Kendig, as it applies to the early and accurate diagnosis of chest disease in children. We are likely to depend too much on modern gadgetry or on the roentgenogram. It is obviously unfair to the radiologist for the pediatrician to request a chest x-ray, noting that the patient has had "cough" and neglecting the result of skin tests or the clinical history. Since the pediatric roentgenologist cannot examine the patient, he should have the advantages afforded the clinician in regard to the family history, the past history, the effect of the disease on growth and development, the findings on physical examination, and the available skin test information. As clinicians we should not attempt to become roentgenologists. On the other hand, the pediatrician should utilize the roentgenogram as another laboratory method to become a better clinician.

This, I believe, is what Dr. Kendig has tried to do in this volume. A distinguished clinician, he has devoted much of his professional life to the study of chest disease in infants and children. He has brought together in this timely volume all that is currently known of those conditions of the chest which are unique to the pediatric age group. He has done this always with the practitioner in mind because he is a practitioner of pediatrics himself. He has carefully selected a group of distinguished collaborators to produce a volume which contains all our newer knowledge in this important field.

As a long-time friend and collaborator, we wish Dr. Kendig and the book every success. We are certain that it will be useful.

AMOS CHRISTIE, M.D.

Preface

Although the past two decades have seen striking developments in the diagnosis and treatment of respiratory tract disorders in children, there has heretofore been no textbook on the subject which might be considered comprehensive and authoritative. We have attempted to meet this need.

The standard textbooks on pediatrics give consideration to the various respiratory tract disorders, but because of space limitation, discussion in real depth is not possible. The present volume, representing the collaborative effort of a number of experienced authorities, was designed and developed to provide an answer to almost any question about respiratory tract diseases in children raised by the practitioner, resident or intern in pediatrics, the chest physician, the roentgenologist, or by the medical student or general practitioner.

In ascribing credit to the many who helped make the book possible, I must naturally speak first of the contributors. Busy people all, and yet they responded vigorously and with dedication to their assignments. For having made my task so much less wearisome than it might have been they have my everlasting gratitude.

I am grateful to Dr. John Chapman, Dr. Rosa Lee Nemir and Dr. Donald Brummer, who have generously read and criticized specific chapters of the book.

Particular gratitude is due Dr. William Laupus, who has read almost the entire manuscript and contributed much valuable advice, and to Dr. Amos Christie, contributor and friend of many years, who wrote the Foreword. Dr. John Kirkpatrick contributed many of the chest roentgenograms, Dr. Richard Lester reviewed some of the other chest x-rays, Dr. Louis Siltzbach provided helpful advice, and Mr. Melvin Shaffer arranged for the preparation of some of the illustrations. Dr. Pinson Neal kindly assisted in the interpretation of many of the x-ray photographs included in Chapters 44 and 67 and provided legends for them. Over the years Dr. Frederick Mandeville has aided in the interpretation of x-ray films for the Medical College of Virginia Child Chest Clinic, some of which appear in this volume.

Mrs. Nellie Gentry has been most helpful in assembling the case material contained in several of the chapters, and Mrs. Nell W. Pargoe and Miss Mary Ellen Brannan have assisted with the proofreading and typing of the manuscripts.

Grateful acknowledgment is made to the staff of the W. B. Saunders Company for their cooperation and assistance.

EDWIN L. KENDIG, JR.

Contents

xi

SECTION VI   GENERAL CONSIDERATIONS IN INFECTIONS OF THE UPPER AND LOWER RESPIRATORY TRACTS

Chapter Eleven

Henry G. Cramblett, M.D.

SECTION VII   INFECTIONS OF THE UPPER RESPIRATORY TRACT

Chapter Twelve

Henry G. Cramblett, M.D.

Chapter Thirteen

Henry G. Cramblett, M.D.

Chapter Fourteen

William E. Laupus, M.D.

Chapter Fifteen

Charles F. Ferguson, M.D.

SECTION IX NONINFECTIOUS DISORDERS OF THE LOWER RESPIRATORY TRACT

Chapter Thirty-One

William Curtis Adams, M.D.

Chapter Thirty-Two

William Curtis Adams, M.D.

Chapter Thirty-Three

William A. Howard, M.D.

Chapter Thirty-Four

Edwin L. Kendig, Jr., M.D.

Chapter Thirty-Five

William Curtis Adams, M.D.

Chapter Thirty-Six

Robert H. High, M.D.

Chapter Thirty-Seven

Douglas C. Heiner, M.D.

SECTION X OTHER DISEASES WITH A PROMINENT RESPIRATORY COMPONENT

Chapter Forty-Eight

Amos Christie, M.D.

Chapter Forty-Nine

Robert H. High, M.D.

Chapter Fifty

Robert H. High, M.D.

Chapter Fifty-One

Robert H. High, M.D.

Chapter Fifty-Two

Edwin L. Kendig, Jr., M.D.

Chapter Fifty-Three

Edwin L. Kendig, Jr., M.D.

SECTION I

The Functional Basis
of Respiratory Pathology

CHAPTER ONE

The Functional Basis of Respiratory Pathology

VICTOR CHERNICK, M.D.,
and MARY ELLEN AVERY, M.D.

A knowledge of normal function is fundamental in considering the effect of pathologic processes on the patient. Over the past twenty-five years pulmonary physiology has been undergoing a revolution in concepts and terminology. As in most revolutions, there have been stages of confusion which precede stages of clarification. Agreement on terminology which ended one aspect of confusion was achieved by a committee of American pulmonary physiologists in 1950. The increasing use of classical physical and engineering concepts has added another order of clarity. And finally, technological advances have increased the precision and availability of measurements of blood gases, pressures and flows, for example, so that functional evaluations are widely available to clinicians.

When tools are available, and physiologic principles elucidated, the translation of the new findings and their ultimate application in illness become the task and obligation of the clinician. The purpose of this opening section of a volume on disorders of the respiratory tract in children is to attempt the translation of relevant physiologic concepts. The principles involved are straightforward. The terminology, once defined, is logical. It is our belief that the physician will find the differential diagnosis of pulmonary problems and the rationale of therapy immensely simplified once he approaches a problem with the question: What is the nature of the functional derangement? Quantification of the functional derangement is most helpful in the evaluation of therapy and in documenting the course of chronic pulmonary diseases.

DEFINITIONS AND SYMBOLS

The principal variables for gases are as follows:

V = gas volume
P = pressure
F = fractional concentration in dry gas
R = respiratory exchange ratio, $\dot{V}$ carbon dioxide/$\dot{V}$ oxygen
f = frequency
D_L = diffusing capacity of lung

The designation of which volume or pressure is cited requires a small capital letter after the principal variable. Thus V_{O_2} = volume of oxygen; P_B = barometric pressure.

I = inspired gas T = tidal gas
E = expired gas D = dead space gas
A = alveolar gas B = barometric pressure

When both location of the gas and its species are to be indicated, the order is $V_{I_{O_2}}$ which means the volume of inspired oxygen. A dot above any symbol represents an amount per unit of time, the $\dot{V}_E$ = amount of air expired per minute.

S.T.P.D. = standard temperature, pressure, dry (0°C., 760 mm. Hg)
B.T.P.S. = body temperature, pressure, saturated with water vapor

A.T.P.S. = ambient temperature, pressure, saturated with water vapor

The principal designations for blood are as follows:

S = percentage saturation of gas in blood
C = content of gas per 100 ml. of blood
Q = volume of blood
Q̇ = blood flow per minute
a = arterial
v̄ = mixed venous
c = capillary

All sites of blood determinations are indicated by lower case initials. Thus Pa_{CO_2} = partial pressure of carbon dioxide in arterial blood. $P\bar{v}_{O_2}$ = partial pressure of oxygen in mixed venous blood. Pc_{O_2} = partial pressure of oxygen in a capillary. (Standardization of definitions and symbols in respiratory physiology is from *Federation Proceedings*, 9:602-605, 1950.)

PROPERTIES OF GASES

Gases behave as an enormous number of tiny particles in constant motion. Their behavior is governed by the gas laws, which are essential to the understanding of pulmonary physiology.

DALTON'S LAW. This law states that the total pressure exerted by a gas mixture is equal to the sum of the pressures of the individual gases. The pressure exerted by each component is independent of the other gases in the mixture. For instance, at sea level, air saturated with water vapor at a temperature of 37° C. has a total pressure equal to the atmospheric pressure (P_B = 30 inches of mercury or 760 mm. Hg), with the partial pressures of the components as follows:
P_B = 760 mm. Hg = P_{H_2O} (47 mm. Hg) + P_{O_2} (149.2 mm. Hg) + P_{N_2} (563.5 mm. Hg) + P_{CO_2} (0.3 mm. Hg).

The gas in alveoli contains 5.6 per cent carbon dioxide, B.T.P.S. If P_B = 760 mm. Hg, then:

$$P_{A_{CO_2}} = 0.056 \ (760 - 47) = 40 \text{ mm. Hg.}$$

The terms "partial pressure" and "tension" are interchangeable for gases.

BOYLE'S LAW states that at constant temperature the volume of any gas varies inversely as the pressure to which the gas is subjected: $PV = k$. Since respiratory volume

measurements may be made at different barometric pressures, it is important to know the barometric pressure, and convert to standard pressure, which is considered to be 760 mm. Hg.

CHARLES'S LAW states that if the pressure is constant, the volume of a gas increases in direct proportion to the absolute temperature (−273° C.). At absolute zero, molecular motion ceases. With increasing temperature molecular collisions increase, so that at constant pressure, volume must increase.

In all respiratory calculations water vapor pressure must be taken into account. The partial pressure of water vapor increases with temperature, but is independent of atmospheric pressure. At body temperature (37° C.), fully saturated gas has P_{H_2O} = 47 mm. Hg.

Gases may exist in physical solution in a liquid, escape from the liquid, or return to it. At equilibrium the partial pressure of a gas in a liquid medium exposed to a gas phase is equal in the two phases (Henry's Law). Note that in blood the sum of the partial pressures of all the gases does not necessarily equal atmospheric pressure. For example, in venous blood: P_{O_2} has fallen from the 100 mm. Hg of the arterial blood to 40 mm., while P_{CO_2} changes from 40 to 46 mm. Hg. Thus the sum of the partial pressures of O_2, CO_2 and N_2 in venous blood equals 655 mm. Hg.

HENRY'S LAW OF DIFFUSION. The diffusion rate for gases in a liquid phase is directly proportional to their solubility coefficients. For example, in water:

$$\frac{\text{Solubility of } CO_2}{\text{Solubility of } O_2} = \frac{0.592}{0.0244} = \frac{24.3}{1}.$$

Therefore carbon dioxide diffuses more than twenty-four times as fast as oxygen.

The diffusion rate of a gas in the gas phase is inversely proportional to $\sqrt{\text{molecular weight}}$ (Graham's Law). Therefore, in the gas phase:

$$\frac{\text{rate for } CO_2}{\text{rate for } O_2} = 0.85.$$

That is, carbon dioxide diffuses slower in the gas phase than oxygen.

Combining Henry's and Graham's Laws for a system with both a gas phase and a liquid phase, e.g. alveolus and blood: carbon dioxide diffuses (24.3 × 0.85 or) 20.7 times as fast as oxygen.

LUNG MORPHOLOGY AND GROWTH

Some aspects of lung growth and morphology are relevant and indeed necessary to the understanding of lung function. For example, the prematurely born infant's survival may be limited by the inability of the lung to distend adequately, retain air at the end of expiration, or be perfused with sufficient blood to permit gas exchange.

Embryology and Histology

The lung arises as an outpouching of gut at twenty-four days, and undergoes progressive bronchial proliferation in the first weeks of fetal life. Inductive interaction between epithelium and mesenchyme occurs. Epithelium, isolated in vitro, does not undergo morphogenesis; when it is recombined with pulmonary mesenchyme, development resumes. Branching proceeds chiefly by a heightened mitotic activity in the epithelium compared with that of the mesenchyme. The mesenchyme differentiates into cartilage, smooth muscle and connective tis-

sue around the epithelial tubes. By the sixteenth week the lung has its full complement of bronchial generations. Bronchial generations are fewer in the upper lobes and more numerous in the lower lobes, where there are twenty-five segmental branches. Before the sixteenth week the glandular appearance of passages lined with cuboidal epithelium predominates. From the sixteenth to the twenty-fourth week a canalicular phase predominates, and thereafter clusters of terminal air spaces with attenuated epithelium appear (Fig. 1). After birth, respiratory passages elongate. It is not until the sixth to eighth week of postnatal life that typical sharply curved alveoli can be identified.

The internal surface of the airways is lined by cells in all phases of lung development. The trachea and bronchi are lined by pseudostratified epithelium of four types: ciliated cells (present from the tenth week), goblet cells (found first at thirteen to fourteen weeks), brush cells, and a short (basal) cell. The bronchioles contain ciliated cells, but here the goblet cells are replaced by another columnar cell with small apical secretory droplets. The last cells to appear in lung develop-

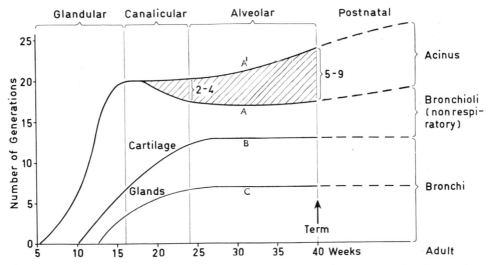

FIGURE 1–1. Intrauterine development of the bronchial tree. Line *A* represents the number of bronchial generations, and *A'* the respiratory bronchioles and alveolar ducts. *B* is the extension of cartilage along the bronchial tree, and *C* the extension of mucous glands. (From U. Bucher and L. Reid: *Thorax*, 16:267, 1961.)

ment are those most specific to the lung, and farthest removed from the pharyngeal area. They are the lining cells of the most terminal air spaces, which are first evident in the sixth month of gestation. At least two types of alveolar lining cells can be distinguished: one an attenuated epithelial cell which may have cytoplasmic continuity with cuboidal cells of the bronchiole (type I cell), the other a more granular cell with many mitochondria, osmiophilic inclusions, Golgi apparatus and other organelles (type II cell). Both alveolar cells rest on a continuous basement membrane (Fig. 2). Macrophages may also be seen fixed to the cell wall or free in the lumen, and these are presumably the cells which can be seen with the light microscope and found by the millions in sputum. Their relation to the granular alveolar lining cell or type II cell remains uncertain.

The larger airways are rich in mucous glands from early development. Acid mucopolysaccharides are abundant in the trachea of an eighteen-week fetus, and persist through the first year of life in relatively greater amount than found in adults.

The pulmonary artery arises from aortic arches and nourishes the lung bud. Capillary proliferation becomes most abundant at twenty-six to twenty-eight weeks of gestation, and it is during this phase of development that the lung becomes the most vascular of all organs of the body. Before that time the pulmonary vascular bed is not able to accommodate the whole of the cardiac output, and it is reasonable to consider the maintenance of life, dependent on the lung for gas exchange, not possible before the stage of capillary proliferation.

Fetal Lung at Term

The fetal lung contains a liquid which differs in composition from blood and amniotic liquid, and therefore is thought to be a secretory product of the lung itself. The pH is about 6.4, the bicarbonate concentration is lower than that of plasma, and hydrogen ion concentration greater. Its protein content is about 300 mg. per 100 ml. The amount of liquid in the fetal lung increases during gestation until at term it is estimated to approximate a functional residual capacity, about 10 to 25 ml. per kilogram of body weight.

The assessment of lung function in early stages of development is based chiefly on measurements in lambs, which provides insight into the direction of changes with time, although exact analogies to the human subject are hazardous. The distensibility of the lung early in gestation is much less than at term. When peak volumes are expressed as milliliters per gram of lung tissue, it is evident that the potential air space is small with respect to lung mass. The ability to retain air at end-expiration, which depends on the presence of the pulmonary surfactant, is not evident until later in the cannicular stage of development. In the lamb it is at 120 to 130 days of a 147-day gestation. In the human being it is probably about the twentieth to twenty-fourth week of gestation, with a wide scatter. The distensibility of the vascular bed likewise increases with fetal age. Little blood flow is possible even at high perfusion pressures in the early fetal lung. As term approaches, the capacity and distensibility of the vascular bed increase. The morphologic counterpart of these changes is seen in the greater wall-lumen ratios in the fetal lung compared to those in postnatal life. After about ten days of extrauterine life the lumens are wider, regardless of the time of birth. The events of birth have little effect on other aspects of lung development, including histochemical changes.

It is useful to remember that the lung has the most abundant lymphatics of any organ of the body. They are located beneath the pulmonary pleura, in perivascular and peribronchial connective tissue sheaths, and within the bronchial walls. They do not form a network around the alveoli, although their endings are within a few microns of the terminal air sacs. They form a plexiform network with sim-

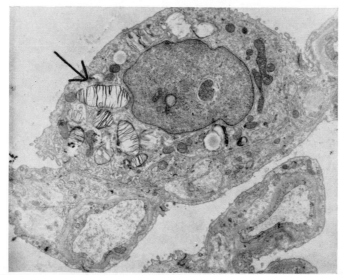

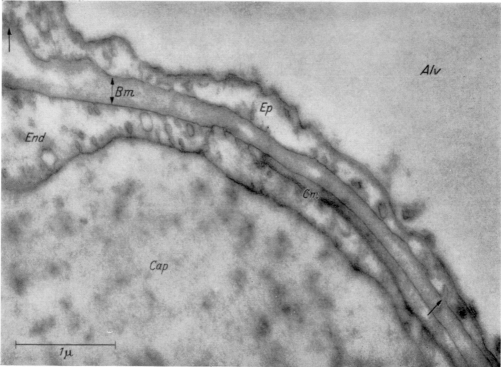

FIGURE 1–2. *Upper,* Electron micrograph of one type of cell which lines the alveolus. This particular cell is from a dog's lung, but is similar to those found in all mammalian lungs. The air space is in the upper portion of the figure. The arrow points to the osmiophilic inclusions that are thought to be associated with the alveolar lining substance. The cell rests on a basement membrane that separates it from the capillary endothelium in the lower part of the picture. (Photograph courtesy of E. S. Boatman and H. B. Martin, University of Washington Medical School, Seattle, Washington.)

Lower, Normal human lung showing the attenuated alveolar cytoplasm. Abbreviations: *Alv,* alveolus; *Ep,* cytoplasmic layer of an epithelial cell; *Bm,* basement membrane; *End,* capillary endothelium; *Cm,* erythrocyte cell membrane; *Cap,* capillary. (Published with permission from H. Schulz: *The Submicroscopic Anatomy and Pathology of the Lung.* Berlin, Springer-Verlag, 1959.)

ple valves which direct flow centripetally. The vessels gain in connective tissue and smooth muscle near the pulmonary hilus and resemble the thoracic duct. They form a closed system and are the main pathway for removal of fine particulate matter and protein from air spaces. Aggregates of lymphoid tissue are located along the bronchi, particularly at sites of branching, but lymph nodes are found chiefly at lobar bronchial branches.

Postnatal Lung

The postnatal growth of the lung continues until approximately eight years of

A

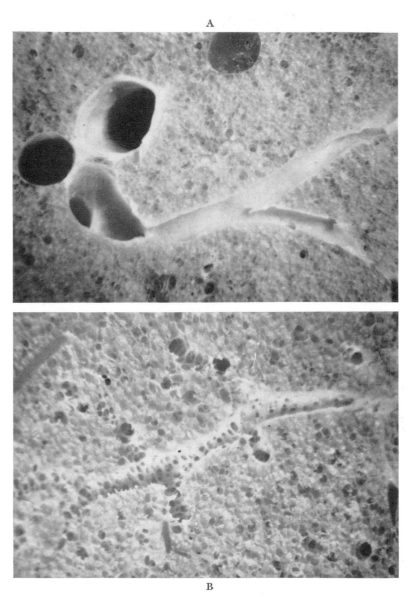

B

FIGURE 1–3. The architecture of the lung. *A*, Fresh frozen cat lung (4×). Segmental cartilaginous bronchus and branches. The pulmonary artery is close to the airway; the pulmonary vein is in a more peripheral location. *B*, Fresh frozen cat lung (4×). Terminal bronchiole with many alveolar ducts arising from it.   (*See facing page for continuation of Figure 1–3.*)

age, with an increase in numbers of alveoli and the dimensions of all the air spaces. Some further increase in dimensions of terminal air spaces may proceed to forty years of age. The lung of the newborn infant is not the miniature of the adult; tracheal diameter approximately triples, alveolar dimensions increase about fourfold, and alveolar numbers increase about tenfold, while body mass increases some twentyfold. The obvious advantage of relatively large airways is to facilitate the movement of air. The relatively smaller alveoli permit a larger surface

C

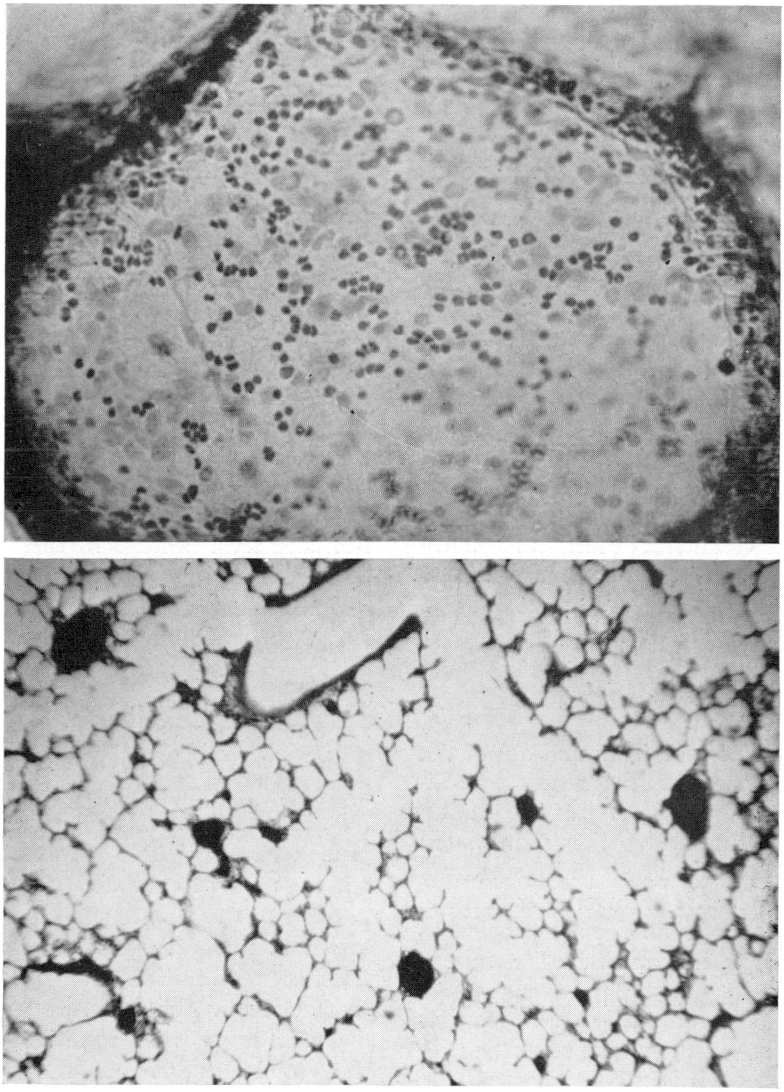

D

FIGURE 1–3. *Continued.* C, Thick section of cat lung (100×). A single alveolar wall is in the plane of focus. Individual red cells in alveolar capillaries are clearly seen. *D*, Guinea pig (15×), fixed thin section. The terminal respiratory unit, with alveoli shown as outpouchings of the alveolar duct, arises from the terminal bronchiole at the top of the picture. Note that 3 vessels, probably pulmonary veins, mark the distal boundaries of the unit. (Reproduced by permission of Dr. Norman Staub, University of California Medical Center, San Francisco. All but *A* appeared in color in *Anesthesiology*, 24:831-54, 1963.)

area per volume of lung, which is essential for gas transfer. Indeed, the internal surface area of the lung bears a close relation to body mass, approximately 1 square meter per kilogram of body weight, which would appear to be a useful design to permit the area for gas exchange to follow changes in amounts of metabolizing tissue.

Other gross anatomic relations of the infant's and child's lung are similar to those of the adult (Figs. 3, 4). The proportion of total lung weight represented by each lobe is remarkably constant from infancy to adulthood. Average values of lung lobe weight expressed as a percentage of total and based on a study of normal human lungs are as follows: right upper lobe 19.52; right middle lobe 8.34; right lower lobe 25.26; left upper lobe 22.48; left lower lobe 24.61. Lobular septa are better developed in the apical regions of the lung and beneath sharp margins than they are near the costal or lateral surfaces and lower lobes. It has been suggested that those areas with many septa would have less collateral ventilation, and hence be more susceptible to atelectasis. Collateral ventilatory pathways, the alveolar pores of Kohn, are also fewer in number in the infant's lung, and increase with advancing age.

Muscles of Respiration

The movement of air in and out of the lungs in normal breathing requires an increase and decrease in size of the thorax which is achieved by the coordinated movements of the muscles which surround it. Their geometric arrangements and the details of their action are so complex as to defy thorough analysis at this time.

The diaphragm is the principal muscle of respiration; however, it is not essential for breathing in the awake state. During deep anesthesia it is essential because the other muscles of respiration become inactive. Its contraction causes descent of its dome, and aids in elevation of the lower ribs in adults. In infants with a very compliant rib cage, descent of the diaphragm may oppose elevation of the lower ribs and

result in subcostal retractions. The force exerted by the diaphragm during maximal inspiration in adults is about 100 cm. of water when its fibers shorten by about 50 per cent of their initial length. Its motor innervation is from the third to fifth cervical roots through the phrenic nerve.

The main portion of the intercostal muscles is arranged to facilitate inspiration by elevating the lower ribs. Contraction of the external intercostals occurs in inspiration; the internal intercostals are active chiefly in expiration. If the intercostals alone are paralyzed, there is little decrease in exercise tolerance.

The abdominal muscles are the most powerful muscles of expiration. The external and internal oblique muscles compress the abdomen, flex the trunk, and help to depress the lower ribs. The recti draw the lower rib cage toward the pubis and further decrease abdominal volume. In most normal subjects there is no participation of the abdominal muscles in quiet breathing. In some persons the abdominal muscles contract at end-inspiration and set a limit to further expansion of the lung.

The scalenes act to elevate the first two ribs even in quiet breathing. Elevation of the sternum is achieved by contraction of the sternocleidomastoid muscles; they are not usually active in quiet breathing in adults. When inspiratory efforts are marked, their activity is significant; in fact, they are considered the most important accessory muscles of inspiration. Elevation and prominence of the upper portion of the sternum is a common observation in infants with respiratory distress, presumably from contraction of the sternocleidomastoid muscles.

Other muscles of respiration include the costal levators and the suprahyoid group. The latter probably stabilize the trachea and larynx when during deep inspiration the descent of the diaphragm acts to draw the lung caudad. It can readily be shown that although the hili do descend slightly during deep inspiration, the larynx barely moves. The action of the sacrospinalis, trapezius, pectorals, and serratus anterior and posterior superior is to enlarge the thorax; the posterior inferior serratus decreases thoracic volume.

Some additional accessory muscles aid inspiration by reducing the resistance to airflow in the upper airway. These in-

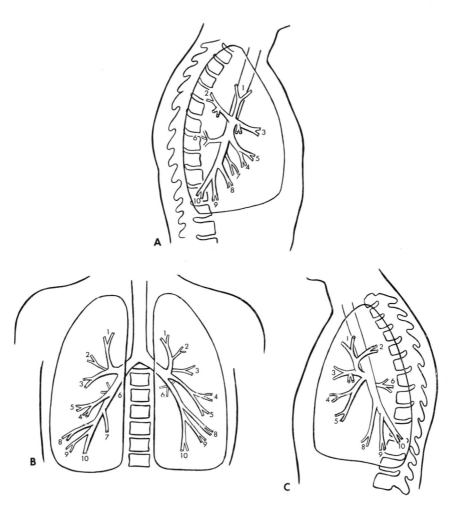

FIGURE 1–4. The nomenclature of bronchopulmonary anatomy, adapted from report by the Thoracic Society in 1950. (Adapted from Negus.)

Right lung
Upper lobe
1. Apical
2. Posterior
3. Anterior
Middle lobe
4. Lateral
5. Medial
Lower lobe
6. Apical
7. Cardiac (medial basal)
8. Anterior ⎫
9. Lateral ⎬ basal
10. Posterior ⎭

Left lung
Upper lobe
1. ⎫
2. ⎬ Apicoposterior

3. Anterior
4. ⎫
5. ⎬ Lingula
Lower lobe
6. Apical
7. —— absent
8. Anterior ⎫
9. Lateral ⎬ basal
10. Posterior ⎭

clude the alae nasi, cheek muscles, platysma, and tongue muscles.

LUNG VOLUMES

Nomenclature

The partition of lung volumes and the nomenclature can be appreciated from Figure 5. The spirogram on the right is a tracing from a rotating drum marked by an ink writer attached to a spirometer.

The concept of lung volumes and capacities, rather than a single volume, derives from the fact that sometimes more or less air is moved, some air is always present in normal lungs, and it is useful to apply labels to the portions of the total gas volume which are under discussion. For example, if it is desired to study lung growth with age, a measure of total lung capacity is appropriate. (A capacity is more than one lung volume.) If an index of the degree of overexpansion of the lungs in chronic lower airway obstructive disease is desired, either the functional residual capacity or residual volume would be helpful. If a patient has a restriction to lung expansion from thoracic disease or a pulmonary fibrotic process, the pertinent measurement would be the largest breath he is capable of taking or his vital capacity.

Methods of Measurement

The tidal volume, inspiratory and expiratory volumes and vital capacity can be measured by asking a patient to breathe quietly, and then take in the biggest possible breath and blow it all out.

The measurement of functional residual capacity and residual volume requires another approach. Since both include the air in the lungs which the patient does

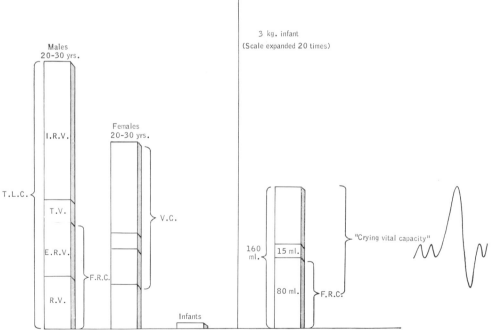

FIGURE 1–5. The lung volumes. A volume is a single subdivision; a capacity is more than one subdivision. Abbreviations: *T.L.C.*, total lung capacity (6 liters in an average male, 4.2 liters in an average female); *I.R.V.*, inspiratory reserve volume; *T.V.*, tidal volume; *E.R.V.*, expiratory reserve volume; *R.V.*, residual volume; *F.R.C.*, functional residual capacity. The spirogram shown on the right is a tracing from a revolving drum attached to a water-filled spirometer. T.V., I.R.V., E.R.V. and vital capacity can be measured from such a tracing.

not normally exhale, they must be measured indirectly. One method uses the principle of dilution of the unknown volume with a known concentration of a gas which is foreign to the lung and only sparingly absorbed, such as helium. The patient breathes from a container with a known volume and concentration of helium in oxygen-enriched air. After sufficient time has elapsed for the gas in his

Table 1. *Normal Values for Lung Volumes (Liters)*

Height Cm.	Males			Females		
	VC	FRC	TLC	VC	FRC	TLC
92	0.68	0.38	0.88	0.66	0.41	0.88
94	0.72	0.40	0.94	0.70	0.44	0.93
96	0.77	0.43	1.00	0.74	0.47	0.99
98	0.82	0.46	1.07	0.79	0.50	1.05
100	0.87	0.49	1.14	0.84	0.54	1.12
102	0.93	0.53	1.21	0.89	0.57	1.18
104	0.98	0.56	1.28	0.94	0.61	1.25
106	1.04	0.60	1.36	0.99	0.64	1.32
108	1.10	0.64	1.44	1.05	0.68	1.40
110	1.16	0.68	1.52	1.11	0.72	1.47
112	1.23	0.72	1.60	1.17	0.76	1.55
114	1.30	0.76	1.69	1.23	0.81	1.63
116	1.37	0.81	1.78	1.29	0.85	1.72
118	1.44	0.85	1.88	1.36	0.90	1.81
120	1.52	0.90	1.98	1.43	0.95	1.90
122	1.59	0.95	2.08	1.50	1.00	1.99
124	1.67	1.01	2.19	1.57	1.05	2.09
126	1.76	1.06	2.29	1.65	1.10	2.19
128	1.84	1.12	2.41	1.73	1.16	2.29
130	1.93	1.18	2.52	1.81	1.22	2.40
132	2.02	1.24	2.64	1.89	1.28	2.50
134	2.12	1.30	2.77	1.97	1.34	2.62
136	2.21	1.36	2.89	2.06	1.40	2.73
138	2.31	1.43	3.03	2.15	1.47	2.85
140	2.42	1.50	3.16	2.24	1.54	2.97
142	2.52	1.57	3.30	2.34	1.61	3.10
144	2.63	1.65	3.44	2.43	1.68	3.23
146	2.74	1.72	3.59	2.53	1.75	3.36
148	2.86	1.80	3.74	2.64	1.83	3.49
150	2.98	1.88	3.90	2.74	1.91	3.63
152	3.10	1.97	4.06	2.85	1.99	3.78
154	3.23	2.05	4.22	2.96	2.07	3.92
156	3.35	2.14	4.39	3.07	2.16	4.07
158	3.49	2.24	4.57	3.19	2.25	4.23
160	3.62	2.33	4.74	3.31	2.34	4.38
162	3.76	2.43	4.93	3.43	2.43	4.54
164	3.90	2.53	5.11	3.56	2.53	4.71
166	4.05	2.63	5.30	3.69	2.62	4.88
168	4.20	2.74	5.50	3.82	2.72	5.05
170	4.35	2.85	5.70	3.95	2.83	5.23
172	4.51	2.96	5.91	4.09	2.93	5.41
174	4.67	3.07	6.12	4.23	3.04	5.59
176	4.83	3.19	6.34	4.37	3.15	5.78
178	5.00	3.31	6.56	4.52	3.26	5.98
180	5.17	3.44	6.78	4.67	3.38	6.17

From Cook and Hamann: *J. Pediat.*, 59:710, 1961.

lung to mix and equilibrate with the gas in the container, the concentration of helium in the container is remeasured. Since initial volume times concentration of helium equals final volume times concentration of helium, the final volume, which includes gas in the lungs, can be calculated. Correction factors can be applied for the volumes of oxygen absorbed or carbon dioxide released during the period of equilibration. Another commonly used method involves measurement of the nitrogen in the lung after it has come into equilibrium with inspired pure oxygen.

If some gas is "trapped" within the lungs, its volume will not be reflected in the helium dilution measurement. There is, however, a method of measurement of total gas volume within the thorax which depends on the change in volume which occurs with compression of the gas with the glottis closed. Practically, this measurement requires the patient to be in a body plethysmograph, and to make a forced inspiration (Mueller maneuver) or forced expiration (Valsalva maneuver) against an obstruction. The change in pressure can be measured in the mouthpiece; the change in volume can be recorded on a spirometer attached to the body plethysmograph: $V = P\Delta V/\Delta P$. This method has the advantage of being repeatable several times a minute. It has the disadvantage of including some abdominal gas in the measurement.

Interpretation

The vital capacity is one of the most valuable measurements which can be made in a functional assessment, although it cannot be interpreted without some additional knowledge of the patient. For example, it is a function of body size and correlates most closely with body height; therefore it should be expressed as a percentage of the predicted value for height (Table 1). It may be decreased by poor patient cooperation, which must be determined by the examiner. It can be decreased by a wide variety of disease processes such as weakness of the muscles of respiration, loss of lung tissue as after lobectomy, obstruction of portions of the airways, changes in lung distensibility as in fibrosis, and space-occupying materials as in effusion, edema and tumors. Thus the vital capacity is not a useful tool to discriminate between types of lesions. Its chief role is to assign a value to the degree of impairment and to document changes with therapy or in time.

The functional residual capacity or the residual volume reflects the degree of distention of lung. Overdistention is usually compensatory for partial lower airway obstruction. When the lung volume is increased, intrathoracic airways enlarge, and widespread partial obstruction may be relieved by the assumption of a large resting lung volume. The increase in the anteroposterior diameter of the chest noted in asthma or cystic fibrosis is accompanied by a large functional residual capacity. A decrease in functional residual capacity is associated with conditions in which alveolar collapse is prominent, such as hyaline membrane disease. Since clinical and roentgenographic signs permit a rough estimate of the functional residual capacity, it is rarely helpful to measure it in infants and children.

MECHANICS OF RESPIRATION

Alterations in the mechanics of breathing account for most of the respiratory complaints and many of the abnormal findings on physical examination. Shortness of breath, tachypnea, stridor, wheezing, retractions and rales are all associated with abnormal ventilatory mechanics. A cough, sometimes deliberate, sometimes involuntary, is associated with a sequence of mechanical events which accelerate the air column and exert a milking action on the tracheobronchial tree.

It is traditional, and useful, to consider mechanical events under two main categories: the static-elastic properties of the lungs and chest wall, and the flow-resistive or dynamic aspects of moving air. Changes in one category may be associated with compensatory changes in the other. Thus many diseases affect both static and dynamic behavior of the lungs. Often the principal derangement is in the elastic properties of the tissues or in the dimensions of the airways, and the treatment or alleviation of symptoms depends on distinguishing them.

Static-Elastic Forces

The lung is an elastic structure which tends to reduce its size at all volumes. It is the elastic recoil of the lung which makes it tend to pull away from the chest wall with a resultant subatmospheric pressure in the pleural "space." The word "space" refers to a potential space; in health the pleural surface of the lung is apposed to the pleura lining the chest wall, held firm by the molecular forces of the thin layers of liquid which cover the two surfaces. The subatmospheric pressure which surrounds the lung (often called negative pressure) is not the same over all surfaces of the lung. Forces are applied to the lung by supporting structures, and gravity. In general, pleural pressures are lower in the apices than the bases. The effect is exaggerated by the height of the person, and further increased during head-forward acceleration.

The elasticity of the lung depends on the structural components (although elastic fibers are not essential for normal performance), the geometry of the terminal air spaces, and the presence of an air-liquid interface. When a lung is made airless, then inflated with liquid, the elastic recoil at large volumes is less than half that of a lung inflated to the same volume with air. Thus the most significant determinant of the elastic properties of the lung is the presence of an air-liquid interface. A further demonstration of the role of the interface is the absence of subatmospheric pleural pressure in the fetus, whose lungs contain liquid, but no air. After the first few breaths pleural pressure is subatmospheric.

The increase of elastic recoil in the presence of an air-liquid interface is from the forces of surface tension. What is surface tension? When molecules are aligned at an air-liquid interface, they lack opposing molecules on one side. The intermolecular attractive forces are then unbalanced, and the resultant force tends to move molecules away from the interface. The effect is to reduce the area of the surface to a minimum. In the lungs, whose surface area in square meters approximates body weight in kilograms, the forces at the air-liquid interface operate to reduce the internal surface area of the lung, and thus augment elastic recoil. A remarkable property of the material at the alveolar interface, the alveolar lining layer or pulmonary surfactant, is the ability to achieve a high surface tension at large lung volumes, and a low tension at low volumes. It is a phospholipid-protein complex which can form insoluble folded surface films of low surface tension on compression, as can be shown on a surface film balance. The ability to achieve a low surface tension at low lung volumes tends to stabilize the air spaces and prevent their closure (Fig. 6). Lacking such a stabilizing substance or emulsifying agent, the smaller alveoli would tend to empty into the larger in accord with the Laplace relationship, which relates the pressure across a surface (P) to surface tension (T) and radius (R) of curvature. For a spherical surface, $P = \dfrac{2T}{R}$. The smaller the radius, the greater is the tendency to collapse.

The elasticity of the lung is described by measuring static volume-pressure relations. These can be done in vivo with a needle in the pleural space to record the transpulmonary pressure at known volumes; alternately, and more safely for the patient, the pressure within the esophagus can be used as an index of pleural pressure. If the changes in pressure at points of no flow are related to the resultant changes in volume, $\triangle V / \triangle P$, it is referred to as the lung compliance, a measure of the elastic recoil of the lung.

The compliance will depend on the initial lung volume from which the change

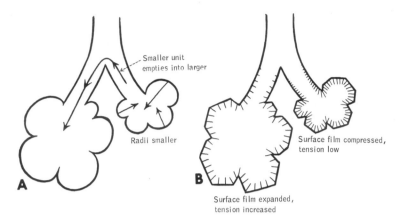

FIGURE 1–6. Schema of terminal ventilatory units and relations between size and surface tension. *A,* Effect of deficient surface film is for smaller unit to empty into larger, since radii are smaller, if surface tension of both units were the same.

$$P = \frac{2T}{r}$$

B, Effect of film is to lessen the role of different radii since surface tension (T) decreases as r decreases. The shape of alveoli tends to be polygonal rather than spherical when the surfactant is present.

in volume is measured, the ventilatory events immediately preceding the measurement, as well as the properties of the lung itself. At large lung volumes the compliance is lower, since the lung is near its elastic limit. If the subject has breathed with a fixed tidal volume for some minutes, portions of the lung are not participating in ventilation, and the compliance may be reduced. A few deep breaths, with return to the initial volume, will increase the compliance. Thus a careful description of associated events is required for interpretation of the measurement.

Changes in lung compliance occur with age (Table 2). Of course, the smaller the subject, the smaller is the change in volume, so that $\Delta V/\Delta P$ is 4 to 6 ml. per centimeter of water in infants, and 125 to 190 ml. per centimeter of water in adults. It is more relevant to a description of the elastic properties of the lung to express the compliance per unit of lung volume, such as the F.R.C. In Table 2 note that the compliance of the lung/F.R.C., or specific compliance, changes very little with age.

The elastic properties of the thorax can be measured by considering the pressure difference between pleural space or esoph-

Table 2. *Lung Compliance* *(C_L) with Age*

	ml./cm. H_2O	C_L/F.R.C.
Newborns		
3 hours	4.75 ± 1.67	0.041 ± 0.01
24 hours	6.24 ± 1.45	0.055 ± 0.01
Infants		
1 month–		
2 years	7.9	0.038
Children		
Average age		
9 years	77	0.063
Young adult		
males	184	0.050
Young adult		
females	125	0.053
Adults over		
60 years	191	0.041

agus and the atmosphere, per change in volume. At resting lung volume (F.R.C.) the elastic recoil of the thorax is equal and opposite to that of the lungs. The lungs tend to reduce their size, the thorax tends to expand.

Significant changes in thoracic compliance occur with age. In the range of normal breathing the thorax of the infant is nearly infinitely compliant. The pressures measured at different lung volumes are about the same across the lung as those measured across lung and thorax together. The functional significance of the very compliant thorax of the fetus is evident if consideration is given to the effect of an outward recoil of the thorax when the lung lacks an air-liquid interface. The fetal lung would then contain an even greater volume of liquid, which would compound the problem of the removal of lung liquid at birth. Alternately, liquid would fill the pleural space, where it would be even more difficult to resorb at birth.

With advancing age the thorax becomes relatively stiffer. Changes in volume-pressure relations are profitably considered only if referred to a reliable unit, either a unit of lung volume or a percentage of total lung capacity. When the compliance of the thorax is considered on a percentage basis, it is evident that it has a decreasing compliance with age. How

much is contributed by changes in tissue properties such as increasing calcification of ribs and connective tissue changes, and how much is a disproportionate growth of the chest wall relative to the lung remain unclear (Fig. 7).

Dynamic Forces

Most of the work of quiet breathing is used to overcome the static-elastic forces which depend on the tissue properties of lungs and thorax. About one third of the total work is expended to overcome the frictional resistance of the movement of air and tissue. In any disease which compromises the airway dimensions, or results in an increased respiratory rate, resistive forces assume much greater importance.

The laws which govern the resistance of flow of gases in tubes apply to pulmonary resistance just as they do in engineering. The equation for calculating the pressure

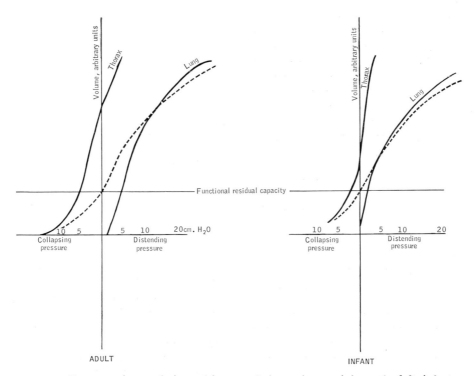

FIGURE 1–7. Pressure-volume relations of lungs and thorax in an adult on the left, infant on the right. The dashed line represents the characteristic of lungs and thorax together. Transpulmonary pressure at the resting portion (functional residual capacity) is less in the infant, and thoracic compliance is greater in the infant.

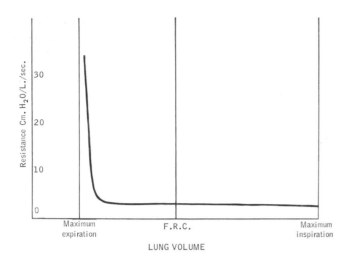

FIGURE 1–8. The relation of airway resistance to lung volume in the normal adult. Resistance remains low through the range of normal breathing, and increases greatly at residual volume, where airways are smallest.

gradient required to maintain streamlined flow of air through a tube is given by Poiseuille's Law:

$$P = \frac{\dot{V}(8l)\eta}{\pi r^4}$$

where P equals pressure; $\dot{V}$, flow; l, length; r, radius of the tube; and η the viscosity of the gas. The viscosity of air is 0.000181 poise at 20° C., 0.0001708 poise at 0° C. The viscosity of water, for comparison, is 0.0100 poise at 20° C., or nearly 100 times that of air. Resistance is pressure/flow. It is clear that the most important determinant of resistance will be the radius of the tube, which is raised to the fourth power in the denominator of the equation. Since flow is not always laminar, but often turbulent, the Poiseuille Law is not strictly applicable to all circumstances. It will underestimate resistance to turbulent flow.

MEASUREMENT OF RESISTANCE. Resistance is calculated from the relation

$$R = \frac{driving\ pressure}{air\ flow}.$$ The pressure must be measured at the two ends of the system—in the case of the lung at the mouth and at alveoli—and the corresponding flow recorded. Alveolar pressure presents the greatest problem. If pleural pressure is substituted, the result is a measure of both airway and lung tissue resistance. In health, tissue resistance is about 20 per cent of the total. Several methods have been used to measure alveolar pressure. The patient is put in a body plethysmograph in which changes in airflow are plotted electronically against the simultaneous changes in pressure in the plethysmograph. The corresponding volume is measured independently by closing the airway to stop flow and measuring pressure changes in the mouth when the patient tries to move air against the obstruction.

Airway resistance changes with lung volumes. At large volumes the airways are distended, and resistance is low. Near the residual volume after forced expiration, resistance becomes infinite as airways are closed by high pleural pressures (Fig. 8).

Estimates of total lung resistance (tissue plus airway) have been obtained on infants by use of dynamic pressure-volume curves. Airflow can be calculated from the slope of the volume tracing versus time, since flow is volume per unit of time. The pressure change is measured on the corresponding esophageal pressure tracing at points of equal volume on inspiration and expiration. That portion of pressure change required to overcome elastic forces is subtracted from the total. Measurements of total lung resistance by this method on infants through the first year of life show a wide scatter, with an average value of 29 cm. of water per liter per second. The average value for airway resistance in infants, measured by the plethysmographic method, is 18 cm. of water per liter per second, suggesting that tissue resistances in the infant are nearly half of the total resistance. By contrast, the adult with larger airways has a much lower airway resistance, 1 to 3 cm. of water per liter per second at resting lung volume.

SITES OF RESISTANCE. The contribution of the upper airway to total resistance is substantial. The average nasal resistance of infants by indirect measurement is 13 cm. of water per liter per second, or nearly half of total respiratory resistance, as is the case in adults. Recent measurements on dogs suggest that nearly all airway resistance is proximal to small bronchioles, or where the total cross-sectional area of the lungs is least. It is hardly surprising that any compromise of the dimensions of the nasal airway in an infant who is a preferential nose-breather will result in retractions and labored breathing. Likewise, even mild edema of the trachea or larynx will impose a significant increase in airway resistance, since the total resistance will increase by at least the fourth power of any reduction in radius of the upper airway.

FACTORS WHICH MAY AFFECT AIRWAY RESISTANCE. The neural regulation of airway dimensions is mediated by efferent impulses over the autonomic nerves to the smooth muscle of the airways. Sympathetic impulses relax, parasympathetic impulses constrict the airways. Bronchi constrict reflexly from irritating inhalants such as sulfur dioxide and some dusts; by arterial hypoxemia and hypercapnia; by embolization of the vessels; by cold; and by some drugs such as acetylcholine and histamine. They dilate in response to an increase in systemic blood pressure through baroreceptors in the carotid sinus, and to sympathomimetic agents such as isoproterenol and epinephrine. The airways are probably in tonic contraction in

health, since in unanesthetized adults atropine or isoproterenol will decrease airway resistance by nearly 50 per cent.

CLINICAL EVALUATION OF AIRWAY RESISTANCE. Careful physical examination can usually provide information on both the degree and site of airway obstruction. Exaggerated inspiratory efforts, with little air flow, are the hallmark of upper airway obstruction. In the absence of veno-arterial shunts, cyanosis in such a situation is reason for urgent intervention with either an oral airway if the obstruction is nasal, or a tracheostomy if it is laryngeal. Indeed, if carbon dioxide retention is evident by an elevation in Pa_{CO_2}, intervention should take place before the appearance of cyanosis which signals serious respiratory failure.

A prolonged expiratory phase, with forced expirations, denotes lower airway obstruction. Usually there is some increase in inspiratory effort as well, associated with retractions of the soft tissues. The principal physiologic derangement is in expiration, when airways are normally of smaller caliber. When pleural pressures are raised in an effort to assist expiration, transmural pressure across the airways may result in their closure. Air trapping ensues, evidenced by an increase in chest volume. The assumption of a larger lung volume promotes distention of the airways, and is a regular compensatory device in patients with lower airway obstruction such as bronchiolitis, asthma and emphysema. Although a larger lung volume is appropriate to distend airways, when extreme, it requires much larger pressures to achieve effective ventilation, since the lungs and thorax are nearer their elastic limit. It is usual to observe an increase in anteroposterior diameter of the chest in patients with lower airway obstruction, associated with an obvious increase in the work of breathing.

Tests of the degree of airway obstruction have extensive use in cooperative subjects. The one-second forced expiratory volume (FEV_1) is a measure of the

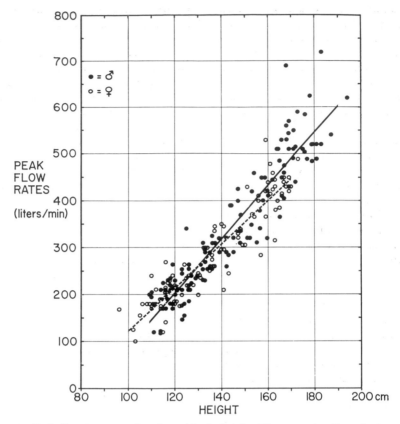

FIGURE 1–9. Peak flow rates as a function of body height. The regression lines for boys (——) and girls (-----) are shown. (From A. B. Murray and C. D. Cook: *J. Pediat.*, 62:186, 1963.)

percentage of the expiratory vital capacity which can be moved by maximal effort in one second. Children can usually expire more than 90 per cent of the total in one second, adults more than 80 per cent of the total. Reduction in the amounts which can be expired per unit of time reflects either poor cooperation, muscle weakness or lower airway obstruction. The maximal inspiratory and expiratory flow rates are more common in organic narume tracing against time. A normal inspiratory flow rate and slow expiratory rate are indicative of weak-walled airways or check valves. Some decrease in both flow rates is more common in organic narrowing of the lumens. Flow meters are available for measurement of the peak expiratory flow rate, and have the advantage over the one-second volume in young children of not requiring a sustained effort (Fig. 9).

Artificial Respiration

A logical outgrowth of recent advances in understanding the mechanics of respiration is the application of the knowledge to assisted respiration. Perhaps the first practical application of the measurement of volume-pressure relations of lungs and thorax was the change in teaching of artificial respiration. No longer is it admissible to try to maintain ventilation by use of the expiratory reserve volume as in the prone back-pressure method of artificial respiration. The pressures applied must be dangerously large to move adequate volumes of air. The inspiratory reserve volume is a more compliant portion of the respiratory system, and is of course the one used in health. Effective assisted breathing requires movement of air into this volume. In the case of the adult with normal lungs, adequate volumes can be moved by tilting as in the rocking bed. The infant, with a shorter abdominal length, cannot be adequately ventilated in this manner.

Active inflation of the lungs can be achieved by a variety of methods, most of which are in everyday use in hospitals. The anesthetist may do it by intubation and the exertion of pressure on a bag of gas which displaces the gas into the chest. The elastic recoil of the distended lungs and thorax raises alveolar pressure, and air is expired, through a valve to prevent rebreathing. In the delivery room it is customary to assist the initiation of breathing either with devices which apply positive pressure to a mask over the nose and mouth, or more effectively in the severely distressed infant by intubation, suction of the trachea, and mouth-to-tube or bag-to-tube application of positive pressure. For patients who require long-term assisted respiration, a variety of respirators are available, some delivering positive pressure to the trachea, others achieving lung expansion by lowering the pressure around the body with respect to that at the nose and mouth. An important consideration in long-term assisted breathing is the ability to give an occasional deep breath to overcome the tendency toward atelectasis with fixed tidal volumes.

PRINCIPLES OF ARTIFICIAL RESPIRATION. Movement of air into the lungs requires that the pressure at the mouth be greater than that in the alveoli. Movement of air from the lungs is passive, since at the beginning of expiration alveolar pressure will exceed mouth pressure. Normally the pressure differences between mouth and alveoli are 4 to 8 cm. of water in adults, probably about 2 to 6 cm. in infants, after the initiation of respiration. Since the movement of air depends only on a pressure difference between two regions, it will be the same regardless of whether the pressure is raised at one point or lowered at another. From the aspect of lung distention, the effect of positive pressure at the mouth is identical with that of negative pressure around the body. The only circumstance in which the effects on the lung could be different is in the event of an air-containing space, such as a cyst or pneumothorax, temporarily not in communication with the airway. With negative pressure around the chest, its volume would temporarily increase; with positive pressure at the mouth, its volume would tend to decrease. This single exception is so unusual, however, that the principle can be emphasized that the effects on airways and alveoli are identical with either positive pressure at the mouth or negative pressure around the body.

The effects of the two kinds of assisted respiration on the circulation are the same, but they differ significantly from the circulatory effects of normal breathing. In normal breathing the decrease in pressure in the thorax, and thus around the heart and great vessels, facilitates return of blood from systemic veins. In positive-pressure breathing, venous return tends to be impeded. Likewise, in body respirators the usual inspiratory augmentation of venous return is not present, since the systemic vessels are also exposed to negative pressure. When the lungs are normal, the applied pressures by either method are not sufficiently great to cause circulatory embarrassment. When the lungs are diseased, and high pressures are required to move air, venous return is reduced, cardiac output falls, and pulmonary blood flow is decreased. Patients in circulatory collapse, as after barbiturate poisoning, in shock, and sometimes infants with severe respiratory distress, may not tolerate artificial respiration without appropriate circulatory support.

The adverse circulatory effects can be reduced if the time of applied pressure is short, less than 50 per cent of the respiratory cycle, and mask pressures during expiration are atmospheric.

APPARATUS. Recently several types of respirators have been designed which overcome most of the problems of older ones. It is imperative that the dead space of the equipment not be excessive. Since the anatomic dead space of a patient is approximately equal in milliliters to body weight in pounds, a mask or tubing of 6 to 8 ml. in an infant will be equivalent to one of 150 ml. in an adult, and significant rebreathing may occur. Either a circle arrangement for the flow of air past an orifice or suitably miniaturized valves can overcome the equipment dead space problem.

Control of the amount of air delivered can be on the basis of a predetermined volume, pre-set pressure limit, or time and flow control. Any one of the three can be effective if the sensitivity of the adjustments is adequate to make the small changes which may be necessary in an infant whose tidal volume is 10 to 20 ml. Usually the volume adjustments depend on a degree of trial and error. Observation of the degree of excursion of the chest wall, the presence of breath sounds bilaterally, and the general response of the infant permit the first estimate of efficacy. Thereafter the only adequate way to evaluate the respirator is to measure the partial pressure of carbon dioxide in arterial or arterialized capillary blood. Hyperventilation is indicated by a low carbon dioxide tension, which can be dangerous at levels under 25 mm. of mercury both because of the associated alkalosis and the decrease in cerebral blood flow. Hypoventilation is indicated by an elevated carbon dioxide tension. Over 50 mm. of mercury the concomitant acidosis, and at higher levels, cerebral depression, are dangerous.

A potentially useful feature available in both positive and negative pressure respirators is a sensing device to permit an infant or child to cycle the respirator. With each inspiratory effort he gets an assist. In the event of apnea, automatic timers trigger the respirator.

Another requirement of a respirator, especially in the young infant, is that it not be so cumbersome that it precludes other supportive and monitoring proce-dures, and that it can be attached to an infant in an incubator, or be itself an integral part of an incubator. The maintenance of environmental temperature sufficient to keep the infant at a normal body temperature without the expenditure of calories for added metabolism is essential in distressed infants. A thermal stress further increases oxygen consumption, and hence ventilatory requirements.

The actual setting of the controls of a respirator cannot be prescribed for all circumstances. The first consideration is whether the need for assisted breathing is due to central respiratory failure or muscle weakness with reasonably normal lungs, or whether pulmonary disease underlies the need. With normal lungs low pressures are adequate. The actual pressure setting depends on where the pressure is measured. If the manometer is far upstream from the mouth, there will be some flow resistance in the tubing, and 10 to 20 cm. of water may be appropriate. If the pressure sensing device is near the mouth, about 10 cm. of water may be suitable. If a patient has diseased lungs, much higher pressures are appropriate, up to 40 cm. at the mouth. If the respirator is adjusted by a volume control, the setting depends on the size of possible leaks. A loose-fitting endotracheal tube allows some advantage in that it effectively lessens the dead space, but the volume setting will have to allow for a variable leak, and may need repeated adjustments. When the inspiratory flow rate and time are pre-set, the pressures and volumes are dependent variables.

ALVEOLAR VENTILATION

The preceding sections have been devoted to the problems of lung growth, volumes, and the mechanical aspects of moving air. Clearly the purpose of the lung is for gas exchange, i.e. the introduction of oxygen and removal of carbon dioxide from the blood which perfuses it. This section and the following ones focus on the fate of air once introduced into the lung, and aspects of gas transport and tissue respiration.

Dead Space

A portion of each inspired breath remains in the conducting airways (consisting of the nose, mouth, pharynx, larynx, trachea, bronchi and bronchioles) where no significant exchange of oxygen and carbon dioxide with blood takes place. The volume of the conducting airways is called the anatomic dead space (V_D anat), and is filled by about 25 per cent of each tidal volume. The remainder of each tidal volume goes to the alveoli, where rapid exchange of oxygen and carbon dioxide occurs, and the proportion of ventilation that undergoes gas exchange is known as the alveolar ventilation (V_A). When some alveoli are relatively underperfused with blood, as in some disease states, a proportion of alveolar air does not undergo gas exchange, but acts as if it were in a dead space. It is called the alveolar dead space (V_D alv). Thus:

$$V_T \text{ (tidal volume)} = V_D \text{ anat} + V_D \text{ alv} + V_A$$

V_D anat $+ V_D$ alv is called the physiologic dead space.

In health anatomic dead space and physiologic dead space are identical, since the distribution of air and blood in alveoli is such that adequate gas exchange takes place (see p. 39). Anatomic dead space in milliliters is roughly equal to the weight of the subject in pounds (for a 7-pound baby 7 or 8 ml.; for an adult 150 ml.) and is normally less than 30 per cent of V_T. In the normal premature infant anatomic dead space is slightly higher than 30 per cent, and physiologic dead space may be over 40 per cent. In the infant with respiratory distress physiologic dead space may be more than 70 per cent of the tidal volume.

Anatomic dead space may be measured by making use of the following argument originally developed by Bohr:

Volume CO_2 expired per breath = volume CO_2 in the dead space + volume of CO_2 in the alveoli

The volume of carbon dioxide is equal to the volume of a compartment times the fractional concentration of carbon dioxide. Thus

$$F_{E_{CO_2}}V_E = F_{D_{CO_2}}V_D + F_{A_{CO_2}}V_A$$

Since the dead space at end-inspiration is filled with air containing no significant amount of carbon dioxide,

$$F_{D_{CO_2}}V_D = 0;$$

and since $V_A = V_E - V_D$,

$$F_{E_{CO_2}}V_E = F_{A_{CO_2}}(V_E - V_D),$$

$$F_{A_{CO_2}}V_D = (F_{A_{CO_2}} - F_{E_{CO_2}})V_E, \text{ and}$$

$$V_D = \frac{(F_{A_{CO_2}} - F_{E_{CO_2}})V_E}{F_{A_{CO_2}}} \text{ (anatomic dead space).}$$

Since normally

$$F_{A_{CO_2}} = Fa_{CO_2}$$

and

$$P_{A_{CO_2}} = F_{A_{CO_2}} \times (P_b - 47)$$

$$V_D = \left(\frac{Pa_{CO_2} - P_{E_{CO_2}}}{Pa_{CO_2}}\right) V_E \text{ (physiologic dead space).}$$

The concentration of carbon dioxide in the alveolus ($F_{A_{CO_2}}$) can be measured from an end-tidal sample, which represents alveolar air. V_E is measured by collecting expired gases, and $F_{E_{CO_2}}$ can be measured on an aliquot of mixed expired air. For physiologic dead space the partial pressure of carbon dioxide in arterial blood is used instead of the end-expired sample. A discrepancy in the two determinations, using end-tidal versus arterial blood, infers the presence of portions of the lung which are ventilated and not perfused.

Another method of measuring the anatomic dead space, Fowler's method, requires that a single breath of oxygen be inspired. On expiration both the volume of expired gas and percentage of nitrogen are measured. The first portion of the expired gas comes from the dead space and contains little or no nitrogen. As the breath is expired the percentage of nitrogen increases until it "plateaus" at the

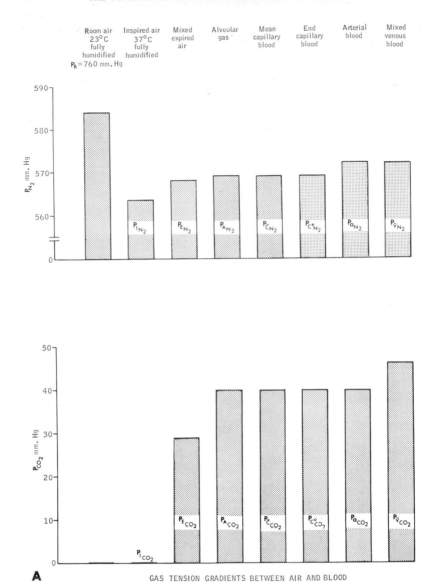

FIGURE 1–10. Partial pressures of nitrogen and carbon dioxide at different portions of the airway and blood. *(See facing page for continuation of Figure 1–10.)*

alveolar concentration. By assuming that all the initial part of the breath comes from the anatomic dead space and all the latter portion from the alveoli, the anatomic dead space can be calculated. The same measurements can be made by monitoring the expired carbon dioxide concentration.

In practice anatomic dead space is difficult to define accurately, since it depends on lung volume (greater at large lung volumes when the airways are more distended) and on body position (being smaller when supine). The physiologic dead space is a more useful measurement in assessing the patient since it reflects the portion of each breath which participates in gas exchange.

From the foregoing discussion it is apparent that a tidal volume must be chosen

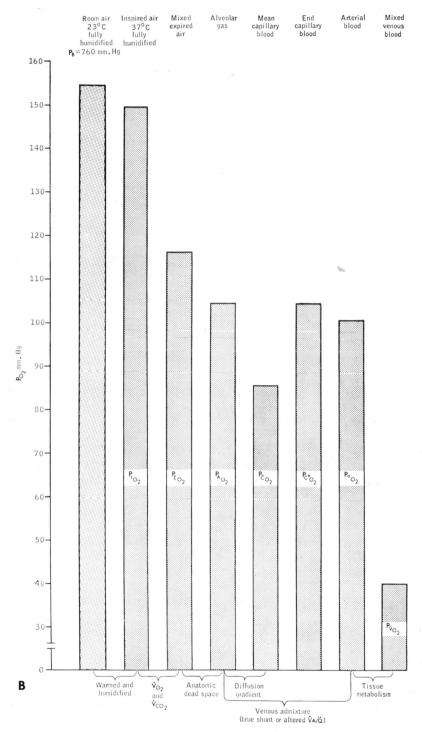

PARTIAL PRESSURE OF OXYGEN AT DIFFERENT PORTIONS OF THE AIRWAY AND BLOOD

FIGURE 1–10. *Continued.*

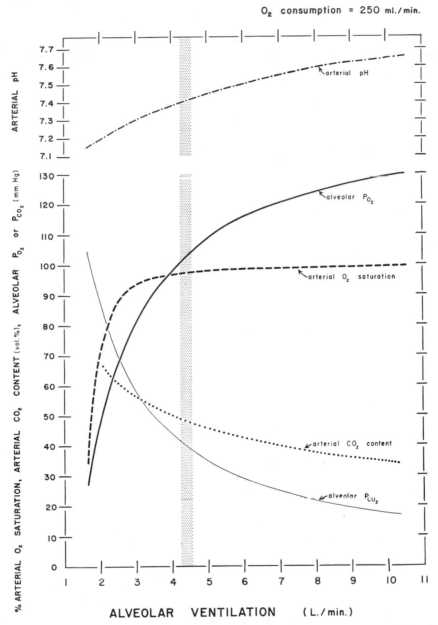

FIGURE 1–11. The effect of changing alveolar ventilation on alveolar gas and arterial blood oxygen, carbon dioxide and pH. (From J. H. Comroe and others: *The Lung.* 2nd ed. Chicago, Year Book Medical Publishers, Inc., 1962.)

which will allow for adequate alveolar ventilation. For example, an adult might breathe sixty times a minute with a tidal volume of 100 ml. for a minute ventilation of 6 liters. Nevertheless alveolar ventilation under these circumstances is zero, since only the dead space is ventilated. When selecting suitable volumes and rates for patients on respirators, it is useful to approximate normal values, and consider adequate alveolar ventilation rather than total ventilation.

Alveolar Gases

The amount of alveolar ventilation per minute must be adequate to keep the alveolar P_{O_2} and P_{CO_2} at values which will promote the escape of carbon dioxide from the venous blood and the uptake of oxygen by venous blood. In health this means that $P_{A_{O_2}}$ is approximately 105 to 110 mm. of mercury and $P_{A_{CO_2}}$ 40 mm. (Fig. 11).

Since inspired air is "diluted" in the alveoli by the functional residual capacity of air containing carbon dioxide and water vapor, the partial pressure of oxygen in alveolar gas must be less than that of the inspired air (cf. Dalton's Law, p. 4). $P_{A_{O_2}}$ may be calculated from the alveolar air equation. When oxygen consumption equals carbon dioxide production, then:

$$P_{A_{O_2}} = P_{I_{O_2}} - P_{A_{CO_2}}$$
$$P_{I_{O_2}} = 0.2093 \times (P_b - 47 \text{ mm. Hg}) = 149 \text{ mm. Hg}$$

If $P_{A_{CO_2}}$ is 40 mm. of mercury, then $P_{A_{O_2}}$ is 109 mm. Usually R is 0.8, or more oxygen is consumed than carbon dioxide eliminated, thereby decreasing $P_{A_{O_2}}$ slightly more than would be expected from the dilution of $P_{A_{CO_2}}$. To account for changes in R a useful form of the alveolar air equation for clinical purposes is:

$$P_{A_{O_2}} = P_{I_{O_2}} - \frac{P_{A_{CO_2}}}{R}$$

When $P_{A_{CO_2}}$ is 40 and R is 0.8, $P_{A_{O_2}}$ is 99 mm. of mercury. Note that 40 per cent oxygen raises $P_{A_{O_2}}$ to 235 mm.

Since the partial pressures of alveolar gases must always equal the same total pressure, any increase in one must be associated with a decrease in the other.

Since Pa_{O_2} is markedly affected by the presence of right-to-left vascular shunts (see p. 4), it is not a good measurement of the adequacy of pulmonary ventilation. Pa_{CO_2} is minimally affected in the presence of shunts because $P\bar{v}_{CO_2}$ is 46 mm. and Pa_{CO_2} 40 mm. of mercury. If one third of the cardiac output is shunted, this raises Pa_{CO_2} to only 42 mm. of mercury. Thus the arterial P_{CO_2} is the optimum

Table 3. *Illustrative Causes of Hypoventilation*

I. *Respiratory Center Depression:* General anesthesia; excessive doses of drugs such as morphine, barbiturates or codeine; severe or prolonged hypoxia, cerebral ischemia, high concentrations of CO_2; electrocution; cerebral trauma; increased intracranial pressure

II. *Conditions Affecting the Airways and Lung:*
  A. *Upper or lower airway obstruction:* Foreign body, large tonsils and adenoids, vocal cord paralysis, croup, endobronchial tuberculosis, chronic bronchitis, emphysema, asthma, bronchiectasis, cystic fibrosis
  B. *Decreased lung compliance:* Vascular diseases such as emboli, polyarteritis, mitral stenosis; parasitic infiltrations; interstitial disease such as sarcoid, Hamman-Rich syndrome, pneumoconioses, lupus, rheumatoid arthritis, berylliosis, histiocytosis X, radiation fibrosis, idiopathic pulmonary hemosiderosis
  C. *Extensive loss of functioning lung tissue:* Atelectasis, tumor, pneumonia, cystic fibrosis, surgical resection
  D. *Limitation of movement of lungs:* Pleural effusion, pneumothorax, fibrothorax

III. *Conditions Affecting the Thorax:*
  A. *Decreased chest wall compliance:* Arthritis, scleroderma, kyphoscoliosis, fractured ribs, thoracoplasty, thoracotomy, pickwickian syndrome, phrenic nerve paralysis
  B. *Diseases of respiratory muscles,* e.g. muscular dystrophy
  C. *Paralysis of respiratory muscles:* Poliomyelitis, peripheral neuritis, spinal cord injury, myasthenia gravis; curare, succinylcholine, botulinus and nicotine poisonings

measurement of the adequacy of alveolar ventilation. Hyperventilation is defined as a reduction in Pa_{CO_2}, hypoventilation as an increase in Pa_{CO_2}. Some of the causes of hypoventilation are listed in Table 3.

DIFFUSION

Principles

The barriers through which a gas must travel when diffusing from the alveolus to the blood include the alveolar epithelial lining, basement membrane, capillary endothelial lining, plasma and the red blood cell. As observed on electronmicrographs of lung tissue, the thinnest part of the barrier is 0.2 micron, but may be as much as three times this distance.

Fick's Law of diffusion modified for gases states:

$$Q/min. = \frac{K \, S \, (P_1 - P_2)}{d}$$

The amount of gas (Q) diffusing through a membrane is directly proportional to the surface area available for diffusion (S), the pressure difference of the two gases on either side of the membrane, and a constant (K) which depends on the solubility coefficient of the gas and the characteristics of the particular membrane and liquid used; and inversely proportional to the distance (d) through which the gas has to diffuse. In the lung of a given subject exact values for K, S and d are unknown. Therefore, for the lung Bohr and Krogh suggested the term "diffusion capacity" (D_L). For oxygen:

$$D_{L_{O_2}} \text{ (ml./min./mm. Hg)} = \frac{\dot{V}_{O_2}}{P_{A_{O_2}} - P\bar{c}_{O_2}}$$

where $P_{A_{O_2}}$ is the alveolar oxygen tension and $P\bar{c}_{O_2}$ is the average capillary oxygen tension. Therefore the denominator represents the average "driving" pressure for oxygen across the alveolar-capillary pathway.

Carbon dioxide diffuses nearly twenty-one times faster than oxygen in a gas-liquid system. Therefore, for all practical purposes, there is never any impairment of diffusion for carbon dioxide from the blood to the alveolus.

Measurement

For the measurement of the diffusing capacity of oxygen in the lung, oxygen uptake and the alveolar oxygen tension are easily determined. The average capillary oxygen tension ($P\bar{c}_{O_2}$) is difficult to assess, however, since we cannot measure it directly. $P\bar{c}_{O_2}$ will vary according to $P\bar{v}_{O_2}$, the diffusing capacity and the time available for diffusion to take place (mean transit time of a red blood cell through a lung capillary has been estimated at rest to be 0.75 second). With a measurement of Pa_{O_2} and a knowledge of the transit time through the pulmonary capillary, a special technique called the Bohr integration procedure can be used to determine $P\bar{c}_{O_2}$. We can easily measure the arterial P_{O_2}, but it is influenced by both the diffusing capacity and the amount of right-to-left shunt present. When low concentrations of oxygen are inspired, the effect of a right-to-left shunt on arterial P_{O_2} is minimal, and any difference between $P_{A_{O_2}}$ and Pa_{O_2} is assumed to be related to a diffusion defect (see p. 29). Therefore $D_{L_{O_2}}$ is measured at two levels of inspired oxygen, room air and 12 to 14 per cent oxygen. Although this method has been extensively used in adults, it has not been used widely in children.

Carbon monoxide (CO), however, has been used extensively in children to test diffusing capacity. The advantage of using carbon monoxide is due to its remarkable affinity for hemoglobin, some 210 times that of oxygen, and therefore the capillary P_{CO} is negligible and offers no back pressure for diffusion. Many different techniques have been used, but the differences between them will not be discussed here.

In order to calculate $D_{L_{CO}}$, one need only know the amount of carbon monoxide taken up per minute and $P_{A_{CO}}$. $D_{L_{CO}}$

is linearly related to lung growth and has been found to be closely correlated with height or total lung capacity.

The reaction rate between hemoglobin and carbon monoxide is affected by the level of alveolar P_{O_2}; if high, this slows down the formation of carbon monoxide hemoglobin; if low, then carbon monoxide and hemoglobin combine more rapidly. If one performs the test at two levels of $P_{A_{O_2}}$, it is possible to separate the $D_{L_{CO}}$ into two components, the membrane diffusing capacity and the red blood cell component. For both children and adults approximately half of the resistance to diffusion of carbon monoxide resides in the alveolar membrane and half in the red blood cell.

Clinically, a reduction in diffusing capacity may be due to an increased thickness of the alveolar-capillary membrane, as seen with interstitial pulmonary fibrosis, sarcoid, pneumoconioses, scleroderma, pulmonary edema or pulmonary hemosiderosis. A reduction in the surface area available for diffusion will reduce the diffusion capacity, as found in patients after lobectomy, or with emphysema when alveolar walls are destroyed. Patients with cystic fibrosis may have much of the lung unavailable for gas exchange and, therefore, a reduced diffusing capacity.

TRANSPORT OF OXYGEN

Dissolved Oxygen and Oxyhemoglobin

Once oxygen molecules have passed from the alveolus into the pulmonary capillary, they are transported in the blood in two ways. A small proportion of the oxygen exists as dissolved oxygen in the plasma and water of the red blood cell. For 100 ml. of whole blood equilibrated with a P_{O_2} of 100 mm. of mercury, 0.3 ml. of oxygen is present as dissolved oxygen. If this represented the total oxygen-carrying capacity of blood, then cardiac output would have to be greater than 80 liters per minute in order to allow 250

ml. of oxygen to be consumed per minute. During 100 per cent oxygen breathing, Pa_{O_2} is approximately 650 mm. of mercury and 100 ml. of blood contains 2.0 ml. of oxygen, and would require a cardiac output of about 12 liters per minute if no hemoglobin were present.

Since 1 gm. of hemoglobin can combine with 1.34 ml. of oxygen, between forty and seventy times more oxygen is carried by hemoglobin than by the plasma and enables the body to achieve a cardiac output at rest of 5.5 liters per minute with an oxygen uptake of 250 ml. per minute.

The recent popularity of hyperbaric oxygen (i.e. oxygen under very high pressures) for a variety of clinical conditions, is due to the fact that at a pressure of 3 atmospheres (absolute) ($P_{A_{O_2}}$ about 1950 mm. of mercury) approximately 6.0 ml. of oxygen is dissolved in 100 ml. of whole blood, and this amount can meet the metabolic demands of the tissues under resting conditions even when no hemoglobin is present.

The remarkable oxygen-carrying properties of blood depend not on the solubility of oxygen in plasma, but on the unusual properties of hemoglobin. Figure 12 illustrates the oxyhemoglobin dissociation curve, showing that hemoglobin is nearly 95 per cent saturated at a P_{O_2} of 80 mm. of mercury. The steep portion of the curve, up to about 50 mm., permits large amounts of oxygen to be released from hemoglobin with small changes in P_{O_2}. Under normal circumstances 100 per cent oxygen breathing will raise the amount of oxygen carried by the blood by only a small amount, since at a P_{O_2} of 100 mm. of mercury, hemoglobin is already 97.5 per cent saturated. Even with air breathing one is on the flat portion of the curve. The presence of a right-to-left shunt markedly affects P_{O_2}, but may reduce the percentage of saturation only minimally. For example, a 50 per cent shunt with venous blood containing 15 ml. of oxygen per 100 ml. will only reduce the oxygen content of 100 ml. of blood from 20 ml. to 17.5 ml. The blood is still 88 per cent saturated, but Pa_{O_2} is now 60 mm. in-

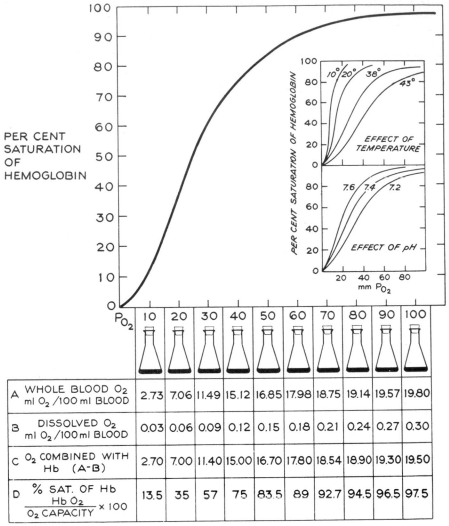

		10	20	30	40	50	60	70	80	90	100
A	WHOLE BLOOD O_2 ml O_2/100 ml BLOOD	2.73	7.06	11.49	15.12	16.85	17.98	18.75	19.14	19.57	19.80
B	DISSOLVED O_2 ml O_2/100 ml BLOOD	0.03	0.06	0.09	0.12	0.15	0.18	0.21	0.24	0.27	0.30
C	O_2 COMBINED WITH Hb (A-B)	2.70	7.00	11.40	15.00	16.70	17.80	18.54	18.90	19.30	19.50
D	% SAT. OF Hb $\frac{Hb\ O_2}{O_2\ CAPACITY} \times 100$	13.5	35	57	75	83.5	89	92.7	94.5	96.5	97.5

FIGURE 1–12. Oxyhemoglobin dissociation curves. The large graph shows a single dissociation curve, applicable when the pH of the blood is 7.40 and temperature is 38°C. The blood oxygen tension and saturation of patients with carbon dioxide retention, acidosis, alkalosis, fever or hypothermia will not fit this curve because it shifts to the right or left when temperature, pH or P_{CO_2} is changed. Effects on the oxyhemoglobin dissociation curve of change in temperature (*upper right*) and in pH (*lower right*) are shown in the smaller graphs. A small change in blood pH occurs regularly in the body; e.g. when mixed venous blood passes through the pulmonary capillaries, P_{CO_2} decreases from 46 to 40 mm. of mercury, and pH rises from 7.37 to 7.40. During this time, blood changes from a pH of 7.37 dissociation curve to a pH of 7.40 curve. (From J. H. Comroe: *Physiology of Respiration.* Chicago, Year Book Medical Publishers, Inc., 1965.)

stead of 100 mm. of mercury. Thus the change in oxygen content is linearly related to the amount of right-to-left shunt, but the change in P_{O_2} is not because of the S-shaped hemoglobin-oxygen curve. It is also apparent that Pa_{O_2} is a more sensi-

tive measure of blood oxygenation because neither percentage of saturation nor oxygen content falls appreciably until P_{O_2} falls from 100 mm. to 60 mm. of mercury.

The oxyhemoglobin dissociation curve is affected by changes in pH, P_{CO_2} and temperature. A decrease in pH, increase in P_{CO_2} (Bohr effect) or an increase in temperature shifts the curve to the right, particularly in the 20- to 50-mm. of mercury range. Thus for a given P_{O_2} the saturation percentage is less under acidotic or hyperpyrexic conditions. In the tissues, carbon dioxide is added to the blood, and this facilitates the removal of oxygen from the red blood cell. In the pulmonary capillaries carbon dioxide diffuses out of the blood, facilitating oxygen uptake by hemoglobin. An increased temperature has a similar effect to an increase in P_{CO_2} and thus facilitates oxygen removal from the blood by the tissues. Note that a patient who is pyrexic with carbon dioxide retention could not have a normal oxygen saturation during air breathing because of the Bohr and temperature effects on the oxyhemoglobin dissociation curve.

The fetal hemoglobin dissociation curve is shifted to the left of the adult curve at a similar pH. Thus, at a given P_{O_2}, fetal blood contains more oxygen than adult hemoglobin. This property ensures that an adequate amount of oxygen will get to fetal tissues, since the fetus in utero has a Pa_{O_2} of 30 to 40 mm. of mercury. The affinity of fetal hemoglobin for oxygen is not a result of the structure of hemoglobin, but depends on an intact fetal red blood cell membrane, for free fetal hemoglobin in solution has the same oxygen-carrying capacity as adult hemoglobin. Fetal hemoglobin disappears from the circulation shortly after birth, and by a few months of age less than 2 per cent is present. Normal fetal development is not dependent on differences in maternal and fetal hemoglobins, since in some species they are identical.

Abnormal hemoglobins differ in their oxygen-carrying capacity. Hemoglobin S has a curve shifted to the right, so that at 100 mm. of mercury P_{O_2} it is only 80 per cent saturated. It is insoluble when deoxygenated, and at low P_{O_2} crystallizes within the erythrocyte. This produces the well known "sickle" cell shape of the cell in this disorder. Hemoglobin H, with twelve times the affinity for oxygen as

hemoglobin A, does not release oxygen readily to the tissues. Hemoglobin M is oxidized by oxygen to methemoglobin, which does not release oxygen to the tissues; a large amount is incompatible with life. The formation of methemoglobin by agents such as nitrates, aniline, sulfonamides, acetanilid, phenylhydrazine or primaquine may also be life-threatening. Congenital deficiency of an enzyme, hemoglobin reductase, is also associated with large amounts of methemoglobin, and these patients are cyanotic in room air. Sulfhemoglobin is, likewise, unable to transport oxygen.

Since carbon monoxide has 210 times more affinity for hemoglobin than oxygen, it is important to note that P_{O_2} may be normal in carbon monoxide poisoning, while oxygen content is markedly reduced.

Cyanosis

The degree of visible cyanosis depends on the amount of unsaturated hemoglobin present in the blood perfusing superficial vessels. In polycythemia adequate amounts of oxygen may be present, but the patient appears cyanotic because not all his hemoglobin is saturated. Conversely, in anemia, a patient may be hypoxic, but not appear cyanotic. The clinical assessment of oxygenation is hazardous in part because a poor peripheral circulation may result in peripheral cyanosis when the arterial blood is well oxygenated.

OXYGEN THERAPY

Increased Inspired Mixtures

Increased inspired mixtures of oxygen are required when tissue oxygenation is inadequate. The response to increased inspired oxygen depends on which cause of hypoxia is present (Table 4). Most of the conditions characterized by hypoxemia respond well to added oxygen. Patients with venous-arterial shunts will respond

Table 4.   *Four Types of Hypoxia and Some Causes*

1. *Hypoxemia (low P_{O_2} and low oxygen content)*
   Deficiency of oxygen in the atmosphere
   Hypoventilation (see Table 3)
   Uneven distribution of alveolar gas and/or pulmonary blood flow
   Diffusion impairment
   Venous to arterial shunt
2. *Deficient hemoglobin (normal P_{O_2} and low oxygen content)*
   Anemia
   Carbon monoxide poisoning
3. *Ischemic hypoxia (normal P_{O_2} and oxygen content)*
   General or localized circulatory insufficiency
   Tissue edema
   Abnormal tissue demands
4. *Histotoxic anoxia (normal P_{O_2} and oxygen content)*
   Poisoning of cellular enzymes so that they cannot use the available oxygen (e.g. cyanide poisoning)

less well, since the shunted blood does not perfuse alveoli. Even so, tissue oxygenation may be improved by the addition of oxygen to the blood which does undergo gas exchange in the lung. A direct attack on the underlying disorder in anemia, ischemia and poisonings is clearly indicated; oxygen therapy may be lifesaving during the time required to treat the disease.

Oxygen therapy can be utilized to facilitate the removal of other gases loculated in body spaces, such as air in pneumothorax, pneumomediastinum and ileus. High inspired oxygen mixtures effectively wash out body stores of nitrogen. With air breathing, the blood which perfuses the tissue spaces has an arterial oxygen tension of 100 mm. of mercury and a venous tension of 40 mm. With oxygen breathing, although arterial tensions rise to 600 mm. of mercury, venous oxygen tensions do not rise above 50 to 60 mm. because of oxygen consumption and the shape of the dissociation curve. With air breathing, arterial and venous nitrogen tensions are the same, about 570 mm. of mercury. If the loculated gas were air at atmospheric pressure, the gradient for the movement of nitrogen to the blood would be very small. After nitrogen washout, with oxygen breathing, the lack of high elevation in venous oxygen tension permits movement of both nitrogen and oxygen into the blood. The increased pressure differences increase the rate of absorption of loculated air some fivefold to tenfold.

Hazards of High Oxygen Mixtures

Hypoxemia in conditions associated with hypoventilation, such as chronic pulmonary disease and status asthmaticus, may be overcome by enriched oxygen mixtures without concomitant lessening of the hypercapnia. The patient may appear pink, but become narcotized under the influence of carbon dioxide retention. In chronic respiratory acidosis, respiration may be maintained chiefly by the hypoxic drive, and correction of the hypoxemia may result in a cessation of respiration. Frequent measurements of arterial gas tensions are invaluable in such patients. Only as much oxygen should be given as is needed to keep the arterial oxygen tension in the range of 40 to 60 mm. of mercury (75 to 90 per cent saturated).

Excessive oxygenation of the blood can be dangerous. Human volunteers in pure oxygen at one atmosphere experience symptoms in about twenty-four hours, chiefly substernal pain and paresthesias. Some animals, exposed for longer periods, die of pulmonary congestion and edema in four to seven days. The toxicity of oxygen is directly proportional to its partial pressure. Symptoms occur within minutes under hyperbaric conditions, and may not be present after one month in pure oxygen at one third of an atmosphere. Some of the effects of oxygen are to decrease minute ventilation and cardiac output slightly, and constrict retinal and cerebral vessels and the ductus arteriosus. Cerebral vasoconstriction may lead to irreversible brain damage. Retinal vasoconstriction does not seem to be a significant problem in mature retinas which are richly vascularized. In premature infants, however, the vasoconstriction may lead to ischemia. After the cessation of oxygen therapy, or with maturation of the infant, neovascularization of the retina occurs. The disorderly growth and scarring may cause retinal detachments and fibroplasia which appears behind the lens; hence the name "retrolental fibroplasia." This manifestation of oxygen toxicity, restricted to prematurely born infants and some animals, depends on the level of oxygen in the arterial blood which perfuses the retina. High oxygen mixtures in infants with large right-to-left shunts do not put the infant at risk of retrolental fibroplasia unless the arterial oxygen tensions are elevated above normal.

Pure oxygen breathing predisposes to atelectasis in the presence of any airway obstruction. Just as it facilitates removal of air from loculated spaces as in pneumothorax, so can it facilitate removal of air from alveoli. The hazard is greater with breathing pure oxygen mixtures at a reduced total pressure, such as the one third of an atmosphere, which is the environment of our space capsules. Absorption of air from the nasal sinuses and middle ear in the event of obstruction may result in painful pressure differences and even hemorrhage.

The mechanism of oxygen's toxic effect on cells is incompletely understood. As an electron acceptor, it goes through a free radical state which is a highly reactive and potent energy releaser. It further has a paramagnetic effect which may affect electron motion of neighboring molecules. Some enzyme systems such as dehydrogenases in the central nervous system do not function in hyperoxic environments, a fact which may underlie the occurrence of convulsions.

Hyperbaric Oxygen

All the toxic effects which may be seen in pure oxygen breathing at one atmosphere are exaggerated and occur sooner under hyperbaric conditions. Nevertheless hyperbaric oxygenation has a role in oxygen therapy of a few disease states such as coronary occlusion and shock, to enhance the effects of radiation in tumor therapy, in the treatment of some infections with anaerobic organisms such as gas gangrene, and in carbon monoxide poisoning. Some gain has been found in cardiac surgery when the period of cardiac arrest can be prolonged. Effective oxygenation by hyperbaric pressure can be achieved even in the face of severe pulmonary insufficiency as in hyaline membrane disease, although it has not been associated with recovery of the patient in that disease.

The procedure requires a rigid chamber capable of withstanding several atmospheres of pressure, and suitable ports for monitoring equipment. For cardiac surgery it also requires space for a complete operating team. Oxygen toxicity and fire are ever-present hazards.

CARBON DIOXIDE TRANSPORT AND ACID-BASE BALANCE

Buffering and Transport

Acids are normally produced in the body at the rates of 15 to 20 moles of carbonic acid and 80 millimoles of fixed acids per day. For the cells to maintain their normal metabolic activity the pH of the environment of the cells must be close to 7.40. The understanding of the regulation of hydrogen ion concentration requires knowledge of the buffering action of the chemical constituents of the blood and the role of the lungs and kidney in the excretion of acids from the body.

The constituents which are of most importance for acid-base regulation are the sodium bicarbonate and carbonic acid of the plasma, the potassium bicarbonate and carbonic acid of the cells, and hemoglobin.

The concentration of carbonic acid is determined by the partial pressure of carbon dioxide, and the solubility co-

CARBON DIOXIDE DISSOCIATION CURVES FOR WHOLE BLOOD

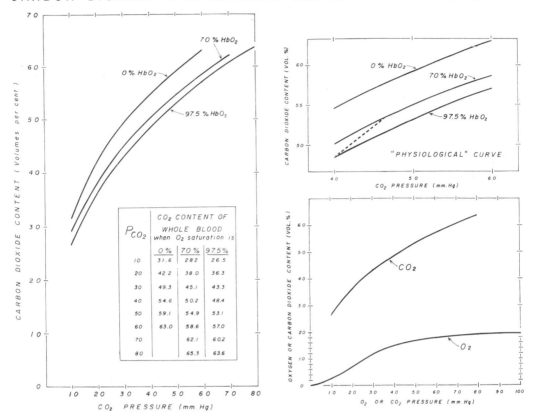

FIGURE 1–13. The carbon dioxide dissociation curve. The large graph shows the relation between P_{CO_2} and carbon dioxide content of whole blood; this varies with changes in saturation of hemoglobin with oxygen. Thus P_{CO_2} of the blood influences oxygen saturation (Bohr effect), and oxygen saturation of the blood influences carbon dioxide content (Haldane effect). The oxygen-carbon dioxide diagram gives the correct figure for both carbon dioxide and oxygen at every P_{O_2} and P_{CO_2}. *Above, right,* Greatly magnified portion of the large graph to show the change that occurs as mixed venous blood (**70 per cent oxyhemoglobin, P_{CO_2} 46 mm. of mercury**) passes through the pulmonary capillaries and becomes arterial blood (97.5 per cent oxyhemoglobin, P_{CO_2} 40 mm. of mercury). Dashed line is a hypothetical transition between the 2 curves. *Below, right,* Oxygen and carbon dioxide dissociation curves plotted on same scale to show the important point that the oxygen curve has a steep and a flat portion and that the carbon dioxide curve does not. (From J. H. Comroe, Jr., and others: *The Lung.* Chicago, Year Book Medical Publishers, Inc., 1963.)

efficients of carbon dioxide in plasma and in red cell water. Carbonic acid in aqueous solution dissociates as follows:

$$CO_2 + H_2O \rightleftarrows H_2CO_3$$
$$H_2CO_3 \rightleftarrows H^+ + HCO_3^-$$

The law of mass action describes this reaction:

$$\frac{(H^+)\,(HCO_3^-)}{(H_2CO_3)} = K$$

In plasma, K has the value of $10^{-6.1}$. Equivalent forms of this equation are

$$pH = pK + \log\frac{(HCO_3^-)}{H_2CO_3}$$

By definition $pH = -\log (H^+)$; $pK = -\log K = 6.1$ for plasma. Applied to plasma, where dissolved carbon dioxide exists at a concentration 1000 times that of carbonic acid, the equation becomes

$$pH = 6.1 + \log\frac{(HCO_3^-)}{0.03P_{CO_2}}$$

This form of the equation is known as the Henderson-Hasselbalch equation.

Just as oxygen has a highly specialized transport mechanism in the blood in order to ensure an adequate delivery to tissues under physiologic conditions, carbon dioxide produced by the tissues has a special transport system to carry it in the blood to the lung, where it is expired. The amount of carbon dioxide in blood is related to the P_{CO_2} in a manner shown in Figure 13. Unlike oxygen, the relation between P_{CO_2} and carbon dioxide content is nearly linear, and therefore doubling alveolar ventilation halves Pa_{CO_2}; conversely, halving alveolar ventilation doubles Pa_{CO_2}. Oxygenated hemoglobin shifts the carbon dioxide dissociation curve to the right (Haldane effect), so that at a given P_{CO_2} there is less carbon dioxide content. This effect aids in the removal of carbon dioxide from the blood in the lung when venous blood becomes oxygenated. The average arterial carbon dioxide tension (P_{CO_2}) in adults is 40 mm. of mercury, in infants closer to 35 mm., and venous levels are normally 6 mm. of mercury higher. Thus the effect of venous admixture on arterial P_{CO_2} is very small.

The processes involved in the uptake of carbon dioxide in the blood and tissues are as follows:

1. Carbon dioxide diffuses into the blood from the tissue. Some carbon dioxide is dissolved in the plasma water in physical solution.

2. Carbon dioxide hydrates slowly in the plasma to form a small amount of carbonic acid.

3. Most of the carbon dioxide enters the red cells. A small amount is dissolved in the water of the red cell. A fraction combines with hemoglobin to form a carbamino compound.

4. A larger fraction in the red cell hydrates rapidly, because of the presence of carbonic anhydrase, to form carbonic acid, which dissociates into H^+ plus HCO_3^-.

5. Bicarbonate diffuses into plasma because of the concentration gradient, and Cl^- ions enter the cell to restore electrical neutrality.

Hemoglobin is important in the transport of carbon dioxide because of two properties of the molecule. First, it is a good buffer. This property permits blood to take up carbon dioxide with only a small change in pH. Second, it is a stronger acid when oxygenated than when it is reduced. Thus when oxyhemoglobin is reduced, more cations are available to neutralize HCO_3^-. Carbon dioxide exists in two forms in the red cell because of this property of hemoglobin as bicarbonate ion and as hemoglobin carbamate ($HbNHCOO^-$).

$$KHbO_2 + H_2CO_3 \rightleftarrows$$
$$HHb + O_2\uparrow + KHCO_3$$
$$KHbO_2 NH_2 + CO_2 \rightleftarrows$$
$$HHb \cdot NHCOOK + O_2\uparrow$$

An enzyme in the red cell, carbonic anhydrase, accelerates the reaction

$$CO_2 + H_2O \rightleftarrows H^+ + HCO_3^-$$

some 13,000 times. A concentration gradient between red cell and plasma causes the bicarbonate ion to leave the red cell. Because the red blood cell membrane is relatively impermeable to Na^+ and K^+, the chloride ion and water move into the red cell to restore electrical neutrality

Table 5. *Carbon Dioxide in the Blood*

| | Arterial Blood | | Venous Blood | |
	mM./L. Bl.	%	mM./L. Bl.	%
Total	21.9		24.1	
Plasma				
Dissolved CO_2	0.66	3	0.76	3
HCO_3^-	14.00	64	15.00	63
Cells				
Dissolved CO_2	0.44	2	0.54	2
HCO_3^-	5.7	26	6.1	25
$HbNHCOO^-$	1.2	5	1.8	7

The table gives normal values of the various chemical forms of CO_2 in blood with an assumed hematocrit level of 46. Approximately twice as much CO_2 exists in the plasma as in the red cells, chiefly as HCO_3^-.

(chloride or Hamburger shift). Thus, although the larger portion of the buffering occurs within the red cell, the largest amount of carbon dioxide is in the plasma as HCO_3^- (Table 5).

Although red blood cells from newborn infants have less carbonic anhydrase activity than adult cells, no defect in carbon dioxide transport is apparent. In patients receiving a carbonic anhydrase inhibitor such as acetazolamide (Diamox) the loss of carbon dioxide from the pulmonary capillaries and the uptake of carbon dioxide from the tissues may be incomplete, leading to an increased arterial and tissue P_{CO_2}. Also, on breathing 100 per cent oxygen less reduced hemoglobin is present in venous blood, and therefore less buffering capacity for H^+ is present, leading to an increased P_{CO_2}. This is an important consideration during hyperbaric oxygenation when the venous blood may remain almost completely saturated with oxygen, H^+ is less well buffered, and tissue P_{CO_2} rises.

Acid-Base Balance

A reduction in pH, acidosis, may be caused by a reduction in HCO_3^- (metabolic acidosis) or an increase in P_{CO_2} (respiratory acidosis). An elevation of pH, alkalosis, may be caused by an elevation of bicarbonate (metabolic alkalosis) or a reduction of P_{CO_2} (respiratory alkalosis) (Table 6).

Metabolic acidosis is found in such conditions as diabetes, in which there is an accumulation of keto-acids, renal failure when the kidney is unable to excrete hydrogen ion, in diarrhea from loss of base, or in tissue hypoxia associated with lactic acid accumulation. When pH falls, respiration is stimulated so that P_{CO_2} will fall and tend to compensate for the reduction in pH. This compensation is usually incomplete, and pH remains below 7.35. The pH, carbon dioxide content $(HCO_3^- + P_{CO_2})$, HCO_3^- and P_{CO_2} are all reduced.

Metabolic alkalosis occurs most commonly after excessive loss of Cl^- in vomiting (as in pyloric stenosis) or after an excessive citrate or bicarbonate load. The carbon dioxide content is elevated, and the P_{CO_2} will be normal or elevated, depending on the chronicity of the alkalosis.

Acute respiratory acidosis is secondary to respiratory insufficiency and accumulation of carbon dioxide within the body. The associated acidosis may be compensated by renal adjustments which promote retention of HCO_3^-. Compensation may require several days. Patients with chronic respiratory acidosis, in whom therapy may improve alveolar ventilation, often have a rapid fall of Pa_{CO_2}. The adjustment in bicarbonate may be much slower, with a resultant metabolic alkalosis of several days' duration. Such a sequence of events has been noted in emphysema and cystic fibrosis.

Similarly, acute respiratory alkalosis, for example, secondary to fever, psychogenic hyperventilation, or a pontine lesion with meningoencephalitis will be associated with a high pH, low P_{CO_2} and normal

Table 6.   *Blood Measurements in Various Acid-Base Disturbances*

	pH	Pa_{CO_2} (mm. Hg)	HCO_3^- (mEq./L.)	CO_2 Content (mEq./L.)
Metabolic acidosis	↓	↓	↓	↓
Acute respiratory acidosis	↓	↑	↔	Slight ↑
Compensated respiratory acidosis ...(↔ or slight ↓)		↑	↑	↑
Metabolic alkalosis	↑	Slight ↑	↑	↑
Acute respiratory alkalosis	↑	↓	↔	Slight ↓
Compensated respiratory alkalosis ...(↔ or slight ↑)		↓	↓	↓
Normal values 7.35-7.45		35-45	24-26	25-28

bicarbonate. Renal compensation in time leads to an excretion of bicarbonate and a return of pH toward normal.

It is important to point out that the lung excretes some 13,000 mEq. of acid per day in the form of carbon dioxide, the kidney 40 to 80 mEq. per day. Thus the lung plays a large role in the acid-base balance of the body, and in fact provides rapid adjustment when necessary. The Henderson-Hasselbalch equation may be thought of as:

$$pH \alpha \frac{Kidney}{Lung}$$

TISSUE RESPIRATION

Aerobic Metabolism

The ultimate function of the lung is to provide oxygen to meet the demands of the tissues and to excrete carbon dioxide, a by-product of metabolic activity. Thus respiratory physiologists have been concerned with the assessment of respiration at the tissue level and the ability of the cardiopulmonary system to meet the metabolic demands of the body.

One method is to measure the amount of oxygen consumed by the body per minute ($\dot{V}_{O_2}$). This is equal to the amount necessary to maintain the life of the cells at rest, plus the amount necessary for oxidative combustion required to maintain a normal body temperature, as well as that used for the metabolic demands of work above the resting level. The basal metabolic rate is a summation of many component energy rates of individual organs and tissues and is defined as the amount of energy necessary to maintain the life of the cells at rest, under conditions in which there is no additional energy expenditure for temperature regulation or additional work.

In practice $\dot{V}_{O_2}$ is measured after an overnight fast, the subject lying supine in a room at a comfortable temperature. This "basal" metabolic rate has a wide variability ($\pm$ 15 per cent of predicted $\dot{V}_{O_2}$). Since absolutely basal conditions are difficult to ensure, the measurement of basal metabolic rate is not widely used at present.

The performance of the cardiopulmonary system can be more adequately assessed and compared with normal measurements under conditions of added work, such as exercise. The healthy lung does not limit the ability to increase oxygen consumption to meet the demands of the body, since even during severe exercise the maximal breathing capacity is not reached. Rather, the inability of cardiac output to exceed a certain level limits exercise tolerance. Performance can be increased by physical fitness, and athletes are able to increase their cardiac output by sixfold or sevenfold. Athletic conditioning also increases the diffusing capacity of the lung and in some manner, not well understood, increases the efficiency of oxygen extraction from the blood in the tissues at a given cardiac output. Few studies have been done in children, but in general the relation between work capacity, ventilation and oxygen consumption is the same as that of the adult. The maximal $\dot{V}_{O_2}$ that can be achieved increases throughout childhood, reaches its peak of 50 to 60 ml. per minute per kilogram between ten and fifteen years of age, and thereafter declines slowly with age.

At the tissue level the ability for a given cell to receive an adequate oxygen supply depends on the amount of local blood flow, the distance of that cell from the perfusing capillary and the difference between the partial pressure of oxygen in the capillary and in the cell. The critical mean capillary P_{O_2} appears to be in the region of 30 mm. of mercury for children and adults. Exercising muscle has ten to twenty times the number of open capillaries as resting muscle.

Anaerobic Metabolism

The adequacy of oxygen supply to the tissues has more recently been assessed by measuring blood lactate, a product of anaerobic metabolism (Embden-Meyerhof pathway). When there is insufficient oxygen supply to the tissues from insufficient blood flow, or a decreased oxygen content of blood, lactic acid concentration within the tissues and blood rises. In the blood this accumulation leads to a metabolic acidosis.

During moderate to heavy muscular exercise the cardiac output cannot meet the demands of the muscles, and an oxygen debt is incurred, which is repaid upon cessation of exercise. During this period lactic acid accumulates, and therefore severe exercise is often associated with a metabolic acidosis. There is an excellent correlation between the serum lactate level and the oxygen debt. Since oxygen debt is not measurable at rest and is difficult to measure during exercise, the adequacy of tissue oxygenation appears to be accurately reflected in the serum lactate level. In adult man blood lactate is less than 1 mEq. per liter, but may rise to 10 or 12 mEq. per liter during very heavy exercise.

Relation Between $\dot{V}_{O_2}$ and $\dot{V}_{CO_2}$

In the normal subject in a steady state the amount of carbon dioxide excreted by the lung per minute is dependent upon the basal metabolic activity of the cells and the type of substrate being oxidized. The volume of carbon dioxide exhaled divided by the amount of oxygen consumed is known as the ventilatory respiratory quotient (R). For the body as a whole the ratio is 1 if primarily carbohydrate is being metabolized, 0.7 for fat, and 0.8 for protein. Normally the ratio is 0.8 at rest and approximately 1.0 during exercise. The ventilatory respiratory quotient may vary considerably with changes in alveolar ventilation and metabolism and therefore must be measured in the steady state, i.e. with a steady alveolar ventilation and a steady metabolic rate. For an individual organ the metabolic respiratory quotient (R.Q.) is nearly constant, but may vary from 0.4 to 1.5, de-

pending on the balance of anabolism and catabolism in a particular organ. Thus the measurement of R represents the resultant of many component metabolizing organs and tissues. In the first few days after birth R falls from nearly 1 to 0.7, indicating a loss of carbohydrate stores, and as feeding is started R approaches 0.8.

Temperature Effects

Increasing emphasis has recently been placed on the relation between metabolism and body temperature, particularly in the newborn infant. Van't Hoff's Law for simple chemical reactions states that the reaction rate is directly proportional to the temperature at which the reaction is taking place. In a biologic system, for each $10°$ C. rise in temperature, reaction rate increases by twofold to threefold (Q_{10} effect). Homeothermic mammals, however, do not obey van't Hoff's Law because as temperature decreases, oxygen consumption increases to maintain a normal body temperature, until hypothermic levels are reached (below $30°$ C. $\dot{V}_{O_2}$ decreases with decreasing temperature). Under a cold stress the adult becomes exhausted after a few hours. Since it is likely that the newborn with a relatively large surface area and poor insulation would fail to maintain a normal body temperature even sooner, the optimum thermal environment for premature and term infants has undergone considerable recent investigation. Evidence that premature infants with a low body temperature have a higher mortality rate has necessitated careful regulation of the environmental temperature.

Normal newborn infants do not exhibit a Q_{10} effect; i.e. they increase $\dot{V}_{O_2}$ with decrease in environmental temperature (Fig. 14). The optimum or neutral environmental temperature, i.e. the temperature at which oxygen consumption is minimal, has been found to be related to the gradient between the skin and deep body temperature. If this does not exceed $1.5°$ C., oxygen consumption remains minimal regardless of the deep body tem-

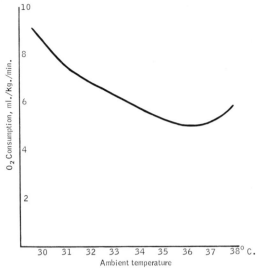

FIGURE 1–14. The relation of oxygen consumption and environmental temperature in a typical infant of 1.5 to 2 kg. of body weight. (Adapted from the data of Mestayn and others.)

perature. If body temperature is low, and the skin temperature is not more than 1.5° C. cooler, body temperature will rise at approximately 1.5° C. per hour until normal temperature is reached. It has been proposed that for premature infants skin temperature be maintained at 36° C. in order to avoid a thermal stress and to reduce mortality.

These considerations are important in a variety of clinical circumstances in which oxygen tents containing cold air are used. A common sight on any pediatric ward is the child with respiratory distress lying in a cold, albeit oxygenated and humidified, environment. The additional thermal stress may be life-threatening.

VENTILATION-PERFUSION RELATIONS

The efficiency of pulmonary gas exchange is remarkable when one considers that air must be properly distributed to several hundred million alveoli in correct proportion to the amount of blood perfusing these alveoli. It is this nearly perfect matching of blood flow ($\dot{Q}$) and alveolar ventilation ($\dot{V}_A$) within millions of respiratory units that enables the healthy lung to maintain blood gas tensions that are nearly constant. For the adult lung as a whole, $\dot{V}_A$ is 4 liters per minute and $\dot{Q}$ 5 liters per minute. The relation between ventilation and perfusion is expressed as the ratio:

$$\frac{\dot{V}_A}{\dot{Q}} = 0.8$$

This ratio reflects the relation of ventilation to perfusion for the lung as a whole. Even in health not all alveoli have a perfect match of $\dot{V}_A$ and $\dot{Q}$. Within an individual alveolus ventilation may be in excess of the blood flow ($\dot{V}_A/\dot{Q}$ greater than 0.8), or blood flow may be in excess of the ventilation ($\dot{V}_A/\dot{Q}$ less than 0.8). What is the effect on alveolar and blood gas tensions of grossly altered $\dot{V}_A/\dot{Q}$? Consider two extreme examples: (a) one lung has normal ventilation, but no blood flow ($\dot{V}_A/\dot{Q} = \infty$); (b) one lung has no ventilation, but normal blood flow ($\dot{V}_A/\dot{Q} = 0$).

In situation a, if one lung receives 2.0 liters per minute of ventilation, but does not receive any blood supply ($\dot{V}_A/\dot{Q} = \infty$), no gas exchange can occur, and the ventilation enters an alveolus which acts as if it were dead space. If the other lung received 2.0 liters per minute alveolar ventilation, half of the total, but now had 5 liters per minute blood flow (instead of

2.5), the blood leaving the lung would have an elevated P_{CO_2} of about 80 mm. of mercury and a P_{O_2} decreased to approximately 60 mm. of mercury (about 80 per cent saturated). If alveolar ventilation is doubled to compensate for the shift in blood flow, the arterial P_{CO_2} and P_{O_2} will return to normal, yet a sample of mixed alveolar gas will not have normal gas tensions. Normally, the alveolar gas from each lung, each with the same P_{CO_2} and P_{O_2}, would mix in the trachea and emerge with a P_{O_2} of 100 mm. and a P_{CO_2} of 40 mm. of mercury. In the above-mentioned example, a, when 50 per cent of the alveolar ventilation goes to alveolar dead space, the mixing of alveolar gas from the two lungs produces a P_{CO_2} of $\frac{40 + 0}{2}$ or 20 mm. of mercury, much lower than the arterial P_{CO_2}. Mixed alveolar P_{O_2} will be higher $\left(\frac{100 + 150}{2} = 125 \text{ mm. Hg}\right)$. Note that Pa_{CO_2} is greater than $P_{A_{CO_2}}$ and $P_{A_{O_2}}$ greater than Pa_{O_2}. These gradients form the basis for the measurement of alveolar dead space (V_D alv) (see p. 23).

In situation b, when one lung has no ventilation and normal blood flow ($\dot{V}_A/\dot{Q} = 0$), while the other lung has a normal $\dot{V}_A/\dot{Q}$, the blood flowing through the nonventilated lung acts as shunted blood, mixes with the arterial blood, and lowers the P_{O_2} and oxygen content (hypoxemia). For example, if mixed venous blood contained 12 ml. of oxygen per 100 ml. of blood and arterial blood coming from the ventilated lung contained 20 ml. of oxygen per 100 ml. of blood, the mixture of equal parts (50 per cent shunt) would have an arterial oxygen content of $\frac{20 + 12}{2} = 16$ ml. per 100 ml. of blood. The arterial oxygen tensions would be reduced from 100 mm. to about 45 mm. of mercury and the saturation reduced to 80 per cent. There is little effect on P_{CO_2}, since arterial-venous P_{CO_2} differences are only 6 mm. of mercury. An increased alveolar ventilation to the one ventilated

and perfused lung, or an increased inspired oxygen concentration would have practically no effect on the oxygen content of the blood coming from that lung, since it was previously nearly fully saturated with oxygen.

The same principles apply to less extreme examples of ventilation-perfusion derangements, such as alveoli which receive slightly more ventilation than perfusion. Here a portion of $\dot{V}_A$ is wasted and acts as if dead space were ventilated. If there is less ventilation than blood flow to an alveolus ($\dot{V}_A/\dot{Q}$ less than 0.8), the blood does not undergo complete gas exchange. The effect is similar to that of an anatomic shunt which permits venous to arterial circulation. The blood from such an alveolus can be considered a mixture of normally arterialized blood and pure venous blood. Indeed, in patients with pulmonary disease the commonest cause of hypoxemia is improper matching of blood and gas in the lung.

Measurement of Distribution of Ventilation

Nitrogen has been used to determine the distribution of inspired gas within the lung because it is poorly soluble and does not pass quickly in large amounts from the pulmonary capillaries to the alveoli. One test requires the inhalation of a single breath of 100 per cent oxygen and measurement of the concentration of nitrogen in the expired air. The concentration of nitrogen at the beginning of expiration is low; as expiration continues, it increases to alveolar tensions and "plateaus" at this value. When there is altered distribution of ventilation, some alveoli get only a small amount of oxygen, while others receive more than their share. Thus there is no representative alveolar nitrogen concentration, and it continues to rise during expiration, since the hypoventilated areas empty last.

Another standard test is to inspire 100 per cent oxygen and watch the fall in alveolar nitrogen concentration that occurs as it is washed out of the lung. For the normal adult, nitrogen concentration should be less than 2.5 per cent after seven minutes of oxygen breathing. With poor distribution of ventilation this value is much higher. In normal children nitrogen concentration falls much more rapidly and is below 2.5 per cent after only two minutes of oxygen breathing. In the normal newborn infant this level is reached in one minute. These two methods measure only the distribution of inspired air to alveoli, without reflecting the relation between $\dot{V}_A$ and $\dot{Q}$.

Several methods are used to examine the distribution of ventilation in relation to perfusion. One of the commonest is the measurement of physiologic dead space. When alveolar ventilation is in excess of blood flow in many areas of the lung, physiologic dead space (anatomic dead space plus alveolar dead space) is elevated.

Another method of assessing $\dot{V}_A/\dot{Q}$, the measurement of a-A nitrogen tension gradients, has recently been developed. Since nitrogen is inert, fluctuations in alveolar nitrogen tension ($P_{A_{N_2}}$) are passive, and depend on changes in oxygen and carbon dioxide tension. Alveolar gas in areas with a low $\dot{V}_A/\dot{Q}$ has a high nitrogen tension because more oxygen is absorbed and less carbon dioxide excreted. On expiration the small amount of ventilation from these areas mixes with a large amount of ventilation from normal areas, and only slightly raises the average $P_{A_{N_2}}$. A relatively large amount of blood from the area of low $\dot{V}_A/\dot{Q}$ in equilibrium with the high $P_{A_{N_2}}$ present mixes with a smaller amount of blood from normal areas, resulting in an elevation of the average Pa_{N_2} that is larger than the average $P_{A_{N_2}}$. Thus the effect of many areas containing a low $\dot{V}_A/\dot{Q}$ is to produce an a-A P_{N_2} gradient. Since nitrogen is inert, P_{N_2} is the same in all biologic fluids. It may be measured, using gas chromatography, in both blood and urine. In normal children the a-A P_{N_2} gradient

averages 3 mm. of mercury (less than 10 mm.). In conditions, however, with severe abnormality in $\dot{V}_A/\dot{Q}$, such as cystic fibrosis, the gradient increases some fivefold to tenfold. Moderate a-A P_{N_2} gradients are found in normal newborn infants during the first day of life, returning to normal by the second day.

The use of radioactive gases such as oxygen, carbon dioxide and xenon has recently enabled investigators to describe $\dot{V}_A/\dot{Q}$ relations of different areas of the lung. Geographic mapping of $\dot{V}_A/\dot{Q}$ from the apex to the base of the lung has supported the previous indirect methods which suggested that $\dot{V}_A/\dot{Q}$ was altered by gravitational forces. Indeed, in normal upright man $\dot{V}_A/\dot{Q}$ may vary from 0.6 at the base to more than 2.0 at the apex. Despite the variance of $\dot{V}_A/\dot{Q}$ in normal man, little effect on blood gases is seen until greater inhomogeneity is present.

Mechanism of Nonuniform Ventilation

The uniformity of ventilation in the normal lung depends on a delicate balance between the resistance and compliance of each ventilatory pathway. A decrease in airway dimensions will increase the time required for air to reach the alveoli; a region with low compliance will receive less ventilation than an area of high compliance. The product of resistance times compliance (time constant) is approximately the same in health for all ventilatory pathways. The unit of resistance times compliance is time. Note:

$$\text{Resistance} = \text{Pressure/Flow} = \frac{\text{cm. } H_2O}{\text{liters/sec.}}$$

$$\text{Compliance} = \frac{\Delta \text{ Volume (liters)}}{\Delta \text{ Pressure (cm. } H_2O)}$$

The product, then, is a unit of time, analogous to the time constant in electrical systems. Almost any disease process in the lung will alter the time constant in the affected areas, and result in uneven distribution of ventilation.

Measurement of the Distribution of Blood Flow

The amount of venous admixture that is present can be estimated from the shunt equation: *

$$\frac{\dot{Q}_s}{\dot{Q}_T} = \frac{Ca_{O_2} - Cc_{O_2}}{C\bar{v}_{O_2} - Cc_{O_2}}$$

where $\dot{Q}_s / \dot{Q}_T$ is the fraction of total cardiac output that is shunted.

In normal subjects up to 6 per cent of the cardiac output may be shunted from right to left primarily through bronchial veins, which empty into the left side of the circulation. A small portion comes from the thebesian veins which drain the coronary circulation directly into the left ventricle. During exercise there is less than 3 per cent venous admixture. An increased venous admixture can be due to low $\dot{V}_A / \dot{Q}$, anatomic right-to-left shunt within the lung, or a cardiac abnormality. Breathing 100 per cent oxygen will obliterate the shunt effect of low $\dot{V}_A / \dot{Q}$, leaving only anatomic shunt, and is used as a test to differentiate between the two effects. Pa_{O_2} should be greater than 500 mm. of mercury during oxygen breathing in the absence of anatomic shunt.

Causes of Nonuniform Pulmonary Blood Flow

1. *Gravity.* Adult man in the upright position does not perfuse the apices of the lung. Since gravity does not greatly affect the distribution of ventilation, the

---

* Since the amount of oxygen in arterial blood equals the amount of oxygen in blood that has passed through pulmonary capillaries (Q_c) plus the amount of oxygen in shunted blood (Q_s), and

Amount of oxygen = content of oxygen/l. (C_{O_2}) $\times$ blood flow ($\dot{Q}$)

Therefore, $Ca_{O_2} \dot{Q}_t = Cc_{O_2} Q_c + C\bar{v}_{O_2} \dot{Q}_s$

(where Q_t = total blood flow)

Since $\dot{Q}_c = \dot{Q}_t - \dot{Q}_s$

$Ca_{O_2} \dot{Q}_t = Cc_{O_2} \dot{Q}_t - Cc_{O_2} \dot{Q}_s + C\bar{v}_{O_2} \dot{Q}_s$

and $\dfrac{\dot{Q}_s}{\dot{Q}_t} = \dfrac{C_{CO_2} - Ca_{O_2}}{C\bar{v}_{O_2} - Cc_{O_2}}$

apices have a high $\dot{V}_A / \dot{Q}$. Children have a relatively higher pulmonary artery pressure and therefore a more uniform distribution of pulmonary blood flow in the upright position.

2. Partial or complete occlusion of the pulmonary artery or arterioles by arteriosclerosis, endarteritis, collagen disease, congenital abnormalities, thrombosis or embolism of blood clots, fats, gas bubbles (caisson disease), tumor cells.

3. Compression of pulmonary vessels by masses, pulmonary exudate, pneumothorax.

4. Reduction in the size of the pulmonary vascular bed.

5. Closure of some pulmonary vessels due to a low pulmonary artery pressure which may occur in shock.

6. Overexpansion of some alveoli and collapse of others.

7. Regional congestion of vessels as in left-sided heart failure.

8. Anatomic pulmonary artery to pulmonary venous shunts, as with pulmonary hemangiomas. The distribution of blood that flows to the capillaries may be uniform, but some mixed venous blood completely bypasses the capillaries and reduces the oxygen content of arterial blood.

Intrinsic Regulation of Regional $\dot{V}_A / \dot{Q}$

Abnormalities of $\dot{V}_A / \dot{Q}$ may be caused by either too much or too little ventilation to an area, although the blood flow may be normal; too much or too little blood flow, although ventilation may be normal; or a combination of both effects. Whatever the absolute amount of regional ventilation and perfusion, the lung has intrinsic regulatory mechanisms which are directed toward the preservation of the "ideal" $\dot{V}_A / \dot{Q}$ of 0.8. In areas where $\dot{V}_A / \dot{Q}$ is high, the low carbon dioxide concentration results in local constriction of airways, and tends to reduce the amount of ventilation to that area. When $\dot{V}_A / \dot{Q}$ is low, the high alveolar carbon dioxide concentration results in local airway dilatation and a tendency to increase ventilation to the area. Furthermore, a low $\dot{V}_A/\dot{Q}$ with an associated low alveolar oxygen concentration causes regional pulmonary vasoconstriction. Effects on airways and vessels from changing gas tensions tend to preserve a normal $\dot{V}_A/\dot{Q}$, but they are limited mechanisms, and derangements are common.

PULMONARY CIRCULATION

The contributions of anatomists, pathologists, cardiologists and respiratory physiologists to our understanding of the pulmonary circulation have been numerous in recent years. The following section cannot be an exhaustive review of the subject, but rather is biased toward those aspects of the pulmonary circulation which are significant in the evaluation of lung function and pathology in the infant and the child.

Anatomy

The main pulmonary arteries and their branches which accompany the cartilaginous bronchi into the lobes of the lung are elastic arteries, characterized by laminations of elastic tissue in the medial layers, similar to the aorta. They branch to form the smaller muscular arteries, with a circular layer of smooth muscle bounded by external and internal elastic laminae. The muscular arteries of the lung have thinner media than their counterparts in the systemic circulation, and range from 100 to 1000 microns in diameter. Arterioles branch from the muscular arteries and are discernible by the lack of a muscular layer. Their walls are composed of some supporting collagen, an elastic layer and a thin adventitia.

Fetal muscular arteries have a thick medial layer which increases during the latter half of gestation; after birth the muscular wall becomes thinner, or the wall-lumen ratio decreases. The adult pattern is reached at different ages in different persons, from two to six months after birth.

The lungs have a double circulation. The pulmonary arteries carry nearly all the cardiac output to the lungs. The nutrient vessels of the lung, the bronchial arteries, are small arteries which arise from the aorta or intercostals and follow the dorsal portion of each primary bronchus. They lose their identity along the respiratory bronchioles; the capillaries they supply drain with the alveolar capillary network into the rich peribronchial venous network which empties into the pulmonary veins. Unlike systemic veins, which usually follow the course of the artery, pulmonary veins follow the interlobular connective-tissue plains. The direct connections of veins to adjacent limiting membranes of lung tissue are the anatomic device which makes their diameters reflect changes in lung volume. Less than 6 per cent of the cardiac output bypasses the alveoli through bronchial vessels and the thebesian veins in the left side of the heart.

Hemodynamics

PRESSURES, FLOWS, RESISTANCES. In the fetal circulation only about 12 per cent of the output of the right ventricle goes to the lungs; the remainder goes through the ductus arteriosus to the aorta. With the initiation of air breathing at birth, pulmonary blood flow increases. The action of increasing oxygen tensions and falling carbon dioxide tensions decreases the tone of the pulmonary vessels, but facilitates closure of the ductus. The changing geometry of the alveoli and vessels which accompanies the creation of an air-liquid interface also promotes increased blood flow.

Left and right ventricular pressures in the fetal heart are nearly the same. Pulmonary artery and aortic pressures in fetal lambs are 50 to 70 mm. of mercury. After birth there is a persistent pulmonary hypertension relative to values at an older age. Mean pulmonary artery pressures in normal term infants are between 20 and 50 mm. of mercury, mean aortic pressures usually 40 to 50 mm. in the first hours of life. During infancy and childhood the tendency is for a gradual increase in systemic pressures and decrease in pulmonary artery pressures.

The pulmonary vessels are capable of dilatation and compression. The degree of distention will depend on the tone of the vessel wall, and the difference in pressure across it, the transmural pressure. In the lung the pressure outside a vessel may vary greatly during the respiratory cycle. The pressure outside the large arteries and veins is pleural pressure, whereas the pressure outside the alveolar capillaries is approximately alveolar pressure. The blood vessels within the lung parenchyma are also subjected to direct forces from the attachments of the pulmonary tissue. Thus the elasticity of the lung tissue exerts a "radial traction" on vessel walls, which increases with lung volume. The pulmonary vascular bed may be thought as existing in two compartments: one which expands with increasing lung volume and presumably includes all vessels outside the alveolar walls, the other which is compressed at large lung volumes and presumably contains alveolar vessels.

It is apparent that evaluations of pulmonary vascular resistance (pressure/flow) will be complicated by the different pressure relations existing across parts of the pulmonary vascular bed. Much of the confusion in the literature about pressure-flow relations in the lung has been overcome by an appreciation of the so-called vascular waterfall phenomenon. The simile implies that upstream pressure and flow are independent of changes downstream in a system of collapsible vessels as long as the downstream pressure is less than that which surrounds the collapsible member. Since the pressure outside the collapsible pulmonary alveolar capillaries is approximately alveolar pressure, when the pressure in the pulmonary veins is less than alveolar pressure, pulmonary blood flow will depend on the difference between pulmonary artery and alveolar pressure. When pulmonary venous pressure is greater than alveolar pressure, pulmonary blood flow will be determined by the difference in pressure between artery and vein.

EFFECT OF GRAVITY. The pressure is not the same in similar vessels in an upright person at the apex of the lung as at the base, and the magnitude of the difference is related to the height of the person. Since the pulmonary artery enters about the midportion of the lung, the systolic arterial pressure of 15 to 20 mm. of mercury is adequate to perfuse the apices during systole, but not during diastole if the distance is greater than the diastolic pressure. The vessels in the lung bases are exposed to pulmonary artery pressure, plus the pressure generated by the weight of the column of blood, which may be another 15 cm. of water. Thus in any situation in which transudation is favored, more fluid will be found in the bases than in the apices in the upright posture. The relative underperfusion of the apices in upright man results in a slightly higher mean alveolar P_{O_2}, and a lower P_{CO_2} in apical alveolar air. One important clinical application of this effect of gravity is that the higher P_{O_2} in apical segments favors the growth of the tubercle bacillus and is thought to be the basis for the apical localization of tuberculosis in adults. The smaller size of the child makes the hydrostatic effects of gravity less and may underlie the random localization of the primary tuberculosis complex in the child. (The physiologic consequences of the forces of gravity on the distribution of the circulation and ventilation are discussed on page 42.)

Movement of Liquid in the Lung

The forces which tend to move liquid from capillary to air space are the positive pressures within the capillary, the negative pericapillary tissue pressures and, in the case of the lung, the pressure exerted by the forces of surface tension at the air-liquid interface. The force which opposes these pressures, and normally keeps liquid in the capillary along its entire length, is the colloid osmotic pressure of the blood (Fig. 15). The amount of edema formation will depend also on the permeability of the capillaries and their filtration area. The area will in turn depend on any nervous, chemical or physical change in blood vessel tone. In general, increased distention of the capillaries will also increase the permeability.

Some of the causes of pulmonary edema are categorized in Table 7. It can be initiated by a variety of insults to several systems, and the mechanism of edema formation may differ accordingly. Most commonly, left ventricular failure and an elevation in capillary hydrostatic pressure underlie pulmonary edema. Humoral agents, vagotomy, alterations in capillary wall integrity and many pharmacologic agents can also induce pulmonary edema.

The pulmonary functional derangements in edema affect both gas exchange and pulmonary mechanics. Usually a diffusion impairment can be demonstrated before there are significant mechanical changes. One of the earliest changes is a thickening of the alveolar-capillary membranes. Arterial hypoxemia is present, and may be ameliorated by forcible inflation of the lungs, suggesting that some of the venous admixture is from blood flow through poorly ventilated portions of the lungs. Edematous lungs lack the pulmonary surfactant, which is either denatured by movement of fluid across alveolar membranes or washed out by the foaming which accompanies acute pulmonary edema. Lung compliance is greatly reduced, airway resistance increased, and respiratory work increases manyfold.

Some water exchange occurs in normal

Table 7. *Some Causes of Pulmonary Edema*

I. Hemodynamic derangements
  1. Coronary occlusion
  2. Left ventricular outflow obstruction
  3. Left atrial occlusion
  4. Mitral valve disease
  5. Hypervolemia
  6. Hemorrhage and shock
  7. Embolism
  8. Pulmonary venous obstruction, high altitude
II. Central nervous system disorders
III. Vagotomy
IV. Respiratory system disorders
  1. Airway obstruction
  2. Hypoxia
  3. Burns
  4. Drowning
  5. Injury
V. Pharmacologic agents
  1. Epinephrine
  2. Histamine
  3. Acetylcholine
  4. Irritant gases
  5. Other agents such as alloxan

lungs. In the resting state net water loss from the lung is about 0.63 to 0.65 mg. per milliliter of oxygen absorbed. Flux of water in the lung is much greater.

Drowning

The inhalation of liquid into the lung is associated with immediate reflex laryngospasm. If this is sustained to the point of severe hypoxia, the larynx opens, and more liquid may enter the lung. The physiologic consequences depend on the nature of the lipid aspirated. If it is fresh water, which is hypotonic with respect to the blood, about 1 ml. per kilo-

FIGURE 1–15. Forces which maintain water balance between alveolus and capillary.

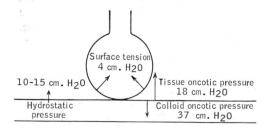

gram is absorbed in two to three minutes. Significant amounts absorbed lead to hypervolemia, hemolysis, hyperkalemia and ventricular fibrillation. If salt water, which is hypertonic with respect to the blood, enters the alveoli, further movement of liquid from blood to lung occurs with pulmonary edema and hemorrhage. Hypovolemia and systemic hypotension ensue.

The physiologic sequelae may be profound even with small amounts aspirated, from reflex irritation of the airways and the obstructive effects of foam. Intermittent positive-pressure breathing may be lifesaving.

Regulation

Some of the passive regulatory events with changes in lung volume have been cited above. Active changes in pulmonary vascular resistance can occur with changes in blood gases, neural stimulation and with drugs. Low oxygen tensions tend to constrict pulmonary vessels, both reflexly and locally. Increased hydrogen ion concentrations potentiate the vasoconstrictive effects of hypoxia, but have little effect in the absence of hypoxia. Reflex vasoconstriction accompanies elevated left atrial pressures, and thus operates to prevent pulmonary edema.

Many drugs affect the pulmonary vasculature, including the arteriolar constrictors norepinephrine, epinephrine, histamine, angiotensin and serotonin. Isoproterenol and acetylcholine are examples of agents which tend to dilate constricted arterioles.

Methods of Evaluation

The chest radiograph remains the most widely used tool to determine the possible presence of pulmonary vascular disease. Prominence of the pulmonary outflow tract, and increased or decreased vascular markings may be noted. Regional pulmonary angiography further delineates localized disturbances in blood flow, although the procedure requires cardiac catheterization. Direct measurements of pulmonary artery and "wedge" or capillary pressures add further information. Occasionally drugs can be infused into the pulmonary artery to evaluate the potential reversibility of pulmonary vasoconstriction.

Recently embolization of a minute but uniformly distributed portion of the pulmonary vascular bed with macroaggregated albumin tagged with I^{131} has permitted direct visualization of regional blood flow. The tagged molecules are metabolized within a few hours, and excreted by six to eight hours. The radioactivity can be recorded with suitable scanners. It has been shown that the density of the radioscan correlates with oxygen uptake. Thus differential lung perfusion can be evaluated, even in infants, with this technique.

Measurements of pulmonary blood flow with an inert gas method are becoming more widely used and are applicable to infants. The method depends on the solubility of nitrous oxide in blood. The patient inspires a mixture of 80 per cent nitrous oxide and 20 per cent oxygen. From the measured volumes and concentrations of the inspired and expired mixtures, the amount absorbed can be calculated. The alveolar nitrous oxide concentration is measured from the end-tidal level read on a continuous analyzer. The formula used is as follows:

$$Q_c = \frac{V_{N_2O} \times f}{[\alpha]^{37° N_2O}} \times F_{A_{N_2O}}$$

where Q_c represents pulmonary capillary blood flow per minute, V_{N_2O} volume of nitrous oxide absorbed per heart beat, f heart rate per minute, and $F_{A_{N_2O}}$ nitrous oxide in the alveolar or end-tidal gas. $[\alpha]^{37°}$ is the solubility coefficient of nitrous oxide in blood at 37° C. and 760 mm. of mercury pressure, and is 0.47 ml. of nitrous oxide per milliliter of blood. The uptake of nitrous oxide will be restricted to those portions of lung which are both ventilated and perfused; thus the measurement is of "effective pulmonary blood flow" and may underestimate total blood flow. In adults the normal value is 5.9 liters per minute, with some increase toward the end of inspiration, and a decrease toward the end of expiration, and is pulsatile during the cardiac cycle.

Estimates from dye studies indicate that about 20 per cent of the total blood volume is in the lungs at any one time, and 6 per cent of the pulmonary blood volume is in the capillary bed.

REGULATION OF RESPIRATION

Over the past fifteen years the classic concepts concerned with the respiratory control system have been challenged and broadened in many areas. It is appropriate for pediatricians to have an understanding of the normal respiratory control mechanisms, since alterations in respiratory frequency or alveolar ventilation are a frequent concomitant of many diseases in childhood.

Two main systems are involved in the regulatory process: (1) a neural system which is responsible for the maintenance of a coordinated, rhythmic respiratory cycle and the regulation of the depth of respiration, and (2) a chemical (neurohumoral) system which regulates alveolar ventilation and maintains normal blood gas tensions.

Neural System

The respiratory center is now recognized to consist of four areas in the brain stem, two pontine and two medullary areas (Fig. 16). The pneumotaxic center is located in the rostral few millimeters of the pons. Section of the pons below this level results in a slowing and an increase in amplitude of respiration. If, in addition, the vagi are cut, respiration stops at a maximal inspiratory position called apneusis. The pneumotaxic center has no intrinsic rhythmicity, but functions to modulate respiratory frequency and depth, since ablation produces respiratory

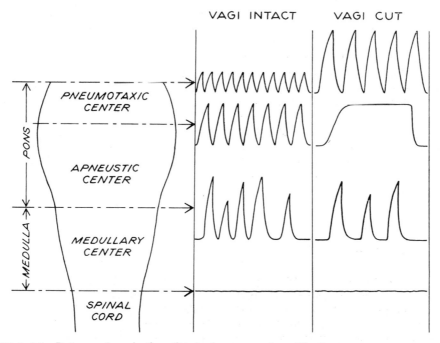

FIGURE 1–16. Patterns of respiration after brain stem sections. The 4 patterns are representative of those which follow complete sections at each level. Section below the medulla results in complete apnea. (From J. H. Comroe: *Physiology of Respiration*. Chicago, Year Book Medical Publishers, Inc., 1965.)

slowing and stimulation accelerates respiration. It is also responsible for periodic inhibition of the apneustic center in the pons.

The apneustic center is located in the middle and caudal pons. This area produces a tonic inspiratory spasm and is modulated through feed-back mechanisms by the pneumotaxic center, medullary respiratory centers and vagal afferent impulses. Total removal of the pons abolishes apneusis and produces rhythmic respirations which are generally gasping and not well coordinated.

The medullary respiratory centers consist of an inspiratory center situated caudally in the ventral portion of the medullary reticular formation, and an expiratory center situated dorsal and cephalad to the inspiratory center. It is now accepted that the medullary centers are intrinsically rhythmic, but are modulated by pontine and vagal discharges.

Proprioceptive vagal impulses from receptors in the lung parenchyma (Hering-Breuer reflex) result in inhibition of inspiration as the lung distends. Cutting the vagi results in slow, deep rhythmic respiration. Therefore vagal reflexes serve to accelerate the central neural mechanism. At slow respiratory rates the stretch receptors increase inspiration slightly, while at rapid frequencies they inhibit inspiration. Thus the peripheral component of the neural system complements the activity of the central neural centers. Stimulation of these receptors in conditions such as pulmonary edema and interstitial pulmonary fibrosis results in tachypnea.

It is worth while noting that brain stem hemorrhage, although usually resulting in apnea, may initially be associated with tachypnea.

The respiratory control areas are also influenced by higher centers. Tachypnea, associated with fever, is presumably mediated by the influence of the hypothalamus on the brain stem centers. Furthermore, voluntary control of ventilation is possible within limits.

It is now apparent that the background of different stimuli through the medullary reticular system is important in maintaining the ability of respiratory neurons to discharge spontaneously. This concept of "neuronal traffic" has been implicated as an important mechanism in the newborn infant who begins to breathe spontaneously in association with the sensory stimuli associated with the birth process, and perhaps explains the lack of rhythmic respiration in utero.

A variety of peripheral reflexes are known to affect respiration. Hyperpnea may be produced by stimulation of pain, temperature or mechanoreceptors in the limbs. Visceral reflexes are usually associated with apnea, e.g. distention of the gallbladder or traction on the gut. Afferent impulses from muscle spindles of the intercostal muscles and diaphragm may play a role in determining the optimum response of the muscles of ventilation to various respiratory stimuli.

Chemical System

The neurohumoral system is primarily concerned with the regulation of alveolar ventilation and blood gases. This chemical control is mediated by two sets of specialized neural structures which are susceptible to changes in pH, P_{CO_2} and P_{O_2}, one, the central receptors, and the other, chromaffin tissue along the great vessels.

The exact location of the central chemoreceptors is uncertain. The most recent evidence suggests that chemoreceptive tissue is located along the ventral lateral medulla near the area postrema. Direct stimulation of this area by increased P_{CO_2} or H^+ produces an increase in ventilation, and, conversely, a decreased P_{CO_2} or H^+ concentration causes a depression of ventilation. It has been suggested that this area is influenced primarily by the the acid-base composition of cerebrospinal fluid and that the delay in ventilatory response to changes in arterial P_{CO_2} and bicarbonate is due to the time required to change the cerebrospinal fluid H^+ concentration. Carbon dioxide, which diffuses into the cerebrospinal fluid in a few minutes, has a rapid effect on the central chemoreceptors. Changes in blood bicarbonate are much less rapidly reflected in the cerebrospinal fluid (twenty-four to forty-eight hours). Thus with acute metabolic acidosis arterial P_{CO_2} falls along with cerebrospinal fluid P_{CO_2}. Hyperventilation is produced by the H^+ stimulation of peripheral chemoreceptors, but this stimulus is inadequate to compensate fully for the metabolic acidosis because of inhibition from the decreased H^+ concentration in the cerebral spinal fluid. After twenty-four hours cerebrospinal fluid bicarbonate falls and restores cerebrospinal fluid pH to normal. There is a further fall in arterial P_{CO_2}, and arterial pH returns toward normal. From these observations it has been suggested that the control of alveolar ventilation is a function of the central chemoreceptors which are under the influence of cerebrospinal fluid H^+, acting in association with the peripheral chemoreceptors, which are directly under the influence of the arterial blood (Table 8).

The peripheral chemoreceptors are embryologic remnants of the primitive gill system of respiration and are found in man along the structures associated with the branchial arches. Two sets of chemoreceptors appear to be of greatest physiologic importance: (1) the carotid bodies, located at the division of the common carotid artery into its internal and external branches, and (2) the aortic bodies, which lie between the ascending aorta and the pulmonary artery. Afferent nerves from the carotid body join the glossopharyngeal (IX) nerve; those from the aortic bodies join the vagosympathetic trunk along with the recurrent laryngeal nerves.

The carotid and aortic bodies are responsive primarily to changes in oxygen tension. At rest they are tonically active, signifying that some ventilatory drive exists at a Pa_{O_2} of 100 mm. of mercury. Inhalation of 33 per cent oxygen reduces ventilation; inhalation of low oxygen mixtures is associated with a significant increase in ventilation when the Pa_{O_2} is less than 60 mm. of mercury. Potentiation of the hypoxic stimulus is achieved by an increase in Pa_{CO_2}. For example, at a Pa_{CO_2} of 50 mm. of mercury, ventilation is significantly increased when Pa_{O_2} is lowered to 80 mm. Hypoxia and hypotension presumably act together to decrease the oxygen supply of the chemoreceptor tissue, resulting in a greater ventilatory response to hypoxia.

The response of the peripheral chemoreceptors to P_{CO_2} is rapid (within seconds), but ventilation increases only slightly until Pa_{CO_2} is increased by 10 mm. of mercury or more. More important than the amplitude of change may be the rate of change of Pa_{CO_2}. Recent evidence supports the hypothesis that the carotid bodies respond more to an oscillating Pa_{CO_2} than to a steady Pa_{CO_2} at the same mean level, because these chemoreceptors adapt to a constant stimulus in the same manner as thermal or touch sensory re-

Table 8. *Acid-Base Relationships in Cerebrospinal Fluid and Arterial Blood*

		pH	P_{CO_2}	HCO_3^-	$\dot{V}_E$
Normal	Arterial blood	7.40	40	25	↔
	Cerebrospinal fluid	7.32	43	21	
Acute metabolic acidosis	Arterial blood	↓↓	↓	↓↓	↑
	Cerebrospinal fluid	↑	↓	↔	
Chronic metabolic acidosis	Arterial blood	↓	↓↓	↓↓	↑↑
	Cerebrospinal fluid	↔	↓↓	↓	
Acute hypoxia	Arterial blood	↑	↓	↔	↑
	Cerebrospinal fluid	↑	↓	↔	
Chronic hypoxia, as at high altitude	Arterial blood	↑↑	↓↓	↓	↑↑
	Cerebrospinal fluid	↔	↓↓	↓	

ceptors of the skin. Part of the hyperventilation of exercise may be accounted for on this basis, since oscillations of arterial P_{CO_2} of about 7 mm. of mercury accompany moderate exercise. The peripheral chemoreceptors play a minor role in the stimulation of respiration when there is central depression because they adapt to the constant Pa_{CO_2}, and respiration is maintained for the most part by the hypoxic drive alone.

The peripheral chemoreceptors, also responsive to changes in arterial pH, increase ventilation in association with a fall of 0.1 pH unit, and produce a twofold to threefold increase with a fall of 0.4 pH unit. Some investigators believe that the peripheral chemoreceptor response is mediated through changes in intracellular hydrogen ion concentration. Direct proof of this hypothesis is lacking.

Response to Hypercapnia and Hypoxia in the Newborn Infant

There is special interest in the control of breathing in the newborn infant, since this is the period of transition from the intrauterine, apneic state to extrauterine existence, which depends on the lung as the organ of gas exchange.

Infants are known to increase ventilation in response to inspired carbon dioxide. When infants (both premature and full term) and adults are compared by ventilation per kilogram of body weight, all infants breathe more at a given P_{CO_2} than adults, presumably because of a higher P_{CO_2} production per kilogram and less buffering capacity of the blood. Yet the change in ventilation per millimeter of mercury change in P_{CO_2} is the same in infants and adults, suggesting that their neurochemical apparatus has the same sensitivity, but that the ventilatory response is a function of body mass. A useful analogy is the thermostat and furnace in a small house; increasing the size of the house does not necessitate a new thermostat, but requires a larger furnace to keep the rooms at the same temperature.

Peripheral chemoreceptors are functional in newborn infants as demonstrated by a slight decrease in $\dot{V}_E$ with 100 per cent oxygen breathing. The effect of hypoxia as a stimulant may differ in the first twelve hours of life; 12 per cent oxygen in the first twelve hours of life fails to stimulate ventilation. Presumably the atypical response reflects persistent fetal shunts which affect the oxygen tensions of blood perfusing the carotid body.

Derangements

PERIODIC BREATHING. Periodic breathing is commonly seen in otherwise normal premature infants. It is characterized by a period of apnea lasting three to ten seconds followed by a period of ventilation for ten to fifteen seconds. The average respiratory rate is 30 to 40 per minute; the rate during the ventilatory interval is 50 to 60 per minute. It is rarely seen during the first twenty-four hours of life and disappears by thirty-eight to forty weeks postconceptual age. Periodic breathing may appear intermittently interspersed by long periods of regular breathing. During periodic breathing infants appear more wakeful, with tremors of the tongue and extremities, and movements of the eyes. This resembles the rapid eye movement stage of sleep in the adult, which can also be associated with periodic or Cheyne-Stokes respiration. Also, as in the adult with Cheyne-Stokes respiration, periodic breathing is associated with mild hyperventilation resulting in slightly alkalotic arterial blood (mean pH 7.44) compared with regular breathers (mean pH 7.39). Average arterial P_{CO_2} is approximately 3 to 4 mm. of mercury lower during periodic breathing. During the apneic period P_{CO_2} increases by 6 to 7 mm. of mercury, and this increased cyclic change in Pa_{CO_2} may be responsible for the slight hyperventilation (cf. peripheral chemoreceptors). It seems probable that immaturity of the central integrating mechanism responsible for the integration of chemical and nonchemical ventilatory stimuli is responsible for periodic breathing, but further evidence is required.

APNEIC SPELLS. Apneic spells, characterized by more than twenty seconds of apnea with bradycardia, occur frequently in distressed premature infants and may be repetitive. They denote serious underlying disease. In one series 70 per cent of premature infants died after a prolonged apneic spell in contrast to 15 per cent of full-term infants. A decrease in arterial oxygen saturation from 95 to 81 per cent follows twenty-five seconds of apnea, with concomitant carbon dioxide retention and acidosis.

The cause is obscure. Some attacks follow feeding and appear to be associated with aspiration; some may be secondary to central nervous system depression. Of those who die, 33 per cent have associated intracranial hemorrhage, but whether the bleeding is primary or secondary to the prolonged apnea remains obscure.

DYSAUTONOMIA (RILEY-DAY SYNDROME). This rare disease, first recognized in 1949, is characterized by some degree of mental and physical retardation, deficient lacrimation, excessive sweating, transient hypertension, postural hypotension, attacks of cyclic vomiting, absent

Table 9. *Some Factors Known to Influence Respiration*

Stimuli	Depressants
Cortical	
Anxiety	Increased intracranial pressure
Pontine lesions	Electrocution
Cerebral hemorrhage	Cerebral hemorrhage
Voluntary control is possible within limits	
Thermal	
Gram-negative septicemia	Hibernation
Fever	Sudden chilling
Sudden chilling	
Chemical	
Arterial P_{CO_2} up to about 80 mm. Hg	Arterial P_{CO_2} over 80 mm. Hg
Rapid rate of change of arterial P_{CO_2}	Arterial pH less than 6.9 or over 7.5
Arterial pH 7.0-7.4	Profound hypoxia
Arterial P_{O_2} less than about 60-80 mm. Hg	
(in adults)	
(Newborn infants with only mild hypoxemia are stimulated by inspired oxygen)	
Pharmacological	
Epinephrine	Morphine
Lobeline	Barbiturates
Nicotine	Chloramphenicol
Salicylates	Neomycin
Picrotoxin	Anesthetic gases, etc.
Nikethamide	
Progesterone	
Pulmonary Reflexes	
Deflation receptors (Hering-Breuer)	Stretch receptors
Stretch receptors (Head's reflex)	Aortic arch and carotid sinus stretch receptors
Pressoreceptors	
Decrease in blood pressure	Increase in blood pressure
Bones and Joints	
Stretch receptors in muscles	Tactile responses
Tactile responses	

knee jerks, absence of the papillae of the tongue, and blotchy skin. It occurs predominantly in Jewish children and may or may not be associated with mental deficiency. Recurrent pulmonary infiltrations are thought to be the result of a defective swallowing mechanism with associated aspiration. Studies of the control of breathing in these patients show that they are less responsive to changes in Pa_{CO_2} and oxygen tensions than normal subjects, perhaps from peripheral chemoreceptor dysfunction. Since they do not have a normal ventilatory drive from changes in arterial P_{CO_2} and P_{O_2}, protection from high altitude and a warning against breath-holding during swimming may be important considerations.

PICKWICKIAN SYNDROME (PRIMARY ALVEOLAR HYPOVENTILATION). This condition, although common in obese adults, is rarely seen in children. It is characterized by extreme obesity and an elevated arterial P_{CO_2} which may result in somnolence. In these patients gastric distention following a meal may acutely elevate the Pa_{CO_2}. The hypoventilation is probably due to the increased work of breathing produced by chest wall obesity or gastric distention; presumably in order to do less respiratory work the body adjusts to an elevated arterial P_{CO_2} with retention of bicarbonate.

Respiratory Stimulants and Depressants

Some of the factors known to influence alveolar ventilation are presented in Table 9.

CLINICAL APPLICATION OF PULMONARY FUNCTION STUDIES

Changing dimensions of lung structure with age, the mechanical properties of the lungs, properties of gases and gas exchange, consideration of blood flow to the lungs, and aspects of the regulation of respiration comprise the substance of this chapter. The preceding sections are a distillate of an extensive literature, largely accumulated since World War II.

It remains to evaluate the role of measurements of lung function, only briefly discussed, in the practice of pediatrics. The pediatrician who approaches a child with respiratory symptoms relies first on an etiologic classification of disorders in differential diagnosis. Are the symptoms the result of an infection, foreign body aspiration, trauma, congenital malformation, allergic manifestation or tumor? Another question concerns the anatomic localization of the disease. Is the upper or lower respiratory tract primarily affected? The majority of respiratory illnesses can be successfully diagnosed and managed without recourse to measurements of lung function.

The role of the pulmonary function laboratory is chiefly to quantify the severity of the derangement. In practice, the most useful measurement is the partial pressure of carbon dioxide in arterial or "arterialized" capillary blood, since the most important question concerns the adequacy of ventilation. An unconscious patient, or one with respiratory muscle weakness or severe pulmonary disease, will need assisted ventilation when the P_{CO_2} rises to narcotic levels. The only way to monitor the efficacy of a respirator is to follow the arterial carbon dioxide tensions. The carbon dioxide-combining power alone is not an adequate determination. Metabolic acidosis is frequently present in conditions which cause respiratory failure, and the carbon dioxide-combining power may be normal or low in combined respiratory and metabolic acidosis.

Measurements of arterial oxygen saturation or tension are of value in assessing the magnitude of venous admixture which may exist with severe ventilation-perfusion imbalance, or anatomic shunts. Oxygen measurements are important in guiding appropriate oxygen administration. Since too little oxygen is lethal and too much is associated with toxicity, serial measurements are of value.

The only other widely used measurement is the vital capacity. Since patient cooperation is required, the measurement has limited usefulness in very sick patients, and is not usually feasible in those under five years of age. Its value is in following the course of chronic pulmonary disease.

The timed vital capacity, or one-second forced expiratory volume, has the same limitations as the vital capacity. It is useful as an index of lower airway obstructive disease. The timed vital capacity and peak flow rate are the most useful measurements to evaluate the role of bronchodilators, e.g. in asthma.

Angiography and cardiac catheterization contribute essential information in delineating malformations of the pulmonary vessels, and the presence of pulmonary hypertension.

Bronchoscopy and bronchography are indispensable tools in localizing abnormalities in the major airways.

The other functional evaluations, such as measurement of diffusion capacity, distribution of ventilation, radioscans, functional residual capacity, compliance and resistance, require more elaborate instrumentation and experience. Such measurements can be done in selected children, and are clinically useful in a few rare situations. For practical purposes, they should be considered research and teaching tools.

It behooves the student of pulmonary diseases to understand the physiologic derangements which contribute to the symptomatology; to appreciate the necessity of measuring blood gases; and to know when further functional evaluations are pertinent. The physician will do his patient a great favor to choose wisely the tests which are helpful, and to refrain from exhausting and exhaustive functional evaluations which do not influence his management of the patient or further elucidate the underlying disease.

REFERENCES

Avery, M. E.: *The Lung and Its Disorders in the Newborn Infant.* Philadelphia, W. B. Saunders Company, 1964.

Aviado, D.: *Lung Circulation.* New York, Pergamon Press, 1965, Vols. I and II.

Bates, D. V., and Christie, R. V.: *Respiratory Function in Disease.* Philadelphia, W. B. Saunders Company, 1964.

Cherniack, R. M., and Cherniack, L.: *Respiration in Health and Disease.* Philadelphia, W. B. Saunders Company, 1961.

Comroe, J. H., Jr.: *Physiology of Respiration.* Chicago, Year Book Medical Publishers, Inc., 1965.

Comroe, J. H., Jr., and others: *The Lung: Clinical Physiology and Pulmonary Function Tests.* 2nd ed. Chicago, Year Book Medical Publishers, Inc., 1962.

Cunningham, D. J. C., and Lloyd, B. B.: *The Regulation of Human Respiration* (J. S. Haldane Centenary Symposium). Oxford, Blackwell Scientific Publications, 1963.

Davenport, H.: *The ABC of Acid Base Chemistry.* 4th ed. Chicago, University of Chicago Press, 1958.

De Reuck, A. V. S., and O'Conner, M. (Eds.): *Ciba Foundation Symposium on Pulmonary Structure and Function.* London, J. & A. Churchill, Ltd., 1961.

Fenn, W. O., and Rahn, H. (Eds.): *Handbook of Physiology*: Section 3, Respiration. Washington, D.C., American Physiological Society, 1964, 1965, Vols. I and II.

Negus, V.: *The Biology of Respiration.* Baltimore, Williams & Wilkins Company, 1965.

Rossier, P. H., Buhlman, A. A., and Wiesinger, K.: *Respiration. Physiological Principles and Their Clinical Applications.* Translated by P. C. Luchsinger and K. M. Moser. St. Louis, C. V. Mosby Company, 1960.

Safar, P. (Ed.): *Respiratory Therapy.* Philadelphia, F. A. Davis Company, 1965.

SECTION II

General Considerations

CHAPTER TWO

The History and Physical Examination

WILLIAM W. WARING, M.D.

THE HISTORY

General Aims

All physicians know that history-taking for disease in any organ cannot be divorced from a general history. When the complaints are primarily pulmonary, however, parts of the general history should be emphasized in order to answer several broad questions:

1. Is the Present Episode a Manifestation of a Chronic or Recurrent Process?

If it is, the closer the symptoms are to birth, the more likely that the process is secondary to a malformation or other congenital disturbance.

2. Is the Process a Life-Threatening One, Either Immediately or Ultimately?

3. What Is the "Inertia" of the Process?

The concept of inertia of a disease is implicit in medicine, but calls for some amplification. Disorders with low inertia begin and end rapidly, either naturally or artificially. Those with high inertia are more ponderous, being slower in onset and harder to stop. The term "inertia"

has nothing to do with severity. Diseases of low inertia can be either serious or mild, as, for example, the common cold and acute lobar pneumococcal pneumonia. On the other hand, severe staphylococcal pneumonia and asymptomatic pulmonary histoplasmosis differ in severity, but both have greater inertia than the first two examples.

4. Can the Process Be Categorized as Mainly Airway Obstructive or Space-Occupying (Restrictive) in the Chest?

5. Does Infection Appear to Be Present?

The most helpful historical criteria of infection are fever, cervical lymphadenitis, and purulent discharges from the nares, ears or lungs (sputum).

6. What Has Been the Effect of Any Prior Treatment?

7. Is the Patient's Disease a Familial One?

If the parents are intelligent and observant, much information can be obtained under these several categories, and the physical examination can then be made with more definite ideas of the nature of the process and its prognosis. Since much of the examination of the chest and lungs consists in inspection of the undisturbed child, it is helpful to take the history in a warm examining room as the child, stripped to the waist, sits on his parent's lap. In this way one can make important observations as he proceeds with the history.

The *chief complaint* serves the prime purpose of initiating the dialogue and also of determining what most disturbs the parents. Chronology is most important, since it yields information on the chronicity and inertia of the disorder. In any detailed chronology the specific symptoms and signs volunteered by the informant should be noted, while additional information is obtained through careful, neutral questions. At each important episode answers should be obtained as to (1) what the patient did, (2) what the family did, and (3) what any "other doctor" did. When the chronologic account has been completed, the informant is psychologically ready for certain "finishing" questions, such as those asked in a review of the cardiorespiratory and other systems. The remainder of the past history follows and, finally, the more intimate family history.

Specific Points of Importance in Present and Past Illnesses

Informants often have information under the following headings, but may not volunteer it.

The Nature of the Cough

Is the cough productive or tight? It is necessary to make clear that expectoration is not the only criterion of a productive cough. Rather, its discontinuous sound informs even the nonmedical observer that fluid (mucus, pus, blood or aspirated liquid) is present in the tracheobronchial tree. Under what circumstances is the cough heard? A nonproductive nocturnal cough suggests an allergic or viral causation. A productive cough, especially on getting up in the morning, indicates the bronchorrhea of chronic bronchitis or bronchiectasis. A paroxysmal cough suggests pertussis or a foreign body. Recurrent cough with wheeze implies tracheobronchial obstruction, as seen in asthma, foreign body, mediastinal tumors or cystic fibrosis. A cough associated with swallowing points toward aspiration of contents into the tracheobronchial tree, due to incoordination of the swallowing and breathing mechanisms, anomaly or mass in the hypopharyngeal area, achalasia of the esophagus or tracheo-esophageal fistula. Cough with aphonia or dysphonia should suggest hypopharyngeal or laryngeal foreign body, papilloma of the larynx, croup (infectious or allergic) or psychoneurosis. Cough with a ringing or "brassy" quality suggests tracheal irritation, as exemplified by the tracheitis of rubeola. The "croupy" cough, which sounds like the bark of a seal or dog, is an indication of involvement of the glottic area. Is the cough heard every day, or may the child be totally free of cough for days or weeks?

Labored Breathing

A history of difficult breathing should first suggest airway obstruction. Has the dyspnea been getting steadily worse, as in bronchiolitis, or does it seem to come and go, as in asthma? Was its onset sudden, as, for example, when a previously well toddler is found suddenly coughing and dyspneic with peanuts in his mouth? Can the dyspnea be consistently related to signs of infection? Perhaps the child has always had labored breathing, as in anomalies of the lungs or heart. Can the child play vigorously without distress, or does he avoid a situation in which increased ventilation would be demanded?

Difficult breathing may also occur in nonobstructive pulmonary disease, such as large pleural effusion, pneumothorax or diaphragmatic paralysis. It may also be produced by pain on chest expansion, regardless of its cause, as in rib fracture or lobar pneumonia.

Noisy Breathing

The informant may have noted various respiratory noises. If so, what sort of noise has been heard and with what phase of respiration has it been associated? Typical *snoring* during sleep may be present in normal children only with acute coryza or may be more or less constant in those with adenoidal hypertrophy, posterior choanal obstruction, nasal polyposis, nasal foreign body or the Pierre Robin syndrome. Most intelligent informants can differentiate the snore of nasal obstruction and the stridor of laryngeal or tracheal origin. The latter is usually described as a "rattling in the chest."

Wheezing

Wheezing is a high-pitched, rather musical sound of varying intensity; it is frequently audible without a stethoscope. It is most common on expiration and indicates partial obstruction in some part of the airway, usually below the larynx. Its paroxysmal occurrence is typical of asthma. Persistent wheezing of sudden onset should suggest an aspirated foreign body. It is most important that this possibility be thoroughly investigated. Slowly progressive wheezing should suggest increasing bronchial obstruction caused, for example, by lymphoma or tuberculous lymphadenitis. If bronchodilators, such as epinephrine, have been administered, information on the response of the patient should be obtained, since prompt disappearance of wheezing after use of a bronchodilator is indicative of a relaxation of the bronchospasm of asthma.

The association of labored breathing and wheezing suggests either a single high obstruction (trachea or main bronchus) or multiple lower obstructions (lobar, segmental or subsegmental bronchi).

Grunting

Grunting is frequently a sign of chest pain and suggests an acute pneumonic process with pleural involvement. It is also seen in pulmonary edema, regardless of its cause.

Cyanosis

The distribution, degree and duration of blueness should be ascertained. In peripheral circulatory stasis, as in a chilled newborn infant, it may have little cardiorespiratory significance. But cyanosis of the lips, mouth, face and trunk almost always indicates cardiorespiratory disease and may demand emergency treatment. It is produced by (1) acute or chronic alveolar hypoventilation (airway obstruction, depressed respiratory center or respiratory muscle weakness), (2) uneven distribution of gas and blood throughout the lungs (bronchopneumonia), (3) anatomic right-to-left shunts of blood (congenital cyanotic heart disease, congenital arteriovenous aneurysms of the lung) or (4) disturbances of alveolocapillary diffusion (interstitial pneumonia or pulmonary fibrosis).

If oxygen was administered to the cyanotic patient, did the informant note that his color improved markedly? If it did not, it is likely that one or more right-to-left shunts are responsible for the cyanosis, since the above-noted other causes of cyanosis respond to increases in the partial pressure of oxygen in the inspired air.

Chest Pain

Older children may have complained of chest pain. The physician should consider disease of the esophagus, pericardium, diaphragmatic and parietal pleuras, or chest wall. In the esophagus foreign body, achalasia, lye stricture and ulceration may be responsible, and the pain is dull, deep and usually referred anteriorly. Parietal pleural pain is usually localized and lies more or less over the involved area. The pain of diaphragmatic pleural irritation may be referred to the base of the neck posteriorly and laterally, or even to the abdomen, where it may cause great diagnostic confusion. Pleural pain is frequently related to respiration, in which case the respirations are rapid and shallow, and there may be an expiratory grunt. Severe chest pain may be produced by the myositis of pleurodynia, by chest wall trauma, or by intercostal neuralgia, as in herpes zoster.

Sputum

The age at which a child can spit out coughed-up sputum varies considerably. Expectoration, literally taken as removal of sputum from the lungs by ciliary activity and cough, certainly occurs at all ages. During infancy such "expectorated" material is universally swallowed and undoubtedly composes at least some of the "cold" or mucus noted in vomitus and stools. Occasionally, older infants with chronic lung disease, e.g. patients with cystic fibrosis, may use their own index fingers to "hook out" viscous mucopurulent material from the oropharynx. Only in the supervised older child, however, will the volume of spit-out sputum approximate the volume ejected from the lungs. Nevertheless the physician should ask for information on the volume, color, viscosity and odor of sputum. Changes in these characteristics are guides to the presence of fresh bacterial infection. The "rusty" sputum of acute pneumococcal pneumonia is unusual in childhood, as is massive pulmonary hemorrhage, but streaks of pink or brownish pink blood are not uncommon in bronchiectasis.

Clubbing

Observant parents may have noted the signs of clubbing and should be directly questioned on progressive changes in the nail curvature and in the shape of the terminal phalanges. The presence of clubbing has etiologic significance, and its duration may throw light on the chronicity of the process.

Bad Breath

A chronically malodorous breath may be noted in children with bronchiectasis, lung abscess, paranasal sinusitis, nasal foreign body, adenoidal infection and allergic rhinitis.

Previous Chest Roentgenograms

If the child has had chest x-rays in the past, it is helpful to elicit the date and interpretation of each. Differentiation may sometimes be clearly made between congenital and acquired diseases by review of former x-ray films. In chest disease of chronic or obscure nature it is essential to locate such roentgenograms for comparison with current films.

Nonspecific Signs of Respiratory Disease

Failure to thrive may be a manifestation of severe, chronic respiratory disease. It may appear as failure to gain or even as loss of weight. Weights at birth and subsequent ages can be requested for plotting on appropriate weight-age graphs. A sudden deviation from the established growth channel of a child may indicate the approximate time of onset of his disease. Stature can be similarly handled if heights at earlier ages are known. Other nonspecific signs include sallowness, pallor, lethargy, subnormal school performance, and emotional disturbances.

The Patient's Environment

The social, psychologic and physical characteristics of the sick child's environment may illuminate the nature of the disease or for other reasons may be important for the physician to know. Information of possible importance includes the status of the parents' marriage, the income of the family and its debts, its recreations and its religion. Where does the family live, and does its location near industry, dump or stable help explain the patient's disease? Has the family lived in areas of endemic fungous infection? Does the patient have his own bed, his own room, and what means exist of heating, cooling, humidifying and dust-freeing the sleeping area, in which he spends a third or more of his life? Is there gross air pollution in the neighborhood or city of residence? Are conditions of crowding, low income, poor nutrition, ignorance, and lack of routine immunizations and skin testing such that infectious disease can quickly spread throughout the family, remain unrecognized for long periods, and be almost ineradicable?

Are there abnormal exposures to the environment, such as that produced by dirt-eating? Is there a possibility that the patient's illness has been caused by "battering," such as thoracic trauma or purposeful exposure to the elements?

Familial Disease

The health of the family should be investigated in all cases because there may be direct or indirect associations between it and the patient's disease. So-called ping-pong infections are frequently seen within the family. Familial disease may be explained by a common genetic background or by exposure to a common group of infectious or physical agents. The same infectious agent commonly has different and nonpulmonary manifestations. For example, a history of breast abscess in the mother or furuncles in siblings may suggest the staphylococcal origin of the patient's pneumonia.

Heredity undoubtedly plays a prominent role in many diseases of the lungs, although the mode of inheritance of so clearly a genetically determined disease as cystic fibrosis is still being debated.

THE PHYSICAL EXAMINATION

The physical examination is traditionally divided into categories of inspection, palpation, percussion-auscultation, and olfaction, for each of which the examiner uses a different organ of sense. Such a division serves basic pedagogic purposes, but in practice one sense is seldom used exclusively. *The senses, as well as the tools actually used, always subserve the goals of examination of the lungs, which are to determine (1) the nature of respiration, (2) the adequacy of gas exchange, and (3) the localization of disease, if it exists.*

The following discussion is in accord-

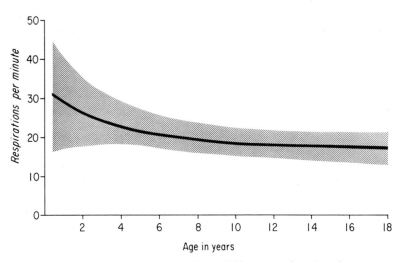

FIGURE 2–1. Normal resting respiratory rates from Table 1 are plotted against age to show more clearly the rapid decrease that occurs during the first 2 years of life. Since there is no significant difference in rates between boys and girls, a single regression is applicable to obth sexes. The shaded area represents the approximate area of normal variation (2 standard deviations above and below the mean at each age). (Iliff and Lee.)

Table 1. *Normal Resting Respiratory Rate per Minute*

Age (Years)	Boys Mean ± SD	Girls Mean ± SD
0- 1 ....31 ± 8		30 ± 6
1- 2 ....26 ± 4		27 ± 4
2- 3 ....25 ± 4		25 ± 3
3- 4 ....24 ± 3		24 ± 3
4- 5 ....23 ± 2		22 ± 2
5- 6 ....22 ± 2		21 ± 2
6- 7 ....21 ± 3		21 ± 3
7- 8 ....20 ± 3		20 ± 2
8- 9 ....20 ± 2		20 ± 2
9-10 ....19 ± 2		19 ± 2
10-11 ....19 ± 2		19 ± 2
11-12 ....19 ± 3		19 ± 3
12-13 ....19 ± 3		19 ± 2
13-14 ....19 ± 2		18 ± 2
14-15 ....18 ± 2		18 ± 3
15-16 ....17 ± 3		18 ± 3
16-17 ....17 ± 2		17 ± 3
17-18 ....16 ± 3		17 ± 3

Data of Iliff and Lee from both fed, sleeping and fasting, awake children. SD = one standard deviation of the mean.

ance with these goals. Emphasis will be placed on the chest and lungs rather than on the upper respiratory tract, and physical findings will be correlated with the causative disturbances of function.

Nature of Respiration

Knowledge of the nature of respiration is best acquired by careful observation of the sleeping or quietly awake child. This general term "nature" includes an evaluation of rate, depth, ease and rhythm of breathing.

Rate of Respiration

The physician should reach a conclusion as to whether the respiratory rate is normal for this patient, abnormally or disproportionately rapid (tachypnea, polypnea) or abnormally slow (bradypnea, oligopnea). Data on the expected rates for age are shown in Figure 1 and Table 1 and indicate a rapid decline from early infancy to about two years, and then a slower, steady fall for the rest of childhood and adolescence. Previously unreported data on normal respiratory rates in both sleeping and awake white subjects from a high socio-economic group in New Orleans are shown in Table 2.

The respiratory rate, when properly observed under controlled conditions, is a simple and useful, although nonspecific, pulmonary function test of thoracic and pulmonary compliance. Diseases of the thorax and lungs that act to stiffen them are associated with significantly higher rates. The course of low-compliance (high stiffness) processes, such as interstitial or other pneumonia, pleural effusion and pulmonary edema, can be simply and accurately evaluated by careful serial observations of rate (Fig. 2). Decreases toward normal indicate improvement,

Table 2. *Respiratory Rates per Minute of Normal Children, Both Sexes, Sleeping and Awake*

Age	Sleeping			Awake			Mean Difference Between Sleeping and Awake
	No.	Mean	Range	No.	Mean	Range	
6-12 months	6	27	22-31	3	64	58-75	37
1- 2 years	6	19	17-23	4	35	30-40	16
2- 4 years	16	19	16-25	15	31	23-42	12
4- 6 years	23	18	14-23	22	26	19-36	8
6- 8 years	27	17	13-23	28	23	15-30	6
8-10 years	19	18	14-23	19	21	15-31	3
10-12 years	11	16	13-19	17	21	15-28	5
12-14 years	6	16	15-18	7	22	18-26	6

whether occurring spontaneously or induced by treatment. Rapid rates are also observed with anxiety, exercise, fever, severe anemia, metabolic acidosis (severe diarrhea, diabetes) and respiratory alkalosis (psychoneurosis, salicylates, central nervous system disturbances).

Bradypnea is less commonly observed, but may be seen, for example, with metabolic alkalosis (pyloric stenosis) and respiratory acidosis due to central nervous system depression (morphine overdosage, increased intracranial pressure).

For ordinary clinical purposes the rate may be counted for a minute, but when the rate is being used to follow the progress of a patient, several resting steady-state counts should be made and the mean rate per minute computed. It is always preferable for the child to be ignorant of the counting process and for the physician to be at a low-anxiety distance. Usually thoracic excursions are sufficiently discrete for counting by inspection, but occasionally a stethoscope must be used.

Depth of Respiration

The physician now attempts to decide whether, for the rate observed, the child is breathing at a normal depth, too deeply (hyperpnea) or too shallowly (hypopnea). Such a clinical estimate of minute volume (the volume of air expired each minute) can be recognized as abnormal only at the extremes. For example, the hyperpnea with metabolic acidosis in the course of diarrhea or diabetes mellitus is easily detected. Similarly, the hypoventilation with metabolic alkalosis can sometimes be sensed, although it is more easily missed because most physicians have not trained themselves to evaluate effortless breathing. Between these extremes much variation may pass undetected.

Hyperpnea occurs with fever, severe anemia, salicylism, metabolic acidosis, respiratory alkalosis, and in those diseases of the lungs in which there is increased dead space. Hypopnea occurs with metabolic alkalosis (pyloric stenosis) and with

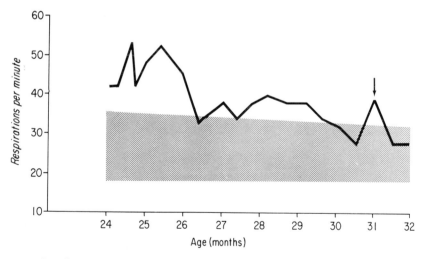

FIGURE 2–2. Respiratory rate per minute in a child with chronic diffuse interstitial fibrosis of the lung (Hamman-Rich syndrome). The diagnosis was confirmed by open biopsy, and treatment has consisted of progressively decreasing oral doses of prednisone. Rates were carefully counted during serial visits to the Chest Clinic. Each point is the mean of 2 or more one-minute counts. Auscultation of the lungs never revealed abnormal breath sounds or rales during the depicted period. The return toward normal of his rate of breathing strongly suggests that the process is in part reversible. The arrow indicates tachypnea produced by an intercurrent, acute respiratory infection with fever.

respiratory acidosis (e.g. bilateral diaphragmatic paralysis or central nervous
system depression).

The depth of respiration is generally
estimated from the amplitude of thoracic
and abdominal excursions. Initial impressions, gained from inspection, may be
reinforced by palpation and auscultation.
The palm of the hand held a short distance in front of the mouth and nose may
reveal increased or decreased tidal volumes. Auscultation of a generalized increase or decrease in intensity of breath
sounds of normal quality similarly helps
to confirm initial impressions. In hyperpnea the faint inspiratory and expiratory
sounds of large tidal volumes can be easily
heard without a stethoscope.

Ease of Respiration

The physician should also evaluate
with what ease respiration is being effected. Effortless breathing (eupnea) indicates that no significant airway obstruction is present. Difficult or labored
respiratory efforts (dyspnea) mean that increased work is being performed by the
muscles of respiration toward ensuring
normal alveolar ventilation. The greatest
increases in work of breathing are caused
by airway obstructions.

Dyspnea is both a sign and a symptom.
If a patient is aware of even the slightest
distress in breathing, he is dyspneic. Such
subtlety is obviously not generally applicable to infants and children, and the
pediatrician accordingly seeks signs of
distressed breathing or extraordinary respiratory effort before deciding that dyspnea is present. These advanced signs include orthopnea, intercostal retractions
and bulging, flaring of the alae nasi, head
bobbing, wheezing and grunting. Each of
these will be briefly discussed.

Orthopnea

Children with pulmonary edema or
asthma, for example, appear unable to
tolerate recumbent positions and will
spontaneously prop themselves upright
with their arms behind in the so-called
tripod position.

Intercostal Retractions and Bulging

The term "retraction" indicates an inspiratory sinking-in of soft tissues in relation to the cartilaginous and bony thorax.
Slight intercostal depressions are normal
and can easily be seen between the lower
ribs, becoming slightly more marked as
the child inspires. In disease, especially
when airway obstruction is severe, retractions may become extreme and extend to
the jugular notch and supraclavicular and
infraclavicular areas. In infants, whose
thoraces are more pliable, the lower sternum may be depressed with each inspiratory effort.

Whether physiologic or pathologic, retractions are produced by differences in
pressure existing at any moment between
the intrapleural space (intrathoracic) and
that outside the thorax (atmospheric)
(Fig. 3, *inspiration*). Greater than normal
decreases of intrathoracic pressure occur
during inspiration with airway obstruction and with increased lung stiffness.
The greater the pressure decrease below
atmospheric, the more the flexible intercostal soft tissues will yield, and the more
conspicuous will be the resulting intercostal soft tissues will yield, and the more
seen only in obstructive lung disease, retractions may extend to the jugular and
clavicular areas. In accord with this concept of retractions, it is not the location
of any obstruction within the respiratory
tract that controls the particular soft tissue
retracted, but rather the degree of that
obstruction, which in turn effects the magnitude of the decrease in intrathoracic
pressure necessary for ventilation.

It is thus clear that retractions, when
abnormal, indicate increased *inspiratory*
effort. It is not generally known, however,
that inspection of the interspaces can also
yield evidence of greater than normal *expiratory* effort, which is common in
asthma, bronchiolitis and cystic fibrosis.

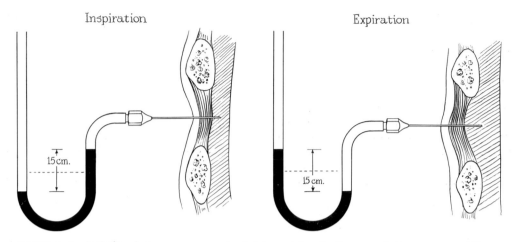

FIGURE 2–3. Relation between movement of intercostal soft tissues and the pressure difference across them. Differences in pressure between the intrapleural space and the atmosphere during obstructed inspiration and expiration are depicted diagrammatically. A simple water manometer is attached to a needle between the parietal and visceral pleuras. Simultaneous pressure differences and movements of the intercostal soft tissues are noted.

Inspiration. During partially obstructed inspiration the intrapleural pressure is shown decreasing to 15 cm. of water below that of the atmosphere. (A normal tidal inspiration does not usually produce a difference of more than 8 cm. of water.) This larger than normal pressure difference, greater on the outside, forces in the pliable intercostal soft tissues, resulting in retractions, which the physician sees on physical examination.

Expiration. During partially obstructed expiration, as in asthma, intrapleural pressure, which is normally always less than atmospheric, may equal or exceed it. In this diagram intrapleural pressure is 15 cm. of water greater than that of the atmosphere. This results in a pressure gradient from inside out, and, as pressure rises, the pliable tissues at first flatten and finally bulge outwards.

Normally, intrathoracic pressure is subatmospheric throughout expiration. With widespread bronchial obstruction, however, increased expiratory muscular effort is required to force air *out* of the lungs. Under such circumstances intrathoracic pressure may exceed atmospheric pressure, and, in obedience to the outward pressure gradient, the intercostal space will be noted to flatten and sometimes to bulge out (Fig. 3, *expiration*). Intercostal bulging is thus always to be taken as a sign of greater than normal expiratory effort.

Movements of intercostal soft tissues are best observed when light is altogether from a direction roughly perpendicular to the plane of the middle ribs, as, for example, from a ceiling light 3 or 4 feet above and in front of the sitting or standing patient. In general, the intercostal spaces that can be observed most satisfactorily are the eighth and ninth in the posterior axillary line.

If the patient is both retracting and bulging his intercostal spaces, a curious flickering bar of light and dark may occur in the same interspace as the space alternately becomes dark with the retraction during inspiration and light with the bulge during expiration. The uninitiated observer may erroneously ascribe this "intercostal flicker" to sudden downward rib movement with expiration. Palpation of the "flickering" interspace will indicate at once that rib movements are too slight and gradual to explain the effect.

Flaring of the Alae Nasi

Flaring of the alae nasi exists when an enlargement of both nares occurs during inspiration. It is due to contraction of the anterior and posterior dilatores naris muscles, which are supplied by the facial nerves. The appearance of flaring indicates that accessory muscles are being recruited for inspiration. Since flaring implies that greater than normal work is required for breathing, it is an excellent sign of dyspnea. In many cases its presence suggests that inspiratory efforts are being abnormally shortened by pain, as in pleuritis or thoracic trauma. Unilateral flaring is a sign of facial paralysis on the opposite side, in addition to its usual significance.

Head-Bobbing

This is a sign of dyspnea best observed in an exhausted or sleeping infant lying in its mother's arms. The head must be unsupported except for the suboccipital area, which rests on the mother's forearm. In synchrony with each inspiration the head is noted to bob forward, owing to neck flexion. The phenomenon is probably explained by contraction of the scalene and sternocleidomastoid muscles, which are accessory muscles of inspiration. Countertraction from the extensor muscles of the neck is insufficient to fix the cervical spine and head. The result is that nonrespiratory work is done in flexing the neck instead of raising the sternum and the first two ribs.

Wheezing and Grunting

Wheezing indicates partial obstruction, usually expiratory, and may be caused by single or multiple points of narrowing within the airways. Usually such obstruction exists in larger (segmental or lobar) bronchi because the necessary critical velocities of air flow for sound production occur only in these larger airways. It is likely that such velocities cannot be reached in the smaller bronchi. For this reason an audible wheeze is not a characteristic sign of bronchiolitis, in which airway obstruction is diffuse and primarily involves the smallest airways. It is commonly heard, however, in patients with asthma or tracheobronchial foreign bodies.

Auscultation at the open mouth may reveal faint wheezes and rales, since sounds from even small bronchi travel easily up the airway.

Grunting, as mentioned above, is associated with pneumonia and chest pain, but in the neonatal period it is commonly observed in the respiratory distress syndrome.

Rhythm of Respiration

Respiration is not absolutely regular in either health or disease. The depth of separate breaths may vary significantly, and the intervals between them are not fixed. Occasional deep breaths, *sighs,* occur in all normal persons and probably serve an important antiatelectatic function.

Periodic breathing occurs so frequently in premature infants as to be considered a normal finding. It usually appears after twenty-four hours and is characterized by acyanotic apneic periods lasting five to ten seconds, followed by periods of ventilation lasting up to fifteen seconds. The phenomenon lacks the crescendo-decrescendo pattern characteristic of Cheyne-Stokes breathing and is probably explained by the immaturity of integrating pathways in the central nervous system.

Premature infants may also show a more serious type of respiratory irregularity, *apneic spells,* that may last more than twenty seconds. Bradycardia is usually present, and cyanosis may occur. Infants with apneic spells have a high mortality.

Classic *Cheyne-Stokes breathing* is characterized by a waxing and waning of the depth of tidal volumes with periods of apnea between each such sequence. The cause is not certain, although it is an abnormal type of respiratory arrhythmia. It is seen in children with congestive heart failure, cerebral trauma and increased intracranial pressure.

Biot's breathing is more ominous and consists of one or several breaths of irregular depth with interspersed apneic periods of varying lengths. It generally signifies severe brain damage.

Adequacy of Gas Exchange

The primary function of the lungs is gas exchange, i.e. getting sufficient oxygen into the body to satisfy metabolic needs and removing carbon dioxide thereby produced. Insufficiency of the lungs' oxygen-supplying role causes hypoxia, and insufficiency of their carbon dioxide-eliminating role causes hypercapnia. In disease both gases may be insufficiently exchanged. Hypoxia may occur without hypercapnia, however, and vice versa. For example, disturbances of distribution of blood and gas throughout the lungs may produce hypoxia without hypercapnia, and oxygen therapy in a patient with over-all alveolar hypoventilation may relieve hypoxia, but it will not lessen hypercapnia.

It would be of inestimable clinical value to be able to detect the presence of hypoxia or hypercapnia, or both, on physical examination. Unfortunately, the recognition of both types of disturbance is difficult, owing to nonspecificity of their manifestations, variations among patients, and differences in the severity and duration of exposure.

The signs and symptoms of hypoxia, listed in Table 3, are cyanosis, tachycardia, exertional dyspnea, and those due to depression of the central nervous system. Dyspnea at rest probably does not occur in hypoxia without hypercapnia. The ability of an observer to perceive cyanosis varies greatly. Some persons may detect cyanosis when arterial oxygen saturation has dropped to 85 per cent from its normal of 96 per cent. The majority of observers, however, will not perceive cyanosis unless arterial oxygen saturation is 80 per cent or less.

The signs of hypercapnia should be especially sought in those clinical situations in which reduction in the depth of respiration is expected or has been observed. Careful studies in adults indicate that signs of hypercapnia appear in relation to an increase in tension of mixed venous carbon dioxide above that which is usual for each person. In other words,

Table 3. *Signs and Symptoms of Hypoxia*

Mild
None or decreased efficiency only

Moderate
Mood changes: euphoria or depression
Decreased efficiency and impaired judgment
Headache
Hypertension
Exertional dyspnea
Hyperpnea, variable
Cyanosis
Tachycardia
Polycythemia (chronic exposure)

Severe
Hypertension or hypotension
Dimness of vision
Somnolence, stupor, coma

chronic mild or moderate elevations of carbon dioxide tension may not be detectable on physical examination, but *acute progressive* elevations of carbon dioxide tension above these levels may be associated with increasingly serious signs; these are listed in Table 4. Although similar correlations have not been reported in infants and children and although differences undoubtedly exist

Table 4. *Signs of Progressive Hypercapnia**

Hot hands (+5)

Rapid bounding pulse (+10)
Small pupils (+10)

Engorged fundal veins (+15)
Confusion or drowsiness (+15)
Muscular twitching (+15)

Depressed tendon reflexes (+30)
Extensor plantar responses (+30)
Coma (+30)

Papilledema (+40)

* Figures in parentheses are the approximate elevations above *usual* levels of mixed venous carbon dioxide tension (mm. Hg) at which each sign may first appear. Thus hot hands may be observed in a patient whose mixed venous P_{CO_2} is only 5 mm. Hg above the value usual for him, whereas the presence of papilledema probably indicates that his P_{CO_2} has risen 40 mm. Hg, or more, above the usual level.

among various age groups, it is probable that the general pattern of signs is sufficiently similar to make Table 4 of value for children.

Localization of Disease

The third main goal of examination of the lungs is to determine the location of disease, if it is present. Considerable information has already been developed on the nature of the process from the history and from judgments made of the nature and adequacy of respiration earlier in the physical examination. Clubbing of the fingers is often a good clue to the presence of significant disease, whereas several other signs are useful in an attempt at its localization.

Clubbing

There is an old physical diagnostic adage that says, "Examination of the lungs begins at the finger tips." There are perhaps two characteristic hallmarks of every examination by a chest physician: careful examination of the ends of the fingers and palpation of the position of the trachea. In the case of advanced clubbing, inspection alone is usually sufficient, but the earliest changes are best observed by holding the child's finger in such a way as to observe the shape of the nail and the angle between the fleshy part of the finger and the nail. An additional characteristic of clubbing is a lifting up of the base of the nail; this produces a hypermobile, "floating" nail. Repeated light pressure over the base of the nail will reveal this "floating" characteristic. The stages of clubbing are shown in Figure 4, and various conditions associated with clubbing are listed in Table 5.

Although the cause of clubbing is not known, a factor common to most diseases in which it occurs is admixture of venous blood with the systemic arterial circulation. In this regard the most attractive hypothesis is that reduced ferritin, normally found in venous blood, may cause

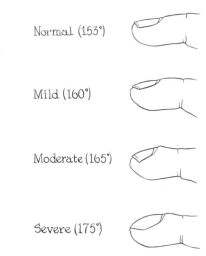

FIGURE 2–4. Stages of clubbing. These profiles are drawn from casts made of the terminal phalanges of children seen in a chest clinic. The number in parentheses for each stage of clubbing represents the angle formed above the finger at the skin-nail junction by straight lines drawn to it from equidistant points in front of and behind the junction. An angle greater than 160 degrees and decided curvature of the nail are good criteria of the presence of clubbing. The "moderate" and "severe" examples are from patients with cystic fibrosis.

Table 5. *Diseases Commonly Associated with Acquired Clubbing in Children*

Pulmonary
Bronchiectasis
Pulmonary abscess
Empyema
Chronic pneumonias, various
Neoplasms, primary and metastatic
Cardiac
Congenital cyanotic heart disease
Subacute bacterial endocarditis
Hepatic
Biliary cirrhosis
Gastrointestinal
Chronic ulcerative colitis
Regional enteritis
Chronic dysentery, amebic and bacillary
Polyposis, multiple
Other
Thyrotoxicosis

clubbing by opening small arteriovenous connections in the tips of the fingers and toes.

Regardless of its precise cause, the observation of nonfamilial clubbing should have a certain significance for the pediatrician. If congenital cyanotic heart disease and the various nonpulmonary causes can be eliminated, it is reasonable to conclude that there exists significant, chronic, organic lung disease that may be either localized or generalized. In such cases saccular bronchiectasis is the most common cause. The appearance of clubbing in "asthma" indicates that either the diagnosis is incorrect or that complicating disease is coexistent, such as atelectasis with bronchiectasis. Observation for clubbing is an absolute essential in the examination of a child with chronic cough, and its discovery is a mandate for extensive additional investigation.

Trepopnea

A child is described as trepopneic if he is more comfortable in one lateral recumbent position than the other. Trepopnea indicates severe predominantly unilateral disease, and the patient prefers to keep uppermost the better functioning lung.

Tracheal Palpation

The trachea can be viewed as the needle of a gauge whose function is the detection of differences in pressure or volume between the two sides of the thorax. The tracheal needle pivots on its fixation in the neck (where differences in thoracic pressure or volume produce little lateral movement) and swings its arrow in an arc at the carina (where lateral movement is maximal). The sign loses sensitivity because the examiner is not able to palpate the position of the trachea at the level of the carina, but must content himself with palpation at the suprasternal notch. Nevertheless, with a little experience in tracheal palpation, it is possible to detect

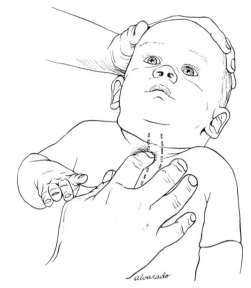

FIGURE 2–5. Technique of determining tracheal position in an infant. The index finger of the palpating hand is placed in the suprasternal notch and gently slid inward in the midsagittal plane. It is essential that the head be fixed in a neutral position, and the neck slightly extended. If the finger consistently slides off one side of the trachea, it can be concluded that the trachea is deviated in the opposite direction. In this illustration the trachea is shifted to the left. This method can also be applied to older children.

relatively small degrees of mediastinal shift.

Discovery of a shift does not alone indicate in which hemithorax the volume or pressure change has occurred, but it does indicate an abnormal inequality between the two sides of the chest. For example, a foreign body in the left main bronchus might completely occlude the bronchus and produce atelectasis of the entire left lung. As air is absorbed from the alveoli of the lung, its volume decreases and intrapleural pressure becomes more negative. The mediastinum with the trachea shifts obediently to the left from an area of higher pressure and greater volume to one of lower pressure and smaller volume. On the other hand, a pneumothorax on the right adds volume to the right hemithorax and makes less negative (increases) intrapleural pressure on that side; the mediastinum and trachea there-

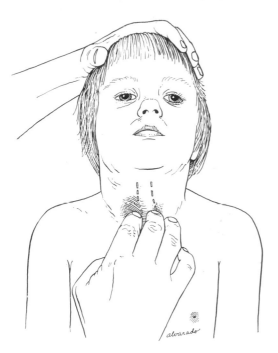

FIGURE 2–6. Technique of determining tracheal position in an older child. Inspection of the suprasternal area may show asymmetry of the fossas bounded laterally by the sternocleidomastoid muscles and medially by the trachea. In this case the fossa on the right is larger than that on the left, as indicated by its larger shadow. It is concluded that the trachea has been shifted to the left. The impression gained from inspection is then tested by two-finger palpation of the relative size of the two fossas. As shown, the index finger fits easily between the right sternomastoid and trachea, but the middle finger is too large for the corresponding space on the left.

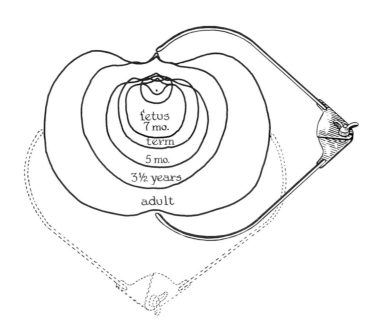

FIGURE 2–7. Changes in chest shape at different ages, and their measurement with obstetrical calipers. The relatively round chest of the fetus and term infant gradually flattens dorsoventrally with age. Measurements should be made in either the recumbent (infants) or standing (children) position, never in the sitting position. Maximum dimensions are measured in both cases without regard to the level or phase of respiration, but care must be taken to place the calipers in a true transverse plane. The distance between the caliper tips is then measured with a steel centimeter rule.

fore still shift to the left. Other portions of the examination should indicate the side responsible for observed shift.

There are two different methods of tracheal palpation. The first is most useful in infants and small children and is performed with one finger (Fig. 5). The other, applicable to older children and adults, involves inspection and two-finger palpation (Fig. 6). In both methods the patient should slightly extend the neck without the slightest lateral tilt or rotation from a midline position. The head of an infant can be fixed in the left hand of the examiner as he palpates with his free right hand.

Thoracic Configuration

As the various characteristics of respiration are being noted the examiner should also evaluate the form and symmetry of the chest. Although palpation and actual measurement may be required to complete such evaluation, especially of the lower costal angle, careful inspection can

Table 6. *Normal Thoracic Dimensions, Boys*

Age Group	Anteroposterior* Mean ± SD (cm.)	Transverse* Mean ± SD (cm.)	Thoracic Index† Mean
0 - 3 months	10.2 ± 0.7	12.1 ± 0.9	0.84
3 - 6 months	11.2 ± 0.8	13.8 ± 0.9	0.81
6 - 9 months	11.6 ± 0.8	14.7 ± 0.9	0.79
9 -12 months	12.0 ± 0.7	15.4 ± 0.7	0.78
1 - 1¼ years	12.2 ± 0.8	15.7 ± 0.8	0.77
1¼- 1½	12.5 ± 0.9	16.1 ± 0.8	0.78
1½- 1¾	12.6 ± 0.8	16.2 ± 0.7	0.78
1¾- 2	12.7 ± 0.7	16.6 ± 0.9	0.77
2 - 2¼	12.7 ± 0.8	16.7 ± 0.9	0.76
2¼- 2½	12.6 ± 0.7	16.7 ± 0.5	0.75
2½- 2¾	12.5 ± 0.8	16.8 ± 1.0	0.74
2¾- 3	12.6 ± 0.7	16.9 ± 0.8	0.75
3 - 3½	12.7 ± 0.6	17.1 ± 0.8	0.74
3½- 4	12.9 ± 0.7	17.4 ± 0.8	0.74
4 - 4½	13.2 ± 0.6	17.6 ± 0.8	0.75
4½- 5	13.3 ± 0.7	17.8 ± 0.8	0.75
5 - 5½	13.6 ± 0.8	18.2 ± 0.9	0.75
5½ -6	13.8 ± 0.9	18.5 ± 1.0	0.75
6 - 6½	14.1 ± 1.0	18.7 ± 1.0	0.75
6½- 7½	14.5 ± 1.0	19.3 ± 1.1	0.75
7½- 8½	15.0 ± 1.1	20.0 ± 1.2	0.75
8½- 9½	15.4 ± 1.1	20.8 ± 1.4	0.74
9½-10½	15.9 ± 1.2	21.6 ± 1.6	0.74
10½-11½	16.3 ± 1.3	22.1 ± 1.7	0.74
11½-12½	17.0 ± 1.5	22.9 ± 1.9	0.74
12½-13½	17.8 ± 1.7	24.0 ± 1.8	0.74
13½-14½	18.6 ± 1.7	25.1 ± 2.1	0.74
14½-15½	19.3 ± 1.7	26.0 ± 2.1	0.74
15½-16½	20.0 ± 1.7	27.0 ± 1.9	0.74
16½-17½	20.7 ± 1.7	27.7 ± 2.0	0.75
17½-18½	21.5 ± 1.7	28.3 ± 1.7	0.76

Data of Meredith for white Iowa City boys.

* Measured at the level of the nipples.

† Thoracic index was obtained by dividing mean anteroposterior diameter by mean transverse diameter.

Table 7. *Normal Thoracic Dimensions, Girls*

Age Group	Anteroposterior* Mean ± SD (cm.)	Transverse* Mean ± SD (cm.)	Thoracic Index† Mean
3 months	10.5 ± 1.0	12.5 ± 0.9	0.84
6 months	11.2 ± 0.8	13.7 ± 1.0	0.82
9 months	11.5 ± 0.8	14.2 ± 0.8	0.81
1 year	11.9 ± 0.8	14.9 ± 0.8	0.80
1¼	12.3 ± 0.7	15.3 ± 0.7	0.80
1½	12.4 ± 0.7	15.5 ± 0.8	0.80
1¾	12.4 ± 0.8	16.0 ± 0.7	0.78
2	12.4 ± 0.7	16.1 ± 0.8	0.77
2¼	12.4 ± 0.7	16.1 ± 0.8	0.77
2½	12.5 ± 0.7	16.3 ± 0.8	0.77
2¾	12.4 ± 0.8	16.3 ± 0.8	0.76
3	12.5 ± 0.8	16.7 ± 0.8	0.75
3½	12.7 ± 0.7	17.1 ± 0.9	0.74
4	12.8 ± 0.7	17.4 ± 1.0	0.74
4½	12.9 ± 0.7	17.6 ± 1.1	0.73
5	12.9 ± 0.8	17.8 ± 1.1	0.72
5½	12.9 ± 0.9	18.1 ± 1.1	0.71
6	13.2 ± 1.0	18.2 ± 1.1	0.73
7	13.4 ± 1.0	18.6 ± 1.2	0.72
8	13.8 ± 1.3	19.2 ± 1.3	0.72
9	14.1 ± 1.2	19.6 ± 1.5	0.72
10	14.5 ± 1.2	20.3 ± 1.4	0.71
11	15.3 ± 1.6	21.1 ± 1.5	0.73
12	16.1 ± 1.6	22.1 ± 1.8	0.73
13	16.8 ± 1.7	23.1 ± 1.7	0.73
14	17.4 ± 2.0	24.1 ± 2.0	0.72
15	17.8 ± 2.3	24.6 + 2.2	0.72
16	18.0 ± 2.1	24.8 ± 2.0	0.73
17	17.8 ± 1.9	24.9 ± 1.8	0.71
18	17.7 ± 1.6	24.7 ± 1.7	0.72

Data of Boynton for white Iowa City girls.

* Measured at the level of the xiphoid.

† Thoracic index was obtained by dividing mean anteroposterior diameter by mean transverse diameter.

detect all but the most subtle changes. Readily seen are absence of the pectoral muscles, pigeon breast (pectus carinatum), funnel chest (pectus excavatum), barrel chest, kyphoscoliosis and left-sided chest bulge due to enlargement of the right ventricle.

The symmetry of inspiration should be noted because those diseases producing unequal ventilation of the two lungs will be manifested by lagging or shallower expansion of the involved hemithorax.

The clinician should ask himself whether the chest shape of a patient devi-ates significantly from normal for that age. Traditionally, such judgments have been based on two generally appreciated facts, that the chests of infants are rounder than those of older children and that chronic diffuse airway obstruction produces an abnormally rounded or "barrel-shaped" chest. It is possible, however, to refine clinical judgment considerably by serial chest measurements that can be made a part of every office visit. Chest circumference, although easily measured, is not a determinant of chest shape. In order to follow changes in shape it is necessary

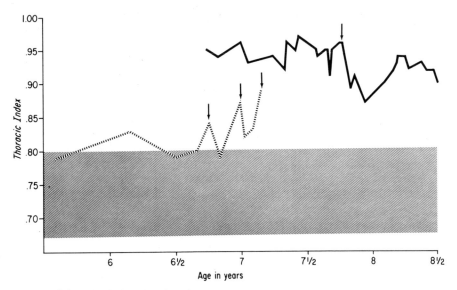

FIGURE 2–8. Thoracic index in chronic obstructive lung disease. Serial measurements of chest depth and width can be made easily in children. In this figure thoracic index (depth-width ratio) is plotted against age for 2 children with severe obstructive lung disease due to cystic fibrosis.

The first patient (broken line) had considerable fluctuation of thoracic index, but the slope is generally upward, suggesting progressive overinflation of the lungs which could be only temporarily relieved by intensive care during hospitalizations (arrows). Death occurred during the last hospitalization.

The second patient (solid line) has more severe overinflation than the first, as shown by higher thoracic indices, but the slope of the serial measurements is generally downward. The rather abrupt decrease in thoracic index beginning at the arrow coincides with a period of intensive combined antibiotic, mucolytic aerosol and physical therapy.

Both patients illustrate the probable value of such measurements for purposes of prognostication and evaluation of therapy in obstructive lung disease.

to measure one or more thoracic diameters. An obstetrical caliper (pelvimeter) and a metal tape measure are the only necessary tools (Fig. 7). Of most importance is a measure of the anteroposterior diameter of the thorax, because overinflation of the lungs affects this dimension more than any other. With a little practice, sufficiently accurate and reproducible results can be obtained. The anteroposterior diameter can be correlated with age, height or another thoracic measure, such as transverse diameter. The thoracic index (depth-width ratio) is obtained by dividing the anteroposterior diameter by the transverse diameter (Tables 6, 7). In severe obstructive lung disease this index or ratio may approach 1.0.

In children with chronic obstructive disease serial determinations of thoracic index or thoracic anteroposterior diameter

may furnish valuable clues to the course of the disease or possibly the efficacy of a treatment regimen (Fig. 8).

Thoracic and Abdominal Respirations

At the time that movements of intercostal soft tissue are being observed the physician should also look for *Litten's phenomenon*. This is not a sign of dyspnea, but an occasionally very helpful sign of diaphragmatic contraction. If the light source is properly adjusted, it can be seen in most normal nonobese children. The phenomenon consists of a slight shadow that moves down the lower intercostal spaces during inspiration, rising upward during expiration. It is related to movements of the diaphragm and is best seen in the posterior axillary line. The sign is probably best explained by the progressive downward extension during inspiration of negative intrapleural pressure as the diaphragm leaves the inner surface of the chest wall. Its absence suggests absolute or relative immobility of the diaphragm (paralysis, eventration, pleural effusion), especially if it is clearly seen on the opposite side. It must be emphasized that this is a subtle sign which can be observed only by looking for it with care.

Inspection of the thorax and upper part of the abdomen of the breathing child indicates the relative importance of thoracic expansion and diaphragmatic contraction. In all normal persons both processes are at work, but in younger ones, especially infants, the role of the diaphragm is of greater importance. Hence the normal infant is seen to protrude the upper part of the abdomen with inspiration, and this movement is larger than that of thoracic expansion. In bilateral phrenic nerve paralysis or diaphragmatic eventration the abdomen may actually sink during inspiration, and the thorax is simultaneously observed to enlarge significantly. In such cases careful inspection for Litten's sign, percussion of the lower lung margins, and palpation of the lower costal angle are indicated to confirm the activity and position of the diaphragms.

Lower Costal Angle

At the xiphoid there exists an angle whose sides are formed by the lower edges of the ribs. Normally, this angle increases with inspiration and decreases with expiration, owing to symmetrical expansion of the lower part of the thorax. Changes in this angle are best appreciated by laying the thumbs along both lower costal margins, their tips meeting at the xiphoid process. The angle changes with respiration, owing to combined action of the diaphragm and of the intercostal and scalene muscles. It increases normally during inspiration because the action of the intercostal-scalene group and the

domed diaphragm all act to elevate the lower ribs. If the diaphragm is flattened by obstructive lung disease, its mechanical advantage acts transversely rather than vertically, and there may be no increase in the angle with inspiration, or occasionally a paradoxical decrease with inspiration. Unilateral diaphragmatic flattening, due to pleural effusion or pneumothorax, causes asymmetrical increase of the lower costal margin on inspiration with less movement on the involved side.

Boundaries and Divisions of the Lungs

By means of percussion the boundaries of the lungs can be clearly delineated and marked with a wax pencil on the skin of the chest (Fig. 9). The divisions within each lung should be mastered if the physician desires to diagnose and treat chest disease in children with any finesse. Fortunately, there is a remarkably constant division of each lung into lobes (Fig. 10), and each lobe into segments (Fig. 11). Although segmental anatomy is most easily learned from a three-dimensional model,* it can also be learned from diagrams. Efforts to remember exact rib and interspace boundaries of the lobes and segments, and their changes with age, are usually wasted because they are soon forgotten. It is much more to the point to be able to transfer the boundaries of the lobes and segments from a figure to a living chest wall so as to get them proportionately within the limits of the lungs, as determined by percussion. The technique is similar to learning how to carve a turkey from a diagram in a book. If the diagram is mastered, the dotted "cut here" lines, proportionately expanded, show up in the mind's eye on the steaming Thanksgiving turkey. Once the examiner has mastered the relative sizes of the segments, he "sees" the dotted lines

---

* For example, the Huber Lung Model, manufactured by the Clay-Adams Company, New York, N. Y.

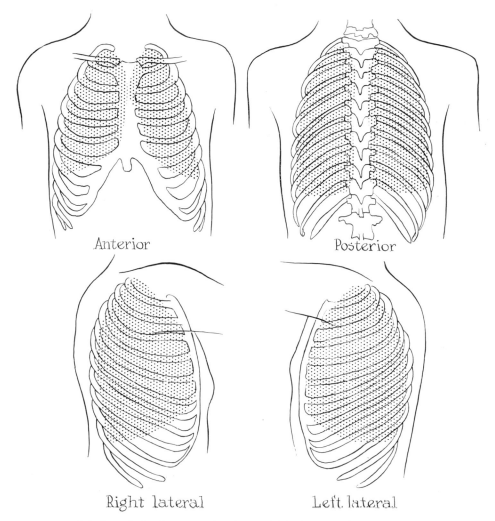

Anterior   Posterior

Right lateral   Left lateral

FIGURE 2–9. Relation of the lungs to the thorax. This figure depicts the approximate areas of resonance produced by air-containing lung tissue within the thorax of an older child. The lungs of infants are of different shapes and proportions, conforming with the previously discussed age changes of the thorax.

that outline the segments on any chest, regardless of its size. He is then able to percuss and auscultate according to the anatomic divisions of the lungs.

Percussion of the chests of children is best done by the indirect method in which a finger tip (plexor) of the examiner's dominant hand taps sharply on a terminal phalanx (pleximeter) of the other hand. The action of the percussing hand is altogether at the wrist; there should be little or no forearm motion. The tap should be just forceful enough to produce

an audible note.* It is a mistaken notion to correlate increases in resonance with increases in amplitude (loudness) of the percussion note. The relation is between increasing resonance and decreasing pitch. In this sense, percussion can be compared to notes on a musical scale with the resonant notes in the bass clef, dull notes in the treble clef, and flat notes even higher.

---

* This is particularly important if the chest of the child is touching another resonating object, such as the mother's chest.

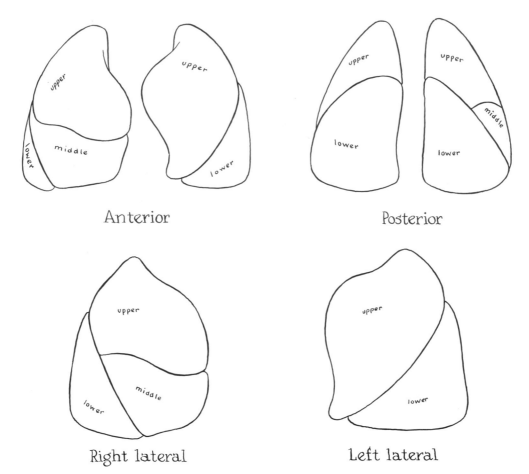

Anterior   Posterior

Right lateral   Left lateral

FIGURE 2–10. Division of the lungs into lobes. The projections here correspond to those of Figure 9. Minor variations in fissures may occur, producing somewhat different lobar proportions, incompletely separated lobes or supernumerary lobes. The patterns above are the most common, however.

There is a physiologic variation in percussion of the normal lung, slightly lower notes being heard toward the base and higher notes toward the apex. The transition is smooth, and sudden changes in pitch should suggest a pathologic state.

Although variably developed among physicians, a sense of touch is also involved in percussion, resonance being more easily felt than dullness.

In lobar or segmental consolidation the transitions from dullness to resonance should correspond to the "dotted lines" that indicate lobar and segmental boundaries. Thus precise anatomic localization of the disease may be possible.

Palpation of the thorax as an aid to localizing disease is generally less helpful in infants than in older children. Areas of increased tactile fremitus may correspond to the topographic anatomy of consolidated lobes or segments. Decreased or absent fremitus may be noted over a hemithorax with pleural effusion or pneumothorax.

Segmental Auscultation

The pediatrician has often been afflicted with acoustically inferior stethoscopes on the grounds of an alleged need for miniaturization. This need has been exaggerated, since his patients extend from the premature through the adoles-

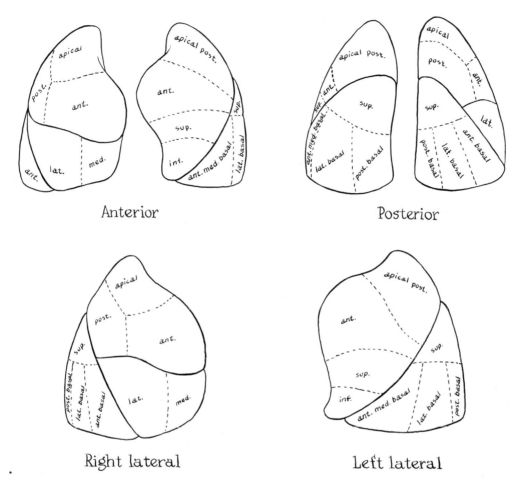

FIGURE 2–11. Division of the lobes into segments. The projections here correspond to those of Figures 9 and 10. The segments of each lung have been labeled. There are 10 segments in the right lung, all of which touch the inner thoracic wall with the exception of the medial basal segment of the lower lobe. On the left there are 8 segments (or 9, depending on notation), all of which touch the thorax, except for the medial portion of the anteromedial basal segment of the lower lobe. The physical diagnostic significance of these facts is that almost all the segments can be percussed and auscultated.

cent, and he must have a stethoscope applicable to all or face the necessity of a stethoscope for each of several age groups. The situation is further complicated by the need for both a bell and a diaphragm in order to extend the range of sound perception to cover both very low and very high frequencies. There are now available greatly improved instruments whose increased cost is easily justified by the very importance and frequency of use of the tool itself. Accordingly, the first and most important rule of auscultation is to procure a bell-diaphragm stethoscope with modern responsiveness.* By proper selection of earpieces it should be made to fit both snugly and comfortably into the external ear canals. Finally, it should be both sturdy and light.

A second rule, almost universally ignored, is to relate auscultation to bronchopulmonary anatomy, as was done for

---

* One such stethoscope is the Littmann, manufactured by Cardiosonics Medical Instruments, Belmont, Massachusetts. The larger model for adults is preferred to the smaller one designed for children because of its superior diaphragm. It works perfectly well on infants and children.

percussion. A busy physician could theoretically listen to every available segment
in both lungs in seventeen respiratory
cycles. In practice, he should listen, preferably with the diaphragm, for one or
two complete respirations over each of
the bronchopulmonary segments, spend-
ing most time on those that the history
and preceding portions of the examination have suggested as sites of disease. It
is convenient to begin auscultation on the
back, since this produces less anxiety for
the child than a frontal approach. The
infant may remain quietly, breast to
breast, in his mother's arms. Every lobe
is covered by listening to each of its various segments before proceeding to another one. The assumption in such segment auscultation is that the relations of
the segments within the lobe and the lobes
within the lung are constant and have
not been grossly disturbed by disease.
This assumption is reasonable in most
instances, since bronchopulmonary segmentation is remarkably constant. It
would obviously be open to error in the
presence of major lung-shifting processes,
such as gross anomalies, large tension
cysts, atelectasis, pneumothorax, pleural
fluid collections, as well as in patients
who have had substantial resections of
lung.

It follows that the physician's records
should indicate by description or diagram
the presumably involved lobe and segment. If a child has persistent rales in the
posterior basal segment of the right lower
lobe, heard on repeated office visits, the
implications are clearly not the same as
those of rales heard in *different* segments
on repeated visits. *Careful, serial recording of anatomically related physical findings is the best means of diagnosing significant, structural lesions in the lungs.*

One of the problems of pediatric pulmonary auscultation is that posed by insufficiently deep breaths. Older children,
like adults, can be shown how to breathe
deeply through the mouth. Smaller children can be asked to "pant like a puppy
dog" or to pretend to blow out candles

on a birthday cake. In others, expiration
may be reinforced by compression of the
thorax between the hand holding the
stethoscope on one side and the remaining
hand on the other. After such an assisted
expiration, especially if well timed, the
next inspiration is usually deeper. This
maneuver may also reveal undetected
rhonchi by increasing expiratory flow
rate. If all else fails, the deep respirations
just before and during crying may produce diagnostically sufficient inspiratory
depths and provide an excellent chance
for careful examination at the height of
inspiration.

Breath Sounds

Since breath sounds are not transmitted
alike through different stethoscopes, an
examiner should always use the same
stethoscope. It requires experience to become familiar with the nature of breath
sounds heard at different ages. The spectrum of breath sounds that range from
vesicular to tracheal exists largely because
of differences in the expiratory phase. The
tubular quality of *tracheal* breathing is
easily learned by placing the diaphragm
over the examiner's own trachea and listening to the high-pitched "tubular"
sound that is audible throughout all of
expiration. This is easily contrasted with
the *vesicular* breath sounds heard in the
examiner's own axilla. The inspiratory
note is softer and lower pitched, and expiration is essentially soundless. Between
these two extremes range both the normal
and abnormal breath sounds of infancy
and childhood.

Bronchovesicular breath sounds are
characterized by a soft, rather low-pitched
expiratory note heard during the early
part of expiration. Breath sounds may
change from vesicular to bronchovesicular
in a child if the depth of ventilation is
increased. The inspiratory note of bronchovesicular breathing is similar to that
of vesicular breathing. *Bronchial breath
sounds* fall between bronchovesicular and
tracheal and are characterized by an audi-

ble tubular note throughout all of expiration, but this tubular quality is less than that heard in tracheal breathing.

As a rule, the closer the stethoscope is to a large airway, the more audible and tubular will be the expiratory note. The bronchial breath sounds of lobar consolidation are based on the transmission through fluid-filled alveoli of sounds made by air moving in the bronchi of that lobe.

If the examiner is in doubt about whether breath sounds in an area are normal or not, he should compare the area in question with a corresponding area of the opposite lung. Clear differences may quickly reinforce his suspicions.

The term *suppressed breath sounds* implies diminished ventilation of that area of the lung being auscultated. Its use is usually based on the amplitude (audibility) of the inspiratory note. Breath sounds may be exaggerated or suppressed without being abnormal in quality. In atelectasis, for example, breath sounds may be vesicular and sharply suppressed over the involved lobe, owing to the relatively great distance from the stethoscope of normally ventilating lung.

Rales and Rhonchi

There exist several conflicting classifications of rales and rhonchi. This author prefers exclusive definitions of the two (Table 8). Rales are discontinuous, nonmusical, crackling or bubbling, soft or loud, inspiratory or expiratory, palpable or impalpable sounds produced by air bubbling through fluid in the lungs. A rhonchus is a continuous, musical, soft or loud, usually expiratory, usually nonpalpable sound produced by air moving with velocity past a fixed obstruction in the airway. The nature of the obstruction may vary, including foreign body, vascular anomaly, bronchospasm, inspissated mucopurulent secretions, or combinations of these. Regardless, it must present a relatively *solid* partial obstruction to airflow.

Table 8. *Classification of Rales and Rhonchi*

Rales
Fine
Medium
Coarse
Rhonchi
Sibilant
Sonorous

Terms such as "crepitant," "dry" and "moist" are apt to be confusing and are better replaced with *fine, medium* and *coarse*. Fine rales imply fluid in or below the terminal bronchioles, whereas medium and coarse rales indicate fluid in the proportionately larger divisions of the airway. Care should be taken to differentiate coarse, frequently palpable, rales from friction rubs.

Rhonchi are either sibilant or sonorous, depending on pitch. Sibilant rhonchi are soft and high-pitched, whereas sonorous rhonchi are louder and lower pitched, such differences being due presumably to differences in caliber of the resonating air columns. In addition to their significance as indicators of obstruction in the airways, the auscultation of rhonchi implies that larger bronchi are involved, because only in the larger bronchi is there sufficient velocity of air movement to produce a musical sound.

REFERENCES

Avery, M. E.: *The Lung and Its Disorders in the Newborn Infant.* Philadelphia, W. B. Saunders Company, 1964.

Banyai, A. L., and Levine, E. R.: *Dyspnea. Diagnosis and Treatment.* Philadelphia, F. A. Davis Company, 1963.

Boynton, B.: *The Physical Growth of Girls.* University of Iowa Studies in Child Welfare, 1936, Volume XII, No. 4.

Cherniack, R. M., and Cherniack, L.: *Respiration in Health and Disease.* Philadelphia, W. B. Saunders Company, 1961.

Comroe, J. H., Jr., and Botelho, S.: The Unreliability of Cyanosis in the Recognition of Arterial Anoxemia. *Am. J. Med. Sc.*, 214:1-6, 1947.

Dawson, J. B.: Auscultation and the Stethoscope. *Practitioner*, 193:315-22, 1964.

Fischer, D. S., Singer, D. H., and Feldman, S. M.: Clubbing, a Review, with Emphasis on Hereditary Acropachy. *Medicine* (Baltimore), 43:459-79, 1964.

Gross, N. J., and Hamilton, J. D.: Correlation Between the Physical Signs of Hypercapnia and the Mixed Venous Pco_2. *Brit. M.J.*, 2:1096-7, 1963.

Hall, G. H.: The Cause of Digital Clubbing. Testing a New Hypothesis. *Lancet*, 1:750-53, 1959.

Howatt, W. F., and DeMuth, G. D.: The Growth of Lung Function. II. Configuration of the Chest. *Pediatrics*, 35:177-84, 1965.

Iliff, A., and Lee, V. A.: Pulse Rate, Respiratory Rate, and Body Temperature of Children Between Two Months and Eighteen Years of Age. *Child Development*, 23:237-45, 1952.

Krahl, V. E.: Anatomy of the Mammalian Lung; in *Handbook of Physiology*, Section 3: Respiration. Washington, D.C., American Physiological Society, 1964, Vol. I, Chap. 6, pp. 213-84.

Landing, B. H.: Anomalies of the Respiratory Tract. *Pediat. Clin. N. Amer.*, 4:73-102, 1957.

Meredith, H. V.: *The Rhythm of Physical Growth*. A Study of Eighteen Anthropometric Measurements on Iowa City White Males Ranging in Age Between Birth and Eighteen Years. University of Iowa Studies, 1935, No. 3, Vol. XI.

CHAPTER THREE

Diagnostic and Therapeutic Procedures

WILLIAM W. WARING, M.D.

It is possible to divide all procedures pertaining to respiratory disease into the categories of prophylaxis, diagnosis and therapy. Only those that are felt to deserve special comment will be discussed in this chapter. Some procedures can be performed without assistance by any physician, while others require specialized skills or other physicians or laboratory workers. Table 1 lists various procedures that may be required to prevent, diagnose or treat lung disease in children. Italicized procedures are discussed below.

DIAGNOSTIC PROCEDURES

Radiologic Examination of the Lungs

The chest roentgenogram deserves its reputation as one of the best diagnostic

Table 1. *Procedures for Prevention, Diagnosis and Treatment of Respiratory Disease**

Prevention

1. Immunization:
   a. Active: influenza, diphtheria, poliomyelitis, pertussis, rubeola
   b. Passive: diphtheria, rubeola, hypogammaglobulinemia
2. Allergic hyposensitization
3. Environmental control: removal of allergens, hospital isolation procedures, ultraviolet irradiation, humidification, urban smog control, education on dangers of smoking, ample living space, etc.

Diagnosis

1. *Roentgenography: routine chest RGs, laminagraphy, fluoroscopy, angiography, bronchography, etc.*
2. *Bronchoscopy*
3. *Lung puncture*
4. *Lung biopsy*

Table 1. *(Continued)*

5. *Pneumoperitoneum*
6. *Pulmonary function testing*
7. Cultures: blood, nasopharyngeal, throat, tracheobronchial (sputum), lung, pleural, and bone marrow for bacteria, fungi, viruses
8. Stained smears: from various loci for eosinophils, macrophages, tumor cells, parasites, bacteria, fungi, etc.
9. Serology: acute and convalescent serums for cold agglutinins, viruses, etc.
10. Electrocardiography
11. Skin testing: for allergy, tuberculosis, atypical mycobacteria, sarcoid, various fungi, etc.
12. Laryngoscopy
13. Nasopharyngoscopy
14. Sweat test: for cystic fibrosis
15. Thoracentesis
16. Gastric washing
17. Protein electrophoresis

Treatment

1. *Bronchial (postural) drainage and physical therapy*
2. *Breathing exercises*
3. *Inhalation therapy: oxygen, aerosol*
4. *Pleural space drainage and intracavitary (Monaldi) drainage*
5. *Transtracheal catheterization and tracheobronchial lavage*
6. *Bronchotomy*
7. *Tracheostomy*
8. *Lung biopsy*
9. *Resection: segmental, lobar, lung*
10. Tonsillectomy; adenoidectomy
11. Myringotomy
12. Bronchoscopy (see No. 2 under *Diagnosis*)
13. Thoracentesis
14. Assisted ventilation

* Italicized procedures are discussed in the text under the same grouping.

tools of chest disease. All children with persistent cough or fever, chest pain, tachypnea or dyspnea should have both posteroanterior and lateral chest roentgenograms. It is surprising how frequently only the posteroanterior view is used. All films should be interpreted both by the radiologist and by the attending physician, since the physician should be in a better position to correlate clinical and radiologic findings. When previous films are available, a careful comparison of them with the current roentgenograms is essential to the diagnosis of most chronic or recurrent lung disease.

The physician should be able to define the projections of the various lobes and segments in both posteroanterior and lateral views. He should know the names and courses of the segmental bronchi (Fig. 1). The pattern of atelectasis for each lobe should be mastered. He should learn to look "through" the heart and the diaphragms in order to see those parts of the lungs concealed by them. "Overpenetrated" chest x-rays are frequently helpful for discovery of otherwise hidden clues to disease.

Acute processes of low inertia may have a lag between the onset of symptoms or signs and significant radiologic findings. A follow-up film in twenty-four hours may reveal the previously unvisualized process, as is notably true in hydrocarbon aspiration pneumonia.

Special views of the lungs are frequently useful. The right posterior oblique overpenetrated view is excellent for inspection of the bronchial tree on that side (Fig. 1, *D*). The left posterior oblique view similarly "opens up" the left bronchial tree (Fig. 1, *E*). Right or left lateral decubitus views are essential if atypical pleural fluid collections are suspected, or if one wishes to confirm possible air-fluid interfaces within the chest. Apical lordotic views for unobstructed visualization of the apices of the lung are less useful in children than in adults, largely because of the different patterns of primary and reinfection forms of tuberculosis. Inspiratory and expiratory films are indicated in any child suspected of having partial mainstem or lobar bronchial obstruction, as with aspirated foreign bodies.

Laminagrams (planigrams, tomograms, stratigrams, body-section roentgenograms) may be useful in certain children old enough to cooperate for them. They may more precisely delineate obscure solid or cystic lesions. Specifically, they may re-

(Text continued on page 86.)

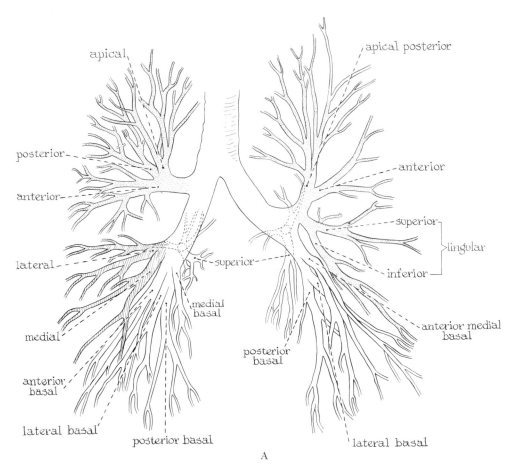

apical

apical posterior

posterior

anterior

anterior

superior

lingular

lateral

superior

inferior

medial
basal

medial

anterior medial
basal

posterior
basal

anterior
basal

lateral basal

posterior basal

lateral basal

A

FIGURE 3–1. Distribution of lobar and segmental bronchi. Upper lobe bronchi are stippled, middle lobe bronchi are diagonally lined, and lower lobe bronchi are outlined only. Segmental bronchi are labeled. *A,* Posteroanterior projection.

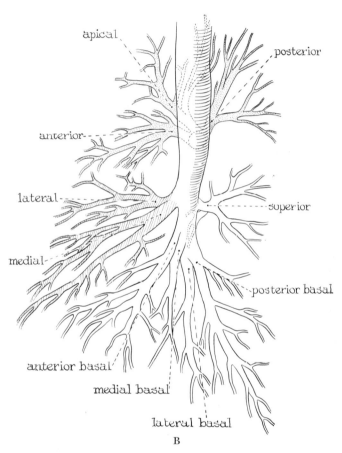

B

FIGURE 3–1. *Continued.* Distribution of lobar and segmental bronchi. Upper lobe bronchi are stippled, middle lobe bronchi are diagonally lined, and lower lobe bronchi are outlined only. Segmental bronchi are labeled. *B,* Lateral projection of right bronchi.

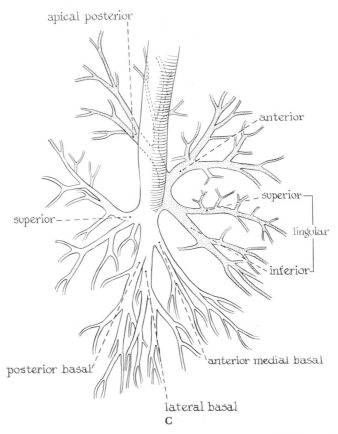

apical posterior

anterior

superior

lingular

inferior

superior

posterior basal

anterior medial basal

lateral basal

C

FIGURE 3–1. *Continued.* Distribution of lobar and segmental bronchi. Upper lobe bronchi are stippled, middle lobe bronchi are diagonally lined, and lower lobe bronchi are outlined only. Segmental bronchi are labeled. *C,* Lateral projection of left bronchi.

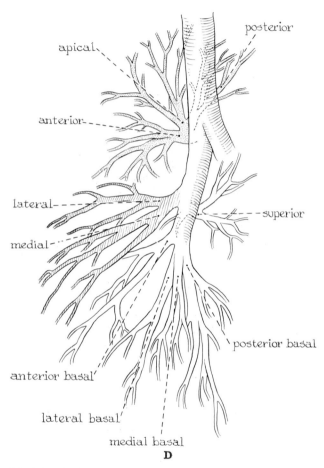

D

FIGURE 3–1. *Continued.* Distribution of lobar and segmental bronchi. Upper lobe bronchi are stippled, middle lobe bronchi are diagonally lined, and lower lobe bronchi are outlined only. Segmental bronchi are labeled. *D,* Right posterior oblique projection of right bronchi.

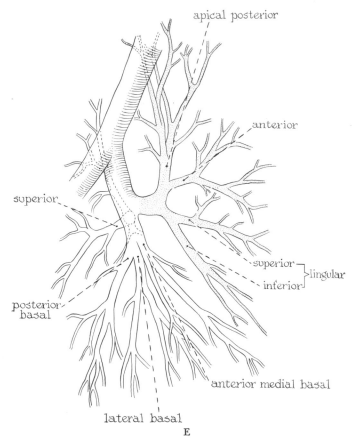

apical posterior

anterior

superior

superior ⎤
inferior ⎦ lingular

posterior basal

anterior medial basal

lateral basal

E

FIGURE 3–1. *Concluded.* Distribution of lobar and segmental bronchi. Upper lobe bronchi are stippled, middle lobe bronchi are diagonally lined, and lower lobe bronchi are outlined only. Segmental bronchi are labeled. *E,* Left posterior oblique projection of left bronchi.

veal bronchial connections with cavities, vascular connections with solid or cystic lesions, confirm the presence and localization of calcification, reveal intrabronchial filling defects, and resolve some lesions from obscuring shadows, as, for example, "separating" a lymph node from other hilar structures. The physician, in consultation with the radiologist, should decide on the most desirable plane and the number of "sections" indicated.

Fluoroscopy may be extremely useful, especially if image intensification and cineradiography are also available. Considerable information can be obtained on diaphragmatic function and regional ventilation of the lungs.

Angiography may reveal anomalies of

the vasculature of the lungs, e.g. an abnormal transdiaphragmatic blood supply to sequestered lung tissue.

Bronchography is usually indicated when significant congenital or acquired bronchial disease is suspected, most frequently bronchiectasis. Even if bronchiectasis is known to exist in only one part of the lungs, complete bilateral bronchographic studies should be performed in order to be certain that significant disease does not exist elsewhere. Specific indications may include persistent rales or recurrent pneumonia in a single segment or lobe, chronic productive cough, or obscure masses within the lungs. If digital clubbing coexists and cannot be explained on a nonpulmonary basis, the above-

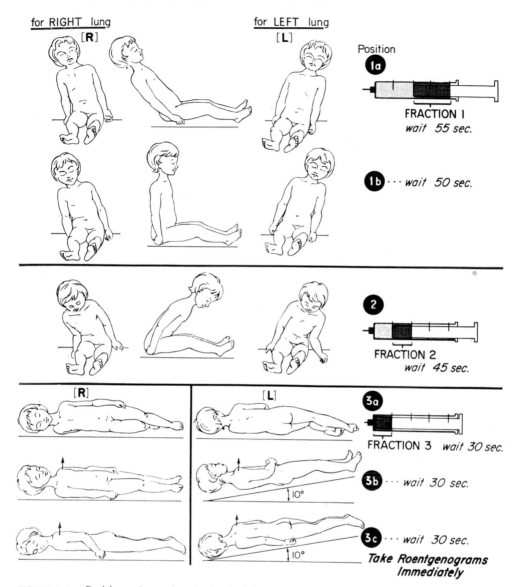

for RIGHT lung [R]

for LEFT lung [L]

Position

1a FRACTION I
wait 55 sec.

1b ··· *wait 50 sec.*

2 FRACTION 2
wait 45 sec.

3a FRACTION 3 *wait 30 sec.*

[R] [L]

3b ··· *wait 30 sec.*
10°

3c ··· *wait 30 sec.*
10°
*Take Roentgenograms
Immediately*

FIGURE 3–2. Positions of a patient for both right (R) and left (L) bronchograms and their relations to times of instillation and fractional doses of contrast medium. The dose of contrast medium for each lung is 1 ml. per year of age (not exceeding 8 ml.), injected in 3 fractions as illustrated. Roentgenograms are exposed, and contrast medium is removed from one lung prior to proceeding with the contralateral bronchogram. (Reproduced from *Pediatrics* with permission of the American Academy of Pediatrics.)

mentioned indications become even more urgent.

The procedure is usually done under general anesthesia in children. A conventional endotracheal tube is then inserted through which the contrast medium is injected from a syringe with attached catheter. Since obstructive or restrictive lung disease is usually present, the procedure is not without hazard. Nice clinical judgment may be necessary in deciding whether and, if so, *when* to do a bronchogram. It is usually possible to perform a complete bilateral bronchogram under brilliant illumination so that the patient's color, respirations and other vital indices

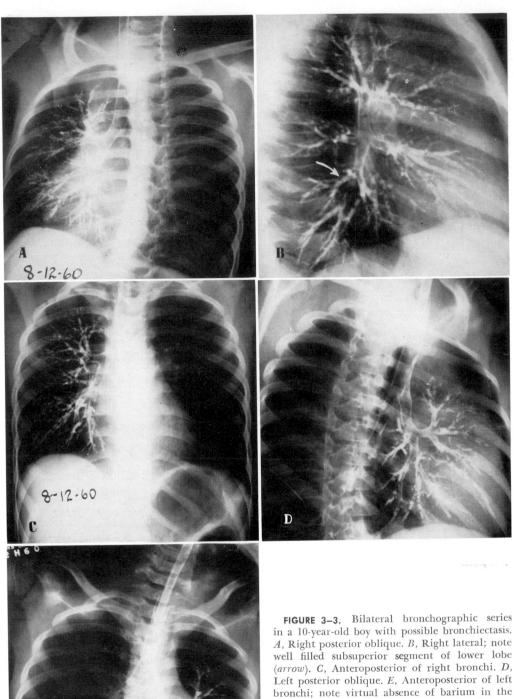

FIGURE 3–3. Bilateral bronchographic series in a 10-year-old boy with possible bronchiectasis. *A,* Right posterior oblique. *B,* Right lateral; note well filled subsuperior segment of lower lobe (*arrow*). *C,* Anteroposterior of right bronchi. *D,* Left posterior oblique. *E,* Anteroposterior of left bronchi; note virtual absence of barium in the previously filled right side. (Reproduced from *Pediatrics* with permission of the American Academy of Pediatrics.)

can be easily and continually monitored.

A satisfactory method of bronchography, shown in Figure 2, uses sequential body positions to ensure entry of the contrast medium into the desired bronchi. Conventional overpenetrated chest roentgenograms give excellent, sharp contrast between the vascular markings and the coated bronchi (Fig. 3). Either the more commonly used iodine-containing compounds or a suspension of barium sulfate in an inert viscous vehicle, such as carboxymethylcellulose, is a satisfactory contrast medium for children.

Bronchoscopy

Bronchoscopy may be both diagnostic and therapeutic. It is frequently useful in determining the cause of bronchial or tracheal obstruction. Secretions or other material removed at bronchoscopy can be cultured or examined histologically. Confirmation of the involved lobes or segments is obtained by visualization of secretions flowing from specific bronchi. Gross tracheobronchial anomalies may be identified. In its more common therapeutic application the bronchoscope is used to remove secretions, tissue, or foreign bodies obstructing those parts of the airway that are directly accessible to it. More distally located causes of obstruction must be removed by other means. The older the child, the farther the bronchoscopic examination can penetrate. It is common practice to subject a patient to bronchoscopy prior to tracheostomy and to leave the bronchoscope in the trachea during the operation until it is time to insert the tracheostomy tube. This is particularly useful in obstructions of the upper airway, since an airway is thus provided until the tracheostomy is operational. Technically, the operation is usually easier with the trachea thus stabilized.

Bronchoscopy may be either an elective or an emergency procedure, and, depending on the circumstances, anesthesia is local, general or necessarily omitted.

Persistent, dependent lobar atelectasis, unresponsive to vigorous medical therapy for two weeks, should be treated by bronchoscopic suction of the affected bronchus. On the other hand, obstruction at the carina or in either main bronchus is usually an indication for immediate bronchoscopy. Atelectasis of the upper lobes is less amenable to bronchoscopic treatment because of the right-angle take off of the upper lobe bronchi.

Careless manipulation of a bronchoscope may be more harmful than helpful. Laryngeal trauma during bronchoscopy may require subsequent tracheostomy, especially in small infants. A desperately ill child with multiple sites of distal bronchial obstruction may obtain no benefit from bronchoscopy and may be further exhausted by the operative manipulations. It follows that this procedure, probably more than most, should be carefully planned, skillfully performed and quickly completed. A "mist tent" (see p. 102) during the immediate postoperative period may lessen laryngeal edema.

Lung Puncture

This diagnostic procedure probably deserves selective, wider application, since it can yield information not otherwise easily obtained. Lung puncture has been used to obtain a lung aspirate for either histologic study or for culture. The technique is simple. A short-bevel 20-gauge needle is attached to a 10-cc. syringe which contains 1 ml. of sterile isotonic saline solution. An intercostal space is locally anesthetized, and a quick stab is made through the space, across the pleuras, and into the lung to a depth of 3 to 4 cm. The saline is injected to assure patency of the needle, and negative pressure is produced in the syringe-needle system by withdrawing the plunger of the syringe. Simultaneously the needle is withdrawn so that tissue fluid is drawn into the needle and syringe. The needle remains in the lung only a few seconds, preferably for less than one respiratory cycle. The contents of the needle and syringe may then be smeared on slides for special staining, or may be transferred to a liquid culture medium by drawing up the medium into the syringe through the aspirating needle and thence returning it to its original container. If the sample is sufficient, both may be accomplished.

Lung puncture may be the only way of obtaining an organism for antibiotic sensitivity testing in children with a deep-seated, subacute or chronic pneumonia. In such patients physical examination and chest x-rays allow the physician to aspirate the most involved segment of the lung. The method has also been of value in diagnosing obscure, interstitial pneumonopathies, such as idiopathic pulmonary hemosiderosis.

The procedure has certain theoretical dangers: pulmonary hemorrhage, empyema and pneumothorax. In practice, the only problem of any significance has been transient, slight pneumothorax when the tap has been made into air-containing lung. Usually this complication can be avoided by choosing a densely consolidated segment for puncture.

Lung Biopsy

Biopsy of the lung is occasionally necessary when protracted pulmonary disease cannot be explained by other means, although careful and intelligent use of less extreme diagnostic procedures makes it rarely necessary. When indicated, lung biopsy is usually performed under general anesthesia with an endotracheal airway, by which normal pulmonary ventilation is maintained and collapse of the lung prevented. Open thoracotomy is performed at a site corresponding to known involvement, and sufficient pulmonary tissue is removed for all required studies. Percutaneous lung biopsy with a Vim-Silverman or Franklin-Silverman needle has been reported in adults, but is not at present recommended for infants and children.

Pneumoperitoneum

The injection of 200 to 300 cc. of air into the peritoneal cavity sharply demarcates the position of the diaphragm on subsequent chest roentgenography. It is occasionally useful in differentiating eventration of the diaphragm from supradiaphragmatic lesions, such as extralobar sequestration. In cases of this type, confirmation of an asymptomatic localized eventration might obviate a formal surgical exploration.

Pulmonary Function Tests

Pulmonary function testing, especially of children, until recently has been an area of little concern to the practicing physician. Such testing has been possible only in research laboratories of children's hospitals or with special and often grudging consent from directors of adult cardiopulmonary laboratories. It is unreasonable to expect practicing physicians to try to become pulmonary physiologists. Nevertheless simple testing equipment, which can be used in any physician's office or carried to the bedside, is available and is helpful in evaluating many acute, recurrent and chronic lung diseases in children.

Although Chapter One deals with the physiologic basis of pulmonary pathology in general terms, we are concerned here with tests that provide a practical means of quantitating lung function in a specific patient.

The respiratory rate of the afebrile, tranquil or sleeping child is a simple, excellent test of lung stiffness. Rapid rates are correlated with diseases that stiffen (reduce the compliance of) the lungs and thoracic cage. Normal values for this "test" are given in the preceding chapter on history and physical examination (p. 62).

Vital capacity is a measure of the effect of those diseases that *restrict* the function of the thorax and lungs. Since restrictive

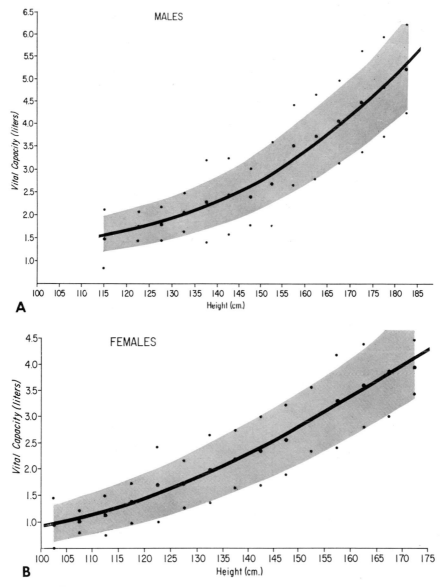

FIGURE 3–4. Vital capacity as a function of height (centimeters) in normal male and female children and adolescents. Gas volumes have been corrected to conditions of body temperature, ambient pressure and saturation with water vapor at 37°C. (BTPS). Data are those of Ferris. *A,* Males; *B,* females.

lung disease is generally associated with decreased compliance, elevated sleeping respiratory rates should correlate with decreases in vital capacity. Cooperative children of five years and older can be shown quickly how to perform the vital capacity test, and compact, relatively inexpensive equipment is available.* Predicted values for vital capacity are shown in Figure 4 and Table 2.

* McKesson Vitalor, McKesson Appliance Co., 2228 Ashland Ave., Toledo, Ohio. This instrument will measure both vital capacity and expiratory flow rates.

Table 2. *Vital Capacity (Liters per Minute) in Relation to Height (Centimeters) for Normal Children and Adolescents**

Male

Height (cm.)	100-105	105-110	110-115	115-120	120-125	125-130	130-135	135-140	140-145	145-150	150-155	155-160	160-165	165-170	170-175	175-180	180-185
No.			7		5	4	5	9	9	9	5	12	13	30	29	16	8
Mean (L.)			1.46		1.64	1.79	2.05	2.27	2.41	2.38	2.69	3.52	3.72	4.07	4.47	4.82	5.24
Std. Dev. (L.)			0.32		0.16	0.18	0.21	0.45	0.41	0.31	0.45	0.44	0.47	0.45	0.55	0.54	0.49

Female

Height (cm.)	100-105	105-110	110-115	115-120	120-125	125-130	130-135	135-140	140-145	145-150	150-155	155-160	160-165	165-170	170-175	175-180	180-185
No.	2	2	7	13	10	15	19	30	19	12	23	38	18	17	6		
Mean (L.)	0.95	1.00	1.12	1.37	1.70	1.70	1.97	2.19	2.32	2.53	2.94	3.28	3.57	3.85	3.91		
Std. Dev. (L.)	0.25	0.10	0.17	0.19	0.35	0.22	0.33	0.27	0.32	0.33	0.30	0.43	0.41	0.44	0.26		

* Data of Ferris. Gas volumes have been corrected to BTPS conditions.

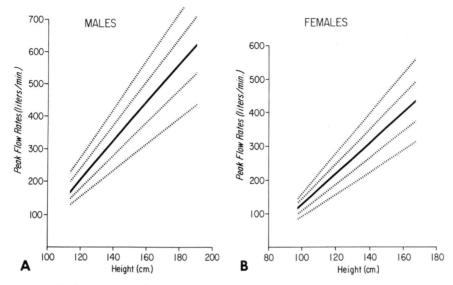

FIGURE 3–5. Peak expiratory flow rate as a function of height (centimeters) in normal male and female children and adolescents. Data are those of Murray and Cook. *A*, Males. Regression equation: PFR (L./min.) = 5.70 × Ht. (cm.) − 480 ± 14.5% (Std. def.). *B*, Females. Regression equation: PFR (L./min.) = 4.65 × Ht. (cm.) − 344 ± 14.3% (Std. dev.).

Neither vital capacity nor respiratory rate is a measure of the severity of obstructive lung disease, and therefore a simple, quantitative test of airway obstruction would be useful. Such a test is the peak expiratory flow rate, for which normal values have been established in children (Fig. 5). Peak expiratory flow rate is measured by a simple, direct-reading device that requires no calculations.* Although the test is open to the criticism that it measures a part of forced expiration that is not maximally dependent on obstruction in the airways, nevertheless it is a useful test, especially in the office and at the bedside. It is also helpful to think of peak flow as correlating with the effectiveness of cough; low flow rates are associated with ineffective coughing. As in most pulmonary function tests, the wide range of normal values makes single observations much more difficult to interpret than patterns established by serial measurements.

Unfortunately, the physician in his office cannot easily quantitate the effects

of respiratory failure: hypoxemia and hypercapnia. Such measurements require more elaborate techniques and samples of arterial blood, although capillary or "arterialized" venous blood may be substituted under certain circumstances. Clues to failure can often be obtained from history, physical examination and the simple tests mentioned above.

It is certain that the coming generations of physicians will learn to depend on objective pulmonary function testing, as the present generation has learned the value of electrocardiography or serum electrolyte determination.

THERAPEUTIC PROCEDURES

Bronchial (Postural) Drainage and Physical Therapy

These methods of treating disease of the bronchi will receive considerable emphasis here because they are neither practiced as effectively nor used as frequently as they should be. Bronchial drainage is indicated in any clinical situation in which excessive fluid in the bronchi is

(Text continued on page 98.)

---

* Wright Peak Flow Meter, Monaghan Company, Denver, Colorado.

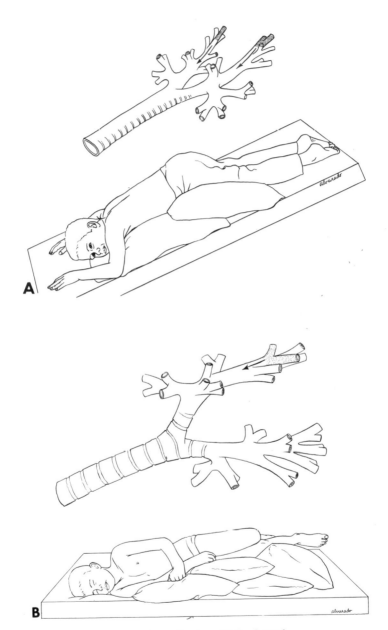

FIGURE 3–6. *See page 98 for legend.*

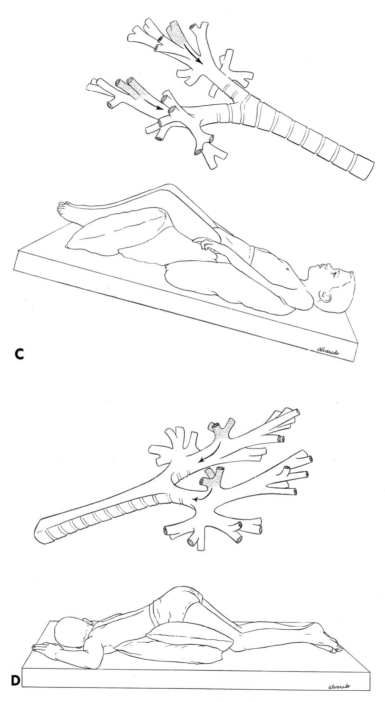

FIGURE 3–6. *See page 98 for legend.*

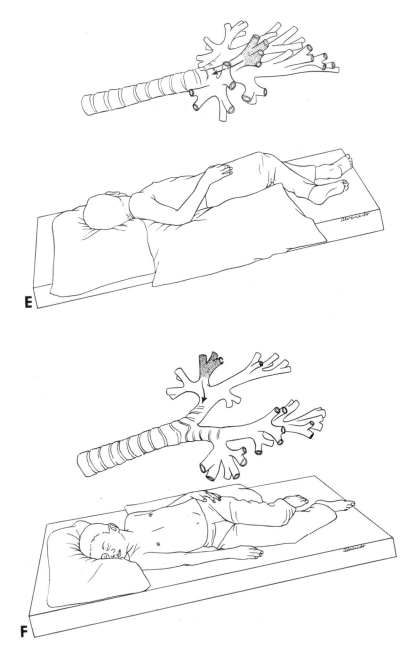

FIGURE 3–6. *See page 98 for legend.*

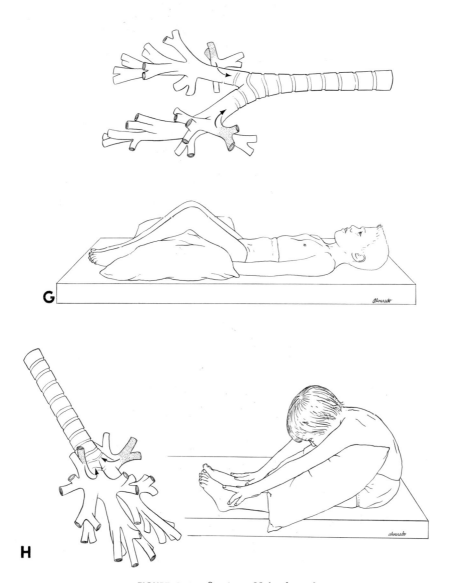

FIGURE 3–6. *See page 98 for legend.*

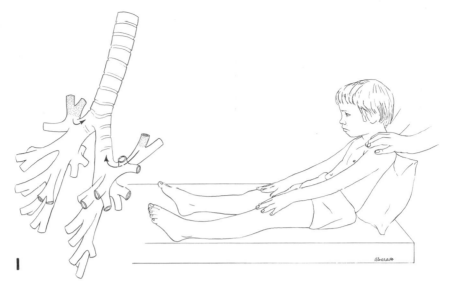

FIGURE 3–6. *Concluded.* Bronchial drainage positions for the major segments of all lobes. In each position a model of the tracheobronchial tree is projected above the child in order to show the segmental bronchus being drained (stippled) and the flow of secretions out of the segmental bronchus (*arrow*). The drainage platform is padded but firm, and pillows are liberally used to maintain each position with comfort. The platform is horizontal unless otherwise noted. *A,* Posterior basal segments of both lower lobes. The platform is tilted to approximately 25 degrees. *B,* Lateral basal segment of the left lower lobe. Drainage of the lateral basal segment of the right lower lobe would be accomplished by a mirror-image of this position (left side down). *C,* Anterior basal segments of both lower lobes. The child should be rotated slightly away from the side being drained. The platform is tilted to approximately 15 degrees. *D,* Superior segments of both lower lobes. Although the platform is flat, pillows are used to raise the buttocks moderately. *E,* Right middle lobe. The platform is tilted to approximately 15 degrees. *F,* Lingular segments of the left upper lobe (counterpart of the right middle lobe). The platform is tilted to approximately 15 degrees. *G,* Anterior segments of both upper lobes. The child should be rotated slightly away from the side being drained. *H,* Posterior segment of right upper lobe and posterior portion of apical-posterior segment of left upper lobe. Drainage moves secretions into main bronchi from which they can be more easily expelled (*curved arrows*). *I,* Apical segment of right upper lobe and apical portion of apical-posterior segment of left upper lobe. Drainage moves secretions into main bronchi from which they can be more easily expelled (*curved arrows*).

(*A, E* and *F* are reproduced with permission from the *Bulletin of the Tulane Medical Faculty,* 23: 141-3, 1964.)

not being removed by normal ciliary activity and cough. Determination of the presence of excessive bronchial fluid and its localization are most easily accomplished by segmental auscultation of the lungs. Persistent rales in a given segment or lobe constitute sufficient indication in themselves for drainage of the involved bronchi.

Examination of the anatomy of the tracheobronchial tree (Fig. 1) indicates that in the erect position the segments of the middle lobe, of the lingular division of the left upper lobe, and of both lower lobes normally must drain against gravity. Only the segments of the right upper lobe and the nonlingular portions of the left upper lobe receive gravitational assistance in erect man. Normally such a situation does not interfere with the body's ability to maintain patency of the tracheobronchial tree. Special loads, however, may be placed on the clearing mechanisms of the relatively small bronchi of children by viscous or excessive mucus and pus. It is axiomatic that infection is ultimately superimposed on bronchial obstruction due to any cause and that infection increases obstruction. Although bronchial drainage may not be the principal or sole therapy, it can be of invaluable assistance. After bronchoscopic removal of a foreign body, after administration of a broncho-dilator to an asthmatic child, or with the resolution of a pneumonia, excessive fluid may remain in one or more lobar or segmental bronchi. The affected bronchi can be identified by the topographical distribution of rales. The physician then can determine the position in which to place the patient that best promotes drainage of involved bronchi (Fig. 6).

Bronchial drainage is carried out three or four times daily, usually before meals and at bedtime, in periods usually not exceeding thirty minutes. Up to four positions may be used, since more than this number tends to exceed reasonable limits of cooperation. The exact arrangements for drainage vary with the situation: the physical therapy department or treatment room if the child is hospitalized, the bedroom if the child is at home. Infants may be positioned on the extended legs of a parent, and small children may be effectively drained on a padded ironing board.

Children with chronic bronchial disease, such as cystic fibrosis or bronchiectasis, may require daily periods of drainage over many months. They will profit from specially constructed tables or platforms, the surfaces of which can be padded for comfort and adjusted to the different angles required to drain all involved segments. Comfort is important because adequate drainage depends on relaxation and cooperation in each position over a period of five to fifteen minutes. Therapy may be discontinued when auscultation reveals that no excessive bronchial fluid remains.

In all cases the exact positions, as well as their order, duration and frequency, should be explained to the person (parent, nurse or physical therapist) who will be working with the child. At least one treatment should be demonstrated on the patient to parents or others who are unfamiliar with the techniques. Positions for drainage are varied subsequently by the physician in conformity with shifting patterns of bronchial disease.

If bronchorrhea is diffuse without any particularly specific localization, it is rea-sonable to recommend positions that will drain major dependent bronchi when the child is in the erect position, i.e. the posterior basal segments, the middle lobe, and the lingula, in that order. Drainage positions for the upper lobes may also be of importance for predominantly recumbent infants.

Certain physical therapeutic maneuvers are of great help when combined with bronchial drainage. Indeed, the modern concept of bronchial drainage implies the use of such maneuvers in addition to simple positioning of the patient. Viscid secretions may not drain from bronchi by gravity alone. The simile is frequently used of a freshly opened catsup bottle. Although the bottle is inverted, i.e. properly positioned for drainage, no catsup may flow until it is ejected by repeated blows on the bottom of the bottle; once started, however, flow may continue with little further agitation.

The maneuvers that may assist the removal of fluid by gravity include deep breathing, reinforced cough, thoracic "squeezing," "cupping" and vibration. Each will be briefly described.

After the child has been placed in position for drainage and has been encouraged to relax, he is asked to take several deep breaths. Since deep inspiration enlarges the tracheobronchial tree, air may penetrate around and through secretions that would not be affected by usual tidal volumes. Expiration following such a deep breath may carry secretions in the desired direction and may even initiate a productive cough.

The child should be taught not to suppress his cough and not to waste his strength with repeated feeble, and therefore ineffective, coughs. Instead, he should take a deep breath and cough once or twice as *hard* as he can. Such anticipated coughs can be reinforced by the hands of the operator encircling and synchronously compressing the sides of the lower half of the chest. The cough may thus be less fatiguing and more effective. Many children are not able to cough well in a dependent position. These children should be allowed to sit up after several minutes of drainage for a further trial of repeated, reinforced coughs. Sputum produced should be spit out into a container so that the productivity of the treatment can be demonstrated to both the child and the physician.

With the child in a bronchial drainage position, another maneuver, the "squeeze," may be tried. The child is asked to take a deep breath and then exhale through the mouth as completely and rapidly as possible, as he would do for a forced expiratory volume determination. The depth of expiration is increased by brief, firm pressure from the operator's hands compressing the sides of the thorax. The goal is to decrease maximally the volume of the tracheobronchial tree. Secretions may thus be expressed from the "open ends" of the bronchi, similar to the squeezing of toothpaste from a tube. The subsequent inspiration may be followed by a most productive cough, which should again be "reinforced" by the operator.

The maneuver known as "cupping" or "clapping" is performed intermittently several times in each drainage position. One or both of the cupped hands of the operator vigorously and repeatedly strike that part of the chest *under which the segment being drained is located*. Although "cupping" should be vigorous, it is painless if performed properly. The patient should wear a light cotton undershirt to avoid irritation of the skin of the chest. Care should be taken not to slap the chest with the fingers or palm, but to make the cupped hand conform exactly to the contour of the chest wall. The entire circumference of the hand should touch the chest at the same instant. A proper "cupping" emits a definitely hollow sound. The effect of "cupping" is related partly to the compression of air between the operator's hand and the patient's chest wall. This compression wave is presumably transmitted to the underlying bronchi and aids the gravitational flow of secretions from them.

Vibration is a more difficult procedure and, therefore, is usually effectively executed only by a physical therapist. A rapid vibratory impulse is transmitted through the chest wall from the flattened hands of the operator by an almost isometric contraction of forearm flexor and extensor muscles. Vibration may be used directly over the involved area, or it may be applied to the sides of the chest in performing the chest "squeeze" maneuver. Conventional electrical mechanical vibrators are not thought to be effective.

If the operator is a parent, he can easily be taught the maneuvers of deep breathing, reinforced coughing, and "cupping." More advanced techniques should be reserved for the trained therapist or for the intelligent parent with a child who requires bronchial drainage over months or years.

Breathing Exercises

Breathing exercises have not been widely applied to children, but are undoubtedly important in certain patients, including those with kyphoscoliosis, cystic fibrosis, asthma and bronchiectasis, as well as those who have had extensive resections of diseased lung. Exercises should be a part of a total therapeutic program that frequently also includes correction of posture, bronchial drainage, and various types of inhalation therapy. Breathing exercises are conveniently done during and after bronchial drainage.

Goals of the exercises include (1) development of more effective diaphragmatic and lower costal breathing, (2) relaxation of all muscles, but especially those of the upper part of the chest, shoulder girdle, and neck, and (3) attainment of a good, easy posture.

The precise manner of proceeding with retraining must depend on the age, motivation and strength of the child, as well as his disease, the extent of the physiologic disturbance, and his emotional reactions to the therapist. In addition to being experienced, the therapist should be cheerful, positive and firmly gentle. A parent should be present for the exercises so that they can be continued correctly at home.

Inhalation Therapy

The term "inhalation therapy" is an inclusive one that covers the theory and practice of treating a patient by certain changes in the composition, volume or pressure of inspired gases. Such alterations include increases in the fractional concentration of oxygen (oxygen therapy), replacement of a part of the nitrogen with another inert gas with more desirable properties (oxygen-helium mixture), increases in the water vapor content of inspired gas (humidification), constant increases in the total pressure of administered gases (hyperbaric therapy), removal of undesirable airborne material, such as dust and bacteria (filtration), the addition of airborne particles with beneficial properties (aerosol therapy), and various means of assisting respiration (intermittent positive-pressure breathing, tank respirator). A full discussion of the indications for these different types of inhalation therapy and of their application to children would require a text in itself. Only certain aspects of this field can be discussed here, but the physician caring for children with respiratory disease is urged to become familiar with the goals of inhalation therapy and with a few, specific items of equipment.

Oxygen therapy is usually administered in the hospital; its use at home is not recommended. Oxygen is indicated when significant reductions in its partial pressure in arterial blood are present and when such reductions can be significantly elevated by increasing alveolar oxygen concentrations. Children with anatomic right-to-left shunts, such as those with tetralogy of Fallot, may neither require nor benefit from oxygen. The presence of cyanosis remains the best single clinical criterion for supplemental oxygen. It is a late sign, however, since a considerable drop in the partial pressure of oxygen in arterial blood must occur before cyanosis is detectable. Oxygen alone will not relieve dyspnea, and, depending on the cause of dyspnea, more rational therapy might be a bronchodilator or mucolytic agent administered in the form of an aerosol.

When oxygen is indicated, it may be given by mask, face tent, nasal catheter, intermittent positive-pressure apparatus or conventional oxygen tent. The method of choice depends on the ventilatory status of the child, the percentage of oxygen desired in the inspired air, and the anticipated duration of need. For most conditions an inspired oxygen concentration of 40 to 60 volumes per cent is satisfactory. Simple open-top tents may give effective concentrations of oxygen for an infant, while a nasal catheter or face tent may be well tolerated by an older child.

The adequacy of oxygen therapy can be monitored by determinations of the concentration of oxygen within a tent* or by more elaborate measurements of arterial oxygen saturation or partial pressure within the patient himself.

Oxygen should not be continued after the indication for its use has ceased. To the extent that it reduces the partial pressure of nitrogen in alveoli, oxygen increases the rate of lung collapse in the event of airway obstruction.

Since oxygen is dry, whether it is supplied from cylinders or from a central hospital system, some provision must be made to humidify it. Even if the oxygen-air mixture in a tent is 100 per cent saturated with water, its water content is obligatorily more than doubled on inhalation. This effect, which results from continued 100 per cent water saturation at relatively high body temperature, causes an insensible loss of water from

---

* Beckman oxygen analyzer (Model D2). This instrument measures oxygen concentration between 0 and 100 per cent, can be operated easily by untrained personnel, and gives oxygen concentration values directly and promptly.

Table 3. *Major Site of Deposition of Various Sizes of Aerosols*

Particle Diameter (microns)	Site
> 8	Mouth, oropharynx
3-8	Trachea and main bronchi
1-3	Bronchioles
0.3-1	Alveoli

the body. The extent of this deficit can be reduced by effective prehumidification or even eliminated by inhalation of fully humidified gas at body temperature (see below).

It is also good practice to measure at regular intervals the temperature of the gases within a tent to avoid an uncomfortably hot environment for a sick child.

The purpose of *aerosol therapy* is to treat respiratory disease by the continuous or intermittent deposition within the airway of particles suspended in inspired air or other gases. Such suspensions are called aerosols. In general, aerosol particles used for therapy range in diameter from less than 1 micron to 20 microns or more. They are usually droplets of water which may also contain sodium chloride, stabilizing agents (propylene glycol, glycerin), or certain medications (e.g. antibiotics, steroids, mucolytics, bronchodilators, vasoconstrictors). Aerosol therapy and oxygen therapy are frequently combined.

It is implicit in all forms of aerosol therapy that the nebulized material is distributed in accordance with flow patterns within the lung. Unventilated areas of the lung thus receive none of the aerosol; this is important in the use of aerosols in obstructive lung disease, especially if atelectasis is present. Other important factors affecting deposition of aerosols are their density and the mean diameter of their droplets. Table 3 indicates the relation between particle size and depth of penetration in the tracheobronchial tree.

Aerosols for clinical use are produced by nebulizers which act as repositories for the solution to be nebulized and also generate visible aerosol mists when connected to a source of gas under pressure (oxygen cylinder, hand bulb, or powered oil-free air compressor).* By suitable internal construction, a nebulizer can be made to baffle out large particles and deliver a spectrum of particles over the desired range of diameters.

The kind of equipment chosen for aerosol therapy is largely dependent on whether the physician wants to treat the patient continuously (hours at a time) or intermittently (twenty or thirty minutes). Equipment suitable for continuous treatment is shown in Figure 7. Such a "mist tent" is used either in the hospital or at home when one desires to thin tracheobronchial secretions that are thickened by disease (cystic fibrosis, bronchiectasis, asthma). A common solution for such "wetting down" is 10 per cent propylene glycol in water or isotonic saline; this mixture forms a more stable aerosol than water or saline alone. The stability imparted by propylene glycol is largely due to its hygroscopicity, which inhibits evaporation of particles after they have been generated by the nebulizer. Acetic acid (0.25 per cent) should be nebulized in such equipment for five minutes daily at some time when the patient is out of the tent; this inhibits bacterial growth within the nebulizers.

When it is desired to administer by aerosol small quantities of an agent for a specific pharmacologic action, the equipment is necessarily different from the "mist tent." A small nebulizer with a capacity of less than 10 ml. is required (nebulizer B, Fig. 8), which should nebulize about 2 ml. per ten minutes. Such a nebulizer for use at home can be powered by a small electric compressor or even a bicycle pump. Hand bulbs are not satisfactory except for bronchodilators. Some patients may require both continuous and intermittent aerosol therapy—i.e. during the night they sleep in a tent for general tracheobronchial wetting and during the

---

* A nebulizer operating on a different principle has recently been marketed (DeVilbiss Company, Somerset, Pa.). Particles are produced by ultrasound in large quantities.

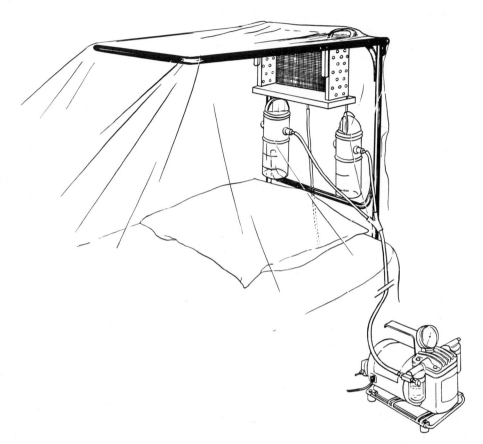

FIGURE 3–7. "Mist tent" for continuous aerosol therapy at home or in the hospital. A light frame of tubular aluminum at the head of the bed supports an ice cannister (with drain) for cooling and 2 nebulizers (Mist-O-Gen MG 11C). Clear, light plastic sheeting covers the frame and tucks snugly under the mattress when the tent is in use. The nebulizers are powered with compressed, filtered air from a portable, continuously running diaphragm-type compressor (Air-Shields Dia-Pump). Two such nebulizers should deliver about 200 ml. of aerosol per 8 hours with a mean particle size of less than 5 microns. They could also be supplied from an intermittently running, stationary, oil-free, tank-type compressor outside the room or from a cylinder of oxygen. The mist should be so dense that it is difficult to see the child inside the tent.

Unfortunately, equipment of the type shown is expensive (about $350), but it is rugged, relatively trouble-free, and delivers a dense mist of the proper distribution of particle sizes.

(This figure is reproduced with permission from the *Bulletin of the Tulane Medical Faculty*, 23: 137, 1964.)

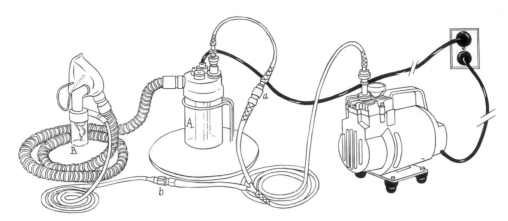

FIGURE 3–8. Equipment for semicontinuous tepid aerosol therapy with provision for addition of special aerosols into the main stream. A single, portable compressor powers both nebulizers (*A* and *B*) by dividing its output through a Y tube. Air flow regulators (*a* and *b*) control the volume of air going to the respective nebulizers. Nebulizer *A* is of large capacity, similar to those shown in Figure 7, and usually contains 10 per cent propylene glycol in water. An immersion heater (electric cord attached) within the nebulizer warms the contained fluid to approximately 140°F. Air passes through regulator *a* and aerosolizes the hot solution. Warm mist thus generated passes through the large-caliber corrugated hose to a light plastic mask over the patient's nose and mouth. The aerosol is cooled in its passage through the tubing, but is inhaled at a temperature above that of the body (100 to 110°F.). Condensation of water occurs in the tubing with cooling; by placement of the mask at a level above nebulizer *A*, fluid thus formed drains back into the nebulizer for reuse.

Nebulizer *B* is of small capacity and is designed to inject unheated agents, such as an antibiotic, into the side of the mask where it mixes and is inhaled with the tepid aerosol.

(The equipment shown is manufactured by the Puritan Compressed Gas Corp., Kansas City, Mo.)

day receive intermittent treatment with an antibiotic or mucolytic agent from a small nebulizer.

Solutions for aerosolization may also be heated so that they are inhaled at temperatures slightly warmer than that of the body (Fig. 8). Such tepid aerosols are fully saturated with water and thus diminish or eliminate the obligatory loss of water from the mucosa of the airway. Tepid aerosols cannot be used in a tent because of their heat, but the attachment of a face tent may allow more prolonged treatments than in the usual intermittent administration of aerosols. Although theoretically more effective than aerosols delivered at ambient temperature, heated aerosols in chronic obstructive lung disease in childhood may be enervating, especially if treatment is prolonged.

The broad application of aerosol therapy is suggested by the situations in which it may be effective (Table 4).

There is a definite relation between aerosol therapy and bronchial drainage.

Table 4. *Various Clinical Situations in Which Aerosol Therapy May Be Indicated*

Asthma
Cystic fibrosis
Laryngotracheobronchitis
Bronchiectasis
Pneumonia, especially with atelectasis
Weakness of muscles of respiration (poliomyelitis, paraplegia, amyotonia, etc.)
Prebronchoscopy and postbronchoscopy
Prebronchography and postbronchography
Prethoracic and post-thoracic surgery
Pretracheostomy and post-tracheostomy

Drainage is much more effective if it follows effective aerosol therapy, of either the continuous or intermittent type.

Pleural Space Drainage and Intracavitary (Monaldi) Drainage

The insertion of a soft catheter between the ribs, for drainage of either the pleural space or of a cavity within the lung, is frequently indicated in certain complications of staphylococcal pneumonia. This procedure may be done in a treatment room, if necessary, but is best performed semielectively in an operating room. Such drainage serves to remove fluid or gas that (1) may restrict pulmonary function, (2) may unduly prolong a septic process, or (3) may cause fibrotic imprisonment of the lung in a partially collapsed state.

Soft rubber catheters are generally used since they are available in a variety of sizes and have the desirable combination of flexibility and relative incompressibility. Several additional holes are cut near the tip so that drainage will not be stopped by occlusion of a single orifice. The catheter is secured to the chest wall and is usually connected to a drainage-suction system that is simultaneously ca pable of removing large volumes of gas, collecting effluvia, and applying a negative pressure of 15 to 18 cm. of water at the catheter holes.

The insertion of such tubes is always indicated in pyopneumothorax, tension pneumothorax and large tension pneumatoceles. Their application to empyema without pneumothorax is less absolute, since some prefer to use intermittent thoracentesis to drain empyemas in childhood. It is true that almost all pleural effusions in the course of acute pneumonias in childhood can be easily drained by one or two needle aspirations, since they are thin and usually sterile. But if the fluid is frankly purulent and is present in more than trace quantities, needle drainage is usually inadequate, and the more effective tube should be inserted.

In empyema without bronchopleural fistula the tube should remain until drainage has ceased and the patient's temperature is essentially normal. In late empyema the tendency of the pus to loculate in various parts of the pleural space may require repositioning of a catheter or insertion of another. In most patients it is possible to discontinue pleural drainage after one week. In pyopneumothorax the tube must remain until the broncho-

pleural fistula has closed; this may require in some cases three weeks or more of suction. Depending on the adequacy of antibiotic therapy, it is usually possible to remove the tube in less than ten days when closure of the fistula is indicated by cessation of bubbling of the underwater portion of the system. Prior to its removal in pyopneumothorax it is wise to clamp the tube for twenty-four hours, at the end of which a chest x-ray will indicate whether the fistula is truly closed or not.

Transtracheal Catheterization and Tracheobronchial Lavage

The development of mucolytic drugs, such as n-acetyl cysteine, has recently led to the exploration of ways in which they can be introduced directly into the tracheobronchial tree. It is presumed that n-acetyl cysteine, for example, is more effective when thus given in large quantities than in the relatively small amounts achievable by aerosol techniques. Two methods of direct delivery of the *fluid* agent will be briefly discussed, although the precise role of each needs clarification.

Transtracheal catheterization is relatively easily performed by threading a small-bore plastic catheter into the lower cervical trachea through a needle, after the pretracheal soft tissues have been anesthetized. The needle is then removed and the catheter fixed by tape or suture, or both. Injection of a minute amount of bronchographic contrast medium allows positioning of the catheter's tip, either above the carina or in either main bronchus. At any time thereafter small quantities (1 to 3 ml.) of diluted mucolytic agent can be injected. Proper positioning of the child at the time of injection ensures delivery of the agent to the desired bronchus (Fig. 2). Such injection is usually followed by a brief, hard paroxysm of coughing which is now more productive than it would be without the agent. Several such injections can be made three or four times daily and can be followed by bronchial drainage and chest "cupping." Since the removal of both the mucolytic agent and the resulting liquefied secretions is largely dependent on the effectiveness of the child's cough, this procedure is contraindicated in children with extreme exhaustion, central nervous system depression, or respiratory muscle weakness due to any cause. It is of definite value in children with atelectasis, especially of an upper lobe, in whom bronchoscopic aspiration may be impossible or unsuccessful.

Tracheobronchial lavage is a more formidable procedure performed in the operating room under general anesthesia. It is reserved for patients with diffuse bronchiectasis whose tenacious mucopurulent secretions cannot be removed by any other means. Large quantities of the mucolytic agent are instilled directly through a conventional anesthesia endotracheal tube. Liquefied secretions are allowed to drain out or are aspirated by catheter through the endotracheal tube. The position of the child is changed regularly so as to wash out all segmental bronchi (Fig. 6). The anesthesiologist assists ventilation throughout the procedure. Results are almost always immediately impressive, but there are differences of opinion on the duration of the cleansing effect. Its widest application thus far has been in children with cystic fibrosis who have not responded to less heroic measures.

Bronchotomy

Occasionally a lobar or segmental bronchus may harbor obstructing material that can be removed only by a direct surgical attack on the involved bronchus at the point of obstruction. Successful bronchotomy demands exact anatomic localization of the pathologic process prior to operation. Such precision is usually possible by combining information from physical examination, chest roentgenography, bronchoscopy and bronchography. It is presumed that the lung distal to the point of obstruction is not permanently damaged,

because, if it were, the treatment of choice would be segmental or lobar resection.

Tracheostomy

Tracheostomy may be a lifesaving procedure, the indications for which may be divided into six categories: (1) mechanical obstruction of the upper airway (croup, foreign body, laryngeal paralysis), (2) disease of the central nervous system (head injury, craniotomy, drug depression), (3) neuromuscular disease (poliomyelitis, tetanus, myasthenia gravis, amyotonia congenita), (4) secretional obstruction (debility with weak cough, painful thoracic or abdominal incision), (5) intrinsic acute or chronic disease with disturbances of gas diffusion or distribution (blunt chest injuries, smoke inhalation, widespread pneumonia), and (6) prophylaxis (radical head and neck surgery).

Tracheostomy may be combined with positive-pressure respiration in children with pulmonary insufficiency (hypercapnia and hypoxia), but in such cases care must be taken not to add excessive dead space by improper selection of equipment.* The management of such patients, especially infants, often calls for serial determinations of arterial P_{CO_2} and pH, as well as P_{O_2} or oxygen saturation, if possible.

The procedure itself is best done on an elective basis, and, even in an emergency, an endotracheal airway (bronchoscope or endotracheal tube) can almost always be inserted prior to the operation. The importance of early tracheostomy has undoubtedly been overemphasized by the expression, "When you begin to wonder whether a tracheostomy is necessary, you should have done it already." Nevertheless the basis of such a statement is the well recognized danger of excessive delay, as opposed to the few risks of an orderly operation. If in doubt, the physician

---

* The Bird Mark 8 respirator, for example, is supplied with a "Q-circle" which has a negligible instrumental dead space. It is thus applicable to very small infants.

should not hesitate to call for emergency consultation. In all cases objective serial observations of the nature of respirations, color, pulse rate and blood pressure should be made and recorded by a trained observer in constant attendance. Increasing pulse and respiratory rates, as recorded every few minutes, are perhaps the best signs of increasing hypoxia. Stridor and retractions may diminish as the child weakens, and, if oxygen is being given, cyanosis may not appear until too late.

The type of tube still most commonly used is the silver cannula with a removable inner liner. If a seal is required between the cannula and the trachea for purposes of positive-pressure ventilation, the conventional silver cannula may be provided with an inflatable rubber cuff. Cuffed tubes of all types are generally considered more hazardous because of greater tracheal irritation. Conventional, flexible endotracheal tubes of the anesthesia type, either cuffed or uncuffed, are not recommended for tracheostomy, because of plugging at the tip and difficulties in proper positioning.

The size of the cannula can be preselected (Table 5), but for all patients the tube must be large enough for effortless gas exchange without excessive pressure inside the trachea. The operator should have cannulas both larger and smaller than the size anticipated. The smaller sizes are available in three lengths and in two angles. Prompt postoperative anteroposterior and lateral roentgenograms are essential; they allow the physician to determine the exact position of the cannula with respect to the trachea and carina,

Table 5. *Dimensions of Tracheostomy Tubes in Relation to Diameter of Tracheal Lumen at Various Ages*

Age	Tracheal Lumen Diameter Sagittal* (mm.)	Number	Outside Diameter (mm.)	Length (inches) Jackson (Regular)	Jackson (Short)	Luer†	Penn Pediatric‡
0- 1 months .	3.6	00	3	1¾	1½	1⅜	1¼
1- 3	4.6	0	4	2	1¾	1⅝	1¼
3- 6	5.0	0	4	2	1¾	1⅝	1¼
6-12	5.6	0	4	2	1¾	1⅝	1¼
1- 2 years ...	6.5	1	5	2¼	2⅛	1¾	1¼
2- 3	7.0	1	5	2¼	2⅛	1¾	1¼
3- 4	8.3	2	6	2½	2¼	2	1¼
4- 6	8.0	2	6	2½	2¼	2	1¼
6- 8	9.2	3	7	2¾	2⅜	2¹⁄₁₆	
8-10	9.0	3	7	2¾	2⅜	2¹⁄₁₆	
10-12	9.8	4	8	3	2½	2⅛	
12-14	10.3	4	8	3	2½	2⅛	
14-16	12.7	5	9	3⅜	2⅝	2¼	
Adult	13-23	5	9	3⅜	2⅝	2¼	
		6	10	3⅝	2⅞	2⅜	
		7	11	4	3	2½	
		8	12	4¼	3⅛	2⅝	
		9	13	4⅜	3¼	2¾	
		10	14	4⅜	3⅜	2⅞	

This table lists suggested tube sizes for children of different ages, as well as for adults. The tube must be individually fitted, however, at the time of operation. Postoperative RGs may call for one of the shorter tubes or one with greater curvature.

* Sagittal diameter is less than frontal. Data from R. E. Scammon, in I. A. Abt (Ed.): *Pediatrics*, Vol. I, p. 257.

† Luer tubes are similar to the Jackson tubes, but are more steeply curved.

‡ Penn pediatric tubes have a steep curve similar to the Luer, but are shorter.

then to make any necessary adjustments or revisions. They also reveal the presence and extent of pneumothorax and pneumomediastinum.

The postoperative care of a child with a tracheostomy is crucial. He requires psychologic and physical support, best supplied by a nurse experienced in tracheostomy care in constant attendance. Vital signs must be regularly monitored. The trachea should be suctioned gently by special sterile catheters. The attendant must be aware of the need to suction the oropharynx occasionally, since vomitus and secretions accumulating there may be aspirated into the lungs between a loose-fitting cannula and the inner wall of the trachea. The inner tube is cleaned and replaced as often as needed, and the outer cannula should be replaced every two days.

A spare cannula and obturator of the proper size should be kept at the bedside in the event that the tube becomes dislodged and requires replacement. A dislodged cannula during the first two days may be extremely difficult to replace. A good light, soft tissue "spreaders" and skill are quickly required in such a circumstance. After two days a tract is usually sufficiently established to allow easy reinsertion.

Provision should be made for humidifying inspired gas, since the wetting, warming and filtering functions of the upper airway are now inoperative. Although plastic "collars" which allow aerosols to be delivered directly to a tracheostomy are available, they are generally not applicable to infants or young children. A "mist tent" (Fig. 7) is probably the best compromise. Instillation of saline, sodium bicarbonate or other solutions into the trachea does not alone prevent drying and crusting within the airway.

The tracheostomy tube should be removed as soon as it is no longer needed. In general, the longer a tube remains in the trachea, the more difficult will be the process of decannulation. Processes of short duration (foreign body, croup) usually permit prompt removal of the tube, whereas others of chronic nature (poliomyelitis) may take much longer.

Although opinions differ on the best way to remove a tube, the more common practice is to reduce the size of the cannula daily. When a small tube (perhaps two or more sizes smaller than the original) is reached without difficulty, it is then plugged. If the child has no difficulty after twenty-four hours, the plugged tube may be removed. Subsequent air leaks through the wound nearly always cease within seventy-two hours. In small infants the mother may partially occlude the tracheostomy tube with her finger while rocking and cuddling the baby. The infant may be thus slowly adapted to decannulation.

The complications of tracheostomy can be divided into immediate (operative) and late (postoperative) categories. Operative complications, usually in children less than five years old, include wound bleeding, pneumothorax, pneumomediastinum, tracheo-esophageal fistula, subcutaneous emphysema, cardiac or respiratory arrest, and apnea immediately after provision of a good airway. Late complications include infection, atelectasis, cannula occlusion, tracheal bleeding, expulsion of the cannula, tracheal ulceration and granulation, tracheal stenosis, aerophagia, and delayed healing of the stoma.

Resection of Lung Tissue

Advances in diagnostic and surgical methods have made it possible to remove diseased segments or lobes, as well as an entire lung. Such operations are indicated when it has been established (1) that the process is creating significant present or potential morbidity, (2) that it is not treatable by other means, (3) that it is sufficiently localized that its resection will leave adequate pulmonary reserve, and (4) that the resection is technically feasible and does not constitute a risk out of proportion to the disease itself.

Surgery should be preceded by adequate bronchograms and, if possible, pulmonary function testing in order to establish the anatomic and physiologic extent of the disease.

The most common indication for resection is bronchiectasis, with or without atelectasis, though asymptomatic bronchiectasis, especially of an upper lobe, and so-called cylindrical bronchiectasis almost never require resection. Other indications include anomalies, tuberculosis and neoplasms.

Postoperative complications are common in small children, especially atelectasis and pneumonia. Unless these complications can be avoided or promptly handled by enlightened management, the procedure may be responsible for more harm than good. Scrupulous attention should be given to maintaining good tracheobronchial toilet. This usually requires continuous or intermittent aerosol therapy and physical therapy (e.g. bronchial drainage, breathing exercises, controlled cough, thoracic "cupping") and may necessitate bronchoscopy, tracheostomy, assisted respiration or transtracheal catheterization.

REFERENCES

Radiologic Examination of the Lungs

Felson, B.: *Fundamentals of Chest Roentgenography*. Philadelphia, W. B. Saunders Company, 1960.

Ferguson, C. F., and Flake, C. G.: Bronchography in the Diagnosis of Pediatric Problems. *J.A.M.A.*, 164:518-21, 1957.

Nice, C. M., Jr., Waring, W. W., Killelea, D. E., and Hurwitz, L.: Bronchography in Infants and Children; Barium Sulfate as a Contrast Agent. *Am. J. Roentgenol.*, 91:564-70, 1964.

Waring, W. W., and Killelea, D. E.: Bronchography in Infants and Children. I. A Nonfluoroscopic Technique. *Pediatrics*, 30:378-88, 1962.

Bronchoscopy

Atkins, J. P.: Bronchoscopic Problems of Infancy and Childhood. *Arch. Otolaryng.*, 79:152-4, 1964.

Lung Puncture

Gellis, S. S., Reinhold, J. L. D., and Green, S.: Use of Aspiration Lung Puncture in Diagnosis of Idiopathic Pulmonary Hemosiderosis. *Am. J. Dis. Child.*, 85:303-307, 1953.

Pulmonary Function Tests

Bernstein, I. L., and others: Pulmonary Function in Children. I. Determination of Norms. *J. Allergy*, 30:514-33, 1959.

Ferris, B. G., Jr., and Smith, C. W.: Maximum Breathing Capacity and Vital Capacity in Female Children and Adolescents. *Pediatrics*, 12:341-52, 1953.

Ferris, B. G., Jr., Whittenberger, J. L., and Gallagher, J. R.: Maximum Breathing Capacity and Vital Capacity of Male Children and Adolescents. *Pediatrics*, 9:659-70, 1952.

Heaf, P. J. D., and Gillam, P. M. S.: Peak Flow Rates in Normal and Asthmatic Children. *Brit. M.J.*, 1:1595-6, 1962.

Heese, J. de V.: Quantitative Investigations of the Forced Vital Spirogram in Healthy Children. I. Normal Values. *Brit. J. Dis. Chest*, 55:131-42, 1961.

Murray, A. B., and Cook, C. D.: Measurement of Peak Expiratory Flow Rates in 220 Normal Children from 4.5 to 18.5 Years of Age. *J. Pediat.*, 62:186-9, 1963.

Nairn, J. R., Bennet, A. J., Andrew, J. D., and Macarthur, P.: A Study of Respiratory Function in Normal School Children. The Peak Flow Rate. *Arch. Dis. Childhood*, 36:253-8, 1961.

Wright, B. M., and McKerrow, C. B.: Maximum Forced Expiratory Flow Rate as a Measure of Ventilatory Capacity, with a Description of a New Portable Instrument for Measuring It. *Brit. M. J.* 2:1041-7, 1959.

Bronchial Drainage and Physical Therapy

Doyle, B.: Physical Therapy in the Treatment of Cystic Fibrosis. *Phys. Ther. Rev.*, 39:24-7, 1959.

Fountain, F. P., and Goddard R. F.: Breathing Exercises for Children with Chronic Respiratory Diseases. *Lovelace Clinic Review*, 1:159-64, 1963.

Miller, W. F.: Physical Therapeutic Measures in the Treatment of Chronic Bronchopulmonary Disorders. Methods for Breathing Training. *Am. J. Med.*, 24:929-40, 1958.

Rattenborg, C. C., and Holaday, D. A.: Lung Physiotherapy as an Adjunct to Surgical Care. *Surg. Clin. N. Amer.*, 44:219-26, 1964.

Reed, J. M. W.: Breathing Exercises and Postural Drainage; in *The "Chesty" Child*. London, The Chest and Heart Association, 1960, pp. 83-92.

Thacker, E. W.: *Postural Drainage and Respiratory Control*. London, Lloyd-Luke (Medical Books), Ltd., 1959.

Oxygen Therapy

Batson, R., and Young, W. C.: The Administration of Oxygen to Infants and Small Children. An Evaluation of Methods. *Pediatrics*, 22:436-48, 1958.

Campbell, E. J. M.: Oxygen Administration. *Anaesthesia*, 18:503-506, 1963.

Comroe, J. H., Jr., and Dripps, R. D.: *The Physiological Basis for Oxygen Therapy.* Springfield, Ill., Charles C Thomas, 1950.

Kory, R. G., Bergmann, J. C., Sweet, R. D., and Smith, J. R.: Comparative Evaluation of Oxygen Therapy Techniques. *J.A.M.A.*, 179:767-72, 1962.

Tizard, J. P. M.: Indications for Oxygen Therapy in the Newborn. *Pediatrics*, 34:771-86, 1964.

Wells, R. E., Perera, R. D., and Kinney, J. M.: Humidification of Oxygen During Inhalational Therapy. *New England J. Med.*, 268:644-7, 1963.

Aerosol Therapy

Denton, R.: The Clinical Use of Continuous Nebulization in Bronchopulmonary Disease. *Dis. Chest*, 28:123-40, 1955.

Halpern, S. R., and Sellars, W. A.: Practical Tips in Aerosol Therapy in Asthma. *Am. J. Dis. Child.*, 107:280-81, 1964.

Olsen, A. M.: Aerosol Therapy in Bronchopulmonary Disease. A Critical Evaluation. *Calif. Med.*, 96:237-44, 1962.

Reas, H. W.: The Use of N-Acetylcysteine in the Treatment of Cystic Fibrosis. *J. Pediat.*, 65:542-57, 1964.

Stamm, S. J., and Docter, J.: Clinical Evaluation of Acetylcysteine as a Mucolytic Agent in Cystic Fibrosis. *Dis. Chest*, 47:414-20, 1965.

Pleural Space Drainage and Intracavitary (Monaldi) Drainage

Greenwood, M. E.: *An Illustrated Approach to Medical Physics.* Philadelphia, F. A. Davis Company, 1963, pp. 99-102.

Rakower, J., and Wayl, P.: Monaldi Drainage in the Management of Postinfectious Pulmonary Cysts. *J. Pediat.*, 52:573-6, 1958.

Webb, W. R.: Chairman: Management of Non-tuberculous Empyema. A Statement of the Subcommittee on Surgery, American Thoracic Society. *Am. Rev. Resp. Dis.*, 85:935-6, 1962.

Tracheostomy

Crawford, O. B.: The Anesthesiologist's Responsibilities in Tracheostomy. *Anesthesiology*, 22:86-92, 1961.

Dugan, D. J., and Samson, P. C.: Tracheostomy: Present Day Indications and Technics. *Am. J. Surg.*, 106:290-306, 1963.

Fennell, G.: Management of Tracheotomy in Infants. *Lancet*, 2:808-809, 1962.

Glas, W. W., King, O. J., Jr., and Lui, A.: Complications of Tracheostomy. *Arch. Surg.*, 85:57-63, 1962.

Head, J. M.: Tracheostomy in the Management of Respiratory Problems. *New England J. Med.*, 264:587-91, 1961.

Oliver, P., Richardson, J. R., Clubb, R. W., and Flake, C. G.: Tracheotomy in Children. *New England J. Med.*, 267:631-7, 1962.

Smith, M. H. D.: Tracheotomy Care; in H. C. Shirkey (Ed.): *Pediatric Therapy.* St. Louis, C. V. Mosby Company, 1964, Chap. 69, pp. 543-5.

Resection

Filler, J.: Effects upon Pulmonary Function of Lobectomy Performed During Childhood. *Am. Rev. Resp. Dis.*, 89:801-10, 1964.

Massion, W. H., and Schilling, J. A.: Physiological Effects of Lung Resection in Adult and Puppy Dogs. *J. Thorac. Cardiovasc. Surg.*, 48:239-50, 1964.

Nanson, E. M.: Pulmonary Resection in Infancy and Childhood. *Canad. M.A.J.*, 87:275-81, 1962.

Quinlan, J. J., Schaffner, V. D., and Hiltz, J. E.: Lung Resection for Tuberculosis in Children. *Canad. M.A.J.*, 87:1362-6, 1962.

CHAPTER FOUR

Age as a Factor in Respiratory Tract Disease

ROBERT H. HIGH, M.D.

The age at which respiratory tract disease is acquired may have significant influences on the symptoms, physical and roentgenographic findings, morbidity, mortality and other manifestations of the disease. The relation of age to these variants can sometimes be explained logically and probably correctly, but in other instances the influence of age on respiratory tract disease is incompletely known. At times no explanation can be offered to support the well recognized observations that some respiratory tract diseases have different patterns in different age groups. The tissues of the respiratory tract have a limited number of responses to disease, and the variation in these responses is often modified in different age groups by some of the factors considered below.

Respiratory tract abnormalities acquired during intrauterine life are usually, though not always, manifest shortly after birth. For example, anomalies such as congenital lobar emphysema or congenital cystic adenomatoid malformation of the lung may not produce symptoms until several months have passed. Some anomalies, such as accessory lobes or fissures of the lungs, may never produce symptoms and are noted as unexpected findings by roentgenographic or autopsy examination.

Infections acquired before or during delivery are likewise usually manifest in the first few days of life. Such is the usual case with pneumonia alba of congenital syphilis or bronchopneumonia secondary to aspiration of infected amniotic fluid. On the other hand, congenital tuberculosis may not produce symptoms until a few weeks after birth.

For a more detailed discussion of the manifestations of respiratory disease in the neonatal period, see the section on Respiratory Disorders in the Newborn.

Attention will not be directed to certain general factors which can affect the manifestations of respiratory tract disease in any age group. Included in these factors is the possible influence of nutrition, host resistance, climate, intensity of the exposure to infectious agents, resistance of the infecting agent to certain drugs, and so forth, because variations in such factors are often equally operative at any age.

Some of the variations in the patterns of respiratory diseases of an infectious origin reflect the immunologic responses of the human organism. At birth the human infant has acquired by transplacental transfer many of the 7S gamma-2 antibodies which were present in his mother's serum. These antibodies help protect him against certain bacterial infections such as diphtheria and pertussis, and certain viral infections such as measles and mumps. Since the 19S gamma-1 antibodies, which are chiefly protective against the enteric organisms such as *E. coli*, do not pass the placental barrier, the infant is susceptible to bacterial infections caused by such organisms. These observations help explain the prevalence of severe infections caused by the gram-negative bacilli in the newborn and the very young infant.

After birth there is a gradual metabolism of the passively acquired antibodies, which are largely destroyed by the time the infant is six to twelve weeks of age. The infant begins to develop antibodies shortly after birth, depending upon the antigenic stimuli to which he is exposed. These two simultaneously occurring immunologic reactions lead to relatively low antibody levels during the first few months of life and seem to be correlated with the occurrence of severe bacterial infections, particularly those caused by enteric organisms, in this age group.

In the first few months of life the infant does not respond as well as he subsequently will to antigenic stimuli, such as the injection of certain vaccines, e.g. D.P.T., but he can nevertheless achieve sufficient response to protect himself against these infections. These observations have led to the recommendation of initiating programs of active immunization in the first or second month of life. The infant's response to naturally and artificially acquired antigenic stimuli gradually increases as he becomes older. The relatively low level of antibodies present during the period of physiologic hypogammaglobulinemia gradually rises during the first year of life, but does not reach its ultimate peak until some years later. The occurrence of severe bacterial infections during the first year or so of life must be related, at least in part, to the relatively low antibody levels present in infancy. The eventual antibody levels are a function of repeated stimulations by ingestion or injection of antigens and by the acquisition of naturally occurring infections and sometimes by reinfection with the same agent. The responses to "boosters" are well known for their continuing protective effects. The long-term resistance to reinfection by some naturally acquired infections, such as measles, is a reflection of a prolonged immune response which may be stimulated by reinfections which can be determined only by serologic studies.

Some infections of the respiratory tract are followed by temporary immunity, so that reinfection can occur after some months. Viral influenza is an example of such an infection. Reinfections following the initial disease are often milder, so that the older child is likely to have less severe disease under such circumstances.

Certain congenital defects in immune responses are often associated with severe bacterial infections in the respiratory tract as well as in other systems. In conditions such as congenital hypogammaglobulinemia and the dysglobulinemias, the Wiskott-Aldrich syndrome, and congenital absence of the thymus or spleen, severe and often recurring bacterial infections in early life are common. These infections seem to be related to the immune defects.

Severe bacterial infections, often of the respiratory tract, are also common in persons with acquired defects in their immune responses. Examples include the occurrence of fatal chickenpox pneumonia or staphylococcal pneumonia in children receiving steroid or cytotoxic drugs, the development of pneumonia, sepsis or meningitis following splenectomy or thymectomy, the acquisition of serious infections in children with the nephrotic syndrome, and the like. Most infections, such as the above-mentioned ones, occur after infancy and are related to the primary disease rather than to age itself.

Some of the variations in the patterns of respiratory tract diseases are related to changes in the anatomic structures which occur with growth and development. Thus middle ear infections and their complications are more common in infancy and early life because the eustachian tube is relatively short, straighter and more patulous during this period. With increasing age this structure becomes longer, relatively more narrow and somewhat more tortuous, thereby increasing the anatomic barriers to the spread of infection from the nasal passages to the middle ear. Similarly, spread of infection from the ethmoid sinuses to the orbital fossa is more common in the younger child. The bony partition, the lamina papyracea, which separates the orbit from the nose is very thin in infants. Thus the thinness of this bony barrier more readily permits extension of infection in the infant than in the older child.

Certain respiratory tract diseases show

variations by age which are related to the internal diameters of the airways. The surface area of a circle, such as a horizontal cross section of the larynx, trachea or bronchi, is calculated by the formula πr^2. As growth progresses the internal diameter of the airway increases, but the surface area increases more rapidly. This anatomic change is one explanation why narrowing of the airway by edema, exudate, and the like, results in a relatively greater encroachment on breathing in the younger patients. This anatomic finding explains why laryngeal edema and infections are commonly more severe in infants than in older children. This same explanation can be applied to the development of bronchiolitis, in which edema and interstitial reaction in the peripheral bronchioles produces a "ball-valve" obstruction or sometimes a complete obstruction to the flow of air. As the internal diameter of the lumen becomes larger with increased growth, such obstructive phenomena become less likely. This factor also helps to explain some of the findings of congenital laryngeal stridor, in which external compression or internal narrowing, secondary to partial collapse, webs, cysts, and so forth, reduces the cross-sectional area of the airway. Increased growth is often followed by the relief of such manifestations.

The localization of pneumonia following aspiration varies somewhat in different age groups because of the anatomic relations within the tracheobronchial structures. In the infant or in an older debilitated child kept in the supine position, aspiration pneumonia most commonly affects the right upper lobe. Anatomic factors of importance are related to the fact that the right main bronchus is more directly in line with the axis of the trachea and is therefore more commonly involved when discrete material is aspirated. Further, the orifice of the right upper lobe is in a dependent position when the patient is in the supine position. An example of such circumstances is the localization of pneumonia in infants with amyotonia congenita. Older,

healthy children who aspirate a foreign body while in the erect position are more likely to have the object lodge in the lower lobe, especially on the right side.

The age at which certain infections are acquired is largely the result of the chance exposure of a susceptible person to the infectious agent. The newborn infant may be immune to some infections such as measles because of transplacentally acquired antibodies. Nevertheless the relative freedom from infection in the newborn infant is largely the result of the isolation technique practiced in the hospital nursery. The occurrence of epidemics of bacterial or viral infections in nurseries, sometimes with attack rates of almost 100 per cent, is ample evidence that the newborn infant is susceptible to many infections, including those of the respiratory tract.

The relatively low frequency of respiratory tract infections in early infancy is also a reflection of our protective practices of infant care. As the infant grows and his personal contacts increase, the chances of exposure increase and more infections are noted. This pattern is particularly prevalent during the preschool years, often culminating in a series of frequent infections, usually including the common contagious diseases, when the child enters school. High has called this pattern "the first grade syndrome," in which the oldest child in the family or an only child has many respiratory infections during this time. The parents and sometimes physicians interpret these infections as exacerbations or a continuation of the initial infection, when in reality the child has contracted, in most cases, a series of new, unrelated, usually viral, infections. Under these circumstances the first-grade child is usually the source for repeated family outbreaks of infections in which most members of his household are involved. The occurrence of secondary infections is usually greatest in the siblings, less in the mother and least in the father.

The presence of the infectious agent in the community also influences the age at which certain respiratory tract illnesses occur. In certain isolated villages outbreaks of some infections occur at widely separated intervals. Under these circumstances it is possible that most of the population, including adults, may be infected with diseases commonly regarded as diseases of childhood in more populous areas. During the 1964 epidemic of German measles, observations of this sort were made in isolated areas of Alaska and elsewhere.

The increasing mobility of our population has tended to reduce the likelihood of the circumstances cited above. The significantly lower rates of measles and mumps occurring in United States military personnel in World War II, in contrast to the experience during World War I, are regarded as being largely a reflection of increased exposure during childhood because of the greater mobility of the population.

The appearance of a new strain of an infecting agent introduces a set of circumstances similar to those in isolated areas, but applicable on a worldwide basis. Everyone is susceptible. The appearance of the Asian strain of influenza virus in 1957 triggered a worldwide pandemic. Under these circumstances persons of all ages are susceptible, and most contract the new infection. Mortality tends to be excessive in infancy and in the elderly.

Of interest, but with inadequate explanation for the observations, are the differences in certain infections in various age groups. Pneumococcal infections, for example, commonly cause bronchopneumonia in any age group, but are especially common in infancy. Pneumococcal pneumonia in children is often of a lobar type, and yet this form is unusual during infancy. The mortality rate of untreated pneumococcal pneumonia in infancy is approximately 30 per cent, whereas in children it is about 8 per cent. The causes for these differences are not completely understood.

Respiratory tract infections caused by the group A beta hemolytic streptococci have different clinical patterns in infancy and in childhood. In the former age group these infections are often manifest as chronic rhinitis with relatively few systemic signs of infection. In the older child such infections are more often acute and often localized in the tonsillar and pharyngeal areas.

Pulmonary tuberculosis (see p. 677) in children shows striking differences in its clinical patterns and mortality, depending upon the age at which it is acquired. When pulmonary tuberculosis develops in an infant, the pulmonary lesions are often extensive, complications such as miliary tuberculosis and tuberculous meningitis are common, and, if the disease is untreated, mortality rates are high. When the disease is first acquired in middle childhood, the pulmonary involvement is less, the frequency of hematogenous complications is less, and the tendency for spontaneous recovery is much greater. On the other hand, pulmonary tuberculosis first acquired in adolescence often mimics the clinical patterns seen in adults, commonly showing progressive destructive and cavitary reactions unusual in younger children.

Additional examples will be cited elsewhere of the variations in the manifestations of infections and other respiratory disturbances according to the age of the individual.

Certain tissue responses to respiratory tract disease are different in different age groups. In tuberculosis or histoplasmosis, for example, pulmonary infections are often associated with hilar adenopathy when the infection is acquired in later infancy or childhood. The same infections first acquired in adolescence or early adult life usually show less and often no demonstrable hilar adenopathy. The greater lymph node reaction in the younger child also is reflected in the greater frequency of atelectasis secondary to external bronchial compression. The right middle lobe most commonly becomes atelectatic under these circumstances, although any lobe can be affected by this mechanism.

The healing responses are also different in the hilar lymph nodes and pulmonary parenchyma, depending upon the age at which tuberculosis is acquired. Those infected in infancy and early childhood are ultimately much more likely to show calcification when healing occurs. On the other hand, tuberculosis acquired in later childhood or adolescence is likely to show less calcification, but more evidence of fibrosis when the disease becomes inactive. Histoplasmosis shows somewhat similar changes.

Age differences in morbidity and mortality of respiratory tract diseases will be discussed in some of the following chapters. In general, most of the infectious diseases of the respiratory tract are more severe in younger persons.

The age at which respiratory tract disease is acquired often has significant influence on its clinical manifestations, severity, and the like. The explanations for some of these variations have been presented above. Regardless of the cause, age is a factor in the variation in the pattern of respiratory tract diseases in different persons.

SECTION III

Respiratory
Disorders in the Newborn

CHAPTER FIVE

Respiratory Disorders in the Newborn

MILDRED T. STAHLMAN, M.D.

The importance of abnormalities in respiration in the newborn cannot be overemphasized. Abnormalities of pulmonary ventilation, whether from intrinsic or extrinsic causes, are associated with most of the morbidity and mortality of newborn babies. During the past two decades a great deal of clinical interest and investigative effort has gone into studies of pulmonary function in both normal and abnormal circumstances, and vigorous attempts are being made to recognize, understand and, if possible, correct abnormalities with rational therapy. This chapter, though not attempting to be all-inclusive, will deal with a number of these conditions in the hope that pediatricians dealing with newborns will be encouraged to assume a more vigorous approach toward the investigation and therapy of respiratory problems in small infants.

An understanding of intrauterine and intrapartum events is vital in the diagnosis of neonatal respiratory distress, and good communication between obstetrician and pediatrician is clearly in the baby's best interest.

EVALUATION OF THE INFANT WITH RESPIRATORY DIFFICULTY

A history of maternal polyhydramnios suggests the possibility of upper gastrointestinal obstruction such as esophageal atresia associated with a tracheo-esophageal fistula. A premature baby of a mother who has had previous premature babies with respiratory distress suggests hyaline membrane disease, as does a maternal history of diabetes or a nonelective cesarean section. The latter especially seems to be true if maternal bleeding has been the indication for section. A history of fetal bradycardia or tachycardia suggests intrauterine distress. This may be associated with the passage of meconium, respiratory depression at birth and subsequent respiratory problems associated with meconium aspiration pneumonia. This becomes even more likely if the pregnancy is abnormally prolonged. The amount and timing of maternal analgesia, sedation and anesthesia are important considerations in the differential diagnosis of respiratory depression, asphyxia and brain hemorrhage. Prolonged and difficult labor, especially if umbilical cord compression is suspected, is often associated with asphyxia, with both metabolic and respiratory acidosis, shock and occasionally pulmonary edema. A history of being the smaller of premature twins might suggest hypoglycemia, while the possibility of baby-to-baby transfusion with either hypervolemia or hypovolemia should be kept in mind. A maternal setup for Rh, ABO or other rare blood factor incompatibility should alert the physician to the possibility of cardiac failure associated with severe anemia as a cause of respiratory distress. A difficult

119

manipulative delivery suggests brain hemorrhage, and so might a maternal bleeding diathesis such as idiopathic thrombocytopenic purpura. Maternal ingestion of iodides can produce thyroid enlargement in the newborn sufficient to embarrass respiration, and reserpine given to the mother can cause enough edema of the nasal mucosa of the newborn to produce severe difficulties in breathing. A history of premature rupture of the membranes, especially if associated with signs of infection in the mother or foul-smelling amniotic fluid, arouses suspicion of intrauterine bacterial sepsis with pneumonia. A history of respiratory depression at birth necessitating positive-pressure resuscitation alerts one to the possibility of pneumothorax or pneumomediastinum as a cause of subsequent respiratory embarrassment.

A complete physical examination is often delayed or only sketchily done in distressed babies, especially in small prematures. Most such babies will be housed in incubators which present a noisy environment and a barrier to careful evaluation of physical signs. Nevertheless inspection usually provides the most valuable information. Such findings as meconium staining or peeling skin on a thin baby bring to mind the likelihood of meconium aspiration pneumonia, or a flat abdomen that of diaphragmatic hernia. Inspection of the respiratory pattern may suggest the difference between central nervous system disease, mechanical obstruction to the airway, intrinsic pulmonary pathology and congenital cardiac disease.

The presence or absence of visible cyanosis can be a deceptive physical sign in the newborn. Many normal newborn babies have venous stasis with cyanosis of the hands and feet for several hours after birth. Because most normal babies are polycythemic by adult standards and appear plethoric, the same number of grams of unsaturated hemoglobin which produce visible cyanosis indicating serious disease in an adult may be associated with mild disorders or even with normal transitional circulation of the newborn. In contrast, a cold baby may appear to have his hemoglobin fully saturated with oxygen in the presence of a lowered arterial oxygen tension by virtue of the shift to the left of the oxygen dissociation curve for hemoglobin which is associated with hypothermia. The normal newborn has a small functioning right-to-left shunt through the foramen ovale for several days, and anatomic closure does not occur for several weeks. Therefore hard crying, breath-holding, or straining with defecation or urination associated with a Valsalva maneuver may increase the functional shunting manyfold and produce transient, visible cyanosis. On the other hand, a newborn who has bled excessively or who is anemic from hemolytic disease may be in serious respiratory distress and even have a high percentage of his arterial blood unsaturated without showing visible cyanosis, because of profound anemia. One of the most characteristic features of severe metabolic acidosis, which may accompany hyaline membrane disease and many other severe respiratory or circulatory disturbances, is the extreme peripheral vasoconstriction which accompanies a very low blood pH and may mask the degree of hemoglobin unsaturation. Such babies are ashen gray rather than blue, and if unheeded, this becomes a poor prognostic sign.

As a part of a routine physical examination of a baby in respiratory difficulties, it is advisable to pass a large-bore catheter into the stomach, introducing air while auscultating over the left upper quadrant in order to identify an intact upper gastrointestinal tract. The stomach is then emptied as completely as possible by suction. Such material as meconium or maternal blood can be identified, and, in the case of suspected amnionitis, the contents may be cultured and examined directly for the presence of polymorphonuclear leukocytes and bacteria.

Physical examination of the chest in a newborn can be deceptive as to the degree and type of pathology inside. Crepitation of air over the upper part of the sternum or in the neck or signs of venous distention in the head and neck are good indications of mediastinal emphysema, but they are frequently absent even though "air block" exists. Inequality of breath sounds, loud on one side, diminished or absent on the other, and interpreted as a sign of pneumothorax, often points to the wrong side of involvement. Rhonchi are frequently heard in newborns with many types of respiratory embarrassment; however, after the oropharynx has been suctioned free of secretions and debris, fine rales are relatively rare, even in the face of widespread parenchymal involvement. When fine rales do occur, they are of significance and are usually associated with bacterial pneumonia. Moist rales are usually heard with pulmonary hemorrhage or frank pulmonary edema, but occur late as a sign of cardiac failure in a newborn. "Poor air entry" is a description of the early auscultatory findings in hyaline membrane disease and is replaced by scratchy, sandpaper to-and-fro sounds late in the disease, as the prognosis becomes poorer. Inspiratory stridor points to partial obstruction in the upper airway, from the oropharynx through the trachea, whereas wheezing respiratory sounds are usually associated with bronchial or bronchiolar obstructive disease, which may be localized or widespread. Expiratory grunt is frequently associated with hyaline membrane disease, but may also occur with meconium aspiration pneumonia, bacterial pneumonia and other causes of severe respiratory distress. It is probably reflex in origin and can frequently be abolished with high oxygen inhalation.

Cardiac murmurs may be difficult to assess in the newborn in respiratory distress. Many murmurs, later clearly audible and associated with congenital cardiac defects, may be inapparent in the newborn because of altered relations in pressure, flow and resistance associated with the transitional circulation. Although the ductus arteriosus is open and may be shunting large amounts of blood for a period of hours, even in the normal newborn or premature, and for many days in distressed infants, until partial constriction

occurs murmurs are rarely heard. Their appearance is usually also associated with a rising systemic and falling pulmonary arterial pressure; they are systolic in time. Only occasionally are typical continuous diamond-shaped murmurs heard with the neonatal closing ductus, and when they occur, they usually persist.

Persistent tachycardia over 160 per minute or bradycardia less than 100 per minute may be present with hypoxia from any cause, and both are frequently relieved by adequate oxygenation. In contrast to the adult, tachycardia may be absent as a physical sign and a clue to severe hemorrhage in the newborn. Bradycardia may also signal hyperkalemia.

An easily palpable liver in respiratory distress may mean many things, ranging from frank cardiac failure to extramedullary hematopoiesis associated with hemolytic disease, liver involvement with cytomegalic inclusion disease, bacterial sepsis or parasites, or emphysema associated with a flattened diaphragm.

Edema may be equally difficult to evaluate. The ability to pit edema requires that the subcutaneous fluid collection be shifted under extrinsic pressure. In the case of the newborn whose skin and subcutaneous tissues are stretched tightly for the first time, pitting may be difficult to demonstrate. Nevertheless a surprisingly large percentage of a baby's body weight may be inapparent edema fluid, most readily diagnosed by observing the shiny, smooth aspect of the skin, especially that of the palms and soles, and the flabby fold of swollen skin along the posterior axillary line, visible when a baby is lying supine. In contrast to this type of generalized edema most frequently seen in premature infants, and most severe in those with hyaline membrane disease, is the anasarca of the hydropic baby, who is more obviously edematous and frequently also shows frank ascites associated with his severe anemia. This also is in striking contrast to the postmature baby who is a good candidate for meconium aspiration pneumonia and shows dry, cracking and peeling integument, but frequently has definite pitting edema of the dorsa of the hands and feet.

Every baby with a respiratory distress which persists or is of any severity deserves a roentgenologic examination. Anteroposterior and lateral portable films can be made with good radiologic technique in an incubator with minimal disturbance to the infant, if the x-ray technicians and nurses are properly oriented as to the positioning and x-ray settings required. Although several clinical entities can produce the same shadows in the lung fields, many others are specific, such as pneumothorax, diaphragmatic hernia and bullous emphysema. Other radiographic pictures, not so specific, must be classified as "compatible with . . ." by the radiologist, and the most likely diagnosis ascribed by the clinician, who has the advantage of a history and physical examination. In the case of specific difficult diagnoses, such as an "H" type of tracheo-esophageal fistula or occult diaphragmatic hernia behind the heart, special roentgenographic techniques using contrast media may aid in the correct diagnosis.

The electrocardiogram is a useful tool in the monitoring and management of many newborns with respiratory difficulties, but only rarely is it of diagnostic aid. Some types of congenital cardiac defects such as endocardial fibroelastosis or tricuspid atresia may have a highly suggestive electrocardiogram, with abnormal left heart preponderance for a newborn. In the case of conduction defects and arrythmias the electrocardiogram is pathognomonic. It is rarely a helpful prognosticator in hyaline membrane disease, except as a valuable index of serum hyperkalemia. The prolonged atrioventricular conduction associated with hyperkalemia in these infants demands prompt and specific treatment.

Arterial blood gas and pH measurements are of tremendous help in differentiating different types of physiologic impairment associated with respiratory distress of varied causes, and repeated measurements are useful both in prog-

nosticating the outcome and in directing therapy.

Many more elaborate tests of pulmonary function have been devised for the newborn, usually as an adaptation from techniques applicable to adults. In research laboratories under trained supervision these can actually pinpoint and quantitate the specific types of physiologic and biochemical abnormalities present in distressed babies. Many of these techniques have recently been summarized. Most clinicians who treat distressed newborns have only their eyes, ears and hands, a roentgenogram and electrocardiogram and perhaps a pH and arterial oxygen tension to help them in their diagnosis and to direct their therapy. Fortunately, each will have his own brain for a computer, and, if the data are programmed correctly, great accuracy can be achieved, and with experience correct correlations can be made.

EFFECTS OF A TRANSITIONAL CIRCULATION ON NEONATAL RESPIRATORY DISTRESS

After birth, with the separation of the infant from the placenta which has served as the fetal lung, and with the onset of respiration, a period of time exists during which the neonatal circulatory pattern undergoes profound adjustments. Normally, with the onset of breathing, pulmonary blood flow is increased manyfold as a consequence of mechanical lung expansion and of progressively better oxygenation to the lung, both of which reduce the pulmonary vascular resistance. This occurs concomitantly with a rise in total systemic vascular resistance consequent to the removal of the large placental run-off. The net effect of these changes is to lower the pulmonary arterial pressure at the same time that the systemic pressure is increased and to reverse the pressure gradient across the ductus arteriosus. A bidirectional ductus arteriosus shunt occurs for a short period and during this time the systemic venous return still exceeds that from the pulmonary veins, and a right-to-left shunt through the foramen ovale persists. As these changes in systemic and pulmonary vascular resistance progress, the shunt through the ductus becomes totally left to right, increasing the amount of pulmonary venous return to the left atrium. This acts to close the foramen ovale valve, which lies on the left side of the atrial septum. As better oxygenation occurs with better pulmonary perfusion, the ductus arteriosus, which is sensitive to oxygen tension, begins to constrict, and shunting through the ductus is progressively diminished and functionally ceases in the normal term infant about twenty-four hours after birth.

The principal differences between the circulation of the newborn and that of an older child or adult are, first, the presence of an anatomically open ductus arteriosus capable of shunting blood in two directions, either into or away from the lungs; second, an unsealed foramen ovale valve which can readily be forced open to allow right-to-left shunting at times when the pressure gradient is in the direction of the inferior vena cava to the left atrium. There is evidence to suggest that the intact valve may be so stretched by an engorged left atrium as to allow left-to-right shunting at the atrial level. Whether or not the unconstricted ductus will allow right-to-left, left-to-right or bidirectional shunting to occur (and, if so, its magnitude and timing) is largely dependent upon the differential pressure gradient between the aorta and the pulmonary artery and on the relative resistances of the systemic and pulmonary circulations. Shunting between the atria, on the other hand, seems to be largely dependent upon their different elasticity characteristics. Situations, therefore, which either increase pulmonary resistance or lower systemic resistance, or do both, will promote resumption of the fetal direction of shunting through both the foramen ovale and the ductus arteriosus.

Pulmonary pathology which itself leads to hypoxia and pulmonary arterial hypertension may thus promote extrapulmonary right-to-left shunting and the maintenance of an unconstricted ductus, resulting in further hypoxemia and the establishment of a vicious cycle.

Many types of pulmonary pathology in the newborn are associated with this type of circulatory maladjustment, especially if inadequate pulmonary oxygenation is present from the moment of birth. Among the more common types of pathologic processes are hyaline membrane disease and intrauterine aspiration pneumonia. Birth asphyxia leading to shock and systemic hypotension or drug depression producing hypoventilation can also be associated with similar maladjustment in the transitional circulation and persistence of the right-to-left direction of fetal shunts. The importance of early and adequate pulmonary oxygenation is stressed in situations in which pulmonary hypoxia produces further hypoxemia from extrapulmonary shunting, since oxygenation can lower pulmonary resistance, raise aortic pressure, decrease right-to-left shunting through both the foramen ovale and the ductus arteriosus, and promote ductus closure.

RESPIRATORY DEPRESSION, ASPHYXIA AND RESUSCITATION

Of the many functions which the placenta serves the fetus in utero, that of gaseous exchange is almost the only one which must be assumed by the infant immediately upon delivery. Infants may survive for hours or days with renal agenesis, atresia of the gut, many extreme forms of cardiac malformations, and even anencephaly; but he must breathe or die. It is still unclear what factor or combination of factors is most important in the initiation of normal respiration by the newly delivered baby, but two main possibilities exist. First, it is possible that the infant in utero lacks the stimuli which induce normal extrauterine respiration, so that the normal circulation on both sides of the placenta maintains fetal blood pH, carbon dioxide tension and oxygen tension at levels incapable of stimulating respiration in utero. In addition, the environmental temperature is stable, and most tactile and painful stimuli are absent. At delivery the separation from maternal blood gas regulation, the abrupt environmental temperature change, the tactile and frequently the painful stimuli and the rising level of chemical stimuli, all may summate to induce respiration. The converse is also possible. It may be that the chemical stimuli capable of initiating and sustaining respiration are continuously present during late pregnancy, but that some substance with a rapid turnover rate elaborated by the placenta is capable of raising the fetal threshold for these stimuli, and that only after the placental source has been withdrawn from the baby does sustained breathing become possible. Failure to breathe promptly after birth might occur under either hypothesis if the turnover rate of the placentally produced depressant were prolonged by asphyxia or if the intrauterine asphyxia itself were of such degree as to cause central depression of respiration.

In the United States by far the commonest causes of neonatal respiratory depression of some degree are maternal analgesia or anesthesia. All the general anesthetics are capable of depressing respiration to some degree, depending upon the depth of anesthesia. Many of the commonly used analgesics such as Demerol or the barbiturates are capable of producing respiratory depression. The amount given, the timing in relation to delivery, the maturity of the infant, and his state of well-being in utero, all may have a profound effect upon the degree to which they depress a given infant.

If an infant, already in some jeopardy in utero because of a compromised placental circulation which impairs his ability to initiate breathing, is further sedated, even lightly, by an inhalation anesthetic which requires pulmonary ventilation for its elimination, the additive effect of moderate asphyxia and mild anesthesia may be enough to suppress breathing completely. Likewise, if drugs which are normally conjugated in the liver, and which, in utero, are metabolized by the mother's liver, happen to be in high concentration in a premature baby's circulation at the moment of birth, and his liver is partially or completely deficient in the enzymes necessary for such a conjugation, owing to immaturity or impaired liver function associated with intrauterine insult, the infant may remain sedated for many hours. Most babies, fortunately, are in an excellent metabolic state in utero, are mature at birth, and tolerate even large amounts of maternal sedation surprisingly well. It is the baby already in jeopardy in utero who requires the most careful judgment in maternal sedation.

Serial studies of the newborn infant's arterial blood immediately after birth have shown that many vigorous infants who have high Apgar scores and who initiate and maintain respiration in a normal fashion may have extremely low aortic oxygen levels at the moment of birth, associated with varying degrees of hypercapnia and lowered pH. Despite prompt respiration and rising arterial oxygen levels, metabolic acidosis continues to develop for several minutes, gradually being corrected over the first hour after birth in the normal infant. It is now clear from these studies, and from those in which blood from the fetal scalp was sampled during labor, that cord blood at delivery reflects changes in the functional relations between mother and fetus during delivery and does not reflect the normal intrauterine state. Serial studies of pH and blood gases of maternal and fetal blood, carried out for many days and using techniques of intrauterine catheterization in sheep which allow for a minimum of disturbance of either ewe or fetus, have shown normal levels of fetal umbilical blood pH and carbon dioxide tension, and high oxygen saturation prior to the onset of labor.

Animal experiments have shown rapid changes in pH and blood gases during acute postdelivery asphyxia, the oxygen content of arterial blood falling to zero in $2\frac{1}{2}$ minutes, the carbon dioxide tension rising at a rate of approximately 10 mm. of mercury per minute, and the pH dropping initially at about 0.1 pH unit per minute. The rapidity with which these changes occur indicates that the period of intrapartum asphyxia of the normal newborn infant must have been very brief.

Carefully controlled studies of asphyxia in newborn monkeys have shown some important considerations relating to resuscitation of the newborn infant. These considerations have been recently summarized. Studies have shown that the longer artificial ventilation is delayed after asphyxia leading to prolonged apnea, the more time will be required for the resuscitation of the infant.

Resuscitation can usually be best carried out in the apneic newborn by introducing an infant-sized laryngoscope, followed by suction of mucus, fluid or debris such as meconium from the airway, and the introduction of a proper-sized endotracheal tube beyond the vocal cords under direct vision. Positive-pressure ventilation can initially be carried out by mouth to endotracheal tube, with an oxygen supply running into the operator's oropharynx. Brief puffs of air into the endotracheal tube sufficient to raise the chest wall can be introduced, but the operator should practice against a water column so that he may learn the approximate effort required to produce 20 to 30 cm. of water positive pressure. If ventilatory assistance is to be required for any period of time in an unresponsive infant, a manually operated infant anesthesia machine with one-way low resistance valves, a carbon dioxide absorber and pressure adjustment can be used more efficiently, and for prolonged use other types of ventilatory aids may be indicated.

The profoundly asphyxiated infant requiring more than a few minutes of positive pressure for the initiation of respiration will almost certainly have bradycardia and be in profound shock. External cardiac massage is indicated once the lungs are expanded. This can readily be applied to the newborn infant with two fingers compressing the chest just to the left of the sternum. Massage should be applied at a rate of 100 to 120 times a minute, and interrupted every five seconds to permit several full inflations of the lung.

The beneficial effects of intravenous buffers and glucose in asphyxiated animals suggest that their use in severely asphyxiated human newborns may be a helpful adjunct to other resuscitative procedures, and such seems to be the case. If buffers such as THAM (Trishydroxymethyl amino methane) or sodium bicarbonate are to be used, it is desirable to be able to monitor the blood pH and to regulate the dosage accordingly.

Evidence seems clear in animals that the length of asphyxia before resuscitative and supportive measures are begun is critical for the development of brain damage. In the newborn infant, knowledge of the extent and length of intrauterine asphyxia is usually inaccessible. Until techniques are developed which allow an accurate assessment of the fetal state in utero and during delivery, the prevention of neurologic damage incident to birth asphyxia must be based upon prompt and vigorous measures directed toward its physiologic and biochemical correction.

INTRAUTERINE ASPIRATION PNEUMONIA (MASSIVE ASPIRATION SYNDROME, MECONIUM ASPIRATION PNEUMONIA)

Except in breech delivery, in which it is considered normal, the presence of meconium staining of the amniotic fluid and fetus should alert the physician to the likelihood of several adverse conditions in the neonate. If the meconium staining is fresh, as indicated by its dark green color, it is indicative of recent, probably intrapartum interruption in blood supply to the fetus, such as cord compression. Such an infant may have profound asphyxia

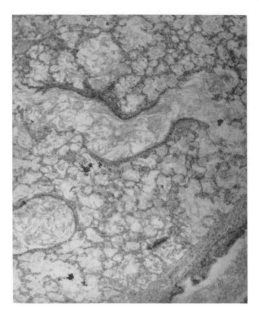

FIGURE 5–1. Photomicrograph of the lung of a postmature infant dying with intrauterine aspiration pneumonia, showing sheets of squamous cells packed into all air passages and scattered meconium pigment.

toward hypoglycemia. The intrauterine passage of meconium is rare in prematurely born infants despite evidence of asphyxia, and yellow staining almost always occurs in postmature infants. Peeling of the integument, which may be extensive in utero when associated with asphyxia of such magnitude as to produce intrauterine gasping, allows the aspiration and, indeed, bronchial and alveolar impaction of sheets of squamous cells, mixed with vernix, meconium and other amniotic debris (Fig. 1). At birth it may be impossible to remove such debris adequately by suction. Severe respiratory distress results. (It should be stated that normal amniotic fluid is not thought to be harmful to the lung; it is rapidly absorbed by the pulmonary vascular bed, and may be partially formed from it.) After initial resuscitation, which is frequently necessary because of central nerv-

and shock at birth, with severe respiratory depression, bradycardia and flaccidity, requiring the most vigorous resuscitative efforts and supportive treatment. In addition to birth asphyxia, such an infant may also have begun to gasp before delivery, thereby sucking large amounts of particulate meconium into his respiratory tree, which, on neonatal gasping or positive-pressure resuscitation, become more distally displaced. This meconium may plug the tracheobronchial tree initially or may cause later respiratory distress referred to as meconium aspiration pneumonia. In other infants the amniotic fluid, skin, cord and nails are not green, but yellow stained. This is indicative of some more remote and perhaps chronic insult to the fetus, since it is almost always associated with other signs of placental dysfunction. These signs include evidence of intrauterine weight loss, with flabby, loose folds of skin, especially about the buttocks and thighs, drawn and pinched facies, loss of vernix, dry, cracking and peeling skin, sparse subcutaneous tissue, and a tendency

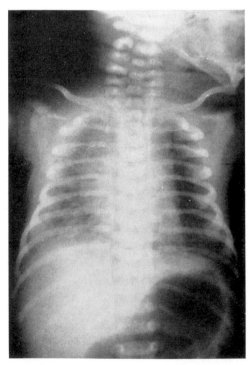

FIGURE 5–2. Anteroposterior x-ray of the chest of a postmature infant with severe intrauterine aspiration pneumonia, showing coarse mottling of the right lung field and emphysema of the left lung.

ous system depression, these babies usually exhibit a strong respiratory effort with deep retraction of the costal margins, loud grunting and appreciable cyanosis. A chest x-ray usually shows patchy and irregular gross densities and radiolucencies, indicative of the inequality of aeration of various portions of the lung (Fig. 2). Intercostal spaces may bulge outward, and the diaphragmatic leaves become flattened by the patchy areas of overdistention produced by the ball-valve airway obstruction. Pneumothorax is a frequent complication of such partial obstruction. Even mildly symptomatic infants may have highly abnormal chest x-rays.

High carbon dioxide tension in arterial blood reflects the degree of pulmonary involvement, and the low oxygen tension reflects the degree of both intrapulmonary and extrapulmonary right to left shunting as well as probable diffusion impairment within the lung. The lowered arterial pH reflects the degree of respiratory acidosis, but this is frequently accompanied by a profound metabolic acidosis, especially if there are signs of prolonged intrauterine distress. Seizures and other evidences of neurologic involvement are common. The use of barbiturates and other analeptic drugs which depress the respiratory center is strongly contraindicated. Dilantin is the drug of choice for the control of neonatal seizures.

Many of these babies may run a course of moderate clinical respiratory distress for several days, requiring only supportive oxygen therapy and perhaps initial intravenous buffering of a lowered pH. The severely ill infants, however, usually require a continuous high oxygen environment, repeated buffering of pH, and some form of ventilatory assistance for several days. Even with vigorous treatment the mortality rate is high, and neurologic residua are common in survivors. The need for new modes of adequate intrauterine assessment is again emphasized by this small but profoundly affected group of babies.

Aspiration of regurgitated feedings is a fairly common occurrence in newborn infants, especially prematures, and such aspirates are capable of causing acute respiratory symptoms and subsequent pneumonia. Such aspiration, if massive and overwhelming, and especially if it consists of large milk curds, may prove immediately fatal to a small, weak premature by occluding the airway completely. Most infants, however, if promptly and adequately suctioned, will recover. Occasionally, subsequent to an aspiration episode, an infant will exhibit signs of respiratory distress consisting of tachypnea, fever and rales. X-ray examination of the chest may show patchy or streaky perihilar densities. Supportive therapy is frequently all that is necessary, although prophylactic antibiotics may be given to prevent secondary bacterial pneumonia. Gradual improvement usually occurs over a three- to four-day period.

EMPHYSEMA, PNEUMOTHORAX AND PNEUMOMEDIASTINUM (AIR BLOCK)

The term "emphysema" implies that some portion of the lung is overdistended with air. Simple emphysema may occur as a compensatory mechanism for filling the chest cavity in conditions in which portions of the lung lose volume, such as lobar atelectasis or pulmonary agenesis. Unaffected portions of the lung then become overdistended simply by the negative pressure within the thorax, inducing them to fill the extra space and lessen the excessive negative intrapleural pressure created by the loss of lung volume. In a number of locations in the newborn's lung air can be found to collect abnormally. Such collections may occur spontaneously in otherwise apparently normal lungs, from iatrogenic cause, or as a complication of intrinsic pulmonary pathology.

Interstitial emphysema is the accumulation of air in interstitial tissue after rupture of alveoli. This air may then penetrate the sheaths of blood vessels and bronchi and progress back along their course into the mediastinum, forming

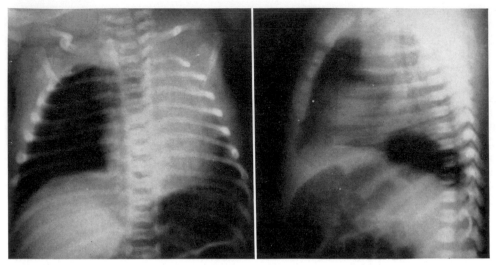

FIGURE 5–3. Anteroposterior and lateral chest x-rays of a postmature infant 2 hours after birth, showing a right tension pneumothorax following resuscitation.

multiple blebs of widely varying size between the heart and the anterior chest wall. Air may also dissect into the supporting tissue of the lung parenchyma, resulting in emphysematous bullae. If dissection occurs toward the periphery of the lung, subpleural blebs will be formed. These are capable of easy rupture into the pleural space, producing pneumothorax.

Iatrogenic interstitial emphysema, pneumothorax or pneumomediastinum can occur in a normal lung with the injudicious use of unmonitored positive-pressure resuscitation, frequently applied by an airtight mask without a clear airway. Both the magnitude and the duration of the application of pressure must be taken into account in order to avoid rupture of alveoli, since "safe" pressures, below 30 cm. of water, may be harmful if applied over a too prolonged period of time. In the case of iatrogenic rupture, symptoms and signs of distress may be present from the onset of respiration at birth. Since respiratory symptoms may be present because of the underlying pulmonary pathology, such as meconium aspiration, which necessitated the resuscitative efforts, every baby with persistent respiratory symptoms following positive-pressure resuscitation deserves antero-posterior and lateral x-ray examination of the chest (Fig. 3).

Since pneumothorax or pneumomediastinum can also occur spontaneously as a complication of pulmonary pathology such as bacterial pneumonia, especially staphylococcal, or in the course of severe hyaline membrane disease, repeat x-ray examination is likewise indicated when, during the course of such a disease process, a sudden deterioration occurs or if respiratory symptoms fail to subside concomitant with other signs of clinical improvement. Pneumothorax or pneumomediastinum may significantly complicate the course of severe hyaline membrane disease, since a lung deficient of surfactant, once completely collapsed, seems almost incapable of re-expansion. A small pneumothorax or pneumomediastinum not associated with increasing tension may go unnoticed, or may be diagnosed only incidentally on chest x-ray. On those occasions when the air accumulation is large, and especially when under progressively increasing tension, respiratory distress may be so severe as to constitute an emergency necessitating immediate relief.

The baby with a large tension pneumothorax or pneumomediastinum is in acute respiratory embarrassment. Vigorous respiratory efforts are maintained as long as central nervous system integrity lasts. Cyanosis is usually marked, and grunting may occur on expiration. The baby frequently lies with head drawn back, using all the accessory muscles of respiration. The chest shows a rather square and bulging appearance, with shoulders drawn back.

In the case of pneumomediastinum, crepitus may occur under the sternum as air dissects into the suprasternal notch and up the neck. Distention appears in the neck veins if cardiac compression and impedance of systemic venous filling occur. Auscultation may be misleading as to the location of the air, but the heart can be shifted to either side by pneumothorax, or heart sounds muffled by overlying air accumulation. In the case of pneumothorax, x-ray films of the chest will usually establish the location of the air collection. An anteroposterior film alone may be inadequate in the case of a modest-sized pneumomediastinum, since only a faint translucency around the heart shadow appears, but a lateral film will confirm its presence. In cases of large accumulations of air in the anterior part of the mediastinum, the chest x-ray will show the air bulging out on both sides of the heart, tempting needle aspiration (Figs. 4, 5). This, however, is usually a futile procedure since the air is not collected in a single large pocket, but in multiple blebs of varying size. Tapping with a needle frequently results in a pneumothorax without relief of the mediastinal pressure. Small and moderate-sized accumulations of mediastinal air, if not life-threatening, can safely be left alone and watched closely by repeated chest x-rays for progression or resolution. Such babies may require supportive measures, such as added oxygen, and deserve alert and constant nursing care. Massive collections of air in the mediastinum which produce severe cardiac and respiratory symptoms and appear to be life-threatening may be treated by incision of the jugular notch and blunt dissection into the anterior part of the mediastinum. Air blebs are ruptured and a drain is left in the mediastinal space when the neck wound is closed.

The treatment of choice of a collection of intrapleural air is largely dependent upon its size and whether or not there exists a tension pneumothorax which reaccumulates after evacuation. Small pneumothoraces may be associated with little

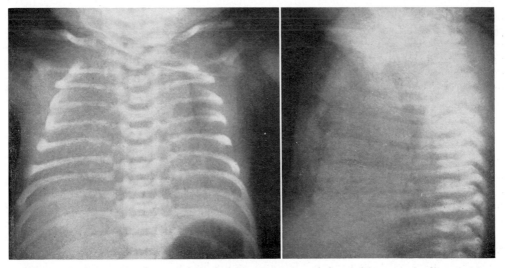

FIGURE 5—4. Anteroposterior and lateral chest x-rays of an infant with severe hyaline membrane disease taken 5 hours after birth, showing reticulogranular pattern with a thin rim of mediastinal air seen just to the left of the cardiac border on the anteroposterior view and between the heart and sternum on the lateral view.

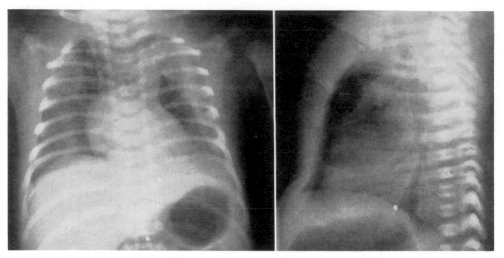

FIGURE 5–5. The same infant 35 hours after birth, showing progression of the pneumomediastinum with a large accumulation of air seen surrounding the heart shadow on the anteroposterior view and posterior compression of the heart on the lateral view. A small rim of pneumothorax is seen on the right. This infant was not resuscitated, and the pneumomediastinum was presumed to be spontaneous.

or no respiratory distress and may be left untreated and observed clinically and roentgenologically. Most will clear spontaneously. A large accumulation of air, however, sufficient to produce respiratory symptoms, should be removed. When initially it is unclear whether or not a tension pneumothorax exists, the side of the chest where the x-ray film shows the air accumulation is tapped with a no. 18 bore needle attached to a 50-cc. syringe by a three-way stopcock, and a rough measure made of the amount of air removed. An x-ray picture is taken to estimate efficacy of the tap, and thirty to sixty minutes later is repeated to see whether air has reaccumulated. If it is apparent that a tension pneumothorax exists, a small-bore catheter with multiple side holes near the end is introduced into the anterior part of the chest and connected to an underwater trap. A ballast bottle is placed in the system and this is connected to one or sometimes two Stedman pumps. Experience has shown that in newborns continuous negative pressure is necessary to prevent the reaccumulation of air and to keep the lung expanded. As long as air bubbles through the trap with respiration, the system is left unchanged.

When bubbling ceases and an x-ray film indicates that insignificant amounts of pleural air remain, the tube can first be clamped for a period of hours, the chest re-evaluated, and if air has still not reaccumulated, the tube removed. In rare instances air continues to accumulate for many days, and in such cases surgical closure of a rent in the lung may be necessary. Infants with chest tubes or repeated pleural aspirations should be placed on wide-spectrum antibiotics, since the opportunities for infection are great. Oxygen, careful nursing and other supportive measures such as intravenous fluid therapy during the acute course may be lifesaving.

HYALINE MEMBRANE DISEASE

The idiopathic respiratory distress syndrome of prematurity, or clinical hyaline membrane disease, is the commonest single cause of respiratory symptoms in the newborn. It is associated with approximately 30 per cent of all neonatal deaths, with 50 to 70 per cent of all deaths in premature infants, and is thought to account for approximately 25,000 deaths per year in the United States alone. It is felt to occur exclusively in prematurely born infants. Even though some babies with the disease have birth weights greater than the arbitrary level of 2500 gm., they have other evidences of immaturity, including low gestational age and absence of palpable breast tissue. Babies of diabetic mothers have an especially high incidence; although many of these infants are large at birth, premature delivery is common. Infants born by cesarean section are also thought to be especially likely to have hyaline membrane disease, although recent evidence suggests that the degree of immaturity of the sectioned baby is a more important factor than the section itself. There are also many suggestions that the indication for the section has great influence on the incidence of the disease; hyaline membrane disease is thirteen times as common when the indication is maternal bleeding as when the cesarean section is an elective one. There are many other suggestions that conditions occurring in late pregnancy or incident to delivery which might be expected to compromise the oxygen supply to the fetus, such as maternal bleeding and hypotension, and birth asphyxia if associated with premature birth, may be important in the pathogenesis.

There seems to be ample evidence that the baby who will subsequently show signs and symptoms of hyaline membrane disease will, on close observation, show some abnormality in respiration at birth, leading to the strong suspicion that the stage is set by intrauterine or intrapartum fetal insult.

These babies frequently have low Apgar scores at birth and require stimulation or resuscitative efforts to establish sustained respiration. The smaller prematures, particularly, may show depression of the central nervous system far beyond that which their maternal analgesic dosage would suggest. Whether this phenomenon is related to the lack of ability to metabolize even light sedation on the part of a baby already in jeopardy in utero, to cerebral hemorrhage which is frequently found at autopsy, or to a central depres-

sion which may be part of the disease process itself, it is a poor prognostic sign.

As soon as respiration is established, an audible expiratory grunt usually appears, along with some degree of labored respiration. In mildly affected babies grunting may quickly disappear as soon as they are placed in an oxygen-enriched atmosphere, but the respiratory pattern usually continues to show tachypnea of 80 to 100 per minute with rapid, shallow breathing, frequently punctuated by irregularities such as cogwheel inspiration. The more severely affected baby will continue to grunt or cry on expiration despite oxygen supplementation. Although the respiratory rate usually increases with warming and oxygenation during the first few hours of life to 70 to 80 per minute, persistent rates above 100 per minute are not so common as in more mildly affected infants. Severely ill babies also show inspiratory retraction of the sternum and lower costal margin, often associated with paradoxical bulging of the abdomen be-

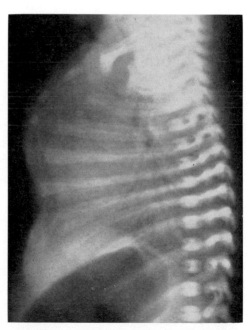

FIGURE 5–6. Lateral chest x-ray of a premature infant made 48 hours after birth, showing the pseudopectus deformity of the chest and air bronchogram associated with severe hyaline membrane disease.

low the diaphragm, creating a seesaw motion and a pseudopectus deformity (Fig. 6). Retraction may be greater and more obvious in smaller babies with weaker chest walls. It is rarely deep in the more mildly affected babies. On auscultation there is only "poor air entry," rales of any kind being rare in the early stage of the disease. Tachycardia above 160 per minute is common in most distressed babies until they have been well oxygenated. It is often striking to observe the disappearance of audible grunting, even in severely ill babies, and the subsidence of tachycardia when they are given high oxygen concentrations to breathe. Edema is common in these infants, being most obvious in the dorsa of the hands and feet, the shiny, full palms and soles, the puffy eyes and the full skin fold in the posterior axillary line of a supine infant. Flaccidity with poor muscle tone and joint relaxation is also characteristic, and the baby assumes a supine frog-leg position with ease.

The x-ray picture is usually character-istic in severe disease, even in the first few hours after birth, but may be only suggestive in more mildly affected infants and become characteristic only if the infant's status worsens. The film of the lung fields shows a diffuse, fine granularity throughout, which, if not prominent, is best distinguished with a bright light (Fig. 7). There is no evidence of gross lobar or lobular atelectasis; the diaphragms are low, and the ribs horizontal. Heavy, diffuse granularity is characteristic of the severe disease (Fig. 8). An air bronchogram extending into the fine radicals can usually be clearly seen. The heart may appear enlarged, especially on the first day of life, and this is often best substantiated by subsequent diminution in size on serial x-ray films. The lateral film may demonstrate the extent of sternal retraction or air in the mediastinum, which occasionally occurs in the course of the disease.

Blood gas studies in mildly affected babies show near-normal arterial oxygen tension even on room air breathing, and

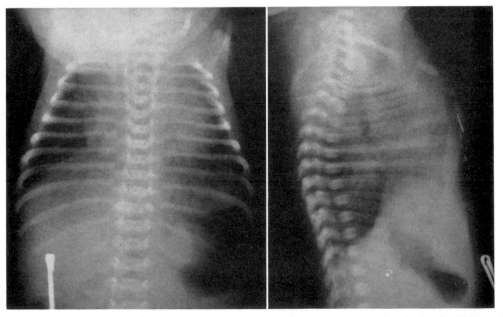

FIGURE 5–7. Anteroposterior and lateral chest x-rays taken at one hour after birth of a 1701-gm. infant in moderately severe respiratory distress due to hyaline membrane disease. They show a diffuse, fine reticulogranular pattern throughout the lung fields and air bronchogram extending into the periphery of the lung fields.

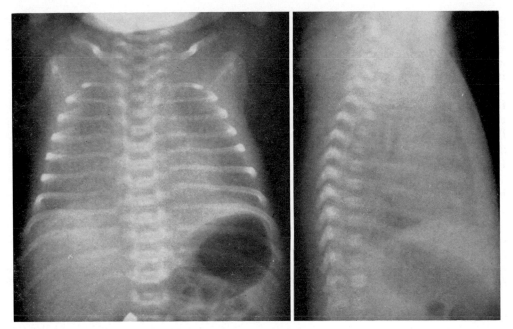

FIGURE 5–8. Anteroposterior and lateral x-rays of the chest of a 1162-gm. infant taken 2 hours after birth, showing the generalized reticulogranular pattern of severe hyaline membrane disease.

on high oxygen inhalation arterial oxygen levels can be raised to 200 to 300 mm. of mercury. Arterial carbon dioxide tension is rarely elevated in these mildly affected babies and may be lowered to the 30's. After the first hour following delivery arterial pH is rarely below 7.25 in mildly ill babies and frequently never falls below 7.30. In contrast, severely ill babies may show a very low arterial oxygen tension on room air; although initially it may be raised above 100 mm. of mercury on high oxygen inhalation, as the disease progresses this no longer becomes possible. Oxygenation becomes progressively more difficult in babies who are going to die, and a persistent level of oxygen tension below 40 mm. of mercury with 100 per cent oxygen inhalation is an ominous sign. The arterial pH in severely ill babies is also low, usually below 7.25, reflecting both respiratory and metabolic acidosis in most instances. The pH, however, can usually be regulated to near-normal levels by the repeated use of intravenous buffers such as sodium bicarbonate, except in moribund babies. The arterial carbon dioxide

tension is usually elevated above 45 mm. of mercury, but only in the depressed babies, those with cerebral hemorrhage, or those who are deteriorating is it above 70 mm. Blood lactic acid levels indicating metabolic acidosis become elevated above 50 mg. per 100 ml. only in the most severely ill babies; levels of this magnitude are considered poor prognostic signs. Blood lactic acid seems to reflect tissue hypoxia associated with poor perfusion rather than anoxemia itself. Serum potassium may rise to dangerously high levels, especially in very small infants, those with occult hemorrhage, and those who have been allowed to undergo hypothermia. Serum protein levels are frequently low, but reflect the size of the baby more closely than the severity of the disease. Serum calcium levels are frequently low, but rarely cause tetany. The blood urea nitrogen and phosphorus levels may be elevated, reflecting a catabolic state, but do not add to the prognostic outlook.

Physiologic measurements of pulmonary function on these infants have shown abnormally low compliance, i.e. a markedly negative intrathoracic pressure necessary to move a normal volume of air. Total ventilation may be greatly increased, but alveolar ventilation is decreased, producing an increased ratio of dead space to tidal volume and an elevated arterial carbon dioxide tension. Abnormal ventilation-to-perfusion ratios exist within the lung, contributing to both the lowered arterial oxygen tension and elevated arterial carbon dioxide tension.

Studies of the cardiovascular system have shown moderate systemic hypotension which can usually be improved by high oxygen inhalation or by the infusion of buffers. Aortic pressure, however, usually increases over the first few days of life except in those babies who will subsequently die. The ductus arteriosus is open, the direction and magnitude of the shunt depending on the pressures and resistances in the systemic and pulmonary arterial systems. Many severely ill infants show bidirectional shunting through the ductus arteriosus and large right-to-left shunts through the foramen ovale. These right-to-left shunts will usually diminish in size with high oxygen inhalation, associated with increasing left-to-right ductus shunting, increased systemic pressure and pulse pressure and increasing arterial oxygen tension. This suggests that pulmonary oxygenation is capable of lowering pulmonary arterial pressure and resistance, thereby decreasing the degree of hypoxemia by decreasing right-to-left shunting through the ductus and foramen ovale. More mildly affected babies may never demonstrate right-to-left ductus arteriosus shunts. Significant left-to-right shunts are common in distressed infants with all degrees of severity. Small to moderate-sized right-to-left shunts through the foramen ovale are also common in babies who do not have extremely large left-to-right shunts through the ductus arteriosus capable of raising left atrial pressure high enough to close the foramen valve.

As babies improve clinically on the third and fourth days after birth, their ductus shunts diminish in size and eventually disappear entirely. Systolic murmurs

frequently become apparent as the ductus constricts, but are rarely heard early in the course of the disease. Such murmurs may persist for weeks or even months in small prematures.

The mildly ill baby usually continues to hyperventilate for thirty-six to seventy-two hours, but is almost never clinically cyanotic in room air; if he is, he requires only moderately elevated oxygen concentrations to restore good oxygenation. Most are edematous and oliguric during this time, but will diurese on the second to third day concomitant with increased alertness, signs of hunger and slowing of respiratory rate. Improvement is rapid thereafter.

The severely ill infant may continue to grunt loudly, although grunting may disappear with 100 per cent oxygen inhalation and buffering. Deep retraction, however, persists for forty-eight to seventy-two hours, and in very severely ill babies for many days to weeks. These babies are frequently both clinically and biochemically worse in their second twenty-four hours of life than in their first, with falling arterial oxygen tensions despite high oxygen inhalation and repeated decline in arterial pH after satisfactory initial pH buffering, indicating progressive worsening of their disease. Scratchy, sandpaper breath sounds are frequently audible. It is at this time that respiratory failure most often begins to be apparent, with physical exhaustion of the baby, and a gradual lessening of the respiratory rate and effort unaccompanied by clinical or biochemical improvement. Irregular respiration may be followed by periods of apnea and bradycardia, ashen cyanosis appears, and death occurs if ventilatory assistance is not given. Constant and experienced nursing and physician attendance are necessary, since respiratory failure demands immediate management. Yet many babies, though clinically and biochemically severely ill, if supported, will be able to survive this second twenty-four hours without ventilatory assistance and gradually begin to show improvement by the third to fourth day. Brief episodes of apnea, frequently associated with excessive mucus, are common during this period, and during this time constant and expert nursing attention is mandatory. Diuresis also occurs on about the third to fourth day in these infants with loss of edema. They gradually become more alert, develop better muscular tone, begin to show hunger, and will suck a pacifier. Small oral feedings can usually be begun by the fourth day of life. As arterial oxygen tension rises, environmental oxygen concentrations can be gradually diminished, and weaning to room air usually completed by the fourth day, occasionally later in the sickest infants. Jaundice is common on the third to seventh day, frequently of alarming degree, being most severe in the most immature babies and in those with suspected occult hemorrhage.

Babies who do not fit into either of these two patterns almost invariably have other complicating factors modifying their course. The commonest of these complications is cerebral hemorrhage. Such a baby will frequently have only mild or moderate respiratory symptoms, mildly abnormal biochemical findings and an x-ray picture not typical of an extremely ill baby; these babies have periods of apnea and bradycardia of increasing length and severity, usually responding at first to mechanical stimulation, but eventually resulting in total and sudden respiratory failure. The outlook for such a baby is poor. Even though he can be adequately oxygenated and ventilated by mechanical means initially, he is frequently unconscious with no respiratory effort of his own, and mechanical ventilation becomes less and less effective. Frank tonic and clonic seizures are rarely seen in prematures, although extensor spasms may occur.

The time of the occurrence of large intraventricular hemorrhage frequently found at autopsy in severely ill infants is unknown, but the onset of cerebral symptoms and respiratory failure in such an infant is frequently in the second twenty-four hours after birth. In such instances

the extreme severity of the disease is probably associated with the pathogenesis of the hemorrhage, and death is almost inevitable.

Extremely small immature babies may also show an atypical course, physical exhaustion playing a role in their early respiratory failure. Persistent hypothermia, profound metabolic acidosis and extreme hyperkalemia leading to early electrocardiographic changes are common. These complications may contribute to their high mortality rate in the face of mildly or moderately severe respiratory symptoms.

Secondary infection, especially pneumonia, has been a cause of late death in some series of babies with hyaline membrane disease, although it can usually be prevented by isolation, aseptic technique and prophylactic antibiotic administration.

The postmortem findings in those babies who die are usually characteristic. The heart when visualized in situ is dilated, and the right atrium and venae cavae are engorged with blood. The liver is also usually large and congested. The lungs are full, solid, airless, dark purplish-red and liver-like in consistency. Pressure-volume curves on excised lungs have shown that pressures higher than normal are required to move a given volume of air. Measurements of surface tension on film from lung homogenates have not shown normal surface properties. This suggests that, in babies who die, the normal amount of alveolar lining layer surfactant necessary for maintaining normal lung stability is either absent or inactivated in some way. The ductus arteriosus is usually unconstricted in babies dying in the first three days of life. Cerebral hemorrhage, especially intraventricular hemorrhage, has been a common finding at autopsy.

Microscopic sections of the lungs of babies dying early in the disease, before eighteen hours, may show a high degree of constriction of the small arterioles adjacent to alveolar ducts and respiratory bronchioles, with beginning sloughing of

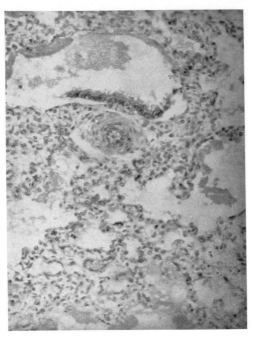

FIGURE 5–9. Photomicrograph of the lung of a premature infant dying 16 hours after birth, showing arteriolar constriction with sloughing epithelium of a respiratory bronchiole adjacent, and early hyaline membrane formation.

the epithelium of these air sacs, protein-containing material in their lumens and a moderate degree of alveolar atelectasis. Scanty, patchy or ill-formed membranes which appear to be made up of sloughed cell debris in a protein-containing matrix may be seen lining some of the dilated respiratory bronchioles and alveolar ducts (Fig. 9). The longer the baby has survived before death, the more well formed and homogeneous these membranes appear, and the less apparent are the cellular components. Also the arteriolar constriction becomes less apparent with time, the alveolar atelectasis more profound, and the dilatation of alveolar ducts more striking by contrast. In babies who have been kept alive for seven to twelve days by mechanical ventilation and who have subsequently died, atelectasis has remained profound, the membranes dense and unresolved, and fibroblasts and macrophages have appeared in their vicinity.

Other babies showing the typical clinical picture of hyaline membrane disease, who have died from unrelated causes at seven to ten days, have shown re-expanding alveoli and varying degrees of resolution of the membranes with considerable fibroblastic and macrophage activity.

Any approach to therapy in a disease process whose cause is in question, but whose pathogenesis is becoming more and more clear-cut, must rely on the correction of those biochemical or physiologic abnormalities which can be demonstrated at any particular stage of development of the disease. If hypoxia is present, normal oxygenation should be attempted; if metabolic acidosis is present, buffers such as sodium bicarbonate or THAM should be useful; if cardiac failure is in evidence, digitalis is indicated; or if hyperkalemia develops, the serum potassium level may be lowered with intravenous administration of glucose and insulin. This approach to therapy has been recently summarized. Whether or not babies with great mechanical problems of maintaining prolonged adequate alveolar ventilation imposed by severe hyaline membrane disease should receive ventilatory assistance of some sort is perhaps open to question, dependent largely upon the safety and efficiency of the method used. Nevertheless, in the face of complete respiratory failure, ventilatory assistance is mandatory and may, indeed, be lifesaving.

If a high pulmonary resistance exists, maintaining the fetal pattern of circulation with right-to-left shunting through the ductus arteriosus and foramen ovale, it may be partially or perhaps completely relieved by high oxygen inhalation and correction of the pH toward normal, especially if these measures are applied early in the disease. Whether or not other pharmacologic means such as acetylcholine infusion or Priscoline are necessary or desirable in an individual case awaits further study. Obviously, one would like to restore lung compliance to normal, but methods so far used have not proved satisfactory. The value of continuous physician supervision and expert individual nursing care cannot be ignored in the over-all therapy of any small or sick new-born. This is especially true in babies with severe respiratory distress, whose status may change from moment to moment and who may require a rapid change of therapeutic approach or just immediate suction of the oropharynx. Nurses experienced in making detailed and frequent observations on distressed infants and capable of acting on them with judgment have proved to be invaluable helpers in the over-all management of the disease.

The ultimate goal in therapy is obviously prevention, but until more of the factors related to etiology, with their interrelation and time sequence, are understood, we can only ask for the best obstetrical care possible, the most judicious conduct of labor and delivery of pregnancies at risk, prompt and adequate resuscitation of the newborn when indicated, and continuity of care and responsibility between the delivery room and the nursery. From this point on rational therapy must be based on the findings in a particular baby at the time the therapy is contemplated, since what may be good or necessary at one time may be harmful at another. Methods for assessing the fetus in utero are at present only rudimentary, and future progress in this important field will probably depend largely upon their development.

INFECTIONS OF THE LUNG

Bacteria may be introduced into the newborn's lung either by aspiration of infected material, such as the intrauterine aspiration of amniotic contents in the presence of amnionitis or the intrapartum aspiration of maternal fecal material; by airborne contamination from hospital personnel such as occurs in some cases of neonatal staphylococcal and streptococcal pneumonia; or as a complication of a more generalized process, such as sepsis. *Intrauterine bacterial pneumonia* occurs almost exclusively in those infants whose mothers' membranes have been ruptured for more than twenty-four hours before delivery. In these instances the mother may show signs of infection such as fever, and the amniotic fluid may be noticeably foul and purulent at delivery. Overt signs of amnionitis may be absent, however.

An infant born after prolonged rupture of the membranes should have cultures taken from the nasopharynx, blood and skin before bathing. Aspiration of the stomach contents and microscopic examination for the presence of excessive numbers of polymorphonuclear leukocytes and especially for the identification of intracellular bacteria may be helpful in the early diagnosis of babies at high risk from intrauterine infection. In the absence of symptoms in either mother or child, prophylactic administration of antibiotics to the infant may be withheld until cultures are positive or symptoms of infection develop. If contamination of the baby's respiratory tract has been recent or occurred intra partum, pneumonia may be the only one of the manifestations of generalized sepsis, which may include meningitis, hepatic and renal abscesses, osteomyelitis and other localizations of blood stream dissemination.

The organisms which most frequently infect the infant in his intrauterine environment are gram-negative rods of the colon bacillus group, proteus organisms and *Pseudomonas aeruginosa*. Many of these organisms are considered to be saprophytes or nonpathogenic "normal flora" in other circumstances, but they are capable of rapidly fatal disease in the newborn infant.

Babies with intrauterine bacterial pneumonia are usually severely ill from birth and may have respiratory distress indistinguishable from clinical hyaline membrane disease. Rales may appear with more regularity, but otherwise the infants retract and grunt, and have cyanosis and air hunger similar to other infants in severe respiratory distress. Fever may be absent or of low grade and may be replaced by hypothermia. The early x-ray appearance of the lung may likewise be

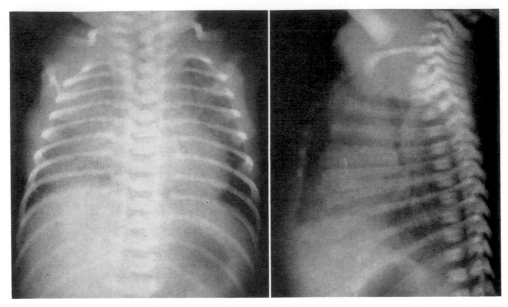

FIGURE 5–10. Anteroposterior and lateral x-rays of the chest of an infant 12 hours after birth, showing diffuse granularity throughout both lung fields. This mother's membranes had been ruptured more than 24 hours before delivery, and *Pseudomonas aeruginosa* was cultured from both blood and lung of the infant.

difficult to distinguish from the generalized reticulogranular pattern seen in hyaline membrane disease (Fig. 10). Later x-ray films may resemble diffuse bronchopneumonia or show early abscess formation (Fig. 11). Respiratory and metabolic acidosis and anoxemia are found on arterial blood gas analysis. Other systemic signs of infection may be apparent if more generalized infection is present and if the infant survives for several days after birth. Among these are opisthotonos and seizures in the case of meningitis, or an umbilical cord with a reddened base and oozing foul-smelling purulent material.

Widespread pneumonia, especially if the blood culture is positive for gram-negative organisms, is a frequently fatal disease and demands prompt and vigorous specific treatment if the infant is to survive. After initial cultures of the amniotic fluid, skin, nasopharynx and blood have been taken, administration of broad-spectrum antibiotics capable of dealing effectively with the most likely organisms should be started promptly. A lumbar puncture may yield an organism which may be promptly identified on smear and Gram stain. Sensitivity to the drugs used may be evaluated when cultures become positive, and changed as indicated. Supportive care in the form of oxygen, buffers and careful nursing are frequently indicated, and ventilatory assistance may be necessary in the face of respiratory failure. Widespread abscess formation is frequently seen at autopsy.

If a newborn infant shows signs and symptoms compatible with bacterial pneumonia several days after birth, the likelihood of a gram-negative organism as the etiologic agent is lessened, and staphylococcal and streptococcal pneumonia occur with increased frequency. Infants exposed to hemolytic streptococci may contract impetigo neonatorum, frequently associated with omphalitis and blood stream dissemination. *Streptococcal pneumonia* rarely occurs in the absence of sepsis. This type of infection can rapidly spread throughout a nursery, and early isolation precautions, specific bacteriologic identification and prompt antibiotic therapy are advisable. Signs and symptoms of pulmonary involvement and x-ray evidence of pulmonary infiltration which appears frequently as bronchopneumonia are usually accompanied or preceded by the appearance of oozing omphalitis or skin blebs filled with thin, purulent material from which organisms may readily be cultured.

Staphylococcal infection in the newborn may likewise take many presenting forms, only one of which is pneumonia. Infants may harbor pathogenic staphylococci in their nasopharynx for many weeks without symptoms, only to present with acute pneumonia later. Omphalitis and skin infection in the form of impetigo neonatorum are likewise common, but pulmonary involvement frequently follows only a carrier state. Such infants are acutely and seriously ill, show severe respiratory symptoms with or without the appearance of rales, and a tendency to bleb formation in the lung, which may rupture and produce sudden pneumothorax. A chest x-ray shows the patchy, mottled appearance of areas of infiltration; emphysema and pleural fluid or air collection are common (Fig. 12). Pneu-

matoceles frequently appear suddenly. Prompt and vigorous antibiotic therapy based on organism sensitivity is indicated. If enough pleural fluid has accumulated to compress functioning lung tissue and produce added respiratory symptoms, thoracentesis is indicated. Surgical drainage may be necessary for encapsulated pus or chronic abscess formation. Pneumatoceles can usually be treated conservatively. Decortication of the lung is occasionally necessary for late restrictive pleural thickening.

Other bacterial organisms occasionally infect the newborn's lungs and must be specifically identified by culture; specific treatment is based on sensitivity studies.

Viral agents such as the parainfluenza group have been occasionally identified in neonatal pneumonia, but their role even in these instances is somewhat questionable. Pneumonic involvement may also occur with cytomegalic inclusion disease. Spirochetal pneumonia may occur with congenital syphilis, but is a rare disease in this country at present. Intrauterine infection with toxoplasma organisms may also occur, and, rarely, widespread fatal

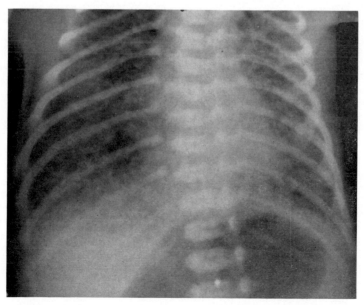

FIGURE 5–11. Anteroposterior x-ray of the chest of an infant 60 hours after birth whose blood culture grew out *E. coli* and from whose lung *E. coli* and *Pseudomonas aeruginosa* were cultured at autopsy. The x-ray film shows coarse, diffuse infiltration throughout both lung fields.

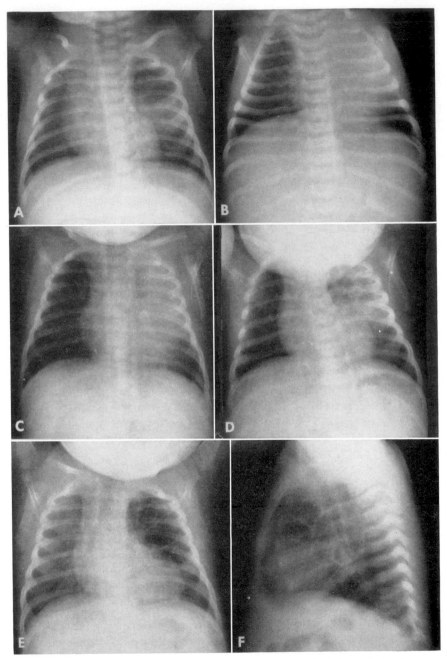

FIGURE 5–12. *A,* Anteroposterior x-ray of the chest of a 3-week-old infant admitted with symptoms of fever and tachypnea whose nasopharyngeal cultures grew out phage type 80-81 staphylococci. Pneumonic infiltrate is seen in the left midlung field. *B,* Anteroposterior x-ray of the chest of the same infant one day later, showing progression of the infiltrate. *C,* Anteroposterior x-ray of the chest one day later, showing beginning resolution of the infiltrate. *D,* Anteroposterior x-ray of the chest one day later, showing further resolution of the pneumonia. *E,* Anteroposterior x-ray of the chest of the same infant 13 days later, showing multiple pneumatoceles in the left upper lung field. *F,* Lateral x-ray of the chest the same day as in *C,* showing the location of the pneumatoceles. These cleared without treatment.

pneumonia results. Other protozoan organisms, such as *Pneumocystis carinii*, may occasionally be found, but in this country their occurrence is rare.

PULMONARY HEMORRHAGE

The occurrence of some extravasated blood in the lungs of newborn infants at autopsy is common, but, to date, the mechanism of its appearance in most instances is unclear. Even in circumstances in which a generalized bleeding diathesis occurs in a newborn with bleeding from many sites, a specific cause is often lacking. Pulmonary hemorrhage as an isolated occurrence is rare, but may appear suddenly from several days of age to several weeks, especially in premature infants, and may be rapidly fatal. More commonly, it is found as a complication of other underlying diseases such as bacterial pneumonia, sepsis, hemolytic disease of the newborn, kernicterus, and central nervous system hemorrhage. A baby may have respiratory distress and bloody tracheal fluid from birth, or at several days of age may bleed with no premonitory signs. The sudden appearance of blood in the mouth and nose accompanied by extreme respiratory distress, often shock and rapid respiratory failure in a previously asymptomatic infant is a distressing and frustrating occurrence. Immediate blood transfusion may combat shock, and ventilatory assistance may tide the baby over the acute episode. Broad-spectrum antibiotics would seem to be indicated in view of the reported high incidence of associated pneumonia. Most cases fail to show specific clotting defects or other hematologic abnormalities, and no specific therapy is known at present.

CONGENITAL LOBAR EMPHYSEMA

Although the name "congenital lobar emphysema" implies prenatal origin (see the chapter on congenital anomalies of the lower respiratory tract), many instances of this entity are almost certainly acquired and have no primary congenital abnormality of the lung involved in their origin. As the name implies, overdistention of one or more lobes occurs, frequently the right upper or right middle lobe, because either intrinsic or extrinsic partial obstruction interferes with deflation of this particular area. Deficiency of the bronchial cartilage involving only one lobe may occur, and this, by failing to supply stability during expiration, produces overdistention of the parenchyma of the lung aerated by that bronchus. Partial intraluminal obstruction with associated lobar emphysema may occur as the result of aspirated foreign material, and extraluminal compression producing partial obstruction may be associated with a large variety of pulmonary and mediastinal masses such as bronchiogenic cysts, teratomas of the anterior mediastinum, neuroblastomas and cysts of the posterior mediastinum. Emphysema of the right lower lobe has also been seen in association with congenital cardiac disease in a newborn when high pressure in the pulmonary artery produced by a ventricular septal defect resulted in a greatly dilated pulmonary artery which, in the presence of a right aortic arch, was responsible for the partial bronchial obstruction.

Regardless of the demonstrable cause or lack of it, symptoms are similar. Wheezing occurs, in some instances from birth, in others only after weeks or months. The degree of respiratory distress depends largely upon compression of normally functioning lung by the overdistended lobe. Herniation of the affected lobe across the mediastinum may occur, the heart may be displaced, and the unaffected ipsilateral lobe may become atelectatic. X-ray examination of the chest shows increased radiolucence of the affected lobe, which, unless lung markings are seen, cannot easily be distinguished from a lung cyst (Figs. 13, 14). Cardiac displacement or atelectasis may be confirmed by x-ray study.

Treatment is dependent upon the severity of the respiratory difficulties. If

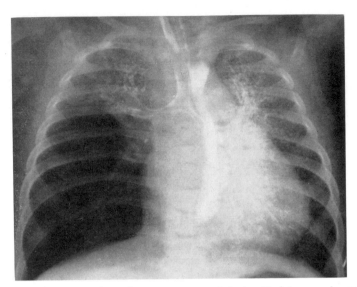

FIGURE 5–13. Bronchogram and esophagogram on an infant with lobar emphysema of the right lower lobe due to congenital heart disease. The infant had a right aortic arch and a large interventricular septal defect with pulmonary hypertension producing enough distention to compress the right lower lobe bronchus between the aorta and the pulmonary artery.

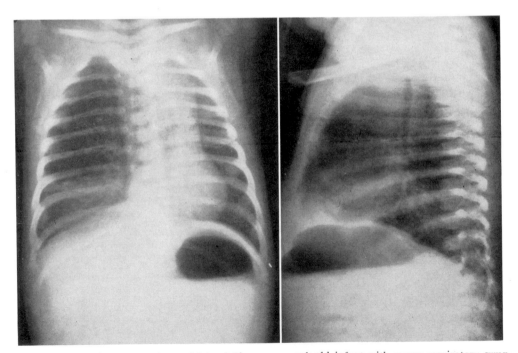

FIGURE 5–14. Anteroposterior and lateral films on a week-old infant with severe respiratory symptoms, showing lobar emphysema of the right upper lobe and compression of the right middle and lower lobes. No cause for the overdistention of the right upper lobe was found at operation.

severe respiratory distress and cyanosis are present, prompt bronchoscopy should be performed in order to remove any intraluminal obstruction. In most cases, however, surgical removal of the affected lobe will be necessary to provide relief. Asymptomatic babies may be watched for progression of the process, since some spontaneously regress.

LUNG CYSTS AND PNEUMATOCELES

Considerable controversy exists concerning the classification of lung cysts in small infants. (See the chapter on congenital anomalies of the lower respiratory tract.) Most agree, however, that true congenital cysts are rare in the newborn, and that most lesions formerly thought to be cysts were, in fact, pneumatoceles, probably resulting from staphylococcal pneumonia. Lung cysts lined with ciliated columnar epithelium do exist, however, but even so, their congenital origin is in doubt.

Bronchogenic cysts may occur in the lumen of a major bronchus, partially occluding it and producing lobar emphysema distally or completely occluding it with atelectasis. If present in the mediastinum, they may not be readily visible on routine x-ray films of the chest, but bronchography will help to identify their location. Wheezing, stridor and frequent bouts of infection are common.

A more common location for congenital cysts is in the periphery of the lung, where they may or may not communicate with bronchi. They may be single or multiple and contain cartilage and elastic tissue in their walls.

If symptomatic, congenital lung cysts should be surgically removed; they may constitute a surgical emergency. If asymptomatic, particularly if there is question of their differentiation from pneumatoceles, they may be followed clinically and roentgenologically and operation delayed until some future time after the infant has attained somatic growth.

Pneumatoceles, often of large size, occur with considerable frequency during the course of staphylococcal pneumonia in infancy. They occasionally occur with pneumonia associated with other organisms. Characteristic are their frequent change in size and their complete regression. Symptoms of lung compression are common, but if pneumatoceles are not infected and pus-containing, or life-threatening because of size or location, conservative management is advisable. The importance of the different natural histories of congenital and acquired lung cysts in infancy is stressed, since unnecessary major surgery can be avoided in many instances.

AGENESIS AND HYPOPLASIA OF THE LUNGS

Complete agenesis of both lungs, a single lobe or a single lung may occur. (See the chapter on congenital anomalies of the lower respiratory tract.) Agenesis of a single lung is more frequent and may be associated with other anomalies. The left lung is more apt to be absent than the right. The remaining lung and mediastinal structures shift into the empty cavity and fill both sides of the chest (Fig. 15). The trachea will be deviated toward the affected side, and evidence of dullness and diminished breath sounds are usually found. As the remaining lung herniates to the affected side, these latter signs may disappear. The existing lung is thought to be hypertrophied rather than emphysematous, and cyanosis will not exist, since no pulmonary vessels perfuse the affected side. No treatment is possible.

Hypoplasia of an entire lung or portion of it is usually associated with other congenital anomalies. With diaphragmatic hernias in which abdominal contents enter the chest cavity during intrauterine life, hypoplasia of the lung on the affected side may result, presumably from interference with lung growth. Pulmonary hypoplasia sometimes accompanies renal agenesis, or Potter's syn-

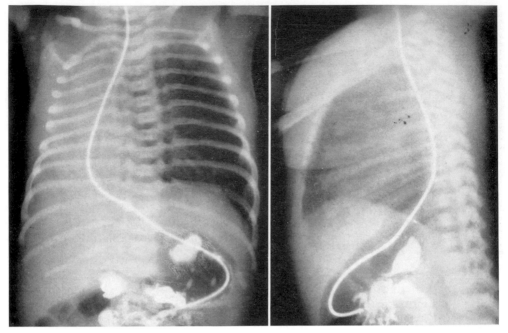

FIGURE 5–15. Anteroposterior and lateral chest x-rays taken on an infant 2 days after birth, showing agenesis of the right lung. A catheter is in the esophagus.

drome. These infants have a characteristic facies with epicanthal folds, flattened nose and low-set ears. Rarely a single hypoplastic lung will exist with systemic arterial blood supply and venous drainage into the inferior vena cava.

CONGENITAL DIAPHRAGMATIC HERNIA

A potentially correctable cause of neonatal respiratory distress is herniation of abdominal viscera into the chest cavity through a defect in the diaphragm. The most frequent site of herniation is the foramen of Bochdalek, situated in the posterior aspect of the diaphragm. The next most common site is the foramen of Morgagni just behind the sternum. The proportion of left-sided herniation is considerably more than on the right side, and both hollow and solid viscera may enter the chest. (See the chapter on congenital anomalies of the lower respiratory tract.)

Symptoms may be present from birth or may appear in the first days of life, or the defect may remain completely asymptomatic. Very early symptoms are related to the compression of pulmonary tissue by the herniated viscera. If parts of the gastrointestinal tract are herniated, vomiting may result, and signs of intestinal obstruction may appear as the lumen fills with gas and fluid.

Physical signs will depend upon the amount and consistency of herniated abdominal contents. In the case of solid viscera, dullness will be present over the affected side, whereas, if dilated loops of bowel fill the chest, hyperresonance may result. Bowel sounds may be heard over the chest on auscultation, and the abdomen is characteristically flattened. X-ray examination will usually be diagnostic, especially if gut is present (Fig. 16). The introduction of contrast medium in the bowel will confirm the diagnosis, but is seldom necessary or advisable.

The treatment is immediate surgical

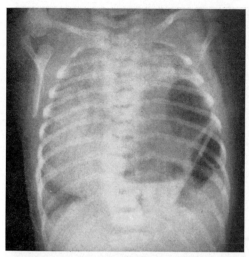

FIGURE 5–16. Anteroposterior x-ray of the chest of a newborn infant in severe respiratory distress, showing a diaphragmatic hernia through the foramen of Bochdalek with abdominal contents in the left chest cavity and displacement of the heart to the right.

replacement of abdominal viscera. The hazards of sudden death with delayed operation are considerable.

VASCULAR RINGS

A great number of variations in the embryologic development of the paired aortic arches occur, and some of them produce partial obstruction to the tracheo-bronchial tree. (See the chapter on congenital anomalies of the lower respiratory tract.) The most common anomalies found to be associated with such symptoms are double aortic arch, right aortic arch with ligamentum arteriosum, anomalous innominate artery, anomalous left common carotid artery and aberrant subclavian artery. Although many of these anomalies may not completely encircle the trachea and the esophagus, each may be capable of partially occluding them because of relatively fixed relations with other structures. Stridor, wheezing respiration and occasionally severe respiratory distress with cyanotic episodes, especially

when the head is flexed, are characteristic of these infants. They tend to lie with the neck hyperextended, a position which presumably allows less restriction of the airway. Partial obstruction of the esophagus is frequently manifested by inability to swallow ingested foods, especially solids, without regurgitation; aspiration pneumonia is a frequent complication. Newborn babies are rarely severely symptomatic, but symptoms appear to become worse in the first few months of life. Diagnosis of the degree of obstruction can be made by x-ray studies during instillation of contrast medium in the esophagus. The exact nature of the vascular anomaly may be elucidated by angiography if the obstruction is not ligamentous in part. Surgical correction of symptomatic lesions should be done early, since the point of tracheal compression may fail to develop properly and tracheal stenosis remain. Asymptomatic lesions may be ignored.

ESOPHAGEAL ATRESIA AND TRACHEO-ESOPHAGEAL FISTULA

Both esophageal atresia and tracheo-esophageal fistulas occur rarely as separate entities, but their occurrence in various combinations is frequent. The various possibilities are (1) esophageal atresia alone, (2) tracheo-esophageal fistula alone, (3) esophageal atresia with (*a*) upper fistula, (*b*) lower fistula or (*c*) double fistula. Type 3(*b*) accounts for 90 per cent of all defects of this sort seen. (See the chapter on congenital anomalies of the lower respiratory tract.)

The diagnosis is frequently first suspected when an alert nurse reports that a newborn infant has excessive mucus and cannot handle his secretions adequately. Suction will provide temporary relief, but secretions continue to accumulate and overflow, usually resulting in aspiration and respiratory distress. Feedings will likewise be regurgitated and frequently aspirated, and the chest be-

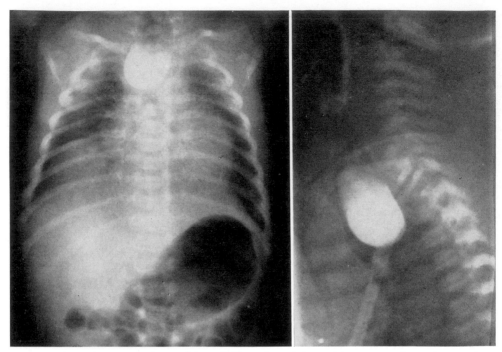

FIGURE 5—17. Anteroposterior and lateral films of an infant with a type 3(*b*) tracheo-esophageal fistula, showing the contrast-filled blind esophageal pouch and secondary aspiration pneumonia.

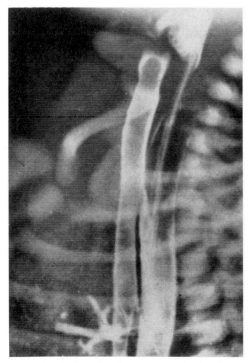

FIGURE 5—18. Simultaneous tracheal and esophageal filling with Lipiodol in an infant with an H type of tracheo-esophageal fistula, demonstrating the communication.

comes filled with rhonchi and coarse rales. In those infants in whom only esophageal atresia exists, the abdomen will remain flat, but if there is a fistula to the lower esophageal segment with or without esophageal atresia, the abdomen usually becomes distended with air, especially if the respiratory effort is great. The diagnosis can be made in those cases with esophageal atresia by attempting to insert a catheter into the stomach and introducing air through it while listening with a stethoscope over the left upper quadrant of the abdomen. If no sound of air entry into the stomach is heard, esophageal atresia is likely. A catheter curling in a blind pouch and thought to be in the stomach may be misleading.

X-ray film of the esophagus using a contrast medium harmless to the lung such as Lipiodol or Hytrast will confirm the presence of a blind pouch of esophagus and occasionally demonstrate the fistula as well (Fig. 17). In the case of a fistula without esophageal atresia the diagnosis may be difficult even after repeated x-ray examination. In such case cinefluorography with both trachea and esophagus simultaneously filled with contrast medium may be necessary (Fig. 18). Immediate surgical correction is indicated, since aspiration pneumonia, if not already present, is inevitable, and secondary infection is common. Even small prematures have survived with corrective surgery and careful postoperative management.

MICROGNATHIA WITH GLOSSOPTOSIS

Congenital hypoplasia of the mandible occurs with several of the so-called first arch defects such as Treacher-Collins syndrome and Pierre Robin syndrome, or may occur as an isolated lesion (see p. 169).

When micrognathia is severe and coupled with glossoptosis, intermittent episodes of dyspnea and cyanosis can occur, especially in association with the supine position. The tongue falls backward over the glottis, effectively obstructing the airway, and the harder the infant struggles, the more firmly the tongue is sucked against the air passage. Aspiration of feedings associated with inability to suck properly is also common. The immediate treatment is to place the infant in the prone position so that the tongue falls forward, and, as soon as is feasible, suture of the tongue to the soft tissue of the floor of the mouth, including the lower gum margin. This effectively prevents cyanotic attacks and allows the infant to feed properly; it can be loosened when the infant grows older and the mandible develops.

CHOANAL ATRESIA

Acute respiratory distress may present at birth if the nasal passages have failed to perforate and either bony or membranous obstruction remains. Such obstruction may be unilateral or bilateral. If it is unilateral, the infant may be symptomless, but if bilateral, mouth-breathing

is obligatory. Such infants usually have episodic bouts of acute respiratory symptoms, most often associated with feeding when mouth-breathing becomes intermittent. Choking spells and aspiration of feedings are frequent. The diagnosis, suspected when no air enters the chest with the mouth held closed, can be confirmed by inability to pass a small catheter through the nose into the nasopharynx and by failure to hear breath sounds on auscultation over the nares. Radiopaque material can be instilled into the anterior nasal cavity with the patient supine, and lateral films will demonstrate the point of obstruction. Tube feedings and an oral airway should be instituted as soon as the diagnosis is made.

Early surgical correction is usually advised in the case of bilateral obstruction, since aspiration pneumonia and respiratory acidosis are almost inevitable complications. This consists in perforation of the obstruction and introduction of obdurators followed by dilatation through either transnasal or transpalatal routes. (See Chapters 6 and 8.)

Surgical correction of unilateral choanal atresia can be deferred until a future elective time.

NONPULMONARY CAUSES OF RESPIRATORY SYMPTOMS IN THE NEWBORN

Central Nervous System Hemorrhage

There are several locations for bleeding into the central nervous system in the newborn which may give rise to respiratory symptoms. *Subdural hematomas* frequently occur in large infants associated with a long and difficult labor or manipulative delivery and are thought to be traumatic in origin. They usually present with focal or generalized signs of central nervous system irritation, such as tonic or clonic seizures, nystagmus or extensor spasms, and, except for apneic attacks of cyanosis associated with seizures, rarely present with respiratory symptoms.

In contrast, both *intraventricular hemorrhage* and widespread *subarachnoid hemorrhage* may present a difficult differential diagnosis with other forms of respiratory distress in the newborn, partly because they are most commonly seen in premature infants who may have asphyxia or hyaline membrane disease or in dysmature infants with signs of intrauterine aspiration pneumonia. Both types of hemorrhage are said to be due to anoxia. This is difficult to assess, since no specific hematologic defects are found in most instances and since respiratory depression and asphyxia at birth could be the result rather than the cause of the hemorrhage. Indeed, in many instances in which large intraventricular hemorrhages are found at autopsy, there seems to be a clear-cut history of the onset of central nervous system symptoms on the second or third day of life.

Irregular and periodic respiration followed by apneic attacks is frequent. Occasionally, however, hyperventilation occurs without x-ray signs of pulmonary disease, usually accompanied by a mottled, ashy gray cyanosis, shocklike picture and metabolic acidosis indicative of vascular collapse. Extensor spasms are common, but frank seizures are rare. As in other cases of central nervous system symptoms in the newborn, barbiturates and other analeptic drugs which depress respiration are contraindicated, and Dilantin is the drug of choice for the control of seizures. The carbon dioxide tension in the arterial blood in the absence of respiratory failure is low as a reflection of the extrapulmonary origin of the hyperventilation, and arterial oxygen unsaturation, if present, can usually be relieved by high oxygen inhalation in the absence of apnea or if ventilation is supported. Complete and sudden respiratory failure frequently occurs, but this may be modified by ventilatory assistance. If the infant with massive cerebral hemorrhage survives for several days, a fall in hematocrit value from the level at birth, jaundice of more than expected degree for the state of prematurity, and hyperkalemia may

be evidence of the amount of blood loss from the intravascular pool and subsequent extravascular blood destruction. Prolonged apneic attacks may lessen over several days to weeks if the infant survives, but the incidence of residual neurologic impairment is high.

When cerebral hemorrhage is an accompaniment of such pulmonary pathology as hyaline membrane disease or intrauterine aspiration pneumonia, the diagnosis is difficult and the prognosis grave. Infants who, because of pulmonary pathology, desperately need to hyperventilate to survive do not tolerate central depression of their respiratory stimuli, such as frequently occurs with cerebral hemorrhage. Understanding of the etiologic mechanisms of production, prevention and management of cerebral hemorrhage in the newborn presents one of the most currently challenging fields of our ignorance.

Congenital Cardiac Disease

Pulmonary Edema and Cardiac Failure

Relatively few congenital cardiac malformations present themselves with acute respiratory symptoms in the neonatal period. Infants with many of the varieties of cyanotic congenital cardiac defects which have severe cyanosis and acute dyspneic episodes associated with diminished pulmonary blood flow later in life are free from such symptoms in early infancy because of the persistence of the ductus arteriosus as a left-to-right shunt. Its persistence promotes the return of adequate amounts of oxygenated blood to the left atrium. Some of the most common cardiac anomalies to present with pulmonary symptoms in the neonatal period are aortic atresia with hypoplastic left heart, postductal coarctation of the aorta, and fibroelastosis. All these may present with moist rales, frank pulmonary edema and x-ray evidence of pulmonary vascular congestion (Fig. 19).

A much more subtle and gradually developing variety of heart failure is that associated with a persistently patent ductus arteriosus with a large left-to-right shunt. Frequently there is a history of respiratory distress in the neonatal period indistinguishable from classic hyaline membrane disease. Such an infant, often a premature, may be without any audible murmur for the first one or two weeks of life. When present, the murmur may initially be only systolic in timing. It usually becomes more typical and continuous as time goes on and the infant grows, expanding his blood volume and adjusting his pulmonary resistance to extrauterine life. The subtle and insidious onset of tachypnea and tachycardia is observable on the infant's graphic record, and dyspnea and fatigue associated with feedings appear. A rapid weight gain may be seen concomitant with clinical signs of edema. Such an infant usually responds well to digitalization, diuretics and, if symptoms are severe, added oxygen. Most such infants can be tided over without surgery at this age, and, if followed up, are, in the majority of cases, found to lose their murmur several months later. An occasional infant will have a persistent murmur with or without symptoms of intractable failure. In the presence of intractable failure, prompt surgical closure of the ductus is indicated.

The occurrence of transient pulmonary congestion and cardiac dilatation associated with birth asphyxia has been described. Serial chest x-rays strongly suggest that such is the case, and frank and sudden pulmonary edema has also been occasionally seen early in the course of severe hyaline membrane disease. It seems likely that intrapartum asphyxial damage to the heart, when followed by high oxygen inhalation associated with prolonged resuscitative measures or early oxygen therapy of severe hyaline membrane disease, could lead to a rapid fall in pulmonary vascular resistance. This, when associated with an unconstricted ductus arteriosus, could rapidly flood the lungs and, in the face of a weakened myocardium, allow left atrial pressure to rise and pulmonary vascular congestion and occasionally frank edema result. The low oncotic pressure of plasma in premature

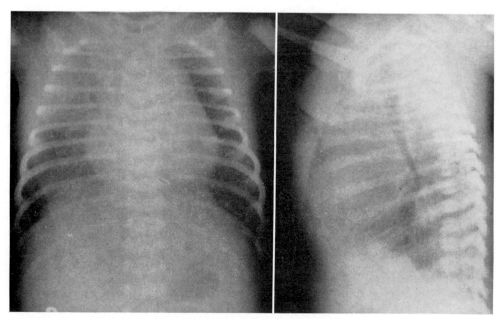

FIGURE 5–19. Anteroposterior and lateral chest x-rays of an infant with aortic atresia and hypoplastic left ventricle, showing pulmonary venous engorgement and pulmonary edema.

infants with low serum proteins would favor this.

Most episodes of pulmonary congestion associated with asphyxia clear as the infant regains acid-base balance and the myocardium improves. Infants with hyaline membrane disease in whom frank pulmonary edema occurs in the first few hours after birth usually run a course typical of severe and often fatal disease.

Acute pulmonary edema in the newborn from whatever cause should be treated with positive-pressure ventilation, oxygenation, correction of acid-base disturbance and rapid digitalization.

Paroxysmal Atrial Tachycardia

Paroxysmal atrial tachycardia can occur in the neonatal period and has even been diagnosed in utero with the fetal electrocardiogram. Most small infants with paroxysmal atrial tachycardia fall into a similar clinical picture. In most cases in this age group no etiologic factors are found. The majority are males. These acutely ill infants frequently present with the picture of pneumonia or septicemia. They are ashen gray with clammy, cold skin and shocklike appearance. Respiration is rapid and labored, and rales are usually heard. The heart is frequently enlarged and the rate so rapid as to be difficult to count. The liver is usually easily palpable, and peripheral and periorbital edema is apparent. The electrocardiogram shows a fixed rate usually greater than 200 per minute, and P waves are rarely identifiable. The QRS complex is normal, resembling that of the ventricular complex with a sinus rhythm, in contrast to that of ventricular tachycardia.

Vagal stimulation by unilateral carotid sinus pressure may be tried, but is only rarely effective in reverting the arrhythmia in small infants in congestive failure. Digitalis is considered to be the drug of choice at this age. Digoxin may be given over a twelve- to eighteen-hour period in a dosage of 45 to 60 micrograms per kilogram intramuscularly in three divided doses, with a maintenance dosage of one eighth the digitalizing dose twice daily

thereafter. Only rarely is it necessary to resort to Prostigmine, quinidine or procainamide, the latter two finding their principal use in paroxysmal ventricular tachycardia.

The change in clinical status in a small, desperately ill infant following digitalization is usually dramatic. The color improves, restlessness and cough disappear, and within twenty-four hours the baby begins to diurese. The heart size and liver size return to normal within a few days. Prophylactic digitalization should be continued for at least one month after reversion to a normal rhythm, at which time cessation can be attempted. If the supraventricular tachycardia recurs, digitalis should be resumed for an additional six months. The prognosis for small infants is usually good, since there is usually no evidence of underlying heart disease.

Pulmonary Symptoms Associated with Hemolytic Disease, Acute Hypervolemia and Hypovolemia

Infants born with severe hemolytic disease of the newborn may present with acute respiratory symptoms from a number of causes. In the case of massive hemolysis associated with hydrops fetalis, the anasarca is considered to be a manifestation of intrauterine heart failure due to extreme anemia. Such infants may, indeed, present in heart failure, the immediate treatment of which is exchange transfusion. Because of an already over-expanded blood volume, such exchanges should be small and frequent, and performed in such a way as to avoid further overloading of a failing cardiovascular system. Leaving a large deficit of blood exchanged in an attempt to lower venous pressure, however, may precipitate shock. In addition to anemia, many of these severely ill and dyspneic infants have profound metabolic acidosis associated with tissue hypoxia, with arterial pH levels below 7.0. Careful addition of buffers such as THAM to the exchange blood will rapidly improve the acid-base balance and help restore the circulatory status toward normal, since shock accompanies such low levels of pH.

An additional cause of respiratory symptoms in the newborn with hemolytic disease may be massive ascites, which, by elevating the diaphragm, severely limits ventilation. If such is apparent, abdominal paracentesis is indicated, care being taken to avoid the enlarged liver and spleen.

In the case of acute blood loss, respiratory symptoms and tachycardia may be disarmingly absent in the newborn until complete cardiovascular collapse supervenes. The treatment is immediate replacement of blood loss and search for its source, which may be obscure. Intrauterine bleeding from the fetal side of the placenta can occur either into the amniotic fluid or into the maternal circulation. In the latter case the presence of fetal hemoglobin in the maternal blood may demonstrate that such an event has occurred. Other occult hemorrhage such as intraventricular, from splenic rupture, or from ulceration of the gastrointestinal tract may occur in the neonatal period and be extremely difficult to diagnose or to localize. A delayed fall in hematocrit value accentuates this difficulty.

In the case of hypervolemia, which may occur as a baby-to-baby transfusion in the case of twins, or simply as a temporary overloading of the circulation with placental blood if the infant cries or gasps vigorously before the cord is clamped, mild to moderate respiratory symptoms may result, the tachypnea and tachycardia usually subsiding in a matter of hours as blood volume adjustments occur. If persistent symptoms of acute hypervolemia of this variety occur, a small phlebotomy may be indicated.

Neuromuscular Weakness as a Cause of Neonatal Respiratory Distress

Unilateral *paralysis of the vocal cords* in the newborn infant is most frequently seen on the left side, presumably from in-

jury to the recurrent laryngeal nerve at the time of birth. Bilateral paralysis is much less common and is thought to be central in origin. Symptoms are hoarseness and stridor, which may persist for several years. Laryngoscopy should be done to identify the lesion and to rule out other causes of stridor. In extreme cases a tracheostomy may be necessary.

Phrenic nerve paralysis also may occur at birth as the result of a difficult delivery. It is frequently associated with brachial nerve palsy, although it may occur as an isolated lesion. The right diaphragm is more often affected than the left. Symptoms, if present, consist of cyanosis, dyspnea and a feeble cry. Fluoroscopic examination for diaphragmatic motion confirms the diagnosis. Complications arise if the atelectatic lung becomes infected and may result in death. Plication of the diaphragm may be necessary in severe cases.

Weakness of the muscles of respiration, including the intercostals and the diaphragm in congenital myasthenia gravis, amyotonia congenita and poliomyelitis of the newborn, may result in severe hypoventilation and its consequences. Myasthenia may be transient if the infant is born to a myasthenic mother or persistent if born to a normal mother. Symptoms in the former may not appear until several days after birth. In either case they consist of weakness, feeble cry, and poor ability to suck and swallow. Ptosis is occasionally seen. A therapeutic trial with Tensilon (edrophonium chloride), 0.1 ml. subcutaneously, will confirm the diagnosis if improvement in strength occurs in ten to fifteen minutes.

Amyotonia congenita is a rare familial disease characterized by generalized and progressive skeletal muscle weakness with sphincter tone and with sensation intact. Involvement of the intercostal muscles and diaphragm leads to retraction and hypoventilation. No treatment is known.

Intrauterine and neonatal infection with *poliomyelitis* virus can likewise affect the muscles of respiration as well as other muscle groups. Central respiratory paralysis is also possible. Those infants with respiratory muscle involvement, if it is not permanent, might presumably be carried by ventilatory assistance much as those with neonatal tetanus, but so far none has been reported.

The prognosis of neonatal *tetanus*, once considered an almost uniformly fatal disease from respiratory failure, has recently been significantly improved by the successful use of ventilatory assistance combined with tracheostomy, curare, antitoxin and careful nursing care. Although a rare disease in the United States, it is extremely common in certain parts of the world where obstetrical practices may include deliberate contamination of the umbilical cord stump by material which frequently is spore-containing. In some instances it is contracted at the time of circumcision. The incubation period is usually short, and the infant begins to have severe tetanic seizures frequently associated with apnea. These become more severe and more prolonged, and the infant usually dies if ventilation is unassisted, despite other therapeutic measures. Positive-pressure ventilation through a tracheostomy combined with curarization has relieved cyanosis and hypoventilation, since the lung is normally compliant if not secondarily infected. Tracheostomies in small infants may become difficult to remove. If successful removal is accomplished after several months, residual deformity of the trachea may be left as a complication.

REFERENCES

Adamsons, K., Jr., Behrman, R., Dawes, G. S., James, L. S., and Koford, C.: Resuscitation by Positive Pressure Ventilation and Tris-Hydromethyl-Aminomethane of Rhesus Monkeys Asphyxiated at Birth. *J. Pediat.*, 65:807, 1964.

Avery, M. E.: *The Lung and Its Disorders in the Newborn Infant.* Philadelphia, W. B. Saunders Company, 1964, pp. 40-54.

Beinfield, H. H.: Ways and Means to Reduce Infant Mortality Due to Suffocation, Importance of Choanal Atresia. *J.A.M.A.*, 170: 647, 1959.

Boss, J. H., and Craig, J. M.: Reparative Phenomena in Lungs of Neonates with Hyaline Membranes. *Pediatrics*, 29:890, 1962.

Burnard, E. D., and James, L. S.: Atrial Pressures and Cardiac Size in Newborn Infants: Relationships, with Degree of Birth Asphyxia and Size of Placental Transfusion. *J. Pediat.*, 62:815, 1963.

Chun, J., and others: The Pulmonary Hypoperfusion Syndrome. *Pediatrics*, 35:733, 1965.

Cohen, M. M., Weintraub, D. H., and Lilienfeld, A. M.: The Relationship of Pulmonary Hyaline Membrane to Certain Factors in Pregnancy and Delivery. *Pediatrics*, 26:42, 1960.

Diament, H., and Kinnman, J.: Congenital Choanal Atresia. Report of a Clinical Series with Special References to Early Symptoms and Therapy. *Acta paediat.*, 52:106, 1963.

Edwards, J.: Malformations of the Aortic Arch System Manifested as "Vascular Rings." *Lab. Invest.*, 2:56, 1950.

James, L. S.: Acidosis of Newborn and Its Relation to Birth Asphyxia. *Acta paediat.* (Suppl. 122), 49:17, 1960.

James, L. S., and Adamsons, K., Jr.: Respiratory Physiology of the Fetus and Newborn. *New England J. Med.*, 271:1352, 1403, 1964.

James, L. S., Weisbrot, J. M., Prince, C. E., Holaday, D. A., and Apgar, V.: Acid-Base Status of Human Infants in Relation to Birth Asphyxia and Onset of Respiration. *J. Pediat.*, 52:379, 1958.

Kirschner, P. A., and Strauss, L.: Pulmonary Interstitial Emphysema in the Newborn Infant. Precursors and Sequelae. *Dis. Chest*, 46:417, 1964.

Nadas, A. S.: *Pediatric Cardiology.* 2nd ed. Philadelphia, W. B. Saunders Company, 1963, p. 236.

Saling, E.: Mikroblutun Tersuchungen am Feten: Klinischer Einsatz und este Ergebniose. *F. Geburtshilfe u. Gynäk.*, 162:56, 1964.

Smythe, P. M.: Studies of Neonatal Tetanus and on Pulmonary Compliance of the Totally Relaxed Infant. *Brit. M.J.*, 1:565, 1965.

Stahlman, M. T.: Treatment of Cardiovascular Disorders of the Newborn. *Pediat. Clin. N. Amer.*, 11:377, 1964.

Stahlman, M. T., Young, W. C., Gray, J., and Shepard, F. M.: The Management of Respiratory Failure in the Idiopathic Respiratory Distress Syndrome of Prematurity. *Ann. New York Acad. Sc.*, 121:930, 1965.

Usher, R., McLean, F., and Maughan, G. M.: Respiratory Distress Syndrome in Infants Delivered by Cesarean Section. *Am. J. Obst. & Gynec.*, 88:806, 1964.

SECTION IV

Disorders of the Nose, Mouth, Pharynx and Larynx

CHAPTER SIX

The Nose

WILLIAM E. LAUPUS, M.D.

The olfactory function of the nose is not highly developed in man, being primarily utilized in distinguishing odors which are pleasing from those which are not. The senses of taste and smell are so interrelated that foods may have an unpalatable flavor when nasal disease interferes with olfaction. Temporary distaste for food, and anorexia, may follow temporary reduction in olfactory acuity, thus accounting in part for the diminished appetite common to nasal disorders.

In conditions of health the nose is admirably adapted for its other functions of controlling the temperature and humidity and for removing the minute foreign substances and bacteria in inspired air. The nose may contribute as much as 1000 ml. of water daily to inspired air in the adult. After passage through the nose in the short time of 0.25 second or less, the air reaching the nasopharynx will have been conditioned to a relative humidity of 75 to 80 per cent and to approximately normal body temperature. The specialized ciliated pseudocolumnar epithelium is covered by a continuous layer of mucus (the "mucous blanket") which collects dust particles, pollens, bacteria and other tiny air contaminants on its surface. The cilia move the mucous blanket toward the pharynx at a rate of 10 mm. or more per minute, providing for replacement of the mucous coating about six times in each hour. Ciliary movement is continuous and little influenced by noxious influences other than removal of the moist mucous surface covering, which rapidly leads to injury of the ciliated cells.

The pH of the nasal secretions is maintained at a nearly constant level of 7; infection or local medication may alter the pH and reduce the effectiveness of natural barriers to infection. Although Fleming described a bactericidal enzyme, a lysozyme, capable of destroying bacteria on contact, present opinion differs as to the importance of the protection afforded by this substance. The principal contributions of the nose to defense against infection appear to be physical in nature: mucus, which separates infectious agents from the underlying mucosal cells, and ciliary action, which rapidly propels the mucus and its entrapped organisms to the pharynx, where it is swallowed and thence eliminated through the gastrointestinal tract.

MALFORMATIONS

Although normal variations in the size and conformation of the nose are great, structural abnormalities are uncommon. When the nasal bones are congenitally absent, the bridge of the nose fails to grow, and *nasal hypoplasia* results. *Hypertelorism,* in which the base of the nose is broad and the eyes are widely separated, results from overdevelopment of the lesser wings of the sphenoid; other congenital anomalies, including mental retardation, are frequently associated with hypertelorism. Congenital absence of the nose, single centrally placed nostril, complete

155

or partial duplication of the nose and other gross abnormalities occur in association with multiple defects in adjacent structures (cyclops, cebocephalus, anterior meningocele, conjoined partial twins and other variations of double monster classification); few, if any, of these latter anomalies are compatible with life.

A number of nasal malformations may result in nasal airway obstruction. *Membranous congenital atresia of the nares* has been described in the newborn. The alae nasi may be thin and so weakly supported that they cause inspiratory obstruction. The anterior septum may project into and occlude the alar opening. *Deviation of the nasal septum,* usually from trauma, varies in degree and is of infrequent clinical significance in childhood. When the nasal bones are narrowly separated, the airway may be sharply constricted. Children with narrow nares and high, narrow hard palates are particularly prone to recurrent and chronic nasal infections, sinusitis and otitis.

Membranous or bony atresia of the posterior choanae causes complete nasal obstruction and is worthy of special mention (see Chap. 8). When choanal occlusion is bilateral, the mouth must be kept open to permit air exchange. Because newborns adjust poorly to mouth-breathing, sucking and swallowing are performed with difficulty, and aspiration frequently occurs. Bilateral occlusion should be suspected whenever persistent mouth-breathing is seen in the newborn or when an infant who is pink and active while crying becomes cyanotic with the mouth closed. The diagnosis is confirmed if a catheter, sound or probe cannot be passed through the nasal passages into the pharynx. After instillation of a radiopaque substance into the nostril, the posterior obstruction will be substantiated radiologically. Unilateral atresia is associated with drainage anteriorly and is usually diagnosed after infection has occurred.

The definitive therapy of both the unilateral and bilateral forms of choanal atresia is surgical. When possible, operative correction should be delayed for several months to facilitate the best result. Such postponement is feasible if the infant tolerates an oropharyngeal airway and gavage feedings for the two or three weeks necessary to learn to mouth-breathe and to suck despite the nasal obstruction. Infants who cannot make these adjustments will require early surgical removal of the obstructing membrane or bone. Postoperatively, polyethylene tubing of appropriate size may be inserted to maintain patency of the new choanal orifice until healing has occurred.

Combined *cleft lip and palate* defects may be associated with multiple nasal deformities such as displacement of the alar cartilage, deficiency of the columella, elongation of the vomer, protrusion of the premaxilla, deviation of the septum and open communication between the nasal and oral passages.

Management and repair of palatal defects has become highly specialized; the timing of the surgical closure should be individualized in accord with the growth of the palate and the nasopharynx. The width of the defect, the palatal tissue available for repair, and the function of the palatal and pharyngeal musculature are factors which determine the time for optimum repair. Closure of the defect facilitates the management of the complications of cleft palate: chronic mechanical, chemical and infectious rhinitis, otitis media and dacryocystitis.

Correction of the cosmetic aspects of nasal septal deviations and other deformities is usually deferred until adolescence when bony, cartilaginous and soft tissue growth has been completed. In selected cases with appreciable nasal obstruction and deformity, conservative surgical procedures directed toward providing an adequate airway and correcting distortion may be undertaken in childhood in order to enable optimum growth of the nose and to prevent the development of greater deformity.

FOREIGN BODIES

Obstruction of one nostril by a small, solid object is a frequent occurrence in childhood. In the usual instance the foreign body is introduced by the child, whose unskilled attempts at removal force the object deeper into the naris, where it may lodge in the anterior vestibule or in the inferior meatus on the floor of the nose. Beads, buttons, stones, peas, beans, erasers, nuts, paper wads, marbles and cherry pits are objects which predominate. Some foreign bodies are hygroscopic and increase in size as water is absorbed.

Rhinoliths are special varieties of foreign bodies composed of insoluble salts derived from the nasal secretions; these salts are incorporated into a calcareous mass about a core such as a blood clot, mucus crust, dried pus or a small foreign body. Larvae of flies have also acted as foreign bodies when deposited in the nasal passages.

Initial symptoms consist in local obstruction with mild or no discomfort. Severe pain is unusual unless the object is large or irregular and sharp. Irritation from the foreign body leads to mucosal swelling and to greater obstruction. Infection often follows and is associated with a purulent or seropurulent discharge with a putrid odor. The drainage may be blood-tinged or frankly bloody if local ulceration and necrosis ensue. Rarely, perforation of the nasal septum may be a late complication of a long-standing foreign body reaction.

The combination of unilateral nasal obstruction and discharge should lead one to suspect the presence of a foreign body; the suspicion can usually be confirmed by examination through a nasal speculum. The foreign body should be removed promptly to minimize the danger of its aspiration into the larynx or tracheobronchial passages and to prevent local infection and necrosis. If the child is cooperative, topical anesthesia should suffice; general anesthesia is occasionally required for the frightened and anxious child who rebels when removal is attempted under local anesthesia. Simple instruments such as "alligator" forceps or a probe with a curved hook at the tip (crochet needle) and nasal suction apparatus suffice for the extraction of most foreign bodies. Saline (0.9 per cent) nose drops instilled four times daily for five days after removal will aid in cleansing the irritated mucous membranes. Most infections will subside spontaneously; if the discharge is persistent and a second foreign body is not identified, culture and appropriate antimicrobial therapy are indicated.

TUMORS

With the exception of nasal polyps, tumors in the nose and nasopharynx occur rarely in childhood. They are primarily of epithelial and mesenchymal origin. The usual signs by which they come to the physician's attention include nasal obstruction, external or locally invasive internal masses, enlargement of regional lymph nodes due to metastases, and occasionally facial asymmetry or disfigurement.

Nasal polyps are not neoplasms; they are pedunculated, edematous, mucosal swellings which present in the nasal cavity as smooth, pale, glistening, grapelike masses arising from the surfaces of the middle turbinates and the ostia of the ethmoid and maxillary sinuses. They may also be found within the maxillary sinus; they occasionally prolapse through the posterior choanae to obstruct one or both choanae. Polyps are of inflammatory (allergic) origin and cause symptoms which are difficult to separate from those of the associated allergic state. They are uncommon in patients with seasonal allergies. Nasal obstruction, excessive secretions and a feeling of pressure within the nasal passage are common complaints. Treatment consists in surgical removal and concomitant correction of the nasal allergy. Polyps frequently recur, especially when the underlying allergies are untreated or prove refractory to therapy.

Papillomas are tumors of epithelial origin arising from the mucosa of the nose or paranasal sinuses. *Adenomas* originate in the glandular portion of the nasal or sinal mucous membranes. When situated in the ethmoid sinus, they may cause bony erosion. Both papillomas and adenomas are nonmalignant, but tend to recur after surgical removal. The usual presenting symptom is nasal obstruction.

Angiofibromas (juvenile nasopharyngeal fibromas) are highly vascular, locally invasive, histologically benign nasopharyngeal tumors which occur almost exclusively in adolescent males. Palatal and facial deformity, including exophthalmos, commonly results from the expanding growth of these locally invasive neoplasms, which bleed easily and may cause severe epistaxis. Metastasis does not occur, but skull x-rays may demonstrate local invasion of adjacent cranial bones. Surgical removal may prove hazardous if excessive bleeding occurs during attempted resection. Irradiation may be helpful in controlling tumor growth, but bleeding may also complicate radiation therapy. The administration of androgens has been proposed as an adjunct to surgery or irradiation, but their value has not been clearly established. Postadolescent regression of the tumor has been rarely reported.

The combination of severe or repeated epistaxis with nasal obstruction in a boy of preteen- or teen-age should lead to the consideration of angiofibroma. The diagnosis can be confirmed by visualizing the tumor with a nasopharyngeal mirror and by biopsy, which should be undertaken only when adequate provision has been made for the control of hemorrhage and for blood replacement.

Nasal gliomas are unusual congenital tumors which histologically contain much glial and fibrous tissue and occasional neurons. When situated on the bridge of the nose, they are characteristically round and smooth and may be freely movable or fixed in the subepidermal tissues. They may superficially resemble hemangiomas. The intranasal gliomas are polypoid in appearance; a few have intracranial connections which qualify them for classification as encephaloceles. Detection of the intracranial component by radiologic and careful pathologic study is important; failure to do so may result in meningitis if the communication between the nose and the cerebral cavity is not recognized and is not properly repaired when surgical removal is undertaken. Incomplete resection is often followed by recurrence.

Lymphoepitheliomas are malignant tumors which infiltrate locally in a diffuse fashion and metastasize to the cervical lymph nodes. Histologically, they may be described as undifferentiated or transitional cell carcinomas or as lymphoepitheliomas; they may be difficult to distinguish from lymphosarcomas. The primary site of the tumor may be difficult to locate; cervical lymphadenopathy is often the earliest sign of the tumor. When the tumor infiltrates diffusely in the nasopharyngeal and palatal areas, change in speech or inability to open the mouth may be the presenting complaint. These tumors are radio-sensitive, and occasional cures have been reported, but the prognosis is generally poor.

Olfactory neuroepithelial tumors cause unilateral nasal obstruction and epistaxis. They are highly malignant, expanding by infiltration in the base of the nose or orbit (with exophthalmos). Histologically, they may resemble neuroblastoma, retinoblastoma or lymphoma. Long-term cures occasionally have followed surgical resection and postoperative irradiation.

Rhabdomyosarcomas may arise in the nasopharynx, but are more likely to originate in the orbit, causing exophthalmos. In young children the histologic appearance of the tumor is that of poorly differentiated embryonal cells. The neoplasm is highly malignant with extensive local invasion and regional and distant metastases. Terminally, the pathologic findings may be difficult to distinguish from acute stem cell leukemia. Combined surgical and irradiation therapy is occasionally successful in eradicating the tumor, but recurrence is much more commonly seen.

Osteomas, calcifying fibromas and teratomas occur even less frequently than the preceding tumors. The epidermoid carcinomas and adenocarcinomas which are the predominating malignancies of the nose and nasopharynx in the adult are seldom seen in childhood.

EPISTAXIS

Nosebleed is a common problem in childhood and occurs with increasing frequency after infancy. Males are more often affected. The source of the bleeding is usually obscure; a tiny bleeding point may be the only visible abnormality. Kiesselbach's vascular plexus on the anterior septum and the mucosa of the anterior turbinates are sites from which bleeding commonly arises. Bleeding originating in the posterior nares is usually of more serious import.

Causes include external trauma and injury from picking of the nose, nasal instrumentation, introduction of a foreign body or forcible blowing of the nose. Rhinitis, sinusitis, nasal allergy, polyps and adenoidal hypertrophy contribute to vascular congestion of the nasal mucosa and to increased frequency of epistaxis. Rheumatic fever, typhoid fever, scarlet fever, varicella, measles, influenza, diphtheria and malaria are associated with heightened susceptibility to nosebleed. Adolescent females occasionally bleed from the nose during menstruation. Vascular abnormalities (telangiectasias, varicosities), arterial hypertension, venous congestion secondary to increased venous pressure, and disorders of hemostasis are causes of serious hemorrhage from the nose. Highly vascular tumors such as angiofibromas may be responsible for serious and repeated epistaxes.

Treatment in most instances is directed toward local control of the hemorrhage, which can be accomplished by compression of the nares or by the insertion of packing. Selvage-edged petrolatum gauze packing ($\frac{1}{2}$ inch in width) is preferred. The gauze is inserted first into the upper posterior nasal cavity and then added anteriorly until the cavity is filled. The packing should be removed in twenty-four to thirty-six hours, and may be reinserted if significant bleeding recurs. Aqueous epinephrine solution (1:1000), topical thrombin and other hemostatic agents such as oxidized cellulose and thromboplastin may be useful occasionally. Placing the patient in an erect or semi-erect position with the head tilted forward facilitates clot formation and eliminates the annoyance of blood trickling posteriorly into the pharynx.

If bleeding is persistent, an anterior nasal pack should be inserted. When the site of bleeding cannot be found or when the bleeding originates in the posterior nares, combined anterior and postnasal or postchoanal packing is indicated. Obliteration of the bleeding site by cautery with silver nitrate or electrocoagulation is useful when bleeding has been controlled, but is seldom helpful when hemorrhage is active. Therapy with estrogens (orally or parenterally, or both) has not been proved to be of value. Ice packs to the nasal area and to the back of the neck are time-honored applications of dubious value in the control of serious hemorrhage. Sedation may be beneficial when anxiety contributes to the patient's discomfort. Hospitalization is indicated when bleeding is severe or underlying disease requires special therapy. Blood transfusion may be required when blood loss has been severe. The use of blood derivatives (platelets, fresh plasma, stored plasma, and the like) may be necessary to control bleeding in patients who have underlying disorders of hemostasis.

Comprehensive care of the patient with nontraumatic and persistent nosebleed implies careful search for underlying and contributing causes of epistaxis. The investigation should include complete history, physical examination and appropriate laboratory studies followed by specific preventive or corrective therapy wherever applicable.

ALLERGIC RHINITIS

The unique and distinguishing feature of the allergic (atopic) person is the capacity to produce antibodies (reagins) to antigens (allergens) to which the normal (nonallergic) person does not respond. The reagins are globulins with molecular weights in the range of 160,000 to 1,000,-000 (gamma$_1$ A and gamma$_1$ M globulin fractions); they are produced by plasma cells, one of the several "wandering" cells of the reticuloendothelial system. The allergens are commonly found in foods, inhalants and contactants. The emergence of allergic symptoms does not appear to be a simple response to a single antigen; rather it seems to depend upon the combination of genetic predisposition with dietary, inhalant, contactant, infectious, irritant and emotional factors, all of which contribute to the patient's reactivity in a seemingly cumulative fashion.

The most common and perhaps most characteristic atopic disorder is *seasonal allergic rhinitis* (hay fever). The common allergens are pollens, molds and house dust. Tree pollens produce symptoms of short duration in the spring of the year, grasses predominate in the summer, and ragweed prevails from August through October; house dust is most troublesome in the winter months, and molds occur throughout the year.

Perennial allergic rhinitis has no special seasonal occurrence. House dust, molds, feathers, danders and wool are the common offending antigens, but foods have also been implicated. In many children this disorder will not be considered to have an allergic basis because the more obvious nasal infections with which it is frequently associated obscure the allergic features. Chronic otitis media is often seen as a complication.

Allergic rhinitis is uncommon in children under five years of age, except in infants with food sensitivity, chiefly due to cow's milk, and in young children with sensitivity to dust and molds. Symptoms vary from mild nasal congestion to the classic combination of sneezing, itching of the nasal mucous membrane and profuse watery rhinorrhea with associated conjunctival involvement. The nasal mucosa is pale and edematous, and the conjunctivae may be reddened and swollen. If infection is present, the nasal mucosa is usually reddened and thickened.

The diagnosis of allergic rhinitis should be considered in any seasonal or perennial nasal disorder producing allergic mannerisms such as "wrinkling" the nose and mouth and rubbing the nose (the "allergic salute"), or complaint of itchy nose or palate. A careful history is fundamental to correct diagnosis, and in chronic or recurrent nasal disorders the family history and past allergic experiences should receive careful attention. The appearance of the nasal mucosa is often characteristic for nasal allergy, but the presence of infection may make differential diagnosis more difficult. Examination of nasal mucus for eosinophilia may be useful. An eosinophilia of 5 per cent or more is seldom seen in nonallergic persons. When infection is present, the eosinophile count is often normal. *Skin tests are useful, but are of little diagnostic value if they do not relate satisfactorily with the patient's history. Negative skin tests do not exclude allergic causation, although such findings decrease the likelihood of allergy.*

Treatment is dependent upon the symptomatology. Mild allergic rhinitis of seasonal nature may be satisfactorily controlled with one of the many available antihistaminic drugs. More severe seasonal or perennial allergic rhinitis will require comprehensive management, including the avoidance of exposure to the offending allergen(s) when possible. Careful attention to detail in evaluating and modifying the patient's environment may lead to the elimination or minimization of allergens in the home. Scratch or intracutaneous skin tests to determine and clarify specific sensitivities are indicated *before* desensitization is begun. Desensitization should be limited to situations in which allergens cannot be avoided or in which the environment cannot be sufficiently "decontaminated" to control symptoms. Allergic rhinitis requiring desensitization will usually be due to windborne pollens (trees, grasses, ragweed, and the like), house dust, molds or animal danders, or to combinations of these allergens. Bacterial vaccines are frequently used, but evaluation of the effect of these materials is difficult, and their value is often questionable. When coexisting infection is present, it should be adequately treated with an appropriate antibiotic for seven to ten days or until the pathogen is eradicated. The use of corticosteroid substances in the treatment of allergic rhinitis in children is *not* recommended. Administration of gamma globulin is indicated only in those situations in which true hypogammaglobulinemia has been demonstrated.

Increased vasomotor reactivity of the nasal mucosa to changes in the physical environment (cold, heat, variations in humidity) is usually designated *vasomotor rhinitis* to distinguish it from allergic rhinitis due to airborne allergens. Clinically, these conditions are similar, and the mucosal response in both is presumed to be mediated in a similar manner. In some patients nasal vasomotor instability and the accompanying sneezing or nasal congestion and rhinorrhea appear to be related to emotional states. Careful his-

tory and examination, extended when indicated to include investigation for infection (sinusitis) and diagnostic skin tests, will usually permit differentiation of these forms of rhinitis. Management of vasomotor rhinitis is often difficult if exposure to the causative elements cannot be avoided or reduced. Antihistaminic therapy is useful for temporary control of symptoms and discomfort.

REFERENCES

Arey, J. B.: Tumors of the Head and Neck. *Pediat. Clin. N. Amer.*, 6:367, 1959.

Boies, L. R., Hilger, J. A., and Priest, R. E.: *Fundamentals of Otolaryngology*. 4th ed. Philadelphia, W. B. Saunders Company, 1964.

Jackson, C., and Jackson, C. L.: *Diseases of the Nose, Throat and Ear*. Philadelphia, W. B. Saunders Company, 1959.

Lowell, F. C., and Franklin, W.: A Double-Blind Study of the Effectiveness and Specificity of Injection Therapy in Ragweed Hay Fever. *New England J. Med.*, 273:695, 1965.

Proctor, D. F.: Physiology of the Upper Airway; in *Handbook of Physiology*, Section 1, Respiration. Washington, D.C., American Physiological Society, 1964, Chap. 8, p. 309.

Vaughan, V. C., III: Allergic Problems in the Upper Respiratory Tract. *Pediat. Clin. N. Amer.*, 4:285, 1957.

Idem: The Allergic Disorders; in W. E. Nelson (Ed.): *Textbook of Pediatrics*. 8th ed. Philadelphia, W. B. Saunders Company, 1964, p. 1453.

Willis, R. A.: *The Pathology of Tumors in Children*. Springfield, Ill., Charles C Thomas, 1962.

CHAPTER SEVEN

The Mouth

LEROY SMITH, M.D.

In order to fully evaluate oral conditions occurring in infancy and childhood, one should not rely upon direct examination alone. A reliable history from the parents and older siblings as to development, habits and environment is helpful. Complete physical examination and x-ray and laboratory studies, including cultures, are necessary.

Direct examination of the oral cavity should progress in an orderly fashion. Beginning with the lips, the inspection proceeds into the mouth. The use of good illumination is of great benefit as one first examines the tongue, floor of the mouth, gums, teeth, cheeks, palate and pharynx. A close observation of muscular function and any areas of tenderness is of importance. With the finger, palpation of the structures will aid in the detection of submucosal masses and points of tenderness which may be hidden from the eye.

The development and the formation of the dental arches and the teeth should always be recorded. Early corrective treatment for dental malformations and disease may prevent a later, more serious problem.

Some of the rarer involvements of the oral cavity have been necessarily omitted in this discussion. For consideration of these, the reader is referred to a more comprehensive text.

CONGENITAL ANOMALIES

Congenital Lip and Commissure Pits

These indentations, apparent at birth, occur most commonly on the lower lip alone, but may be seen on both lips. They are usually bilateral and occur at an equal distance from the midline. In the beginning the pits are only 2 or 3 mm.

in depth, but because the mucosa at the base of the pit is rigidly attached to the underlying musculature by dense fibrous tissue, the indentation becomes deeper as the child grows. The invaginated mucosa appears to be normal. At the commissure the pits are usually smaller in diameter, although the depth may be greater. Treatment is necessary only from a cosmetic standpoint and consists in the surgical removal of the indented mucosa with primary closure of the wound. The results are usually satisfactory.

Congenital Fissures of the Commissure

A congenital fissure of the commissure of the mouth may be either unilateral or

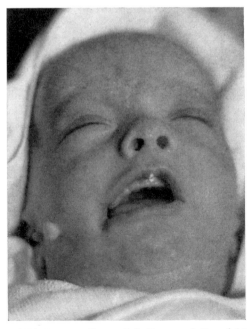

FIGURE 7–1. Congenital fissure of the right oral commissure.

162

bilateral, and may vary in size from that of a small separation to a cleft extending as far as the ear. In the latter condition the entire oral cavity on the affected side may be exposed. When the cleft is large enough to affect the function of the orbicularis oris, the child's ability to nurse or to retain fluids within the oral cavity is markedly reduced. Because of this feeding handicap, these deformities should be surgically corrected as early as possible.

Mandibular Cleft Lip

Separation of the two halves of the lower lip in the midline is rare and may involve either the lip or the lip and the bone. These children frequently have difficulty in retaining food or fluid in the mouth and become feeding problems. The treatment, which should be carried out as early as possible, consists in surgical closure of the cleft; if the mandible is involved, bone grafts to the center arch may be necessary.

Cleft Lip and Cleft Palate

Cleft of the upper lip with or without an associated cleft palate occurs in about

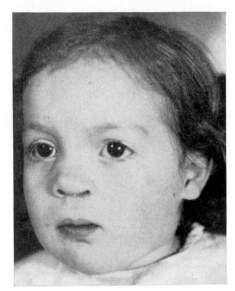

FIGURE 7–3. Repaired cleft lip.

one in every 800 to 900 births in the United States. It is more prevalent in the white race and slightly more frequent in males than in females. A family history of this deficit is obtained in approximately one fourth of the patients. In our experience the deformity seems to occur more often in children born of young parents and in the first child of the union. The occurrence of other congenital anomalies in those children with a cleft lip and cleft palate varies from 15 to 20 per cent. Complete rehabilitation of the child so affected will depend on the combined efforts of the pediatrician, the surgeon and the family. Not only must the deformity be corrected, but also satisfactory psychologic adjustment for the parents, and later for the patient, must be accomplished.

The formation of the face begins about the fourth week of pregnancy and is complete by the end of the twelfth week. Interference with the normal development of the fetus during this period may lead to cleft lip or cleft palate.

Cleft Lip

No universally accepted classification has been given to grade the degree of de-

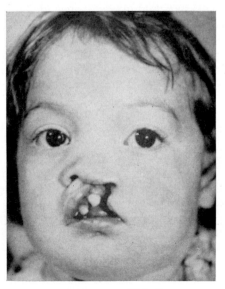

FIGURE 7–2. Cleft lip.

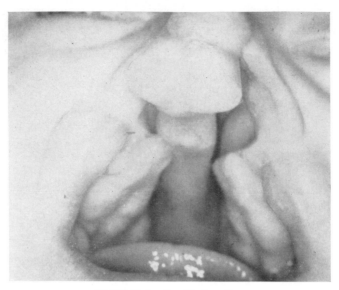

FIGURE 7–4. Double harelip.

formity encountered. The amount of deficient closure may vary from a small notching of the vermilion border to those clefts that extend into the nostril floor and through the alveolar ridge. The defect may be unilateral or bilateral (Figs. 2, 3, 4). In bilateral cases defects may be similar or dissimilar, with varying degrees of malformation on either side.

If the separation of the lip extends past the mucocutaneous junction, the child is usually unable to nurse at the mother's breast, and artificial means of feeding must be carried out by the use of some form of dropper technique. The mother should be carefully instructed in regard to the recommended method of feeding. It is often necessary for badly affected babies to be fed by a nasogastric tube during the first two to three weeks of life in order to prevent aspiration.

Repair of a cleft lip is usually accomplished at four to six weeks of age, although some surgeons operate during the first week of life and others wait until twelve weeks of age. Suffice it to say that the child should be in good general physical condition at the time of operation. Surgical revision is sometimes necessary later.

Cleft Palate

The formation of the hard and soft palates occurs some time between the seventh and twelfth weeks of pregnancy. Insult to the fetus during that period may result in cleft palate. The cleft in the palate may be either single or double and may or may not be associated with a cleft lip. The optimum time for surgical repair is not yet settled, but most surgeons prefer to operate when the child is twelve months to two years of age. Many surgeons now carry out preliminary procedures including prosthetic devices and bone grafting to close and stabilize the alveolar ridge in the young infant with cleft palate involving the alveolar ridge.

Speech therapy is usually indicated and, if so, should be instituted by the time the child is five years of age. At the first sign of the eruption of teeth, the child with a repaired cleft palate should be referred to a pedodontist. Psychologic treatment may be necessary.

Before closure of the defect in the palate, chronic irritation of the nasal mucosa by food is common. Secondary nasal infection, often with otitis media and lacrimal duct involvement, is a frequent

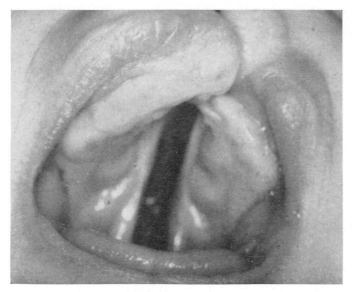

FIGURE 7–5. Cleft palate.

complication which may become chronic and troublesome to the patient.

Congenital Paralysis of the Palate

This condition is probably due to faulty innervation (glossopharyngeal). It is usually unnoticed for the first twelve to twenty-four months of life, since the development of the palate is not interfered with during this time. The first symptoms are the regurgitation of fluids through the nasal cavity and, as speech begins, a nasal quality of the voice. On physical examination an attempt at the elicitation of the gag reflex shows an inability of one side of the palate to be raised to the normal level. Treatment consists in a palatopharyngoplasty. In rare instances there may be a perfectly functioning soft palate which has not developed normally in length. Children with this condition also have a tendency toward a nasal voice and an inability to maintain fluids in the oral cavity when swallowing. Surgical correction by means of a pharyngeal flap is usually effective.

Congenital Anomalies of the Tongue

Ankyloglossia

The most common deformity of the tongue is ankyloglossia, or tongue-tie. In this condition there is a shortening of the lingual frenum so that the tip of the tongue is tied to the floor of the mouth or to the posterior surface of the lower anterior alveolar arch. Movement of the tip of the tongue may be so restricted by the tongue-tie that speech is or will be impaired; in such instances surgical release of the tie will be necessary. Milder forms will usually not require treatment.

Microglossia

This is a relatively uncommon condition in which there may be varying degrees of underdevelopment of the entire structure of the tongue. There is usually also an underdevelopment of the entire lower jaw and associated difficulty in sucking and in swallowing. Nasogastric feed-

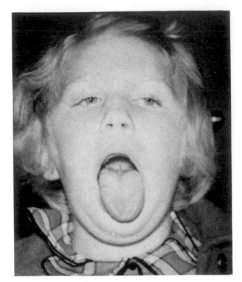

FIGURE 7-6. Macroglossia.

tongue begins to show definite signs of growth between twelve and eighteen months of age and in most instances will achieve normal size. Rarely, microglossia may continue into adult life.

Macroglossia

This is more common than microglossia and usually involves generalized muscular hypertrophy of the tongue. The hypertrophy may be so great that the patient is unable to contain the tongue within the oral cavity, and the tip protrudes beyond the lips while the mouth is held in an open position. In the more severe cases control of the tongue may be a problem. There may be hindrance to nursing and, in older children, to speech. Hemihypertrophy (Fig. 7) may also occur, but this is more frequently caused by defective lymphatics or by hemangiomas within the tongue musculature. These should be sought for and eradicated when found. In the management of generalized macroglossia the approach is a conservative one. When the hypertrophy is slight, there is usually no particular problem, but in severe cases resection of the excess musculature is indicated.

ings should be carried out until such time as the tongue has developed and normal swallowing can be accomplished; in some cases this may require several months. Strangulation and aspiration may be encountered, and, if this danger cannot be obviated by adequate nursing care, surgical attachment of the tongue in an anterior position will be necessary. Usually the

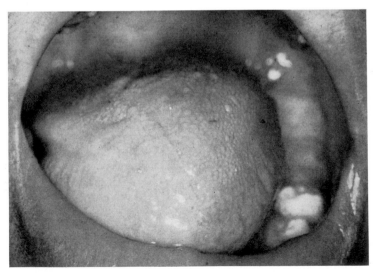

FIGURE 7-7. Congenital hemihypertrophy of tongue. (Courtesy of Dr. Richard P. Elzay, Medical College of Virginia School of Dentistry.)

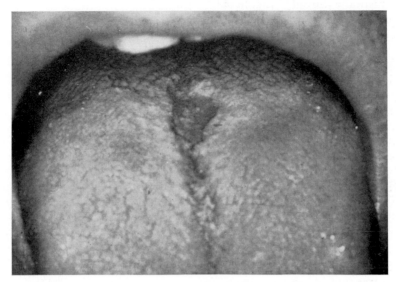

FIGURE 7–8. Median cleft of the tongue. (Courtesy of Dr. Richard P. Elzay, Medical College of Virginia School of Dentistry.)

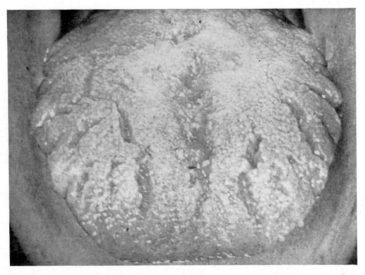

FIGURE 7–9. Fissures of tongue (scrotal tongue).

Thyroglossal Duct Cyst

A thyroglossal duct cyst may occur anywhere along the tract of the thyroglossal duct, which begins at the thyroid gland and passes medially through the hyoid bone and on upward to end in the foramen caecum of the tongue. Such a cyst may occur at any age. Although the majority appear in the portion of the duct below the hyoid bone, the duct occasionally becomes cystic in the posterior portion of the tongue. As the cyst enlarges, the tongue begins to project anteriorly. On examination there is a firm mass in the posterior portion of the tongue which cannot be reduced on pressure and, if sufficiently large, may actually interfere with swallowing. Treatment of this condition is surgical excision, which should be done as soon as possible.

Cleft of the Tongue

This is a rare anomaly in which there has been a failure in union of the two halves of the tongue, resulting in a shallow or sometimes rather deep cleft in the midportion of the tongue (Fig. 8). The cleft rarely may be complete. The tip is usually not involved. Symptoms are usually few, but in some instances food may become lodged in the deep fissure, causing some local irritation. In such an event surgical removal of the fissure is advisable. Multiple large crevices may occur in the tongue, and this condition is sometimes described as a scrotal tongue (Fig. 9). No treatment is required for this abnormality.

Median Rhomboid Glossitis

This congenital anomaly of the tongue is an oval or rhomboid-shaped, slick, reddish patch in the midline of the posterior portion of the tongue just anterior to the circumvallate papillae. Heavy coating of the papillae of the surrounding normal tongue mucosa makes this readily apparent; there are no papillae in the anomalous area, and such coating does not adhere to its surface. Actually, there is no infection, and therefore the term "glossitis" is a misnomer. There are no symptoms, and no treatment is necessary.

Hypertrophied Maxillary Frenum

This is an abnormal widening of the mucosa in the central portion of the upper lip where the maxillary labial frenum normally occurs. The excessive

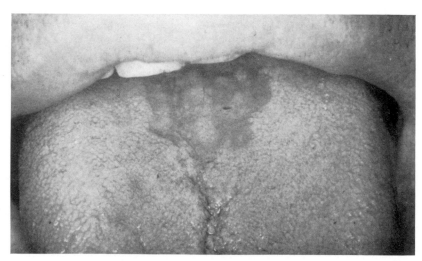

FIGURE 7—10. Glossitis rhomboidea mediana. (Courtesy of Dr. Richard P. Elzay, Medical College of Virginia School of Dentistry.)

width is frequently associated with a shortening of the frenum. At its gingival termination there is a hypertrophied band of fibrous tissue which extends across the gingival arch, and if the hypertrophy is extensive, there may be a resultant separation between the upper central incisor teeth when they erupt. The amount of separation depends upon the width of the arch and the size of the teeth. If nothing is done to correct such a marked hypertrophy of thick, fibrous tissue, the permanent teeth may be abnormally separated. If indicated, operation should be performed before the time of eruption of the permanent teeth. Some pedodontists disagree with this approach, preferring to delay operation until the central incisors have erupted and the degree of separation can be visualized.

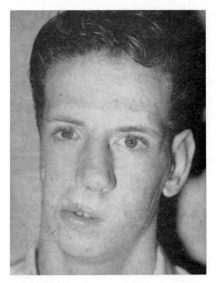

FIGURE 7–11. Congenital absence of the right half of the mandible and right ear.

Variations of Mandibular Development

Growth of the mandible occurs from the condylar cartilages. Practically no growth occurs at the chin. Disturbances at the growth site, whether congenital, the result of faulty blood supply or birth trauma, may lead to various deformities which usually make their appearance during infancy.

Henognathia

This denotes the absence of a part or all of either jaw. There may be absence of the condyle, ramus and condyle or absence of the entire half of the mandible. Complete absence of the mandible is rare. If an entire half of the mandible is missing, there is almost inevitably some defect in the external ear (Fig. 11). As development occurs there is distortion of the entire half of the face. There are no feeding difficulties. Correction of the absence of a portion of the mandible should be carried out by a bone graft around the age of ten years, but further correc-

tion is usually necessary when the patient attains adult life.

Micrognathia

In this condition either the mandible or the maxilla may be too small, but the mandible is more frequently involved. Although micrognathia is often observed at birth, in most instances the mandible seems to grow more rapidly and the lower jaw reaches normal size by the time the child is five to ten years of age. When the condition persists to such an extent that occlusion and the cosmetic appearance are grossly defective, corrective measures should be carried out. Orthodontic therapy should first be instituted, and if this is not successful in overcoming all the deformity, bilateral osteotomies, through the rami or sometimes through the body of the mandible, will usually correct the occlusion as well as the cosmetic deformity. When hypoplasia of the mandible is severe, there may be posterior displacement of the tongue. When there is an associated cleft palate, the condition is known as the Pierre Robin syndrome. Congenital hypoplasia of the mandible may also be present with the

Treacher-Collins syndrome (mandibulo-facial dysostosis). (See also Micrognathia with Glossoptosis, page 147.)

Macrognathia

When the jaws are larger than normal, the condition is termed macrognathia. Most frequent is involvement of the lower jaw, or prognathism. This may result from a generalized hyperplasia of the mandible or may be due to an increase in size of one portion of the mandible. The cause of macrognathia is not known, although heredity plays an important role. As the mandible increases in size, so do all the structures of the lower jaw. The difference in size of the two jaws usually continues to increase until early adult life, and rare cases have been reported in which the excessive growth of the mandible has been so great that mastication and speaking have become seriously affected. Surgical repair may be necessary, and if so, the most opportune time for correction is during the midteens.

Hemihypertrophy of the Mandible

This condition is usually associated with hemihypertrophy of the entire face and often of the entire body. Both jaws are usually affected, but the mandible may show greater enlargement than does the maxilla. In mandibular involvement one side develops at a much faster rate than the other, the teeth erupt sooner, the bone is thicker and wider, and there is frequently malocclusion on the hypertrophied side. There is no specific treatment. Orthodontia will be necessary, and surgical reduction of the bony hypertrophy may be helpful.

TUMORS OF THE ORAL CAVITY

Papillomas

These are benign tumors arising from the epithelium of the mucous membrane of the oral cavity. They may be flat or pedunculated, but are usually small, wartlike projections. They may occur on any portion of the epithelium, but in children they are most frequently found around the mucous membrane of the lips and on the surface of the tongue (Fig. 12). They may be either single or multiple. Irritation of a papilloma frequently causes bleeding and occasionally may result in infection. Although it has been asserted that these papillomas may be of

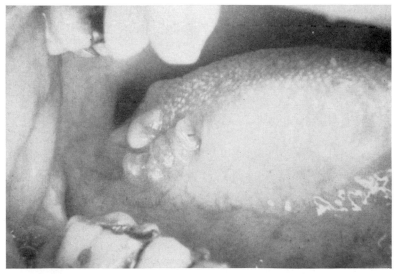

FIGURE 7–12. Papilloma of the tongue. (Courtesy of Dr. Charles Vincent, Medical College of Virginia School of Dentistry.)

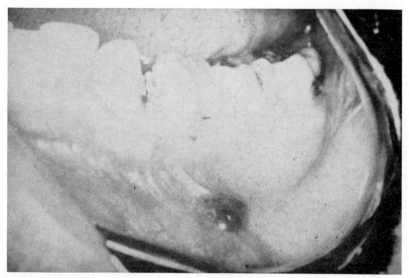

FIGURE 7–13. Nevus of the buccal sulcus. (Courtesy of Dr. Richard P. Elzay, Medical College of Virginia School of Dentistry.)

viral origin, there is no evidence to show that they can be transmitted from one person to the other. They may disappear spontaneously. Treatment consists in surgical excision or electrocoagulation, and in either event the pedicle at the mucous membrane level should be destroyed in order to prevent recurrence.

Pigmented Nevus

This does not usually occur on the mucous membrane; however, when it does occur, the most frequent sites are the lips and the palate. The more common types are the intradermal or the junctional nevus (Fig. 13), but occasionally amelanotic moles are found. The pigmented variety are usually brownish red with a slick surface and usually are only slightly elevated above the mucous membrane surface. The percentage of malignancy in these tumors has not been established, but malignancy is rare, particularly before the advent of puberty. Treatment is by surgical excision.

Fibromas

These benign tumors arise in the submucosal layers and in any of the connective tissues of the oral cavity (Fig. 14). They may lie completely beneath the surface of the mucous membrane or present as pedunculated, round, firm masses. They usually follow some chronic irritation or trauma to the submucous tissues. They are not painful, but continue to grow. The treatment is surgical incision.

Giant Cell Epulis

These connective tissue tumors derive from the periodontal membrane or from the periosteum of the bone surrounding the teeth and are usually due to chronic irritation of the tissues. Growth is rapid, and constant trauma may produce ulceration. If considerable size is attained, the tumor may extend along the gingival border surrounding several teeth so that the origin of the pedicle of the growth is obscured. There are no symptoms except for the occasional case in which ulceration occurs and secondary infection follows. The treatment includes removal of the growth and the tooth from which it originates. If the tumor is incompletely removed, recurrences are frequent.

Epulis granulomatosum tumors originate at sites of trauma or chronic irritation. These differ from the giant cell

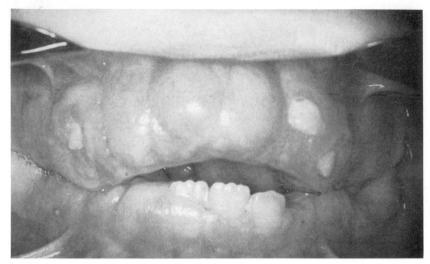

FIGURE 7–14. Fibroma of the gingiva. (Courtesy of Dr. Charles Vincent, Medical College of Virginia School of Dentistry.)

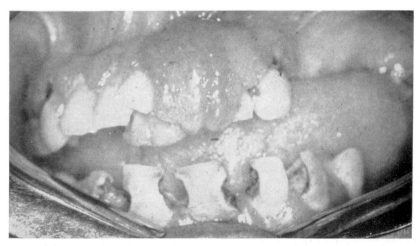

FIGURE 7–15. Giant cell epulis. (Courtesy of Dr. Charles Vincent, Medical College of Virginia School of Dentistry.)

tumor only in that the covering of the epulis granuloma is the same as that of the gingiva, while the giant cell tumor takes on a pinkish-red appearance and is highly vascular. The treatment is the same as that for the giant cell epulis.

Lipomas

These tumors consist of fatty tissue proliferation and may originate anywhere where fat is found in the oral cavity. The most frequent sites are the cheeks and the lips (Fig. 16). They are rare in children. The lesion is a slow-growing, rather firm, freely movable mass beneath the mucous membrane which produces no symptoms. Treatment is surgical incision. Recurrence is rare, although multiple lipomas may occur under the mucous membrane of the cheeks.

Hemangioma

Most hemangiomas are congenital and, although the oral cavity is not the usual site, may involve any portion of the mucous membrane or submucosal tissues (Fig. 17). They may vary in size from a small surface mucosal lesion to one which

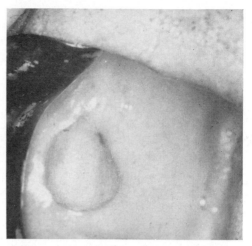

FIGURE 7–16. Lipoma of the cheek. (Courtesy of Dr. Richard P. Elzay, Medical College of Virginia School of Dentistry.)

covers practically all of the oral cavity. There have been many classifications of hemangiomas, but for clinical simplicity they may be grouped into two main categories—those of capillary origin and those which are cavernous (venous).

Capillary Hemangiomas

These angiomas are the result of the proliferation of small capillaries which occur in both the mucosal and submu-

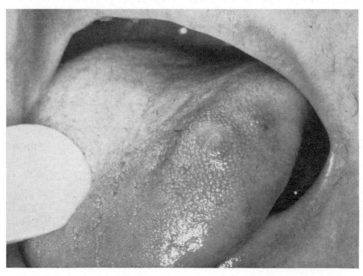

FIGURE 7–17. Hemangioma of mucosa and submucosa of tongue.

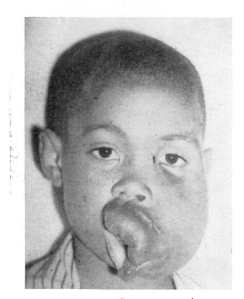

FIGURE 7–18. Cavernous angioma.

plished with little discomfort to the patient. Such treatment should be carried out every four to six weeks until the tumor has disappeared. Surgical excision should be used when the tumor is small or when there is submucosal involvement. Small submucosal tumors may be treated by the injection of sclerosing agents. The solution most often used is sodium tetradecyl sulfate (Sodium Sotradecol). Irradiation is effective, but the danger of excessive radiation and of local slough makes this a less desirable method of treatment.

Cavernous Angiomas

These tumors are composed of large, dilated venous lakes which have extremely thin walls. They may extend into the surrounding tissue, involving muscle, bone and in some instances the entire thickness of the cheek or lip (Fig. 18). These tumors do not undergo spontaneous resolution and, if untreated, cause widespread destruction of the soft tissue and the bone. If any portion of the tumor is traumatized from the inside of the oral cavity, serious hemorrhage may result. Whenever possible, the best treatment is surgical excision. If this is not practicable, the injection of sclerosing agents into the tumor may be effective. In some instances a combination of the two may be used.

cosal layers. The majority are present at birth, and between 85 and 90 per cent make their appearance by the end of the first year of life. The tumor is slightly raised and intensely red or bluish-red. On palpation it is soft and warm, and if extension has occurred into the submembranous layers, a noticeable bulge of the underlying tumor can be demonstrated. The chief characteristic of the capillary angiomas is rapid growth. If untreated, they will often double in size within a period of four to six weeks. If traumatized, profuse bleeding may result. Although it is true that capillary hemangiomas will undergo spontaneous involution, one is never certain as to when or whether this will take place. Since the oral cavity is a self-limited space, excessive growth of tumor may cause interference with feedings and the maintenance of an adequate airway.

The destruction of capillary angiomas may be accomplished in several ways— surgical removal, irradiation, the local use of carbon dioxide snow, and injection with sclerosing agents. If the lesion is superficial, the simplest treatment is the local application of carbon dioxide snow. If it is treated properly, little scarring results, and the procedure can be accom-

Lymphangioma

These tumors are benign and occur in lymphatic vessels. They may be simply a proliferation of lymphatic endothelial-lined spaces, or they may be cavernous. The simple lymphangioma is most common. This may involve the mucosa in any part of the mouth, but most frequently occurs on the tongue and the lips. The tumor appears as a group of small, raised vesicles covering a portion of the surface of the mucosa. Some are grayish, others translucent, and some are hemorrhagic. The growth of the tumor is slow as compared with that of the hemangioma. Occasionally the submucosal layers are involved and, particularly when there is involvement of the tongue, may cause considerable enlargement. Cavernous angiomas are more frequently found in the floor of the mouth and on the cheek. When present in the floor of the mouth, they may attain such considerable size that they affect the mobility of the tongue. The treatment of lymphangiomas is limited to surgical eradication, since irradiation is not effective. In the cavernous variety, sclerosing agents may be tried, but they are usually not successful. When there is such extensive involvement of the superficial membranes that surgical removal cannot be effectively carried out, destruction of the tumor by electrocoagulation may be adequate, although recurrences are frequent after this technique.

Benign Tumors of Bony Origin

Osteoma

Although simple osteomas do occur in the maxilla, palate or mandible (Fig. 19), they are not common. Clinically, this tumor presents as a bony prominence usu-ally placed along the normal cortical edge or plate of the bone. It is asymptomatic. Growth is slow, and x-ray film reveals a well defined, dense, bony nodule with no evidence of matrix. The treatment is surgical excision. If the tumor is completely removed, there is no recurrence.

Osteoid Osteoma

This is a benign tumor, possibly caused by trauma, which rarely occurs in the oral cavity. It is occasionally seen in children under the age of ten years (Fig. 20). Males are affected more often than females. The overlying mucosa is frequently tender and sometimes red. On x-ray examination there is a circular, dense area of bone with a translucent center. As growth continues, the surrounding sclerotic bone increases in size, and the center becomes larger. Calcification may arise in the translucent area in tumors of long standing. The treatment is surgical incision.

Fibro-osteoma

This is one of the most common benign tumors of the bone in children. It may

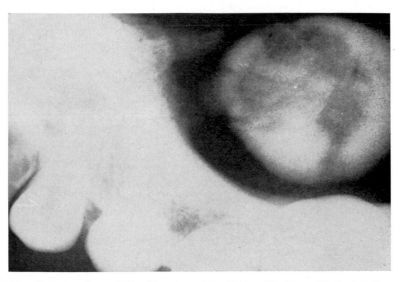

FIGURE 7–19. Osteoma of mandible. (Courtesy of Dr. Richard P. Elzay, Medical College of Virginia School of Dentistry.)

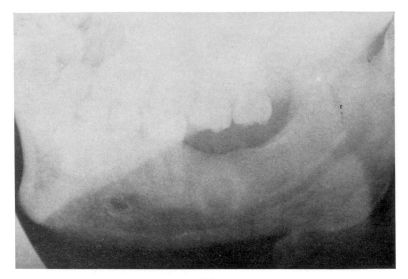

FIGURE 7–20.   Osteoid osteoma of mandible. (Courtesy of Dr. John I. Bowman, Jr.)

affect the maxilla and the mandible, but occurs most frequently in the mandible. The tumor grows somewhat slowly and usually involves the bone where teeth are present. One of the early symptoms is loosening of the teeth at the tumor site. As growth continues, there is a noticeable change in contour with asymmetry of the cortex as it is thinned out by the neoplasm. If the maxilla is involved, the tumor will frequently involve the maxillary sinus and cause an increased asymmetry in the cheek as the anterior walls of the sinus give way to the growth. In early tumors x-ray examination shows a translucent area within a well circumscribed, thin cortex wall. In more mature tumors small foci of bony trabeculae occur. As these increase, they produce an increasing reabsorption. Treatment is conservative surgical excision.

Bone Cysts of Dental Origin

A simple classification of odontogenic cysts is as follows:

1. Follicular cysts
    a. Primordial
    b. Dentigerous
2. Periodontal cysts
    a. Apical
    b. Lateral
3. Gingival cysts

All these cysts may occur in children.

Primordial Cysts

Multilocular or unilocular cysts result from some malformation in a normal enamel organ before any enamel forms. There are no appreciable symptoms until adjacent teeth become sensitive or loose. On x-ray examination the cyst presents a clear-cut margin and appears where a tooth should be, usually in the third molar area. Surgical removal is the treatment of choice, and there should be no recurrence.

Dentigerous Cysts

These cysts are the result of some malformation of the enamel organ after some portion of the enamel has formed. Usually only the crown of the tooth is present. The symptoms are the same as those of the primordial cyst. On x-ray examination some part of the tooth can be demonstrated within the cystic cavity. The treatment is surgical removal with extraction of the malformed tooth.

Apical or Periodontal Cysts

These cysts, sometimes called radicular cysts, occur around the root end of an erupted tooth. They result from infection, usually involving the pulp of the tooth. As growth occurs, the lesion may or may not give pain, depending upon its viability, but as the cyst increases in size, the affected tooth will inevitably become loose. The cortex of the bone may be eroded away as the tumor develops, and clinical examination may reveal a bulge. X-ray examination demonstrates that the borders of the cyst are clear-cut and surround the root of the tooth. Treatment is surgical removal, preceded by the extraction of the involved tooth. When a similar cyst develops after extraction of the tooth, it is termed a residual cyst, and the treatment is the same.

Radicular cysts may originate along the sides of a tooth, owing to periodontal infection. These are also called lateral cysts. The symptoms, development and the treatment are the same as for those of the apical cyst.

The gingival cysts (Fig. 22) arise from the dental lamina and are usually found in early infancy. They occur in the soft

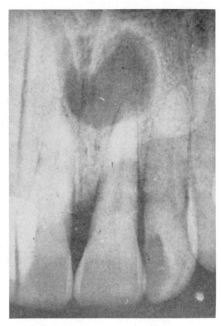

FIGURE 7–21. Apical cyst. (Courtesy of Dr. Charles Vincent, Medical College of Virginia School of Dentistry.)

tissue of the gingiva. They may occur on either side of the gum and appear as round nodules covered with normal-appearing epithelium. The treatment in older children is surgical removal. In infants, however, they usually undergo spontaneous degeneration and disappear.

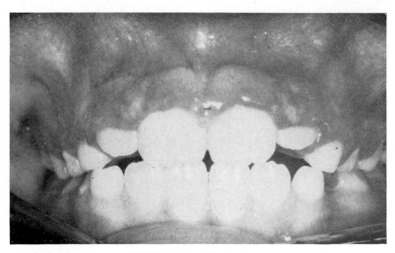

FIGURE 7–22. Gingival cysts.

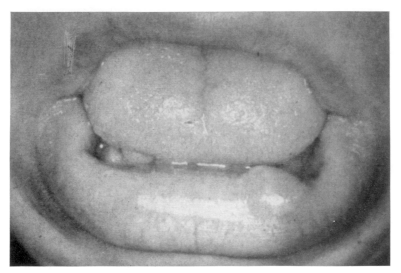

FIGURE 7–23.   Mucocele of the lower lip.

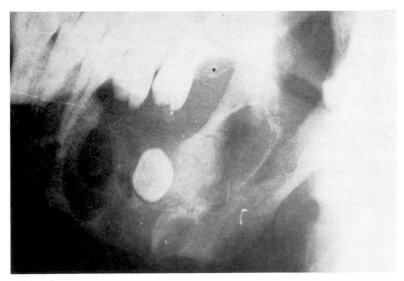

FIGURE 7–24.   Ameloblastoma of the mandible. (Courtesy of Dr. Phillip Peters, Medical College of Virginia School of Dentistry.)

Cysts of the Soft Tissues

Mucocele

These cysts result from closure of the duct of a mucous gland, leading to the retention of secretions of the gland and forming a cystic mass elevated above the overlying mucous membrane of the mouth (Fig. 23). If they are traumatized, hemorrhage may occur within the sac. The cysts may rupture spontaneously and disappear, only to recur after a varying period of time. Treatment is surgical removal.

Ameloblastoma

This tumor originates from the enamel organ of a tooth (Fig. 24). It usually occurs in persons between thirty and forty years of age, but is occasionally seen in children. The distribution between sexes is approximately equal. This tumor appears four times as often in the mandible as in the maxilla. When the maxilla is involved, the tumor usually occurs in the molar area or in the floor of the nose. When the mandible is involved, the ramus is most often affected.

Most pathologists consider the ameloblastoma to be a benign tumor, although malignancies occurring within the lesion have been reported. Clinically, the tumor may appear as a cyst or as a solid tumor. Growth is insidious, and there is usually no pain. Nevertheless, as the tooth-occupying bone is involved, the teeth may become painful and loose. It is a bone-destroying tumor, and as the growth breaks through into the soft tissues surrounding the involved bone, the cortex is usually thinned out, or in advanced cases an area may be completely eroded. Roentgen examination shows either a cystic tumor with multilocular areas throughout the involved bone and thinning of the cortex, or a solid tumor with the same picture except that the translucent appearance of the tumor on x-ray film is not as clear. Treatment consists in surgical removal of the neoplasm, with some area of the cortex left behind so that regeneration of the bone may occur. Recurrence after conservative surgical management is frequent, and some advocate a more radical treatment in which the entire surrounding normal bone is removed and the defect corrected with a bone graft at a later date.

Ranula

This is a retention cyst in either the submaxillary or sublingual ducts (Fig.

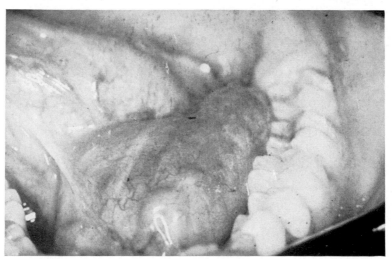

FIGURE 7–25. Ranula of the floor of the mouth. (Courtesy of Dr. S. Elmer Bear, Medical College of Virginia School of Dentistry.)

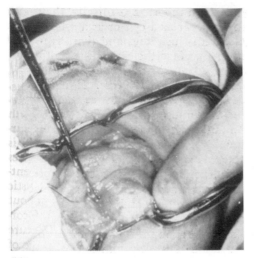

FIGURE 7–26. Dermoid cyst of the floor of the mouth.

25) and, therefore, occurs only in the floor of the mouth. Clinically, it is characterized by a slow-growing mass on one side or the other of the lingual frenum. As it bulges under the lining, it usually has a slightly bluish color. Except for its size, there are no particular symptoms. Treatment is by surgical marsupialization.

Dermoid

Dermoid cysts rarely occur in the oral cavity, but occasionally may be found in the floor of the mouth (Fig. 26). They are usually round, discrete nodules, beneath the mucous membrane and attached to the periosteum of the mandible. Growth is slow, and they cause no symptoms unless they attain considerable size. Treatment is surgical excision.

Fibromatosis of the Gingiva

This is a rare malady. Most of the reported cases seem to be hereditary, although this is not necessarily the case. It usually makes its appearance when the permanent teeth are erupting, but a few cases have been reported in early infancy. In the majority of instances both arches are affected, although, clinically, the upper arch seems to be affected earlier. At the onset there is a slow, progressive thickening of the gingival structure, and as time passes, the teeth are partially covered. In some instances the entire palatal area may be involved. Examination reveals a rigid, hard, nontender mass involving the entire gingival structure. The mucous membrane appears to be normal or slightly hyperemic. As the deciduous teeth are shed, there is a delay in the eruption of the permanent teeth because of the enlargement of the gingiva. Microscopic examination shows a dense, fibrous network overlying the bone and covered with apparently normal epithelium. If no treatment is undertaken, the child has difficulty in eating, and general debilitation ensues. Surgical excision of the excessive amount of fibrous tissue is the treatment of choice, but recurrence may be expected.

Malignant Tumors of the Oral Cavity

Most of the malignancies which occur in adults have been reported in children. Fortunately, they are rarely seen in the oral cavity. Early recognition and the prompt institution of appropriate therapy are paramount.

Fibrosarcoma

As in all cases of sarcoma, this tumor is found in the younger age groups. Although it may appear in any portion of the body, approximately one fifth of the cases reported are in the head and the neck. This neoplasm may occur anywhere in the oral cavity, and, though the rate of growth varies, it usually is fairly rapid in its invasion of the surrounding tissue (Fig. 27). The tumor is a solid, smooth mass adjacent to the overlying mucous membrane and is so firmly attached to the surrounding tissues that the borders of the growth are difficult to establish. Ulceration of the mucous membrane is

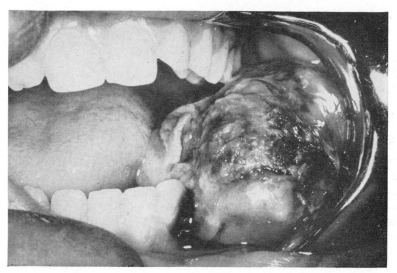

FIGURE 7–27. Fibrosarcoma of buccal sulcus. (Courtesy of Dr. S. Elmer Bear, Medical College of Virginia School of Dentistry.)

infrequent, but when it does occur, hemorrhage and secondary infection may follow. There are relatively few symptoms unless ulceration takes place. The tumor itself is not painful, and only after it has attained sufficient size to interfere with the function of the involved structures is there any complaint. Metastasis in fibrosarcoma apparently occurs late, thus giving it a much more favorable prognosis than that in most malignancies. The treatment is radical surgical removal of the tumor. If the tumor is readily accessible, one should expect a cure in 30 to 40 per cent of the cases.

Hemangioendothelioma

This neoplasm is of mesenchymal origin and is derived from the endothelial cells. It may occur anywhere in the body, and primary lesions of the oral cavity are occasionally seen. Because of similarity to the hemangioma, it is often misdiagnosed. The tumor resembles a capillary angioma and shows prominent capillaries extending along the surface of the mucous membrane with invasion of the submembranous tissues. The borders of the lesion are not circumscribed as they are in benign hemangiomas, and

the rate of growth is much faster. If the tumor is adjacent to bone, there frequently is early invasion. Metastases are infrequent, and the prognosis is fair. Treatment is radical surgical excision where the tumor is accessible, or the administration of x-ray.

Osteogenic Sarcoma

This is a rare neoplasm, but it may involve the bones of the face, particularly the mandible. It occurs in two forms, one an osteoplastic or sclerosing type and the other osteolytic. In the former there is an attempt at bone formation within the tumor, whereas in the latter there is no attempt at bone regeneration. Both tumors occur in young people. Occasionally there is a history of trauma before the onset of the tumor, but there is some question as to whether or not this is a factor in the causation. From the onset there is bone destruction at the periphery of the tumor, and in the osteoplastic type there are some attempts at bone formation within the tumor substance as represented by spotty spicules of calcification laid down throughout the mass. In the osteolytic type there is no evidence of this new bone formation, and therefore the diagnosis is not as clear-cut. A positive diagnosis can be made only by tissue biopsy. Metastasis in these tumors occurs early both by blood stream and by the lymphatic system. The prognosis, therefore, is extremely poor. Treatment is always by radical surgical excision.

Lymphosarcoma

This tumor is common to all age groups, and a relatively large number of cases occur in children. The majority of them occur in the male, the ratio being approximately two to one. About one fifth of all lymphosarcomas occur in the head and the neck. In the oral cavity the most frequent sites are the tonsils, palate, gingiva, buccal mucosa and the floor of the mouth. At the onset the tumor appears to be a single mass beneath the mucous membrane, showing invasive characteristics by the fact that it is early attached to the underlying structures. It is not painful at first, and the rate of growth is fairly rapid. In most instances, by the time the nodule is seen, there has already been evidence of lymph node metastasis. Pain does not occur until the tumor reaches considerable size. If invasion of the gingiva occurs, the teeth become loose and the gums bleed easily. Although ulceration does not occur until late, it will be seen eventually. These ulcers have irregular borders and become secondarily infected early, giving rise to a necrotic foul-smelling mass. At this time the tumor begins to grow above the level of the surrounding mucous membrane in a fungating pattern and is exceedingly friable, with hemorrhage from the growth resulting from the slightest trauma. The prognosis is generally hopeless in children. Because the tumor is extremely radio-sensitive, x-ray is the best method of palliative therapy.

Rhabdomyosarcoma

This malignant tumor arises in the skeletal muscle. Although it is rare, the majority of cases occur in children. The neoplasm may originate anywhere within the oral cavity where striated muscle exists, but the soft palate seems to be the most common site. The tumor first makes its appearance as a small, round, nontender nodule beneath the mucous membrane, and is fixed to the underlying muscle. As growth ensues, the mucous membrane overlying the tumor will be slightly lighter than that of the surrounding lining and, as infiltration of the tissues occurs, nodules appear. The growth of the tumor is relatively slow, and metastasis may occur at any time. Extension occurs by way of the lymphatics or by the blood stream. There are practically no local symptoms unless sensory nerves are involved, and in that case there may be soreness associated with the growth of the neoplasm. The accepted method of treatment is one of surgical excision. Early recognition of tumors of this type increases the chance of cure. Recurrences occur in 10 to 20 per cent of the cases.

INFECTIONS OF THE ORAL CAVITY

Syphilis

Acquired syphilis in children has become relatively rare since the advent of penicillin, but there are still cases which may demonstrate any one of the three intraoral manifestations. The primary stage is represented by a chancre which may occur on any part of the surface of the mucous membrane, but is more frequently present on the lip or tongue. This is a shallow, well circumscribed, painless ulcer, often with a bright red base. If no treatment is instituted, the chancre usually disappears in two to three weeks. The secondary or metastatic stage of the disease is represented by the so-called mucous patch. Whereas no part of the mucous membrane surface is exempt from these lesions, most of them are found on the lips or buccal mucosa. The lesion appears as a simple erosion of the mucous membrane surface covered by a silver-gray membrane and surrounded by a small area of inflammatory reaction. It is not painful. When the membrane is removed, the presence of the *Treponema pallidum* in the lesion can be demonstrated by darkfield examination. Other lesions of the secondary stage are condylomata (Fig. 28), which occur in the sulcus of both jaws and lips. These vary in size and are frequently detached by trauma with resultant mild bleeding at the point of attachment to the mucous membrane. Fissures occur at the angles of the mouth, and there may or may not be maceration of the skin and mucous membrane. All lesions of this phase disappear spontaneously. In late stages of syphilis, gummas may occur. These are found more frequently in the tongue and the tonsils. They are often confused with other tumors because they are submembranous and adhere to the underlying tissue. On palpation there is little tenderness, and they increase in size fairly rapidly. Ulceration of the gumma may occur, giving rise to a necrotic ulcer which causes pain when the secondary infection occurs. A positive diagnosis of any one of the three stages is best made from serologic examinations and, when possible, from darkfield studies.

Herpes Zoster

Herpes zoster (shingles) is an acute infection characterized by crops of vesicles. It is usually confined to a dermatome, and there is neuralgic pain in that area. The disease itself is relatively uncommon, but there is involvement within the oral cavity in approximately 15 per cent of the cases. Herpes zoster usually occurs in adults, and is relatively uncommon under ten years of age. The onset is usually associated with pain, and later burning and vesicular eruption on the membrane of the soft palate, tongue or buccal mucosa. It may be difficult to distinguish the vesicles from those of herpes simplex, but their occurrence over the distribution of the nerve is helpful. The lesions begin on a reddened mucosal surface, and as

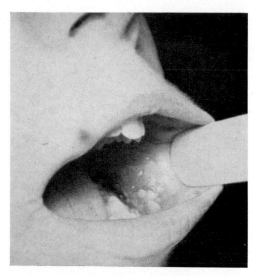

FIGURE 7–28. Condylomata of the left cheek.

the eruption continues, tiny vesicles measuring 2 to 3 mm. in diameter emerge from the surface membrane. These rupture, leaving shallow ulcerations which frequently become secondarily infected and thereby increase the pain already present. The duration of herpes zoster is usually measured in weeks, and if secondary infection has taken place, there is further delay in the healing. Treatment of the disease is symptomatic. Suitable antimicrobial therapy is suggested for any secondary infection.

Moniliasis

Moniliasis (thrush) is caused by the fungus *Candida (Monilia) albicans.* This fungus is a saprophyte in the normal oral cavity except in the newborn infant. The organism becomes pathogenic whenever there is sufficient impairment of tissue resistance; thus the disease is seen more often in weak, undernourished infants and children. Maternal vaginal moniliasis seems to be the main cause of infantile moniliasis, but cross-infection may result from poor nursery technique. Suppression of the normal flora of the oral cavity by long-term antibacterial therapy, especially with broad-spectrum antibiotics, may pro-

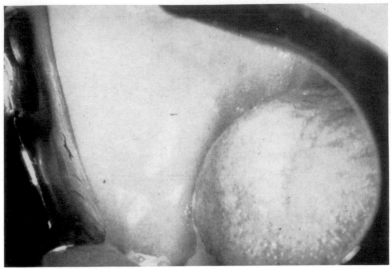

FIGURE 7–29. Moniliasis of the cheek. (Courtesy of Dr. Charles Vincent, Medical College of Virginia School of Dentistry.)

mote any fungal growth. Thrush develops on any membranous surface of the mouth and is characterized by soft, white, elevated plaques. These patches vary in size and frequently join to form large areas of involved membrane. A raw surface remains when the plaques are forcibly removed. The lesions are painless. Systemic symptoms are prominent only if the infection spreads beyond the oral cavity. Pneumonitis and esophagogastritis may occur, but extensive spread of the infection usually occurs only in infants with an underlying debilitating condition.

There is no completely effective therapeutic agent. Mycostatin, in a dosage of 200,000 units per milliliter applied locally with a soft cotton swab three or four times daily (with the remaining portion swallowed by the infant), the local application of 1 per cent aqueous gentian violet, or the local application of 1:1000 aqueous solution of benzalkonium chloride (Zephiran) is usually effective, but there may be recurrence with each of these therapeutic approaches.

Herpes Simplex

It has been estimated that *Herpesvirus hominis* is present in approximately 90 per cent of the adult population. The virus is usually latent, but infection may become manifest in two forms: (1) primary herpes simplex and (2) recurrent or secondary herpes simplex. In the former the first exposure of a susceptible host results in a subclinical infection without symptoms or in a general systemic reaction. Systemic infection usually occurs in a newborn infant or in a severely malnourished one. An infant with generalized disease may show fever or hypothermia, dyspnea, vomiting, jaundice, lethargy or convulsions. There may be hepatosplenomegaly, purpura and circulatory collapse. The disease is usually fatal; survivors may have chorioretinitis and mental retardation (see Aphthous Stomatitis, p. 186).

In the secondary (recurrent) form the lesions are localized, and little or no systemic reaction occurs. These lesions are considered to be the result of the activation of latent virus by such stimuli as gastrointestinal disturbances, emotional upsets, febrile reactions, foods, changes in environment or menstruation. They occur only in persons who have already had a primary infection.

The vesicular lesions, which occur more often about the lips, may appear gradu-

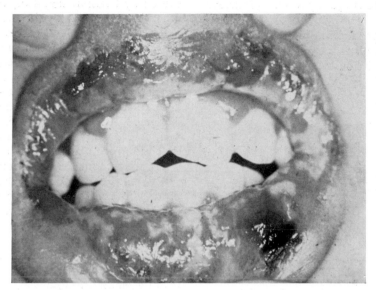

FIGURE 7–30. Herpes simplex. (Courtesy of Dr. Charles Vincent, Medical College of Virginia School of Dentistry.)

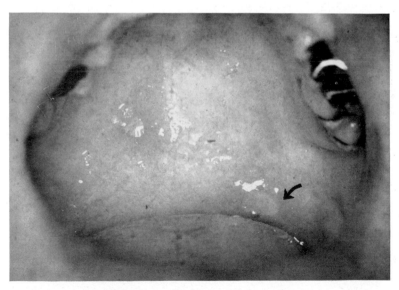

FIGURE 7–31. Recurrent aphthous ulcer.

ally over a period of several days. The vesicles rupture, and shallow ulcers are left. In time crusts cover the ulcerated areas, and healing takes place. The course of the disease is usually seven to fourteen days.

When the vesicles appear on the buccal mucous membrane, they may simulate recurrent aphthous ulcers (Fig. 31).

Treatment is symptomatic.

Aphthous Stomatitis

This condition is probably another manifestation of primary infection with *Herpesvirus hominis.* It is the commonest form of stomatitis in children between one and three years of age. The onset may be acute or insidious. There is pain, fetor oris, excessive salivation, fever, irritability, and refusal to eat.

The vesicular lesion ruptures early and leaves an ulcer covered with a yellowish-gray membrane. There is an associated gingivitis and regional adenopathy. The usual duration of the disease is ten to fourteen days, but the acute phase does not persist quite so long.

Gangrenous Stomatitis or Noma

Noma is a relatively rare disease which occurs in debilitated children. It may be caused by fusospirochetal organisms, but other bacteria such as the Streptococcus and Staphylococcus may be involved. The onset is sudden, and the lesion more often begins on the gingival border, but may occur on the buccal mucosa or mucocutaneous border. In the beginning there is a small ulcer. The tissues then become edematous, hard and grayish-blue with a line of demarcation between the gangrenous process and the normal tissue. The gangrenous process continues to spread until the cheeks are perforated; it attacks both soft tissue and bone. Specific antibacterial therapy should be intensive and prolonged until all necrotic tissue has sloughed. Supportive therapy is a necessity, and plastic surgery will usually be indicated when there has been complete healing of the process.

Pyogenic Granuloma

The exact cause of this disease is not known; it has been suggested, however,

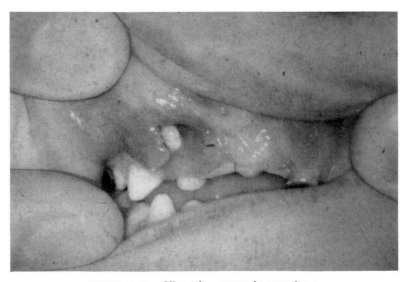

FIGURE 7–32. Ulcerating pyogenic granuloma.

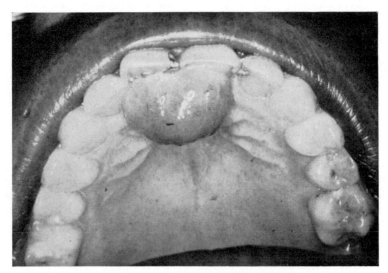

FIGURE 7–33. Pyogenic granuloma of maxillary arch.

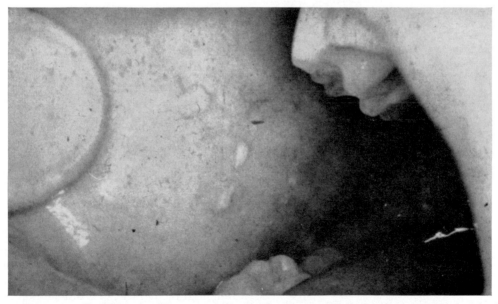

FIGURE 7–34. Koplik's spots. (Courtesy of Dr. Charles Vincent, Medical College of Virginia School of Dentistry.)

that it may be due to traumatic irritation of the mucous membrane whereby bacteria, such as the Staphylococcus or Streptococcus, may reach the deeper layers of the mucosa and then cause an overproduction of highly vascularized fibrous tissue (Fig. 32). Any age group may be involved. Clinically, there is a smooth, slightly elevated, pedunculated or flat mass on the surface of the mucosa (Fig. 33). As development ensues, the superficial layers desquamate, leaving a rather shallow, irregular, dirty gray membranous ulcer. Depending upon the degree of vascularity, irritation may or may not produce easy bleeding. The intact mucous membrane around the lesion becomes a red or reddish-purple. The granulomas develop rapidly for a short period and persist for long periods of time. They are rarely tender. Treatment consists in surgical excision and improvement of the oral hygiene.

ORAL MANIFESTATIONS OF SYSTEMIC DISEASES

Measles (Rubeola)

In the prodromal phase of the disease there is a generalized swelling of the soft palate with a red mottling over the hard and soft palates. So-called Koplik's spots precede the appearance of that rash by one or two days. These Koplik's spots, the pathognomonic sign of measles, are bluish-white or grayish-white dots (Fig. 34) surrounded by an area of hyperemia. They are not elevated. The lesions tend to occur on the buccal mucous membrane opposite the lower molars, but may occur anywhere on the buccal mucosa. They disappear rapidly.

Chickenpox (Varicella)

The mucosa of the oral cavity is frequently involved in chickenpox. The pharyngeal wall is usually involved first, and later there may be involvement of much of the mucous membrane of the oral cavity. The lesions may first appear as small clear vesicles approximately 1 mm. in size. These rupture, and the resulting ulcerations are covered with a yellowish membrane. The mucous membrane between the lesions is intensely red, and the whole area becomes extremely painful. As the lesions spread over the entire oral cavity, the child usually refuses to eat or drink. These lesions gradually subside in seven to ten days. No local treatment is indicated.

Diphtheria

See the chapter on The Pharynx, page 201.

Metabolic Diseases

Vitamin A

The oral manifestations of vitamin A deficiency are primarily hyperplasia and keratinization of the gums. If this deficiency occurs to a serious degree before the sixth year, disturbance of tooth formation may occur.

Vitamin B Complex

The oral manifestations of vitamin B deficiency are usually those of the entire vitamin B complex. There is usually dryness, increased pain, and then burning of the lips. Fissures appear at the angles of the mouth, and the lining within the oral cavity becomes increasingly red and thickened. The tongue is somewhat swollen. Generally, the papillae are swollen and mushroom in shape, but as the deficiency increases, the papillae take on an atrophic appearance. Swallowing becomes increasingly painful. Superficial ulcerations along the margins of the tongue may occur. They vary in size and have irregular borders. The gums bleed easily, and secondary gingivitis is a common finding.

Vitamin C

Vitamin C deficiency is characterized by hypertrophy of the gums, which are soft and spongy and bluish red. These changes are most noticeable when the teeth have erupted. Slight pressure or irritation of the gums may cause bleeding. The teeth become loosened, and if the deficiency persists, actual loss of several or all of the teeth may occur.

Vitamin D

Vitamin D deficiency will produce enamel hyperplasia and hypertrophic gingivitis.

Vitamin E

There is no known oral manifestation of vitamin E deficiency.

Vitamin K

Vitamin K deficiency gives rise to increased bleeding whenever there is trauma to the oral cavity.

ACUTE INFECTIONS OF FASCIAL SPACES

Acute infections of the oral cavity are common. If the bacteria are extremely virulent or are resistant to antibiotics, any focus within the mouth may readily spread to the soft tissues of the face and neck. Acute cellulitis with gross edema and firmness of the tissues ensues. The invading organism is usually either a Staphylococcus or a Streptococcus. Within a matter of hours the patient becomes acutely ill with high fever. When cellulitis is not controlled, septicemia and death may result. Sometimes acute inflammatory processes begin in and are confined to the fascial spaces surrounding the oral cavity. Such involvement requires prompt diagnosis and treatment.

REFERENCES

Abramson, P. D.: Bilateral Congenital Cleft of the Lower Lip. Surgery, 31:761, 1952.

Allen, A. C.: Juvenile Melanomas of Children and Adults and Melanocarcinomas of Children. Arch. Dermat., 82:325, 1960.

Archer, W. H.: Lymphangioma of the Lips. Oral Surg., Oral Med. & Oral Path., 4:170, 1952.

Austin, L. T., Jr., Dahlin, D. C., and Royer, R. Q.: Giant-Cell Reparative Granuloma and Related Conditions Affecing the Jawbones. Oral Surg., Oral Med. & Oral Path., 12:1285, 1959.

Bauer, W. H., and Bauer, J. D.: The So-Called "Congenital Epulis." Oral Surg., Oral Med. & Oral Path., 6:1065, 1953.

Bernick, S.: Growths of the Gingiva and Palate. I. Chronic Inflammatory Lesions. II. Connective Tissue Tumors. III. Epithelial Growths. Oral Surg., Oral Med. & Oral Path., 1:1029, 1098, 1948; 2:217, 1949.

Bhaskar, S. N.: Oral Tumors in Infancy and Childhood. A Survey of 293 Cases. J. Pediat., 63:195-210, 1963.

Bhaskar, S. N., and Akamine, R.: Congenital Epulis (Congenital Granular Cell Fibroblastoma). Oral Surg., Oral Med. & Oral Path., 8:417, 1955.

Blackfield, H. M.: Lateral Facial Clefts. Plast. & Reconstr. Surg., 6:68, 1950.

Blair, V. P.: Surgery and Diseases of the Mouth and Jaws. A Practical Treatise on the Surgery and Disease of the Mouth and Allied Structures. 2nd ed. St. Louis, C. V. Mosby Company, 1913.

Blair, V. P., and Brown, J. B.: The Dieffenbach-Warren Operation for Closure of the Congenitally Cleft Palate. Surg., Gynec. & Obst., 40:309, 1934.

Boies, L. R., Peterson, R. G., and Waldron, C. W.: Osteogenic Sarcoma of the Maxilla; Report of a Case. J. Oral Surg., 4:56, 1946.

Broadbent, T. R., and Swinyard, C. A.: The Dynamic Pharyngeal Flap. Plast. & Reconstr. Surg., 23:301, 1959.

Bromberg, B. C., Pasternak, R., Walden, R. H., and Rubin, L. R.: Evaluation of Micrognathia with Emphasis on Late Development of the Mandible. Plast. & Reconstr. Surg., 28:537, 1961.

Brown, J. B., McDowell, F., and Byars, L. T.: Double Cleft of the Lip. Surg., Gynec. & Obst., 85:20, 1947.

Bruce, K. W., and McDonald, J. R.: Chondroma of the Tongue. *Oral Surg., Oral Med. & Oral Path.*, 7:1281, 1954.

Bruce, K. W., and Royer, R. Q.: Lipoma of the Oral Cavity. *Oral Surg., Oral Med. & Oral Path.*, 7:930, 1954.

Brucker, M.: Studies on the Incidence and Cause of Dental Defects in Children. III. Gingivitis. *J. Dent. Res.*, 22:309, 1943.

Brunner, H.: Eosinophilic Granuloma of Mouth, Pharynx, and Nasal Passages. *Oral Surg., Oral Med. & Oral Path.*, 4:623, 1951.

Burford, W. N.: Lymphosarcoma of the Soft Palate. *Am. J. Orthodont. & Oral Surg.*, 33:24, 1947.

Burket, L. W.: *Oral Medicine*. Philadelphia, J. B. Lippincott Company, 1946.

Burket, L. W., and Hickman, G. C.: Oral Herpes Manifestations. *J.A.D.A.*, 29:411, 1942.

Burnett, G. W., and Scherp, H. W.: *Oral Microbiology and Infectious Disease*. 2nd ed. Baltimore, Williams & Wilkins Company, 1962.

Cadham, F. T.: Vincent's Disease: Infection Due to Fuso-spirillary Invasion. *Canad. M.A.J.*, 17:556, 1927.

Cahn, L. R., and Bartels, H. A.: Apthae and Herpetic Gingivostomatitis. *Am. J. Orthodont. & Oral Surg.*, 28:140, 1942.

Callister, A. C.: Hypoplasia of the Mandible (Micrognathia) with Cleft Palate: Treatment in Early Infancy by Skeletal Traction. *Am. J. Dis. Child.*, 53:1057, 1937.

Calnan, J. S.: Movements of the Soft Palate. *Brit. J. Plast. Surg.*, 5:286, 1953.

Campbell, J. A. H.: Congenital Epulis. *J. Path. & Bact.*, 70:233, 1955.

Canick, M. L.: Cleft Lip and Cleft Palate—A Review of Embryology, Pathologic Anatomy and Etiology. *Plast. & Reconstr. Surg.*, 14:30, 1954.

Chapple, C. C.: Abnormalities of Infants Resulting from Non-genetic Factors. *Postgrad. Med.*, 7:323, 1950.

Christensen, R. W.: Lymphangioma of the Tongue; Report of a Case. *Oral Surg., Oral Med. & Oral Path.*, 6:593, 1953.

Christiansen, G. W.: Lymphosarcoma of the Jaws and Palate. *J.A.D.A.*, 25:728, 1938.

Christopherson, W. M., Foote, F. W., Jr., and Stewart, F. W.: Alveolar Soft-Part Sarcomas. *Cancer*, 5:100, 1952.

Comerford, T. E., Jr., and others: Nevus of the Oral Cavity. *Oral Surg.*, 17:148-51, 1964.

Converse, J. M.: *Reconstructive Plastic Surgery*. Philadelphia, W. B. Saunders Company, 1964.

Conway, H., and Goulian, D., Jr.: Experiences with the Pharyngeal Flap in Cleft Palate Surgery. *Plast. & Reconstr. Surg.*, 26:590, 1960.

Cook, T. J.: Oral Tumors, Benign and Malignant. *Oral Surg., Oral Med. & Oral Path.*, 4:2, 1951.

Cooke, B. E. D.: The Giant-Cell Epulis: Histogenesis and Natural History. *Brit. D.J.*, 93: 13, 1952.

Coventry, M. B., and Dahlin, D. C.: Osteogenic Sarcoma. *J. Bone & Joint Surg.*, 39A:741, 1957.

Crikelair, G.: Early Orthodontic Movement of Maxillary Segments Prior to Cleft Lip Repair. Presented at American Society for Cleft Palate Rehabilitation, Montreal, Canada, 1961.

Cronin, T. D.: Surgery of the Double Cleft Lip and Protruding Maxilla. *Plast. & Reconstr. Surg.*, 19:389, 1957.

Dahlin, D. C., Coventry, M. B., and Scanlon, P. W.: Ewing's Sarcoma. *J. Bone & Joint Surg.*, 43A:185, 1961.

Davis, A. D.: Median Cleft of the Lower Lip and Mandible. *Plast. & Reconstr. Surg.*, 6:62, 1950.

Davis, A. D., and Dunn, R.: Micrognathia: Suggested Treatment for Correction in Early Infancy. *Am. J. Dis. Child.*, 45:799, 1933.

Davis, J. S.: The Incidence of Congenital Clefts of the Lip and Palate. *Ann. Surg.*, 80:363, 1924.

Davis, J. S., and Ritchie, H. P.: Classification of Congenital Clefts of the Lip and Palate. *J.A.M.A.*, 21:322-3, 1922.

Davis, W. B.: Harelip and Cleft Palate. *Ann. Surg.*, 87:536, 1928.

Dodd, K., Johnston, L. M., and Buddingh, G. J.: Herpetic Stomatitis. *J. Pediat.*, 12:95, 1938.

Dorrance, G. M., and Bransfield, J. W.: Cleft Palate. *Ann. Surg.*, 117:1, 1943.

Idem: The Push-Back Operation for the Repair of Cleft Palate. *Plast. & Reconstr. Surg.*, 1: 159, 1946.

Douglas, B.: The Treatment of Micrognathia Associated with Obstruction by a Plastic Procedure. *Plast. & Reconstr. Surg.*, 1:300, 1946.

Dunn, F. S.: Management of Cleft Palate Cases Involving the Hard Palate. *Plast. & Reconstr. Surg.*, 9:108, 1952.

Englart, R. J., and Leuin, I. S.: Diffuse Osteofibromatosis: A Symptom Complex. *Oral Surg.*, 7:837, 1954.

Epstein, C. M., and Zeisler, E. P.: Chancre of the Gingiva. *J.A.D.A.*, 20:2228, 1933.

Farber, S.: The Nature of "Solitary or Eosinophilic Granuloma" of Bone. *Am. J. Path.*, 17:625, 1941.

Fogh-Anderson, P.: *Inheritance of Harelip and Cleft Palate*. Copenhagen, Nyt Nordisk Forlag, Arnold Busck, 1942.

Foss, E. L., Dockerty, M. B., and Good, C. A.: Osteoid Osteoma of the Mandible. *Cancer*, 8:592, 1955.

Foster, T. D.: Maxillary Deformities in Repaired Clefts of the Lip and Palate. *Brit. J. Plast. Surg.*, 15:182, 1962.

Fraser, F. C., and Fainstat, T. D.: Causes of

Congenital Defects. *Am. J. Dis. Child.*, 82: 593, 1951.

Freiberger, R. H., Loitman, B. S., Helpern, M., and Thompson, T. C.: Osteoid Osteoma: A Report on 80 Cases. *Am. J. Roentg., Rad. Ther. & Nucl. Med.*, 82:194, 1959.

Garn, S. M., and Hatch, C. E.: Hereditary General Gingival Hyperplasia. *J. Hered.*, 41:2, 1950.

Glickman, I.: Fibrous Dysplasia in Alveolar Bone. *Oral Surg., Oral Med. & Oral Path.*, 1:895, 1948.

Idem: Acute Vitamin C Deficiency and Periodontal Disease. *J. Dent. Res.*, 27:201, 1948.

Graber, T. M.: The Congenital Cleft Palate Deformity. *J. Am. Dent. A.*, 48:375, 1954.

Green, M. C. L.: Speech Analysis of 263 Cleft Palate Cases. *J. Speech & Hearing Dis.*, 25: 43, 1960.

Hagerty, R., and Hoffmeister, F. S.: Velopharyngeal Closure. An Index of Speech. *Plast. & Reconstr. Surg.*, 13:290, 1954.

Harkins, C. S., Berlin, A., Harding, R. L., Longacre, J. J., and Snodgrasse, E. M.: A Classification of Cleft Lip and Palate. *Plast. & Reconstr. Surg.*, 29:31, 1962.

Hiatt, W. H., and Orban, B.: Hyperkeratosis of the Oral Mucous Membrane. *J. Periodont.*, 31:96, 1960.

Hine, M. K.: Fibrous Hyperplasia of Gingiva. *J. Am. Dent. A.*, 44:681, 1952.

Holdsworth, W. G.: *Cleft Lip and Palate*. 3rd ed. New York, Grune & Stratton, Inc., 1963.

Hollander, L., and Goldman, B. A.: Syphilis of the Oral Mucosa. *D. Digest*, 40:135, 1934.

Huebsch, R. F.: Gumma of the Hard Palate, with Perforation; Report of a Case. *Oral Surg., Oral Med. & Oral Path.*, 8:690, 1955.

Hutter, R. V. P., Worcester, J. N., Jr., Francis K. C., Foote, F. W., Jr., and Stewart, F. W.: Benign and Malignant Giant Cell Tumors of Bone. A Clincopathological Analysis of the Natural History of the Disease. *Cancer*, 15:653, 1962.

Idem: Stomatitis and Gingivitis in the Adolescent and Preadolescent. *J.A.D.A.*, 44:37, 1952.

Ivy, R. H.: Congenital and Acquired Defects and Deformities of the Face and Jaws: Review of Literature for 1936. *Internat. Abstr. Surg.*, 64:433, 1937.

Johnson, A. E., Stenstrom, K. W., and Waldron, C. A.: Multiple Lymphosarcoma (Lymphoblastoma) of the Oral and Cervical Regions. *J. Oral Surg.*, 4:159, 1946.

Jolleys, A.: A Review of the Results of Operations on Cleft Palates, with Reference to Maxillary Growth and Speech Function. *Brit. J. Plast. Surg.*, 7:229, 1954.

Keith, A.: Congenital Deformities of the Palate, Face, and Neck. *Brit. M.J.*, 2:310, 1909.

Kernahan, D. A., and Stark, R. B.: A New Classification for Cleft Lip and Cleft Palate. *Plast. & Reconstr. Surg.*, 22:435, 1958.

Kerr, D. A.: Stomatitis and Gingivitis in the Adolescent and Preadolescent. *J. Am. Dent. A.*, 44:27, 1952.

King, J. D.: Nutritional and Other Factors in "Trench Mouth," with Special Reference to the Nicotinic Acid Component of the Vitamin B_2 Complex. *Brit. D.J.*, 74:113, 1943.

Kiskadden, W. S., and Dietrich, S. R.: Review of the Treatment of Micrognathia. *Plast. & Reconstr. Surg.*, 12:364, 1953.

Krogman, W.: The Problem of the Cleft Palate Face. *Plast. & Reconstr. Surg.*, 14:370, 1954.

Kruger, G. O.: *Textbook of Oral Surgery.* St. Louis, C. V. Mosby Company, 1959.

LeMesurier, A. B.: A Method of Cutting and Suturing the Lip in the Treatment of Complete Unilateral Clefts. *Plast. & Reconstr. Surg.*, 4:1, 1949.

Idem: The Operative Treatment of Cleft Palate. *Am. J. Surg.*, 39:458, 1938.

Lichtenstein, L., and Jeffe, H. L.: Eosinophilic Granuloma of Bone. *Am. J. Path.*, 16:595, 1940.

Lighterman, I.: Hemangioendothelioma of the Tongue; Report of Case. *J. Oral Surg.*, 10: 163, 1952.

Litzow, T. J., and Lash, H.: Lymphangiomas of the Tongue. *Proc. Staff Meet., Mayo Clin.*, 36:229, 1961.

Logan, W. H. G., and Kornfeld, R.: Development of the Human Jaws and Surrounding Structures from Birth to the Age of Fifteen Years. *J.A.D.A.*, 20:379, 1933.

Love, F. M., and Fashena, G. F.: Eosinophilic Granuloma of Bone and Hand-Schuller-Christian Disease. *J. Pediat.*, 32:46, 1948.

Meyer, G., Roswit, B., and Unger, S. M.: Hodgkin's Disease of the Oral Cavity. *Am. J. Roentg., Rad. Ther. & Nucl. Med.*, 81:430, 1959.

Moore, O., and Grossi, C.: Embryonal Rhabdomyosarcoma of the Head and Neck. *Cancer*, 12:69, 1959.

Moran, R. E.: The Pharyngeal Flap Operation as a Speech Aid. *Plast. & Reconstr. Surg.*, 7:202, 1951.

Olin, W. H.: *Cleft Lip and Palate Rehabilitation.* Springfield, Ill., Charles C Thomas, 1960.

Padgett, E. C.: The Repair of Cleft Palates Primarily Unsuccessfully Operated Upon. *Surg., Gynec. & Obst.*, 63:483, 1936.

Padgett, E. C., and Stephenson, K. L.: *Plastic and Reconstructive Surgery.* Springfield, Ill., Charles C Thomas, 1948.

Peer, L. A., Strean, L. P., Walker, J. C., Bernhard, W. G., and Peck, G. C.: Study of 400 Pregnancies with Birth of Cleft Lip-Palate Infants. *Plast. & Reconstr. Surg.*, 22:442, 1958.

Pindborg, J. J.: Fibrous Dysplasia or Fibroosteoma. *Acta. Radiol.*, 36:196, 1951.

Pruzansky, S., and Richmond, J. B.: Growth of the Mandible in Infants with Micrognathia. *Am. J. Dis. Child.*, 88:29, 1954.

Rappaport, I., and others: The Significance of Oral Angiomas. *Oral Surg.*, 17:263-70, 1964.

Rise, E. N.: Dermoid Cyst of the Tongue and Floor of the Mouth. *Arch. Otolaryng.* (Chicago), 80:12-15, 1964.

Robin, P.: Glossoptosis Due to Atresia and Hypotrophy of the Mandible. *Am. J. Dis. Child.,* 48:541, 1934.

Rush, B. F. J., Chambers, R. G., and Pavitch, M. M.: Cancer of the Head and Neck in Children. *Surg.,* 53:270-84, 1963.

Schour, I., and Massler, M.: Gingival Disease (Gingivosis) in Hospitalized Children in Naples (1945). *Am. J. Ortho. & Oral Surg.,* 33:757, 1947.

Shafer, W. G., Hine, M. K., and Levy, B. M.: *A Textbook of Oral Pathology.* 2nd ed. Philadelphia, W. B. Saunders Company, 1963.

Ship, I. I., Ashe, W. K., and Scherp, H. W.: Recurrent "Fever Blister" and "Canker Sore." Test of Herpes Simplex and Other Viruses with Mammalian Cell Cultures. *Arch. Oral Biol.,* 3:117, 1961.

Ship, I. I., Merritt, A. D., and Stanley, H. R.: Recurrent Aphthous Ulcers. *Am. J. Med.,* 32:32, 1962.

Smith, J. B.: Cancer of the Floor of the Mouth. *J. Oral Surg.,* 6:85, 1948.

Smith, J. L., and Stowe, F. C.: The Pierre Robin Syndrome (Glossoptosis, Micrognathia, Cleft Palate). A Review of Thirty-Nine Cases with Emphasis on Associated Ocular Lesions. *Pediatrics,* 27:128, 1961.

Stammers, A. F.: Vincent's Infections: Observations and Conclusions Regarding the Aetiology and Treatment of 1,017 Civilian Cases. *Brit. D.J.,* 76:147, 1947.

Stark, R. B.: Pathogenesis of Harelip and Cleft Palate. *Plast. & Reconstr. Surg.,* 13:20, 1954.

Stark, R. B., and Ehrmann, N. A.: The Development of the Center of the Face, with Particular Reference to Surgical Correction of Bilateral Cleft Lip. *Plast. & Reconstr. Surg.,* 21:13, 1958.

Stewart, W. J.: Congenital Median Cleft of the Chin. *Arch. Surg.,* 31:813, 1935.

Sutton, R. L., Jr.: Recurrent Scarring Painful Aphthae. *J.A.M.A.,* 117:175, 1941.

Tanger, J.: Oral Manifestations of Hurler-Pfandler and Pierre-Robin Syndromes. *Oral Surg.,* 17:453-6, 1964.

Thoma, K. H., Holland, D. J., Woodbury, H. W., Burrow, J. G., and Sleeper, E. L.: Malignant Lymphoma of the Gingiva. *Oral Surg., Oral Med. & Oral Path.,* 1:57, 1948.

Thomas, K. H.: Vincent's Infection or Fusospirochetosis. *Am. J. Orthodont. & Oral. Surg.,* 27:479, 1941.

Tondury, G.: On the Mechanism of Cleft Formation; in S. Pruzansky: *Congenital Anomalies of the Face and Associated Structures.* Springfield, Ill., Charles C Thomas, 1961, p. 85.

Topazian, R. G., and other: Macrotomia with Auricular Appendages. *Oral. Surg.,* 22:313-17, 1964.

Trusler, H. M., Bauer, T. B., and Tondra, J. M.: The Cleft-Lip Cleft Palate Problem. *Plast. & Reconstr. Surg.,* 16:174, 1955.

Veau, V.: Discussion on the Treatment of Harelip. *Proc. Roy. Soc. Med.,* 21:1868, 1927.

Waldron, C. W.: Management of Unilateral Clefts of the Palate. *Plast. & Reconstr. Surg.,* 5:522, 1950.

Wardill, W. E. M.: Cleft Palate. *Brit. J. Surg.,* 16:127, 1928.

Warkany, J.: Congenital Malformations and Pediatrics. *Pediatrics,* 19:725, 1957.

Wolbach, S. B.: Pathologic Changes Resulting from Vitamin Deficiency. *J.A.M.A.,* 108:7-13, 1937.

Wolbach, S. B., and Bessey, O. A.: Tissue Changes in Vitamin Deficiencies. *Physiol. Rev.,* 22:233, 1942.

Woolf, R. M., Georgiade, N. G., and Pickrell, K. L.: Micrognathia and Associated Cleft Palate (Pierre Robin Syndrome). *Plast. & Reconstr. Surg.,* 26:199, 1960.

CHAPTER EIGHT

The Pharynx

CHARLES F. FERGUSON, M.D.

The pharynx is a common passageway from the nasal and oral cavities to the larynx and the esophagus, conducting air into and out of the lower respiratory tract, and fluid, food and saliva into the upper digestive system. Traditionally, it is divided into three component parts, all of which are in direct continuity: namely, the nasopharynx, the oropharynx (or mesopharynx) and the hypopharynx (or laryngopharynx) (Fig. 1).

The *nasopharynx* extends from the vault at the basal process of the occipital bone just beneath the sphenoid sinus, downward to the free edge of the soft palate, opening anteriorly into the nasal cavities through the posterior choanae, and laterally into the tympanic cavities through the eustachian tubes. It contains the pharyngeal tonsil ("the adenoid").

The *oropharynx (mesopharynx)* extends from the soft palate to the hyoid bone or upper edge of the epiglottis, directly communicating above with the nasopharynx, anteriorly with the buccal cavity, and inferiorly with the hypopharynx. It contains the palatine tonsils, lying laterally in the fauces between the anterior and posterior pillars, which separate the oropharynx from the oral cavity.

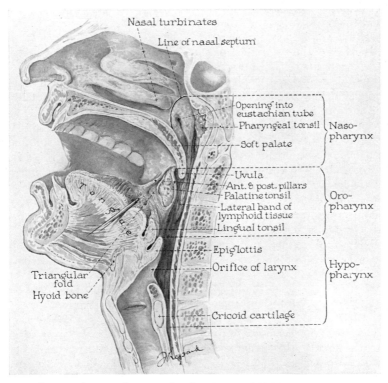

Nasal turbinates

Line of nasal septum

Opening into eustachian tube

Pharyngeal tonsil — Naso-pharynx

Soft palate

Uvula

Ant. & post. pillars

Palatine tonsil — Oro-pharynx

Lateral band of lymphoid tissue

Lingual tonsil

Epiglottis

Orifice of larynx — Hypo-pharynx

Tonsil

Triangular fold

Hyoid bone

Cricoid cartilage

FIGURE 8–1. Sagittal section of pharynx, showing its 3 subdivisions. (From Jackson and Jackson: *Diseases of the Nose, Throat and Ear.*)

On the anterior wall it also contains the lingual tonsil along the base of the tongue, and the lateral bands of lymphoid tissue running downward behind the posterior pillars.

The *hypopharynx* (*laryngopharynx*) is a continuation of the oropharynx downward, extending from the upper edge of the epiglottis to the lower border of the cricoid cartilage at the sixth cervical vertebra, and merging directly into the esophagus posteriorly. It also connects directly with the larynx and trachea anteriorly.

Surrounding the entrance to the upper air and food passages is a complete circle of lymphoid structures designated as Waldeyer's ring. This includes the pharyngeal tonsil (or adenoid mass) superiorly, the two palatine tonsils laterally, and the lingual tonsil inferiorly. Together these structures, along with the many solitary lymphoid nodules on the posterior pharyngeal wall and the lateral bands, form this important ring of lymphoid tissue so strategically located about the entrance to the respiratory and digestive tracts. It is essential to remember that this tissue, or many of its component parts, usually undergoes hypertrophy in early childhood, during the period when exposure to infections is frequent and the immune processes are being developed. This hypertrophy reaches a peak at four to six years of age. Later on these structures begin to undergo involution and decrease greatly in size around puberty, unless chronic infection is present. In fact, in most instances, after adolescence the adenoid for all practical purposes gives no further trouble, either from gross enlargement or from infection.

MALFORMATIONS

The pharynx, like all other areas of the body, is not infrequently the site of congenital malformations due to errors of embryologic development. At one stage in early fetal life the nasal cavity is completely separate from the nasopharynx, and persistence of this separation into postnatal life results in congenital choanal atresia. It is a well documented cause of fatality during the very early neonatal period. In early embryonic life the pharynx has a direct communication with the central nervous system by way of the craniopharyngeal canal, and from this area tumors may arise. Likewise the path of the primitive notochord may be the source of later difficulties. Maldevelopment of the branchial arches with their intervening clefts and pouches may result in a cervical cyst, or a sinus tract still retaining its communication with the tonsillar fossa. In the midline of the neck a draining sinus may persist as a patent thyroglossal duct, and its related cyst is often misdiagnosed as an abscess, lymph node or dermoid, unless the process of embryologic development is recalled.

Nasopharynx

Choanal Atresia

One of the commonest malformations of the nasopharynx is an atresia of the posterior choanae, separating completely the nasal cavities from the nasopharynx itself. (See also page 156.) It is important to recognize this anomaly at birth, especially if the atresia is bilateral, since it is a preventable cause of neonatal mortality. The newborn infant will suffocate if an adequate airway is not immediately established, since mouth-breathing is always a necessarily acquired ability. The harder the infant with complete nasal obstruction tries to breathe, the tighter his mouth closes until asphyxia results. The bucconasal membrane, which separates the primitive oral cavity from the primitive nasal cavity, should rupture between the thirty-fifth and thirty-eighth days of fetal life. Failure to do so will produce atresia, and in most instances this is a solid bony obstruction. Persistence of the more posterior embryonic membrane (the buccopharyngeal membrane) may result in a membranous atresia which can be easily perforated if it is recognized sufficiently soon.

Passage of a catheter through each nostril into the pharynx should be part of the routine examination of every infant immediately after birth. If patency is not apparent, a plastic pharyngeal airway should immediately be inserted, or a nipple with a large hole strapped into the mouth. Then a more thorough investigation should be made as soon as possible. (See Section on Respiratory Disorders of the Newborn.)

From the therapeutic point of view, the large-hole rubber nipple securely strapped into the mouth of such an infant (according to the McGovern technique) will serve for feeding purposes, as well as an airway, until the patient learns satisfactory mouth-breathing. Frequently in the past, immediate intranasal perforation of the atresia was done, using various techniques, but such openings have a great tendency to close rapidly.

With constant nursing care, and the use of the McGovern nipple technique, satisfactory mouth-breathing will be acquired at the end of a week or ten days in almost every case. Tracheostomy is rarely indicated in choanal atresia, and generally it is to be avoided, since other methods of handling the situation are more effective, and the often troublesome problem of extubation does not arise. When the infant is larger and stronger and well over the immediate neonatal pe-riod, more definitive surgical removal of the atresia can be done more completely. This is preferably done through a direct transpalatal approach, and the atretic wall removed under direct vision, along with the posterior portion of the septum. This has proved to be the most successful method of handling a large series of cases of congenital choanal atresia.

Persistent Craniopharyngeal Canal

In 1839 Rathke described a case of cerebral herniation through an opening in the sphenoid bone which he considered the result of hydrocephalus prior to closure of this embryologic passageway which now bears his name. Since that time there has been great confusion over malformations, tumors or cysts which originate in or near this region. In fetal life the craniopharyngeal canal extends from the pharynx, often through the vomer or septal area of the sphenoid sinuses to the sella turcica beneath the hypophysis (Fig. 2). Instances of persistence of this canal have been reported, and since the anterior lobe of the pituitary gland develops from the dilated cranial portion of Rathke's pouch, embryonic rests of pituitary tissue have been found in the pharynx. According to Wilkerson, an incomplete canal ending in the septum is more common than a persistent canal which goes all the way into the pharynx. The persistent canal has been demonstrated by probes and by radiologic studies with contrast-medium injection, but ordinarily this anomaly in

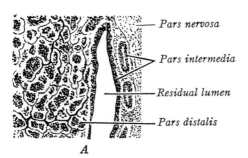

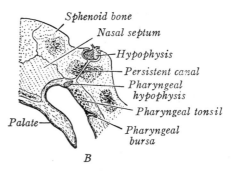

Pars nervosa

Pars intermedia

Residual lumen

Pars distalis

A

Sphenoid bone

Nasal septum

Hypophysis

Persistent canal

Pharyngeal hypophysis

Pharyngeal tonsil

Palate

Pharyngeal bursa

B

FIGURE 8–2. *A,* Hypophysial region at 8 months. *B,* Persistent craniopharyngeal canal in newborn. (From Arey: *Developmental Anatomy.*)

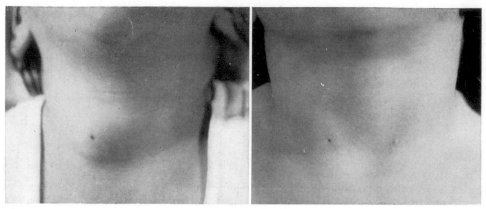

FIGURE 8–3. Branchiogenic sinus and cyst in 2 children. (From Gross: *Surgery of Infancy and Childhood.*)

itself produces no symptoms and is discovered accidentally. (See Craniopharyngioma, p. 197.)

Oropharynx

Branchiogenic Sinus or Cyst

The commonest malformation associated with the oropharynx is the branchiogenic sinus, which connects the base of the tonsillar fossa or the posterior pillar externally with the neck. In the embryo during the first two or three weeks there are four or five parallel grooves externally in the lateral aspects of the neck, and these grooves are lined with ectoderm. Each groove is matched by a corresponding pouch or outpocketing of the foregut and lined with entoderm. Between the grooves and clefts lie the branchial arches.

The first pouch gives rise to the eustachian tube, the tympanic cavity and the mastoid, and the first cleft produces the auditory canal and drum. A preauricular fistula is not an uncommon anomaly, and originates from this first pouch and cleft.

Anomalies of the second cleft, however, are about six times more frequent. From this cleft arise the cervical fistulas which open into the tonsillar area. The external opening is always just anterior to the sternomastoid muscle, and in most instances fairly low down in the neck.

Branchiogenic cysts occasionally occur, but they are somewhat higher than a fistula, and often appear later (Fig. 3). A constant discharge of saliva from the side of the neck may direct attention to such a cervical sinus tract. Many of these fistulas remain dry for years, but at times repeated infections may result in complete closure. Blind cysts may occur with no external opening in the neck, but still retaining a communication internally with the tonsillar fossa, or the posterior pillar. Dissection of the complete tract, or removal of the intact cyst, is necessary for a satisfactory and permanent cure.

Thyroglossal Duct Cyst

The thyroglossal duct opens internally into the foramen caecum at the base of the tongue. A cyst which originates from this duct is always in the midline and usually about the level of the isthmus of the thyroid or just above it (Fig. 4). It ordinarily passes through the center of the hyoid bone, and is the tract provided by migration of the thyroid gland from its origin at the base of the tongue outward into the neck. Removal of a thyroglossal duct cyst should always include the central portion of the hyoid bone, and the tract must be dissected back as far as possible to the foramen caecum, or recurrence may be anticipated.

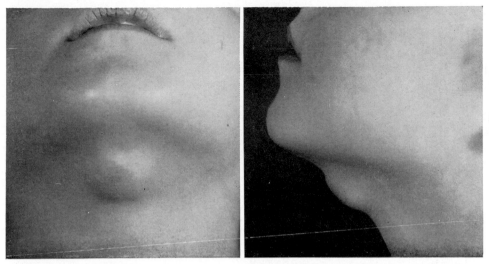

FIGURE 8–4. Thyroglossal duct cyst. (From Gross: *Surgery of Infancy and Childhood.*)

TUMORS AND CYSTS

Nasopharynx

Craniopharyngioma

These tumors, although technically in the region of the sella turcica rather than in the nasopharynx, arise from a persistent craniopharyngeal canal (see p. 195). They are not uncommon, and craniopharyngiomas are reported as comprising 10 to 13 per cent of all intracranial growths in children (Wilkerson), 4 per cent of all intracranial tumors generally, and 30 per cent of all pituitary tumors (Leve and Marshall). Craniopharyngiomas may be solid, but more frequently are cystic. They are histologically benign, but the operative mortality rate is high, and cures are limited. Symptoms produced by such tumors include increased intracranial pressure, with headache and separation of the sutures, visual disturbances, with papilledema, optic atrophy from pressure on the chiasm, and narrowing and restriction of the visual fields. There are also hypopituitary symptoms. Radiation has not been successful, and the best method of treatment is by craniotomy.

Chordoma

The chordoma is a relatively rare tumor seen in the nasopharynx, and develops from remnants of the notochord which often persist in this region near the base of the skull. It may be adherent to the wall of the sphenoid or the base of the occipital bone. The tumor obliterates the adenoid fissures or actually displaces the adenoid mass. It may be seen with a mirror, Yankauer speculum or nasopharyngoscope, or may be directly palpated. It is a solid tumor which contains a great deal of connective tissue, and is usually benign, although occasionally it may show malignant changes and even develop into a sarcoma. Ulcerations may occur, but bleeding is not too common. It may extend into the skull or dura.

Tornwaldt Cyst

A more cystic type of structure is encountered lower in the nasopharynx, especially in the adolescent age group or in young adults. Technically, this structure is neither a tumor nor a malformation. In 1895 Tornwaldt originally described a cyst which he considered to arise from in-

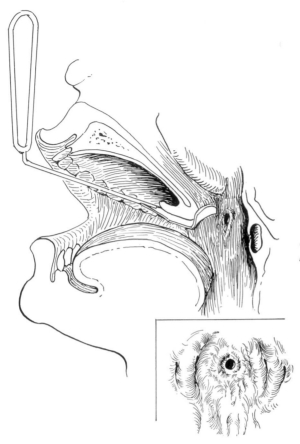

FIGURE 8–5. Sagittal section of naso-pharynx with Yankauer speculum in place, showing nasopharyngeal bursa and its small midline opening (Tornwaldt cyst). (From Boies: *Fundamentals of Otolaryn-gology*.)

flammation of the nasopharyngeal bursa because of infection. It is questionable whether this bursa is due to adhesions of the fetal notochord to the pharyngeal ectoderm, or possibly remnants of the hypophysial duct. Since the hypophysial duct should be at a much higher level in the nasopharynx, it is still a confused situation. Such a structure might even result from obstruction of a deep adenoid crypt with constant exfoliation of the mucosal lining, producing a retention type of cyst. The true Tornwaldt cyst occurs much lower down than the craniopharyngeal canal or Rathke's pouch anomalies (Fig. 5).

A true bursa may exist as a central depression in the midline of the adenoid mass. Frequently this bursa becomes infected and then may be associated with a persistent postnasal discharge with a great deal of scab formation and crusting, along with an unpleasant odor to the breath. The midline groove between the two halves of the adenoid may be converted into a canal by adhesions. This lining membrane may grow in along a path formed by the degenerating notochord. When infection takes place, an abscess may form, or if the fluid is sterile, a midline cyst may result. Caseous, putty-like material is extruded from time to time. Removal by ordinary adenoid curets is relatively simple.

Angiofibroma

The most important tumor of the nasopharynx in the later pediatric age group is the juvenile angiofibroma. (See the chapter on The Nose.) Although this is histologically a benign tumor, it may be invasive, and its removal may be fraught with serious hemorrhage. It occurs almost entirely in males, and is usually noted at the time of puberty or early adolescence. It originates from the fibrous periosteum of the vault of the nasopharynx. Because of its dense fibrous tissue component, it is a solid tumor, and the many large blood vessels it contains lack normal contractibility. This is the reason why hemorrhage may be profuse and serious. The chief symptoms are obstruction and bleeding, but fullness in the ears, tinnitus and pain are not uncommon.

Radiation therapy has been used, because surgical removal produces many hazards. Sometimes removal is easier after radiation has reduced the size of the mass. Hormone therapy has also been used without dramatic results. When cryosurgical procedures are better developed, it is hoped that by this method the hazard of bleeding will be minimized and the tumor more safely removed.

Neurofibroma

The neurofibroma may be encountered in the nasopharynx. It is ordinarily well encapsulated and not particularly vascular. It may be deeply embedded in the posterior wall of the nasopharynx, or extend downward into the pharyngeal area, where it is visible.

Polyps

True benign polyps arising in the nasopharynx are rare. Occasionally polyps are seen in the nasopharynx, but in most instances they originate in the paranasal sinuses and merely prolapse backward through the choanae, hanging into the nasopharynx as they become more edematous. In any case of polyps, either nasal or nasopharyngeal, in a child under ten years of age, cystic fibrosis must always be suspected and appropriate diagnostic measures carried out.

Oropharynx

Papilloma

The papilloma is the commonest tumor of the pharynx. It may occur anywhere, but is most often seen at the base of the uvula, along the faucial pillars, or on the tonsil itself. Often bits of papilloma are implanted elsewhere in the mucosa of the mouth or pharynx by manipulation. It is a benign tumor, composed of masses of stratified squamous epithelium in papillary formation. It does not invade or metastasize. Simple superficial removal is usually satisfactory, but recurrences are not infrequent.

Cysts

Cysts of the vallecula or the lingual surface of the epiglottis may occur, but are rare in children. They are removed by simple dissection, but complete removal is essential, since incision and drainage will result only in refilling of the cyst. Otherwise secretion continues from the remaining epithelial lining, and nothing has been accomplished. Occasionally the cyst may be exteriorized and the lining membrane cauterized, but complete destruction of all the epithelium is necessary to prevent recurrence.

Adenoma, Fibroma and Hemangioma

Adenoma, fibroma and hemangioma are other benign oropharyngeal tumors, but in childhood are rare.

Malignant Tumors

Of the malignant tumors of this region in childhood, the commonest (although still rare) is the *lymphosarcoma*. In the adult it is the transitional-cell carcinoma, or the lymphoepithelioma. The lymphosarcoma is highly malignant and very rapidly growing. It usually originates in the nasopharynx, but may also arise lower down in the oropharyngeal wall. This tumor causes rapid nasal obstruction, and early cervical metastasis occurs. Cases are seen even in infants, and the prognosis is very poor. Recently at the Children's Hospital Medical Center in Boston we saw an epidermoid carcinoma of the nasopharynx in a husky, well developed fourteen-year-old boy whose only complaint was progressive unilateral cervical glandular enlargement of one month's duration. The nodes were not tender, he ran no fever, and there were no other symptoms. Nasopharyngoscopy was essentially negative, except for two or three tiny bits of apparently normal-appearing lymphoid tissue. Because of a definite diagnosis of metastatic epidermoid carcinoma from a cervical biopsy, these bits of lymphoid tissue were carefully removed, and histologic study showed the adenoid as the primary source of the epidermoid carcinoma. In the adult such a tumor is relatively common, but at this age is most unusual.

PHARYNGEAL TONSIL

Before leaving the nasopharynx, the importance of adenoid in children must be stressed. Although it is not within the scope of this chapter to go into a discussion of the adenoid in its relation to conductive deafness or recurrent otitis media, it must be stated here that the commonest cause of these conditions in childhood is enlargement or infection of the adenoid mass. Proper functioning of the eustachian tube throughout childhood is essential if chronic catarrhal deafness in later life is to be prevented. This obstructive tissue must be removed in children who have a history of conductive hearing impairment or recurrent otitis media, to permit proper functioning of the eustachian tubes. It must be done before irreversible middle ear changes become permanently established. (See the chapter on The Ear.)

PHARYNGEAL MANIFESTATIONS OF INFECTIOUS DISEASE

Acute Tonsillitis

Acute tonsillitis (see also Chap. 13) is an extremely common respiratory disease and frequently attacks children of any age, but is relatively uncommon during the first year of life. It may be caused by various bacteria or viruses, but the beta hemolytic streptococcus is the commonest infectious agent. It is a specific infectious disease, and should be distinguished from acute generalized pharyngitis and the ordinary acute upper respiratory tract infection. Ordinarily it is of sudden onset, with relatively high fever and even chills. Younger children rarely complain of a sore throat, but refusal of feedings and dysphagia are frequently noted. In the older child, pain may be referred to the ear.

The white blood cell count is elevated, with a preponderance of polymorphonuclear leukocytes. The sedimentation rate is also increased. Bacteriologic cultures usually show the beta hemolytic streptococcus, but frequently the pneumococcus and the coagulase-positive staphylococcus are causative organisms.

Examination of the throat shows red, edematous tonsils, with acutely inflamed pillars, and often the tonsils are covered with a whitish, spotty exudate. This exudate, however, can easily be removed when the culture is taken, without producing bleeding. The tonsillar nodes at the angle of the jaw are tender as well as enlarged, and sometimes this glandular involvement is the presenting symptom.

Penicillin is ordinarily the drug of choice, and should be used until cultures and sensitivity tests indicate otherwise. If the organism is resistant to penicillin, one of the broad-spectrum antibiotics should be given. Warm saline throat irrigations and warm compresses to the neck are helpful in older children, but generally are refused and impractical in the younger age group. Aspirin will reduce fever and relieve pain. A high fluid intake and light diet are indicated. The disease is usually self-limited, and if it is treated properly, complications today are negligible.

Scarlet Fever

At present there is a great question as to whether scarlet fever (scarlatina) is a specific entity. Many authorities consider the disease an acute streptococcal tonsillitis or pharyngitis, followed by a diffuse erythematous rash, which is presumed to be a sensitivity reaction to a specific hemolytic streptococcus. The exotoxin liberated by the particular strain of the organism produces a characteristic punctiform scarlet blush which is most evident in the skin folds, but more or less generalized. It appears in twenty-four to forty-eight hours. There is usually circumoral pallor. The throat is very sore, swallowing is difficult, and there is high fever, headache, vomiting and occasionally chills. Two to five days' incubation period is usual. In this stage examination shows a diffuse punctate rash over the palate, and the tonsils and entire pharynx show an acute inflammatory reaction. There may be exudate in the crypts of the tonsils, typical of acute tonsillitis. The tongue may show enlarged, red papillae which produce the characteristic "strawberry tongue." The anterior cervical lymph nodes, especially at the angle of the jaw, are enlarged and tender. Direct throat cultures are positive for the beta hemolytic streptococcus. The Dick test (an intradermal injection of dilute scarlet fever streptococcus toxin) gives a positive reaction, but is seldom used today.

Penicillin therapy in full doses for a ten-day period is specific for this disease; the response is usually rapid and complete. Today, complications of scarlet fever, such as otitis media, severe mastoiditis or nephritis, are infrequent if treatment is prompt and thorough.

Diphtheria

Diphtheria is a rare disease today, but must always be considered in any acute throat infection, since prompt and proper therapy *early in its course* before complications arise is imperative. Early diagnosis and treatment of such cases will prevent serious complications, such as postdiphtheritic paralysis and myocarditis. The history of a negative Schick test is not always reliable, since on occasions so-called permanent immunity runs out, and if the organism is particularly virulent, the patient may contract the disease. The incubation period is two to five days.

The presenting symptom is sore throat, which is usually not as severe as that in scarlet fever. The fever is much lower than in scarlet fever, and rarely goes above 101 degrees, although the pulse rate may be proportionately more rapid. Low-grade temperature elevation and throat infection may persist for several days, and significant cervical adenitis is always present. Along with these symptoms, headache, nausea and general malaise are common.

Examination shows a characteristic coalescent, grayish membrane formation over the tonsils, extending onto the pillars or even onto the soft palate. At first this may resemble ordinary cryptic exudate, but in a day or two it forms a tough membrane which, when disturbed with a culture swab, bleeds on attempted removal, leaving an oozing base. It is a firm fibrinous structure, and rapidly reforms over the bleeding surface. This membrane has a characteristic musty odor. Direct cultures should always be obtained, with a specific request for incubation on a Klebs-Loeffler medium. If at first diphtheroids are reported, further investigation must be carried out by the bacteriologist, using the various sugar media to determine whether the organism is actually the diphtheria bacillus or not. This should be accompanied by a virulence test carried out by injection into a guinea pig. Ulcerations are not common, and sloughing to any great extent is never encountered.

Meanwhile, as the diagnosis is being made in the laboratory, a patient suspected of having the disease should be adequately treated with diphtheria antitoxin to neutralize the circulating toxin produced by the bacillus. Otherwise late complications of a serious nature may ensue while the final diagnosis is being delayed. It is unfortunate that penicillin, the commonest antibiotic used in throat conditions, is effective in eradicating the organisms and relieving the symptoms, since it is ineffective against the diphtheria toxin. Penicillin will apparently "cure" diphtheria clinically, but the patient may die of cardiac complications later on, unless specific antitoxin has been given to neutralize this circulating toxin. If antitoxin is used, penicillin is not necessary. Postdiphtheritic paralysis of the soft palate, eye muscles, diaphragm or extremities may ensue in 15 to 20 per cent of the cases, or the more serious complication of diphtheritic myocarditis may develop, and fatality ensue.

Vincent's Angina

Sometimes a differential diagnosis of the sore throat of acute tonsillitis, agranulocytosis or Vincent's angina is difficult to make on inspection alone, since all these conditions produce a pharyngeal membrane or pseudomembrane. In Vincent's angina a dirty white, grayish-yellow membrane covers the tonsils or fossae, and the underlying tissues show a bleeding tendency when the false membrane is removed. Removal is much easier than when dealing with the diphtheritic membrane, since it is not so adherent. In Vincent's angina there usually are also ulcerated lesions. These ulcerations are often deep and sharply punched out, and there may be considerable sloughing. Surrounding the ulcerations is a band of inflammatory reaction and edema. Presenting symptoms are sore throat, dysphagia, cervical glandular enlargment and a char-

acteristic odor to the breath. The lesions also involve the mucosa of the pharynx, as well as the tonsils, and often the gingiva and buccal membranes, producing gingivitis and stomatitis. Fever is usually of a low grade.

Cultures show a combination of a fusiform bacillus and a characteristic long, thin spirochete. There has been considerable discussion as to whether these organisms, which are sometimes found in the normal mouth, are the causative agents. When they are found in symbiosis, however, the diagnosis is most probable. It has also been suggested that Vincent's angina may be due to an anaerobic streptococcus.

Penicillin is usually effective, as are also the tetracyclines. Oxidizing agents, such as hydrogen peroxide, or sodium perborate applied locally as a paste, give good results. Ten per cent silver nitrate or copper sulfate (10 per cent) may be applied locally to the lesions. The disease is self-limited, but highly contagious, and therefore deserves adequate precautions and proper treatment.

Fungous Infections

In the very young child fungus infections of the mouth and pharynx are frequent. Poor hygiene in the newborn, along with improper sterilization of nipples and bottles, may lead to rapid spread of this infection throughout nurseries. In older children orally administered antibiotics may disturb the normal flora of the mouth and give the ever-present fungi a chance to overgrow. Thrush, which is due to *Candida albicans*, is manifested by small, whitish, curdlike patches or plaques adherent to the gums, buccal mucosa, tongue, lips or pharynx. Moniliasis may involve the entire respiratory tract, and often the entire gastrointestinal tract becomes infected; improvement and recovery are slow.

Treatment consists in elimination of oral antibiotics, if they are being used, and the local use of 1 per cent aqueous gentian violet. Mycostatin may be used by dropping 1 cc. of an aqueous suspension containing 100,000 units per cubic centimeter into the mouth four or five times daily.

Viral Infections

See Chapter 13.

PHARYNGEAL MANIFESTATIONS OF SYSTEMIC DISEASE

Agranulocytosis

Agranulocytosis is often first manifested by symptoms of sore throat, as in acute pharyngitis or acute tonsillitis. Unless a blood examination is obtained, the correct diagnosis is often missed. The mouth, tongue, pharynx and tonsils may show a grayish white or yellowish exudate, which looks not unlike that of Vincent's angina or other exudative throat infection. Later this area may become necrotic; glandular enlargement is common, and mucosal hemorrhages are frequent. The throat is very painful, and dysphagia is frequently present. The patient is usually prostrated, even though the fever may be only slight. In fulminating cases fever may be very high. In contrast to the lesion in Vincent's infection, there is rarely a surrounding red inflammatory reaction, although ulceration may be extensive and the mucosal areas may be diffusely involved.

The disease is due to depression of the granulocytic series of white blood cells, with a granulocytic leukopenia of 2000 cells or less. It signifies a toxic bone marrow depression following sensitization to certain drugs, especially those with benzine rings such as aminopyrine, some of the sulfonamides, chloramphenicol, penicillamine and occasionally some of the antihistamines.

After discontinuation of the offending drug, large doses of penicillin are usually effective in preventing the secondary infection which is the serious sequela. In some patients transfusion is indicated. Pentnucleotide (1 to 2 Gm. intravenously daily) has been used with questionable benefit.

Acute Infectious Mononucleosis

This is an acute systemic infectious disease presumed to be due to a virus. It is usually manifested first by pharyngeal symptoms and occurs for the most part in young adults; as "glandular fever" it is recognized not infrequently in children. It is relatively contagious, and may spread rapidly through schools or other institutions. Fever and general malaise are common as the sore throat develops into a true pharyngitis or tonsillitis. Small patches of superficial exudate may be noted; occasionally even membrane formation is found with superficial ulceration, but there is no underlying bleeding surface as in diphtheria. Early in the course of the disease the cervical glands become enlarged and tender; this is followed by a generalized lymphadenopathy, including enlargment of the liver and spleen. Jaundice may develop on rare occasions.

Blood studies by the fourth or fifth day show a high white blood cell count with a preponderance of large lymphocytes and monocytes. The abnormal large lymphocytes (or Downes cells) are characteristic of the disease. On rare occasions there may be a leukopenia. By the second week the Paul-Bunnell heterophile antibody test becomes positive and may remain so for many weeks.

The disease usually persists for several weeks with slow recovery; complications are rare. Supportive and symptomatic treatment only is indicated, and antibiotic therapy should be reserved for the rare bacterial complications. Corticosteroids may shorten the period of indisposition, but routine use of these drugs in this otherwise self-limited disease is open to question.

Acute Leukemia

Examination of the pharynx may give the first clue to this serious systemic blood disease; the pharyngeal disease is often confused with the sore throat, fever and cervical adenitis of an ordinary bacterial infection, but ulcerations of the tonsils or pillars may be apparent, and the oral and gingival mucous membrane may show similar ulcerations, not unlike those seen in agranulocytosis. The onset is usually acute. Nosebleeds are common, and bleeding from any mucosal surface may occur and be persistent. The mucosa shows pronounced pallor, and cervical nodes, spleen and liver are usually enlarged. The blood smear and white blood cell count will usually provide the diagnosis. This disease should always be suspected when an apparently ordinary throat infection fails to respond properly to treatment. The white blood cell count is usually very high, except in the aleukemic stages. The blood smear shows myeloblasts, lymphoblasts or monoblasts, depending on the type of leukemia, and there is inevitably an associated anemia and thrombocytopenia. At present various chemotherapeutic agents establish and prolong remissions, but so far the disease is always fatal.

REFERENCES

Arey, L. B.: *Developmental Anatomy*. 7th ed. Philadelphia, W. B. Saunders Company, 1965.

Boies, L. R., Hilger, J. A., and Priest, R. E.: *Fundamentals of Otolaryngology*. 4th ed. Philadelphia, W. B. Saunders Company, 1964.

Coates, G. M., and Schenck, H. P.: *Otolaryngology*. W. F. Prior Company, 1956.

Flake, C. G., and Ferguson, C. F.: *Ann. Otol., Rhinol. & Laryngol.*, 73:458, 1964.

Gross, R. E.: *The Surgery of Infancy and Childhood*. Philadelphia, W. B. Saunders Company, 1963.

Jackson, C., and Jackson, C. L.: *Diseases of the Nose, Throat and Ear*. 2nd ed. Philadelphia, W. B. Saunders Company, 1959.

CHAPTER NINE

The Larynx

WILLIAM E. LAUPUS, M.D.,
and PETER N. PASTORE, M.D.

The principal functions of the larynx are protective and phonatory in nature, although the larynx also takes part in respiration, deglutition, coughing and other complex activities. Its phylogenetic oldest and primary role is in safeguarding the lower airway from the aspiration of foreign bodies and liquid substances. Laryngeal participation in phonation and communication is generally considered to be a secondary function.

The larynx has a somewhat triangular funnel shape with the broad opening superiorly. Structurally, it has a cartilaginous framework which begins with the epiglottis at the base of the tongue and ends in the cricoid ring cartilage at its junction with the upper part of the trachea. The major cartilages are four in number: the thyroid cartilage anteriorly, the two arytenoids superiorly and posteriorly, and the cricoid inferiorly. The epiglottic and the paired cuneiform and corniculate cartilages are termed the accessory group. The cartilages are united by various ligaments and membranes. The mucous membrane is continuous with that of the pharynx and the trachea and is of the ciliated pseudocolumnar type except for the stratified squamous epithelium of the vocal cords. The mucous membrane is loosely attached to the areolar tissue of the submucosa; edema of the submucosa tends to be poorly confined and may seriously narrow the airway, causing extensive or complete obstruction. The most constricted area of the laryngeal airway is at the site of approximation of the vocal cords.

The larynx is located at a higher cervical level in infancy, remaining slightly higher in the female at all ages. As the neck elongates with growth, the larynx gradually assumes its adult position approximately two vertebral bodies lower than in infancy. Laryngeal growth is gradual throughout childhood until puberty, when the rate is accelerated in both sexes, especially in the male, in whom voice change and the prominent "Adam's apple" become common.

The valvular closure of the larynx with deglutition is accomplished by strong adduction of the true vocal cords assisted by approximation of the false vocal cords and of the aryepiglottic folds and by movement of the epiglottis in a posterior and downward direction. Contrary to popular opinion, the epiglottis is not essential to deglutition; other than deflecting the bolus of food and shielding the false vocal cords, closure of the airway by the epiglottis is incomplete and affords little protection from aspiration.

Infants and children with severe laryngeal disease often appear anxious and apprehensive; cyanosis is unusual except when the airway is greatly constricted. The signs of laryngeal involvement are variable and range from noisy breathing to inspiratory wheezing or stridor with laryngeal "crowing," barking cough, dyspnea and inspiratory retraction in the intercostal, subcostal and supraclavicular spaces. Hoarseness or aphonia may be present. If secretions are abundant, the noisy respirations may have a "gurgling" quality, present both in inspiration and expiration. Feeding difficulties, including choking and aspiration, are commonly associated with obstructive laryngeal diseases, and undernutrition may develop in infants with chronic respiratory difficulty. Superimposed respiratory infections usually increase the degree of the pre-existing signs.

The small size of the pharynx and the larynx in the infant makes direct laryngoscopy technically somewhat more difficult than in older children and adults; the child's size, however, should seldom be the reason for deferring this procedure if the signs of laryngeal obstruction are severe. Direct laryngoscopy should be performed by a skilled laryngoscopist under optimum circumstances, and this should include adequate provision for handling laryngospasm, which occasionally occurs during instrumentation.

MALFORMATIONS

Malformations of the larynx are relatively common. Although present at birth, partially obstructive laryngeal lesions may not become evident for several days or weeks when tidal airflow becomes insufficient and respiratory effort is compensatorily increased.

Congenital webs of the larynx are rare. Generally, the webs are incomplete and are confined to the anterior vocal cord area; they may also be found in supraglottic or subglottic locations, and subglottic webs have been reported in four members of one family. They may cause stridor, dyspnea and hoarseness or other abnormal qualities to the voice; if small, they may cause no signs referable to the airway or larynx. Complete, or nearly complete, webs can be responsible for asphyxia in newborns; early recognition by direct laryngoscopy and surgical incision of the web have proved lifesaving. Webs are difficult to remove surgically and frequently recur after excision. Dilatation may be more useful than surgery in the smaller webs and may prevent reformation after excision of the larger ones.

Congenital subglottic stenosis, sometimes also involving the true cords, has been reported to cause stridor and other signs of respiratory embarrassment without hoarseness or other changes in the quality of the voice. The stenosis may be so severe that tracheostomy is required.

Atresia of the larynx, a cause of complete obstruction in newborns, has been associated with bilateral absence of the eyes, but may also occur without other malformations. Immediate tracheostomy is required to establish an airway.

Duplication of the vocal cords is another anomaly capable of causing stridor.

Congenital laryngeal stridor is the most frequent abnormality in childhood, occurring in variable and usually transient form in otherwise healthy infants. The condition is usually ascribed to abnormal flaccidity of the epiglottic and supraglottic structures (laryngomalacia), to exaggeration of the normal shape of the epiglottis ("omega" epiglottis) or to generalized flabbiness of the laryngeal and tracheal cartilages (chondromalacia). In the latter two variations the airway may be seen to constrict considerably with inspiration and to expand with expiration, the reverse of the normal changes with respiration. Stridor due to these conditions is self-limited, being most pronounced during the first year of life and gradually subsiding spontaneously by the age of two years.

Similar signs of airway obstruction are seen in a variety of extralaryngeal problems which must be differentiated from the intrinsic causes of congenital stridor. These disorders include true macroglossia, the Pierre Robin syndrome (micrognathia, cleft palate, retrodisplaced tongue), subglossal tumors, neurogenic paralyses of the palate and pharynx, aortic arch and great vessel anomalies ("vascular rings" impinging on the trachea), and the "H type" of tracheo-esophageal fistula, which

by chronic aspiration may simulate the signs of laryngeal and laryngotracheal obstructive lesions. Rarely, branchial cleft cysts, thyroglossal duct cysts and congenital goiter may compress the airway, causing stridor. In the neonatal period laryngospasm associated with low-calcium tetany and laryngeal edema due to aspiration or to trauma relatable to endotracheal intubation during resuscitation may be responsible for transient stridor.

Although benign and self-limited, congenital laryngeal stridor causes great parental concern. Many of these babies are difficult to feed; they are prone to aspirate at any time when respirations are rapid and breathing and swallowing are difficult to coordinate. Feeding must be given slowly and carefully by nipple or dropper. *Breck feeders and similar devices are unsafe and should not be used.* Feeding by nasogastric tube or gastrostomy may be helpful in unusually severe forms of congenital stridor. The noise associated with breathing, and to some extent the dyspnea, may be helped by positioning the baby on his side with the neck hyperextended. Many of these babies naturally assume an opisthotonic posture as the position of maximal comfort. Respiratory infections are likely to cause exaggeration of the signs of airway obstruction, and exposure to "colds" and similar illnesses should be avoided whenever possible. Moist oxygen may be helpful in the management of superimposed respiratory infection. In rare instances tracheostomy may be required and will be lifesaving. Unfortunately, removal of the tracheostomy tube may prove difficult if the respiratory distress is aggravated when the lumen of the tube is partially occluded in preparation for its removal in the routine, graduated manner. Often the tracheal airway is only slightly larger than the tracheostomy tube; in such circumstances partial occlusion of the tube critically narrows the total available airway, causing exacerbation of the respiratory difficulty. It should also be appreciated that stridor may be temporarily increased after the tracheostomy tube has been taken out because of local edema and increased secretions. Tracheostomy, therefore, should be reserved for urgent situations with severe obstruction, tachypnea and cyanosis unrelieved by proper positioning and oxygen.

STENOSIS

Acute laryngeal stenosis is the term applied to sudden or rapidly progressive laryngeal obstruction of many and varied origins. (See also Chapter 18.) The causes include trauma, benign and malignant neoplasms, angioneurotic edema, and supraglottic, glottic and subglottic infections (*H. influenzae*, type B, group A streptococcus, *C. diphtheriae* among others). Foreign bodies may in themselves be obstructive or may induce reactive mucosal edema which produces the constriction. Bilateral midline abductor paralysis in which the vocal cords are in apposition and cannot be moved laterally (abducted) is another cause for stenosis.

The common pathologic feature is severe narrowing of the laryngeal airway which greatly interferes with the intake of air. Increase in respiratory effort and obstructive dyspnea follow. Infants and children usually become visibly apprehensive and anxious. Inspiratory stridor, dilatation of the alae nasi and retraction of the suprasternal, supraclavicular, intercostal, xiphoid and subcostal areas are evidences of obstruction of severe degree. Skin pallor which may vary from a dusky (cyanotic) hue to an ashen gray color and restlessness are signs of oxygen deficit.

Proper treatment consists in prompt management of the underlying cause, but in many situations immediate low tracheostomy may be the only reasonable immediate measure. Moist oxygen in high concentration is always indicated, but it is unwise to rely solely on this form of therapy. Sedation for the restless, dyspneic patient is contraindicated; the hazard of barbiturates and other sedatives lies in inducing sleep which may abolish the voluntary respiratory efforts and thereby

critically reduce the air exchange, leading to a fatal outcome. Once an adequate airway and air exchange have been reestablished, diagnostic laryngoscopy and additional therapeutic procedures can be carried out in comparative safety.

Chronic laryngeal stenosis is uncommon in childhood. It formerly was a frequent sequel to improperly placed tracheostomy (so-called high tracheostomy) in which the cricoid cartilage or first tracheal ring was incised. Intraluminal procedures, including intubation in small infants, and operations on the vocal cords may occasionally be followed by cicatricial stenosis. Congenital webs are by nature stenotic. Laryngeal diphtheria, syphilis and tuberculosis are now rarely seen and are of decreasing importance in the causation of this lesion. External direct trauma to the larynx is now the most important cause, but serious chronic laryngeal stenosis may be avoided or lessened by appropriate management of the acute injury (see Trauma, below). Hoarseness, stridor, dysphagia and dyspnea are the usual presenting complaints. Direct laryngoscopy and x-ray examinations, including laryngography and cinelaryngography using contrast media, are helpful in establishing the extent of the stenosis and its location. Correction involves surgical excision of scar tissue, plastic remodelling of the laryngeal cartilages and lumen and the use of an internal mold as a splint for several months while healing and maximum postoperative contraction takes place. The results of these procedures are encouraging.

TRAUMA

Internal trauma to the supraglottic and glottic structures is fortunately rare. Occasionally surgical procedures on the vocal cords in which the mucosa was injured or denuded have resulted in cicatricial web formation. Foreign bodies with sharp edges may cause perforating wounds leading to perichondritis. Pressure on the cricoid cartilage from an improperly fitted tracheostomy tube or from a firm naso-gastric feeding tube (reported only in adults) may produce necrosis and peri-chondritis of the cricoid and collapse of the subglottic space. Endolaryngeal burns from inhaled smoke and flame or caustic vapors occasionally occur in children, but are more often seen in firemen and in-dustrial workers.

External direct trauma to the larynx is far more common; most of these injuries are associated with automobile, athletic and industrial accidents. The cartilages may be contused, lacerated, perforated, fractured or dislocated. The glottic and thyroarytenoid folds may be torn; the intrinsic muscles may be injured; the re-current laryngeal nerves may be dam-aged, causing bilateral abductor paralysis. Hematomas, when present, are most fre-quently found in the supraglottic submu-cosa and mucosa. Gross internal laryngeal bleeding may be present and difficult to control. Trauma to other regions of the body often overshadows the laryngeal in-volvement until serious interference with breathing has developed.

The symptoms produced by direct trauma to the larynx are variable and are dependent upon the degree of distor-tion of the lumen from primary changes in the cartilaginous supporting structures and upon the extent of mucosal edema, hemorrhage and soft tissue injury. Im-mediate respiratory difficulties include laryngospasm which, if not quickly al-leviated, may cause death. Alone or in combination, stridor, hoarseness or apho-nia, obstructive dyspnea, dysphagia and pain on swallowing, and hemoptysis are indicative of potentially serious laryngeal injury.

Treatment involves immediate provi-sion of an adequate airway, by means of a tracheostomy, and the control of asso-ciated traumatic problems such as hemor-rhage and shock. Direct laryngoscopy aids in assessing the extent of the laryngeal injury; if fracture or dislocation of the cartilage is found, anatomic reduction and internal splinting are carried out as soon as the patient's condition permits.

Reconstructive surgery is then under-taken and usually involves several months of internal support by an indwelling luminal mold to prevent cicatrization. Chronic stenosis of the larynx is the most frequent sequel to trauma and may de-velop insidiously in the patient who has apparently recovered quickly and spon-taneously after laryngeal injury. It is wise in such patients to evaluate anatomically the larynx by palpation and endoscopy several weeks after injury to ascertain whether the larynx has fully recovered.

Birth trauma is occasionally associ-ated with congenital laryngeal problems. *Dislocations of the cricothyroid or cri-coarytenoid articulations* may lead to hoarseness, wheezing or stridor. Direct laryngoscopy is required to establish the diagnosis; treatment consists in laryngeal dilatation and other endoscopic manipu-lations. Tracheostomy may be needed if significant airway obstruction is present. Unilateral and bilateral *midline abductor laryngeal paralyses* are sometimes due to birth injury, especially in difficult in-strument deliveries. Although central nervous system signs of hypoxia and hem-orrhage predominate, the actual area of injury is more likely to be found in the vagus or inferior laryngeal nerve leading to flaccid palsy of the vocal cords. Al-though obstructive symptoms and signs may be short-lived, a tracheostomy airway is usually necessary until recovery takes place. (See Laryngeal Paralysis, p. 212.)

TUMORS

Epitheliomas, fibrosarcomas and *carci-nomas* of the larynx have been reported in childhood and adolescence, but malig-nant tumors are exceedingly rare in the first two decades of life. Hoarseness, dis-comfort, pain on swallowing or talking, dyspnea and stridor are symptoms which direct attention to these tumors. Diagnosis is made at direct laryngoscopy and is confirmed by biopsy. Therapy is depend-ent upon the location and the extent of lesion. Radical surgical excision and irradiation have been the procedures generally used.

Benign tumors are considerably less rare, but may be lethal if they cause respiratory obstruction. *Hemangiomas* in the subglottic region are occasionally responsible for stridor and dyspnea in early infancy. Hemangiomas elsewhere, particularly in the head and the neck, are found in many of these infants. Treatment is difficult and hazardous; irradiation may temporarily increase the size of the tumor, causing greater obstruction. Tracheostomy is usually necessary. The natural history of regression in the size of hemangiomas and the gradual increase in the size of the airway with growth favor ultimate improvement, but the mortality is high in infancy. The combination of tracheostomy, irradiation and later surgical excision has been successful in several instances. *Lymphangiomas* and *neurofibromas* have also been rarely found in the larynx.

Vocal nodules ("screamer's nodes") are occasionally responsible for slight hoarseness or "husky" voice in children. They are usually found on the free margins of the vocal cords at the junction of the anterior and middle thirds. Histologically, the nodules are inflammatory, with thickened epithelium covering fibrous and loose vascular tissue. Regression of the nodules follows vocal rest. Definitive therapy, when indicated, consists in surgical removal with special cupped forceps under direct laryngoscopic visualization.

Congenital embryonal cysts are sometimes found on the anterior surface of the epiglottis as well as on the vocal cords.

Aryepiglottic cysts may be responsible for increasing inspiratory stridor and serious respiratory obstruction in early infancy. These thick-walled mucus-retention cysts are technically difficult to excise. Recurrence usually follows partial excision, which may also be complicated by local hemorrhage which is controlled with difficulty. Periodic needle aspiration performed under direct laryngoscopic visualization may be helpful in reducing the size of the cystic mass until either spon-taneous regression takes place or surgical excision can be performed with safety.

Small *mucous cysts of the cord* are occasionally mistaken for vocal nodules. Treatment is surgical; superficial removal under direct laryngoscopy usually suffices.

The most common laryngeal neoplasms in childhood are *papillomas*. These benign tumors of epithelial origin are found in all parts of the larynx and less frequently in the trachea and bronchi; they usually occur as multiple lesions. Recurrence after surgical removal is common; malignant change is rare; spontaneous regression at or near puberty is frequent, and it is uncommon for adults with laryngeal papillomas to have had the disease as children. Hoarseness and dry cough are the initial symptoms; tachypnea, dyspnea, stridor and other signs of airway obstruction develop as the tumors enlarge.

At laryngoscopy papillomas are seen to resemble pink, irregular, verrucous-like growths; some have a filiform appearance. Tentative diagnosis can be made from the physical appearance of the tumors at direct or mirror laryngoscopy, but confirmation by biopsy is necessary. Treatment consists in the removal of these superficial growths with an appropriate grasping forceps through an endoscope. General anesthesia is necessary. The surgeon must exercise great care to avoid injury to underlying normal tissues; severe scarring of the larynx will result if these tissues are traumatized. Repeated excision is associated with a higher incidence of laryngeal fibrosis, and chronic huskiness of the voice is common in the patients with multiple recurrences. Tracheostomy is often necessary in children with severe papillomatosis. Contrast laryngography may be helpful in determining whether all papillomas have been removed, particularly when subglottic and upper tracheal lesions are present. Irradiation was sometimes used in treating these lesions in the past, but the lesions are generally resistant, and the growing larynx is particularly susceptible to radiation injury; hence present opinion is against radiation therapy. Vaccine preparations, based on the postulation that these papillomas are of viral origin, have not been particularly helpful. Ultrasonic therapy is now under study in several centers; preliminary results suggest that it may be useful in the control of these tumors.

Laryngeal polyps, considered to be of inflammatory or allergic origin, are occasional causes of hoarseness in children. These benign tumors vary in size and shape and may be either sessile or pedunculated in type. They usually arise on the free margin of the anterior half of the true vocal cord. Hoarseness is the usual presenting complaint. Treatment is simple excision by direct laryngoscopy.

The *laryngocele* is a congenital anomaly consisting of an air-containing sac communicating with the laryngeal ventricle. The sac may herniate through the thyrohyoid membrane and become visible in the neck between the hyoid bone and the thyroid cartilage, where it can be seen to bulge on coughing or straining. They may be identified within the larynx. Occasionally laryngoceles are of traumatic origin, the sac protruding through the fracture site. They may be associated with impairment of the voice. If they present externally, excision is indicated.

Laryngoscopy is an invaluable tool in the diagnosis and treatment of laryngeal tumors in childhood. The patient's age and size are not factors which should enter into the decision to carry out direct laryngoscopy; small infants can be safely subjected to laryngoscopy (or bronchoscopy) by physicians skilled in this procedure. Hoarseness, stridor, obstructive dyspnea and the other presenting complaints of laryngeal disease should be promptly investigated to establish a clear-cut cause for the symptomatology. Procrastination may permit the development of increasing respiratory difficulty, eventuating in complete laryngeal obstruction from a benign and easily eradicable cause.

FOREIGN BODIES

Aspiration of a foreign object is relatively common in childhood. In general, the area of lodgment is determined by the size, shape and density of the foreign body. Small ones, which easily pass through the glottis, are found in the lower respiratory passages; those which are larger than the diameter of the larynx at the vocal cords and those with sharp or pointed features tend to lodge above the cords or in the aperture between them. The local reaction produced by the object depends upon its composition, its shape and the degree of obstruction produced. Irritant substances of vegetal origin and sharp or irregular-surfaced materials will cause severe local mucosal edema, and penetration of the object beyond the mucosa may lead to submucosal inflammation and to perichondritis. Pressure necrosis, ulceration, bleeding, and mucosal or submucosal infection are often consequences of chronic foreign body lodgment.

The first symptoms of foreign body aspiration are choking, gagging, respiratory distress, cough, temporary aphonia and wheezing. Laryngospasm of a few seconds' duration is common. A symptom-free period may follow, or poorly localized pain may be present. Subsequent symptoms are relatable to the site where the foreign body lodges. Large objects may occlude the airway completely. If the object is smaller and remains in the larynx, hoarseness or aphonia and a "croupy" cough (a sign of subglottic edema) are usually present; wheezing, with or without dyspnea, and cyanosis are common. Progressive signs of obstruction may follow as mucosal edema increases and contributes to the narrowing of the airway; total obstruction resulting in a fatal outcome may ensue if the object is not promptly removed or tracheostomy performed. Radiopaque substances may be identified by x-ray examination. Anteroposterior and lateral views of the neck will generally show the foreign body to be lodged anteriorly and to lie in the sagittal plane. Because of lack of contrast, radiolucent materials are rarely identifiable on x-ray films.

The nature of the aspirated foreign body is dependent upon the child's age, his environment and parental example (e.g. placing tacks and pins in the mouth). Although few instances occur under six months of age, thumbtacks from bassinets and small safety pins pose the principal hazard. Safety pins continue to be most frequent until two years of age; coins, small plastic toys and all kinds of hardware predominate thereafter. Nuts, especially peanuts, and nut shells are serious threats to children from one to five years. The two-year-old is especially prone to aspiration; small metal and plastic objects and nuts which are potential foreign bodies should be kept from his environment.

Direct laryngoscopy is the procedure of choice for identification and removal of laryngeal foreign bodies. If respiratory obstruction or dyspnea is present, tracheostomy prior to x-ray studies and laryngoscopy will decrease the risk of total airway obstruction during endoscopy. Whenever possible, instrumentation for the removal of foreign bodies in the larynx and elsewhere in the tracheobronchial tree should be performed under optimum conditions, preferably in the operating room, by physicians skilled in the management of these problems.

Tracheal foreign bodies may produce signs and symptoms similar to those of laryngeal lodgment; often, however, they are relatively symptomless for long periods after the initial aspiration. The presence of a dry cough or asthma-like wheezing in a child with a history of choking or gagging on nuts, grass or other substance is worthy of investigation for foreign body; the absence of such history by no means excludes the possibility.

The classic clinical signs of tracheal foreign bodies include an inspiratory and expiratory *audible wheeze* heard best by listening to the breath sounds at the pa-

tient's open mouth, the *audible slap* and the *palpatory thud*. The sudden stopping of the foreign body as it is propelled against the glottis in expiration or in coughing produces the slapping sound, which, like the wheeze, is best heard through the patient's open mouth. The thud is the palpable component of the slap and is felt by palpating the thyroid cartilages. Laryngeal signs of hoarseness and croupy cough are the result of trauma from the foreign body striking the larynx. Auscultatory findings in both lungs may be produced by a foreign body at the bifurcation of the trachea.

Radiopaque substances can be seen by x-ray film, but most foreign bodies are of vegetal or plastic origin. Peanuts, dry beans, and seeds may cause immediate and severe mucosal edema, whereas bones, shells, inorganic substances and grasses give rise to more insidious mucosal reaction and to a secondary infection which ultimately leads to suppurative pulmonary disease if the foreign body is not detected.

A history of choking, gagging, wheezing or protracted coughing is helpful, but the possibility of aspiration cannot be discarded if the history is atypical or devoid of a suspicious initial episode. When the patient's presenting symptoms and physical signs lead to the suspicion of foreign body aspiration, the diagnosis should be confirmed or eliminated promptly. X-ray studies may be helpful, but normal findings do not exclude the many nonopaque foreign body possibilities. Although it has been estimated that 2 per cent of the tracheal foreign bodies are spontaneously expelled by coughing, so long as the alien material remains in the trachea the patient is in danger of total airway obstruction from impaction of the foreign body at the glottis. Removal of the foreign body by peroral bronchoscopy is, therefore, mandatory; diagnostic bronchoscopy should be carried out as quickly as possible under optimum circumstances, and in children this will usually involve general anesthesia in the hospital operating room.

Postbronchoscopy care will depend upon the nature of the foreign body and the difficulty with which it is removed.

LARYNGEAL PARALYSIS

The frequency of laryngeal paralysis in childhood is not known with any certainty. Flaccid paralysis of the abductor musculature (*midline abductor paralysis*), a lower motor neuron lesion, is seen in both the bilateral and unilateral forms in newborns, in whom these problems are usually related to birth trauma associated with difficult instrument deliveries. Paralysis may be transitory, lasting a week or two, or may less commonly be permanent. Unilateral abductor paralysis is the most common variety and is almost always left-sided. Stridor and hoarse cry are the usually observed signs in unilateral disease; dyspnea, cyanosis and other findings of respiratory obstruction are found in bilateral involvement when the failure of the cords to abduct results in closure of the glottis and promotes asphyxia. In the newborn bilateral abductor paralysis is an emergency, requiring immediate attention. Direct laryngoscopy will reveal the failure of abduction, and an endotracheal or bronchoscopic airway will permit adequate air exchange and alleviation of hypoxia. If the vocal cords resume the closed position as the bronchoscope is removed, then the bronchoscope should be reinserted and a low tracheostomy performed with the bronchoscope in place. Moist oxygen should be provided throughout the procedure. Direct laryngoscopy is then repeated at intervals until laryngeal function returns and the tracheostomy can be safely removed.

Abductor paralysis, usually unilateral, is also seen in older children; trauma, perforating injuries which damage the inferior laryngeal nerve, and pressure on the nerve by tumors, adenopathy and enlarged left atrium are the leading causes.

Adductor paralysis, usually due to an upper motor neuron (central) lesion, is seldom reported in childhood, but may be more commonly present, especially in conjunction with severe head trauma. It may be an unrecognized contributor to breathing difficulty in newborns with intracranial bleeding and edema. The patient is without voice because the glottis is continuously open; the cough tends to be weak and wheezy. Treatment depends on the underlying cause. Chronic tracheobronchitis and chronic food aspiration are the main complications.

Other varieties of laryngeal paralysis are described in adults: total, transitory adductor, cricothyroid muscle paralysis, and others. Although these entities are not reported in childhood, it seems likely that careful examination of all children with stridor will ultimately reveal the full spectrum of adult laryngeal disease of neurogenic origin.

REFERENCES

Boies, L. R., Hilger, J. A., and Priest, R. E.: *Fundamentals of Otolaryngology.* 4th ed. Philadelphia, W. B. Saunders Company, 1964.

Holinger, P. H., Johnson, K. C., and Schiller, F.: Congenital Anomalies of the Larynx. *Ann. Otol., Rhin. & Laryng.,* 63:581, 1954.

Jackson, C., and Jackson, C. L.: *Diseases of Nose, Throat and Ear.* Philadelphia, W. B. Saunders Company, 1959.

Rabe, E. F.: Infectious Croup. I. Etiology. II. "Virus" Croup. III. Hemophilus Influenzae Type B Croup. *Pediatrics,* 2:255, 415, 559, 1948.

SECTION V

The Ear

CHAPTER TEN

The Ear

G. DOUGLAS HAYDEN, M.D.,
and GAYLE G. ARNOLD, M.D.

ANATOMY

External Ear

The external ear consists of the auricle and the external auditory canal. Cartilage and skin make up the entire auricle except for the lobule, which contains no cartilage. The muscles that attach the auricle to the head are innervated by the seventh cranial nerve. The lymphatic drainage of these structures is anteriorly, inferiorly and posteriorly. Postauricular lymphadenopathy in patients with external otitis or scalp lesions may confuse the examiner, and one has to examine the middle ear and hearing carefully to differentiate this from a subperiosteal abscess. The sensory nerve supply is from the great auricular nerve, the lesser occipital nerve, auricular branch of the vagus nerve (Arnold's nerve) and the auriculotemporal nerve (V).

External Auditory Canal

The external canal is oblique, so that its superior wall is about 5 mm. shorter than its anterior inferior wall. This accounts for the oblique position of the tympanic membrane. Furthermore, the canal bends, and it is necessary to straighten it by upward traction on the auricle before the ear drum can be easily examined in most patients. The outer half of the ear is cartilaginous and the inner half bony, except in the infant, in whom

ossification has not yet occurred. The skin lining the cartilaginous canal is thick and contains fine hairs, sebaceous glands and special glands that produce cerumen. Epithelium lining the bony half of the ear canal is very thin and contains no hair or glands. Therefore wax found next to the tympanic membrane probably has been pushed there. The epithelium is very delicate, and the slightest trauma may produce a hematoma.

Middle Ear

The middle ear is a roughly oblong cavity lined by mucous membrane. All its walls, except the lateral wall, are bony. The inferior part of the lateral wall is the tympanic membrane. Anteriorly, the eustachian tube leads downward and medially to the nasopharynx. The middle ear opens posteriorly and superiorly into the mastoid antrum. The auditory ossicles, malleus, incus and stapes are located in the posterior-superior part of the middle ear. The tensor tympani muscle attaches to the malleus, and the stapedial muscle to the stapes. The seventh cranial nerve crosses the medial wall of the middle ear in close proximity to the stapes.

Eustachian Tube

The eustachian tube connects the middle ear and the nasopharynx, providing an air passage from the nasopharynx to the middle ear through which the pressure in the middle ear is equalized with that of the external ear. The tube is normally closed and opens during swallowing, but not with every swallow. When pus is under pressure in the middle ear, drainage is naturally accomplished by perforation of the ear drum rather than by way of the eustachian tube, which has been closed by swelling. The eustachian tube can have anatomic changes which diminish its caliber and thus predispose to lack of aeration in the middle ear, thereby initiating the development of chronic otitis media and its consequences. At the opening of the tube in the nasopharynx, adenoid tissue surrounds the ostium, so that enlarged or swollen lymph tissue here can also cause poor drainage of the middle ear.

Mastoid

The mastoid portion of the temporal bone provides an attachment for the sternocleidomastoid and digastric muscles. At birth the mastoid process is present, but is small and filled with diploic bone. During the first two to six years of life the diploic bone is gradually replaced by air cells which bud off from the mastoid antrum in pneumatic mastoids. In some cases pneumatization does not occur, and the mastoid is classified as a sclerotic or acellular mastoid.

The nerve supply of the middle ear is from branches of the fifth, seventh, ninth and tenth cranial nerves. Branches of these nerves form the tympanic plexus on the promontory of the middle ear. Disturbance of other areas supplied by these nerves, such as teeth, tongue, tonsils and larynx, may cause referred pain to the ear.

Inner Ear

The inner ear is that portion of the ear composed of the end-organ receptors for hearing (the cochlea) and equilibrium (the labyrinth). These structures are protected by extremely hard bone (otic capsule) and are surrounded by fluid (perilymph) and filled with fluid (endolymph).

The cochlea is shaped like a small snail and makes $2\frac{1}{2}$ turns. The basal turn makes up the promontory of the middle ear. The neural end-organ for hearing is the organ of Corti, which extends the length of the cochlea. When its hair cells are bent or distorted, the mechanical force of sound is converted into an electrochemical impulse which is interpreted in the temporal cortex as understandable sound. High-pitched sounds stimulate the basal portion of the cochlea, and low-pitched sounds the apical end.

Vestibule

The vestibular portion of the inner ear is composed of the utricle, saccule and three semicircular canals. Both ends of each of the semicircular canals open into the utricle, and near the utricle each canal has an enlargement known as the ampulla. In each ampulla is found the specialized neuroepithelium (cristae) which is the end-organ for equilibrium. Additional specialized epithelium is present in the utricle. The axons from the utricle, saccule and semicircular canals join to form the vestibular portion of the eighth cranial nerve.

PHYSIOLOGY

When the utricle or semicircular canals are stimulated, nystagmus, past pointing and loss of equilibrium are expected to occur. Motion of the endolymph stimulates the hair cells of the cristae, which set up a series of reflexes causing contraction in the extraocular muscles, the neck muscles and the muscles of the trunk and extremities. In normal persons these reactions restore the body position when any force throws it out of balance. Artificial stimulation (caloric test) or a malfunctioning labyrinth will cause vertigo.

DEVELOPMENTAL ABNORMALITIES

Congenital malformations of the external ear result from developmental failure of the first and second branchial arches and grooves. For the patient with aural atresia, the establishment of useful hearing is the most desired result of any operative procedure. The best basis for comprehending the problems encountered in aural atresia is knowledge of the embryology of the ear.

Embryology

The components of the ear are derived from all three embryonic primordial layers, ectoderm, mesoderm and entoderm. Early in the third week of intrauterine development the superficial ectoderm thickens on both sides of the neural plate. This thickening (auditory placode) invaginates during the fourth week to form the auditory pit. Later the auditory vesicle differentiates into the vestibular and cochlear portion of the membranous labyrinth, and by the third month an almost adult configuration exists. While the membranous labyrinth has been taking shape, the surrounding mesenchyme has been transformed into cartilage and is separated from the membranous labyrinth by the perilymphatic space. The cartilage capsule is converted into bone by the spreading of multiple centers of enchondral ossification. On the outside of the embryonic head, between the first and second branchial arches, a branchial groove becomes the outer part of the external canal; the inner portion is not formed until the sixth or seventh fetal month. Toward the end of the second fetal month a solid epithelial cord grows inward from the primitive meatus, ending in a dishlike extension close to the epithelium of the developing tympanic cavity from which it is separated by the thin layer of connective tissue, which will become the fibrous layer of the tympanic membrane. This epithelial cord begins to canalize at its medial end in the seventh fetal month, forming the outer surface of the tympanic membrane and then proceeding outward to open into the primitive meatus.

The dorsal end of the first pharyngeal pouch, through gradual extension, becomes the eustachian tube, the tympanic cavity, epitympanic recess, the mastoid antrum and mastoid air cells. The entodermal layer of the pouch becomes the epithelium of the mucous membrane of the middle ear. The auditory ossicles are derived from cartilaginous supports of the branchial arches. The malleus and incus are derived from Meckel's cartilage of the first branchial arch which also forms the mandible. The stapes is partially derived from Reichert's cartilage of the second branchial arch and partially from the otic capsule. The muscles and ligaments of the middle ear which are associated with the ossicles arise from the mesoderm in which these cartilages are embedded.

The epithelium at the depth of the first branchial groove is separated from the entoderm of the first pharyngeal pouch by mesodermal tissue. Together these form the tympanic membrane, which separates the external ear from the middle ear.

The auricle is formed by growth of the mesenchymal tissue flanking the first branchial grove. By about the sixth week six knoblike evaginations appear which coalesce by the third month. Their further development molds the pinna of the ear, the tragus coming from the first branchial arch and the remainder from the second branchial arch. At the site where the hillocks of these two arches join, an epithelium-lined pit may persist as a congenital preauricular cyst or fistula.

Malformations of the outer end of the middle ear result from disturbances in development. Disturbance in differentiation of the first and second branchial arches may result in microtia or anotia. Failure of the first branchial groove to develop may cause atresia of the external auditory meatus. Failure of the first branchial arch to differentiate may result in malformation of the malleus and incus. Malformation of the stapes results from developmental failure of the second branchial arch or of the otic capsule.

The development of the membranous labyrinth is independent of the development of the middle ear. Therefore, in the majority of cases of impairment of hearing due to congenital malformation, only the sound-conducting apparatus (ossicles, drum) or only the neurosensory apparatus (labyrinth, cochlea) is involved.

Abnormalities of the Auricle

Minor Variation in Shape

There is a wide variation in the shape of the auricle, and no two human beings have ears exactly alike, and the ears are not exactly identical in one person. The ears of many children appear unduly prominent until the mastoid process has developed. Parental anxiety concerning the so-called bat ears or lop ears is understandable, but correction should be delayed until the mastoid process has developed and the true configuration of the ear deformity can be determined.

True Deformities of the Auricle

Anotia (absence of the auricle) is usually part of a first arch syndrome involving agenesis of other elements. Reconstructive plastic surgery seldom, if ever, succeeds in building an auricle which can be considered an improvement upon the modern artificial prosthesis. *Microtia,* in varying degrees, is seen in conjunction with atresia of the external meatus and other mandibular arch anomalies.

Congenital Aural Fistula, Preauricular

Defective closure of the first branchial cleft may result in a persistent fistula, opening in most cases close to the anterior border of the ascending limb of the helix, but they may be found elsewhere. Aural fistulas are lined by stratified squamous epithelium and often follow a complex course inward, as far as the tympanic ring, where they end abruptly. Fistulas seldom give rise to symptoms unless they become infected. Nothing short of complete excision of the tract will result in cure of infection with chronic discharge or recurrent abscess.

First-Arch Syndrome

Different types of anomalies affecting the head and neck have been attributed to a single, hereditary, first-arch syndrome caused by a dominant gene.

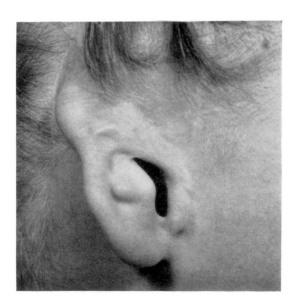

FIGURE 10–1. Abnormal pinna.

TREACHER-COLLINS SYNDROME. This syndrome consists of notched lower eyelids and hypoplasia of the malar bones; other associated anomalies include agenesis of the mandible, poorly developed eyelashes in the medial part of the lower lid, abnormalities of the external ear and middle ear, deafness, and drooping of the outer canthus, giving an antimongoloid obliquity of the palpebral fissures. The term "mandibulofacial dysostosis" is applicable to this combination of abnormalities. Treatment is regional. Each case requires separate otological assessment of the functional and cosmetic problems concerned.

PIERRE ROBIN SYNDROME. Hypoplasia of the mandible may be associated with posterior displacement of the tongue and cleft palate.

DEFORMITIES OF THE EXTERNAL EAR AND MIDDLE EAR. In general, the greater deformity of the auricle, especially in the direction of anotia, the greater is the likelihood of associated meatal and middle ear deformities.

CONGENITAL DEAF-MUTISM. Although most frequently perceptive in type, congenital deaf-mutism can occur in severe abnormalities involving the conductive apparatus. Failure to gain normal speech in a child with first arch anomalies demands careful diagnostic assessment of the type of deafness present.

Conductive deafness is remediable by surgery or a hearing aid and normal development of speech ensured if the conductive deafness is recognized early as a cause of mutism. It is equally important to recognize perceptive deafness as the cause of mutism and encourage audiologic evaluation and speech therapy.

Atresias

Isolated Atresia

Although atresia commonly occurs in association with microtia and abnormalities of the middle ear, there are some patients whose congenital deformity consists solely of a failure of complete canalization

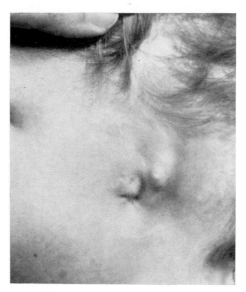

FIGURE 10–2. Anotia and atresia.

of the ectodermal core which fills the dorsal end of the first branchial cleft during the eighth to twenty-eighth week of fetal life. In such cases the deep part of the meatus is canalized, but the outer part is replaced by bone or fibrous tissue, or by an extremely narrow passage with an hourglass constriction. Sometimes the canal will end in a blind pouch, and beneath will be a bony atretic plate blocking the passage of sound to the middle ear.

Atresia with Microtia and Abnormal Middle Ear

A combination of congenital defects of the ear is most commonly encountered. An abnormal auricle and an absent or rudimentary meatus usually involves a middle ear defect, especially when x-ray films reveal a small sclerotic mastoid. Defects may vary from a complete lack of the middle ear to various malformations of the ossicles.

Atresia with Inner Ear Affected

Although the development of the inner ear is nonbranchiogenic, it is not exceptional for inner ear anomalies to be com-

bined with congenital abnormalities of
the external ear and middle ear. The
presence or absence of normal inner ear
auditory function has an important bearing on treatment, and appropriate tests,
including radiographic studies, must always be carried out as part of the routine
assessment of all cases of atresia.

Pathophysiology

Microtia and congenital atresia are
noted immediately or soon after birth,
and attention is focused first on the deformity rather than on the hearing problem. If the malformation is unilateral,
the hearing becomes of secondary importance if the hearing in the opposite ear is
normal. In typical cases hearing tests show
a conductive type of impairment and
often relatively good hearing of the spoken voice. Even in bilateral atresia with
normal cochlear function, the spoken
voice is understood when it is loud enough
and speech development is not necessarily
impaired severely. These children, therefore, do not become "deaf mutes."

Treatment

Reconstructive surgery is justified when
reasonable success can be expected after
appropriate investigation of the cochlear
function and radiologic studies of the
middle ear and mastoids. When possible,
in bilateral meatal atresia, the operation
should be postponed until the child is six
or seven years old when the mastoid process has become well pneumatized and the
middle ear has completed its development. Unilateral aural atresia with normal hearing in the other ear does not
present an urgent hearing problem; hence
operation may be postponed until later.
Still, the advantages of binaural over
monaural hearing may persuade the surgeon to attempt early correction.

Abnormalities of the Tympanic Membrane

Rudimentary tympanic membrane is
usually found with congenital defects of
the meatus and middle ear. Defects in the
drum may be corrected with the use of
skin or fascia grafts.

Abnormalities of the Middle Ear and Mastoid Process

Congenital fixation of the stapes may
occur in the absence of other obvious associated abnormalities. A presumptive
diagnosis is based on the presence of severe congenital conductive deafness in an
otherwise normal ear. The recommended
treatment is stapedectomy and replacement of the stapes with a prosthesis made
from stainless steel wire or Teflon.

Natural dehiscence may occur in the
tympanic portion of the fallopian canal,
thus accounting for some cases of facial
nerve palsy in association with middle ear
infections. Bony deficiencies may also
occur in the tegmen tympani which, together with persistence of embryonic connections between small vessels of the dura
mater and tegmen, predispose to intracranial spread of infection from the middle ear and mastoid antrum. Absence of
mastoid air cells is not considered an abnormality.

Congenital Cholesteatoma

Primary or congenital cholesteatomas
are tumors, believed to arise from epithelial cell rests in the temporal bone. These
epidermoid tumors are rare compared
with the secondary cholesteatomas of the
middle ear. From an aberrant epidermal
rest, keratinizing stratified epithelium begins to form a tumor composed of material shed from the epithelium and
arranged in laminated whorls. Enlargement of the cholesteatoma is accompanied by slow destruction of structures in

and around the petrous bone. The labyrinth and facial nerve may be eroded, as well as the middle ear structures.

Clinical Features

The majority of cases of congenital cholesteatoma present with symptoms referable to the seventh cranial nerve, either as twitching of the face or progressive facial weakness and severe deafness in the affected ear. If the tumor erodes the membrane and becomes infected, the patient may present with an acute complication of otitis media; i.e. meningitis, because the intratemporal erosion is likely to have extensive exposure of the dura.

X-ray films of the temporal bone and skull will suggest some abnormality or outline a spherical defect.

Treatment

Surgical removal to prevent further destruction of the temporal bone, to attempt the restoration of the facial nerve function and to forestall the possible complication of infection and subsequent meningitis is the treatment of choice.

DISEASES AND INFECTIONS OF THE EXTERNAL EAR

Foreign Bodies

Foreign bodies in the external auditory canal are found most commonly in children who, out of boredom or curiosity, are wont to push beads, food or any small object that comes to hand, into the ear. Insects, kernels of corn, sand, gravel and other material may be encountered at any age on otoscopic examination; the foreign body may be asymptomatic or responsible for symptoms of irritation and pain. Vegetable foreign bodies, such as beans, tend to swell and become macerated, causing local inflammation of the skin. A foreign body in this area may be the primary cause of a chronic, nonpro-

ductive, persistent cough; removal of the foreign body leads to immediate subsidence of the cough. The reflex cough is by way of Arnold's nerve, a branch of the tenth cranial nerve.

If the foreign body lies external to the isthmus, it may be removed with either forceps or a hook. Observation of the foreign body will help in determining the best instrument to use. Any round or hard object is likely to be forced deeper into the meatus if an attempt is made to grasp it with forceps. A right angle hook is helpful in most cases. If the foreign body cannot be removed by forceps or hook, use of an ear syringe may be indicated. The solution used in syringing must pass between the foreign-body and the meatal wall to build up an expulsive pressure. Use of a suction apparatus sometimes succeeds where other methods fail. The child must be held firmly, but if he is uncooperative, attempts at removal without general anesthesia must be abandoned. Once the skin of the meatus is injured, the procedure becomes painful, and when the patient struggles, the risk of damage to the tympanic membrane is added. If the object lies internal to the isthmus and appears to fill the meatus, it is wise not to attempt removal without an anesthetic. Smaller objects, however, may be flushed out.

Insects may be drowned and removed by syringing. If living, they may first be killed by instilling chloroform or ether. The discovery of a foreign body in one ear calls for examination of the other ear and nasal passages, for some children tend to secrete objects in more than one orifice.

External Otitis (Otitis Externa)

The skin normally offers strong resistance to infection. An intact stratum corneum is an effective barrier against the entry of organisms, particularly if it maintains a skin pH from 3.0 to 5.0.

External otitis is difficult to classify because of the secondary infection and inflammatory change. Pure fungous disease, for example, may become complicated by bacterial invasion and an eczematoid reaction and simple bacterial infection may be modified through secondary involvement of fungus and other bacteria. When the ear is examined, one should acquire the habit of inspecting the external ear and meatal opening before inserting the ear speculum. Swelling about the meatal orifice or pain on traction of the pinna is suggestive of an acute external otitis. Purulent exudate in the canal does not necessarily denote middle ear disease.

It is the responsibility of the physician to see the tympanic membrane, and careful and gentle removal of all exudate and debris is necessary for both diagnosis and treatment of ear disease. This may be effected by using aural spot suction or cotton-tipped aural probes moistened with a solution such as Cresatin, or careful use of curets and syringing. Canals filled with caseous debris are often seen in small infants; if the child permits thorough and gentle cleaning of the canal without crying or moving, it is almost diagnostic of chronic external otitis. Often he appears to enjoy the cleansing.

Diffuse Otitis Externa (Swimmer's Ear)

A great many cases of otitis externa present clinically as a diffuse infection of the whole external meatus with symptoms of irritation, discharge and swelling. Cultures usually grow *Staphylococcus aureus, P. pyocyaneus* and Proteus. Fungi may sometimes be identified. There is little evidence to support the contention that bathing in fresh or sea water causes sufficient maceration of the horny layer to allow entry of organisms, but it is possible that vigorous drying with a twisted and perhaps dirty towel corner is a factor.

Typical clinical features of the acute phase are a burning sensation in the ear followed by aural discharge and swelling of the soft tissues with resultant pain. On examination the skin of the meatus at first

appears red and moist, while the intact tympanic membrane may at times look opaque. Later the appearance of the meatus reflects the intense exudation and exfoliation, while swelling may hinder adequate examination.

In the chronic phase there may be a scanty discharge along with a mild irritation and pruritus. The risk of reinfection and acute flare-up is great. Examination of the meatus sometimes reveals a gray, boggy, swollen appearance of the skin, or a scaly appearance with a tendency to bleed if the scales are pulled off.

In the treatment, careful and gentle removal of all exudate and debris with a cotton-tipped ear applicator and with an aural spot suction apparatus, when indicated, is absolutely necessary. The cotton-tipped applicator may be moistened with Cresatin, or if the canal is too inflamed, sterile liquid paraffin renders the cotton less abrasive. Local medication such as VoSol otic solution with hydrocortisone will clear up the majority of cases if the preliminary cleansing has been thorough.

In all cases, whenever practical, culture for bacteria and fungi should be taken from the meatus when the patient is first seen. Local antibiotics should then be used in accordance with the results of the culture and the sensitivity of the organism to the various antibiotics. If the cleansing has been thorough, the use of ear drops such as those containing drying agents, antibiotics and steroids will usually produce an excellent result even though the culture report is not available.

If considerable edema occludes the canal, a wick soaked in VoSol (1,2 propanediol diacetate 3.0 per cent, acetic acid 2.0 per cent, benzethonium chloride 0.02 per cent, in propylene glycol) solution should be inserted into the canal. The drop solution should then be applied four times daily and the patient scheduled for returns at 24- to 48-hour intervals for changing of the wick. A wick thoroughly saturated with Mycolog (Mycostatin, neomycin-gramicidin, triamcinolone acetonide) is effective and does not require the instillation of additional drops. Removal of the wick, cleansing of the canal and insertion of another wick are carried out at 48-hour intervals until the canal shows no exudate, desquamation, edema or erythema. Systemic therapy with an antibiotic or chemotherapy may be helpful in promoting more rapid healing.

During the local treatment of otitis externa, general measures to assist natural healing and prevent reinfection are advisable. It is most important to keep the ear canals dry and avoid local trauma; skin disorders such as furuncles and nail-bed infections which may lead to reinfection should be adequately treated.

Otomycosis

The fungi account for only a small percentage of the causative factors of external otitis. They may secondarily invade a primary bacterial infection or seborrheic dermatitis and lead to chronicity and apparent resistance to treatment. The fungi most commonly found are *Aspergillus niger, Aspergillus fumigatus* and *Candida (Monilia) albicans*. When present among debris, the *Aspergillus niger* may be identified by the black-headed conidiophores. The conidiophores of *Aspergillus fumigatus* may be pale blue or greenish. *Candida albicans* may be seen as white or cream-colored desposits, but are difficult to differentiate from squamous debris.

In the moist stage of otitis externa, mycelial threads or conidiophores are not visible to the naked eye; unless the exudate is examined microscopically in the laboratory, the fungus will not be identified. Suspected debris may be placed on a drop of 10 per cent caustic potash on a slide and covered with a cover slip, warmed slightly and examined. The discharge is commonly scanty and usually colorless. Irritation in the ear canal may be intense, but meatal swelling is rare. In the acute state the canal is clogged with a mass of pultaceous debris which on removal reveals a magenta-colored epithelial surface studded with small, glistening white deposits. In less acute cases asper-

gillus clusters may be seen with the otoscope. Candida infections generally appear as white deposits on magenta-colored skin.

With these facts in mind and the knowledge that the entity exists, treatment for otomycosis should be given an immediate trial in any suspicious case.

In treating otomycosis, thorough cleansing as previously described for external otitis, followed by application of a medication such as Cresatin drops, Vioform or Mycostatin ointment, will correct the majority of cases rapidly.

Furunculosis

Furunculosis occurs only in the outer cartilaginous portion of the canal where there are hair follicles. This inflammatory reaction in the depths of the hair follicle begins with discomfort which increases to severe pain about the ear. The boil is noted in the meatal area in various stages from a slight painful swelling, sensitive to the touch of a probe or speculum, to a large swelling with occlusion of the meatal opening.

If the furuncle is on the posteroinferior segment of the meatus, the edema may obliterate the postauricular sulcus, causing protrusion of the auricle. The physician must be certain that an acute mastoid infection is not present; the history and examination are usually sufficient to exclude mastoid involvement. The cardinal signs and symptoms of otitis are deep earache, deafness and otorrhea. The latter may appear within a few hours after the onset of pain, with subsequent symptomatic relief. In furunculosis the pain may last several days, without deafness, before the furuncle and pus appear in the canal. Traction on the pinna accentuates pain when a furuncle is present, and the lymph node anterior to the tragus may be enlarged and tender to pressure. These findings are not noted with mastoiditis (Fig. 3). History of recent otitis media suggests the possibility of mastoiditis. The signs of acute mastoiditis vary with the extent

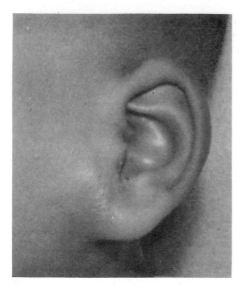

FIGURE 10–3. Furuncle, external canal, with preauricular lymph node.

of the disease. There may be retroauricular edema and tenderness, pus on the ear canal and sagging of the posterosuperior meatal wall; on the other hand, there may be only slight tenderness or pressure over the retroauricular area, an opaque membrane with some conductive deafness, and radiologic evidence of the coalescence of air cells.

Treatment

Incision should be postponed until central necrosis has occurred and pus can be seen about to burst through the skin. If incision is made too early, there is risk of spreading the infection and causing a perichondritis. A medicated wick such as a cotton wick with Mycolog ointment is recommended along with adequate doses of penicillin or a broad-spectrum antibiotic. The wick should be changed daily for five or six days and the canal cleansed gently of debris and pus. Opiates or similar medications are needed in most cases for the relief of pain.

The skin surrounding a previous furuncle must be disinfected or it will harbor *Staphylococcus aureus* and predispose to

recurrent furunculosis. The control of recurrent furunculosis is based upon elimination of the Staphylococcus from the skin of the auditory canal and from carrier sites such as the nasal vestibules. Aural discharge from chronic otitis media predisposes to furunculosis and should be diagnosed and treated.

EXAMINATION OF THE MIDDLE EAR

To the physician the examination of the middle ear of an infant or child may be the most profitable part of a general physical examination. He may find the primary cause of the presenting complaint in a surprisingly great number of children. The presenting complaint may be fever, cough, vomiting, diarrhea, sleeplessness, crying, irritability, personality change, deafness or earache. Any or all of these may be due to middle ear disease.

The physician looks down the external auditory canal at the tympanic membrane to answer the question: What is in the middle ear? The membrane is a window which provides a view into the middle ear, and the answer to the foregoing question may be air, fluid, pus, blood, scar tissue or congenital anomaly. The diagnosis of otitis media is tenable only when something other than air is in the middle ear.

The tympanic membrane of a premature or newborn infant is difficult to see and evaluate because of detritus in the external canal. Once the drum is visible, however, visual diagnosis is possible. The light reflex is not prominent, the drum has a gray or silvery appearance, and in the very young menisci of clear fluid may be seen. The infant is peculiarly prone to middle ear disease because of the anatomic closeness to the nasopharynx and the straight, short eustachian tube. Prematures may have middle ear disease as part of the clinical syndrome of sepsis. A recent postmortem study of the middle ear structures of prematures showed a high percentage of middle ear infection which had not been suspected clinically. When the diagnosis is questionable in a tiny baby with sepsis, a diagnostic myringotomy may be indicated.

When the examiner has sufficiently cleaned the external canal of wax and debris and the tympanic membrane is easily visible, the drum may appear to be too close to the otoscope speculum and none of the usual landmarks may be visible. If, in addition, the surface of the presenting membrane has a strawberry-like appearance or single or multiple bullae bulge into the external canal from the surface of the drum, bullous myringitis is probable. These bullae are extremely painful; in spite of all symptomatic measures, they are the commonest form of middle ear disease to give parents and child a sleepness night. It is our practice to break these bullae to give relief from the severe pain and to enable the examiner to visualize the ear drum and determine whether or not otitis media is present. Rarely bullous myringitis or influenzal myringitis will be seen in which the drum or canal shows one or more hemorrhagic bullae with no middle ear disease. Treatment is similar, and may then be followed by an anesthetic, hygroscopic ear drop for local relief of pain.

When inspection of the drum shows a glistening, transparent membrane, with a normal-sized light reflex, the examiner can be certain that the middle ear contains only air. The commonest error made by physicians is to mistakenly call an ear normal when there is actually very thin fluid present; if the middle ear cavity is full "to the top," no fluid level will be visible. Much experience is necessary to differentiate a catarrhal otitis media from a slightly scarred or retracted drum. Audiometry is helpful. All physicians can easily use the Weber test by simply placing a 512 cps tuning fork on the child's forehead, and then asking where the sound is heard. In unilateral conduction deafness it is heard in the obstructed ear (Fig. 4). By using the

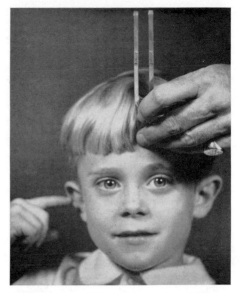

FIGURE 10–4. The Weber test. "Where do you hear it?"

same fork, bilateral conduction deafness can be suspected when bone conduction is equal to or greater than air conduction. Normally, in an unobstructed ear, air conduction is much greater than bone conduction.

Figure 5 shows the otoscopic findings and the corresponding pathology in the middle ear. The circular diagram represents an ear drum, seen through a speculum, and the cut-away diagram represents a sagittal section through the middle ear at the same time.

As treated catarrhal or purulent otitis media subsides, frequent examination may show these stages in reverse, as the process heals.

If there is unsatisfactory improvement after a reasonable period of adequate medical management, myringotomy and the suctioning of pus from the middle ear should be carried out. Often the fluid in the middle ear is of gluelike consistency and will not drain through a simple myringotomy incision. Myringotomy and suctioning may be necessary many times, and if the infection is chronic, involvement of the mastoid must be suspected.

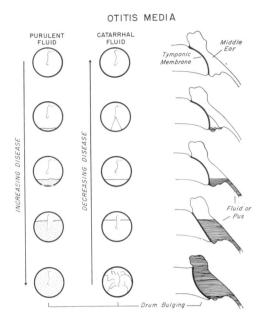

OTITIS MEDIA

PURULENT FLUID   CATARRHAL FLUID

Middle Ear

Tympanic Membrane

INCREASING DISEASE   *DECREASING DISEASE*

Fluid or Pus

— Drum Bulging —

FIGURE 10–5. Otoscopic findings in the middle ear.

DISEASES OF THE MIDDLE EAR

Acute Otitis Media

Otitis media is an inflammation of part or all of the mucoperiosteal lining of the middle ear cleft. The middle ear cleft is the collective anatomic term for the eustachian tube, tympanic cavity, mastoid antrum and mastoid air cells. As long as the inflammatory process is confined to the mucoperiosteal lining of these air spaces, otitis media is uncomplicated. If the inflammatory process affects any part of the bony walls or spreads beyond these walls into adjacent structures, the disease becomes otitis media with a complication. As long as the inflammation is confined to the lining of the cleft, it is a relatively safe and easily managed condition, but once the inflammation has spread beyond the middle ear cleft confines, the condition is dangerous and difficult to correct. For this reason, treatment aims at confining the disease to, and eradicating it in, the middle ear cleft.

Otitis media is most frequently a complication of an upper respiratory tract infection, and the health of the middle ear cleft is intimately related to the health of the nose, throat and sinuses. The inflammatory reaction of the columnar ciliated epithelium of the lower tympanic cavity and eustachian tube is similar to that of the nose. Thus infection with a common cold virus may result in mucosal engorgement and profuse exudation, while infection with pyogenic bacteria results in pus formation. The middle ear mucosa may also share in an allergic reaction to inhalant or other antigens with consequent edema and effusion.

The reaction of the pavement nonciliated epithelium of the attic, mastoid antrum and air cells is, on the other hand, different. The reaction is proliferative with a tendency toward chronic granulation tissue formation. Resolution is impeded by restricted drainage because of the ossicles and ligaments, and the infection may sometimes remain quiescent and confined to the mucoperiosteum of the attic with no symptoms except loss of hearing. At other times suppuration and bone necrosis may proceed rapidly.

Differential Diagnosis

Otitis media, in the stage of eustachian tube occlusion, is indistinguishable from occlusion due to other causes such as adenoids, viral infection or allergic swelling of the lining membrane. All that can be said at this stage is that the signs and symptoms indicate air absorption, mucosal thickening and perhaps nonpurulent effusion. Since these may also be the early changes of suppurative otitis media, the ear requires close observation until the cause is clear.

In the presuppurative stage the diagnosis is seldom in doubt as long as trouble has been taken to ensure that the whole of the membrane has been inspected. The red discoloration of acute suppurative otitis media and the associated acute earache denote inflammation.

The suppurative stage again offers little difficulty in diagnosis, provided the tympanic membrane can be wholly visualized. A patient with a meatal furuncle may have pain, loss of hearing and fever, and the meatus may be so swollen as to exclude a view of the membrane. Careful attention to the history and careful inspection of the canal with the knowledge that a meatal furuncle is most likely to be found in an ear that is quite painful to the slightest traction or touch of the ear speculum will assist in the diagnosis.

Treatment

STAGE OF TUBAL OCCLUSION. When signs and symptoms are indicative only of tubal occlusion, it is not necessary to prescribe antibiotics for the ear alone, but frequently the ear disease is a complication of a generalized respiratory infection which does require antibiotic therapy. Tubal occlusion does not in itself prognosticate suppuration, and it is undesirable to risk the use of an antibiotic at this time. To promote passive tubal opening, the use of a local decongestant, such as ephedrine hydrochloride (0.5 per cent) in normal saline or an oral decongestant containing a synthetic ephedrine and an antihistamine, is indicated.

STAGE OF PRESUPPURATION. Once the membrane shows evidence of middle ear infection (Fig. 5), segmental or complete, the indication for antibiotic therapy and analgesics is clear.

Antibiotic Therapy. At this stage the selection of antibiotics cannot be assisted by laboratory tests. The compelling presumption in every new case of acute suppurative otitis media is that the causal organisms are the gram-positive *Streptococcus pyogenes* (hemolytic), *Staphylococcus pyogenes* (*aureus*) or *Diplococcus pneumoniae*. It should be noted that many question the occurrence of Staphylococcus as the cause of primary bacterial otitis media even though the organism is often cultured from the ear canal.

No antibacterial agent against these organisms is superior to penicillin by injection. If a patient is sensitive to penicillin, erythromycin or a broad-spectrum antibiotic such as tetracycline is often effective. It should be the rule always to give an apparently curative antibiotic for seven to ten days. Premature withdrawal of an antibiotic encourages growth of the persistent or resistant strains of bacteria, which may produce a subclinical necrosis of mastoid air cells, and an extradural abscess with such little local disturbance in the mastoid process that mastoiditis may be masked with the attendant danger of belated recognition.

Delayed Resolution. It is uncommon for an inflamed membrane not to return to normal after an adequate course of penicillin or tetracycline. Occasionally, redness may persist, especially in the posterosuperior segment. The cause may lie with an organism unaffected by the antibiotic. In general, a gram-negative organism such as *E. coli, H. influenzae, Bordetella pertussis* or *B. proteus,* or an antibiotic-resistant organism such as *Staphylococcus aureus* is implicated. In this instance x-ray films of the mastoid should be obtained, and if the radiologic appearance of the mastoid is normal, a course of another more suitable antibiotic may be prescribed.

STAGE OF SUPPURATION. Advance of the disease to the stage of suppuration brings into consideration surgical intervention to provide drainage.

Indications for Myringotomy. Myringotomy is indicated when (1) pain is not quickly relieved by antibiotics. (2) Bulging of the membrane (independent of pain) if not quickly relieved by antibiotics. A convex membrane under tension is liable to perforate spontaneously, allowing destructive necrosis with loss of tissue. Use of myringotomy reduces the long-term risk of hearing loss. (3) Resolution is delayed despite antibiotics.

Failure of resolution may be associated with the continual drainage of pus through a perforation, with the appearance of effusion (purulent or otherwise) beyond a "full" opaque membrane, or with persistent mucosal engorgement, accompanied in each case by residual deafness.

Persistent Otorrhea

Assuming that the patient has received an effective initial course of antibiotic, the discharge should cease in about seven to ten days. Persistence of the discharge after this, whether following spontaneous rupture or myringotomy, demands bacteriologic assay of the organisms present with determination of antibiotic sensitivities and the institution of a further course of the appropriate antibiotic. At the same time the exudate should be suctioned from the middle ear and the canal carefully cleansed and dried daily.

After a second or third course of antibiotic many ears will become dry. If each course lasts five to seven days, there will remain at the end of the third course a residue of cases in which otorrhea has continued unchecked for about three weeks. X-ray films of the mastoids may indicate a coalescence of air cells, i.e. a mastoid reservoir, as the explanation of the otorrhea, and an exploratory mastoidectomy should be considered.

It is the object of all treatment to eradicate the disease entirely and to secure conditions for full recovery of hearing. Simple mastoidectomy is a safe and occasionally necessary operation whose place in elective treatment has by no means been eliminated by the advent of antibiotics.

Persistent "Full" Middle Ear

A course of antibiotic sometimes succeeds in attenuating an infection without curing it. Effusion may persist because of inadequate tubal drainage. It is reasonable to prescribe one or two further courses of antibiotic and continue the use of decongestants in an effort to reduce the edema in the eustachian tube.

If the patient is still deaf, if the mastoid air cells are normal by x-ray, and if the membrane is still opaque and "full" at the end of three weeks, a myringotomy with suction removal of the exudate or, better still, an exploratory tympanotomy should be performed.

Failure of Antibiotic Treatment

Otologists see many ears in which the infection continues in subclinical form as hidden or masked mastoiditis, a new phenomenon noted only since the introduction of the antibiotics and sulfonamides.

Typically, the patient has been diagnosed as having acute otitis media, in the presuppurative stage, and an antibiotic has been prescribed. The response to treatment was dramatic, but the inconvenience of maintaining administration of the antibiotic on a regular schedule, especially at night, when the child has apparently been cured, led to the discontinuation of the treatment by the parents after two to three days. Two or three weeks after the initial illness the child becomes listless and complains of headache or of slight tenderness behind the ear. Examination reveals the membrane to have a lackluster and thickened appearance, and on careful examination conductive deafness is present. The danger inherent in this situation should not be underemphasized. When the mastoid is incised, it is not uncommon to find the air cells replaced by pale, mushy granulation tissue. There may be a defective bone plate over the dura mater of the lateral sinus or beneath the dura mater of the middle cranial fossa, with granulation tissue sprouting from the dura.

It should, therefore, be a firm rule of antibiotic treatment for acute suppurative otitis media that the prescribed dosage should be faithfully administered for a minimum of seven to ten days, regardless of apparent cure, after which the ear should be re-evaluated.

Chronic Suppurative Otitis Media

The changes in chronic infection take place slowly, but even though the pathologic advance may be chronic, the mode of presentation may at times be acute. A facial nerve palsy or an attack of vertigo, for example, may be the first indication of the long-standing presence of progressive disease.

The disease may be potentially very serious, requiring urgent intervention. For this reason chronic suppurative otitis media is described as consisting of two main clinical types: a dangerous type and a benign or safe type. The line of demarcation between these types conforms to the embryonic pattern of development. Chronic infection in that part of the middle ear cleft originally derived from the tubotympanic recess, lined by columnar ciliated epithelium, seldom if ever gives rise to a complication. But if the cleft above the level of the chorda tympani nerve and lined by pavement type of epithelium becomes the seat of chronic infection, the risk of complications merits the designation "dangerous."

The presenting symptom of chronic otitis media is chronic purulent otorrhea, while the principal sign is the observation of pus coming from the middle ear through a perforation.

The "safe ear" (tubotympanic) infection is one in which the area of infection lies between the eustachian tube opening in the nasopharynx and an anterior or central perforation of the pars tensa of the tympanic membrane.

The activity of the infection is related closely to the health of the upper respiratory tract. The discharge is mucopurulent, and though it may be extremely profuse, it is seldom fetid. The ossicular chain is not involved, and the hearing loss is not severe.

The "dangerous ear" (attic-antral) infection is one in which the area of infection lies in the attic or antrum between a posterior marginal perforation of the pars tensa or a perforation of the pars flaccida (Shrapnell's membrane) and the posterior "blind end" of the middle ear cleft.

This area is lined by cuboidal (pavement) epithelium, and drainage is poor, being impeded by the head of the malleus and the body of the incus. Since the underlying bone of this portion of the middle ear cleft invests vital structures, such

as the dura mater, membranous labyrinth and facial nerve, complications are relatively frequent.

Every case of chronic otitis media when first seen should be identified as being in the safe or dangerous category, and every ear showing an attic or posterior marginal perforation should be designated as dangerous. Thick, scanty, fetid pus along with moderate or severe conductive loss of hearing is typical of a "dangerous ear" with cholesteatoma formation.

Cholesteatoma

Epidermoid cholesteatoma is a baglike cystic structure lined by stratified squamous epithelium. Cholesteatoma is most commonly attributed to suction of the pars flaccida into the attic because of negative pressure in the middle ear. The development of the negative pressure has been considered to be due either to faulty aeration of the mastoid or to subclinical attacks of otitis media, especially with undetected effusions leading to fibrosis or with chronic eustachian tube occlusion.

Congenital cholesteatoma is usually not connected anatomically with the middle ear cleft. It arises in an embryonic cell rest in any of the cranial bones and may remain undetected for years, when symptoms of facial nerve paralysis or other complications develop.

Treatment

The degeneration, destruction and fibrosis accompanying chronic infection, together with granulation and polyp formation, and the development of cholesteatoma, most often require some form of surgical treatment. Medical treatment, using antibacterial and anti-inflammatory agents, is disappointing in chronic otitis media. The fibrotic changes tend to isolate pockets of infection from an effective blood supply. Topical antibiotic application has proved more useful, but is used primarily with the aim of preparing the ear for a tympanoplastic procedure. The tympanoplasty will consist of surgical removal of all chronic disease followed by reconstruction of the middle ear and tympanic membrane in an attempt to restore a useful, safe and functioning ear.

Safe types of otitis media often show a rapid response to treatment and later relapse. Investigation frequently discloses diseased tonsils, adenoids or maxillary antra which should be treated appropriately. If the perforation remains, a myringoplasty should be considered for the protection of the middle ear and improvement of the patient's hearing.

Allergic effusions are not uncommon at any age. After all local causes of chronic otitis media have been excluded, an investigation of possible allergy, especially to ingestants, e.g. eggs, milk or chocolate, may be rewarding. Skin tests are not as useful as a careful history, food diary, and withdrawal of various suspected foods. Severe pollen allergy may also be the cause of secretory otitis.

A "mastoid reservoir" of infection is not uncommon in children. Repeated otitis media increases the risk of a left-over tidal pool of infection in mastoid air cells, especially when the otitis media has been inadequately treated with antibiotics.

Bacterial resistance to antibiotics is common in childhood. The high incidence of acute upper respiratory tract infections, including viral diseases, undifferentiated tonsillitis and acute otitis media, has resulted in antibiotic practices which favor undertreatment of potentially serious bacterial infections. The emergence of resistant strains of bacteria is thus encouraged and the causes for chronic infection are increased.

Cholesteatomas are not uncommon in children, and in the absence of infection this disease is often overlooked. Minute retraction of the attic membrane is an indication of negative pressure, and unless corrected, an expanding bag of cholesteatoma may form. Tympanotomy is a useful procedure for the removal of disease from the attic and the correction of any negative pressure tendency. At the same time a polyethylene tube may be inserted through the drum and into the middle ear space for temporary help in improving aeration of the middle ear.

Acute Nonsuppurative Otitis Media

Acute secretory otitis media, or acute nonsuppurative otitis media, is essentially the sudden appearance of nonpurulent effusion in the middle ear.

Etiology

Eustachian tube obstruction is thought to interfere with replacement of tubal air which is continuously being absorbed from the middle ear under normal circumstances. A potential or real vacuum formation results, and the effusion of fluid into the middle ear follows. This hypothesis helps to explain many of the cases; others derive from upper respiratory tract infections of a viral origin. The adenoviruses and rhinoviruses may include some with a proclivity for involvement of the mucosa of the middle ear cleft. Allergic upper respiratory tract reactions due to various inhalant or ingestant allergens are often responsible for a clear effusion of the middle ear.

The signs of effusion are first, a conductive deafness (Fig. 3); second, a retracted membrane; third, moving bubbles visible through the drum; fourth, a darker, lackluster appearance of the membrane (Fig. 5).

Treatment

The return to normal depends on drainage of the effusion. Natural cure may occur through drainage of the effusion down the eustachian tube, and medical management aims at encouraging this natural process. The medical measures generally found useful are as follows: (1) inflation of the middle ear by Valsalva's maneuver or politzerization; (2) shrinkage of the mucosa of the eustachian tube orifice with vasoconstrictive nose drops, e.g. ephedrine hydrochloride (0.5 per cent), Neo-Synephrine (0.25 per cent); (3) systemic antihistamine therapy; (4) elimination of bacterial upper respiratory tract infection with antibiotics. If the effusion is persistent after medical treatment has been carried out for two or three weeks, recourse to surgical treatment may be indicated. (5) A myringotomy with suction removal of all exudate in the middle ear will rapidly correct the condition. Recurrence can usually be prevented by the insertion of a small polyethylene tube into the myringotomy opening.

Chronic Nonsuppurative Otitis Media (Chronic Secretory Otitis Media)

In this condition the effusion appears gradually. It is more commonly seen in children than is the acute type. The cause of chronic effusion is similar to that of acute effusion.

The general management of chronic effusion closely follows that of the acute condition. Chronic secretory otitis media typically involves persistent conductive deafness. A myringotomy and suction or tympanotomy with the direct removal of all exudate in some cases are necessary to remove the mucoid, tenacious (glue) effusion. Polyethylene drainage tubes are helpful if all exudate has been removed. General treatment in the form of antibiotics, antihistamines, surgical removal of tonsils and adenoids and nasal decongestants are often disappointing. Unless repeated observations are made and the exudate is completely removed, the child may have permanent conductive deafness.

Chronic Adhesive Otitis Media

Adhesive otitis media may result from suppurative otitis media or nonsuppura-

tive otitis media due to organization and fibrosis of undrained effusions. With improved operating techniques there should be less reluctance to explore the middle ears in children whose hearing has not returned to normal after adequate medical treatment.

The only symptom is deafness of a varying degree. The tympanic membrane is noted to have a more dull, dense, retracted appearance and lacks mobility, as confirmed with Siegle's apparatus.

Treatment

The management of this problem is complicated and difficult. The aim is to restore the middle ear space and mobility to the ossicular chain and drum. Exploratory tympanotomy should be done to correct any abnormality present in the middle ear. The best treatment is prevention. Middle ear infection in infancy and childhood is the most important cause, and prophylactic treatment should be aimed at the elimination of residual effusion in the tympanic cavity. To this end the following rules are advised:

1. Continue antibiotics in the patient with otitis media for ten days, even though the response seems immediate and recovery complete in a shorter length of time.

2. Perform myringotomy and suction removal of any residual effusion. (The important signs of effusion are opacity and "fullness" of the membrane with conductive deafness.)

3. Perform an exploratory tympanotomy in all cases of residual conductive deafness present eight weeks after an attack of acute otitis media.

Complications of Suppurative Otitis Media

Suppurative otitis media becomes complicated when the infection spreads out of the middle ear cleft and into the surrounding areas; the complications may be listed as follows:

Nonmeningeal	*Meningeal*
Mastoiditis	Extradural abscess
Petrositis	Subdural abscess or
Facial paralysis	effusion
Labyrinthitis	Venous sinus thrombo-
Brain abscess	phlebitis
	Meningitis

DISEASES OF THE MASTOID

Infection of the mastoid bone occurs in two main forms: acute and chronic. In acute mastoiditis coalescence of air cells secondary to hyperemic osteoporosis and pressure necrosis of the bony cell walls is associated with the retention of pus (empyema). The acute mastoid infection arises by direct extension from an acute otitis media. Chronic mastoiditis is the invasion of bone by granulation tissue arising from a chronic otitis media. "Masked" mastoiditis is a variant of acute mastoiditis occurring as a "cold" coalescence of air cells in an infection not completely eliminated by antibiotics.

Acute Mastoiditis

It is rare for otitis media to proceed unhindered to acute mastoiditis with the

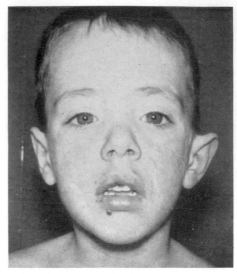

FIGURE 10–7. Auricle protrusion in acute mastoiditis.

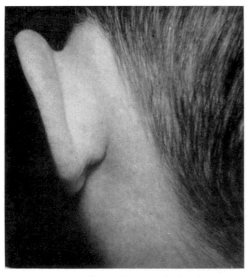

FIGURE 10–6. Loss of postauricular crease secondary to mastoiditis.

antibiotics now available. In the untreated case, pain and tenderness are present over the mastoid along with increased otorrhea and fever. In infants and young children there may be gastrointestinal disturbances.

Signs of acute mastoiditis vary with the extent of the disease. In the preantibiotic days the presence of acute mastoiditis was readily recognized by the appearance of retroauricular edema and tenderness (Figs. 6, 7). Otoscopic examination revealed pus in the canal, along with a sagging of the posterosuperior meatal wall. The patient was acutely and seriously ill, and the diagnosis was seldom in doubt.

In the less dramatic but no less serious mastoiditis appearing after apparent resolution of otitis media treated with antibiotics, there may be no retroauricular edema, pus in the canal or sagging of the meatal wall, and the patient may not appear to be very ill. The only signs may be slight tenderness on pressure, an opaque membrane with some conductive deafness, and radiologic evidence of the coalescence of air cells.

Treatment

In most instances acute mastoiditis responds well to parenteral penicillin or other antibiotic therapy. If a subperiosteal abscess is present after antibiotic treatment, the patient should have a simple mastoidectomy. The occurrence of such an abscess is infrequent.

Chronic Mastoiditis

The precursor of true chronic mastoiditis is conversion of the lining membrane of the middle ear or antrum into granulation tissue. Chronic mastoiditis is seen only in acellular mastoids and is secondary to the neglect of chronic suppuration in the middle ear. The absence of air cells eliminates the possibility of escalating symptoms such as are seen in acute mastoiditis.

Persistent otorrhea and severe conductive deafness are the two main symptoms, but in chronic otitis media with cholesteatoma there is an increased risk of chronic mastoiditis, owing to the erosive capacity of cholesteatoma.

Treatment

Local treatment will often control the infection temporarily, and should be used. A tympanoplasty should be performed in most instances to eradicate the disease permanently. A tympanoplastic procedure has two primary aims: (1) removal of all infection in the middle ear and mastoid and (2) reconstruction of the middle ear in order to restore hearing, if possible.

Complications

GRADENIGO'S SYNDROME. When the petrous tip cells become infected, the syndrome of Gradenigo may occur, i.e. sixth cranial nerve paralysis and pain in the area supplied by the fifth cranial nerve. Treatment is the same as that outlined for acute mastoiditis. Mastoidectomy may be necessary.

FACIAL NERVE PARALYSIS. Paralysis of the facial muscles due to inflammatory swelling of the facial nerve sheath may occur during the course of acute or chronic suppurative otitis media. In acute otitis media the paralysis will most likely disappear if the disease is controlled with antibiotics. In chronic otitis media the palsy is due to penetration of cholesteatoma granulation tissue, and a radical mastoidectomy, with decompression of the facial nerve, is required.

OTITIC MENINGITIS. Meningitis, although now not commonly seen, is a serious complication of otitis media, and should be treated with specific antibiotics and medical management. Consideration should be given to the elimination of the mastoid focus by surgical means.

Other complications are brain abscess and lateral sinus thrombophlebitis with thrombosis. These complications require coordinated medical and surgical care and are considered dire emergencies.

Extradural abscess is an accumulation of pus between the dura mater and tegmen tympani or between the dural covering of the lateral sinus and the bony sinus plate. It is most often diagnosed at the time of operation in the patient with "masked" or chronic mastoiditis.

LABYRINTHITIS. Labyrinthitis may occur as a complication of otitis media in various degrees of severity. Perilabyrinthitis is associated with a fistula formation in the bony labyrinth, and the patient may have vertigo if the ear is syringed or cleansed. More often vertigo may occur on movement of the head or change of body position.

Evidence of fistula formation is an indication for possible surgical intervention.

Serous and suppurative labyrinthitis may occur as complications of active suppurative otitis media. The patient with suppurative otitis media who has spontaneous nausea, vomiting and vertigo and retains some or most of his vestibular and auditory functions most likely has serous labyrinthitis. The end-organs of hearing and balance are destroyed by suppuration, and a nonfunctioning labyrinth results.

Labyrinthitis is rarely a complication of acute otitis media unless cholesteatoma invasion has made the labyrinthine structures vulnerable. Operation should be considered in all cases of labyrinthitis.

THE EUSTACHIAN TUBE

The eustachian tube consists of a bony portion which is normally patent and a cartilaginous portion which is normally closed, but opens when one yawns or swallows and air passes into the middle ear. When the eustachian tube is obstructed, the air in the middle ear is absorbed and the drum becomes retracted. This development of excessive negative pressure tends to promote exudation from the blood and lymphatic vessels of the middle ear mucosa. Patients with cleft palate are prone to otitis media because the eustachian tube fails to function normally; the tensor palati muscles are unable to open the tube in the absence of an intact palate.

Examination of the nasopharynx and the tubal orifices should be carefully performed to rule out any extrinsic tubal cause of obstruction. Utilization of a Shepard drain tube through the tympanic membrane is of some benefit, but the patient must have repeated examinations because of the tendency for expulsion of the tube from the middle ear.

Congenital stenosis of the eustachian tube is occasionally noted, but most of the stenosis is related to chronic infection. Partial stenosis may be treated with inflation techniques, politzerization or Valsalva's maneuver. Also, insertion of a flanged Teflon tube (Shepard drain tube) through the tympanic membrane will act as a safety valve and help prevent recurrences of negative pressure and exudation, as long as they remain in place.

Chronic salpingitis in children is an especially difficult problem and is due to hypertrophic or adhesive changes in the tubal lining. Attacks of otitis media are followed by persistent retraction of the tympanic membrane with conduction deafness, despite every measure, including adenoidectomy, tympanotomy and tubal inflation.

Adenoidal hypertrophy is a common cause of eustachian tube obstruction in children, owing to lateral compression of the torus tubarius. Adenoidectomy is the treatment of choice if there have been repeated attacks of otitis media. If the infections continue to recur after careful surgery and there is excessive lymphoid tissue in the fossae of Rosenmuller, the use of x-ray therapy to this area should be considered; the danger of x-ray-induced malignancy must, however, be kept in mind and weighed against the threat of deafness.

DEAFNESS

Speech is acquired by imitation, and a child born with a severe degree of irremediable deafness so as to prevent the perception of ordinary speech is destined to mutism unless auditory training is given at an early age. A child who is deaf needs to be brought up to the level of other children by early diagnosis, early medical treatment and early auditory training.

Prenatal Deafness

Prenatal deafness is conveniently grouped according to the chronologic sequence of the cause.

Hereditary Group

This group consists of those whose perceiving or conducting apparatus fails to develop normally or later degenerates, owing to inherited defects of maturation or maintenance.

Pregnancy Group

The deafness occurring in this group is perceptive in type, the development of the normal epithelium being adversely affected by the toxic effects of maternal rubella or other influences. It is to be noted, also, that the degree of deafness in this group will be related to the stage of development reached when the arrest of development or degeneration occurs.

Birth Group

This group will also have a perceptive deafness and need early auditory training.

Postnatal Deafness

Cases of prenatal deafness, with the exception of otosclerosis and branchial malformations, are exclusively perceptive in clinical type. The causes of postnatal deafness may be conveniently grouped under conductive and perceptive deafness types and occasionally psychogenic deafness. It is important that the various types be properly differentiated so that the appropriate treatment can be instituted.

The following is a list of the types of inner ear perceptive deafness:

Congenital

Complete or partial maldevelopment may follow when the mother contracts rubella or ingests Thalidomide during the first trimester of pregnancy. Usually no predisposing cause is found.

Hereditary

ABIOTROPHY. This presenile familial deafness presents as a progressive cochlear degeneration in late childhood. Congenital syphilis must be ruled out. It may occur alone or with other deformities as retinitis pigmentosa, renal abnormalities, ear-pits, branchial fistulas and congenital familial anhidrosis.

PENDRED SYNDROME is an inherited perceptive deafness with hypothyroid goiter.

WAARDENBURG SYNDROME may be characterized by a white forelock, prominent epicanthal folds, eyes of different colors, and deafness.

Delayed Congenital

KERNICTERUS may affect the dorsal and ventral auditory nuclei and cause nerve deafness, with or without auditory imperception (aphasoid). Pure auditory imperception may be found without nerve deafness.

CONGENITAL SYPHILIS. Secondary syphilis becomes manifest in the first two years. Tertiary syphilis becomes manifest in the eighth to twentieth years. Hutchinson's triad occurs with tertiary disease and consists of labyrinthitis, interstitial keratitis and notched teeth.

Traumatic

CONCUSSION. Deafness, tinnitus and vertigo may follow. Return to normal is usual, but persistent loss can occur.

SKULL FRACTURE. Head injury associated with loss of consciousness and hearing, and blood in the middle ear (seen as a blue tympanic membrane) should be considered to be due to basilar skull fracture regardless of the x-ray findings. Cerebrospinal fluid leak may be a troublesome complication. Manipulation of the ear during the acute phase should be discouraged for fear of introducing infection. Broad-spectrum antibiotic coverage for at least one week is recommended.

BLAST INJURY. A cap pistol fired close to the ear may cause such an injury. This loss can be transient. Further trauma should be carefully avoided.

Infection

The most frequent diseases which may cause deafness are measles, whooping cough, influenza, mumps (unilateral loss), suppurative infection and cholesteatoma associated with chronic otitis media and mastoiditis.

Allergic

VOGT-KOYANAGI SYNDROME (HARADA'S DISEASE). This is thought to be an allergic response of pigmented tissue characterized by neurosensory deafness (temporary), uveitis, poliosis (crops of white hair), vitiligo and alopecia (loss of hair).

Toxic

ACUTE. With streptomycin, vestibular sensation may be abolished first.

Dihydrostreptomycin is ototoxic and should not be used.

Neomycin, kanamycin, vancomycin, Viomycin, Ristocetin, Framycetin and polymyxin B may be ototoxic.

CHRONIC. Salicylates used in high dosage as in rheumatoid arthritis commonly cause tinnitus and deafness. Recovery is usual when the drug is discontinued.

Tobacco, alcohol and quinine are the most common offenders.

Heavy metals, e.g. lead, mercury.

Fumes of benzene, carbon monoxide, carbon disulfide.

Medications, e.g. caffeine, barbiturates, oil of chenopodium (anthelmintic), ergot, iodine, iodiform, morphine, Novocain, strychnine, scopolamine and Chloroquin.

In ototoxicity, deafness is likely to be preceded by tinnitus. Audiometric tests should be done when tinnitus occurs, and the suspected ototoxic drug should be discontinued.

Metabolic or Nutritional

PERNICIOUS ANEMIA.

LEUKEMIA. Hemorrhage or infiltration into the cochlea can occur.

NIEMANN-PICK AND HAND-SCHUELLER-CHRISTIAN DISEASE. The ear is frequently affected with suppuration and granulation of the temporal bone. Middle ear and mastoid infection may be the presenting picture.

AVITAMINOSIS such as beriberi.

CHRONIC NEPHRITIS.

HYPOTHYROIDISM.

MÉNIÈRE'S DISEASE. Episodic vertigo and tinnitus with fluctuating neurosensory deafness may occur.

Spontaneous, Idiopathic

Sudden deafness with tinnitus and vertigo may occur in an otherwise healthy patient.

Vascular

Perceptive deafness may be associated with unilateral vasomotor rhinitis, or unilateral gustatory sweating, or migraine and ocular symptoms or acrocyanosis in a young female.

One must not confuse central disorders that might resemble inner ear disturbances:

EPILEPSY may present with vertigo, but loss of consciousness should alert the clinician that this is not an inner ear problem.

DISSEMINATED SCLEROSIS. Nystagmus is a common finding, but other neurologic signs are present.

VASCULAR ACCIDENTS. Loss of hearing and vertigo may occur in cases of a subarachnoid hemorrhage from a leaking berry aneurysm.

POSTERIOR FOSSA TUMORS. Other neurologic signs will be present; gliomas as well as the commonly associated cerebellopontine angle tumors predominate.

EIGHTH CRANIAL NERVE NEUROMA, which may be part of neurofibromatosis (von Recklinghausen's disease), may be present very early in life, causing vertigo or neurosensory deafness.

Early Diagnosis

Hearing is a primary sensation, and the newborn responds to loud sounds entirely by reflex, such as the "startle" reflex noted in the first six months. If a small bell is rung gently in front of the ear, but outside the range of vision, an infant may suddenly "freeze," and sometimes the eyes will move toward the side of the bell. During the first three months an artificial noise such as a whistle or squeaker is a better stimulus than the voice.

SECOND SIX MONTHS. The child turns its head toward sources of interest such as his mother's voice, or the opening and closing of doors. The vocalizations of the normal child increase at this period, and he babbles "mum mum" or "da da." By comparison, the deaf child's vocalization gradually diminishes, and the sounds he makes are few and toneless.

SECOND YEAR. It is during this period that parental doubts about the hearing are generally resolved. It may be taken as a general rule that a child who has not uttered a recognizable word by the age of sixteen months should receive prompt investigation for possible deafness.

The high-tone deafness present in many congenitally deaf children may have a selective effect on the vocabulary. Such speech sounds as s, sh, f, th, fr, k, ch, may not be heard and, therefore, are not imitated, making speech unintelligible. A reliable pure-tone audiogram may be obtained in a child who has reached the mental age of four.

The real difficulties in differential diagnosis arise in connection with cerebral conditions, in which, for example, mental retardation rather than deafness may be the cause of delay in speaking. Otologic testing must be thorough and often repeated; intelligence testing will often be helpful in distinguishing the retarded group.

Early Medical Treatment

It is unfortunately still true that few cases of perceptive deafness can be medically or surgically treated successfully; it is of no benefit to the patient or parents if false hopes are encouraged in such instances. Acceptance of this disability is not easy for parents, and sympathetic support by the physician is a necessary part of the total case. The child should be referred to a hearing and speech center for therapy.

Patients with prenatal conductive deafness, i.e. atresia, or acquired conductive deafness due to middle ear disease or eustachian adenoid obstruction have remediable problems. Early and accurate diagnosis is essential for maximal improvement in hearing in these circumstances.

REFERENCES

Best, T. H., and Anson, B. J.: *The Temporal Bone and the Ear.* Springfield, Ill., Charles C Thomas, 1949.

Brennemann's Practice of Pediatrics, 1964, Vol. IV.

Cawthorne, T. E.: *Medical Press,* 25:560, 1953.

Chalmers, B. J.: *Deafness.* London, Churchill, 1960.

Conference, American Academy for Cerebral Palsy: *Kernicterus and Its Importance in Cerebral Palsy.* Springfield, Ill., Charles C Thomas, 1961.

DeWeese and Saunders: *Textbook of Otolaryngology,* St. Louis, C. V. Mosby Company, 1960.

Diarmant, M.: *Arch. Otolaryng.,* 68587, 1958.

Gray's Anatomy: 31st ed.

Holt, E. L., Jr., and McIntosh, R.: *Pediatrics.* 12th ed. New York, Appleton-Century-Crofts, Inc., 1960.

Mawson, S. R.: *Diseases of the Ear.* London, Spottis, Ballantyne & Co., 1963.

McNalley, W. J.: Five Lectures on the Physiology of the Ear. *Ann. Otol., Rhin. & Laryng.,* 38:1163, 1959.

Nelson, W. E. (Ed.): Symposium on Respiratory Disorders. *Pediat. Clin. N. Amer.,* 4:1-312, 1957.

Proctor, B.: The Development of the Middle Ear Spaces and Their Surgical Significance. *J. Laryng. & Otol.,* 78:631, 1964.

Schuhnecht, H. F.: *Laryngoscope,* 65:40, 1955.

Transactions of the American Otological Society, May, 1940, pp. 126-7.

Wilson, T. G.: *Diseases of the Ear, Nose and Throat in Children.* London, Heinemann, 1955.

SECTION VI

General Considerations in Infections of the Upper and Lower Respiratory Tracts

CHAPTER ELEVEN

General Considerations in Infections of the Upper and Lower Respiratory Tracts

HENRY G. CRAMBLETT, M.D.

The respiratory tract of infants and children is subject to infection with a large number of pathogens, including fungi, bacteria, rickettsiae, Mycoplasma (PPLO) and viruses. In most instances these agents do not produce a specifically recognizable syndrome which enables the physician to make a precise etiologic diagnosis without resorting to laboratory tests—tests that are often expensive or unavailable.

From a practical standpoint, it is helpful to establish an anatomic diagnosis in respiratory illness; once this is done, sufficient epidemiologic data are available to the physician for etiologic considerations. Respiratory infections often overlap in anatomic involvement, and the anatomic diagnostic approach is most useful when utilized from the standpoint of the initial and most prominent region of localization. Table 1 lists the principal recognized etiologic agents of rhinitis (nasopharyngitis, coryza, common cold), tonsillitis, pharyngitis, laryngitis (croup), bronchitis, pneumonia and bronchiolitis.

In following sections, clinical complexes which are helpful in differentiating between viral and bacterial infections are emphasized. In general, rhinorrhea, complaint of sore throat without much objective erythema, and hoarseness are indicative of the onset of a nonbacterial respiratory infection.

241

Table 1. *Etiologic Agents of Rhinitis, Tonsillitis, Pharyngitis, Laryngitis,
Bronchitis, Pneumonia and Bronchiolitis*

I. Upper respiratory tract illnesses
  A. Rhinitis
    1. Bacterial (rare if ever)
    2. Viral
      a. Rhinoviruses
      b. Adenoviruses
      c. Enteroviruses
      d. Influenza viruses
      e. Parainfluenza viruses
      f. Respiratory syncytial virus
    3. Mycoplasma
      a. Mycoplasma pneumoniae
  B. Tonsillitis or pharyngitis
    1. Bacterial
      a. Group A beta hemolytic
        streptococci
      b. Corynebacterium diphtheriae
      c. Staphylococci and pneumococci
        (rarely in debilitated patients)
    2. Viral
      a. Adenoviruses
      b. Influenza viruses
      c. Enteroviruses
      d. Parainfluenza viruses
      e. Respiratory syncytial virus
        (?)*
      f. Rhinoviruses (?)*
      g. Reoviruses (?)*
      h. Presumed viral: infectious
        mononucleosis
    3. Mycoplasma
II. Lower respiratory tract illnesses
  A. Laryngitis: laryngotracheobronchitis
    1. Bacterial
      a. Hemophilus influenzae, type B
      b. Corynebacterium diphtheriae
      c. Staphylococci (?);* streptococci
        (?);* pneumococci (?)*
    2. Viral
      a. Parainfluenza viruses, types 1,
        2 and 3
      b. Adenoviruses

      c. Influenza viruses
      d. Respiratory syncytial virus
      e. ECHO viruses
      f. Coxsackie viruses
  B. Bronchitis or pneumonia
    1. Bacterial
      a. Pneumococci
      b. Hemophilus influenzae, type B
      c. Streptococci
      d. Staphylococci, coagulase-posi-
        tive
      e. Mycobacterium tuberculosis
    2. Viral
      a. Respiratory syncytial virus
      b. Parainfluenza viruses
      c. Rhinoviruses
      d. Influenza viruses
      e. Adenoviruses
      f. Psittacosis
    3. Mycoplasma
      a. Mycoplasma pneumoniae
    4. Fungi
      a. Histoplasma capsulatum
      b. Cryptococcus neoformans
      c. Coccidioidomycosis
      d. Blastomycosis
      e. Nocardiosis
    5. Rickettsiae
      a. Q fever
    6. Protozoa
      a. Pneumocystis carinii
  C. Bronchiolitis
    1. Bacterial
      a. Hemophilus influenzae, type
        B (?)*
    2. Viral
      a. Respiratory syncytial virus
      b. Parainfluenza viruses
      c. Adenoviruses
      d. Rhinoviruses*
    3. Mycoplasma
      a. Mycoplasma pneumoniae*

* Organisms in which there is suggestive but not conclusive evidence of etiologic association
with the respective respiratory syndrome.

SECTION VII

Infections of the Upper Respiratory Tract

CHAPTER TWELVE

Acute Rhinitis (Acute Nasopharyngitis; Common Cold; Coryza)

HENRY G. CRAMBLETT, M.D.

Acute rhinitis is the most common respiratory illness of infants and children. Although it is certain that many viruses cause the common cold, the recent recovery and characterization of the rhinoviruses have provided a significant advance in our understanding of the causation of the syndrome.

Incidence

It is estimated that each child has an average of three to six episodes of acute rhinitis, common cold or undifferentiated upper respiratory tract disease each year.

Etiology

Bacteria rarely, if ever, cause primary rhinitis. A wide variety of viruses, including the rhinoviruses, adenoviruses, enteroviruses, influenza viruses, parainfluenza viruses and respiratory syncytial virus, have been shown to cause this anatomic syndrome. To date, in adult studies, the rhinoviruses have proved to be the most important agents in the causation of acute rhinitis. Although these viruses also cause an important portion of upper respiratory tract disease in infants and children, the exact importance of this group in the origin of all respiratory illnesses in children is unclear. There is nothing in the clinical picture which would help one to differentiate the common cold due to one virus from that due to another.

Pathogenesis

The primary focus of infection in this disease is in the mucosa of the nose. Initially there is mononuclear infiltration which later may be followed by a polymorphonuclear infiltrate. Ordinarily other portions of the respiratory tract, including the pharynx, larynx, the tracheobronchial tree and occasionally the accessory sinuses, are involved in the illness.

Clinical Manifestations

The child with acute nasopharyngitis differs from the adult with the same disease in that the child usually has accompanying fever, whereas the adult is usually afebrile. In infancy a frequent presenting sign of acute nasopharyngitis is fever. This may precede the onset of a serous or seromucoid nasal discharge and other signs of coryza, including cough and sneeze, by several hours. In older children, fever may not be as prominent, and the initial complaint may be a feeling of dryness of the nose or the nasopharynx followed by a profuse watery, serous or seromucoid nasal discharge.

245

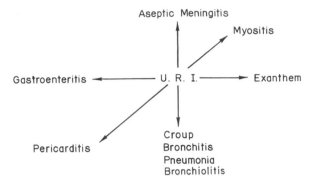

FIGURE 12–1. Schematic representation of biphasic viral illnesses in which the initial disease is an upper respiratory illness. (From H. G. Cramblett: Viral Respiratory Illnesses of Infants and Children. *Bacteriol. Rev.*, 28:431-8, 1964.) ,

Cough may occur because of postnasal drainage or because of actual involvement of other portions of the tracheo-bronchial tree. In infancy, vomiting and diarrhea, usually not severe, may accompany the respiratory symptoms.

Diagnosis

In considering the diagnosis of primary acute rhinitis, one must rule out the existence of other diseases which are viral and biphasic in nature and in which the minor illness may be rhinitis. These diseases with more major manifestations include exanthematous disease, aseptic meningitis, pneumonia and croup (Fig. 1). There is nothing distinctive about naso-pharyngitis caused by one virus as opposed to that caused by another virus.

Complications

The most frequent complication of acute rhinitis in infancy and childhood is the development of otitis media. Although this may begin as a serous otitis media, it frequently develops into purulent otitis media with inflamed, bulging ear drums. In addition, either primary or secondary pneumonia may occur. Moreover, secondary purulent bacterial rhinitis may follow a primary viral rhinitis.

Treatment

Since nasopharyngitis is due entirely to viruses, there is no specific therapy. Symptomatic therapy of infants with this disease includes the judicious use of Neo-Synephrine nose drops or spray, adequate hygiene to the nose, and the use of a vaporizer. In some infants in whom the nasal discharge becomes so thick and profuse that it interferes with feeding it may be necessary to irrigate the nasal passages gently with normal saline solution by means of an ear-bulb syringe. In case of secondary purulent rhinitis, the use of a nasal spray with neomycin or bacitracin, after careful cleansing of the nose, may be helpful.

Symptomatic measures which may be of value include the use of acetylsalicylic acid and one of the antihistamines.

REFERENCES

Cramblett, H. G.: Viral Respiratory Illnesses of Infants and Children. *Bacteriol. Rev.*, 28: 431-8, 1964.

Hamparian, V. V., Leagus, M. B., and Hilleman, M. R.: Additional Rhinovirus Serotypes. *Proc. Soc. Exp. Biol. & Med.*, 116:976-84, 1964.

CHAPTER THIRTEEN

Pharyngitis and Tonsillitis

HENRY G. CRAMBLETT, M.D.

Although pharyngitis frequently heralds the onset of a biphasic illness in which the principal manifestation is aseptic meningitis, gastroenteritis or exanthem, this chapter will deal only with those infections in which involvement of the pharynx or tonsils is the primary manifestation of disease.

Etiology

The principal bacterial cause of pharyngitis is the group A beta hemolytic streptococcus. In the nonimmunized person *Corynebacterium diphtheriae* causes sporadic cases of disease. In the debilitated patient or the patient with underlying disease such as leukemia or cystic fibrosis of the pancreas, staphylococci or pneumococci may occasionally be recovered in pure culture from patients with a pseudomembranous type of tonsillitis. In the otherwise healthy child these organisms are unlikely causes of primary pharyngitis.

Many viruses have been associated with pharyngitis, including adenoviruses, influenza viruses, Coxsackie viruses and parainfluenza viruses. Other viruses in which the proof of etiologic association is not conclusive include respiratory syncytial virus, rhinoviruses and reoviruses. Pharyngitis may occur early in the course of infectious mononucleosis, a disease presumed to be of viral origin.

Manifestations

From the clinical standpoint, in order to assess possible causation, it is helpful to divide pharyngitis into severe, moderate and mild categories depending upon the presence of certain physical findings.

SEVERE PHARYNGITIS. Severe pharyngitis includes the unequivocal findings of fever, exudate, and erythema of the pharynx, or fever and erythema of the pharynx associated with a scarlatinal rash. Most studies indicate that about 90 per cent of the patients with severe pharyngitis have this disease as the result of infection by group A beta hemolytic streptococci. It is not unusual for the exudate to appear after the onset of erythema or the actual complaint of sore throat (Fig. 1). Early in the course of streptococcal pharyngitis the younger patient may complain of headache accompanied by vomiting before the obvious signs of severe pharyngitis are present. The peripheral white blood cell count is usually elevated during the first two days of illness. In addition, other physical findings may include edema and petechiae of the soft palate and uvula and tender, enlarged tonsillar lymph nodes.

MODERATE PHARYNGITIS. In moderate pharyngitis there are two of the three characteristics of fever, erythema and exudate. From the etiologic standpoint, approximately 50 per cent of the patients with moderate pharyngitis have this disease as a result of infection with group A beta hemolytic streptococci, and in the other 50 per cent the disease is due to a virus. Factors favoring a viral origin of moderate pharyngitis include a normal white blood cell count, absence of regional lymphadenopathy, and the presence of hoarseness. Hoarseness rarely if ever occurs in streptococcal infections. Moreover, in viral pharyngitis (with the exception of infectious mononucleosis) there is usually little or no edema of the soft palate.

MILD PHARYNGITIS. Mild pharyngitis

247

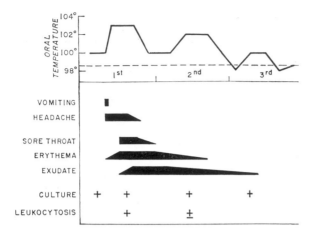

FIGURE 13–1. Typical clinical pattern of streptococcal pharyngitis in school-age children. (From H. L. Moffet, H. G. Cramblett and A. Smith: Group A Streptococcal Infections in a Children's Home. II. Clinical and Epidemiologic Patterns of Illness. *Pediatrics*, 33:11-17, 1964.)

is defined as the subjective complaint of sore throat or evidence of mild pharyngeal erythema on physical examination, without fever or exudate. Such patients commonly have minor complaints of cough or rhinorrhea. From the etiologic standpoint, at least 85 to 90 per cent of the cases of mild pharyngitis are due to a virus. There is nothing clinically distinguishable between mild pharyngitis due to one virus from that due to another, except in herpangina caused by Coxsackie A viruses; in this disease vesicular or ulcerated lesions may be present in the pharynx.

Table 1 lists the diagnoses in school-age children from whose throat cultures ten colonies or more of group A beta hemolytic streptococci were recovered. It should be stressed that in younger children there may be an undifferentiated febrile illness in which there are no signs or symptoms of pharyngitis. In the study from which the data in Table 1 were de-

Table 1. *Diagnoses Associated with Recovery of More Than 10 Colonies of Group A Beta Hemolytic Streptococci*

| | Children | Positive Cultures | |
Clinical Diagnosis	(no.)	(no.)	(%)
Pharyngitis, severe	99	87	88
Pharyngitis, moderate	83	44	53
Undifferentiated febrile illness	46	13	23
Acute otitis media	33	5	15
Pharyngitis, mild	65	8	12
Headache only	30	3	10
Vomiting without fever	88	9	10
Vomiting with fever	34	3	9
Nausea	24	2	8
Bronchitis or pneumonia	27	2	7
Febrile rhinitis	16	1	6
Other*	51*	3	6
Diarrhea	23	1	4
Cough only or rhinitis	73	2	3
	692	182	

* Other: otitis externa, 16; laryngitis, 11; conjunctivitis, 10; asthma, 5; sinusitis, 3; urinary tract infections, 3; herpes simplex, 2; arthralgia, 1.

rived it was concluded that the carrier rate of streptococci in the children studied was approximately 10 per cent. Hence those diseases from which 10 per cent or less of the positive cultures were obtained probably have no etiologic importance.

Diagnosis

Since the only significant bacteriologic cause of pharyngitis is the group A beta hemolytic streptococcus, a precise diagnosis may be made by culture of the pharynx. A dry swab may be rubbed over the tonsillar and pharyngeal areas and then plated on 5 per cent sheep blood agar. Although immediate plating of the specimen is optimum, it has been shown that swabs taken in this manner, if kept in a tightly stoppered container, may be kept overnight in the refrigerator or at room temperature and plated the following morning. The characteristic beta hemolytic streptococcal colonies can be recognized with little practice. In order to assure that the beta hemolytic streptococcus is indeed group A, the organism may be subcultured onto a plate containing a bacitracin disk. At least 95 per cent of group A beta hemolytic streptococci are sensitive to bacitracin, whereas nongroup A beta hemolytic streptococci are usually resistant.

Prognosis

It has been demonstrated that patients with streptococcal pharyngitis need not be treated immediately in order to prevent the complications of rheumatic fever or glomerulonephritis. As a matter of fact, if therapy is instituted within six days after the onset of symptoms of streptococcal pharyngitis, there will be ample time to prevent these complications. Figure 1 presents a diagrammatic representation of the typical clinical pattern of streptococcal pharyngitis in school-age children. Many patients improve rapidly and are well within twenty-four hours without specific antibiotic therapy.

Treatment

If cultures are not obtained for the purpose of therapy, all patients with severe pharyngitis should be considered to have streptococcal infection. As indicated above, of those with moderate pharyngitis, approximately half will have disease caused by streptococci, and in the other half disease will be the result of virus infection. It is usually impossible to differentiate between these two groups, and unless throat cultures or leukocyte counts are available to aid in differentiation, they should probably all be treated as if they are caused by the streptococcus. Those patients with mild pharyngitis who do not have throat cultures should be considered to have virus infection and not be subjected to treatment.

For those patients who are not allergic to penicillin, this antibiotic is the agent of choice for the treatment of streptococcal pharyngitis. One of the three following regimens may be chosen for the treatment of streptococcal pharyngitis: (1) intramuscular injections of procaine penicillin on days 1, 4, 7 and 10 in 300,000- to 600,000-unit doses, depending upon the age of the child; (2) oral administration of penicillin, 200,000 units (125 mg.) three times daily for ten days; or (3) intramuscular injection of Bicillin, 600,000 units for children under six years of age, 900,000 units between six and nine years, and 1.2 million units over nine years of age. In order to achieve a rapid level of penicillin in the blood and therefore more rapid clinical improvement, administration of three doses of an oral penicillin such as phenoxymethyl penicillin in the amount of 200,000 units each may be given to those patients receiving Bicillin. Of the three regimens, the one utilizing Bicillin is preferable. The only disadvantage is that an injection must be given, which is sometimes painful. With the oral regimen the child improves rapidly, and there is a tendency for the parent to disregard the instructions to administer the ten days of therapy necessary to completely eradicate streptococci and to prevent recurrence of the streptococcal infection.

If the patient is allergic to penicillin, erythromycin may be given. Erythromycin estolate given in doses of 10 to 20 mg. per kilogram per day for ten days has been shown to produce results comparable to those achieved with a ten-day course of phenoxymethyl penicillin.

REFERENCES

Moffet, H. L., Cramblett, H. G., and Black, J. P.: Group A Streptococcal Infections in a Children's Home. 1. Evaluation of Practical Bacteriologic Methods. *Pediatrics*, 33: 5-10, 1964.

Moffet, H. L., Cramblett, H. G., and Smith, A.: Group A Streptococcal Infections in a Children's Home. 2. Clinical and Epidemiologic Patterns of Illness. *Pediatrics*, 33:11-17, 1964.

CHAPTER FOURTEEN

Chronic Rhinitis

WILLIAM E. LAUPUS, M.D.

Chronic rhinitis and chronic hypertrophic rhinitis are descriptive terms broadly used for the thickening and edema of the nasal mucous membranes which occur perennially or for prolonged periods and which are, in most instances, manifestations of underlying disease of the nasal or paranasal cavities. In young children chronic rhinitis is usually associated with adenoidal hypertrophy, chronic sinus infection, and nasal deformities, including deviated septum. *Although the problem may appear to be primarily infectious, nasal allergies are fundamentally involved in many instances.* Occasionally hypothyroidism may be causative.

Temporary and self-limited hypertrophy of the nasal mucosa occurs in some adolescent girls and adult women at the time of the menses. More prolonged hypertrophy is seen at puberty in both sexes; endocrine factors are suspected, but actually little is known about the precise hormonal relations to nasal mucosal hypertrophy.

Atrophic rhinitis may develop during adolescence, either as an end-stage of chronic hypertrophic rhinitis or chronic infectious rhinitis or as a primary disease in which hereditary features predominate. Bacterial infection, particularly involving Klebsiella and similar organisms, is commonly associated with atrophic rhinitis, but is not generally considered to be its cause.

The principal complaint is nasal obstruction. Mouth-breathing is common, and pharyngeal dryness or soreness may be troublesome. Lethargy, poor appetite, headaches, and abdominal and leg pains are often present. The turbinates are red and swollen, and the posterior pharynx often shows many small foci of lymphoid hypertrophy. The mucous membranes are firm and thickened, and a thick, tenacious secretion may be seen in the nasal airway or as a postnasal discharge. With diphtheria, syphilis or unilateral foreign body, the discharge may be blood-tinged or frankly bloody. In atrophic rhinitis the tenacious and crusted mucopurulent secretions frequently occlude the nares. An offensive odor is present and is troublesome to the patient. The underlying mucosa is glistening, pale and atrophic; the turbinates are small. The nasopharynx and the pharynx may also be involved in the atrophic process.

Successful management of chronic rhinitis requires a comprehensive approach to the contributory causes. Foci of infection in the adenoids, sinuses, tonsils and middle ears should be eradicated. House dust and mold sensitivities are frequently found in patients with chronic sinus and nasal disorders, and the allergic aspects warrant careful investigation and treatment. Environmental control of dust and inhalant allergies, appropriate dietary restrictions and desensitization when indicated are the usual antiallergic measures taken. Nose drops containing deconges-tants, antihistamines or both may be of temporary benefit, but prolonged use may provoke irritative mucosal changes which perpetuate the chronic rhinitis. Prolonged antibiotic therapy may be helpful in selected instances after culture has been carried out and bacterial sensitivity to a specific antimicrobial agent has been demonstrated. The atrophic form of chronic rhinitis is often refractory to therapy; removal of crusted secretions, cleansing irrigations and local or systemic administration of estrogenic substances appear to be the most useful ministrations.

CHAPTER FIFTEEN

Pharyngeal Abscesses

CHARLES F. FERGUSON, M.D.

RETROPHARYNGEAL ABSCESS

The common throat abscess of infancy and *early* childhood is the retropharyngeal abscess. Early in life the potential retropharyngeal space between the posterior pharyngeal wall and the prevertebral fascia contains several lymph glands of Henle, which tend to disappear after three or four years of age. These glands drain the nasopharynx and eustachian tube areas, as well as the posterior nasal passages, and frequently become secondarily infected in the young. When these glands break down and suppuration ensues, pus is formed in the loose areolar tissue of the retropharyngeal space, producing a bulge of the posterior wall. Symptoms are high fever, stertorous respirations, refusal of feedings, and dysphagia. The infant may lie with his head considerably extended if the swelling is near the larynx. Respirations are labored, and mucus accumulates in the mouth because of the difficulty in swallowing. Serious respiratory obstruction may result, especially when the abscess is situated low in the hypopharyngeal region. Rupture may cause aspiration of pus into the tracheobronchial tree, with asphyxia or with the development of pulmonary infection. A retropharyngeal abscess in the nasopharynx will cause nasal obstruction with bulging forward of the soft palate. Palpatation of any throat abscess is risky, unless the patient is in Trendelenburg position and suction is available in case of rupture.

If the abscess is fluctuant, it should be adequately incised in the Trendelenburg position; thereafter the opening should be probed daily to prevent sealing until drainage is complete. In most instances today the child is seen before fluctuation has developed, and the gland is merely in the inflamed presuppurative state, with the swelling tender but firm. Adequate antibiotic therapy will usually cause satisfactory resolution, and surgical drainage does not often become necessary. Local therapy, such as the use of gargles or warm throat irrigations, is not practical at this age. In inadequately treated patients, infection may extend laterally into the parapharyngeal or pharyngomaxillary space, or descend downward into the posterior mediastinum.

LATERAL PHARYNGEAL ABSCESS

Lateral pharyngeal abscess is the common throat abscess of *childhood*, much as the retrophargyngeal abscess is the common one of *infancy*. As the name implies, the localization is in the lateral pharyngeal wall. Although the entire tonsil, the soft palate and the uvula may be considerably displaced medially and the pharynx has an asymmetrical appearance, the tonsil itself is not involved and trismus (from spasm of the pterygoid muscles) is absent. The entire pharyngeal wall is displaced medially. The swelling is localized behind the posterior pillar. There is usually considerable cervical adenitis as well.

Since most abscesses of the throat are caused by the beta hemolytic streptococcus, the drug of choice in any abscess, unless individual sensitivity precludes its use, is penicillin in large parenteral doses. This drug should be continued for at least a week or ten days *in full dosage*. Frequently, warm saline irrigations to localize the infection, and hot compresses externally to the involved side of the neck are comforting in older children. Aspirin will be helpful in alleviating the discomfort and fever. Culture and sensitivity tests should be carried out; if a resistant staphylococcus is the causative organism, methicillin or sodium oxacillin should be given.

As in the retropharyngeal abscess, most of the cases will go on to satisfactory resolution, but occasionally instances of inadequate or tardy treatment will require incision and drainage. If general anesthesia is used, the abscess should be evacuated with the patient in the Trendelenburg position, preferably using intratracheal fluothane; adequate suction should always be available.

PERITONSILLAR ABSCESS

True peritonsillar abscess (quinsy sore throat), which is the common throat abscess of adults, is rare in children under ten to twelve years of age. In this condition pus localizes in the supratonsillar region, or works up into this area from behind the tonsil, or behind a tonsillar remnant. The anterior pillar and the soft palate overlie the site of localization. Because of the proximity of the pterygoid muscles, severe trismus occurs. These findings are rarely seen in children, and the suspected peritonsillar abscess usually turns out to be a lateral pharyngeal abscess.

CHAPTER SIXTEEN

Sinusitis

WILLIAM E. LAUPUS, M.D.,
and PETER N. PASTORE, M.D.

Although the nasal accessory sinuses are present in complete or precursory form at birth, only the maxillary antra and the anterior and posterior ethmoidal cells are sufficiently well differentiated and pneumatized to be involved in nasal infection in young infants and children. The frontal sinuses are derived from anterior ethmoidal cells and are incorporated into the growing frontal bone after the second year of life; they become pneumatized slowly and are of clinical importance after the sixth year. The sphenoid sinus is intranasal until about the third year, when, through absorption of intervening cartilage and growth, it becomes surrounded by the sphenoid bone; it is rarely of clinical significance before the fourth or fifth year of age. Variations in size, shape, position and *number* of sinuses are common, especially in the ethmoid and frontal groups. Ethmoidal infection early in life may prevent or impair the development of the frontal sinuses, which may then be small, unilateral or even absent.

The mucosal lining of the sinuses is continuous with that of the nasal passages, and acute nasal infections of the "common cold" type involve the sinuses as well as the nose. Such infections, though properly included in the category of acute sinusitis, are short-lived and subside concomitantly with the nasal infection.

Acute suppurative sinusitis caused by pyogenic bacteria is most commonly seen as a complication of an acute viral rhinitis. Although knowledge of respiratory infections is incomplete, the available evidence supports the postulate that bacterial infection gains entrance to the mucosal cells of the upper respiratory tract after viral infection has interfered with normal defense mechanisms. When the sinal mucous membrane becomes infected, narrowing of the ostium of the involved sinus may interfere with the movement of mucopurulent secretions from the sinus, leading to stasis and producing an *empyema* if the ostium is obstructed. If the sinus orifice is partially open, the purulent discharge drains into the nasal cavity. Pus seen superior to the middle turbinate usually originates from the sphenoid or posterior ethmoid sinuses, whereas secretions seen in the region of the middle meatus arise in the anterior sinuses (maxillary, frontal or anterior ethmoid sinuses). In infants and small children periorbital edema or cellulitis may be seen with infection in the ethmoid cells. Older children with acute sinusitis complain of pain in particular locations: in the temporal region or above or between the eyes with anterior ethmoiditis; in the postauricular (mastoid) region with posterior ethmoiditis; in the face or upper teeth with maxillary antritis; in the forehead with either frontal or maxillary disease, alone or in combination; and in the suboccipital area with sphenoiditis. Fever, nasal congestion, sensation of fullness or pain, tenderness over the sinus and facial paresthesias are common complaints in acute sinus infections.

Nasoscopy usually reveals red, thickened, edematous nasal mucosa and purulent discharge in the nasal passages. Transillumination in older children may be helpful in delineating frontal and maxillary disease. X-ray films are not usually necessary to establish the diagnosis of acute sinusitis, but, when taken, may show increased opacity of the involved sinus or sinuses.

Pneumococci and group A hemolytic

(beta) streptococci are the predominating bacterial organisms in acute sinusitis; *Hemophilus influenzae* type B and the coagulase- and pigment-producing hemolytic staphylococci are less common offenders; other organisms, including those generally considered to be nonpathogens, may occasionally be involved.

Treatment is directed to promoting drainage of the infected sinus and to specific antimicrobial therapy of the infection. Instillation of nasal vasoconstrictors at regular intervals and gentle aspiration are helpful in shrinking the nasal mucosa, opening the sinal ostia and keeping the airway clear, but the use of nose drops should not be prolonged. Nasal aspiration may be beneficial. Blowing of the nose should be avoided. Culture of the nasopharynx aids in the selection of the proper antimicrobial agent, which should be administered in full therapeutic dosage until the nasal symptoms have cleared, usually seven to ten days. Undertreatment in terms of dosage and duration of antimicrobial therapy is common and may lead to recrudescence of the infection or to subacute or chronic sinusitis. Penicillin is effective in streptococcal and pneumococcal infections and in staphylococcal infections if the organism does not produce penicillinase. Erythromycin and lincomycin (Lincocin) may be used if the patient is allergic to penicillin. For staphylococci resistant to penicillin, erythromycin, oxycillin (Prostaphlin), methicillin (Staphcillin), nafcillin (Unipen) or cephalosporin (Keflin) may be used if the organism proves to be sensitive to one of these agents. A tetracycline or ampicillin (Omnicillin, Polycillin) is advocated for the *H. influenzae* infections.

Most acute sinus infections will respond satisfactorily to the combination of vasoconstrictive nose drops and appropriate antibiotic therapy. Patients with true empyema of the maxillary sinus may be benefited by surgical drainage, either by cannulation of the natural orifice or rarely by puncture of the nasoantral wall. Irrigation is commonly used in conjunction with drainage procedures. Instilla-

tion of antibiotic solutions into the sinus cavity is often practiced, but seems to be of questionable value. The sphenoid and frontal sinus orifices can also be cannulated, but these procedures should be reserved to the skilled rhinologist, who will make use of them in unusual situations when drainage cannot otherwise be established or when serious complications threaten.

Complications of acute sinusitis include otitis media, orbital cellulitis, meningitis, brain abscess, osteomyelitis (especially of the frontal bone), cavernous sinus thrombosis, oroantral fistula formation, and nephritis. Aspiration of the purulent discharge may occasionally lead to lung abscess. Virulent acute infections may rarely give rise to bacteremia and to metastatic infection in bones, joints, kidneys, lungs and endocardium.

Subacute or chronic suppurative sinusitis is most commonly seen in association with local or systemic conditions which prevent eradication of the offending infection. Search should be made for such abnormalities as nasal deformity (deviated septum), hypertrophied adenoids, foreign body, infected upper posterior teeth and nasal allergy. Children with cystic fibrosis commonly have chronic sinusitis, as do children with hypogammaglobulinemia, hypothyroidism, Down's syndrome (mongolism) and nutritional deficiencies.

Nasal allergies as predisposing factors in chronic sinal infections are deserving of special mention. Inhalant sensitivities to dust and molds (alternaria and hormodendron especially) are often overlooked in consideration of specific therapy in children with sinusitis. Food allergies, particularly to milk and chocolate, may occasionally be important in chronic nasal and paranasal disease.

The manifestations of chronic sinus infection are variable. The most frequent are low-grade fever with late afternoon temperature elevation, anorexia, malaise, easy fatigability, and decline in school performance with accompanying complaints of poorly localized headache and abdominal or leg pain. Sneezing, nasal obstruction and discharge, purulent post-nasal obstruction and discharge, dry "sore" throat, frequent dry cough and persistent mouth-breathing are common. Chronic bronchitis, occasionally with bronchiectasis, is the most important and frequent complication.

Chronic sinusitis should always be considered in the differential diagnosis of preschool and older children with unexplained fever (fever of unknown origin).

Treatment is directed to the correction of underlying local anatomic or general health problems as well as to the eradication of the infecting organism. Nasopharyngeal culture with antimicrobial sensitivity testing is mandatory to the selection of the appropriate antibiotic agent. Vasoconstrictive nose drops have little value; prolonged use may lead to local irritation and chronic congestion of the nasal mucosa. Saline nose drops are of benefit in thinning the secretions.

Drainage is facilitated by the method and positioning described by Parkinson.* Cannulation of the natural sinus orifice or direct puncture of this sinus may be necessary in some instances. A careful history for familial incidence of allergy and detailed study of the patient from an allergic standpoint, including skin testing when indicated, may contribute to the comprehensive care of the problem.

---

* In the Parkinson method the child lies on his side with the shoulder elevated by a firm pad such as a folded blanket, and the head is bent down to a dependent position. The nasal solution which is then instilled can be expected to have contact with the various sinal ostia on both sides. The child should breathe through the mouth to prevent drawing the medication into the pharynx. The position is maintained for five to six minutes, and the face is then turned downward for a few moments to permit drainage of the nasal contents, or the child may sit up and place his head down between his knees.

From W. E. Nelson (Ed.): *Textbook of Pediatrics*. 8th ed. Philadelphia, W. B. Saunders Company, 1964, p. 812.

CHAPTER SEVENTEEN

The Tonsils and Adenoids
WILLIAM A. HOWARD, M.D.

The faucial and pharyngeal tonsils are part of a mass of lymphoid tissue encircling the nasal and oral pharynx known as Waldeyer's ring. Acute infections and conditions involving these tissues have been described elsewhere. In this chapter, interest is centered on the possibility of chronic and persistent tonsil and adenoid involvement and the desirability or necessity of surgical removal of these structures as a method of treatment.

Pathogenesis

The lymphoid tissue of Waldeyer's ring undergoes physiologic hypertrophy and hyperplasia, usually greatest between two and five years of age, in response to infections in this general area. Such hyperplasia is associated with an increase in lymphocytes in these tissues and with increased immunologic activity of the host in response to specific infections. These infections of the tonsils and adenoids are most prevalent during these early years, and as increasing resistance to infection develops, the frequency and severity of respiratory infections diminish rapidly, usually with a corresponding decrease in the size of the lymphoid mass. Under the stress of acute infection tonsils and adenoids may undergo rapid enlargement, but as infection subsides, they generally return to their former state. One should not judge the tonsil by viewing it only under the stress of acute infection.

Clinical Manifestations

Chronic infection in the tonsils and adenoids may be associated with a variety of clinical manifestations. There may be recurrent bouts of acute infection manifested by a sore throat or a more or less continuous low-grade involvement, with or without fever. Some degree of cervical adenitis is often present, and there may be a history of recurring middle ear infections, with or without some degree of hearing loss. Mouth-breathing may occur as a result of adenoid enlargement, and a heavy, fetid breath may be noted in the morning. Though less common than formerly, peritonsillar and retropharyngeal abscesses may develop adjacent to the chronically infected tonsil.

A variety of other symptoms have been ascribed to diseased tonsils and adenoids, including fatigue, loss of appetite, failure to gain weight, so-called growing pains, difficulty in swallowing, chronic cough, frequent upper respiratory tract infections, postnasal drip, "clearing of the throat" and many others.

Physical findings generally relate to the size of the tonsils, which may be large or small, and of the adenoids, which are usually enlarged. The chronically infected tonsil cannot be diagnosed by a single, simple inspection, and usually a careful chronologic history is essential for a proper evaluation of the nature and degree of infection present. Additional findings will include varying degrees of cervical adenitis, nasal obstruction, occasional hearing loss, and rarely a collection of serous fluid behind the tympanic membrane, the so-called serous otitis media. When nasal obstruction has been present for a considerable period of time, there may be a thoracic deformity, usually a simple funnel chest of varying depth, involving the lower portion of the sternum,

the xiphoid and the neighboring rib cartilages. Some depression also may be noted at the level of attachment of the diaphragm. Malocclusion of varying degree, associated with enlarged adenoids and nasal obstruction, may help in producing what is termed the adenoid facies.

Many of these signs and symptoms can be produced by other causes, the most common of which is allergic involvement of the upper respiratory tract. It should be emphasized again that a careful history is most important in making a decision about the removal of tonsils and adenoids.

Indications for Adenotonsillectomy

Based upon an abundance of available evidence, a few salient facts may be noted.

Although a more conservative attitude has developed toward adenotonsillectomy, the operation is still extremely common, and probably is performed much too frequently.

The wide variation in the reported incidence of adenotonsillectomy in different groups rated according to age, geographic location, socio-economic status, medical insurance and educational levels is such that one cannot escape the conclusion that the operation must at times be performed for reasons other than those purely medical.

Indications for operation vary greatly, emphasizing the lack of understanding of the basic function of this lymphoid tissue and the consequences of its early removal.

It is extremely difficult to assess the results of adenotonsillectomy because of the wide variety of indications for its performance and the lack of long-term follow-up by those who perform the operation, and because it is usually done at an age when gradual but spontaneous improvement in response to exposure to infection is to be expected.

Adenotonsillectomy is not without danger, 200 to 300 deaths being reported each year from this elective procedure.

Tonsillectomized persons are neither more nor less susceptible to streptococcal infections, nor is the clinical course of streptococcal disease modified. There is also no effect on the development of rheumatic fever or rheumatic valvular heart disease. Streptococcal infections are less readily recognized in tonsillectomized children, who may thereby escape adequate treatment. Although the occurrence of bulbar poliomyelitis in recently tonsillectomized persons may once have been a main consideration, this now seems much less important in view of the high percentage of persons who have received adequate immunization against this disease.

With due consideration of the foregoing discussion it is possible to give a brief résumé of the various situations which have been considered indications for adenotonsillectomy.

PERITONSILLAR ABSCESS. Once this complication has been diagnosed, there is fairly general agreement that a second attack should not be risked, and that adenotonsillectomy should be done as soon as feasible.

RECURRENT TONSILLITIS. Recurrent acute tonsillar infections, with fever, cervical adenitis and possibly otitis media, may constitute a sound indication for operation, especially if there is persistent evidence of chronic involvement between acute attacks. There exists the possibility, however, that such attacks represent new infections with differing etiologic agents, and that they constitute an immunologic experience that might occur regardless of the presence or absence of the tonsils.

RECURRENT "COLDS." Recurrent upper respiratory tract infections resembling the common cold generally are not controlled by adenotonsillectomy, and operation is not recommended.

RECURRENT OTITIS MEDIA. If ear infections are frequent, and there is any evidence of hearing loss, adenoidectomy alone should be considered the operation of choice. Removal of the tonsils should not be done at the same time unless there are specific indications.

HYPERTROPHIED TONSILS. Tonsillar enlargement alone, especially under the age of five to six years, is seldom if ever sufficient indication for operation.

ADENOID ENLARGEMENT. If adenoid enlargement is sufficient to cause noisy mouth-breathing, snoring, and persistent low-grade nasal congestion and discharge, removal of the adenoids is considered proper, provided one can be assured that the symptoms are not produced by allergic involvement in the same area.

CERVICAL ADENITIS. Chronic infection in the cervical lymph nodes, with frequent acute flare-ups, are fundamentally an indication of persistent infection in the pharyngeal area. Depending on the appearance of the tonsils and the degree of infection present, cervical adenitis may then constitute a valid indication for tonsillectomy.

In considering the indications for adenotonsillectomy, it becomes apparent that there will be many instances in which removal of the adenoids may be the only surgical procedure indicated, and that results may be more satisfactory and much less disturbing if tonsillectomy is avoided. Also, in making a decision about operation, the possibility of an allergic cause of the signs and symptoms must be considered. Nasal obstruction, frequent upper respiratory tract involvement resembling "colds," serous otitis media, enlargement of tonsils and adenoids and diminished hearing may all appear on the basis of nasal allergy. Adenotonsillectomy may be indicated in the allergic child as well, but the indications for operation should be at least as stringent as those for the nonallergic child, if not more so. It is the consensus among pediatric allergists that adenotonsillectomy should not be undertaken in the allergic child until there has been a period of definitive treatment of the underlying allergy, and adequate treatment of any accompanying infection. After three to six months of such treatment the indications for operation may have lessened a great deal or even may have disappeared entirely. Removal of tonsils and adenoids in a child with untreated nasal allergy may be followed by the development of bronchial allergic symptoms.

Complications

Complications from adenotonsillectomy are relatively infrequent with the exception of postoperative hemorrhage. Blood loss occasionally may be sufficient to warrant replacement by transfusion. Pneumonia, lung abscess, atelectasis and septicemia have occurred. As indicated earlier, death may occur, usually as a result of cardiac arrest, hemorrhage or infection. The psychologic reaction to the trauma of hospitalization and operation should not be overlooked.

Results from Adenotonsillectomy

Although the incidence of epidemic respiratory infections is not altered by virtue of the removal of the tonsils and adenoids, there may be a decrease in the number and severity of throat infections, and in the amount of fever which accompanies them. Obstructive symptoms may be relieved, especially by adenoidectomy, but relief from recurrent otitis media is variable. There is generally a gradual disappearance of cervical adenopathy, and bouts of acute adenitis are decreased or absent. There may be gain in weight and apparent benefit to general health and appetite, but multiple factors may be involved in this general improvement. It is unwise to promise too much as a result of adenotonsillectomy.

REFERENCES

Bakwin, H.: The Tonsil-Adenoidectomy Enigma. *J. Pediat.*, 52:339, 1958.

Canby, J. P.: Acquired Fibrinogenemia. An Unusual Cause of Post-Tonsillectomy and Adenoidectomy Hemorrhage. *J.A.M.A.*, 183:282, 1963.

Chamovitz, R., Rammelkamp, C. H., Jr., Wannamaker, L. W., and Denny, W. F., Jr.: The Effect of Tonsillectomy on the Incidence of Streptococcal Disease and Its Complications. *Pediatrics*, 26:355, 1960.

Chobot, R.: Infectious Aspects of Asthma in Children; in S. Prigal: *Fundamentals of Modern Allergy*. New York, McGraw-Hill Book Company, Inc., 1960.

Clein, N.: Influence of Tonsillectomy and Adenoidectomy on Children, with Special Reference to the Allergic Implications. *Ann. Allergy*, 10:568, 1952.

Howard, W. A.: Childhood Complications of Respiratory Allergies. *Clin. Proc. Child. Hosp, D.C.*, 8:210, 1952.

Idem: Diagnosis and Treatment of Nasal Obstruction in Children. *Postgrad. Med.*, 21:136, 1957.

Lelong, M.: Asthma et amygdalectomie. *Lille Med.*, 9:77, 1964.

Ravenholt, R. T.: Poliomyelitic Paralysis and Tonsillectomy Reconsidered. *A.M.A. J. Dis. Child.*, 103:658, 1962.

Sherman, W. B., and Kessler, W. R.: *Allergy in Pediatric Practice*. St. Louis, C. V. Mosby Company, 1957.

Sobel, G.: Adenotonsillectomy in the Allergic Child; in S. Prigal: *Fundamentals of Modern Allergy*. New York, McGraw-Hill Book Company, Inc., 1960.

SECTION VIII

Infections of the
Lower Respiratory Tract

CHAPTER EIGHTEEN

Croup (Epiglottitis; Laryngitis; Laryngotracheobronchitis)

HENRY G. CRAMBLETT, M.D.

Croup is a syndrome in which there is inspiratory stridor, cough and hoarseness due to varying degrees of laryngeal obstruction. The obstruction in infectious croup is due to inflammatory edema and spasm. In this chapter infections involving the epiglottis, the vocal cords or the subglottic area will be considered together.

Incidence and Etiology

The true incidence of croup is difficult to determine. Undoubtedly this syndrome is responsible for a significant number of emergency calls to the physician, particularly at night. From an etiologic standpoint, viral croup occurs in at least 85 per cent of all cases.

The various bacteria and viruses which have been demonstrated to cause croup are outlined in the table of Etiologic Classification of Primary Respiratory Tract Illnesses (p. 242). To date the parainfluenza viruses have been recovered from patients with croup more commonly than any other virus or group of viruses. *Hemophilus influenzae* type B is responsible for the majority of cases of bacterial croup. Ordinarily, *Hemophilus influenzae* causes epiglottitis, but may involve other areas of the larynx, or the infection may extend into the tracheobronchial tree.

With present immunization procedures *Corynebacterium diphtheriae* is a rare cause of croup, but this possibility must be kept in mind in dealing with a non-immunized patient. It is extremely doubtful whether or not pneumococci, streptococci or staphylococci play a significant role in the causation of croup. In most carefully controlled studies the incidence of recovery of these potential pathogens is little greater in patients with croup than with similarly matched controls who do not have croup.

As far as the cause of viral croup is concerned, it has become increasingly apparent that the importance of any given virus in the origin of croup will vary from season to season, from year to year and from geographic area to geographic area. In his early studies Rabe showed that no more than 14.7 per cent of patients had disease as a result of infection with bacteria, with the inference that the remainder were caused by viruses. Table 1 summarizes the results of three different etiologic studies of viral croup. It is apparent from the table that the parainfluenza viruses are the most important ones yet recovered from patients with this disease. Yet, as additional studies are performed and virologic techniques are improved, it is possible that this picture will change. Over-all, using diagnostic

261

Table 1. *Etiology of Nonbacterial Croup*

Virus	Per Cent Reported		
	McLean	Parrott	Cramblett
Adenovirus ...	..	9	4
Influenza (A + B)	1.5	8	6
Parainfluenza 1.	30	21	8
Parainfluenza 2.	0.5	8	6
Parainfluenza 3.	4	10	14
Respiratory syncytial	..	8	..
ECHO viruses .	0.2	..	10
Coxsackie viruses	..	..	2
No virus recovered	64	36	50

techniques presently available, it is possible to recover viruses from as many as 65 per cent of the patients with croup.

Pathogenesis and Predisposition to Croup

Patients with viral croup may have a preceding infection of the upper respiratory passages with primary involvement of the mucous membranes of the nose. After three to four days the infection may progress to the area of the larynx where the true cords and subglottic structures become inflamed and edematous. Associated with viral croup, especially in those children with so-called spasmodic croup, there is an additional element of spasm which contributes to the laryngeal obstruction. In the past "spasmodic croup" was classified separately from infectious croup, but there are now data which indicate that this form of the disease results directly or indirectly from virus infection. Figure 1 is a diagrammatic presentation of the fact that edema and spasm may be present in varying degrees in infectious croup.

In infections due to *Hemophilus influenzae* type B the primary site of inflammation is the epiglottis, which becomes enlarged because of inflammatory edema. This is a serious disease (see Diagnosis). Inflammation may spread to involve the remainder of the supraglottic as well as the subglottic area. With *Hemophilus influenzae* infections the inflammation commonly extends downward into the respiratory tract, involving the trachea and bronchi. If this occurs, the prognosis is worse.

In croup due to *Corynebacterium diphtheriae* it is usual to have inflammation and infection of the upper respiratory tract, including pharyngitis and rhinitis, preceding the signs and symptoms of laryngeal inflammation. There is usually "membrane" formation in the pharynx, or even in and around the larynx, which may give rise to complete, sudden obstruc-

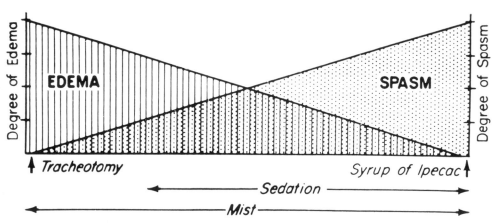

FIGURE 18–1.   A schematic representation of the pathogenesis and treatment of croup. (From H. G. Cramblett: Croup—Present Day Concept. *Pediatrics, 25*:1071, 1960.)

tion if it becomes dislodged from the mucous membrane surface.

Regardless of the direct precipitating cause of croup, a number of factors are of importance in predisposing an individual child to the development of the syndrome. Even though some of these factors are poorly understood, they are worthy of consideration.

Age is an important factor. The majority of patients with viral croup are between the ages of three months and three years. Hemophilus influenzal and diphtheritic croup occur most commonly in children between the ages of three and seven years.

The incidence of croup is higher among males than among females. Even in children with postoperative or traumatic croup, the same sex incidence prevails. There is no obvious explanation for this.

Most cases of croup occur during the cold season of the year. This is in all probability a reflection of the increased incidence of all respiratory infections during this period.

All the factors thus far mentioned which predispose to croup are those which have been statistically proved by the analysis of large series of cases. In addition to these, it has frequently been postulated that there are certain "endogenous factors" that predispose a given child to croup. Evidence for this includes the fact that croup tends to be recurrent in a child who has had one episode. Further, recent virologic studies reveal that all the viruses which have been associated with croup cause other types of clinical disease. There has been no one virus yet identified which causes only croup. The question why one child suffers croup as the result of a particular viral infection while another child has only a minor upper respiratory tract infection or involvement of the lower tracheobronchial tree without laryngeal involvement is still unanswered.

It has been postulated that an "anatomically defective larynx" or an "immaturity" of the larynx may be a factor. There is no evidence to suggest that these are important considerations. What constitutes the host factor in the pathogenesis of croup is unknown, but the concept must be accepted.

Evidence that "allergic" factors predispose to the development of croup is inconclusive. In one study the family history of allergic disorders in children with croup and in a group of randomly selected children were analyzed. There was no difference. Among children with allergic diseases there does not appear to be an increased incidence of croup.

Clinical Manifestations

Croup due to *Hemophilus influenzae* type B epiglottitis is usually rapid in onset and tends to run a fulminating course. The initial symptom may be throat discomfort, and after this the signs and symptoms of toxicity and acute inspiratory obstruction may develop out of proportion to the duration of illness. Fever is present early. The total duration of the disease from the onset to hospitalization with extreme stridor may be only a few hours. The patients appear markedly apprehensive and exhibit supraclavicular, suprasternal and subcostal retraction.

Children with croup due to viral infections usually give a history of upper respiratory tract infection one to three days preceding the onset of croup. Although these children show apprehension and restlessness, they do not show the same degree of toxemia as do children with the same disease due to *Hemophilus influenzae*. Approximately 50 per cent of the children with viral croup have no fever. This is in contradistinction to those patients with *Hemophilus influenzae* type B epiglottitis.

In croup due to *Corynebacterium diphtheriae* there is usually a preceding upper respiratory tract infection of three to four days' duration before the onset of symptoms of croup. A frequent sign in children with diphtheria is a serosanguineous nasal discharge. In addition, a membrane may be present in the posterior pharynx. The symptoms of croup usually develop slowly. Signs of severe obstruction may occur suddenly, however, if the membrane becomes dislodged and obstructs the laryngeal airway. The patients appear quite toxic.

Diagnosis

The diagnosis of *Hemophilus influenzae* type B epiglottitis may be established by observing a fiery red, swollen, edematous epiglottis on physical examination. It is to be stressed that before the patient is manipulated, and especially before efforts are made to visualize the epiglottis, the observer must be prepared to establish an airway either by intubation, tracheostomy, or the placing of a large-caliber needle through the skin into the lumen of the trachea. The addition of the trauma of the examination to the patient's apprehension and the compromised airway may be enough to cause complete respiratory obstruction. Thus, although the diagnosis can be easily established by physical examination, this procedure is not one to be undertaken without due caution. In the establishment of an etiologic diagnosis, blood cultures are positive as often as are nasopharyngeal cultures or cultures taken directly from the epiglottis. A peripheral leukocyte count will show an increase in the total count with a preponderance of polymorphonuclear cells.

In diphtheritic croup the presence of a serosanguineous nasal discharge and a membrane in the absence of a history of immunization against diphtheria are suggestive of the diagnosis.

In viral croup the diagnosis is most often made by exclusion of infections due to *Corynebacterium diphtheriae* and *Hemophilus influenzae* type B. The child who has a "spasmodic croup" or is afebrile most certainly has a virus infection. On the other hand, if the course of disease is not fulminating, but the child is febrile, there is a marginal possibility that the disease is caused by *Hemophilus influenzae* type B. When available, throat washings for inoculation into tissue culture may provide an etiologic viral diagnosis. The parainfluenza viruses grow in monkey kidney cell cultures, where their presence is most easily recognized by hemadsorption of guinea pig erythrocytes. Influenza viruses may be similarly grown, or an alternate method is inoculation of the patient's secretions into embryonated hens' eggs. Adenoviruses and respiratory syncytial virus may be grown in continuous cell cultures of HeLa or Hep-2. The enteroviruses grow well and produce cytopathic effects in monkey kidney cell cultures.

Prognosis

The necessity for tracheostomy and the prognosis of croup vary according to the involvement of the various anatomic structures. In Rabe's series, 0.6 per cent of the cases with laryngitis required a tracheostomy, whereas 16.3 per cent of those with laryngotracheitis required this procedure. The important statistic is that 47 per cent of those with laryngotracheobronchitis had need for the establishment of an adequate airway by tracheostomy. In another series of patients with epiglottitis, 43 per cent of the patients required tracheostomy. In this same series 12 per cent of the patients were dead on arrival at the hospital or died after admission.

Treatment

Because patients with croup are extremely apprehensive, it is important that they be handled with a minimum of activity in order not to aggravate their respiratory distress. The patient should be immediately placed in an atmosphere with high humidity and oxygen. The oxygen will help alleviate anxiety, apprehension and increased respiratory efforts. All diagnostic and nursing procedures should be kept to a minimum. Under no circumstances should a sleeping child with croup be awakened. In order to decrease apprehension and restlessness, it is helpful at times to sedate the patient cautiously. The same caution should be exercised in the administration of sedatives to these patients as that which is observed in any patient with respiratory difficulties. Phenobarbital may be used in a dosage of 6 mg. per kilogram per 24 hours in three or four divided doses.

In order that the child be minimally disturbed, it is advisable to administer fluids intravenously. Intravenous administration of fluids obviates the frequent arousal of the child, which may result in the exaggeration of symptoms, and at the same time ensures adequate hydration.

In those instances in which spasm of the larynx is more prominent than edema, administration of syrup of ipecac may produce prompt relief of symptoms. It is assumed that ipecac has a relaxing effect upon the larynx by means of a vagal response. Ipecac is given in subemetic doses, but frequently the full therapeutic effect of the drug is not achieved without vomiting. The usual dose is 1 drop per month of age up to two years. Children two years of age or older may be given 1 ml. per year of age. Any infant or child who receives ipecac should be closely observed in the hour following its administration to prevent aspiration of gastric contents in case emesis does occur. If symptoms subside, one can assume that the croup is at least partially caused by spasm, and valuable information is thus obtained without resort to laryngoscopy. If there is no response and the patient does not vomit, the same dosage may be repeated. Caution should be exercised to be certain that fluid extract of ipecac is not erroneously substituted for syrup of ipecac. The former is fourteen to twenty times as potent as the latter and may cause serious toxicity. Figure 1 diagrammatically relates certain therapeutic measures to pathogenesis.

Although corticosteroids are occasionally recommended for the therapy of croup, evidence from those controlled studies in which precise etiologic diagnoses have been made does not support their use. Moreover, the course of croup is so variable that any attempt at evaluation of the use of corticosteroids is most difficult.

In the patient with *Hemophilus influenzae* type B croup, either tetracycline

or chloramphenicol may be administered. All strains of *Hemophilus influenzae* type B are uniformly sensitive to these antibiotics. More important than the choice of the antibiotic is the mode of administration, which should be intravenous. The dose of tetracycline for intravenous therapy is 12 mg. per kilogram per twenty-four hours, and that of chloramphenicol is 50 to 75 mg. per kilogram per twenty-four hours. In patients with infections due to *Corynebacterium diphtheriae* the immediate therapy is the administration of antitoxin followed by the use of penicillin.

The decision as to the need for tracheostomy must always be based on the individual circumstances. If the signs and symptoms of laryngeal obstruction increase in spite of the aforementioned measures, the procedure will be necessary. Extension of the inflammatory process down into the tracheobronchial tree may likewise provide an indication if secretions are excessive. Careful timing of the procedure is important. Therefore it is desirable to have an otolaryngologist see the patient as soon as possible after admission so that he may follow the progress of the disease carefully. Because of the sequelae and the difficulty in management, tracheostomy in infants is avoided whenever possible. As an emergency procedure, intubation with the insertion of an airway or the placing of a large-bore needle (14 g. or greater) through the skin into the lumen of the trachea may be lifesaving and also may provide the opportunity for a carefully performed tracheostomy later.

REFERENCES

Berenberg, W., and Kevy, S.: Acute Epiglottitis in Childhood: Serious Emergency, Readily Recognized at Bedside. *New England J. Med.*, 258:870-74, 1958.

Cramblett, H. G.: Croup—Present Day Concept. *Pediatrics*, 25:1071-6, 1960.

McLean, D. M., Bach, R. D., Larke, R. P. B., and McNaughton, G. A.: Myxoviruses Associated with Acute Laryngotracheobronchitis in Toronto, 1962-1963. *Canad. M.A.J.,* 89:1257-9, 1963.

Parrott, R. H.: Viral Respiratory Tract Illnesses in Children. *Bull. New York Acad. Med.,* 39:629-48, 1963.

Rabe, E. F.: Infectious Croup. I. Etiology. *Pediatrics,* 2:255-65, 1948.

Turner, J. A.: Present-Day Aspects of Acute Laryngotracheitis. *Canad. M.A.J.,* 70:401, 1954.

CHAPTER NINETEEN

Bronchitis

J. A. PETER TURNER, M.D.

The term "bronchitis" is traditional in the language of laiety and medical profession alike. Despite clearer definition and increased understanding of pulmonary problems, it remains a comfortable cliché whenever one is confronted with the common symptom of cough. In Great Britain and Australia the word is used with much greater frequency than it is in North America. This is particularly true in adult literature with relation to chronic bronchitis, but the disparity exists in pediatric publications as well.

In childhood, bronchitis occurs as a component of many conditions in which the primary problem exists in the upper or lower respiratory tract. In an attempt to embrace the multiple areas involved, our terminology has become complicated by such combinations as sinobronchitis, laryngotracheobronchitis, asthmatic bronchitis, bronchiolitis, capillary bronchitis, bronchopneumonitis, and others. Pure bronchitis exists in very few situations. The bronchial tree, however, may be the presenting area of symptoms, if not of primary disease, under many circumstances.

It is the purpose of this chapter to outline the diseases in which inflammation of the bronchi plays a significant role. The following classification based on etiologic factors will be followed:

1. Infection
   a. Viral agents
   b. Bacterial agents
   c. Fungal agents
2. Allergic factors
3. Chemical factors

INFECTION

Viral Infections

Acute bronchitis closely follows the pattern of upper respiratory tract infection in childhood. Since most such infections are viral in origin, it follows that involvement of the bronchial tree is likewise due to viral agents in the same proportion. Viral cultures carried out on hospitalized patients have yielded results which suggest that such infections occur in both a seasonal and an epidemic pattern. The common agents isolated are the myxoviruses, the respiratory syncytial virus and the adenoviruses. Measles is responsible for a specific inflammatory reaction of the tracheobronchial tree.

Since mortality rates in such diseases are low, pathologic material is scanty. One may assume from the few studies available that there is catarrhal inflammation of the bronchial mucosa, along with a stringy mucus, only scantily mixed with leukocytes. In most instances such a reaction is self-limited. Clearing occurs with reduction in the inflammatory reaction and with thinning of the mucus, which may then be raised by ciliary action.

Clinical signs vary with the age of the child. In the young infant, below one year of age, infection with viral agents will be responsible for the clinical picture of bronchiolitis. The bronchial lumen is small, and therefore the mucosal reaction or mucus production is sufficient to produce obstruction both on inspiration and on expiration. The detailed clinical picture of this disease, together with the specifics of treatment, will be found in the following chapter.

In the older infant the same pathologic process may manifest itself as asthmatic bronchitis, i.e. respiratory distress with the obstructive phenomenon most evident in the expiratory phase. This feature may be explained by the physiologic reduction in size of the bronchial lumen on expiration which is exaggerated under conditions of inflammatory edema. These infants may present a clinical picture as acute as the foregoing. Indeed the two terms "asthmatic bronchitis" and "bronchiolitis" may be interchangeable. The age of the child is important in the clinical manifestation of viral infections of the bronchi. A common infecting agent, parainfluenza 1, has been isolated from contemporary patients in the hospital, presenting as bronchiolitis in the young infant, acute laryngotracheitis in the older infant and young child, and acute bronchitis in the older child. These differences may be explained by the variations in airway size according to age.

In the older child viral agents produce the picture of acute bronchitis, which is universally manifested by the common symptom of cough. In the early stages this cough is associated with coryza, but may progress to the dry, hacking, unproductive type, so familiar to the clinician. Although there may be pyrexia in association with this illness, a normal temperature or very low-grade fever may be present. The cough may be painful with the pain centered in the substernal area. Auscultation may reveal only roughened breath sounds. Not infrequently, however, coarse rales or rhonchi may be present. These are, as a rule, inconstant and change with coughing.

The most common complication of viral bronchitis is pneumonia, either as an extension of the primary viral infection or because of secondary bacterial invasion. Occasionally pulmonary interstitial emphysema, mediastinal emphysema or pneumothorax may ensue, particularly in the infant or young child. Anoxia, due to obstruction of the airway in infancy, is not uncommon. Cardiac failure may occur in the younger age groups.

The treatment of bronchitis depends largely on control of the cough. The *Vademecum,* 1965, lists fifty-seven antitussives. Many of these preparations contain a combination of expectorant, sedative and antihistaminic agents in the same mixture—a true "shotgun" approach. One may state two general principles in terms of cough control: (1) If secretions of the tracheobronchial tree are thinned, then physiologic ciliary action may take place with beneficial results. (2) Effective sedation may depress the cough reflex designed to clear the airway of the small child. This, in turn, may result in bronchial obstruction with its complications of secondary infection and distal atelectasis. In general terms, then, expectorant therapy, particularly in the young child, is to be desired. A simple agent which we have found useful is syrup of hydriodic acid in doses of 1 minim (1 drop or 0.06 ml.) per kilogram of body weight four times daily. Humidification of inspired air is beneficial, both in reducing inflammatory edema and in liquefying bronchial secretions. Although steam has, for years, been a ready source of moisture, there is reason to doubt its efficacy in the treatment of true bronchial disease. The droplet size from an ordinary steam kettle is too large to reach beyond the upper respiratory passages, and the heat of the steam may lead to eventual drying of secretions. Cold moisture is to be preferred whenever possible, and from a vaporizer yielding a droplet size of 0.5 to 0.3 micron. Such humidification should be continuous until clinical improvement occurs. Adequate hydration of the patient is of equal importance in maintaining thin bronchial secretions. This may be achieved by increasing oral fluid intake or, if necessary, by parenteral fluid therapy.

If viral infection is suspected, expectant therapy may be sufficient in the older child who has a simple upper respiratory tract infection complicated by bronchitis. In the infant and the young child, however, and particularly if fever is present, it is wise to use antibiotics as prophylaxis against secondary infection. In these cases the tetracycline drugs are preferred because of their additional effect against certain of the viral agents.

Bacterial Infections

The older medical literature contains many references to acute suppurative bronchitis in childhood. It is entirely possible that many of these cases were due to cystic fibrosis. Others were due to secondary infections of the bronchi following primary viral disease. The paucity of such cases now, in clinical practice, probably reflects the widespread use of chemotherapeutic agents for upper respiratory tract disease. Unlike viral infection, primary bacterial invasions of the tracheobronchial tree occur rarely. These agents manifest their effects only when some derangement of the normal bronchial defenses pre-exists. Such underlying disturbances as a primary viral bronchitis or allergic bronchitis may permit implantation, growth and invasion of the bacteria with the production of suppurative changes.

Hemophilus influenzae, chiefly type B, is commonly associated with bacterial infection of the bronchi. Staphylococcus, Streptococcus and occasionally gram-negative enteric organisms are other agents which may be isolated. *Bordetella pertussis* should be mentioned as a specific primary cause of bronchitis. This organism produces an acute inflammatory reaction of the tracheobronchial mucosa, together with the secretion of thickened tenacious mucus which is difficult to mobilize. Although the course of pertussis may be modified by vaccine, it is possible for this infection to be acquired after pertussis immunization. Such an infection may be responsible for the symptoms of bronchitis, with a cough of several weeks' duration.

Primary tuberculosis in childhood may produce an endobronchitis by the extrusion of infected caseous material from contiguous lymph nodes through the bronchial wall. Although this disease will be dealt with more fully in the chapter on tuberculosis (p. 656), it should be noted here that tuberculous infection of the bronchi may produce symptoms indistinguishable from those caused by other agents. A Mantoux test is therefore an important diagnostic tool in any child with cough of bronchial origin.

Children suffering from bacterial infection of the bronchial tree exhibit clinical signs consistent with the causative organism. Fever, tachycardia and even prostration may occur as a result of such invasion. The findings on chest examination are similar to those mentioned under viral infection. In the older child purulent sputum may be produced on coughing.

The complications of secondary infection of the bronchial tree depend upon bacterial spread to adjacent structures and to the blood stream. Bacterial pneumonia as an extension of suppurative bronchitis is common in most instances in which pathogenic bacteria are involved. Retrograde spread to the paranasal sinuses is a common accompanying feature.

Treatment of suppurative bronchial disease depends upon drainage and antibiotic therapy. Drainage of the tracheobronchial tree is best accomplished by posturing and physiotherapeutic clapping of the posterior thorax. Bronchoscopic suction may be necessary in the more severe cases. Effective antibiotic therapy depends on the culture of the offending organism and its sensitivity to the appropriate chemotherapeutic agent. Penicillin remains the drug of choice for gram-positive infections. Ampicillin, methicillin and more recently cephaloridine and nafcillin hold promise for the treatment of penicillin-resistant infections. With newer antibiotics available, chloramphenicol is indicated only occasionally. Inspired moist air and hydration are important for mobilization of secretions. Cough control, again, depends upon thinning of the bronchial mucus, and expectorant cough therapy is therefore indicated. Pertussis specifically requires cough sedation, particularly in the unmodified case. Codeine or dihydrocodeinone is useful in this infection.

Fungal Infections

Fungi may produce bronchial disease in childhood, but are rarely responsible for bronchitis alone. Monilia may invade the bronchial mucosa as a phenomenon secondary to oropharyngeal thrush. This may occur in the neonate, in infants and children who are debilitated, or in those receiving prolonged broad-spectrum antibiosis or antileukemic chemotherapy.

ALLERGIC FACTORS

It is well recognized that the bronchial mucosa is a sensitive end-organ in the allergic state. This is demonstrated most convincingly in asthma, in which spasm of the smooth muscles of the bronchi, edema of the bronchial mucosa and exudation of mucus produces the obstructive phenomenon so familiar to the clinician. Less well understood, however, is the role of allergy in the recurrent bronchitis of childhood. Many children, from infancy on, suffer an exaggerated response to each minor upper respiratory tract illness. With the onset of every cold there is a moderate to severe cough which is protracted and is accompanied by the finding of rhonchi or coarse rales in the chest. Ultimately these cases may show bronchospasm or frank asthma. Many years may pass, however, and many such episodes may occur before the typical allergic end-organ response becomes manifest.

The pathogenesis of this situation is obscure, but probably relates to an underlying hypersensitivity of the bronchial mucosa. Under the trigger of upper respiratory tract infection there is produced a degree of edema and secretion sufficient to cause symptoms of bronchitis without producing true asthma. In infants and young children this may be manifested by bronchiolitis or asthmatic bronchitis. Follow-up studies of such patients have revealed an incidence of asthma significantly higher than that expected in the general population.

The common complication of this condition involves secondary infection. As mentioned previously, the underlying derangement of bronchial mucosa renders it susceptible to bacterial invasion leading to suppurative bronchitis. Local obstructive phenomena may predispose to segmental collapse, and ultimately to bacterial pneumonia.

E.B. was an eight-year-old boy with a history of recurrent colds with protracted cough for one year. For five months before admission the cough was more prolonged and was associated with frequent episodes of vomiting. Purulent sputum was noted several times by the mother. Treatment had consisted of antibiotics on numerous occasions. Examination showed a well nourished, well developed boy who had minimal pharyngeal injection and moderate enlargement of the tonsils. The chest revealed rhonchi on both inspiration and expiration, heard throughout both lung fields; occasional coarse rales were heard bilaterally at the bases, but these cleared on coughing. There was no bronchospasm. X-ray examination (Fig. 1) showed only some increase in the peribronchial markings with some streaking evident in the right lung base. Bronchoscopic examination showed edematous bronchial mucosa with much purulent exudate. Cultures of pus revealed pyogenic staphylococcus sensitive to all antibiotics. Sweat chlorides and protein electrophoretic pattern were both normal.

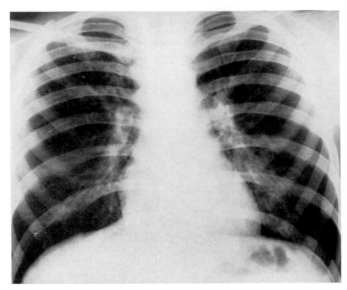

FIGURE 19–1.   Allergic bronchitis with secondary suppurative changes.

Treatment in the hospital consisted of intramuscular and then oral administration of penicillin with resultant improvement. Allergy skin testing showed positive reactions to twenty common inhalants and eight foods. The boy was placed on environmental control and hyposensitization plus prophylactic erythromycin at the time of upper respiratory tract infections. He has been completely well for eleven months.

The management of such children involves recognition of the underlying hypersensitive state. Examination of nasal mucous smears for eosinophils may be helpful. Diagnostic allergy skin tests should be carried out in order to elucidate the problem. Environmental control and hyposensitization procedures should then be instituted. Sulfonamide-antihistamine preparations are valuable if initiated early in the course of upper respiratory tract infections in order to minimize their trigger effect (see Chap. 41).

CHEMICAL FACTORS

There is a growing interest in air pollution with relation to both chronic and acute chest disease in man. Although this has been, for some years, of great concern in Great Britain, it has only recently received increasing attention in North America. Paralleling this experience has been the demonstration of significant statistics on cigarette smoking and bronchitic change. Although most of the collected data have concerned themselves with the adult population, one must suspect that children suffer the same effects from these environmental factors. With evidence of the increasing smoking habits of children from nine years of age upward, we must consider the possibility of cigarette irritation as a cause of chronic cough or indeed of repeated respiratory illness with bronchitis in the older child.

Inhalation of smoke, as from a burning house, is responsible for acute bronchial edema, with or without the added features of heat damage. Although such an exposure may be responsible for full-blown pulmonary edema, it should be recognized that, in lesser exposures, only bronchial irritation may result. Such damage to bronchi may predispose to more serious complications. Recent experience has indicated that a combination of steroid therapy and broad-spectrum an-

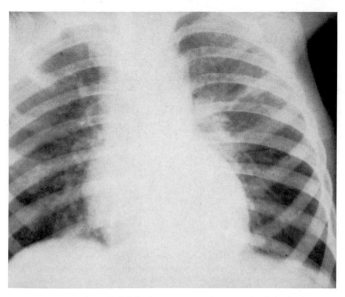

FIGURE 19-2. Initial chest x-ray after smoke inhalation.

tibiotic coverage, instituted as soon as possible after exposure, may dramatically reduce such complications.

L.E., a six-year-old boy, was trapped in his room in a frame house which caught fire. When removed by firemen, he had second-degree burns of the face and was in severe respiratory distress. Initial examination revealed respiratory difficulty on both inspiration and expiration with poor air entry into all areas of the chest. No rales were heard, and a few coarse rhonchi were referred from the laryngeal area. Initial laryngoscopy showed extensive slough involving both the false and true vocal cords. For this reason tracheostomy was performed. Bronchoscopy through the tracheostomy wound showed much thick fibrinous exudate with extensive edema of the tracheobronchial mucosa. Initial x-ray examination (Fig. 2) revealed increased peribronchial markings with light mottling in the central regions. The boy was placed on intravenous hydrocortisone, aqueous penicillin and chloramphenicol therapy for five days. These drugs were then given by mouth for a further week. After forty-eight hours he required bronchoscopy through the tracheostomy incision for removal of crusts and secretions. Subsequent bronchoscopic examination after sixteen days revealed only minimal tracheobronchial erythema. The laryngeal area was normal, and therefore he was extubated. He remained well thereafter with

no residual signs in the chest on physical examination or by x-ray. Total hospitalization was twenty days.

Environmental exposure to noxious gases (NO_2 in silo-fillers disease), or such pulmonary irritants as mouldy hay, cotton fibers, and the like, are usually considered to be occupational hazards, and are most frequently associated with frank pulmonary disease. It should be considered, however, that initial exposure to such factors may produce only bronchial irritation without lung involvement, and may resemble an attack of constrictive bronchiolitis. This is particularly the case in children so exposed.

REFERENCES

Anderson, D. O.: Smoking and Respiratory Disease. *Am. J. Pub. Health*, 54:1856-63, 1964.

Balchum, O. J., Felton, J. S., Jamison, J. N., Gaines, R. S., Clarke, D. R., Owan, T., and the Industrial Health Committee, the Tuberculosis and Health Association of Los Angeles County: A Survey for Chronic Respiratory Disease in an Industrial City. *Am. Rev. Resp. Dis.*, 86:675-85, 1962.

Eisen, A. H., and Bacal, H. L.: The Relationship of Acute Bronchiolitis to Bronchial Asthma, a 4 to 14 Year Follow-up. *Pediatrics*, 31: 859-61, 1963.

Feingold, B. F.: Infection in Bronchial Allergic Disease: Bronchial Asthma, Allergic Bronchitis, Asthmatic Bronchitis. *Pediat. Clin. N. Amer.*, 6:709-24, 1959.

Fletcher, C. M.: Chronic Bronchitis. *Am. Rev. Resp. Dis.*, 80:483-94, 1959.

Forbes, J. A., Bennett, N. M., and Gray, N. J.: Epidemic Bronchiolitis Caused by a Respiratory Syncytial Virus; Clinical Aspects. *Med. J. Aust.*, 2:933-5, 1961.

Garrow, D. H., and Taylor, C. E. D.: An Investigation of Acute Respiratory Disease in Children Admitted to Hospital in the South West Metropolitan Region. *Arch. Dis. Childhood*, 37:392-7, 1962.

High, R. H.: Bronchiolitis (Acute Asthmatic Bronchitis, Acute Capillary Bronchitis). *Pediat. Clin. N. Amer.*, 4:183-91, 1957.

Hinshaw, H. C., and Garland, L. H.: *Diseases of the Chest*. 2d ed. Philadelphia, W. B. Saunders Company, 1963.

Lewis, F. A., Rae, M. L., Lehman, N. I., and Ferris, A. A.: A Syncytial Virus Associated with Epidemic Disease of the Lower Respiratory Tract in Infants and Young Children. *Med. J. Aust.*, 2:932-3, 1961.

Lincoln, E. M., and Sewell, E. M.: *Tuberculosis in Childhood*. New York, McGraw-Hill Book Company, Inc., 1963.

Linhartova, A., and Chung, W.: Bronchopulmonary Moniliasis in the Newborn. *J. Clin. Path.*, 16:56-60, 1963.

MacKeith, R.: Respiratory Disorders in Infants and Young Children, with Specific Reference to Recurrent Stress Bronchitis. *Practitioner*, 175:692-9, 1955.

MacLean, D. M., Bach, R. D., Larke, R. P. B., and McNaughton, G. A.: Myxoviruses Associated with Acute Laryngotracheobronchitis in Toronto 1962-63. *Canad. M.A.J.*, 89:1257-9, 1963.

MacLean, D. M., Morison, J. B., Medovy, H., and

MacDonell, G. T.: Health Education and Cigarette Smoking; A Report on a 3-Year Program in the Winnipeg School Division, 1960-63. *Canad. M.A.J.*, 91:49-56, 1964.

Marshall, G., and Perry, K. M. A.: *Diseases of the Chest*. London, Butterworth & Co., 1952.

May, J. R., and Delves, D.: Treatment of Chronic Bronchitis with Ampicillin. *Lancet*, 1:929-33, 1965.

Mork, T.: International Comparisons of the Prevalence of Chronic Bronchitis. *Proc. Roy. Soc. Med.*, 57:975-8, 1964.

Mortensen, E.: Follow-up on Children with Asthmatic Bronchitis with a View of the Prognosis. *Acta paediat.* (Stockholm), Supplement, 140:122-3, 1963.

Olson, E. T.: Occurrence of Silo-Fillers' Disease in Children. *J. Pediat.*, 64:724-7, 1964.

Parrott, R. H., Kim, H. W., Vargosko, A. J., and Chanok, R. M.: Serious Respiratory Tract Illness as a Result of Asian Influenza and Influenza Infections in Children. *J. Pediat.*, 61:205-13, 1962.

Parsons, C.: The Child with Chronic Lung Disease. *Practitioner*, London, 174:407-13, 1955.

Reid, D. D.: Air Pollution as a Cause of Chronic Bronchitis. *Proc. Roy. Soc. Med.*, 57:965-8, 1964.

Robbins, S. L.: *Textbook of Pathology*. 2d ed. Philadelphia, W. B. Saunders Company, 1962.

Seal, R. M. E., Thomas, G. O., and Griffiths, J. J.: Farmer's Lung. *Proc. Roy. Soc. Med.*, 56:271-3, 1963.

Speer, F. (Ed.): *The Allergic Child*. New York, Harper & Row, 1963.

Williams, A.: Bronchitis, Asthma and Emphysema in Childhood. *Med. J. Aust.*, 1:781-2, 1957.

Williams, S.: Aetiology and Diagnosis of Bronchial Asthma, Bronchitis and Emphysema in Children. *Med. J. Aust.*, 1:782-3, 1957.

CHAPTER TWENTY

Bronchiolitis

E. O. R. REYNOLDS, M.B.

Acute bronchiolitis, or capillary bronchiolitis, may be defined as an acute illness, mainly affecting infants, in which the principal lesion is an inflammatory obstruction of the small airways.

Incidence

This illness affects males and females equally and occurs almost exclusively in infants of less than two years. The majority are less than six months of age. Bronchiolitis is probably the main lower respiratory tract disease causing hospital admission in infants of less than one year. It is most often seen in the winter or early spring and may occur as an epidemic illness associated with upper respiratory tract infections in the community.

Etiology

Engel and Newns in England in 1940, and Adams in the United States in 1941, were probably the first to differentiate bronchiolitis from bronchopneumonia and to suggest that since inclusion bodies could be demonstrated in the bronchiolar mucous membrane, a virus might be responsible. No virus was implicated with any regularity, however, until Chanock and his co-workers in 1957 isolated the previously unknown respiratory syncytial virus and subsequently showed that this organism could often be isolated from infants with bronchiolitis. This finding has been confirmed in several other laboratories, and it is likely that the respiratory syncytial virus is an important cause of the illness. Nevertheless other viruses can produce the same clinical picture, and included among these are parainfluenza 3, the Eaton agent and the adenovirus. Since a rising titer of antibodies to *Hemophilus influenzae* can often be demonstrated in babies with bronchiolitis, Sell has suggested that this organism plays some role, possibly acting in combination with a virus in the causation of the disease. At present, however, bronchiolitis should be considered principally a viral illness.

Pathogenesis and Pathophysiology

Histologically, the most important lesion is bronchiolar obstruction. This may be caused by thickening of the bronchiolar walls with edema, lymphocytic cellular infiltrate and occasionally by actual proliferation of cells, and also by obstruction of the lumen with mucus and cellular debris. In very severe cases there may be sloughing of the bronchiolar epithelium. Peribronchiolar infiltration and spread to the lung parenchyma may be remarkably slight even when the bronchiolar walls are enormously swollen. Characteristically, the lesions vary in intensity in different regions of the lung, and the bronchi are much less severely affected.

Because the size of airways is greater during inspiration than in expiration, air is trapped beyond the bronchiolar lesions and emphysema results. If the obstruction becomes complete, absorption atelectasis may take place. If so, the lungs may show areas of both emphysema and collapse, with emphysema predominant. Because resistance (R) to airflow in a tube is related to the inverse of the fourth power of the radius (r) (fifth power if the airflow is turbulent)

$$R \, \alpha \, \frac{1}{r^4}$$

it follows that thickening of the bronchiolar wall in the small airways of an infant will cause a far greater increase in resistance to airflow than in the larger airways of an adult. This may explain the particular vulnerability of small infants to diseases, such as bronchiolitis, causing airway obstruction. Measurement of the degree of airway obstruction, desirable so that therapy can be accurately evaluated, has proved difficult, probably because of the lack of uniformity of the lesions, which may include some bronchioles with complete obstruction, while others, unaffected by the disease process, are abnormally wide open.

An important effect of the widespread airway obstruction is interference with gas exchange. In twenty-five patients with bronchiolitis between three weeks and seven months of age studied by the author in which the arterial oxygen and carbon dioxide tensions were measured when the babies were breathing room air, it was found that hypoxemia was almost always present and that this was very severe in some infants. In the most severely hypoxemic infants there was carbon dioxide retention as well. It can be demonstrated that babies with bronchiolitis have large alveolar to arterial oxygen differences (see Chap. 1). It appears likely that abnormal gas exchange is produced in the following manner. In the mild case partial obstruction of the small airways leads to underventilation of a proportion of the alveoli and a rise in the carbon dioxide tension of the blood perfusing them. Because an abnormally large amount of carbon dioxide can be removed by hyperventilation in the alveoli with relatively less obstructed airways, the carbon dioxide tension of the arterial blood, representing the mixture of blood from both poorly and well ventilated alveoli, remains normal. The arterial oxygen tension cannot be maintained at a normal level in a similar fashion for the following reason: the oxygen tension of blood perfusing underventilated alveoli is low, and only a small amount of extra oxygen is added to the blood perfusing hyperventilated alveoli because of the nature of oxygen dissociation; the net effect is insufficient to compensate for the low oxygen tension of blood from underventilated alveoli, and arterial hypoxemia results. In the more severely affected infant airway obstruction becomes more widespread and severe, and as the arterial oxygen tension decreases, the total volume of ventilation becomes insufficient to maintain normal arterial carbon dioxide tension. In consequence, increased hypoxemia is accompanied by carbon dioxide retention.

Clinical Manifestations

Frequently another member of the immediate family has a respiratory infection at the time the infant becomes ill. The first sign of illness in the infant is usually coryza with a serous nasal discharge and sneezing. The nasal signs may last several days or be rapidly followed by a cough, which in the small baby may be paroxysmal and indistinguishable from that of whooping cough. The infant is often irritable and cannot sleep. He has diffi-

culty with feedings and may vomit. The temperature is usually below 100°F. and may even be subnormal. Tachycardia is present, and the respiratory rate rises, in a severely affected infant to 80 per minute or more. (The normal respiratory rate is variable in infancy, but a sustained rate of above 40 per minute should be definitely abnormal.) The more severely affected infants are cyanotic.

Because the respiratory rate and the observation of cyanosis are used as clinical indices of the severity of the disease, it is instructive to compare these signs with the simultaneously recorded arterial blood gas tensions. From Figure 1 it can be seen that the respiratory rate and the arterial oxygen tension are significantly correlated and that in general the most hypoxemic infants are those with the most rapid respiratory rates. Too much reliance should not be placed on this physical sign, however, because infants with slow rates may have appreciable hypoxemia, in part because severe hypoxemia causes depression of the respiratory center. Figure 2 demonstrates that respiratory rates above 60 per minute are usually associated with carbon dioxide retention. The observation of cyanosis depends on a number of factors, including the amount of reduced hemoglobin in circulation and the skin blood flow; it is a difficult sign to rely on in infants. Figure 3 shows the relation between the arterial oxygen tension and the presence or absence of cyanosis in babies with bronchiolitis. It can be seen that cyanosis is not necessarily present with an arterial oxygen tension as low as 50 mm. of mercury, a figure which is barely above the oxygen tension of normal venous blood; the absence of cyanosis, although a useful clinical sign, does not rule out serious hypoxemia.

The accessory muscles of respiration are brought into use in babies with bronchiolitis, and the chest wall retracts with each inspiration. Because of the comparative flexibility of the rib cage, retraction is particularly obvious in the smallest infants. When the chest becomes overin-

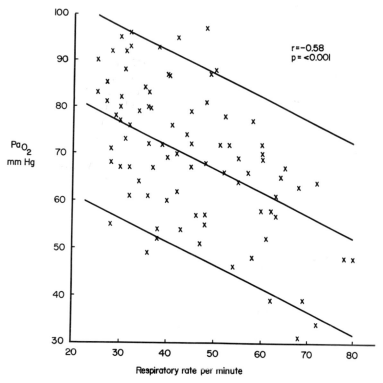

FIGURE 20–1. The relation of the respiratory rate to the arterial oxygen tension (Pa_{O_2}) in babies with bronchiolitis aged from 3 weeks to 7 months ($\pm$ 2 standard deviations).

flated, the anteroposterior diameter is increased and hyperresonance can be detected on percussion; cardiac dullness and liver dullness are diminished. The overinflation of the lungs displaces the liver and spleen downward, so that they become easily palpable; these signs in an infant with bronchiolitis do not necessarily indicate heart failure. In fact, at present there is no definite evidence that heart failure occurs in bronchiolitis, although heart failure may occasionally be present in very severely ill infants.

The most characteristic finding on auscultation is widespread, fine rales (crepitations) occurring on both inspiration and expiration. There may also be sibilant rhonchi, but if air entry is very poor, no adventitious sounds may be heard. Unlike asthma, the expiratory phase of the respiratory cycle is not necessarily prolonged, because the airway obstruction is not uniform and rapid air flow occurs in the unobstructed airways.

Babies with bronchiolitis frequently become dehydrated because of their inability to drink and the loss of water from the lungs associated with the rapid respiratory rate.

The chest x-ray in a mild case may occasionally appear deceptively normal, but there is nearly always hyperinflation, particularly well seen in lateral films (Fig. 4), in which an obvious increase in the anteroposterior diameter of the chest and depression of the diaphragm can be seen. The lung fields appear abnormally translucent, and there are sometimes small areas of collapse. The thickened bronchioles may be visible as abnormal linear shadows; it has been suggested that areas of consolidation may be mimicked by large numbers of affected bronchioles seen superimposed upon one another, together

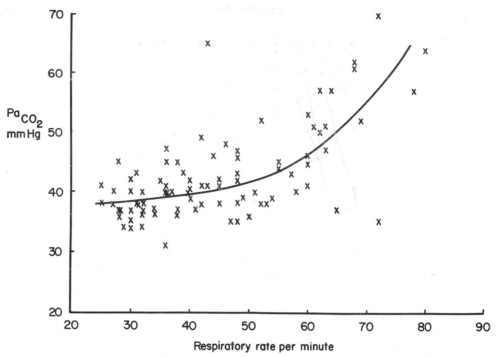

FIGURE 20–2. The relation of the respiratory rate to the arterial carbon dioxide tension (Pa_{CO_2}).

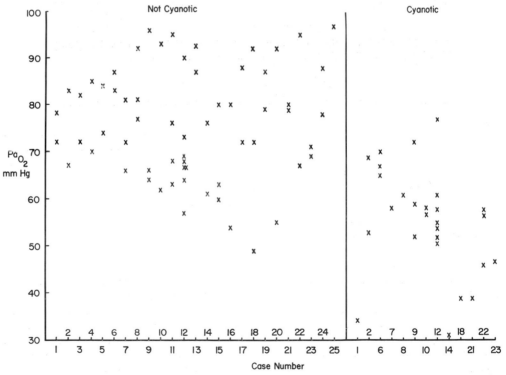

FIGURE 20–3. The relation between the observation of cyanosis and the arterial oxygen tension (Pa_{O_2}). Multiple observations were made on 25 infants, 13 of whom appeared cyanotic at some stage of their illness.

276

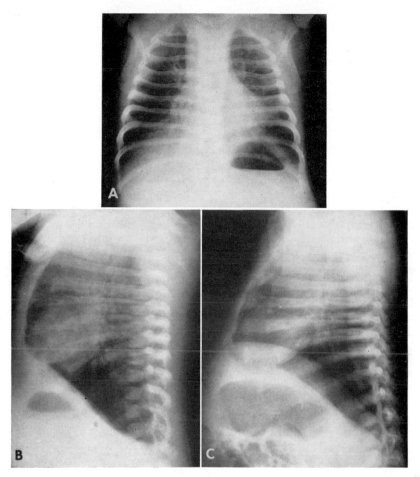

FIGURE 20–4. *A, B,* Chest x-rays from a 10-week-old infant with bronchiolitis. There is obvious severe hyperinflation and abnormal markings caused by inflamed airways and patchy atelectasis. *C,* Lateral chest film from the same infant on recovery one week later. Hyperinflation is no longer present, and the contrast with *B* is striking.

with areas of collapse. Films taken in expiration as well as inspiration are sometimes helpful because areas of hyperinflation in the lungs may then be more readily visible.

Bacterial pathogens are frequently isolated from the throat in patients with bronchiolitis; *Staphylococcus aureus, H. influenzae* and pneumococci are particularly common. The usual rapid recovery from the illness suggests that these organisms do not often play a serious pathogenic role. Secondary bacterial infection does, however, sometimes occur. The white blood cell count is normal unless there is a secondary bacterial infection,

when a neutrophile leukocytosis may appear.

Diagnosis

It is sometimes impossible to make a clear distinction between bronchopneumonia and bronchiolitis in the infant. The signs of obstructive emphysema are much less obvious in bronchopneumonia than in bronchiolitis. Also, in bronchopneumonia the fever is commonly higher than in bronchiolitis, and there may be a neutrophile leukocytosis. X-ray films in bronchopneumonia are more likely to show areas of consolidation, but again the distinction from bronchiolitis may be difficult or impossible. Secondary bacterial infection in a patient with bronchiolitis produces bronchopneumonia, making it pointless to try to make any distinction between the two illnesses at this stage. Primary pneumonias caused by infections with specific bacterial pathogens, except for staphylococcal pneumonia, are not very common in infancy, and can be identified by chest x-rays and appropriate cultures. Acute bronchitis causes less severe obstruction and therefore less interference with gas exchange than bronchiolitis; rhonchi rather than fine rales are heard on auscultation. Acute bronchitis may develop into bronchiolitis; thus bronchiolitis forms part of a spectrum of pulmonary disease, merging with bronchopneumonia on the one hand, and acute bronchitis on the other.

Whooping cough in the small infant is clinically identical with bronchiolitis, but may be distinguished from it by the white blood cell count. A lymphocytosis of more than 15,000 cells per cubic millimeter is most unusual in bronchiolitis and strongly suggests whooping cough. Measles may be followed by bronchiolitic involvement, and similar lesions have been reported during epidemics of severe influenza. Tuberculosis can be excluded by cultures, x-ray films and a tuberculin skin test.

Asthma poses a diagnostic dilemma. In general, asthma is rare in infancy, but a number of babies with clinically apparent bronchiolitis do suffer asthma in later life. Convincing prospective follow-up studies are needed, but 10 per cent (some authors have suggested 30 per cent) of these patients may subsequently have asthma. It seems likely, therefore, that some infants who have a diagnosis of bronchiolitis are really suffering from asthma, or, conversely, that bronchiolitis predisposes to the later development of asthma. Points in favor of a diagnosis of asthma are a positive family history, repeated attacks of respiratory disease, sudden onset of illness, markedly prolonged expiration, eosinophilia and an obvious response to bronchodilator therapy.

Cystic fibrosis needs to be considered in the differential diagnosis, but it can usually be distinguished by the history, physical findings and a sweat chloride determination.

Croup causes hoarseness and stridor, usually affects a somewhat older age group and can be readily distinguished from bronchiolitis. Foreign bodies in the tracheobronchial tract and congenital abnormalities can usually be easily excluded.

In the severely ill child, seen for the first time, heart failure may be surprisingly difficult to differentiate from bronchiolitis. Many of the physical signs of heart failure in infancy, such as an easily palpable liver and spleen, are also found in bronchiolitis, and there is frequently costal retraction and an increase in the anteroposterior diameter of the chest. A most important point in the diagnosis of heart failure is the taking of a careful history for previous episodes of illness. Growth retardation, an enlarged heart (rare in bronchiolitis) and cardiac murmurs may be present, and additional information may be obtained from a chest x-ray and an electrocardiogram.

Complications

One of the principal complications of bronchiolitis is secondary bacterial infection, which most commonly occurs on the second to the fifth day, but, unless severe, rarely causes prolonged illness. Secondary bacterial infection may be diagnosed when there is a rising temperature and neutrophile leukocytosis. Often a bacterial pathogen can be isolated from the larynx, and areas of consolidation are frequently on x-ray examination. Otitis media may also occur if there is bacterial infection.

Pneumothorax and mediastinal emphysema have both been reported in bronchiolitis, but are distinctly uncommon.

Sudden attacks of apnea, identical with those sometimes seen in whooping cough, are occasionally observed in small babies with bronchiolitis (especially those less than six weeks of age) and are probably reflex in origin. Respirations usually begin again spontaneously in about thirty seconds, but the attacks may be repetitive. Cessation of respiration may also occur in the severely ill and exhausted infant, in whom apnea of this sort is often much more prolonged and difficult to overcome.

Course and Prognosis

Infants with bronchiolitis may become severely ill within a few hours after the onset of coryza, or several days may elapse before the infection reaches the lungs. It should be remembered that any upper respiratory tract infection in a small infant may progress to bronchiolitis; parents should be warned to watch for increasing respiratory rate and the signs of rib retraction and cyanosis, so that appropriate treatment may be given. A remarkable feature of this illness is that although an infant may appear desperately ill, the severe phase of airway obstruction usually lasts no more than a day or two, and recovery is almost always complete, or nearly so, within two weeks. Figure 5 shows arterial oxygen and carbon dioxide ten-

sion measurements and the respiratory rate in a typical case of severe bronchiolitis. It can be seen that the carbon dioxide tension had returned to normal by the fifth day and that the oxygen tension was almost normal by the eleventh day. This course of events is usual. Table 1 shows the results of blood gas tension measurements made on twenty-five babies with bronchiolitis at the height of their illnesses and again fourteen days later. By fourteen days all had normal carbon dioxide tensions and only five still had arterial oxygen tensions of less than 75 mm. of mercury. Of these five, three had severe secondary bacterial infections, sufficient to account for prolonged hypoxemia.

The mortality rate is usually very low; it is probably below 1 per cent if infants with associated factors such as prematurity or congenital heart disease are excluded; higher rates have been reported in some epidemics.

The prognosis seems excellent, and no permanent sequelae have so far been reported. It is, however, common to find that a child with chronic respiratory disease had severe bronchiolitis as an infant. Since actual sloughing of the bronchiolar

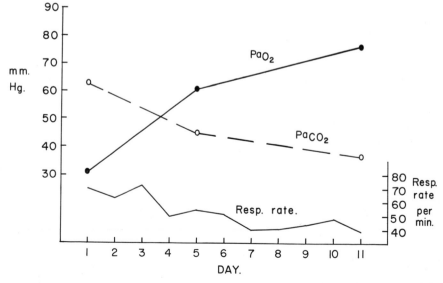

FIGURE 20–5. The arterial oxygen (Pa_{O_2}) and carbon dioxide (Pa_{CO_2}) tensions, and the respiratory rate during the illness of a 5-week-old infant with severe bronchiolitis.

Table 1.   *Number of Babies with Respiratory Rates Above 40 per Minute, Arterial Oxygen Tension (Pa_{O_2}) below 75 mm. Hg. and Carbon Dioxide Tensions (Pa_{CO_2}) Above 48 mm. Hg at the Height of the Illness and 14 Days Later (Total No. of Cases, 25)*

	Respiratory Rate > 40/min.	Pa_{O_2} < 75 mm. Hg	Pa_{CO_2} > 48 mm. Hg
At height of illness	25 (100%)	21 (84%)	11 (44%)
14 days later	4 (16%)	5 (20%)	0

Reproduced by courtesy of the Editor and publishers of *The Journal of Pediatrics.*

walls has been reported in babies dying from bronchiolitis, it is tempting to speculate that this kind of lesion may occasionally lead to permanent bronchiolar damage with the subsequent development of recurrent respiratory infections and chronic emphysema. At present there is no evidence to support this hypothesis.

Treatment

Because of the difficulty of making a clear distinction between bronchiolitis and other illnesses such as bronchopneumonia and asthma, it is not possible to be dogmatic about treatment. Also, since no simple objective measurements of the degree of airway obstruction are available at present, there is no certain way of assessing the results of the many forms of therapy.

In the planning of the therapy of bronchiolitis, it is most important to remember that although the illness may appear extremely severe, the mortality rate is low. Further, the serious phase is short, lasting from hours to a day or two. Treatment should be aimed at tiding the infant over this phase.

Because there is often hypoxemia which is difficult to detect clinically, humidified oxygen should be given to all but the mildest cases. It has been shown that oxygen corrects the hypoxemia of these infants and that a concentration of 40 per cent is usually sufficient. There are theoretical disadvantages in the use of high concentrations of oxygen in treatment. Nearly all babies with bronchiolitis are beyond the immediate neonatal period

when retrolental fibroplasia may be produced by inhalation of oxygen, but there is good evidence in experimental animals that the breathing of a high concentration of oxygen damages the lungs if it is continued for many hours or days.

If oxygen is administered to patients with chronic hypoxemia and carbon dioxide retention such as those with chronic emphysema, respiration may be severely depressed. This occurs because the respiratory center has become relatively insensitive to the raised carbon dioxide tension, and the stimulus to breathe is being derived from the low arterial oxygen tension, by means of the chemoreceptors. In bronchiolitis, however, there is no evidence that respiratory depression occurs during oxygen breathing, probably because this is an acute illness and sufficient time has not elapsed for the respiratory center to become insensitive to the raised carbon dioxide tension. Measurements made on eight babies with severe bronchiolitis showed them to have an average arterial carbon dioxide tension of 59 mm. of mercury (range 51 to 69 mm.). After oxygen breathing for twelve to forty minutes the mean arterial carbon dioxide tension was 58 mm. of mercury (range 50 to 70 mm.). No change had occurred, giving evidence that the level of alveolar ventilation was unaltered. Therefore, on present evidence, oxygen can be administered without risk of producing respiratory depression.

The conventional oxygen tent, unless carefully tended, is not a good way of administering oxygen. Any small opening in the tent will cause a sharp drop in the oxygen concentration inside, even with a fast flow rate of oxygen. A better (and less expensive) method of administering oxygen is to place a bottomless transparent plastic box over the baby and run humidified oxygen in through the side. No significant accumulation of carbon dioxide occurs inside the box. In a warm environment steps may have to be taken to keep the interior reasonably cool; this is not generally a problem. The flow rate of oxygen into the box can be regulated so that the desired concentration of oxygen (usually about 40 per cent) in the inspired gas is obtained. The concentration can easily be monitored with one of the several inexpensive oxygen analysers on the market. If the flow rate is increased, the top of the box can be opened for short periods for nursing care while the baby still breathes a sufficiently high concentration of oxygen. When necessary, oxygen can also be administered by means of a face mask or funnel. A particularly satisfactory way of giving oxygen if the baby is being transported, or must be removed from his box or tent, is the use of a disposable adult-sized plastic face mask, which fits comfortably around the front of the baby's head. While oxygen is being given by mask there should be close observation in case the mask becomes displaced or the flow of gas interrupted.

When the baby lies flat with the head inclined downward, the abdominal contents tend to encroach on the thoracic cavity. For this reason it is probably best to feed babies with bronchiolitis in a semi-sitting position, unless there is vomiting.

Mild dehydration is common, and in some infants fluid may have to be given for a day or two either by a gastric tube or intravenously.

Babies with bronchiolitis are commonly placed in mist, but there is no evidence that this is beneficial. It is conceivable, however, that secretions may be liquefied to some extent and loss of water through the lungs reduced. Because bronchiolitis is a viral illness, antibiotics are generally not indicated and have not been shown to influence the course of the illness. At the first sign of secondary bacterial infection, however, a broad-spectrum antibiotic should be given. In the severely ill infant the risks associated with contracting a secondary infection are high, and an antibiotic should in these circumstances be used prophylactically.

Bronchodilator drugs such as epinephrine, isoproterenol and aminophylline are commonly used in bronchiolitis, but they do not seem to be beneficial in more than an occasional infant. The use of bronchodilators is based on the assumption that there is an element of bronchospasm present which can be relieved. When one considers the microscopic appearance of the lesions, with thickening of the bronchiolar walls and plugging of the lumen, it is easy to understand why bronchodilators have no great effect. Of course, since bronchiolitis cannot be clearly distinguished from infantile asthma, in which bronchodilators are useful, it appears reasonable to try the effect of these bronchodilator drugs, particularly in infants with a family history of asthma or allergy, but they should not be continued unless a therapeutic response, such as improved air entry, diminution of chest retraction, reduction of cyanosis and slowing of the respiratory rate, is observed.

Corticosteroids have been advocated by some authors, but again there is no real evidence that they are useful. It is possible that these agents may cause a reduction in inflammation or bronchospasm, but because of the well known dangers of corticosteroid therapy present knowledge suggests that they should be withheld or reserved for the occasional very severely ill infant.

Babies with bronchiolitis often appear extremely restless, and it is tempting to use sedatives, but these should rarely, if ever, be given because of the risk of respiratory depression. Restlessness in bronchiolitis is caused partly, at least, by hypoxemia, which will be better relieved by oxygen therapy than by sedation.

Digitalis is usually not indicated (no evidence exists that babies with bronchiolitis suffer heart failure). In the very seriously affected infant with progressive tachycardia, whose liver and spleen show definite enlargement rather than displacement, the use of digitalis is permissible, but this situation is rare.

In the desperately ill infant or child the possibility of bronchoscopy or tracheostomy arises. Neither of these maneuvers can be expected to deal with the principal problem, namely, obstruction of the small airways. In rare instances secretions collect in the upper respiratory tract, and under these conditions it is reasonable to do a bronchoscopy. Beneficial results have been reported from this procedure, but it must be stressed that this situation is exceedingly unusual. If apneic attacks occur and become life-threatening, tracheostomy should be avoided if possible. It is often difficult to remove a tracheostomy tube from an infant because of tracheal damage, and subsequent tracheal stenosis is common. The apneic infant can usually be maintained with an endotracheal or nasotracheal tube for a period long enough to tide him over the critical phase. Although respiratory stimulants such as nikethamide, which work by causing a general arousal rather than by any specific effect on the respiratory center, may be tried in an occasional baby, such use certainly should not be continued if no response is obtained. A negative-pressure tank respirator which does not require tracheostomy may be used if sustained assisted ventilation is required.

To sum up, hypoxemia is common in bronchiolitis, and should be corrected by oxygen administration. There is no evidence that any other therapy is useful in more than an occasional infant. Because withdrawal of oxygen may lead to a precipitous drop in arterial oxygen tension, it is important that oxygen therapy should not be interrupted, particularly for the administration of less effective forms of treatment.

REFERENCES

Adams, J. M.: Primary Virus Pneumonitis with Cytoplasmic Inclusion Bodies. *J.A.M.A.*, 116: 925, 1941.

Boesen, K.: Asthmatic Bronchitis in Children. Prognosis for 162 Cases Observed 6-11 Years. *Acta paediat.* 42:87, 1953.

Chanock, R. M., and Finberg, L.: Recovery from Infants with Respiratory Illness of Virus Related to Chimpanzee Coryza Agent (CCA). *Am. J. Hyg.*, 66:291, 1957.

Engel, S.: *Lung Structure*. Springfield, Ill. Charles C Thomas, 1963.

Engel, S., and Newns, G. H.: Proliferative Mural Bronchiolitis. *Arch. Dis. Childhood*, 15:219, 1940.

Eisen, A. H., and Bacal, H. L.: The Relationship of Acute Bronchiolitis to Bronchial Asthma. A 4 to 14 Year Follow-up. *Pediatrics*, 31:859, 1963.

Henderson, A. T., and Rosenzweig, S.: Bronchiolitis in Infancy. *U.S. Armed Forces Med. J.*, 2:943, 1951.

High, R. H.: Bronchiolitis. *Pediat. Clin. N. Amer.*, 4:183, 1957.

Koch, D. A.: Roentgenologic Considerations of Capillary Bronchiolitis. *Am. J. Roentgenol.*, 82:433, 1959.

Krieger, I.: Mechanics of Respiration in Bronchiolitis. *Pediatrics*, 33:45, 1964.

Morrison, B.: Anoxia in the Acute Infections of Childhood: Its Recognition and Treatment. *Lancet*, 2:737, 1955.

Morrison, B., and others: Acute Lower Respiratory Infections in Childhood. *Lancet*, 2:1077, 1957.

Parrott, R. H., Vargosko, A. J., Kim, H. W., and Chanock, R. M.: Clinical Syndromes Among Children. *Am. Rev. Resp. Dis.*, 88:73, 1963.

Reynolds, E. O. R.: The Effect of Breathing 40% Oxygen on the Arterial Blood Gas Tensions of Babies with Bronchiolitis. *J. Pediat.*, 63: 1135, 1963.

Idem: Recovery from Bronchiolitis as Judged by Arterial Blood Gas Tension Measurements. *J. Pediat.*, 63:1182, 1963.

Sell, S. H. W.: Some Observations on Acute Bronchiolitis in Infants. *Am. J. Dis. Child.*, 100:7, 1960.

Wittig, H. J., Cranford, N. J., and Glaser, J.: The Relationship Between Acute Bronchiolitis and Childhood Asthma. *J. Allergy*, 30:19, 1959.

Ziegra, S. R., Keily, B., and Morales, F.: Cardiac Catheterization in Infants with Bronchiolitis. *Am. J. Dis. Child.*, 100:528, 1960.

CHAPTER TWENTY-ONE

Bacterial Pneumonias

MARGARET H. D. SMITH, M.D.

PNEUMOCOCCAL PNEUMONIA

The incidence of full-blown pneumococcal pneumonia has decreased notably since the early 1940's, owing almost certainly to the widespread use of antimicrobial drugs in the treatment of incipient respiratory infections.

Bacteriology and Immunity

The pneumococcus (*Diplococcus pneumoniae, Streptococcus pneumoniae*) is a gram-positive coccus, most often oval-appearing under the microscope, with pointed ends, usually arranged in pairs or short chains. It grows readily in fresh meat infusion broth with added peptone, especially under reduced oxygen tension (e.g. candle jar), or in the presence of a reducing agent such as cysteine or thioglycollic acid; the addition of blood to the medium increases viability, probably by providing catalase to destroy the hydrogen peroxide which otherwise accumulates. Filter paper disks containing bile or optochin serve as a useful means of identifying pneumococci in the diagnostic laboratory; dropped onto a blood agar plate streaked with a culture of "viridans" streptococci, they will selectively inhibit the growth of pneumococcus, but not of other similar streptococci.

Immunologic classification of pneumococci into some 80 types depends on the production by all virulent strains of complex type-specific polysaccharide antigens which can be identified by the use of type-specific antiserums* in slide agglutination tests, or by observing capsular swelling ("Quellung") under the microscope.

---

*Available from the Statens Seruminstitut, Copenhagen S. Denmark.

Types 1 through 8 account for 80 per cent of the cases of lobar pneumonia in adults, whereas in children types 14, 1, 6 and 19 have most frequently been associated with disease.

Resistance to pneumococcal infection seems to be determined both by nonspecific factors such as the mucous secretions and ciliary action of the intact respiratory mucous membranes, a lively cough reflex, and phagocytosis, as well as by type-specific humoral antibodies which facilitate phagocytosis by combining with capsular polysaccharide.

Antipneumococcal immunity varies with age. The pneumococcidal power of whole defibrinated blood for types 1, 2 and 3, as well as the level of mouse protective antibodies, is high during the first month of the newborn infant's life, owing to passive transfer of maternal antibody; rare or absent between one and fifteen months, these same antibodies rise to a peak titer in late adolescence.

Epidemiology

Healthy carriage of one or up to five types of pneumococcus simultaneously is observed in 40 to 70 per cent of the normal human population. Only a very small percentage of carriers, particularly of the higher types of pneumococcus, ever displays overt disease. Abundant evidence, however, attests to the contagiousness of pneumococcal pneumonia. Lobar pneumonia due to the same type in twins, transmission from mothers to newborn infants, outbreaks of pneumococcal pneumonia within families, as well as spread to contacts outside the family, and both explosive and endemic pneumococcal infections in orphanages, schools and dormitories have all been described. Children appear to be relatively more susceptible than adults, as shown by a higher attack rate for type 1 infections among infants, and children under four years of age. Seasonal variations are well known and appear to be similar in both adults and children, with March the month of peak incidence. Since seasonal variations in the virulence of the pneumococcus seem unlikely, crowding and antecedent viral infections are probably the determining factors in precipitating overt disease.

Pathology and Pathogenesis

Pneumococcal pneumonia can be readily produced experimentally in rats and dogs by promoting aspiration of infected upper respiratory tract secretions through anesthesia, or narcosis with drugs such as morphine or alcohol. Viral infections, which greatly increase the volume of nasopharyngeal secretions, are probably frequently accompanied by aspiration. If aspiration is indeed such an important factor in pneumococcal pneumonia, then the straightness of the right main stem bronchus may account for the greater frequency of right-sided pneumonia, and for the more frequent involvement of the right upper lobe in small infants who spend most of the time recumbent. Cardiac failure, nephrosis and inhalation of smoke or kerosene promote fluid accumulation in the bronchioles and alveoli and probably predispose to pneumonia in the same way.

The characteristic lung lesion in pneumococcal pneumonia, whether localized ("lobar pneumonia") or disseminated ("bronchopneumonia"), consists of an outpouring of edema fluid into the alveoli; enormous numbers of leukocytes and some erythrocytes follow, pack the alveoli, and ingest the bacteria ("surface phagocytosis"); opsonizing antibodies, detectable several days after the onset of infection, hasten phagocytosis, but are not a necessary prerequisite. Later, macrophages reach the site and remove cellular and bacterial debris. In the meantime, how-ever, the process may have extended further within the same segment or lobe, or may have been spread by infected bronchial fluid to another part of the chest. The pulmonary lymphatics are probably involved early in the process: the lymphatics and the thoracic duct probably serve as the route by which pneumococci reach the blood stream in some 10 to 25 per cent of patients with pneumococcal pneumonia. The lymphatics are probably also the route of spread to the visceral pleura, which is frequently involved, reacting with an outpouring of edema fluid, followed by fibrin deposition which in some cases is exuberant. The effusion may be sterile; or, if bacteria are present, leukocytes and macrophages follow. Tissue necrosis is not a feature of uncomplicated pneumococcal pneumonia; hence rapid and complete resolution is the rule, unless the pneumonia is superimposed on an underlying lesion such as an aspirated foreign body, or is accompanied by atelectasis or by a massive fibrinous pleurisy in which bacteria are trapped and protected from the action of phagocytes, antibodies and antibacterial drugs ("pleuropneumonia").

Clinical Features

The onset of pneumonia in infants and children is usually preceded by a relatively mild upper respiratory tract infection of some days' duration, and occasionally by a purulent unilateral conjunctival discharge in which pneumococci can be demonstrated, or by otitis media.

In *infants* pneumonia is often ushered in by an abrupt rise in temperature to 103 to 105° and a generalized convulsion, accompanied in some cases by vomiting or diarrhea. Restlessness, apprehension, flaring of the alae nasi, rapid, shallow, grunting breathing, abdominal distention, slight circumoral cyanosis, tachycardia, with a pulse rate of 160 per minute or more, splinting of one side of the chest, are all characteristic of the full-blown picture of pneumonia. Cough is frequently absent. Percussion is rarely helpful because the lesions are often patchy in distribution, and the chest is small. Auscultatory findings may be misleading: on auscultation, suppression of breath sounds is frequently detectable, but the showers of fine rales characteristic of early pneumonia in older patients are not to be relied on. The breath sounds are often exaggerated on the healthy side and so bronchial in quality as to suggest tubular breathing; hence the great importance of inspection in determining the affected side. Even over the area of dullness in an infant with empyema, the breath sounds are not, however, always suppressed, because of the relatively small size of the chest, the inevitable thinness of the layer of fluid, and the short path of transmission for the breath sounds. When dullness to percussion is readily detectable in an infant, pleural effusion or empyema should be suspected. Abdominal distention is frequent and, when severe, is a poor prognostic sign; moreover, it may be impossible to ascertain the presence of peritonitis. Enlargement of the liver is important to assess, since this is usually the earliest sign of cardiac failure; but it is also often difficult to differentiate clinically between actual enlargement of the liver and downward displacement of the liver due to splinting of the diaphragm. If the liver edge is palpable more than three fingerbreadths or so below the right costal margin, and if the heart rate exceeds 160, or if a gallop rhythm or embryocardia is present, it is wise to assume that cardiac failure is complicating the pneumonia. Stiffness of the neck often accompanies pneumonia in infants; lumbar puncture is then mandatory to differentiate meningismus (normal spinal fluid under increased pressure) from very early meningitis (normal spinal fluid which on culture, however, yields pneumococcus) or from overt pneumococcal meningitis.

Older children display a clinical picture more like that associated with pneumonia in the adult. The initial phase, with headache, fever, malaise and possibly gastrointestinal symptoms, is followed within a few hours by high fever, often drowsiness, interrupted by periods of restlessness, hacking, shallow cough and maybe delirium. The facies is anxious and lined and may be flushed, often with a tinge of circumoral cyanosis and dry lips. Occasionally the cheek on the side of the pneumonia lesion is markedly flushed and the homolateral pupil dilated.

The older child often complains of chest pain and lies on the affected side in bed, with the knees drawn up. Chest findings, even in older children, are not quite like those characteristic of classic lobar pneumonia in adults; suppression of breath sounds over the affected area, often with no perceptible change on percussion, and few if any fine rales, characterize the initial stage in children. Later, during resolution, rales are often readily heard. A friction rub is rare in children. Chest pain, when present, is sometimes referred to the abdomen. If the right leaf of the diaphragm is involved, acute appendicitis may be suspected; sometimes the prostration, high fever and abdominal tenderness may simulate the picture of acute liver abscess. Subdiaphragmatic abscess, which occasionally comes in question in adults under such circumstances, is so exceedingly rare in children that it can almost be disregarded. Although the spleen is usually enlarged at autopsy in fatal cases, it is so rarely palpable in children with acute pneumococcal infections as to cast doubt upon the diagnosis. Rashes sometimes occur; transient patches of erythema, or a few urticarial wheals, or a usually rather sparse petechial eruption. Herpes simplex, which is so frequent in adults, is not seen in children. Jaundice, osteomyelitis, prolongation of the coagulation time, decrease in the circulating platelets during the acute illness and urinary chloride retention have all been observed in children, but have been better studied in adults.

The entire clinical course of pneumococcal pneumonia has undergone a great change since the widespread use of antimicrobial drugs. The initial diagnosis is often rendered difficult by the fact that the patient has received some drugs before the diagnosis of pneumococcal pneumonia is seriously entertained, but the dose may have been insufficient or the duration of treatment too short for cure. Once the diagnosis is suspected and effective treatment instituted, an abrupt drop in the temperature usually ensues within a few hours, with concomitant improvement in the patient's appearance. Only under exceptional circumstances (e.g. remoteness from medical care) would a patient nowadays run the five- to ten-day febrile course, usually with high sustained fever, characteristic of untreated pneumococcal pneumonia, whether localized or disseminated.

Laboratory investigation usually reveals a leukocytosis of 18,000 to 40,000 cells with a shift to the left. White blood cell counts of less than 10,000 per cubic millimeter are a poor prognostic sign. A slight anemia is often present, especially during convalescence, as well as transient albuminuria. The pneumococcus can usually be readily cultured from the nasopharynx, less often from the throat; these cultures, as well as a blood culture, should

be obtained prior to the institution of therapy.

Roentgenographic Appearance

Complete lobar consolidation is not common in infants and children. The distribution of the pneumonic consolidation is more often "patchy bronchopneumonia." The bronchi and the interstitial tissues are not involved, nor are the hilar lymph nodes usually notably enlarged. The pleura, however, frequently *is* involved, although the pleural lesions are often obscured early in the disease by the shadows of the alveolar consolidation. Although the lung lesions often clear within a week or so, roentgenographic improvement usually lags behind clinical improvement, and the residual pleural changes may persist for weeks. Lateral as well as frontal projections are essential for a proper understanding of the pathologic process. *Most important of all is for the physician to be sure that a technically satisfactory pair of films, obtained during convalescence, is clear;* i.e. that the patient is not discharged from follow-up with some underlying process such as atelectasis, foreign body or tuberculosis.

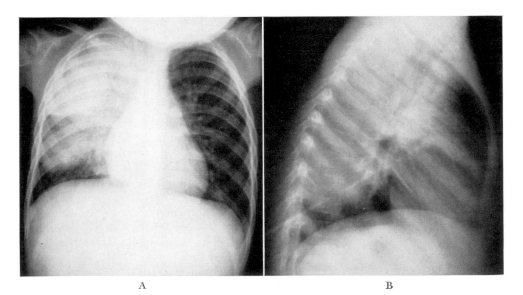

| A | B |

FIGURE 21–1. Pneumococcal lobar pneumonia in a 4-year-old boy. Consolidation of right upper lobe and of superior segment of right lower lobe. *A,* Frontal view. *B,* Right lateral view.

Diagnosis

The diagnosis is suspected on the basis of characteristic history, clinical picture and initial roentgenographic findings. It is confirmed by the recovery of the etiologic agent from the blood stream or, rarely, from empyema fluid. Isolation of pneumococci from the nasopharynx, particularly if present in large numbers or in pure culture, is strongly suggestive evidence. The correct diagnosis is substantiated in retrospect by the prompt response to antimicrobial drugs and complete roentgenographic clearing of the pneumonic process.

The differential diagnosis of pneumococcal pneumonia includes first and foremost pneumonia due to other infectious agents such as *Hemophilus influenzae, Klebsiella pneumoniae, Staphylococcus aureus,* streptococcus, *Mycoplasma pneumoniae* and the respiratory viruses. Acute pneumonia with splenomegaly should suggest the possibility of ornithosis or psittacosis, or of tuberculosis, particularly if the hilar lymph nodes are definitely enlarged. Endothoracic tuberculosis in children predisposes to secondary infection with respiratory pathogens, and it may be the latter which brings the patient to medical attention. Other underlying pulmonary lesions upon which pneumococcal pneumonia may be superimposed are atelectasis due to foreign body aspiration, bronchiectasis and fungal infections. If abdominal pain is pronounced, the differential diagnosis may include acute appendicitis or liver abscess. With severe prostration and abdominal distention. acute peritonitis must be considered. In infants with convulsions or stiffness of the neck, meningitis may be present, either alone or in combination with pneumonia.

Management

Hospitalization is usually advisable, at least during the first two or three days of illness, to facilitate laboratory procedures and the parenteral administration of drugs.

The pneumococcus is sensitive to most of the commonly used *antimicrobial agents,* and particularly so to penicillin G, which is the drug of choice. The pneumococcus is, in fact, so sensitive to penicillin that the optimum dosage schedule is difficult to define. The effective dose is probably much smaller than that ordinarily used today; moreover, the interval between injections can probably be much longer. Intramuscular injection of 50,000 units per kilogram of aqueous crystalline penicillin G twice a day, or, in very ill patients, administration of the same amount in a continuous intravenous drip, is recommended. Twenty-four to forty-eight hours later, after satisfactory initial response, intramuscular administration of procaine penicillin may be substituted. Benzathine penicillin G alone probably cannot be relied on in the treatment of pneumococcal pneumonia, nor can the oral penicillin preparations. In a patient known to be sensitive to penicillin, an initial injection of sodium sulfadiazine (50 mg. per kilogram) followed by 100 mg. per kilogram per twenty-four hours divided into four oral doses is usually satisfactory, as are also chloramphenicol and the newer semisynthetic penicillins. Strains of pneumococcus highly resistant to erythromycin and the tetracyclines have been described, however, rendering these drugs less desirable in the treatment of pneumococcal infections.

Antimicrobial therapy should be continued for several days after defervescence and until clearing is present on the roentgenogram. If pneumonia is complicated by otitis media, drug therapy must be considerably prolonged.

Supportive therapy includes administration of humidified oxygen whenever indicated for cyanosis and restlessness; occasionally the use of one or two doses of codeine or Demerol for patients with severe pleuritic pain or intractable hacking cough which prevents sleep. Rapid digitalization may be indicated to relieve cardiac failure. Abdominal distention can be serious; oxygen administration, a semi-sitting position, evacuation of the stomach with a stomach tube, a small enema with the rectal tube left in place, and heat applied externally to the abdomen usually help. Sedation is potentially dangerous, since it may decrease respiratory efforts, thereby contributing to carbon dioxide narcosis; however, a single dose of barbiturate may occasionally be used in an irritable patient with impending convulsions. Measures to lower the body temperature should be resorted to only if essential to relieve cardiac strain or prevent convulsions; then a tepid alcohol sponge, aimed at reducing the temperature no more than 2 to 3 degrees Fahrenheit, may be beneficial, and may be repeated.

Complications

Otitis media and *sinusitis* are now uncommon complications of pneumonia when treatment is early and intensive. *Empyema,* which formerly occurred in about 5 per cent of children with pneumococcal pneumonia, is now rarely seen; commonest during the second and third years of life, it should be treated in the same manner as staphylococcal empyema (see p. 289) and usually responds well. *"Pleuropneumonia"* refers to the syndrome of thick fibrinous pleurisy encasing all or most of a lung, seen occasionally in a patient under three years of age, who exhibits a high continuous or remitting fever, usually with intermittent pneumococcal bacteremia; though this syndrome is seen even less frequently than in the prechemotherapy era, it is still refractory even to high doses of penicillin, and relapses are frequent. *Meningitis* should be considered in any patient seriously ill with pneumonia, at any stage of the disease.

Prognosis

Although the death rate prior to chemotherapy was estimated at 20 to 30 per cent in infants, it was never high in older children and is now very much below 5 per cent.

STREPTOCOCCAL PNEUMONIA

Infections due to the group A streptococci decreased strikingly in the 1940's and early 1950's; now they are on the increase again, but it is not clear whether the greater number of cases is due to the population increase or to some change in the characteristics of the microorganism itself. The incidence of streptococcal pneumonia is very difficult to evaluate. A 1942 report on 4849 cases of streptococcal disease seen in the pediatric service at the New Haven Hospital mentions fifteen patients with empyema, but only one with "pneumonia." On the other hand, the Children's Medical Center in Boston admitted ninety-three patients with pneumonia between June 1958 and June 1959; eleven cases were attributed to the beta hemolytic streptococcus on the basis of positive cultures from nose, throat, pleural fluid or blood.

Streptococcal pneumonia, more often than other bacterial pneumonias, seems to complicate viral infections such as influenza, measles, chickenpox, German measles; or bacterial infections such as pertussis or pneumococcal pneumonia; or it may accompany other streptococcal illnesses such as pharyngitis, erysipelas or scarlet fever.

The salient pathologic changes comprise necrosis of the mucosa of the tracheobronchial passages with formation of ragged ulcers, thickened bronchioles filled with exudate, patchy hemorrhagic interstitial bronchopneumonia, often symmetric, with extensive involvement of lymphatic channels both toward the draining lymph nodes and toward the pleural surfaces. Owing presumably to the production of streptokinase by group A streptococci, streptococcal exudates have a low fibrin content as compared to pneumococcal exudates; the very liquid consistency of streptococcal exudate is further assured by the deoxyribonucleases produced by these organisms.

The *clinical features* of streptococcal pneumonia are extremely variable. The onset may be sudden and accompanied by chills and pleuritic pain, or the disease may start as an insidious exacerbation of an underlying process, with gradual rise in fever and intensification of cough. A scarlatiniform rash or purpuric lesions of the extremities are rarely present. Empyema accompanied the pneumonia in six out of eleven children reported by Kevy and Lowe, and sixteen of fifty-five patients of all ages described by Keefer and associates. The white blood cell count varies in reported cases from 7000 to 59,000 per cubic milliliter. Bacteremia occurs in perhaps 10 per cent of the patients, mainly in the severely ill ones.

The *roentgenologic picture* closely resembles that seen in pneumonia due to *Mycoplasma pneumoniae* or *Staphylococcus aureus:* even the pneumatoceles described in the latter are occasionally found. Enlargement of the hilar lymph nodes can be striking, especially in young children, a feature which is not shared with pneumococcal pneumonia.

Diagnosis is established by the recovery of the beta hemolytic streptococcus group A from nose and throat cultures, from empyema fluid if present, or occasionally from the blood. Useful in retrospect, or as an adjunct, is a rise in the antistreptolysin-O titer: it does not, however, occur so

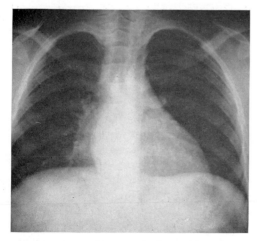

FIGURE 21–2. Pneumonia due to beta hemolytic streptococcus.

regularly in the very young child as in the older one.

The mainstay of *treatment* is aqueous penicillin G administered parenterally at first, with rather prolonged oral administration during convalescence to prevent relapse. Some 20 per cent of group A beta hemolytic streptococci are resistant to tetracyclines, so that this group of drugs should not be relied on. Erythromycin is probably the drug of choice for patients who are sensitive to penicillin.

STAPHYLOCOCCAL PNEUMONIA

Staphylococcal disease has been referred to as "probably the foremost parasitic cause of death in many modern communities." As the ravages of streptococcosis and the other epidemic respiratory diseases associated with the industrial revolution were brought under control by immunization and antimicrobial drugs, the versatile staphylococci, uncurbed by vaccines and readily able to produce variants resistant to antimicrobials, have again come to the fore. The fact that most births nowadays occur in hospitals, and that the rapidly rising birth rate forces serious overcrowding in nurseries, favors heavy exposure of infants at a susceptible age, so that they and their mothers, as well as hospital visitors and attendants, serve as foci for dissemination of staphylococci in the community.

Bacteriology and Immunity

Staphylococcus aureus and *Staphylococcus epidermidis* are the two species which constitute a genus within the family of Micrococcaceae. Although mucoid, encapsulated strains have been described, they are rare, and encapsulation seems unrelated to pathogenicity. Able to grow readily on conventional culture media, *Staphylococcus aureus* frequently produces clear hemolysis on media containing blood. L-forms have been described; of practical importance may be the fact that these forms can develop in the presence of high concentrations of the penicillins; on other hand, they tend to be more sensitive than the parent forms to erythromycin, tetracyclines and lincomycin.

Typing of *Staphylococcus aureus* has been attempted by serologic differentiation of strains; unfortunately, because of the multiplicity of antigens produced and their overlap, this approach to classification has proved disappointing. Identification is usually by "bacteriophage typing," in which susceptibility to a standard set of four groups of lytic phages (each group containing one to nine phages), plus two "miscellaneous" ungrouped phages, is determined. Determination of antimicrobial sensitivity patterns may be a useful epidemiologic adjunct to phage typing.

Coagulase formation characterizes almost all pathogenic strains of *Staphylococcus aureus*, whereas nonpathogenic strains rarely display this property. Free staphylocoagulase interacts with a "coagulase-reacting factor" present in plasma to produce an active principle similar to thrombin. Coagulase-reacting factor levels are notably lower in children than in adults, and lower also in certain disease states such as viral pneumonia and infectious hepatitis. Several antigenically distinct coagulases have been described. Anticoagulases are found in the serums of children recovering from staphylococcal infections, as well as in monkeys after experimental infection. Active immunization with coagulase has been thought to confer some protection against staphylococcal disease in rabbits, but the role of coagulases and anticoagulases in human infection is far from clear. Other substances isolated from staphylococci include at least three hemolysins; also a "lethal toxin" and an enterotoxin; leukocytotoxic substances, hyaluronidase, staphylokinase. Many strains, especially those lysed by the bacteriophages in group III, produce penicillinase, an enzyme which opens the beta-lactam ring of the penicillin molecule; penicillinase production is increased not only by the presence of the penicillin substrate, but also by exposure to some of the synthetic penicillins. Relative resistance to phagocytosis characterizes many strains of *Staphylococcus aureus*; on the other hand, many, if phagocytized, survive long periods of time within leukocytes, protected from antimicrobial drugs and possible immune substances within the surrounding body fluids. In this respect their behavior differs markedly from that of pneumococcus and *Klebsiella pneumoniae*. Although it is difficult to define the antistaphylococcal antibodies responsible for immunity, the falling incidence of staphylococcal pneumonia and sepsis with increasing age certainly suggests that immunity is important; in most reported series of staphylococcal pneumonia and empyema in children, some 30 per cent occur in infants three months of age or less, and 60 to 70 per cent in children under one year. Not only the incidence, but also the relative mortality, is much higher in infants.

Epidemiology

Staphylococcal pneumonia in infants actually seems to have become more frequent in recent years. Phage type 80/81 has frequently been associated with epidemics; these strains are usually hospital-acquired, and are resistant to penicillin G and often to streptomycin and tetracyclines. More common in boys than in girls, 70 per cent of the cases occur in the six winter months.

Transmission can be by the airborne route or by direct personal contact, especially by the hands of personnel. As many as 90 per cent of newborns are carriers of *Staphylococcus aureus*, the carrier rate falling to 20 per cent during the first two years of life and rising slowly thereafter to some 30 to 50 per cent. Most infants, even though carriers, are not infectious to others; a small number of infants, who behave as though surrounded by "clouds" of bacteria, have been dubbed "cloud babies" and are deemed important in the dissemination of *Staphylococcus aureus*. Eichenwald's data suggest that "cloudiness" is determined by simultaneous infection with certain respiratory viruses, such as adenovirus type 2 and ECHO virus type 20. Not only do respiratory viruses seem to favor transmission of *Staphylococcus aureus*, but also they seem to precipitate overt disease; epidemics of influenza in particular have long been associated with staphylococcal pneumonia.

Pathogenesis and Pathology

Staphylococcal pneumonia can occur as a primary "bronchogenic" infection of the upper respiratory tract, seemingly alone, although it is not clear how often it is really concomitant with a viral infection. That approximately one third of the cases of primary bacterial pneumonia in infants under two years of age can be due to *Staphylococcus aureus* was shown in a study by Disney. Staphylococcal pneumonia can also complicate measles, chickenpox or mucoviscidosis. In 15 to 20 per cent of cases septic lung lesions arise secondary to staphylococcal infection elsewhere in the body.

There are few descriptions of the pathologic findings in staphylococcal pneumonias in children. MacGregor studied ten cases in the prechemotherapy era. Characteristic were "one or more areas of massive consolidation, sharply defined, intensely hemorrhagic." There was a "strong tendency to suppuration, especially in the bronchi, where the walls were destroyed." Grumbach and Blondet studied an infant who died after several weeks of penicillin treatment and found bullous cavities lined with a thick, pearly-looking, connective tissue membrane; they demonstrated a tiny bronchial fistula plugged with mucus, and epithelialization of the interior of the communicating cavity. Elsewhere a bronchus opened widely

into the bullous cavity through a necrotic stoma. They postulate the development of a necrotic staphylococcal lesion, characteristic of staphylococcal lesions wherever they occur in the body, which either disappears by healing, with development of a bulla in the area left vacant, or a tearing of the weakened area by the neighboring elastic traction of the normal lung. That some bullae collapse and heal rapidly, whereas others remain distended for long periods of time, may depend on whether or not epithelialization of the cavity takes place from the adjacent bronchus. Brown and associates believe that the annular or elliptical shadows often seen in staphylococcal pneumonia are "small Staph. abscesses and that the cystic spaces are the same lesions in their natural course of cavitation, thinning and ultimate disappearance." Hay, however, suggests that these lesions are septic infarcts and that the annular lesions are due to cyst formation from "obstructive emphysema."

Experimental staphylococcal pneumonia of the "secondary" type, produced in rabbits by intravenous injection of *Staphylococcus aureus* cultures from patients, was studied by Herbenval and Debry. Here the fundamental lesion is a microbial arterial embolus which may develop as a "cuff" near an arteriole, and may rupture because of pressure changes in the surrounding air, with an implosion of pus into the surrounding tissues. It may bear no relation to a bronchus, or, if the lesion should arise adjacent to a bronchus, there may be bronchial necrosis; there may be infarction of a blood vessel.

The importance of widespread, non-suppurative vascular lesions described in staphylococcal septicemia should not be overlooked. Consisting of focal hemorrhages, fibrin thrombi in blood vessels, infarction with arterial or venous occlusion, renal cortical necrosis, they undoubtedly account in large part for the shock and prostration seen especially in older children.

In summary, the available data from human and experimental sources suggest that *Staphylococcus aureus,* whether it reaches the lung through the tracheo-bronchial tree or by way of the blood-stream, gives rise to typical lesions either in the bronchial wall (in which case plugging of the bronchus by pus may occur, or evacuation of the abscess into the bronchus, or a bronchial fistula into the lung), or in a blood vessel (with sub-sequent infarction or implosion of the abscess into lung tissue), or in the lung tissue itself. The characteristic bullous lesions, pneumatoceles or abscesses which have been evacuated into the bronchus are kept open by the pus and fibrin plastered over their walls, and later by epi-thelialization from the bronchus. Pneu-mothorax and pyothorax probably result from rupture of necrotic lesions near the pleura. Widespread vascular lesions, when they occur, may account for the extreme degree of shock and prostration.

Clinical Features

The clinical features of staphylococcal pneumonia are as variable as the fore-going discussion would suggest. Some-times there is no evidence of predisposing disease, staphylococcal or other; some-times the pneumonia is secondary to skin lesions, osteomyelitis, mucoviscidosis, hy-pogammaglobulinemia or treatment with immunosuppressive drugs. At the onset a mild upper respiratory tract infection may lead to a clinical picture typical of pneumonia, with fever, cough and rapid, grunting respirations; or the course may be fulminating, with prostration, cyano-sis, dyspnea, shock and excessively high temperature. In the 329 cases reported by Rebhan and Edwards from the Hospital for Sick Children in Toronto, 13 per cent had had symptoms for only one day, 50 per cent for four days, the remainder for up to six weeks: fever was the commonest

symptom, followed by cough, dyspnea, evidence of upper respiratory tract infection, anorexia, grunting, irritability and vomiting. Physical findings are often misleading, especially in the smaller in-fants, in whom the breath sounds may be well heard even in the presence of a mas-sive pyopneumothorax. Mediastinal shift may be noted, or it may be absent despite a large pleural effusion. Tachypnea and cyanosis may be striking and may seem disproportionate to the meager physical signs and roentgenographic changes noted early in the disease. Abdominal disten-tion is often pronounced, and the liver palpable below the costal margin, owing either to true engorgement of the liver itself or to its downward displacement. The leucocyte count in a series of twenty-four patients reported by Pryles varied from 2800 to 72,700 cells, averaging 24,-100 per cubic milliliter; polymorphonu-clear cells predominated in all but one patient. Anemia often develops rapidly. Bacteremia was present in 41 per cent of Forbes's patients under two years of age and in 20 per cent of the older children. Pyopneumothorax may develop abruptly, with acute respiratory difficulty, shift of the mediastinum toward the opposite side, cyanosis and prostration: aspirations of air and pus by syringe may be lifesaving. The disease almost always runs a long and stormy course, the duration of hospitaliza-tion averaging a month or more.

Roentgenographic Appearance

The admission roentgenogram in Reb-han's series of 329 patients disclosed in-volvement of the right lung alone in 65 per cent, and of both lungs in 17 per cent. There was infiltration in 83 per cent, pleural effusion in 55 per cent, pneumo-thorax in 21 per cent, abscess or pneu-matocele formation in 13 per cent. Characteristic is the rapid change in appearance of the lesions at the start of illness; often minimal at first, even in an extremely ill child, they progress from

A   B

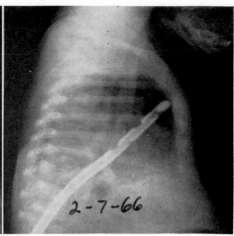

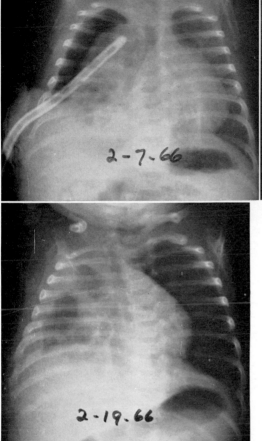

FIGURE 21–3. Staphylococcal pneumonia. *A* (2/7/66), Frontal view. Tube with waterseal drainage in place for 6 days. Persistent bronchopleural fistula and pneumothorax. "Swiss cheese" appearance of the basal segments of the right lower lobe due to pneumatoceles. *B* (2/7/66), Right lateral view. *C* (2/19/66), Diminished volume of entire right hemithorax, hyperaeration of the left lung, persistent pneumatoceles and pleural thickening. Patient clinically well, receiving orally antistaphylococcal drugs only.

C

small, focal infiltrative lesions with faint mottling or haziness of the parenchyma to patchy consolidation to pneumatocele formation to empyema or pneumothorax, all within a few hours. Pneumatoceles, true abscesses and loculated areas of pyopneumothorax may be indistinguishable from each other. Pneumothorax may arise spontaneously from rupture of a small subpleural lesion, or it may follow a diagnostic thoracentesis; it may be self-limited or, arising from a larger area of

necrosis in the visceral pleura which constitutes a bronchopleural fistula, it may steadily increase in size and constitute a so-called tension pneumothorax with great shift of the mediastinum. This picture is seen particularly in early infancy, and sudden death may result. Although at the onset of the illness the patient often appears much sicker than the chest x-ray alone would lead one to expect, clinical improvement usually precedes roentgenographic clearing by many

A B

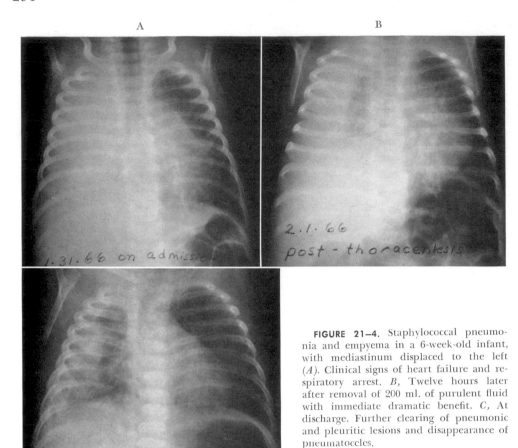

C

FIGURE 21–4. Staphylococcal pneumonia and empyema in a 6-week-old infant, with mediastinum displaced to the left (*A*). Clinical signs of heart failure and respiratory arrest. *B,* Twelve hours later after removal of 200 ml. of purulent fluid with immediate dramatic benefit. *C,* At discharge. Further clearing of pneumonic and pleuritic lesions and disappearance of pneumatoceles.

days or even weeks. The pneumatoceles in particular may persist as thin-walled asymptomatic "cysts" for several months.

Diagnosis

Staphylococcal pneumonia is a likely possibility in every infant under one year of age with pneumonia, and particularly in those under three months. Prostration, cyanosis and respiratory difficulty with minimal roentgenographic changes; lower respiratory tract infection with total involvement of one hemithorax; pneumonia with pneumatocele or abscess formation, or pyopneumothorax are all typical pictures of staphylococcal pulmonary disease. In an older child with abrupt onset of prostration, shock, tachypnea and a temperature of 106° or over, staphylococcal pneumonia should be considered in the differential diagnosis (along with meningococcal bacteremia and Shigella infection). Empyema which on thoracentesis yields pinkish or anchovy-colored pus is usually staphylococcal in origin, although the pus may be whitish or yellow. The presence of mucoviscidosis, or of foci of staphylococcal infection elsewhere in the patient or his family, may provide a useful clue to diagnosis.

To be considered in the differential diagnosis are pneumonia due to pneumococcus, *Hemophilus influenzae* (particularly in small children) or *Klebsiella pneumoniae;* progressive primary tuberculosis with cavity formation; aspiration of nonradiopaque foreign body with subsequent abscess formation; diaphragmatic hernia with loops of bowel in the thorax.

The diagnosis can be immediately, albeit tentatively, confirmed by demonstrating clusters of gram-positive cocci in the pleural fluid obtained on thoracentesis, if fluid is present. Final diagnosis is established by isolating coagulase-positive *Staphylococcus aureus* from the blood, empyema fluid or lung puncture. Suitable specimens should be obtained and cultured immediately, before administration of antimicrobial drugs is begun. Determination of the sensitivity of the organism to *all* potentially useful antistaphylococcal drugs is an essential part of the initial bacteriologic diagnosis. Isolation of coagulase-positive *Staphylococcus aureus* in pure culture from the nasopharynx is highly suggestive evidence, as is also the presence of single or multiple abscesses or pneumatoceles on the roentgenogram of a tuberculin-negative child. Lung puncture or bronchoscopic aspiration is sometimes useful in confirming the diagnosis in certain complicated situations such as the following: a patient with underlying tuberculosis has a fresh pneumonic lesion which might be due to either staphylococcal or tuberculous infection. In such a situation, particularly if *Staphylococcus aureus* is strongly suspected, but not recovered upon culture of readily available sites, then cultures of lung aspirate or bronchoscopic washings may yield the answer.

Management

Hospitalization is mandatory whenever staphylococcal pneumonia is seriously considered. Only in the hospital can the proper bacterial cultures of nasopharynx, throat and blood be obtained and studied for sensitivity to antimicrobial agents; and only the hospital is equipped to deal with the abrupt occurrence of bronchopleural fistula and the need for prolonged parenteral drug administration.

Antimicrobial therapy must be instituted immediately after cultures have been obtained. Large doses of one or more of the penicillins are the backbone of treatment. A successful initial regimen in our experience has included aqueous penicillin G (50,000 units per kilogram per twenty-four hours, divided into four to six "stat" intravenous doses); methicillin (100 to 150 mg. per kilogram per twenty-four hours, also divided into four to six "stat" intravenous doses) (remember that methicillin solution is very labile and should be freshly prepared every eight hours!); and a third drug such as chloramphenicol, cloxacillin, nafcillin, novobiocin or oxacillin which is administered parenterally at first, later orally. As soon as the pattern of the infecting organism is known, either penicillin G or methicillin is dropped, and the "third drug" is changed if need be. Bacitracin, cephalothin, erythromcycin, lincomycin and kanamycin are all useful antistaphylococcal agents which may be given, depending on special circumstances. Administration of at least two drugs to which the particular strain of staphylococcus is shown to be sensitive should be continued until the patient has been afebrile for at least a week, with oral administration of the "third drug" continued for at least two further weeks. Intrapleural administration of antimicrobial agents has never been shown to be beneficial.

Supportive therapy should include elevating the patient's shoulders and trunk in case of dyspnea and abdominal distention; oxygen administration and humidification of the atmosphere for cyanosis and severe dyspnea; aspiration of gastric contents if partial paralytic ileus is present; transfusion for the anemia which not infrequently develops during the course of the disease. Maintenance of fluid and electrolyte balance is essential, and the cation content of the penicillins must be taken into account: 15 million units of potassium penicillin G is equivalent to 25 mEq. of potassium and 4 gm. of methicillin to 10 mEq. of sodium. The question of whether or not to use steroids has been discussed by Oleson and Quaade, who observed that pneumothorax accompanied staphylococcal pneumonia in four of nineteen adult patients treated *with* steroids, but occurred in none of the twenty-six patients who did not receive such drugs in addition to antimicrobial therapy. No satisfactory data are available with respect to children. Severe shock, however, accompanying acute staphylococcal pneumonia and sepsis should probably be treated with large amounts of intravenous plasma and hydrocortisone, perhaps also with chlorpromazine or dibenzyline, according to the best evidence available today.

SURGICAL CONSIDERATIONS. Shift of the mediastinum may supervene abruptly, owing to development of a tension pneumothorax, in which case removal of air by syringe may be lifesaving; or it may develop slowly owing to collection of fluid or pus in the pleural cavity, in which case thoracentesis should be performed; occasionally shift of the mediastinum may be due to a large pneumatocele. In any of these situations insertion of a chest tube (red rubber urethral catheter, 10 to 14 French) combined with water-seal drainage often precipitates almost unbelievable improvement within minutes of insertion of the tube. The tube should be left in place, never clamped, and on continuous gentle suction (8 to 10 cc. of water) until bubbling and purulent discharge have ceased. Then it should be withdrawn a short distance each day. If in doubt, it is better to remove the tube rather than to leave it too long *in situ*, where it may serve as a foreign body and as a portal

of entry for secondary bacterial invasion. Sometimes, while one tube is in place, a new lesion will appear (e.g. pneumatocele), requiring placement of a second or even a third tube; each lesion and each tube should be handled separately. Daily roentgenograms, including both postero-anterior and lateral views, are indispensable during the early phase of the illness in assuring that the tube (or tubes) is properly located and not kinked. Should the tube stop draining satisfactorily early in the course of illness, gentle irrigation with sterile saline may restore patency.

Enzymatic débridement with streptokinase-streptodornase, instilling 10,000 to 20,000 units of streptokinase and 2500 to 5000 units of streptodornase directly into the pleural cavity, has been found useful in some patients with extremely thick fibropurulent discharge. Since, however, sharp febrile reactions, cyanosis and dyspnea frequently accompany such instillations (also sometimes the appearance of a bronchopleural fistula), extreme caution is recommended, especially in young infants.

Resection of pneumatoceles and decortication are rarely if ever indicated, even though pneumatoceles or fibrothorax may persist for many months before clearing.

Prognosis

Although the reported mortality rate has varied considerably from one series to another, the deaths in well managed groups of patients at present probably do not exceed 10 per cent. The younger the patient, the graver the outlook. Long-term follow-up studies are few. Three or four years after a bout of staphylococcal pneumonia, resolution is almost always complete, with the disappearance of pneumatoceles and no apparent residual bronchiectasis. Hoffman, however, who carried out bronchograms on ten infants who recovered from staphylococcal empyema, demonstrated "minimal to moderate segmental dilatations" in one, whereas among seven older children he found one with gross bronchiectasis and two with minimal lesions.

REFERENCES

Pneumococcal Pneumonia

Austrian, C. R., and Austrian, R.: Pneumococcal Pneumonia; in *Tice's Practice of Medicine*. Hagerstown, Md., W. F. Prior and Co.

Eagle, H., Fleischman, R., and Musselman, A. D.: Effect of Schedule of Administration on Therapeutic Efficacy of Penicillin: Importance of Aggregate Time Penicillin Remains at Effectively Bactericidal Levels. *Am. J. Med.*, 9:280, 1950.

Finland, M.: Recent Advances in Epidemiology of Pneumococcal Infections. *Medicine*, 21: 307, 1942.

Gillmore, B. B., and Anderson, G. W.: A Community Outbreak of Type I Pneumococcus Infection. *Am. J. Hyg.*, 28:345, 1938.

Heffron, R.: *Pneumonia, with Special Reference to Pneumococcus Lobar Pneumonia.* New York, Commonwealth Fund, 1939.

McLeod, C. M.: The Pneumococci; in *Bacterial and Mycotic Infections of Man.* R. J. Dubos and J. G. Hirsch (Eds.): 4th Ed. Philadelphia, J. B. Lippincott Company, 1965.

Schaedler, R. W., Choppin, P. W., and Zabriskie, J. B.: Pneumonia Caused by Tetracycline-Resistant Pneumococci. *New England J. Med.*, 270:127, 1964.

Sutliff, W. D., and Finland, M.: Antipneumococcic Immunity Reactions in Individuals of Different Ages. *J. Exper. Med.*, 55:837, 1932.

Tillet, W. S., McCormack, J. E., and Cambier, M. J.: Treatment of Lobar Pneumonia with Penicillin. *J. Clin. Invest.* 29:161, 1950.

Tumulty, P. A., and Zubrod, G.: Pneumococcal Pneumonia Treated with Aqueous Penicillin at Twelve-Hour Intervals. *New Engl. J. Med.*, 239:1033, 1948.

Walker, I. C., and Hamburger, M.: Pneumococcal Lobar Pneumonia Treated with One Injection of Dibenzyl-Ethylenediamine Dipenicillin G, a Report of 49 Cases. *Antibiotics & Chemotherapy*, 4:76, 1954.

Wood, W. B.: Pneumococcal Pneumonia: in *Textbook of Medicine.* 11th ed. P. B. Beeson and W. McDermott (Eds.): Philadelphia, W. B. Saunders Company, 1963.

Streptococcal Pneumonia

Boisvert, P. L., Darrow, D. C., Powers, G. F., and Trask, J. D.: Streptococcosis in Children, a Nosographic and Statistical Study, *Am. J. Dis. Child.*, 64:516, 1942.

Keefer, C. S., Rantz, A., and Rammelkamp, C. H.: Hemolytic Streptococcal Pneumonia and Empyema: A Study of 55 Cases with Special Reference to Treatment. *Am. Int. Med.*, 14:1533, 1941.

Kevy, S. V., and Lowe, B. A.: Streptococcal Pneumonia and Empyema in Childhood, *New Engl. J. Med.*, 264:738, 1961.

Rantz, L. A., Maroney, M., and DiCaprio, J. M.: Antistreptolysin O Response Following Hemolytic Streptococcus Infection in Early Childhood. *Arch. Int. Med.*, 87:360, 1951.

Tillett, W. S.: Studies on the Enzymatic Lysis of Fibrin and Inflammatory Exudates by Products of Hemolytic Streptococci, *Harvey Lectures*, series 45 (1949-1950), 1952, p. 149.

Staphylococcal Pneumonia

Blair, J. E., and Williams, R. E. O.: Phagetyping of Staphylococci. *Bull. World Health Organ.*, 24:771, 1961.

Boake, W. C.: Antistaphylocoagulase in Experimental Staphylococcal Infections. *J. Immunol.*, 76:89, 1956.

Brown, M., Buechner, H. A., Ziskind, M., and Weill, H.: Septicemic (Pyemic) Abscesses of the Lung. *Transactions of the 22nd Research Conference in Pulmonary Diseases*, 1963.

Disney, M. E., Wolff, J., and Wood, B. S. B.: Staphylococcal Pneumonia in Infants. *Lancet*, 1:767, 1956.

Eichenwald, H. F., Kotsevalov, O., and Fasso, L. A.: The *"Cloud Baby"*: An Example of Bacterial-Viral Interaction. *Am. J. Dis. Child.*, 100:161, 1960.

Fisher, J. H., and Swenson, O.: Surgical Complications of Staphylococcic Pneumonia. *Pediatrics*, 20:835, 1957.

Forbes, G. B.: Staphylococcal Empyema: The Importance of Pyopneumothorax as a Complication. *J. Pediat.*, 29:45, 1946.

Forbes, G. B., and Emerson, G. L.: Staphylococcal Pneumonia and Empyema. *Pediat. Clin. N. Amer.* 4:215, 1957.

Grumbach, R., and Blondet, P. L.: Etude anatomique d'une pneumopathie bullouse extensive staphylococcique. *Presse Méd.*, 64:542, 1956.

Hay, D. R.: Pulmonary Manifestations of Staphylococcal Pyemia. *Thorax*, 15:82, 1960.

Hendren, W. H., III., and Haggerty, R. J.: Staphylococcal Pneumonia in Infancy and Childhood. *J.A.M.A.*, 168:6, 1958.

Herbenval R., and Debry, G.: Le poumon staphylococcique expérimental. *Presse méd.* 64:-542, 1956.

Hewitt, H. L.: Penicillins: Review of Strategy and Tactics. *J.A.M.A.* 185:264, 1963.

Hoffman, E.: Empyema in Childhood. *Thorax,* 16:128, 1961.

Huxtable, K. A., Tucker, A. S., and Wedgwood, R. J.: Staphylococcal Pneumonia in Childhood. *Am. J. Dis. Child.,* 108:262, 1964.

Kagan, B. M.: Staphylococcal L-Forms. Ecologic Perspectives. *Ann. New York Acad. Sc.,* 128: 81, 1965.

Kanof, A., Kramer, B., and Carnes, M.: Staphylococcus Pneumonia. *J. Pediat.,* 14:712, 1939.

Lillehei, R. C., Longerbeam, J. K., Block, J. H., and Manax, W. G.: The Modern Treatment of Shock Based on Physiologic Principles. *Clin. Pharmacol. & Therap.,* 5:63, 1964.

MacGregor, A. R.: Staphylococcal Pneumonia. *Arch. Dis. Childhood,* 11:195, 1936.

Madoff, M. A., and Weinstein, L.: Studies of Staphylococcal Coagulase-Reacting Factor and Anticoagulase in Man. *Am. J. Hyg.,* 75:212, 1962.

Mortimer, E. A., Jr., Lipsitz, P. J., Wolinsky, E., Gorezaza, A. J., and Rammelkamp, C. H., Jr.: Transmission of Staphylococci Between Newborns. Importance of Hands of Personnel. *Am. J. Dis. Child.,* 104:289, 1962.

Oleson, K. H., and Quaade, F.: Pneumothorax Accompanying Staphylococcic Pneumonia in Patients Treated Without Steroids. *Lancet,* 1:535, 1961.

Parker, M. T., and Jevons, M. T.: Hospital Strains of Staphylococci; in R. E. O. Williams and R. A. Shooter (Eds.): *Infection in Hospitals.* Oxford, Blackwell.

Powell, D. E. B.: Non-suppurative Lesions in Staphylococcal Septicaemia. *J. Path. & Bact.,* 82:141, 1961.

Pryles, C. V.: Staphylococcal Pneumonia in Infancy and Childhood. An Analysis of 24 Cases. *Pediatrics,* 21:609, 1958.

Rammelkamp, C. H., Jr., and Lebovitz, J. L.: The Role of Coagulase in Staphylococcal Infections. *Ann. New York Acad. Sci.,* 65:144, 1956.

Rammelkamp, C. H., Jr., Hezebicks, M. M., and Dingle, J. H.: Specific Coagulases of *Staph. Aureus. J. Exper. Med.,* 91:295, 1950.

Ravenholt, R. T., and Ravenholt, O. H.: Staphylococcal Infections in the Hospital and Community: Hospital Environment and Staphylococcal Disease. *Amer. J. Pub. Health,* 48:3, 1958.

Rebhan, A. W., and Edwards, H. E.: Staphylococcal Pneumonia, Review of 329 Cases. *Canad. M.A.J.,* 82:513, 1960.

Rogers, D. E.: The Current Problem of Staphylococcal Infections. *Ann. Int. Med.,* 45:748, 1956.

Rogers, D. E., and Tompsett, R.: The Survival of Staphylococci Within Human Leukocytes. *J. Exper. Med.,* 95:209, 1952.

Tager, M.: Problems in the Coagulation of Plasma by Staphylocoagulase. *Ann. New York Acad. Sc.,* 65:109, 1956.

Velarde-Frias, R., and Shaffer, M. F.: Anticoagulase in Sera of Children with Staphylococcal Infections. *Pediatrics,* 34:401, 1964.

Williams, R. E. O.: Healthy Carriage of *Staphylococcus Aureus*: Its Prevalence and Importance. *Bact. Rev.,* 27:56, 1963.

CHAPTER TWENTY-TWO

Pneumonia Due to Hemophilus Influenzae and to Klebsiella (Friedlaender's Bacillus)

MARGARET H. D. SMITH, M.D.

PNEUMONIA DUE TO HEMOPHILUS INFLUENZAE

Nonencapsulated, so-called rough strains of *H. influenzae* are frequently present in the upper respiratory tract of normal persons, but appear to be of low pathogenicity. What relation they bear to the more pathogenic encapsulated strains a through f, and particularly to type b, which is responsible for almost all cases of frank hemophilus infection, is not clear. A synergistic action between certain respiratory viruses and members of the Hemophilus group has been partially substantiated by the experiments of several investigators. Clinical observations during epidemics of influenza also suggest that simultaneous infection with *H. influenzae* and influenza virus may be more serious than either alone.

The pneumonia produced by *H. influenzae* may be either focal ("lobar pneumonia") or disseminated ("bronchopneumonia"). Microscopic examination of the lungs in fatal cases has shown circumscribed areas of consolidation, consisting mainly of polymorphonuclear leukocytes, with destruction of bronchial and bronchiolar epithelium, interstitial pneumonitis and hemorrhagic edema. The degree of edema produced by *H. influenzae* is often striking and is typified by acute epiglottitis and acute bronchiolitis caused by this organism. Neither on the basis of anatomic changes, nor by roentgenogram or clinical picture, however, can *H. influenzae* pneumonia be differentiated with certainty from pneumo-coccal pneumonia. Some observers believe that the onset of *H. influenzae* pneumonia is apt to be more insidious; characteristic in the experience of others is a diffuse bronchopneumonia, accompanied by bronchiolitis and displaying on roentgenogram a "shaggy" appearance. Infants are more often affected than older children, and seem more prone to bacteremia, empyema and concomitant pyarthrosis than older patients, or than infants in the same age group with pneumococcal pneumonia. Adults with *H. influenzae* pneumonia are said to display "apple green" sputum; discharge from sinuses and bronchi in older children with *H. influenzae* infection may also be green, but this is not a reliable diagnostic point. Prolonged, pertussis-like cough sometimes accompanies the disease. Leukocytosis is almost invariably striking (18,000 to 70,000 cells), with relative or even absolute lymphocytosis. The other features of the disease do not differ from those described under Pneumococcal Pneumonia.

Diagnosis is established by finding *H. influenzae* in the blood culture or in the empyema fluid, if present. Very suggestive is the isolation of a near-pure culture of *H. influenzae* from the nasopharynx.

Management includes the administration of appropriate antimicrobial drugs such as sulfadiazine, chloramphenicol and ampicillin, alone or in combination, in adequate dosage; initial treatment should be parenteral until clinical improvement, when oral preparations may be used for some five to seven days longer. Supportive therapy and the treatment of

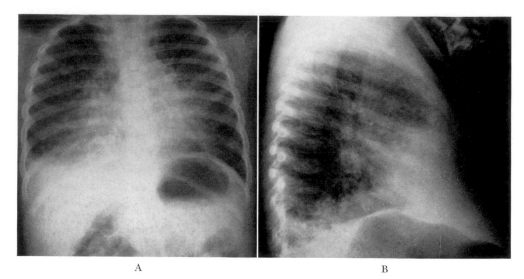

A   B

FIGURE 22–1. Pneumonia due to *Hemophilus influenzae. A,* Frontal view. Lobar consolidation of right lobe with overlying localized pleuritis (or small pleural effusion); also bronchitis and patchy bronchopneumonia. *B,* Right lateral view.

empyema are as described for Pneumococcal and Staphylococcal Pneumonia (pp. 287, 295).

PNEUMONIA DUE TO KLEBSIELLA (FRIEDLAENDER'S BACILLUS)

The *Klebsiella* group of bacteria (variously known as *K. pneumoniae, K. aerogenes,* Friedlaender's bacillus, pneumobacillus, *Bacillus mucosus capsulatus*) are short, nonmotile, gram-negative bacilli whose component polysaccharides have permitted their differentiation into more than seventy types. Organisms of this group are frequently found in the respiratory, gastrointestinal and urinary tracts of normal human beings as well as of many animals and insects. Klebsiella pneumonia is well recognized in adults, in whom it occurs particularly in older people and in diabetics. In infants it is seen infrequently, but its epidemic occurrence has several times been described in nurseries for premature and newborn infants. In recent years cases have occasionally been seen in older children, particularly as a secondary infection in patients who have received humidified

oxygen for some other disease, such as croup.

The *clinical picture* is indistinguishable from that seen in other types of acute bacterial pneumonia, although the presence of copious, thick mucous secretions is suggestive. Cystic changes in the lung on roentgenogram, due to areas of necrosis analogous to those which characterize staphylococcal pneumonia, are seldom reported in infants, despite the fact that they are a common feature of Klebsiella pneumonia in adults. Bacteremia, empyema and residual pleural thickening have all been seen in association with Klebsiella pneumonia in infants.

Diagnosis depends on nasopharyngeal and blood cultures, which should be taken routinely in patients with acute pneumonia. Any microorganism of the *Klebsiella* group recovered from nasopharynx or blood should immediately be tested for sensitivity to *all* potentially useful antimicrobial agents.

Initial *antimicrobial therapy,* in a patient suspected of Klebsiella pneumonia because of a current outbreak of the disease, or because of having received prior oxygen therapy, should include kanamycin in high dosage (for newborns 10 to 15 mg. per kilogram per twenty-four hours divided into two doses intramuscularly or intravenously; for older infants and children 25 mg. per kilogram per twenty-four hours divided into two doses). Cephalothin, chloramphenicol, colistimethate, polymyxin B, streptomycin and sulfonamides are other drugs which can be useful in Klebsiella infections.

Supportive and surgical management of empyema follows in general the same principles described for staphylococcal pneumonia (see p. 295). In cases in which copious purulent secretions are present, humidification of the air, face-down position and frequent suction are important.

REFERENCES

H. Influenzae Pneumonia

Alexander, H. E.: The Hemophilus Group; in R. J. Dubos and J. G. Hirsch (Eds.). *Bacterial and Mycotic Infections of Man.* 4th ed. Philadelphia, J. B. Lippincott Company, 1965.

Bang, F. B.: Synergistic Action of *Hemophilus Influenzae Suis* and the Swine Influenza Virus on the Chick Embryo. *J. Exper. Med.*, 77:7, 1943.

Buddingh, G. J.: Bacterial Dynamics in Combined Infection. A Study of the Population Dynamic of Strains of *Hemophilus Influenzae* Type b in Combined Infection with Influenza C Virus in Embryonated Eggs. *Am. J. Path.*, 43:407, 1963.

Crowell, J., and Loube, S. D.: Primary *Hemophilus Influenzae* Pneumonia. *Arch. Int. Med.*, 93:921, 1954.

Nyhan, W. L., Rectanus, D. R., and Fousek, M. D.: *Hemophilus Influenzae* Type b Pneumonia. *Pediatrics*, 16:31, 1955.

Shope, R. E.: Old, Intermediate and Contemporary Contributions to Our Knowledge of Pandemic Influenza. *Medicine*, 23:415, 1944.

Pneumonia Due to Klebsiella (Friedlaender's Bacillus)

Ferguson, J. A., and Tower, A. A.: Pneumonia in Infants Due to Bacillus Mucosus-Capsulatus. *Am. J. Dis. Child.*, 46:59, 1933.

Kauffmann, F.: The Differentiation of *Escherichia and Klebsiella Types.* Springfield, Ill., Charles C Thomas, 1951.

Miller, B. N., Orris, H. W., and Taus, H. H.: Friedländer's Pneumonia in Infancy. *J. Pediat.*, 31:521, 1947.

Obrinsky, W., Dormont, R. E., Fowler, R. E. L., and Ruhstaller, F.: Friedländer-Aerogenes Infections in Infancy. *Am. J. Dis. Child.*, 80:621, 1950.

Steiner, B., and Putnoky, G.: *Klebsiella Pneumoniae* (Friedländers Bacillus) Infections in Infancy. *Arch. Dis. Childhood*, 31:96, 1956.

Thaler, M. M.: Klebsiella-Aerobacter Pneumonia in Infants. *Pediatrics*, 30:206, 1962.

CHAPTER TWENTY-THREE

Giant Cell Pneumonia

SAMUEL STONE, M.D.

Giant cell interstitial pneumonia was first described by Hecht, who in 1910 reported autopsy findings in twenty-seven children. In nineteen of these cases there was an antecedent history of measles. Clinically, the disease cannot be distinguished from other pneumonias. The diagnosis depends solely upon the histologic examination of lung tissue.

Pathologically, the lungs show an interstitial pneumonia characterized by the presence of epithelial giant cells with intranuclear and intracytoplasmic inclusions. There is a preponderance of mononuclear cells in the infiltrate, squamous metaplasia of the bronchial and bronchiolar epithelium, and proliferation of alveolar lining cells. Occasionally giant cells

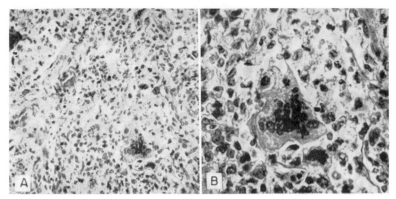

FIGURE 23–1. Photomicrographs from a lung section of a baby with primary pneumonitis, illustrating a low- (*A*) and a high-power (*B*) magnification of the general pathologic state with characteristic multinucleated giant cells. (J. M. Adams and D. T. Imagawa: *Pediat. Clin. N. Amer.*, 4:193, 1957.)

may appear in organs other than the lungs.

The nature of the etiologic agent has remained obscure until recently. In many cases there has been a history of measles immediately preceding the pneumonia. In the absence of clinical evidence of measles the disease has been referred to as Hecht's pneumonia. Some observers have found morphologic similarities between giant cell pneumonia and the pneumonia found in fatal measles. Other investigators have also been impressed with the morphologic and certain clinical similarities between giant cell pneumonia in human patients and distemper infections in animals. Up to 1958 it was the impression of workers that when clinical measles was present in association with giant cell pneumonia, the lesions were directly attributable to the measles virus. But since not all patients dying with giant cell pneumonia had clinical measles, the pneumonia was often referred to as Hecht's pneumonia, and another virus was felt to be the cause.

The most valuable contribution in elucidating the causation of this disease was made by McCarthy, Enders, Mitus and their group. A virus indistinguishable from the measles virus was isolated at autopsy from each of three cases of giant cell pneumonia. There had been no clinical manifestations of measles in these patients. All had other serious illnesses such as mucoviscidosis, leukemia and Letterer-

Siwe disease. This report suggests that in cases of giant cell pneumonia occurring in the course of other serious disease, but with no clinical measles, the host response to the measles infection is altered. Although giant cell pneumonia in patients who did not have clinical measles has been called "Hecht's pneumonia," there are no morphologic differences between such cases and the giant cell pneumonia of measles. It is likely that "Hecht's pneumonia" is caused by the measles virus in persons who do not exhibit the rash. The reason for this atypical host response is not clear, although it has been reported in patients already affected with chronic debilitating disease and with impaired immune response.

These observers also reported four children with leukemia who had typical measles followed by pneumonia; two of these children died, and autopsy showed typical features of giant cell pneumonia which had been provisionally diagnosed during life. Agents identified as measles virus were isolated during life and from tissues taken at autopsy. In these two cases the measles virus persisted for an unusually long period in the upper respiratory tract, and the patients also failed to respond in the normal manner by formation of specific antibodies. The virus persisted in these two cases for several weeks after the onset of the measles rash. This is in sharp contrast to the rapid disappearance of the agent from the throats of normal children suffering from measles. As a rule, attempts to isolate the virus from normal children forty-eight hours or longer after the rash are unsuccessful. In the two survivors measles virus persisted for an unusually long period in one, and the antibody response was depressed in both. Presumably giant cell pneumonia was also present in these two children.

From the practical standpoint, laboratory diagnostic methods now available for the detection of measles virus may permit the clinical recognition of giant cell pneumonia. It is especially important to make this diagnosis regarding therapy and prevention of measles in contacts, since the virus may persist and be a source of contagion for considerable periods after the initial infection. The survival of two patients who received large doses of gamma globulin at the time of exposure suggests that this material may be of value in the modification of subsequent measles pneumonitis. Furthermore, it is possible that large quantities of antibody administered intravenously in the form of measles convalescent plasma may mitigate this condition. Since, in children with acute leukemia, measles infection may present as a mild disease typical in course or as a fatal giant cell pneumonia, it is important to offer these children protection. Administration of attenuated live measles vaccine of Enders to children with acute leukemia appears to be contraindicated.

Use of an inactivated measles vaccine is preferable for immunization.

REFERENCES

Adams, J. M., and Imagawa, D. T.: The Relationship of Canine Distemper to Human Respiratory Disease. *Pediat. Clin. N. Amer.*, 4:193-201, 1957.

Enders, J. F., McCarthy, K., Mitus, A., and Cheatham, W. J.: Isolation of Measles Virus at Autopsy in Cases of Giant-Cell Pneumonia. *New England J. Med.*, 261:875, 1959.

Hecht, V.: Die Riesenzellenpneumonia im Kindesalter, eine historische-experimentelle Studie. *Beitr. z. path. Anat. u.z. allg. Path.*, 48:263, 1910.

Janigan, D. T.: Giant-Cell Pneumonia and Measles: An Analytical Review. *Canad. M.A.J.*, 85:741, 1961.

Koffler, D.: Giant Cell Pneumonia. Fluorescent Antibody and Histochemical Studies on Alveolar Giant Cells. *Arch. Path.*, 78:267, 1964.

McCarthy, K., Mitus, A., Cheatham, W., and Peebles, T. C.: Isolation of Virus of Measles from Three Fatal Cases of Giant-Cell Pneumonia. *Am. J. Dis. Child.*, 96:500, 1958.

McConnell, E. M.: Giant-Cell Pneumonia in an Adult. *Brit. M.J.*, 2:289, 1961.

Mitus, A., Enders, J. F., Craig, J. M., and Holloway, A.: Persistence of Measles Virus and Depression of Antibody Formation in Patients with Giant-Cell Pneumonia After Measles. *New England J. Med.*, 261:882, 1959.

Mitus, A., Holloway, A., Evans, A. E., and Enders, J. F.: Attenuated Measles Vaccine in Children with Acute Leukemia. *Am. J. Dis. Child.*, 103:413, 1962.

Pinkerton, H., Smiley, W. L., and Anderson, W. A. D.: Giant-Cell Pneumonia with Inclusions. *Pediatrics*, 10:681, 1952.

CHAPTER TWENTY-FOUR

Interstitial Plasma Cell Pneumonia (Pneumocystis Carinii Pneumonia)

SAMUEL STONE, M.D.

Within recent years interstitial plasma cell pneumonia has been reported with increasing frequency. Although originally described in continental Europe in 1938, many cases have been reported subsequently from North America, Australia and the Middle East. *Pneumocystis carinii* has been associated most frequently with "plasma cell" pneumonia. The inability to cultivate the organism in artificial media, chick embryos or tissue culture and the difficulty in demonstrating its presence in body fluids ante mortem have contributed to the difficulty in diagnosis.

The Organism

Pneumocystis carinii is an organism whose taxonomic classification is controversial. Some observers believe this organism to be a protozoan; others regard it as a fungus. A viral origin for the pulmonary lesion has been proposed with *Pn. carinii* as a secondary invader.

The most characteristic form of this parasite is a cyst 7 to 10 microns in diameter which contains eight bodies each measuring 1 to 2 by 1 micron surrounded by a mucoid capsule. Smaller cysts containing fewer bodies also are present. *Pneumocystis carinii* can be stained by the Giemsa method, which reveals excellent morphologic detail in both smears and tissue sections. The capsule stains with methenamine silver or with periodic acid-Schiff stain. Both techniques are useful for screening tissue sections.

Clinical Features

The clinical significance of Pneumocystis infection in the premature and debilitated infant has been known for some time. Its occurrence has been noted in young children with hypogammaglobulinemia or dysgammaglobulinemia. It has been recognized in postmortem findings in adults who suffered from other debilitating diseases, especially lymphomatous lesions, in which prolonged treatment with antibiotics, steroids and antimetabolites had been given.

The disease usually has its onset between the sixth and sixteenth weeks of life, though infants of six months and older may be affected. The illness occurs most frequently in premature and debilitated infants and is encountered chiefly in hospitals. It may be contagious, and epidemics of the disease have been reported. The incubation period is about forty days. The onset is insidious, and the first signs are poor feeding, failure to thrive, languor and irritability. Tachypnea, which may rise to 80 and more per minute, cyanosis and sometimes cough appear gradually and increase in severity. The temperature is either normal or slightly elevated. Physical findings are slight; there may be little or no impairment of resonance; auscultation may show good air exchange with occasional scattered rales and rhonchi. The disease may run a rapid course, and the infant may die within a few days after onset, usually from respiratory failure. Occasionally the disease may last for many months. Death may occur in 20 to 50 per

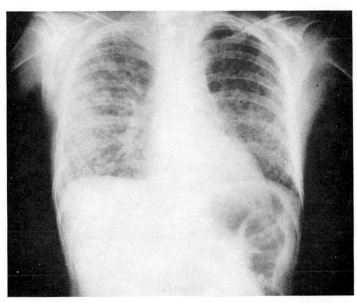

FIGURE 24–1. Child, 8 years old with leukemia, who had received antimetabolites. Roentgenogram shows diffuse, bilateral infiltration radiating from hili. Autopsy revealed *Pneumocystis carinii* pneumonia. (Courtesy of Dr. Charles Hilton, San Antonio, Texas.)

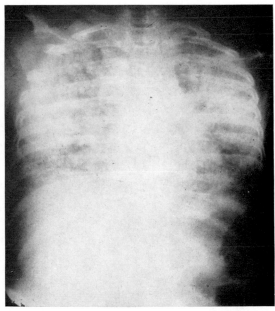

FIGURE 24–2. Roentgenogram of advanced stage of interstitial plasma cell pneumonia in same child. Confluent infiltrate in both lung fields. (Courtesy of Dr. Charles Hilton, San Antonio, Texas.)

cent of the cases. Those who survive recover slowly.

Roentgenologic examination shows a characteristic infiltration radiating bilaterally from the hili without hilar adenopathy. The peripheral lung fields, especially the bases, are relatively spared.

The white blood cell count is elevated to between 15,000 and 20,000 per cubic millimeter, though a normal count is commonly reported. Eosinophilia may be present.

Pathologic Findings

At necropsy the lungs are voluminous and completely fill the chest. The pleural surfaces are smooth without pleuritis. There may be areas of parenchymal interstitial and mediastinal emphysema.

Microscopy reveals the alveolar walls to be thickened with a great interstitial infiltration of lymphocytes and plasma cells. The alveoli are lined by large cuboidal epithelial cells which are often packed with a foamy material resembling a honeycomb. The foamy alveolar contents consist of innumerable Pneumocystis organisms. Vacuoles of parasites may be seen occasionally in alveolar septa.

Diagnosis and Treatment

The only reliable way to diagnose *Pn. carinii* pneumonia is by lung biopsy. A needle biopsy may be used, or open thoracotomy may be done. The organism has been demonstrated in sputum, hypopharyngeal material, tracheal aspirates, bronchial washings and rarely in thick smears of peripheral blood. The organism has not been found in gastric washings, urine or feces. Material should be specifically examined for the parasite with the use of special silver stains. A complement fixation test for the diagnosis of Pneumocystis infection has been developed in Europe.

Isolated cases must be differentiated from lipoid pneumonia, primary atypical pneumonia, pulmonary hemosiderosis, pulmonary alveolar proteinosis, diffuse pulmonary fibrosis of the Hamman-Rich type and histiocytic reticuloendotheliosis.

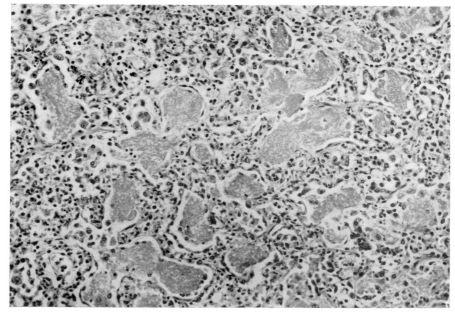

FIGURE 24–3. Section of lung. Alveolar spaces and ducts are filled with foamy material containing *Pneumocystis carinii*. (H. E. stain. × 150.) (Courtesy of Dr. Renata Dische, Department of Pediatric Pathology, New York University School of Medicine.)

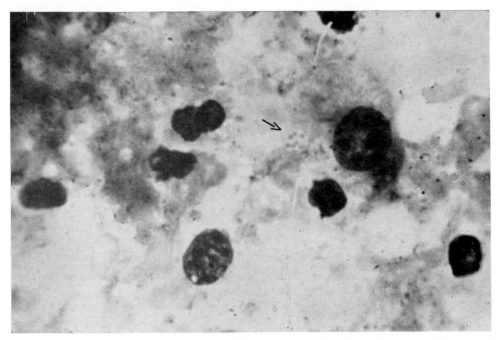

FIGURE 24–4. "Spores" of *Pneumocystis carinii*. One cyst with 8 "spores" (arrow). (Giemsa stain, magnification × 1500.) (Courtesy of Dr. Renata Dische, Department of Pediatric Pathology, New York University School of Medicine.)

Treatment consists in nursing care, and administration of oxygen and humidity for the cyanosis; gavage feeding may be necessary. Antibiotics, blood, gamma globulin or steroids have not been found to influence the disease. Antiprotozoal and antifungal agents have been used. The aromatic diamidines and pentavalent antimony compounds, e.g. neostibosan, pentamidine isothionate and stilbamidine, have been reported as being successful in treatment and are deserving of further trial.

REFERENCES

Burke, B. A., Krovetz, L. J., and Good, R. A.: Occurrence of Pneumocystis Carinii Pneumonia in Children with Agammaglobulinemia. *Pediatrics*, 28:196, 1961.

Erchul, J. W., Williams, L. P., and Meighan, P. P.: Pneumocystis Carinii in Hypopharyngeal Material. *New England J. Med.*, 267: 926, 1962.

Gajdusek, D. C.: Pneumocystis Carinii: Etiological Agent of Interstitial Plasma Cell Pneumonia of Premature and Young Infants. *Pediatrics*, 19:543, 1957.

Gerrard, J. W.: Pneumocystis Pneumonia. *Pediat. Clin. N. Amer.*, 5:323-35, 1958.

Ivady, G., Paldy, L., and Unger, G.: Weitere Erfahrungen bei der Behandlung der interstitiellen plasmazellularen Pneumonie mit Pentamidine R. *Monatschr. f. Kinderh.*, 111: 297, 1963.

Marshall, W. C., Weston, H. J., and Bodian, M.: Pneumocystis Carinii Pneumonia and Congenital Hypogammaglobulinaemia. *Arch. Dis. Childhood*, 39:18, 1964.

Robbins, J. B., Miller, R. H., Arean, V. M., and Pearson, H. A.: Successful Treatment of Pneumocystis Carinii Pneumonia in a Patient with Congenital Hypogammaglobulinemia. *New England J. Med.*, 272:708, 1965.

Sheldon, W. H.: Pulmonary Pneumocystis Carinii Infection. *J. Pediat.*, 61:780, 1962.

Vanek, J., and Jirovec, O.: Parasitare Pneumonia. "Interstitielle" Plasmazellen- Pneumonia der Frühgeborenen, verursacht durch Pneumocystis Carinii. *Zentralbl. f. Bakt.*, 158:120, 1952.

Weintraub, H. D., and Wilson, W. J.: Pneumocystis Carinii Pneumonia in Wiskott-Aldrich Syndrome. *Am. J. Dis. Child.*, 108:198, 1964.

CHAPTER TWENTY-FIVE

Viral Pneumonia

HENRY G. CRAMBLETT, M.D.

Recent data from etiologic studies of respiratory disease in infants and children indicate that a large number of viruses may cause pneumonia in infants and children.

Incidence

There are no definitive etiologic studies to date which enable one to compare the incidence of children hospitalized with viral pneumonia with that of children admitted because of pneumonia due to bacteria or *Mycoplasma pneumoniae*. Likewise, there are no data to allow one to generalize about the frequency of viral pneumonia in children of various ages. Meaningful data will be derived only from carefully designed studies from different geographic areas encompassing more than a one-year experience. Undoubtedly, the importance of the various viruses in the causation of pneumonia will vary from year to year in each geographic area.

Etiology

Many viruses have been etiologically associated with pneumonia in infants and children. These include respiratory syncytial virus, parainfluenza viruses, rhinoviruses, influenza viruses, adenoviruses and psittacosis virus. Although the agent of psittacosis is not considered to be a "true" virus, it is listed here for the sake of completeness.

There are many indications that an infant's or young child's first infection with many of the respiratory viruses may give rise to great expressivity in clinical disease. Data at present indicate that illnesses accompanying recurrent infections with a given virus are usually less severe

and are more likely to involve the upper respiratory tract. Thus it is not surprising that viral pneumonia appears to be more frequent in infants and younger children than in older children. Of the respiratory viruses thus far recovered, respiratory syncytial and the parainfluenza viruses are the ones most likely to cause pneumonia.

Pathogenesis

Frequently the viral infection will involve the mucous membranes of the upper respiratory passage prior to involvement of the lung parenchyma. In the lungs the lesion usually consists of an interstitial mononuclear infiltrate. The infiltrate may have a peribronchial distribution.

Clinical Manifestations

In an individual patient there are no readily available means to differentiate between pneumonia due to a virus and that due to a bacterium or *Mycoplasma pneumoniae*. Ordinarily, upper respiratory symptoms of several days' duration, including fever, coryza, hoarseness, sore throat and cough, precede the pulmonary illness. After this there may be a second febrile period in which the symptoms of cough and fever are exaggerated and there is the concomitant appearance of physical findings suggestive of viral pneumonia. Clinically, such a biphasic illness suggests that the causative organism of the disease is viral.

Diagnosis

A specific virus diagnosis may be established by the culturing of respiratory secretions and the recovery of the specific viral agent by tissue culture techniques. Serologic tests are also available for the diagnosis of adenovirus, respiratory syncytial and parainfluenza virus infection.

From the radiologic point of view, the infiltrates in viral pneumonia tend to be diffuse, ill-defined and hazy. It is not uncommon to have more than one lobe involved simultaneously. Pleural effusions and consolidation do not occur in primary viral pneumonia.

Treatment

Antibiotics are of no value in the treatment of viral pneumonia. Symptomatic therapy, including bed rest, acetylsalicylic acid for fever, and the use of humidity for younger children and infants, may be of value.

CHAPTER TWENTY-SIX

Infections of the Respiratory Tract Due to Mycoplasma Pneumoniae (Eaton Agent; Primary Atypical Pneumonia)

HENRY G. CRAMBLETT, M.D.

With the recovery and recent characterization of *Mycoplasma pneumoniae*, much of the confusion over the syndromes variously termed "primary atypical pneumonia," "Eaton agent pneumonia," "cold-agglutinin-positive pneumonia" and "viral pneumonia" has been dispelled. *Mycoplasma pneumoniae* is a pleuropneumonia-like organism, and studies to date indicate that many of the respiratory syndromes mentioned above are due to this agent.

Incidence

It has been estimated that *Mycoplasma pneumoniae* is responsible for 9 to 20 per cent of the hospital admissions of infants and children with pneumonia. Moreover, in 24 to 30 per cent of adults hospitalized with pneumonia, the disease is caused by *Mycoplasma pneumoniae*. In general, pneumonia caused by *Mycoplasma pneumoniae* occurs most often in persons ten to twenty-five years of age and least often in children less than five years.

Etiology

Mycoplasma pneumoniae was first isolated in 1944 by Eaton and his colleagues, and the organism has subsequently been called Eaton's agent. In early studies the agent was thought to be a virus, but the

observation that broad-spectrum antibiotics shortened the course of the disease
suggested that Eaton's agent was not a
virus. Liu in 1957 used fluorescent microscopy to demonstrate that infections with
this agent resulted in cold-agglutinin-
positive pneumonia and that patients exhibited a rise in antibody titer during
convalescence. The successful cultivation
of the Eaton agent on cell-free media and
its positive definition as a PPLO or Mycoplasma was accomplished by Chanock,
Hayflick and Barile in 1962.

Mycoplasma pneumoniae is 180 to 220
millimicrons in diameter as measured by
filtration. The organism appears either as
a very small coccus or coccobacillus. The
colonies are 10 to 50 microns in diameter
and usually appear as small spheres with
a "fried egg" appearance submerged in
agar. The agent can be propagated aerobically on specially prepared media containing yeast extract and horse serum, or in
chick embryos by amniotic inoculation.
Mycoplasma pneumoniae produces pneumonia in both cotton rats and hamsters
and grows in a variety of tissue cultures.
Mycoplasma pneumoniae may be differentiated from other known human mycoplasma by demonstrating that it is able to
cause lysis (beta hemolysis) of red blood
cells.

Pathogenesis

The incubation period has been established by human volunteer experiments
as seven to fourteen days in those patients
who had pneumonia and from one to
nineteen days in those who had other
types of respiratory illness. Frequently, at
onset the disease shows involvement of
the upper respiratory tract with rhinitis
and pharyngitis. The principal pathologic
changes occur in the lower respiratory
tract with inflammation of the tracheal
and bronchial mucosa. There may be obstruction of terminal bronchioles with alternating atelectasis and emphysema. The
parenchymal interstitial infiltration is
composed largely of round cells.

Clinical Manifestations

Clinically, there is little to distinguish
pneumonia due to *Mycoplasma pneumoniae* from that caused by bacteria or viruses. Ordinarily, the onset is abrupt with
constitutional symptoms of fever, chills,
myalagia, headache and malaise. These
symptoms usually precede the initial respiratory symptoms of rhinitis and sore
throat. After this there is a dry, hacking
cough, which eventually is productive of
a seromucoid or, later, a mucopurulent
sputum. Substernal pain or "pressure"
and abdominal pain are late symptoms.

The initial physical examination may
reveal amazingly few signs in comparison
with the symptoms or the appearance of
the chest roentgenogram. If not present
initially, eventually fine, inspiratory
"sticky" rales will be heard on auscultation of the lungs. Later in the course of
the disease, atelectasis may produce signs
suggestive of consolidation. Fever may be
remittent and intermittent and frequently
subsides by lysis.

Although to date pneumonia has been
present in the majority of patients from
whom *Mycoplasma pneumoniae* has been
recovered, other patients have been observed who have had febrile rhinitis,
bronchitis, bronchiolitis and bullous myringitis.

Diagnosis

On roentgenogram, the findings in
pulmonary infections due to *Mycoplasma
pneumoniae* may resemble those of bacterial bronchopneumonia. But because
the parenchymal infiltrate is peribronchial
and not exudative, the shadows are usually softer and "fluffier" and tend to be
ill defined. There are increased bronchovascular markings, areas of atelectasis and
rarely interlobar fluid. The densities are
frequently wedge-shaped, radiating out
from the hilus (Fig. 1). The lower lobes
are most frequently involved, and in at
least 50 per cent of cases there is involvement of more than one lobe.

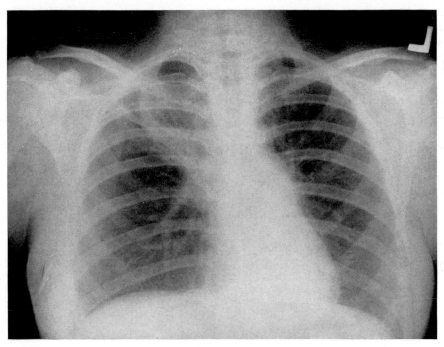

FIGURE 26–1. Chest roentgenogram of a 13 year-old girl hospitalized with cough, dyspnea, headache and anorexia of one week's duration. Illness began 2 weeks before admission with malaise, sore throat and headache. Cold agglutinins were present in a titer of 1:512 at time of hospitalization. The wedge-shaped infiltrate with a linear radiation in the right upper lobe is characteristic of infections due to *Mycoplasma pneumoniae*. (Roentgenogram courtesy of Dr. Frank Stroebel.)

The simplest serologic test for the diagnosis of *Mycoplasma pneumoniae* infection is the demonstration of at least a fourfold rise in cold agglutinins in the patient's convalescent serum, as compared with the level in the serum taken during the acute phase of the disease. Cold agglutinins usually do not develop until seven to ten days after the onset of symptoms. In addition to the diagnostic fourfold rise in titer in the convalescent serum, a randomly selected serum with a titer of 1:32 or greater carries similar diagnostic importance. Blood for the test must be allowed to clot at room temperature, since clotting at a lower temperature permits autoadsorption of antibody. Unfortunately, however, even though the test is simple to perform, it is relatively nonspecific. To date studies indicate that no more than 50 to 60 per cent of patients with *Mycoplasma pneumoniae* infections develop cold agglutinins. Those with the

more severe illnesses are more likely to develop cold agglutinins than those with less severe illness. Further, as many as 17 per cent of those patients with pneumonia due to adenoviruses or those from whom no etiologic agents can be recovered also develop rises in cold agglutinins. False-positive reactions also occur in hepatitis, cirrhosis, hemolytic anemia, infectious mononucleosis and sepsis. The Streptococcus MG test is also nonspecific, and the same deficiencies characteristic of the test for cold hemagglutinins apply.

The definitive diagnosis may be established only by the recovery of the organism or by the demonstration of a specific antibody response. *Mycoplasma pneumoniae* may be recovered from the sputum, washings of pharyngeal swabs in cotton rats, embryonated eggs, tissue culture and on cell-free artificial media. The infection may be prolonged, and the recovery of *Mycoplasma pneumoniae* as late as forty-five days after the onset of symptoms has been reported. The use of artificial media for propagation of these organisms is being adapted to the routine clinical diagnostic microbiology laboratory. The fluorescent antibody test has been extensively evaluated, but the technique is difficult to perform and is usually available only in research laboratories. There is an indication that there may be a complement fixation procedure which would be adaptable for use in the routine diagnostic laboratory.

Complications

Although the complications are few, recovery may be protracted. Otitis externa and inflammation of the tympanic membrane (bullous myringitis), pericarditis and erythema nodosum have been reported.

Course

The course of untreated pneumonia due to *Mycoplasma pneumoniae* may be long. It is not unusual for abnormal roentgenographic findings, cough and rales to persist for seven to twenty-one days after the onset, but fever, headache, malaise and fatigue rarely persist more than ten days. The chest roentgenogram may show actual progression of the pulmonary infiltrate between the fourth and sixteenth days of illness. This finding is in contrast to that in other types of pneumonia due to viruses in which the maximal roentgenographic involvement is usually demonstrable on the initial film.

Prognosis

Although the course of the infection and the illness may be protracted, recovery is the usual result.

Treatment

Few carefully controlled studies of the efficacy of antibiotics in the therapy of *Mycoplasma pneumoniae* infections have been reported since the means of establishing a precise etiologic diagnosis have become available. In-vitro sensitivity tests indicate that there are a number of potentially useful antibiotics, including the tetracyclines, chloramphenicol, erythromycin and oleandomycin. In one controlled study in which the specific diagnosis was established, the efficacy of demethylchlortetracycline was proved. In all probability, other tetracyclines will prove to be equally effective.

REFERENCES

Clyde, W. A., Jr., and Denny, F. W., Jr.: The Etiology and Therapy of Atypical Pneumonia. *Med. Clin. N. Amer.*, 47:1201-18, 1963.

Chanock, R. M., Hayflick, L., and Barile, M. F.: Growth on Artificial Medium of an Agent Associated with Atypical Pneumonia and Its Identification as a PPLO. *Proc. Nat. Acad. Sc.*, 48:41-9, 1962.

Grayston, J. T., and others: Mycoplasma Pneumoniae Infections: Clinical and Epidemiologic Studies. *J.A.M.A.*, 191:369-74, 1965.

Rytel, M. W.: Primary Atypical Pneumonia: Current Concepts. *Am. J. M. Sc.*, 247:84-104, 1964.

CHAPTER TWENTY-SEVEN

Influenza

ROBERT H. PARROTT, M.D.

For many years influenza viruses were the only laboratory-defined nonbacterial agents proved as respiratory tract pathogens. They are members of the myxovirus group and fulfill all the original criteria for inclusion in this group: hemagglutination of fowl red blood cells; association of receptor-destroying enzyme with the virus; destruction of virus red cell receptors by receptor-destroying enzyme; removal of a normal inhibitor from the serum by receptor-destroying enzyme; growth, at least under laboratory conditions, in the amniotic cavity of hens' eggs; size in the range of 80 to 200 millimicrons; ether sensitivity, stability at $-70°$C. and acid lability. More specifically, influenza viruses are comprised of a virion 80 to 120 millimicrons in diameter. They contain a ribonucleic acid nucleoprotein, central helix which is approximately 9 to 10 millimicrons in diameter, surrounded by an envelope of lipoprotein. The envelope has periodic projections or spikes which house the hemagglutinating activity of the agent.

There are three distinct serotypes of influenza virus: A, B and C. Within the A and B serotypes there is significant antigenic variation in structure which favors the appearance of several subtypes. This variation accounts for the ability of influenza to produce epidemics even in populations of persons who have previously experienced influenza infection or immunization. Indeed, the importance of recognizing antigenic changes among current strains is not that there is any significant difference in the clinical response, but that there are serious epidemiologic implications concerning the preparation and availability of effective vaccines.

Influenza infection often occurs in epidemics which may sweep through a community in a matter of one or two months. Morbidity in a susceptible population may be high and is particularly severe in infants and very old patients. The incidence of infection and illness is, however, highest in childen of school age. Type and subtype specific immunity after natural infection is not of high order; children may become infected several times within a matter of years, owing to the same or related strains. Detectable type-specific antibodies, however, do occur and persist. There is evidence that antibody developed against earlier strains may rise during a subsequent infection with a related strain of influenza virus. Perhaps this is why the incidence of influenza infection and clinical illness is lower in older children, young adults and adults than in school-age children.

Laboratory proof of influenza virus infection may include either recovery of the virus from throat washings and swabbings or evidence of a rise in antibody during convalescence from illness. Chick embryo has been the traditional laboratory host for isolation of influenza viruses. The clinical specimen is preferably inoculated into the amniotic sac of thirteen- to fourteen-day-old chick embryos. The amniotic fluid is harvested in two or three days and tested for hemagglutinins with chicken red blood cells. The inoculation of monkey kidney tissue cultures, however, and the subsequent development of hemadsorption, which occurs with myxovirus-infected tissue culture, seems to be a simpler and more sensitive method. Type-specific serums are used to identify the virus recovered in egg or tissue culture. Serums obtained early and about three weeks after the onset of illness are tested for antibodies to influenza

313

virus by complement fixation, hemagglutination inhibition or tissue culture neutralization methods.

One of the predominant pathogenic characteristics of influenza viruses in susceptible hosts such as chick embryo, ferret or man is a peculiar affinity for epithelial cells of the respiratory tract mucosa. Typically, influenza virus infection destroys ciliated epithelium, and there is metaplastic hyperplasia of the tracheal and bronchial epithelium plus edema. The alveoli may become distended with a hyaline-like material.

Infection and the damage to respiratory tract epithelium in man may be subclinical or be accompanied by mild, moderate or severe clinical manifestations. In most cases of overt illness the throat and nasal mucous membranes are dry, and there is a dry cough with a tendency toward hoarseness. There is fever of sudden onset accompanied in a child by a flushed facies, photophobia with retrobulbar pain, myalgia, hyperesthesia and sometimes prostration. In uncomplicated cases these symptoms last for four or five days.

In some influenza outbreaks children have a severe clinical reaction. For example, in 1957 and 1958, of forty hospitalized patients wtih influenza A-2 (Asian) or B infection, 50 per cent had bronchopneumonia, 27 per cent had the croup syndrome, and 23 per cent had severe bronchitis. Bacterial infection due to *H. influenzae,* beta hemolytic streptococci, or *Staphylococcus aureus* may complicate influenza infection, apparently with a higher frequency than in other viral illnesses. Pneumonia is the principal clinical manifestation of bacterial invasion.

There is no specific *therapy* for influenza virus infection. Many clinicians caution against widespread use of antibiotics during the influenza epidemic because antibiotic-resistant bacteria become a secondary problem. Experimentally, the drug amantadine has been shown to have some effect in preventing and possibly ameliorating influenza virus infection. More studies are required, however, to assess the chemotherapeutic value of this drug in influenza infection.

A multivalent inactivated influenza virus vaccine is available for immunization. The composition of the vaccine can be changed according to current antigenic variants. The number of severe cases of influenza is relatively few, but they do occur. Since there is no specific therapy, routine influenza immune *prophylaxis* for children might seem advisable. A majority, however, recommend that such prophylaxis be limited to children at unusual risk of severe complications, because local and systemic febrile reactions to egg-grown influenza vaccine occur much more often in children than in adults; specific protection is conferred for only a year or less; there is also doubt that protection is afforded against strains other than those included in this vaccine, particularly in the very young who have had no previous antigenic experience with influenza viruses. Therefore the decision to use influenza vaccine routinely must take into account the likelihood that such vaccines in children will reduce no more than 5 per cent of respiratory tract illness requiring hospitalization.

REFERENCES

Curnen, B. C.: Influenza and the Use of Killed Virus Vaccines for Its Prevention in Children; in *Viral Infections of Infancy and Childhood.* New York, Paul B. Hoeber, Inc. 1960, Chap. 11.

Davenport, F. M.: Current Knowledge of Influenza Vaccine. *J.A.M.A.,* 182:11, 1962.

Francis, T.: Influenza. *Med. Clin. N. Amer.,* 43:1309, 1959.

Parrott, R. H., Kim, H. W., Vargosko, A. J., and Chanock, R. M.: Serious Respiratory Tract Illness as a Result of Asian Influenza and Influenza Type B Infections in Children. *J. Pediat.,* 61:205, 1962.

CHAPTER TWENTY-EIGHT

Bronchiectasis

ROSA LEE NEMIR, M.D.

Bronchiectasis, meaning dilatation of bronchi, was first described by Laennec in 1819 in his *Traité de l'Auscultation Médiate.* Since this first report, extensive literature has accumulated giving the natural history of the disease based on both clinical and experimental observations. Currently, reports on effective surgical procedures are appearing.

Incidence

The true incidence of bronchiectasis is not reflected by any statistical report, and an accurate statement of its frequency is difficult. Bronchography, the most reliable diagnostic test, is not used often enough in those asymptomatic patients whose history suggests the possibility of bronchial damage; nor is it applied to many of those recovering from such infections as pertussis and measles in whom continuing symptoms and persistent roentgenographic findings suggest an underlying pulmonary pathology.

Clark, reviewing the experience in Great Britain, suggested an annual incidence in 1951 of 1.06 per 10,000 children. In the United States, Ruberman and others reviewed 1711 patients with pneumonia and studied by bronchography sixty-nine children whose chest x-rays showed residual findings. Bronchiectasis was present in twenty-nine, or 1.7 per cent. In Copenhagen, in a follow-up study of 151 patients who had pneumonia or pertussis possibly complicated by pneumonia, Biering found only one child with bronchiectasis.

Certainly children with the classic symptoms of bronchiectasis have not been commonly seen during the past decade. The decreased incidence is probably the result of two factors: a decrease in the incidence of such childhood infections as pertussis and measles, which are commonly associated with the development of bronchiectasis; and the effective use of antibacterial agents in preventing and promptly curing the common lower respiratory tract infections.

Factors Associated with the Development of Bronchiectasis

Congenital bronchiectasis, long a subject of discussion, is now generally accepted as existent and responsible for a small percentage of recognizable disease. It is thought to be the result of developmental arrest. In postnatal developmental arrest the involved areas may result in the formation of cysts which retain fluid or air and which may become infected, resulting in saccular bronchiectasis. The signs of disease usually appear early, but are contingent on the frequency of the predisposing respiratory infections.

ACQUIRED BRONCHIECTASIS. Most of the patients belong in this group. Many clinical studies involving large numbers of children have established that the three most frequent antecedent infections are pertussis, measles and pneumonia. Other predisposing factors are those associated with bronchial obstruction: foreign body aspiration, enlarged bronchopulmonary nodes of primary tuberculosis or other causes, and mediastinal masses and tumors.

In 1933 Kartagener described a syndrome consisting of the triad of bronchiectasis, sinusitis and situs inversus. The greater frequency of bronchiectasis in such instances has been documented by many reports. According to Adams and Churchill and Olsen, who also described an accompanying nasal polyposis in many of his cases, the frequency of bronchiectasis in congenital dextrocardia is from 15 to 20 per cent. The rarity of this triad among all patients with bronchiectasis is apparent in Perry and King's report of 400 patients, only six of whom were found to have the Kartagener syndrome.

The familial nature of bronchiectasis is indicated by a report of two children in one family, and the genetic factor, postulated by Cockayne and developed by Torgersen, is supported by its presence in identical twins. The cause of the high incidence of bronchiectasis among the Maoris in New Zealand has not been determined, but among the sixty-five described by Hinds, none had dextrocardia or cystic fibrosis.

It is understandable that the diffuse, frequent respiratory infections in patients with cystic fibrosis of the pancreas may produce extensive bronchial damage resulting ultimately in pulmonary complications such as bronchiectasis. The pathology and pathogenesis of the pulmonary lesions have been well described. The frequency of cystic fibrosis was surprisingly high in one study from Australia with fifty-seven cases among 241 patients studied (1959).

Similarly, patients with agammaglobulinemia have acquired bronchiectasis. Collins and Dudley reported the pathologic findings in two such cases and Visconti in another. Nevertheless gamma globulin deficiency does not appear to be commonly associated with bronchiectasis. Pittman, for example, studied the gamma globulin concentrations in fifty-two patients with long-standing bronchiectasis. She failed to find any with agammaglobulinemia, but found one patient with hypogammaglobulinemia whom she treated over a four-year period.

Asthma and chronic sinusitis are frequently present in patients with bronchiectasis, whether as antecedent or complication is not yet clear. Today, with the liberal use of antibiotics, sinusitis is less common and, when it occurs, is usually amenable to medical therapy. The causal or sequential relationship should soon become apparent.

REVERSIBLE AND IRREVERSIBLE BRONCHIECTASIS. The type of pneumonia preceding bronchiectasis is more often interstitial or bronchopneumonic. Such infection is associated with bronchial pathology because of peribronchial infiltration and endobronchial edema, mucosal swelling, and obstruction by mucosecretions. Serial bronchograms in patients with prolonged atypical pneumonia have demonstrated that bronchial dilatation may clear within two to three months in many instances.

The term *reversible bronchiectasis* is generally applied to this pathologic state, and Blades and Dugan called these cases *pseudobronchiectasis*. It has become clear that bronchial dilatation described as cylindrical may be reversible, but saccular bronchiectasis is irreversible. Lees has shown that cylindrical bronchiectasis is relatively common after pertussis in which viscid secretions are abundant. This concept of reversible bronchiectasis, entailing the disappearance of the compensatory bronchial dilatation following the expansion of a previously collapsed portion of the lung, is important to the clinician, pointing up the need for a follow-up bronchogram before pulmonary resection is recommended. Nelson and Christoforidis, for example, reported four patients who were thought to have cylindrical bronchiectasis shortly after pneumonia, but were spared operation by a second bronchogram, interpreted as normal.

Pathogenesis

A number of experimental studies and extensive publications have thrown new light on the long controversy over the pathogenesis of bronchiectasis. It is now generally agreed that infection and obstruction of the bronchi are the two important etiologic factors in the production of acquired bronchiectasis. It is also clear that mechanical stress and obstruction alone may not result in permanent damage to the bronchi. It is still not certain in which order these two underlying causes need to occur. Certainly they complement each other in the development of damaged bronchi.

In atelectatic areas produced by the obstruction of major bronchi or peripheral bronchi where the dilatation compensates for the decreased parenchymal lung volume, the retained bronchial secretions favor anaerobic growth which results in damage to bronchial walls. The pressure of tuberculous bronchopulmonary nodes damages the bronchi early, often eroding the bronchus and injuring its elastic tissue and muscular wall. Stenosis alone may occur, or bronchiectasis may develop later.

In patients with pneumonia, severe bronchial infection may produce abnormal physiology associated with decreased ciliary action and necrosis of the bronchial walls. These factors, together with retained bronchial secretions, may lead to weakening of the walls of the bronchi and resultant dilatation.

Clinically and experimentally, atelectasis over a period of time may occur without subsequent ectasia of the bronchi. Lees, in a report of 150 children with pertussis, found atelectasis in sixty-five, or 43 per cent, and yet found only four cases of bronchiectasis, three reversible and one showing possible permanent damage on follow-up. On the other hand, similar observations by others in children with bronchiectasis have stressed atelectasis as an antecedent factor.

Anspach described the triangular shadow adjacent to the heart as atelectasis of the lower lobe of the lung and pointed out the direct relation of the long duration of such obstruction to the development of bronchiectasis. Indeed, necropsies in infants dying early in the course of such lower lobe collapse failed to show bronchial dilatation even though thick exudate filled the smaller bronchi.

The well known experimental work in rabbits done by Tannenberg and Pinner showed that ligation of the bronchi alone did not lead to bronchiectasis. They concluded that the mechanical forces operating when air is absorbed after bronchial occlusion tend to constrict, not dilate, bronchi and that uncomplicated pulmonary atelectasis would not cause bronchiectasis unless accompanied by infection. Such an infection may produce, within three to four weeks, an extensive saccular bronchiectasis in an atelectatic lung.

Experimental work on dogs by Croxatto and Lanari also demonstrated the effect of bronchial ligation on dilatation of the bronchi by retained secretions. Within two months the bronchial dilatation became stabilized. "Infection superimposed to the dilatation produced by retained secretions led to the production of bronchiectasis and . . . in some cases, even though the dilating material was extracted, the bronchus remained dilated." Clearly, in some instances, the bronchial dilatation was reversible.

A controlled experimental study was done by Cheng, who subjected rats to both sham and actual bronchial ligation, using antibiotic therapy in some. From his investigation Cheng suggested that bronchitis and stagnation of the accompanying secretions and exudate are two essential factors in the development of bronchiectasis. He concluded that bronchiectasis is apparently due to the pressure of accumulated stagnant secretions on bronchial walls weakened by inflammation.

Parenchymal collapse of varying extent occurs early in bronchiectasis on the basis of bronchial obstruction alone, extrinsic or intrinsic, and late in the disease on the basis of resultant bronchial wall pathology. The normal flexibility of the bronchi is lost when the elastic and muscular tissues are destroyed and replaced by fibrous tissues.

Pathology

Until several decades ago the pathology of bronchiectasis was based on postmortem specimens of advanced disease. Large ectatic bronchi filled with purulent material were grossly characteristic of the disease, and the adjacent parenchyma was usually infected, showing diffuse pneumonia or abscesses and sometimes emphysema. Such pathologic features are seen less frequently today because antibiotic therapy has prevented many advanced inflammatory lesions, and surgical resection, in suitable cases, has cured many patients. Surgery has also made available for pathologic study ample material which reflects the stages in the development of bronchiectasis, so that mild, moderate and severe instances may be analyzed. Macroscopically, in acquired bronchiectasis, there are dilated bronchi, whether fusiform, cylindrical or saccular; often parenchymal collapse of the involved lobe; and usually pleural thickening with strong adhesions. If the disease is early, cylindrical or fusiform bronchi are found; if late, the saccular variety occurs, often filled with mucopurulent material. Occasionally an accompanying bronchopneumonia or fibrosis and patchy emphysema in the area distal to the diseased bronchi may be found.

Microscopically, the chief lesion is found in the bronchi; the duration of infection determines the tissue reaction. There is relatively severe bronchial destruction with inflammatory changes. The progression of bronchial wall damage is, first, destruction of elastic tissue; next, damage to the muscular coat; and finally, damage to the cartilage of the bronchi. Calcifications have also been described in the cartilage. These sequential changes have been especially well analyzed by Whitwell, who used 200 consecutive specimens from the bronchial epithelial lining. The columnar cells are replaced by cuboidal and then by squamous cells which are sometimes heaped into layers. Notably, long-standing bronchiectasis is associated with epithelial cells which show absence of or scanty cilia. The bronchial lining may be ulcerated, fibrosed or denuded, sometimes immediately overlying distended blood vessels. Such areas may lead to hemoptysis. Ogilvie described these and other lesions and emphasized, as did Whitwell, the pronounced increase in size of the bronchial glands, lymphoid hyperplasia, and hypertrophy of mucous glands

which may obstruct the bronchi. Important changes in the vascular structure of both bronchial and pulmonary arteries may occur in the diseased lung. In human beings there may be enlarged aneurysmal structures often associated with a history of hemoptysis. The walls of the bronchial arteries may be thickened, and there may be hyperplasia of the intima.

Other pathologic findings may be related to the etiologic factor of an associated disease such as tuberculous hilar or bronchial lymph nodes, evidence of cystic fibrosis of the pancreas, of asthma or of situs inversus.

SITE OF BRONCHIECTASIS. The left lower lobe is most frequently involved, with both lower lobes more often involved than the upper lobes. The right middle lobe is the common site of foreign body aspiration and of collapse from the pressure of tuberculous bronchial lymph nodes. When bronchiectasis is bilateral, it is usually patchy; the most common pattern is a combination of left lower lobe and lingula and right middle and lower lobes. Perry and King reported a 54 per cent incidence of left lower lobe bronchiectasis (usually including the lingula as well) in 400 patients of all ages. In children, Strang and later Clark also reported that bronchiectasis occurred more often in the left lower lobe. Swierenga, in a critical analysis of 221 children under sixteen years of age with bronchiectasis, related the site of the disease to the history and found that the right side predominated when tuberculosis or aspiration of a foreign body was responsible.

The predisposition of the left lower lobe to atelectasis and bronchiectasis may be due to the fact that the left main bronchus is two thirds the size of the right main bronchus and, secondly, that the left main bronchus crosses the mediastinum at an acute angle behind the aorta, by which it can be readily compressed. Whitwell, who also found the left lower lobe involved three times more frequently than the right in 200 consecutive resection specimens, explained the bilateral lesions as follows: "Clinical evidence is against the view that bronchiectasis spreads from one lobe to another; a more likely explanation is that at the onset of disease the bronchi are subjected to varying degrees of injury."

Clinical Features

Bronchiectasis may present a broad spectrum of clinical features from the full-blown classic picture of the chronically ill patient to the healthy-appearing, fully active child whose only evidence of pulmonary pathology is found in the bronchogram. The former group is rare today. The majority present minimal symptoms and physical findings.

ONSET. The onset may be acute, immediately following an infection such as pneumonia, pertussis or measles, in which continued bronchial obstruction producing collapse suggests the possibility of bronchiectasis in a child who fails to recover or whose chest roentgenograms fail to clear. Another group of patients are those with recurring and chronic pulmonary disease such as asthma, bronchitis and pneumonia in whom increasing or persistent symptoms of illness suggest the need for complete investigation, often including a bronchogram.

It is commonly recognized that tuberculous hilar adenopathy often leads to long-standing parenchymal atelectasis and subsequent bronchial dilatation, but these dilatations usually remain free from disturbing secondary bacterial infection. Consequently they are usually asymptomatic, detectable only on bronchographic study.

In earlier studies the average age of the patient at onset was in childhood, before the age of five years. In these reports percentages varied from 66 to 80 per cent; in more recent reports they are much lower. In Clark's study of 116 children, thirty-five gave a history of symptoms for five years and only twenty-five had symptoms for less than one year.

The nature of the initial illness varies according to authors, the composition of the population (such as the peculiar susceptibility to bronchiectasis seen among the Maoris), and the geographic areas by countries. In Scotland, Clark observed 116 children between 1946 and 1955 and ascribed the illness in more than half to pneumonia, pertussis and measles.

The findings of Williams and O'Reilly in Melbourne included several unusual features: the frequency of cystic fibrosis of the pancreas, and the greater number of patients whose bronchiectasis dated from bronchiolitis or interstitial pneumonia in early childhood. Indeed, those authors grouped their patients clinically into two categories which also differed in response to surgery, the first favorably, the second less successfully. The first group included those patients with subacute pyogenic collapse occurring at all ages, usually beginning as an acute illness associated with pathogenic organisms, and terminating in a unilateral bronchiectasis. In these the genetic history for chronic respiratory disease was negative. The second group consisted of those with nonspecific infectious bronchiolitis, or interstitial pneumonia, occurring under three years of age, unassociated with culturable pathogens, and terminating in diffuse disease and positive bronchographic findings. There appeared to be a strong genetic factor in this latter group; the family history revealed definite bronchiectasis in 14 per cent and probably in an additional 38 per cent. It must be remembered that this series was heavily weighted by patients with cystic fibrosis, in which the genetic factor is known to exist.

The importance of pneumonia as an antecedent to bronchiectasis is well recognized. In the United States 28 per cent of the 400 patients reported by Perry and King had a history of pneumonia, and approximately two thirds of the children in an earlier study by Raia had pneumonia, with or without pertussis, and measles. One third of the series of patients seen by Avery and others between 1940 and 1960 gave a history of pneumonia at onset, but rubeola held a less conspicuous position than in earlier studies.

SIGNS AND SYMPTOMS. The most frequent symptom of bronchiectasis is a cough which may be dry or productive of sputum varying in amount, but greatest in the early morning. Foul-smelling sputum has seldom been encountered in children during the last two decades. Franklin, in his six-year-long observations of 171 children in the Meath School of Recovery for bronchiectatic children, noted that there was no relation between the degree of health and the amount of sputum and cough. Patients with saccular bronchiectasis produce more sputum. Hemoptysis resulting from erosion of the bronchi, particularly in the well advanced saccular variety, is not common (Field), even though bronchiectasis is the most frequent cause of hemoptysis. Irregular episodes of fever may indicate infection in the diseased lung and may be associated with bronchitis or pneumonia. Disturbances of nutrition are seen occasionally in the severe cases. In general, the patients appear well. Dyspnea on exertion, and fatigability are found in those with severe chronic disease.

Clubbing of the fingers varies in frequency from 25 to 50 per cent. Most observers believe that its occurrence is correlated with the activity of disease, but Whitwell found no correlation between the presence of clubbing of the fingers and the extent or severity of pulmonary lesions; nor was there correlation with the nature of the patient's sputum. Long-term observations have demonstrated that clubbing of the extremities is reversible in both medically and surgically treated patients.

Occasional medium moist rales over the ectatic lung, which vary in relation to the bronchial drainage of retained secretions and to the extent of such secretions, may be present. When the bronchi are filled, there may only be some diminution of breath sounds and impairment of resonance. After complete clearing for a period of time there may be no abnormal physical findings. Patients with asthma and bronchiectasis are more apt to have abnormal lung findings, and also have more diffuse pathology with bilateral signs. Such patients are more difficult to treat successfully. Atelectatic areas are often undiagnosed by physical findings, and the collapsed segments of the lung are diagnosed only by chest roentgenograms.

As the child approaches adolescence, he shows improvement. Even patients with known extensive disease may become asymptomatic for a period, sometimes indefinitely; they may have no more respiratory infections than the average adult. But others show greater susceptibility to colds, influenza, sinusitis and chronic bronchitis. Frequent cough, lingering on after the acute episode, is the distinguishing feature of bronchiectasis.

Diagnosis

Three particular categories should lead to further investigation of the bronchial tree: a history of chronic cough, the persistence of atelectasis from whatever cause, and the failure of the chest roentgenogram to clear after respiratory infections or, particularly, after pertussis, measles, bronchiolitis and interstitial pneumonia. Bronchoscopy may be especially indicated for patients with prolonged or recurrent atelectasis, or with abnormal localized lung findings. Occasionally an unsuspected foreign body, such as timothy grass in summer, may be aspirated, or the cause of obstruction may be intrabronchial mucous plugs or the pressure of surrounding tissue such as lymph nodes.

DIAGNOSTIC AIDS. Since the introduction of radiopaque contrast media for the visualization of the bronchial tree by Sicard and Forestier in 1922, a definitive diagnostic tool has been available. Bronchography, as done by the trained physician, is safe, provided a test is given for the rare case of sensitivity to the dye used, and provided the procedure is instituted only after the acute infection has subsided and after a period of proper postural drainage of the bronchial tree. Bronchograms made shortly after acute inflammation show some cylindrical dilation, probably due to the loss of muscle tone secondary to the infection. The lung should be free of secretions and relatively clear from treatable bacterial infections when a bronchogram is performed. Therefore a period of appropriate antimicrobial therapy may be indicated prior to bronchography. If these methods fail to clear the tracheobronchial tree, preliminary bronchoscopy may be desirable before bronchography is attempted. Some authorities recommend that bronchoscopy precede a bronchogram. Bilateral bronchograms may be obtained at one time, except when there is definite impairment of respiratory function; in this case the lung with the greater pulmonary disease should be observed first. Differences in the size of the bronchioles during the inspiratory and expiratory phases in the bronchograms of patients with bronchiectasis as compared with normal subjects have been noted by Isley and others. The patient with bronchiectasis shows a decease in size during forced expiration.

The ordinary roentgenogram of the chest is helpful in suggesting bronchiectasis in some cases, although the four tenets described by Andrus are not always found in bronchiectasis: namely, an increase in pulmonary markings, chronic pneumonia, ring shadows, and displacement of heart and mediastinum. The last, of course, applies only when there is accompanying atelectasis. Lateral and oblique views are needed to clarify and often to diagnose pulmonary collapse. Negative chest roentgenograms may be found in some patients with bronchiectasis.

The honeycombed lung is characterized by areas of circular or polygonal translucencies surrounded by dense fibrous bands. This characteristic finding of advanced disease is correlated in pathologic specimens with pronounced peribronchial fibrosis and emphysema.

In most cases flat plates of the chest and bronchograms are adequate for diagnosis. In some cases in which better understanding of parenchymal shadows at the periphery of bronchi is desired tomobronchography may be helpful. This procedure is rarely indicated in children, and the advisability of additional irradiation must be weighed in determining its use. Pulmonary function studies are helpful in the management of the patient and in deciding on the suitability of surgical therapy.

The microbial flora in the patient with bronchiectasis is varied and in many instances has no causal relation to the disease symptoms or even to the exacerbations. A mixed flora of bacteria, pneumococci, streptococci and staphylococci, fusiform bacilli, and spirochetes has been described. The *Hemophilus influenzae* has repeatedly been isolated by many workers, recently by Allibone and others. The search for infectious agents in 137 Naval recruits with cylindrical bronchiectasis by Rytel and others included cultures for mycoplasma and bacteria grown from material obtained by bronchoscopy from the diseased lung. Viral tissue culture studies and complement fixation tests for adenovirus infections also were made. This study resulted in an unusually small percentage of *Hemophilus influenzae* (5.5 per cent); the finding of a high incidence of antibody titer to adenovirus of 1:64 or greater (present in 46 per cent of those with bronchiectasis as compared to 27 per cent with bronchopneumonia), although a virus (influenza B) was isolated in only two patients; and finally, the failure to isolate mycoplasma from a single case.

Disease States Associated with Bronchiectasis

SINUSITIS. The frequent association of sinusitis with bronchiectasis has been noted by clinicians, especially in the earlier studies. More recent observers find that sinusitis is much less frequent and troublesome.

The interrelation of sinusitis and lower respiratory tract infection associated with chronic productive sputum is apparent. The determination of the identity of the original offender required study. Ormerod contributed evidence that iodized poppy seed oil (Lipiodol) could be found in the nasal passages shortly after use of the oil in bronchography. Previously

McLaurin had demonstrated Lipiodol in the bronchial tree twenty-four to forty-eight hours after injection into the sinuses.

The continuity of the epithelial lining of the upper and lower respiratory tract facilitates the spread of infection from one area to another. The antibiotic era is associated with the decreased incidence of persistent infection in sinuses. Since the organisms most commonly cultured from the sinuses (*Staphylococcus aureus*, coagulase-positive, or Streptococcus) are usually susceptible to antimicrobial therapy, effective clearing of infected sinuses may be accomplished, even though Hogg and Brock have suggested that severe bronchiectasis will continue to reinfect the sinuses.

There is a cycle of infection between upper and lower tract infection until the bronchiectasis is cleared. In many instances the edematous sinuses reflect an allergic state which underlies the bronchiectasis.

ASTHMA.   The frequency of asthma in patients with bronchiectasis has varied in different groups. Wheezing, a common finding in bronchiectatic patients, does not always denote allergic asthma. In Field's group a high proportion of children were found to have asthma, and she emphasized the poorer prognosis in this group. The seriousness of asthma as a diffuse disease underlying bronchiectasis when the two coexist is illustrated by the pulmonary function studies made by Strang, who found that abnormal pulmonary function tests associated with obstruction to air flow persisted between attacks of overt wheezing, suggesting an association with either bronchial obstruction or pulmonary fibrosis or a combination of both.

Gomez and Filler found that the specific tidal volume during an attack differed from that of normal children, owing to the presence of obstacles to the diffusion of molecules in the gaseous phase of the lung.

TUBERCULOSIS. The association of childhood tuberculosis with bronchiec-

tasis has been indicated repeatedly and is related to the bronchial obstruction by the hilar and mediastinal lymph nodes. The greater frequency of right lung pathology has also been noted.

Respiratory infections occur more often in children with *serum protein deficiency, dysgammaglobulinemia* and *agammaglobulinemia*. The bronchial damage and resultant bronchiectasis will depend on the sequence and the type of infection.

CYSTIC FIBROSIS.   Similarly, the diffuse bronchial epithelial pathology of the uncontrolled patient with fibrocystic disease of the pancreas makes these patients fertile ground for the development of bronchiectasis. Diarrheal episodes in patients with bronchiectasis, especially early in life, should lead to an investigation of the chlorides by sweat tests and other suitable methods (see Cystic Fibrosis, p. 541).

SYSTEMIC DISEASES.   An increasing volume of literature indicates the association between bronchiectasis and such systemic diseases as xanthomatosis, tuberous sclerosis, scleroderma, and cystic lung disease with fibrotic changes. The bronchiectasis in all these diseases is not distinctive, and pathologic specimens of the lungs do not suggest these underlying disease states.

Medical Treatment

Once the diagnosis of bronchiectasis is established, it should be determined whether or not the damage is irreversible, remembering the tendency of the bronchial tree to dilate after certain pneumonias and to produce cylindrical reversible or "pseudo"-bronchiectasis. Drainage of the retained secretions is essential and is usually accomplished by postural drainage, but sometimes requires bronchoscopy. Postural drainage exercises, occasional use of positive-pressure breathing, and warm, moist inhalations are helpful in promoting drainage.

Relief of atelectasis, which entails investigation of its cause, is essential for the ultimate success of bronchiectasis therapy.

Bronchoscopy is indicated for the persistent segmental or lobar atelectasis that fails to respond to postural drainage.

The possibility of sinusitis coexisting with bronchiectasis should always be remembered. Attention should be given to the general health of the patient, and tests should be made for the study of any underlying predisposing pathology as described in the preceding section. Antibiotics and chemotherapy may be used for the acute episodes, as indicated by bacterial cultures and antibiotic resistance determinations.

The introduction of penicillin marked the beginning of a new era in the medical treatment of bronchiectasis. In 1945 Kay and Meade reported the value of penicillin in preoperative treatment, and its effectiveness in reducing sputum in some patients after parenteral therapy. After many studies, chiefly in adults, long-term administration of antibiotics, whether continuous or interrupted, is not generally recommended. Relatively short courses of a few days to several weeks are desirable if needed. Many infections, especially in young children, are of viral origin and are not responsive to such therapy. The possibility of side effects from the long-standing use of such medication, as well as interference with microbial balance and the possible subsequent invasion by mycotic infections, is also an important consideration.

Surgical Treatment

Before surgical treatment is considered for any patient, a period of observation while on medical treatment is essential to determine the degree of possible improvement, to make certain that the bronchiectasis is not reversible (if cylindrical type), and to clear the airways of as much secretion as possible. Pulmonary resection is seldom an emergency measure. The indications for surgery in bronchiectasis are extensive or repeated hemoptysis; a history suggesting foreign body aspiration; and a well localized saccular or advanced fusiform bronchiectasis with associated re-

current pneumonia or bronchitis. A patient without symptoms need not be subjected to resection even though bronchiectasis is apparent in the bronchogram. Patients with upper lobe lesions where the site of the lesion favors drainage rarely fail to respond to adequate medical therapy. Patients with extensive bilateral disease offer a problem, in part because of limited pulmonary reserve, and should be carefully evaluated. Bilateral resection in two stages has been successfully achieved, taking full cognizance of the pulmonary function prior to surgery. The more severely damaged area is removed first. Sometimes improvement is so great that the second operation may be unnecessary. When bilateral bronchiectasis is part of a general systemic disease, conservative treatment is usually preferable. Bronchiectasis in patients with tuberculosis usually responds well to medical treatment. A child should be at least eight years of age, and preferably ten to fifteen years of age, before such an elective operative procedure is carried out.

To summarize, *medical treatment* is preferred for patients whose disease is minimal and asymptomatic, for patients with far advanced disease who may not tolerate surgery well because of other associated diseases or much diminished pulmonary function, and for patients whose bronchiectasis has been diagnosed too recently to determine the degree to which it can be cleared by adequate medical treatment.

Surgical resection is preferred when the lesion is localized to one segment or lobe and the patient is symptomatic, as when there is persistent or recurring bronchial obstruction; when there is failure to control localized infection by antimicrobial therapy; or when, despite medical treatment over a period of time, the patient fails to do well. There are always patients who do not fall into clear-cut categories and whose treatment requires painstaking evaluation. Carefully accumulated facts and knowledge of the individual case over a fairly long observation period are essential in making a wise choice between surgical resection and medical treatment.

Complications

In patients with extensive disease the medical complications which were more common before the use of antibiotics are abscess of brain or lung, empyema, bronchopleural fistula, emphysema and severe, sometimes fatal pneumonia. In addition, there is always the possibility of hemoptysis and, in those with advanced chronic disease, cor pulmonale with fatal outcome, and amyloidosis.

For the past two decades, atelectasis has been the most frequent postoperative complication. The changed picture, with its improved surgical results for both mortality and complications, is illustrated by Ochsner and others who present multiple factors which have influenced the improved results in ninety-six patients (105 resections) from 1933 to 1945, but a change in surgical techniques and better control of infection have markedly improved this picture.

Chest deformity is minimal in children because of the compensatory growth of the remaining pulmonary tissues. Modern physiotherapy has also added to the improved results following surgery in childhood.

Prognosis

The outlook for patients with bronchiectasis has greatly improved in the past few decades, owing in large measure to a decrease in the predisposing childhood infections (especially measles and pertussis) and to the control of bacterial infections of the respiratory tract made possible by antimicrobial therapy. Even associated diseases such as cystic fibrosis are better controlled. The management of the asthmatic patient still remains a challenge, and patients with asthma and bronchiectasis have the poorest prognosis.

As compared with earlier reports from the preantibiotic period, recent studies have shown that the general health of the patients has been improved and that re-sponse to medical treatment has been rewarding. Such observations in children correspond to long-term studies chiefly in adults, in whom asymptomatic bronchiectasis has been found not uncommonly in those fifty years of age and over and even in older age groups (seventy to eighty years). The need for eradicating segments of the lung or a lung in which the bronchial tree is damaged or ectatic is no longer urgent or even necessary to maintain health, and is compatible with a normal span of life.

Although the only real cure for bronchiectasis is eradication of the diseased lung by surgical resection, the patient may remain asymptomatic for very long periods of time. It has been repeatedly shown that bronchiectasis is not progressive, but remains localized. Its apparent spread to adjacent areas postoperatively is thought to be in reality residua of a previously infected area reactivated after surgery. Evidence for this statement may be found in long-term studies of children and adults.

The postoperative fatality rate is low. Davis and others reviewed their experience with 433 patients having bronchiectasis seen between the years 1950 and 1960 and ranging from four years to eighty-four years of age (approximately 13 per cent were under twenty years of age). The surgical case fatality rate was 1.7 per cent in the 175 patients who were so treated. A comparable report of surgical therapy in 215 patients from Finland is that of Peräsalo and others based on observations between 1953 and 1958 with a 1.6 per cent surgical fatality rate and a 16 per cent incidence of postsurgical complications and infections, such as bronchopleural fistula and empyema.

Pulmonary function studies from the Children's Service at Bellevue Hospital made by Filler on fifteen adolescents who had surgical resections showed that these patients made good physiologic and functional adjustments after operation. When the lung resections were small (bisegmentectomies or right middle lobectomy), there was no reduction in lung volume or in respiratory capacity. In those with

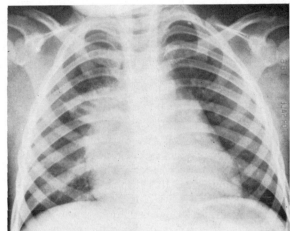

FIGURE 28–1. Case 1. Irregular triangular density extending out from the hilus and above the fissure line to the right upper lobe, which is displaced upward.

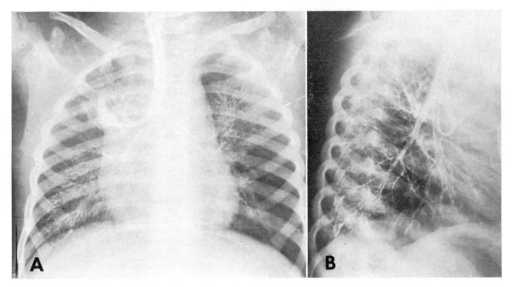

FIGURE 28–2. Case 1. *A,* In the right upper lobe there are crowding of the bronchi and irregular dilatations. *B,* Irregularly enlarged and tortuous bronchi of the posterior segment of the right upper lobe are demonstrated in the lateral view.

more extensive surgery (removal of one fourth to one third of the lung) the decrease in vital capacity was less than anticipated, perhaps because of the overdistention of the remaining lung tissue. No reduction in maximal breathing capacity was observed. Follow-up observation of most of these patients in the Chest Clinic of New York University Medical Center has revealed normal-functioning youths who exercise and pursue an unmodified school program.

Prevention

Control of the childhood diseases underlying the development of bronchiectasis is the essence of prevention. Already pertussis vaccine has had a great impact on the reduction of this disease in both frequency and severity. Measles vaccine is now rapidly showing its value as a preventive measure. Interstitial or viral pneumonias, unlike bacterial pneumonias, still offer a therapeutic challenge, particularly since parenchymal atelectasis occurs frequently. Attention to segmental collapse, especially if persistent or recurrent, using proper therapeutic measures, is essential in the prevention of bronchiectasis. Because of the urgency for prompt therapy by bronchoscopy, foreign body aspiration must always be remembered.

Case Reports

CASE 1. Tuberculosis was diagnosed in a two-year-old Negro boy one year before admission to the Children's Chest Service, Bellevue Hospital. A right upper lobe infiltrate was found, and isoniazid therapy was begun. He was admitted to the Hospital in August 1962 because of recent weight loss, a persistent pulmonary shadow and a history of irregular isoniazid medication.

Physical examination was not remarkable except for undernutrition and an enlarged liver, an infected pharynx and cervical adenopathy. All gastric cultures and culture from bronchoscopic aspiration were negative for acid-fast bacilli.

Bronchoscopy one month after admission showed a nipple of granulation tissue inside the right upper lobe bronchus at the carina between the segmental orifices. Figure 1 shows the chest x-ray one day previously. A bronchogram two weeks later (Fig. 2) showed a saccular bronchiectasis of the anterior and posterior segments of the right upper lobe.

Shortly afterwards the child was discharged home and was followed up regularly in the Bellevue Hospital Children's Chest Clinic. He has received isoniazid and PAS therapy for eighteen months. One episode of persistent low-grade fever required inpatient study in the winter of 1965. All cultures for acid-fast bacilli were negative. Bronchoscopy of the right upper lobe revealed a patent and normal bronchus, but the mucosa was red and swollen at the segmental spurs. The lungs were clear, and there was no cough and no weight loss.

CASE 2. Repeated attacks of pneumonia throughout childhood resulted in saccular bronchiectasis of the right upper lobe in a nine-year-old girl. A successful lobectomy was followed by improved pulmonary function, loss of clubbing of fingers, and improved health. Follow-up for seven years shows no recurrence of bronchiectasis. (See Figure 3.)

CASE 3. A 5½-year-old girl was seen at Bellevue Hospital Children's Chest Out-Patient Department approximately five months before her death in the Hospital on January 29, 1960. A premature baby whose first year of life was marked by failure to thrive, she was the subject of many attacks of pulmonary disease throughout her short life, beginning at two years of age with her first attack of asthma. She had four bouts of pneumonia, including the terminal one. She was considered to be an asthmatic child, although no allergen was found to which she was sensitive. (See Figures 4–9.)

Gamma globulin studies and sweat tests gave essentially normal results. During her first admission to the Children's Service for respiratory distress she was found to have bronchopneumonia and bronchiectasis of the right middle lobe with impaired pulmonary function. There was decreased oxygen saturation and some carbon dioxide retention. The fingers showed clubbing. After two months she recovered sufficiently to return home and receive ambulatory care. The terminal diffuse pneumonia occurred two months later.

Autopsy revealed bilateral interstitial pneumonia and cylindrical bronchiectasis of the right middle lobe and a portion of the right lower lobe.

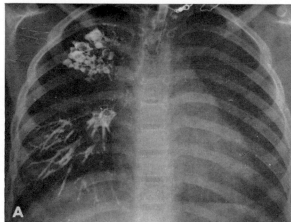

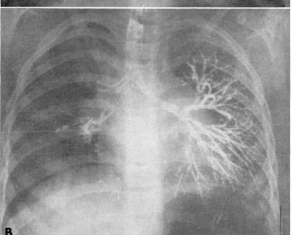

FIGURE 28–3. Case 2. *A*, Broncho-gram taken 2 months before operation shows a saccular bronchiectasis in a shrunken right upper lobe. *B*, Normal left lung demonstrated shortly after operation.

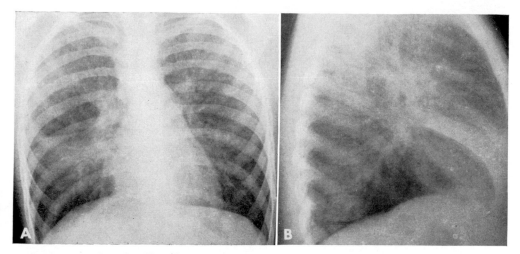

FIGURE 28–4. Case 3. Diffuse bronchopneumonia one month before death. Note collapse of right middle lobe, especially well visualized in the lateral view (*B*).

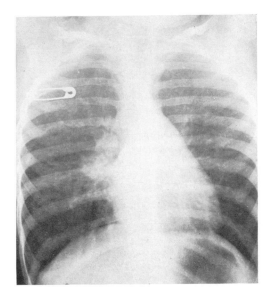

FIGURE 28–5. Case 3. Four days before death there is distention of the lungs and diffuse increase in bronchial markings with bilateral mottling in the upper third and hyperaeration at the bases. The large right root in the right middle lobe appears to have expanded.

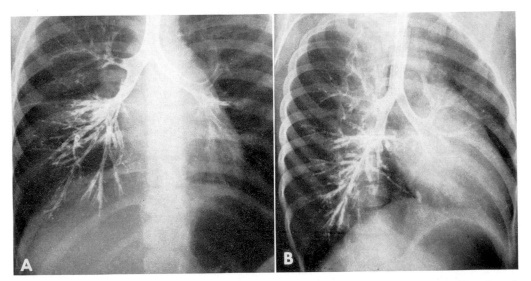

FIGURE 28–6. Case 3. *A*, Bronchogram taken 3 months before death shows cylindrical dilatation of the right middle and adjacent right lower lobe bronchi with some crowding of these bronchi. A fine horizontal pleural line is visible on the right. *B*, The lateral view shows the sudden stublike termination of some of these bronchi.

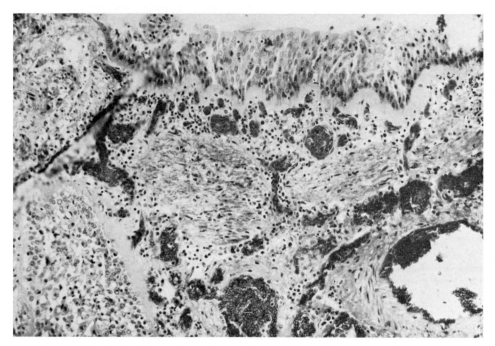

FIGURE 28–7. Case 3. A microscopic section of the bronchus (× 500) shows a thick basement membrane beneath the epithelial lining. There is extensive inflammation involving the muscular tissue as well, where there is also some destruction of muscle.

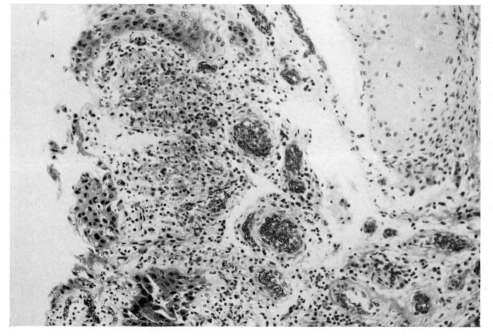

FIGURE 28–8. Case 3. Squamous cell metaplasia of the lining epithelium of the bronchus is illustrated. There is also destruction of smooth muscle and beginning alteration of the cartilage. × 500.

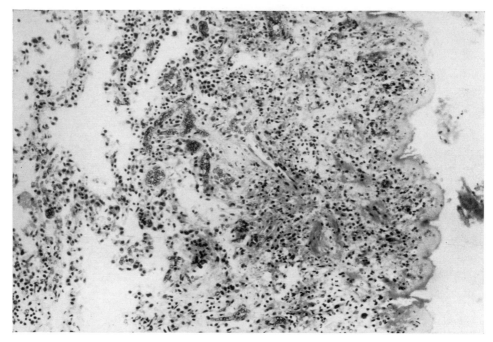

FIGURE 28–9. Case 3. A microscopic section of a bronchiole (× 500) shows the destruction of the wall. There is loss of mucosa and a thickened basement membrane.

REFERENCES

Adams, R., and Churchill, E. D.: Situs Inversus, Sinusitis and Bronchiectasis. Report of 5 Cases, Including Frequency Statistics. *J. Thoracic Surg.,* 7:206, 1937.

Allibone, E. C., Allison, P. R., and Zinnemann, K.: Significance of H. Influenzae in Bronchiectasis of Children. *Brit. M.J.,* 1:1457, 1956.

Andrus, P. M.: Bronchiectasis, an Analysis of Its Causes. *Am. Rev. Tuberc.,* 36:46, 1937.

Idem: Chronic Nonspecific Pulmonary Disease. *Am. Rev. Tuberc.,* 41:87, 1940.

Anspach, W. E.: Atelectasis and Bronchiectasis in Children. Study of 50 Cases Presenting Triangular Shadow at Base of Lung. *Am. J. Dis. Child.,* 47:1011, 1934.

Idem: Bronchiectasis, Collapsed Lung, and the Triangular Basal Shadow in the Roentgenogram, and their Inter-relationship. *Am. J. Roentgenol.,* 41:173, 1939.

Aronson, S. M., and Wallerstein, L.: Protein Nature of Scleroderma. Note on Pulmonary Changes. *New York State J. Med.,* 50:2723, 1950.

Avery, M. E., Riley, M. C., and Weiss, A.: The Course of Bronchiectasis in Childhood. *Bull. Johns Hopkins Hosp.,* 109:20, 1961.

Bachman, A. L., Hewitt, W. R., and Beekley, H. C.: Bronchiectasis—A Bronchographic Study of Sixty Cases of Pneumonia. *Arch. Int. Med.,* 91:78, 1953.

Berg, G., and Nordenskjöld, A.: Pulmonary Alterations in Tuberous Sclerosis. *Acta Med. Scand.,* 125:428, 1946.

Bergstrom, W. H., Cook, C. D., Scannell, J., and Berenberg, W.: Situs Inversus, Bronchiectasis and Sinusitis; Report of a Family with Two Cases of Kartagener's Triad and Two Additional Cases of Bronchiectasis Among Six Siblings. *Pediatrics,* 6:573, 1950.

Biering, A.: Childhood Pneumonia, Including Pertussis Pneumonia, and Bronchiectasis. A Follow-up Study of 151 Patients. *Acta paediat.,* 45:348, 1956.

Blades, B., and Dugan, D. J.: Pseudo Bronchiectasis in Atypical Pneumonia. *J. Thoracic Surgery,* 13:40, 1944.

Boyd, G. L.: Bronchiectasis in Children. *Canad. M.A.J.,* 25:174, 1931.

Bradshaw, H. H., Myers, R. T., and Cordell, A. R.: Bronchiectasis: A Fourteen-Year Appraisal. *Ann. Surg.,* 145:644, 1957.

Bremer, J. L.: Postnatal Development of Alveoli. Publ. No. 459, Carnegie Inst. of Washington, July 1935.

Brock, R. C.: Problem of Sinusitis in Bronchiectasis. *J. Laryng. & Otol.,* 65:449, 1951.

Broman, I.: Zur Kentniss der Lungenentwicklung. *Verh. Anat. Ges.,* 32:83, 1923.

Carter, M. G., and Welch, K. J.: Bronchiectasis Following Aspiration of Timothy Grass. *New England J. Med.,* 238:832, 1948.

Cheng, Kwok-Kew: The Experimental Production of Bronchiectasis in Rats. *J. Path. & Bact.*, 67:89, 1954.

Cherniach, N. S., Vosti, K. L., Dowling, H. F., Lepper, M. H., and Jackson, G. G.: Long-Term Treatment of Bronchiectasis and Chronic Bronchitis. A.M.A. *Arch. Int. Med.*, 103:345, 1959.

Clark, N. S.: Bronchiectasis in Childhood. *Brit. M.J.*, 1:80, 1963.

Cockayne, E. A.: The Genetics of Transposition of the Viscera. *Quart. J. Med.*, 7:479, 1938.

Collins, H. D., and Dudley, H. R.: Agammaglobulinemia and Bronchiectasis. A Report of Two Cases in Adults, with Autopsy Findings. *New England J. Med.*, 252:255, 1955.

Corpe, R. F., and Hwa, E. C.: A Correlated Bronchographic and Histopathologic Study of Bronchial Disease in 216 TBC Patients. *Am. Rev. Tuberc.*, 73:681, 1956.

Croxatto, O. C., and Lanari, A.: Pathogenesis of Bronchiectasis. Experimental Study and Anatomical Findings. *J. Thoracic Surg.*, 27:514, 1954.

Davis, A. L., Grobow, E. J., Tompset, R., and McClement, J. H.: Bacterial Infection and Some Effects of Chemoprophylaxis in Chronic Pulmonary Emphysema. I. Chemoprophylaxis with Intermittent Tetracycline. *Am. J. Med.*, 31:365, 1961.

Davis, M. B., Jr., Hopkins, W. A., and Wansker, W. C.: The Present Status of the Treatment of Bronchiectasis. *Am. Rev. Resp. Dis.*, 85:816, 1962.

Diamond, S., and Van Loon, E. L.: Bronchiectasis in Childhood. *J.A.M.A.*, 118:771, 1942.

Dickey, L. B.: Pulmonary Diseases Associated with Cystic Fibrosis of the Pancreas. *Dis. Chest*, 17:153, 1950.

Dyggve, H., and Gudbjerg, C. E.: Bronchiectasis in Children. *Acta paediat.*, 47:193, 1958.

Edwards, F. R.: The Long-Term Results of the Surgical Treatment of Bronchiectasis. *Acta chir. Belgica*, 46:668, 1954.

Ellis, W. B.: Atelectatic Bronchiectasis in Childhood. *Arch. Dis. Childhood*, 8:25, 1933.

Engel, S.: *The Child's Lung*. London, E. Arnold & Co., 1947.

Farber, S.: Pancreatic Function and Disease in Early Life. V. Pathologic Changes Associated with Pancreatic Insufficiency. *Arch. Path.*, 37:238, 1944.

Field, C. E.: Bronchiectasis in Childhood. I. Clinical Survey of 160 Cases. *Pediatrics*, 4:21, 1949.

Idem: Bronchiectasis in Childhood II. Aetiology and Pathogenesis, Including a Survey of 272 Cases of Doubtful Irreversible Bronchiectasis. *Pediatrics*, 4:231, 1949.

Idem: Bronchiectasis in Childhood. III. Prophylaxis, Treatment and Prognosis. *Pediatrics*, 4:335, 1949.

Idem: Bronchiectasis. A Long-Term Follow-up of Medical and Surgical Cases from Childhood. *Arch. Dis. Childhood*, 36:587, 1961.

Filler, J.: Effects upon Pulmonary Function of Lobectomy Performed During Childhood. *Am. Rev. Resp. Dis.*, 89:801, 1964.

Findlay, L.: Atelectasis or Compensatory Bronchiectasis. *Arch. Dis. Childhood*, 10:61, 1935.

Findlay, L., and Graham, S.: Bronchiectasis in Childhood. *Arch. Dis. Childhood*, 2:71, 1927.

Finke, W.: The Reversibility of Early Bronchiectasis. Its Implication for Therapy and Prevention. *New York J. Med.*, 5:1163, 1951.

Fleischner, F.: Reversible Bronchiectasis. *Am. J. Roentgenol.*, 46:166, 1941.

Franklin, A. W.: The Prognosis of Bronchiectasis in Childhood. *Arch. Dis. Childhood*, 33:19, 1958.

Gandevia, B.: Combined Tomography and Bronchography (Tomobronchography) in the Investigation of Pulmonary Disease. *Med. J. Australia*, 2:813, 1957.

Getzova, S.: Cystic and Compact Pulmonary Sclerosis in Progressive Scleroderma. *Arch. Path.*, 40:99, 1945.

Ginsberg, R. L., Cooley, J. C., Olsen, A. M., Kirklin, J. W., and Clagget, O. T.: Prognosis of Bronchiectasis After Resection. *Surg., Gynec. & Obst.*, 101:99, 1955.

Gómez, D. M., and Filler, J.: An Analysis of the Distribution of Specific Tidal Volume in Children with Bronchial Asthma. *Ztschr. f. d. ges. exper. Med.*, 139:513, 1965.

Good, C. A.: Some Remarks Concerning the Roentgenologic Diagnosis of Bronchiectasis. *Proc. Staff Meet., Mayo Clin.*, 20:22, 1945.

Gottlieb, O., and Storm, O.: The Results of Surgical Resection for Bronchiectasis. *Acta Chir. Scand.*, 3:228, 1956.

Graham, S., and Hutchinson, J. H.: Absorption Collapse in Primary Tuberculous Infection in Childhood. *Arch. Dis. Childhood*, 22:162, 1947.

Gray, I. R.: Atelectasis as a Complication of Pulmonary Lobectomy. *Thorax*, 1:263, 1946.

Gudbjerg, C. E.: Roentgenologic Diagnosis of Bronchiectasis. *Acta Radiol.*, 43:209, 1955.

Idem: Bronchiectasis. Radiologic Diagnosis and Prognosis After Operative Treatment. *Acta Radiol.*, 143:11, 1957.

Helm, W. H., and Thompson, V. C.: The Long-Term Results of Resection for Bronchiectasis. *Quart. J. Med.*, 27:353, 1958..

Heusfeldt, E.: Bronchiectasis: Etiology, Surgical Treatment and Prevention. *Acta Chir. Scand.*, 245 (Suppl.): 76, 1959.

Hinds, J. R.: Bronchiectasis in the Maori. *New Zealand M. J.*, 57:328, 1958.

Hogg, J. C.: Discussion on the Role of Sinusitis in Bronchiectasis. *J. Laryng. & Otol.*, 65:442, 1951.

Hutchinson, J. H.: The Pathogenesis of Epituberculosis in Children, with a Note on Obstructive Emphysema. *Glasgow M.J.*, 30:271, 1949.

Isley, J. K., Jr., Bacos, J., Hickam, J. B., and Baylin, G. J.: Bronchiolar Behavior in Pulmonary Emphysema and in Bronchiectasis. *Am. J. Roentgenol.*, 87:853, 1962.

Jennings, G. H.: Re-expansion of the Atelectatic Lower Lobe and Disappearance of Bronchiectasis. *Brit. M.J.*, 2:963-965, 1937.

Johansson, L., and Silander, T.: Surgery for Bronchiectasis. Primary Results in 61 Cases. *Acta Chir. Scand.*, 124:419, 1962.

Jones, E. M., Park, W. M., and Willis, H. S.: Bronchiectasis Following Primary Tuberculosis. *Am. J. Dis. Child.*, 72:296, 1946

Jones, E. M., Rafferty, T. N., and Willis, H. S.: Primary Tuberculosis Complicated by Bronchial Tuberculosis with Atelectasis (Epituberculosis). *Am. Rev. Tuberc.*, 46:392, 1942.

Jones, E. M., Peck, W. M., Woodruff, C. E., and Willis, H. S.: Relationship Between Tuberculosis and Bronchiectasis. A Study of Clinical and of Post-mortem Material. *Am. Rev. Tuberc.*, 61:387, 1950.

Jones, O. R., and Cournand, A.: The Shrunken Pulmonary Lobe with Chronic Bronchiectasis. *Am. Rev. Tuberc.*, 28:293, 1933.

Kartagener, M.: Zur Pathogenese der Bronchiektasien: Bronchiektasien bei Situs Viscerum inversus. *Beitr. z. Klin. d. Tuberk.*, 83:489, 1933.

Kartagener, M., and Horlacher, A.: Zur Pathogenese der Bronchiecktasien; Situs Viscerum inversus und Polyposis nas: in einem Falle familiärer Bronchiectasien. *Beitr. z. Klin. d. Tuberk.*, 87:331, 1935.

Kay, E. B.: Bronchiectasis Following Atypical Pneumonia. *Arch. Int. Med.*, 75:89, 1945.

Kay, E. B., and Meade, R. H., Jr.: Penicillin in the Treatment of Chronic Infections of the Lungs and Bronchi. *J.A.M.A.*, 129:200, 1945.

Laennec, R. T. H.: *De l'auscultation médiate, un traité du diagnostie des maladies des poumons et de coeur, fondé principalement sur ce noveau moyen d'exploration.* Paris, Brosson et Chaude, 1819.

Lander, F. P. L.: Bronchiectasis and Atelectasis: Temporary and Permanent Changes. *Thorax*, 1:198, 1946.

Lees, A W.: Atelectasis and Bronchiectasis in Pertussis. *Brit. M.J.*, 2:1138, 1950.

Liebow, A. A., Hales, M. R., and Lindskog, G. E.: Bronchiectasis and Abnormal Changes in Pulmonary Bronchial Vessels, *Am. J. Path.*, 25:211, 1949.

Lindskog, G. E., and Hubbell, D. S.: An Analysis of 215 Cases of Bronchiectasis. *Surg., Gynec. & Obst.*, 100:643, 1955.

Logan, W. D. Jr., Abbott, O. A., and Hatcher, C. R. Jr.: Kartagener's Triad. *Dis. Chest*, 48:613, 1965.

Lorenz, T. H.: Bronchiectasis. *Am. J. M. Sc.*, 221:522, 1951.

McLaurin, J. G.: Review of Interrelationship of Paranasal Sinus Disease and Certain Chest Conditions, with Especial Consideration of Bronchiectasis and Asthma. *Ann. Otol., Rhin. & Laryng.*, 44:344, 1935.

Idem: Interrelationship of Upper and Lower Respiratory Infections Emphasizing Routes of Infection. *Ann Otol., Rhin. & Laryng.*, 52:589, 1943.

McNeil, C., MacGregor, A. R., and Alexander, W. A.: Studies of Pneumonia in Childhood: Bronchiectasis and Fibrosis. *Arch. Dis. Childhood*, 4:170, 1929.

Mayer, E., and Rappaport, I.: Developmental Origin of Cystic, Bronchiectatic and Emphysematous Changes in the Lungs. *Dis. Chest*, 21:146, 1952.

Nelson, S. W., and Christoforidis, A.: Reversible Bronchiectasis. *Radiology*, 71:375, 1958.

Norman, P. S., and others: Long-Term Tetracycline Treatment of Chronic Bronchitis. *J.A.M.A.*, 179, 833, 1962.

Ochsner, A., DeBakey, M., and De Camp, P. T.: Bronchiectasis: Its Curative Treatment by Pulmonary Resection. An Analysis of Ninety-Six Cases. *Surgery*, 25:518, 1949.

Ogilvie, A. C.: The Natural History of Bronchiectasis: A Clinical, Roentgenologic and Pathologic Study. *Arch. Int. Med.*, 68:395, 1941.

Olsen, A. M.: Bronchiectasis and Dextrocardia. Observations on the Aetiology of Bronchiectasis. *Am. Rev. Tuberc.*, 47:435, 1943.

Palley, A.: Factors Leading to the Production of Bronchiectasis in Childhood and Its Prevention. *South African Med. J.*, 22:169, 1948.

Pastore, P. N., and Olsen, A. M.: Absence of Frontal Sinuses and Bronchiectasis in Identical Twins. *Proc. Staff Meet., Mayo Clin.*, 16:593, 1941.

Peräsalo, O., Scheinin, T. M., and Pantzar, P.: On the Surgical Treatment of Bronchiectasis. *Acta Chir. Scand.*, 119:198, 1960.

Perry, K. M. A., and King, D. S.: Bronchiectasis: A Study on Prognosis Based on a Follow-up of 400 Patients. *Am. Rev. Tuberc.*, 41:531, 1940.

Pittman, H. S.: Gamma Globulin Concentrations in Ambulatory Patients with Bronchiectasis. *Am. Rev. Resp. Dis.*, 81:251, 1960.

Prolonged Antibiotic Treatment of Severe Bronchiectasis. A report by a Subcommittee of the Antibiotics Clinical Trials (Non-Tuberculous) Committee of the Medical Research Council. *Brit. M.J.*, 2:255, 1957.

Raia, A.: Bronchiectasis in Children with Special Reference to Prevention and Early Diagnosis. *Am. J. Dis. Child.*, 56:582, 1938.

Ruberman, W., Shauffer, I., and Biondo, T.: Bronchiectasis and Acute Pneumonia. *Am. Rev. Tuberc.*, 76:761, 1957.

Rytel, M. W., Conner, G. H., Welch, C. C., Kraybill, W. H., and Edwards, E. H.: Infectious Agents Associated with Cylindrical Bronchiectasis. *Dis. Chest*, 46:23, 1964.

Sant'Agnese, P. A. di: The Pulmonary Manifestation of Fibrocystic Disease of the Pancreas. *Dis. Chest*, 27:654, 1955.

Sauerbruch, F.: *Chirurgie der Brustorgane.* Berlin, Julius Springer, 1929, Vol. I, pt. 1, p. 869.

Idem: *Arch f. klin. Chir.,* 180:312, footnote 17, 1934.

Sicard, J. A., and Forestier, J.: Iodized Oil as Contrast Medium in Radioscopy. *Bull. et Mém. Soc. Méd. hôp. Paris,* 46:463, 1922.

Smith, K. R., and Morris, J. F.: Reversible Bronchial Dilatation. Report of a Case. *Dis. Child,* 42:652, 1962.

Spain, D., and Thomas, A. G.: The Pulmonary Manifestations of Scleroderma. *Ann. Int. Med.,* 32:152, 1949.

Spain, D. W., and Lester, C. W.: Time Demand in the Development of Irreversible Bronchiectasis. *J. Pediat.,* 32:415, 1948.

Strang, C: The Fate of Children with Bronchiectasis. *Ann. Int. Med.,* 44:630, 1956.

Strang, L. B.: Abnormalities of Ventilatory Capacity in Children with Asthma and Bronchiectasis. *Arch. Dis. Childhood,* 35:224, 1960.

Strang, L. B., and Court, S. D. M.: Studies of Lung Function in Children. *Postgrad. M.J.,* 36:276, 1960.

Swierenga, J.: Childhood Bronchiectasis. *Dis. Chest,* 32:154, 1957.

Szpunar, J., and Okrasinka, B.: Sinusitis in Children with Bronchicctasis. The Influence of Allergy on Its Development. *Arch. Otolaryng.,* 76:352, 1962.

Tannenberg, J., and Pinner, M.: Atelectasis and Bronchiectasis. An Experimental Study Concerning Their Relationship. *J. Thorac. Surg.,* 11:571, 1942.

Temple, A. D., Smoling, L., and Aubeit, E.: Long-Term Antibiotic Therapy in Chronic

Chest Disease. *Med. Serv. J., Canada,* 19:473, 1963.

Torgersen, J.: Transposition of Viscera—Bronchiectasis and Nasal Polyps. Genetical Analysis and Contributions to Problem of Constitution. *Acta Radiol.,* 28:17, 1947.

Van Creveld, S., and Ter Poorten, F. H.: Reticuloendotheliosis Chiefly Localized in the Lungs, Bone Marrow and Thymus. *Arch. Dis. Childhood,* 10:57, 1935.

Visconti, R. J.: Agammaglobulinemia with Bronchopulmonary Manifestations. *Dis. Chest,* 48:530, 1965.

Whitwell, F.: A Study of the Pathology and Pathogenesis of Bronchiectasis. *Thorax,* 7:213, 1952.

Williams, H., and Anderson, C.: Bronchiectasis and Bronchostenosis Following Primary Tuberculosis in Infancy and Childhood. *Quart. J. Med.,* 22:295, 1953.

Williams, H., and O'Reilly, R. N.: Bronchiectasis in Children: Its Multiple Clinical and Pathological Aspects. *Arch. Dis. Child.,* 34:192, 1959.

Willson, H. G.: Postnatal Development of the Lung. *Am. J. Anat.,* 41:97, 1928.

Wynn-Williams, N.: Bronchiectasis: A Study Centered in Bedford and Its Environs. *Brit. M.J.,* 1:1194, 1953.

Idem: Observations on the Treatment of Bronchiectasis and Its Relation to Prognosis. *Tubercle* (London), 38:133, 1957.

Zuckerman, H. S., and Wurtzebach, L. R.: Kartagener's Triad. Review of the Literature and Report of a Case. *Dis. Chest.,* 19:92, 1951.

Zuelzer, W. W., and Newton, W. A.: The Pathogenesis of Fibrocystic Disease of the Pancreas. *Pediatrics,* 4:53, 1949.

CHAPTER TWENTY-NINE

Pulmonary Abscess

ROBERT H. HIGH, M.D.

Pulmonary abscess develops when a portion of the pulmonary parenchyma is infected and subsequently becomes suppurative and necrotic. Occlusion of the bronchial segments leading to the involved area often occurs. The frequency with which lung abscess is noted has decreased in children, owing in part to the more prompt and effective treatment of pneumonia and to the more widespread use of endotracheal intubation during anesthesia, especially for surgical procedures in the oropharynx.

Pulmonary abscess may be multiple or single. In the former instance septicemia, especially staphylococcal, is commonly the cause. Septicemia occurring in children who have had shunts of cerebrospinal fluid, in particular those using the ventriculojugular route with a valve in the drainage system, is likely to produce multiple pulmonary abscesses. Multiple abscesses may also complicate extensive pneumonia, especially that caused by staphylococci or Friedlaender's bacillus. Multiple abscesses often develop in the presence of chronic suppurative bronchopulmonary disease associated with cystic fibrosis of the pancreas, extensive bronchiectasis or congenital hypogammaglobulinemia. In the latter group pulmonary abscesses often develop during the terminal phase of the disease.

Single lung abscesses often follow the aspiration of infected material or a foreign body, and they may also be produced by infected emboli. Many times solitary lung abscesses develop during the course of acute pneumonia, especially that caused by staphylococci. Occasionally, anomalous cysts or sequestered lobes become infected with the subsequent development of pulmonary abscess.

Abscesses which follow the aspiration of secretions or a foreign body are often caused by a variety of bacteria, chiefly those of the oral cavity, including fusospirochetal organisms, bacteroides species and streptococci which are not of the group A type. Such abscesses are often called anaerobic or putrid abscesses.

Pulmonary abscesses which complicate the course of pulmonary tuberculosis and that of the pulmonary mycotic infections are considered elsewhere.

In response to the infecting material the pulmonary parenchyma undergoes intense acute inflammatory changes, thrombosis of the vascular supply and edema, with resulting obstruction of the bronchi draining the area. Necrosis and central liquefaction of the involved area occur. After about ten days the abscess is likely to rupture into a bronchus, and the contents may be evacuated by coughing; sometimes the material is aspirated, producing a widespread bronchopneumonia. After evacuation of an abscess the granulation tissue lining the walls may bleed. In the older child such hemorrhage may be manifested by hemoptysis, but this is not likely in the younger patient. After evacuation of a pulmonary abscess, fibrosis often occurs; many abscesses heal spontaneously, often with no sequelae.

Pulmonary abscesses located near the periphery of the lung are likely to cause inflammation of the overlying pleura with a resultant plastic pleuritis. Sometimes such peripheral abscesses rupture into the pleural cavity, and a bronchopleural fistula associated with a pyopneumothorax develops. These latter circumstances are serious consequences of a pulmonary abscess, particularly if the abscess is produced by anerobic organisms.

Aerobic (nonputrid) pulmonary abscesses secondary to septicemia, pneumo-

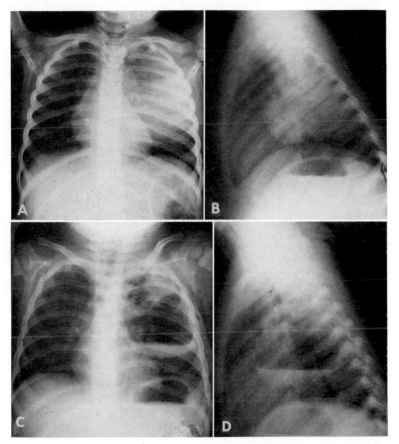

FIGURE 29–1. Solitary pneumococcal abscess. *A* and *B,* Preaspiration and (*C, D*) postaspiration films (same day). The outcome was complete recovery.

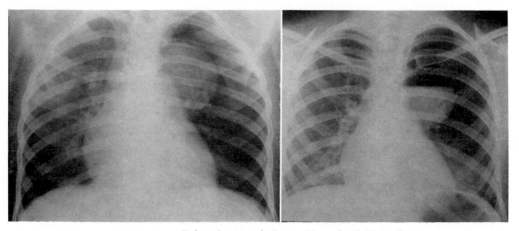

FIGURE 29–2. Infected congenital cyst. Note the fluid levels.

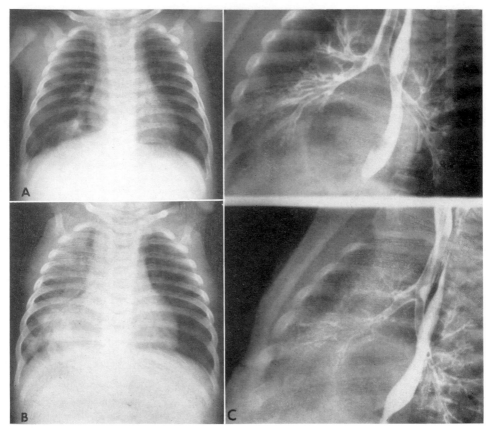

FIGURE 29–3. *A*, Recurrent pulmonary abscess, right lower lobe (7/26/65). *B*, Extension of abscess (9/17/65). *C*, Demonstration of lack of filling by bronchography (9/23/65). Subsequent thoracotomy revealed sequestered lobe. Removal was followed by cure.

nia, cystic fibrosis of the pancreas, and the like, may be difficult to recognize because of the manifestations of the primary disease. Physical examination may suggest the presence of pulmonary consolidation. Roentgenographic examination shows segmental areas of pneumonia which resolve slowly. When the abscess communicates with the bronchial tree, air will displace some or all of the purulent material, and a cavity with or without a fluid level will be apparent. An area of inflammatory reaction will be noted surrounding the abscess. If the abscess ruptures into the pleural space, the physical and roentgenographic findings will be those of pyopneumothorax.

In *putrid (anaerobic) pulmonary abscesses* there is often a history of aspiration of secretions or of a foreign body, recent

tonsillectomy, general anesthesia, or the like, but such is not always the case. After aspiration a latent period of a few days may be noted before symptoms and signs of pulmonary infection develop. Occasionally the onset is insidious, but more commonly it is sudden with the appearance of fever, cough, chest pain, dyspnea, tachypnea, occasionally hemoptysis in the older child, as well as general manifestations of infection such as malaise and anorexia. Leukocytosis is often marked. The cough is usually dry and nonproductive in the early stages of the disease. After the abscess has liquefied and communicates with the bronchial tree, a large amount of purulent material may be raised by coughing.

Physical examination of the chest may suggest the presence of consolidation of the lung. Occasionally a pleural friction rub may be heard. Sometimes, especially if the diseased area is surrounded by normally aerated lung tissue, localized changes cannot be detected by physical examination. Under such circumstances the diagnosis of pulmonary disease is suggested by the presence of such findings as cough, chest pain, and dyspnea.

Symptoms and abnormal physical findings tend to subside after the contents of the abscess have been evacuated. If the abscess persists for several weeks, clubbing of the fingers may develop.

Roentgenographic examinations show changes similar to those described above (aerobic pulmonary abscess).

Antimicrobial treatment of the basic disease, when such is present, is imperative. In the presence of acute pneumonia or septicemia such therapy may be all that is required. Most of the bacteria causing pulmonary abscess are the common pathogens of the respiratory tract. Infections with Friedlaender's bacilli are fortunately uncommon in children. Accordingly, penicillin G should be administered in large doses initially by parenteral routes and later by the oral route. Whenever staphylococci are suspected of causing the abscess, initial therapy should include the administration of one of the semisynthetic penicillin preparations which are resistant to degradation by

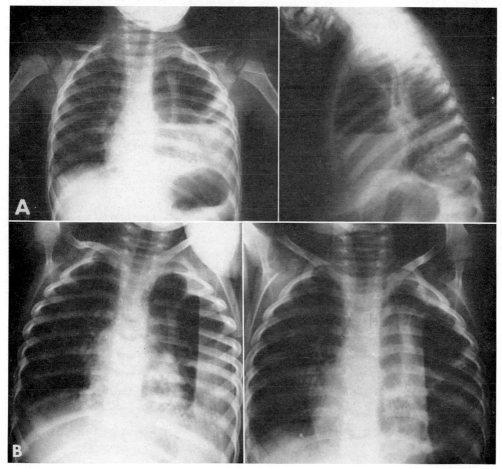

FIGURE 29–4. A 2-year-old male child with staphylococcal pulmonary abscesses and pyopneumothorax. Note the fluid levels and shift of fluid with change in position. The outcome was complete recovery.

staphylococcal penicillinase. (See Staphylococcal Pneumonia.) Streptomycin, kanamycin, colistin or ampicillin may be given in addition to penicillin until the results of cultures and sensitivity tests are available. Sulfonamide drugs are not recommended when purulent collections are present.

When an abscess has formed, bronchoscopic examination should be performed to aspirate as much of the purulent material as possible, to remove a foreign body or to exclude its presence and, of much importance, to secure material for culture and sensitivity tests. Cultures should be made for pyogenic bacteria, fungi and mycobacteria. Subsequent therapy may be guided by the results of such cultures. Bronchoscopic aspirations should be repeated until the amount of purulent material is minimal. Some recommend the instillation of proteolytic enzymes or antimicrobial agents or both, during the bronchoscopic examination. The efficacy of such topical applications is difficult to evaluate, but theoretical considerations favor their use.

Postural drainage, aided by appropriate physical therapy to the chest (see p. 93) should also be used.

The aerosol administration of antibiotics and agents which help to liquefy mucus, such as N-acetylcystine, may also be recommended. Systemic absorption of antibiotic agents is minimal after aerosol administration, and systemic toxic reactions are infrequent. Aerosol therapy is an addition to, but not a substitute or alternative for, intensive systemic therapy.

In those instances in which the foregoing measures fail to provide adequate and prompt drainage of a pulmonary abscess, direct aspiration under biplane fluoroscopic guidance is recommended. After aspiration of as much purulent material as possible, instillation of antibiotics and proteolytic enzymes may be made directly into the abscess cavity. Repeated aspirations and instillations may be made in those instances in which resolution is slow.

In most instances a pulmonary abscess will resolve when treated as outlined above. Those caused by staphylococci or pneumococci, in general, respond well. In those patients in whom abscess closure does not occur after a trial of conservative treatment of perhaps a month's duration, surgical removal of the involved lobe or portion of a lobe is indicated.

Children who have healed pulmonary abscesses should be observed for the possible development of bronchiectasis in the involved area.

REFERENCES

Burnett, W. E., Rosemond, G. P., Caswell, H. T., Hall, J. H., and Bucher, R. M.: The Topical Treatment of Lung Abscess. *Pennsylvania M.J.,* 52:719, 1949.

Cook, C. D.: Pulmonary Abscess; in S. S. Gellis and B. M. Kagan (Eds.): *Current Pediatric Therapy* 1966-1967. Philadelphia, W. B. Saunders Company, 1966, pp. 150-51.

High, R. H.: Pulmonary Abscesses; in H. C. Shirkey (Ed.): *Pediatric Therapy* 1966-1967. 2nd ed. St. Louis, C. V. Mosby Company, 1966, p. 564.

Pickett, L. K.: Pulmonary Abscess; in W. E. Nelson: *Textbook of Pediatrics.* 8th ed. Philadelphia, W. B. Saunders Company, 1964, pp. 868-9.

Thomas, D. M.: Management of Postoperative Pulmonary Complications. *J. Kentucky M.A.,* 61:869-70, 1963.

CHAPTER THIRTY

Diseases of the Pleura

ROBERT H. HIGH, M.D.

Inflammatory diseases of the pleura may be separated into three major groups: (1) dry or plastic pleurisy, (2) serofibrinous pleurisy or pleurisy with effusion, and (3) purulent pleurisy or empyema. Separation of pleurisy into these groups is somewhat arbitrary and often is best done at the onset of the pleural reaction, since many children who initially have plastic pleurisy ultimately have an effusion; conversely, as serofibrinous pleurisy undergoes resolution, a stage occurs when plastic pleurisy is present. The frequency of the occurrence of serofibrinous pleurisy has decreased in proportion to the decrease in the number of pulmonary infections with tuberculosis in children. Purulent pleurisy has likewise become less common because of the early treatment of bacterial pneumonia with antimicrobial agents.

History and physical examination may sometimes be sufficient to establish the diagnosis of pleural disease, but in most instances roentgenographic studies, including examination in the prone and upright positions as well as in the lateral projection, are necessary. Fluoroscopic examination may also be required, although such examinations are performed less frequently than formerly in order to reduce the patient's exposure to irradiation.

In many instances thoracentesis must be performed in order to distinguish between purulent and serofibrinous pleurisy. When aspiration yields air, frank pus or blood, the diagnosis of the type of pleural disease is readily made. When aspiration yields clear or slightly yellowish fluid, appropriate examination should be performed to attempt to distinguish between pleural exudates and pleural transudates, although such differentiation cannot always be made. Exudate usually has a protein content greater than 0.3 gm. per 100 ml. and has a specific gravity above 1.015. The sediment from pleural exudates when stained appropriately is apt to show polymorphonuclear leukocytes instead of mesothelial cells, and Gram stains may reveal bacteria. Particular attention should be directed to opalescent aspirates, which suggest the possibility of chylothorax. Such aspirates should be overlaid with an organic solvent, such as ether, to which a fat-soluble dye such as Sudan 3 is added. If, after such a preparation has been shaken and permitted to stand, the dye becomes concentrated in the solvent layer while the original fluid loses its opalescence, a presumptive diagnosis of chylothorax is justified. It is advisable to have the pleural fluid cultured for pyogenic bacteria, fungi and *Mycobacterium tuberculosis*. Nonpurulent fluid should also be studied by appropriate pathologic techniques for cell characteristics, clumps of neoplastic cells, bacteria, and so forth.

DRY OR PLASTIC PLEURISY

Dry or plastic pleurisy most often occurs in association with bacterial or viral pneumonia, but sometimes is noted with upper respiratory tract infections. Occasionally dry pleurisy is noted with tuberculosis, rheumatic fever, systemic lupus erythematosus and other mesenchymal diseases. It may also be secondary to inflammatory disease in the abdomen or chest wall.

The symptoms of dry pleurisy are often overshadowed by those of the primary disease. The principal symptom is chest pain which is made worse by coughing and straining. The pain may be localized to a portion of the chest wall, but may radiate to other areas, depending on the area of involvement. Thus the pain from pleural disease over the middle or lower lobe is often referred to the abdomen. The pain from pleurisy involving the diaphragm may be referred to the abdomen, but is often referred to the shoulder area, whereas pleurisy of the apical areas may have pain referred to the arm. Pain is lessened by shallow breathing and the avoidance of coughing. The patient may lie on the affected side.

Physical examination will reveal the findings of the primary disease. The presence of plastic pleurisy is revealed by a "leathery" friction rub which is heard in both phases of respiration. The friction rub is more apparent if there is no underlying pneumonia. Pleural friction rubs subside as the underlying disease improves and are commonly detectable for only a day or so. Roentgenographic examination may reveal areas of thickening of the pleura, especially in the interlobar areas.

Plastic pleurisy must be distinguished from other diseases which cause similar pain, such as fractured ribs, epidemic pleurodynia, herpes zoster, other lesions of the dorsal root ganglions, intraspinal disease, trichinosis, intra-abdominal disease, and the like.

Treatment is first directed to the primary disease. The only significant symptom of dry pleurisy which requires treatment is the chest pain. In most children the pleural pain is relieved by the administration of analgesics such as aspirin, but occasionally codeine or similar drugs will be required for short periods of time. The local application of heat or cold may provide some symptomatic relief. Strapping the chest with adhesive plaster is apt to be a source of annoyance to many children and is not generally recommended.

SEROFIBRINOUS PLEURISY

Serofibrinous pleurisy or pleurisy with effusion is usually a reaction to pulmonary disease or to inflammatory disease in the abdomen. It may also be a manifestation of a systemic disease such as rheumatic fever or lupus erythematosus. Occasionally it is a reaction to primary or metastatic intrathoracic neoplasms, although such diseases often cause hemothorax. In the past most patients with serofibrinous pleural effusions had pulmonary tuberculosis, but at present this is less likely to be the case. Tuberculosis must obviously still be considered in the differential diagnosis of serous pleural effusions.

The clinical manifestations of serofibrinous pleurisy will be superimposed on those of the primary disease. If plastic pleurisy was previously present, the development of an effusion is often associated with decrease in pleural pain. The severity of the symptoms depends upon the amount of fluid present in the pleural space. Small effusions often do not produce any symptoms. Large effusions cause cough, dyspnea, tachypnea, orthopnea and sometimes cyanosis. The abnormalities noted by physical examination are related to the extent of the effusion. They include a decrease in the percussion note ranging from dull to flat; decrease or absence of the breath sounds is commonly noted, although sometimes in infants with large effusions the breath sounds are relatively unchanged. If pneumonia is present, rales are often heard despite the presence of the effusion. Palpable fremitus is decreased. In large effusions the heart and mediastinal structures are shifted toward the uninvolved side, and occasionally the interspaces between the ribs bulge outward. The involved side often shows a lag in expansion during inspiration. Scoliosis, with the concavity away from the involved side, may be noted. If the pleural fluid is not loculated, the physical examination will reveal shifting signs as the patient's position is changed, and the abnormal signs are most audible over the dependent areas. (See the chapter History and Physical Examination.)

Roentgenographic examinations should be made in both the prone and upright positions. The area of effusion is manifested by a more or less homogenized density which obliterates the normal markings in the underlying lung. Small effusions may be manifested by obliteration of the costophrenic or cardiophrenic sulci. Small effusions may also be seen as widening of the interlobar septa. Large effusions are associated with a shift of the heart and mediastinal structures to the opposite side. Occasionally, in the presence of extensive pleural effusions, the intercostal spaces on the involved side are widened and may bulge toward the chest wall.

Serofibrinous pleurisy cannot regularly be distinguished from purulent pleurisy or from hydrothorax by any means other than direct examination of the pleural fluid. Accordingly, a diagnostic thoracentesis is almost always indicated when fluid is present in the thorax. Occasional exceptions may be made, e.g. in the presence of minimal effusions occurring with typical pneumococcal lobar pneumonia in children who are responding favorably to therapy. As a rule, however, the best management requires that thoracentesis be performed and any aspirated fluid be studied as described above. A large pericardial effusion may simulate a pleural effusion, especially on the left side of the thorax. Appropriate cardiac studies usually permit differentiation between the two. If such studies do not permit resolution of the diagnosis, thoracentesis or pericardial aspiration may be necessary.

Serofibrinous effusions resolve as the primary disease improves, the resolution being most rapid when associated with acute bacterial pneumonia. The disappearance of pleural fluid is less rapid when it is caused by tuberculosis. As the effusion is absorbed, adhesions may develop between the visceral and parietal layers of the pleura, but these adhesions do not cause any functional impairment of the lung. The roentgenographic abnormalities often clear less rapidly than the patient's clinical course would suggest. Residual pleural thickening may persist for long periods of time, often producing peculiar densities over the lungs. Occasionally, calcification develops in the pleura after the effusion has been absorbed. In many instances, however, the abnormalities caused by the effusion will disappear entirely, leaving no evidence of the previous pleural disease.

The treatment of serofibrinous pleurisy is basically that of the primary disease. Occasionally the pleural effusion becomes so large that respiratory distress occurs because of compression of the lung. Oxygen therapy may occasionally be necessary. Usually there is relief of respiratory distress after removal of the fluid. Occasionally the pleural effusion may reaccumulate to such an extent that repeated thoracenteses must be performed. Under such circumstances an intensive search must be made for the possible presence of an intrathoracic malignancy, a subdiaphragmatic abscess or chylothorax.

Pain in the chest is usually not a prominent symptom of serofibrinous pleurisy.

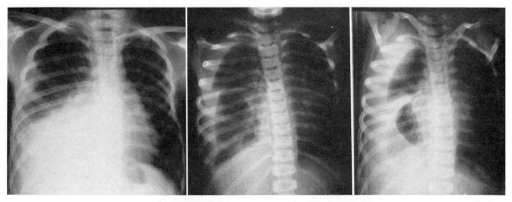

FIGURE 30–1. Massive pleural effusion secondary to pneumococcal pneumonia. Note shift of effusion with change of position. Outcome—recovery.

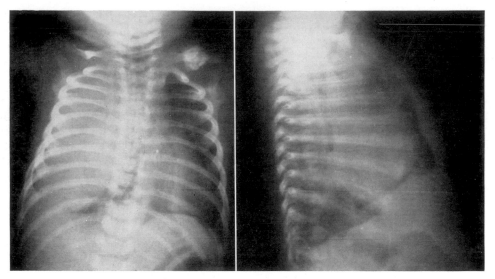

FIGURE 30–2. Tension empyema secondary to staphylococcal pneumonia.

PURULENT PLEURISY

When present, it is treated as described above. The painful manifestations of dry pleurisy usually disappear when a pleural effusion develops.

Purulent pleurisy or empyema is a collection of purulent material in the pleural cavity or occasionally in both pleural cavities. In most instances empyema is secondary to bacterial pneumonia, especially staphylococcal (see p. 289), but may be secondary to lung abscess (see p. 334), bronchiectatic abscesses (see p. 315), cystic fibrosis of the pancreas (see p. 541), mediastinitis, and penetrating trauma of the chest wall, or may follow cardiac or thoracic surgery. Empyema may also develop secondary to an intra-abdominal abscess.

Empyema can be loculated in the pleural space or in the interlobar fissures, but more commonly occupies a large portion of the pleural cavity. Empyema of a small amount may resolve with antimicrobial treatment. Such may be noted occasionally with pneumococcal empyema. Larger collections of pus may drain spontaneously through the lung by the establishment of bronchopleural fistulas, through the chest wall *(empyema necessitatis)* or through the diaphragm. Such spontaneous drainage is rarely curative. Without drainage there is a tendency for thick-walled cavities to develop or for the empyema to collapse the lung. If drainage of the empyema is not accomplished, the thick, organized exudate which maintains the lung in a collapsed position must be removed by decortification of the lung if re-expansion is to occur.

The manifestations of empyema follow those of the primary disease, usually bacterial pneumonia. Under these circumstances the patient fails to respond to treatment and often rapidly worsens. A rapidly progressive deterioration is often noted in infants who have empyema secondary to staphylococcal pneumonia. Increasing evidence of respiratory distress appears, often associated with chest pain, cough and recurrent fever. Occasionally patients who have been treated with antimicrobial drugs, but without complete eradication of their pulmonary infection, will have a latent period of a week or longer between the original infection and the development of the manifestations of empyema.

The findings by physical and roentgenographic examination are similar to those described under serofibrinous pleurisy. Patients with empyema generally tend to appear sicker than those having pleural effusions and usually have more severe systemic response to the infection; fever, leukocytosis and respiratory distress tend to be worse.

The diagnosis of empyema is made when purulent material is obtained after a thoracentesis. Occasionally, in the early course of staphylococcal pneumonia in infants, the initial aspiration yields serous fluid from which staphylococci are cultured. Subsequent aspirations are likely to show obviously purulent material. Empyema should be suspected in every patient with pneumonia who fails to improve rapidly.

Therapy of empyema includes continuing the treatment of the primary disease and the prompt and complete drainage of the pleural cavity. As much purulent material as possible should be removed at the time of the initial thoracentesis, and antimicrobial drugs such as penicillin G or one of the semisynthetic antistaphylococcal penicillins (methicillin, oxacillin or nafcillin) should be instilled into the pleural cavity. An occasional patient with a small or loculated empyema may be successfully drained by repeated thoracentesis accompanied by the instillation of appropriate antibiotic agents and proteolytic enzymes such as streptokinase-streptodornase mixtures or pancreatic dornase. This method is too traumatic for most infants and children in whom more than a few thoracenteses are necessary. It is not recommended for patients with pyopneumothorax or for those with extensive purulent collections.

The preferred method of drainage of empyema in infants and children is the continuous, closed drainage system which may be controlled by an underwater seal or by continuous suction. (See standard surgical texts for the details of these techniques.) As large a tube as possible should be inserted through an intercostal space. Local anesthetics are usually infiltrated into the site prior to the insertion of the tube; general anesthesia should not be necessary for this procedure. The lung tends to expand rapidly after removal of the purulent collection, and respiratory distress is often dramatically improved after the initial drainage.

After the initial instillation of antibiotics as described above, the subsequent choice of agents for local and systemic use should be made according to the results of bacterial cultures and sensitivity studies.

Closed pleural drainage is continued until the empyema cavity has been evacuated and the lung has re-expanded, usually a period of about seven to ten days. Many recommend instillation of appropriate antibiotics intrapleurally along with proteolytic enzymes several times a day during the first few days of treatment. These agents are introduced through a three-way stopcock installed in the drainage system as close to the chest wall as is practical. After the intrapleural instillation of antibiotics and enzymes, the chest drainage tube is completely clamped for at least an hour. During this period the patient's position is changed frequently to promote penetration of these agents into the entire pleural cavity.

The systemic administration of antimicrobial drugs is continued until the primary disease, usually pneumonia, has cleared completely.

Empyema which develops secondary to causes other than pneumonia may require special therapy. When empyema is secondary to penetrating wounds of the chest, mediastinitis, rupture of the esophagus, transdiaphragmatic spread of an intra-abdominal abscess or the occurrence of bronchopleural fistula, the infection is commonly produced by a mixture of organisms, often including coliform species. The initial selection of antibiotics should include an agent active against such bacteria. Moreover, in these situations, tetanus toxoid or antitoxin should be administered. Surgical treatment, in addition to drainage of the empyema, may also be indicated.

In addition to surgical drainage and antibiotic therapy, general supportive measures are often necessary, especially during the first few days of treatment. These measures often include the administration of oxygen, parenteral fluids, analgesics, and so on. Sedation is usually contraindicated.

Prompt, complete evacuation of empyema coupled with intensive systemic and intrapleural therapy should result in the re-expansion of the lung and eradication of the pleural infection. Such a program almost completely avoids the necessity for subsequent pulmonary surgery such as evacuation of the empyema by thoracotomy or decortication of the lung.

PUTRID EMPYEMA

Putrid empyema, a variant of purulent empyema, is sometimes classified as a separate clinical entity. In this situation the pleural infection is caused by anaerobic hemolytic streptococci, often in combination with bacteroides species, nonhemolytic streptococci, fusospirochetes, and others. The usual source of the pleural infection is the rupture of a lung abscess which has developed secondary to aspiration of infected material (see p. 334). The systemic manifestations of infection may be more severe than ordinarily observed with other causes of empyema. The aspirated purulent fluid has a foul odor.

The general principles of treatment are similar to those described above (see p. 343): namely, intensive systemic and topical antibiotic treatment and adequate pleural drainage. In addition, early surgical drainage or resection of the underlying abscess may be necessary.

Empyema which develops from the transdiaphragmatic spread of the intra-abdominal abscess may on rare occasions be caused by *Entameoba histolytica*, although such instances of empyema are more commonly caused by those bacterial species which are normally present in the intestinal tract. Under these circumstances the antibiotic therapy must be altered according to the infecting organisms, and the intra-abdominal abscess may also have to be drained, often by an open technique.

HYDROTHORAX

Hydrothorax is a noninflammatory reaction of the pleural cavity in which fluid collects as a transudate. The fluid has a specific gravity lower than 1.015 and a protein content less than 3.0 gm. per 100 ml. Hydrothorax is usually associated with the collection of fluid in other areas such as the peritoneal cavity and subcutaneous tissues. The most frequent cause of hydrothorax is cardiac failure or a variety of renal diseases. It may be noted with severe nutritional edema, beriberi, and other states. Hydrothorax may be unilateral or bilateral, but the right side is more often involved.

The symptoms of hydrothorax are those secondary to compression of the lung from the collection of fluid. Some dyspnea and orthopnea may result. The principal symptoms are those of the primary disease. Physical examination of the chest reveals findings similar to those described under serofibrinous pleurisy (see p. 340).

The treatment of hydrothorax is directed basically at the relief of the underlying disease. Occasionally thoracentesis must be performed to relieve the pulmonary compression. Sleeping in the semierect position may provide some comfort for certain children, but is not very practical for small children and infants.

HEMOTHORAX

Hemothorax or massive bleeding into the thorax is not common in children. The usual causes are trauma to the chest wall, injuries of a vessel at the time of operation or erosion of a vessel by inflammatory or malignant processes. In some instances hemothorax may be associated with a hemorrhagic disease. Hemorrhage from aneurysms is rare in children, but has occasionally been noted in children with Marfan's syndrome.

The symptoms are chiefly those of the primary disease and of blood loss. Some respiratory distress may occur from compression of the lungs. Physical examination of the lungs reveals findings similar to those noted in patients with empyema.

Treatment is, as in many pleural diseases, directed at the cause. Small amounts of blood in the pleural cavity require no treatment, since the blood will soon be absorbed. A massive hemothorax should be aspirated as completely as possible. If the blood has clotted, removal can be facilitated by the intrapleural instillation of a fibrinolytic enzyme preparation such as streptokinase-streptodornase mixtures. Fever and an increased amount of chest pain often follow the injection of this material. Thoracentesis should be repeated about eighteen hours after the intrapleural instillation, and at this time aspiration of the liquefied blood can be performed. If no further bleeding has occurred and if the blood has not been removed completely, additional instillations of the enzyme mixtures can be made. Occasionally, closed continuous chest drainage is required.

If active bleeding continues within the thoracic cavity, surgical exploration may be necessary to find and ligate the bleeding areas.

When hemothorax is secondary to a malignant process, irradiation or chemotherapy may result in temporary relief.

Transfusion of whole blood and measures to relieve pain may also be indicated.

CHYLOTHORAX

Chylothorax is a rare condition in infants and children and results from leakage of chyle from the thoracic duct or its branches into the pleural space. The most common causes include trauma to the chest, injury to the thoracic duct or its branches during cardiac or thoracic surgery, pressure from enlarged mediastinal lymph nodes and leakage from lymphangiomas of the mediastinum. It has been noted when a lymphangioma of the neck, so-called cystic hygroma, has grown into the mediastinal structures. In some instances no cause can be found, as is often the case in chylothorax of the newborn.

Symptoms and the findings of the physical examination are related to the amount of chyle which has collected. They are similar to those described under serofibrinous pleurisy (see p. 340) secondary to the loss of nutrients, chiefly fat and proteins, into the fluid. Wasting is sometimes severe, especially if recurrent collections require repeated pleural aspirations.

Roentgenographic examination is indicated to demonstrate the extent of the chylothorax, the presence of lymphadenopathy, and the like. A few efforts at lymphangiography have been made, but these are often not useful diagnostically because the lymphatic drainage from the extremities usually does not enter the thoracic duct system.

The diagnosis is established by obtaining milky opalescent fluid when thoracentesis is performed. This fluid is usually distinctive in appearance and suggests the diagnosis of chylothorax, but sometimes in serofibrinous pleurisy there may be some accumulation of fatty material, so-called pseudochylous effusion. The fluid should be treated as noted earlier (see p. 341). An additional diagnostic study can be performed by feeding a fat-soluble dye, such as D.C. #6 green, with some fatty food. Thoracentesis is repeated twelve to twenty-four hours later, at which time the chylous fluid is noted to be greenish-tinged.

When chylous fluid continues to accumulate in the pleural space, repeated thoracenteses may be necessary to relieve the respiratory distress. Under these circumstances serious nutritional depletion can occur, and nutritional supplements must be given parenterally to replace these losses. The intravenous injection of the aspirated fluid is no longer recommended because of the frequency and severity of reactions to the chylous fluid.

Approximately half of the patients with chylothorax will recover after repeated aspiration. If the leakage of chyle continues, surgical exploration of the mediastinum is indicated. Localization of the site of leakage of chyle may be identified more readily if the patient is fed a fat-soluble dye, such as D.C. #6 green, pre-operatively. At operation the green dye will stain the area where the leak has occurred.

In some instances no therapeutic measures are effective, and the patient dies from inanition.

REFERENCES

High, R. H.: Pleural Diseases; in S. S. Gellis and B. M. Kagan (Eds.): *Current Pediatric Therapy* 1966-1967. Philadelphia, W. B. Saunders Company, 1966, pp. 152-6.

Kinsey, D. L., and others: Simplified Management of Malignant Pleural Effusion. *Arch. Surg.,* 89:389-92, 1964.

Nelson, W. E.: Pleurisy; in W. E. Nelson (Ed.): *Textbook of Pediatrics.* 8th ed. Philadelphia, W. B. Saunders Company, 1964, pp. 870-72.

Idem: Hydrothorax; Hemothorax; Chylothorax; in W. E. Nelson (Ed.): *Textbook of Pediatrics.* 8th ed. Philadelphia, W. B. Saunders Company, 1964, pp. 875-6.

Pickett, L. K.: Purulent Pleurisy; in W. E. Nelson (Ed.): *Textbook of Pediatrics.* 8th ed. Philadelphia, W. B. Saunders Company, 1964, pp. 872-4.

Stead, W. W., and others: Pleural Effusion. *Disease of the Month,* July, 1964, pp. 1-48.

SECTION IX

Noninfectious Disorders
of the
Lower Respiratory Tract

CHAPTER THIRTY-ONE

Aspiration Pneumonia

WILLIAM CURTIS ADAMS, M.D.

The aspiration of foreign substances into the tracheobronchial tree may result in a variety of clinical situations depending upon the specific substance, the host reaction and the amount of the substance aspirated. Immediate death from suffocation or anaphylaxis is one extreme, and complete physiologic acceptance is the other. Between these extremes are the interrelated findings of pulmonary edema, emphysema and aspiration pneumonia The clinical picture is often indistinct, and in many instances elements of all these may be present.

Anatomic malformations may be associated with aspiration, e.g. cleft palate, tracheo-esophageal fistula and esophageal obstruction. Problems of deglutition, whether due to debilitation, or whether psychic or of central or peripheral nervous origin, e.g. prematurity or chronic or acute illness, may contribute to the aspiration of foreign substances (Figs. 1, 2).

The instillation of improper substances such as oily nose drops into the nose, and the use of such substances as zinc stearate powders have caused aspiration pneumonia.

The aspiration pneumonia resulting from forced feeding (Breck type feeder) and the feeding of crying children warrants specific mention. Oily substances such as cod liver oil, castor oil and mineral oil are easily aspirated when administered under the best of circumstances. Their use either in a forced feeding mechanism or for a crying child should be seriously questioned.

In some parts of the world, including parts of the United States of America, both turpentine and kerosene are used as folklore oral medications. Kerosene and turpentine rank high among the potentially toxic substances "accidentally" ingested by children and on the mortality lists resulting from such ingestion.

The pathogenesis of the pulmonary lesions resulting from the ingestion of lipids and hydrocarbons is subject to conflicting interpretations. Many investigators believe that aspiration of the lipids and hydrocarbons during the time of swallowing, vomiting or gastric lavage is the cause of most of the pulmonary problems. Others feel that the substance reaches the lungs after absorption from the gastrointestinal tract and "excretion" into the lung fields. It would seem obvious that both occur. Extensive pulmonary changes have been noted on x-ray examination shortly after ingestion, whether or not the ingestion has been accompanied by coughing, spluttering or vomiting. In contrast, roentgenographic evidence of pulmonary involvement has been demonstrated in experimental animals after absorption under conditions in which aspiration was impossible. Furthermore, selected cases will show an increase in roentgenographic evidence of pulmonary involvement on the third day with or without changes in symptomatology (Figs. 3 through 7). Probably both these routes of entry are important in producing the pulmonary reaction seen on x-ray examination.

Various lipid substances vary in the se-

(*Text continued on page 355.*)

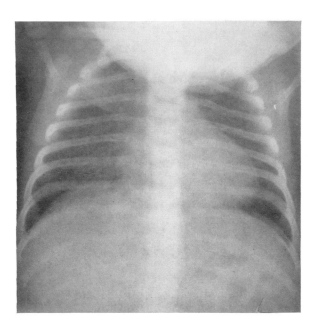

FIGURE 31–1. Three-year-old infant with respiratory symptoms following feeding. Note evidence of aspiration in the right upper lobe. (Courtesy of John Kirkpatrick, M.D., St. Christopher's Hospital for Children and Temple University School of Medicine.)

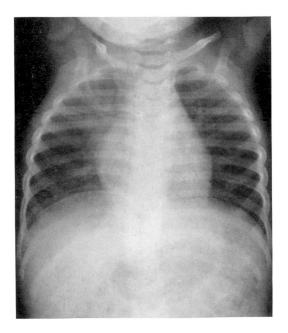

FIGURE 31–2. Eighteen-month-old retarded male child with respiratory symptoms following feeding. Note evidence of aspiration pneumonia in right upper lobe. (Courtesy of John Kirkpatrick, M.D., St. Christopher's Hospital for Children and Temple University School of Medicine.)

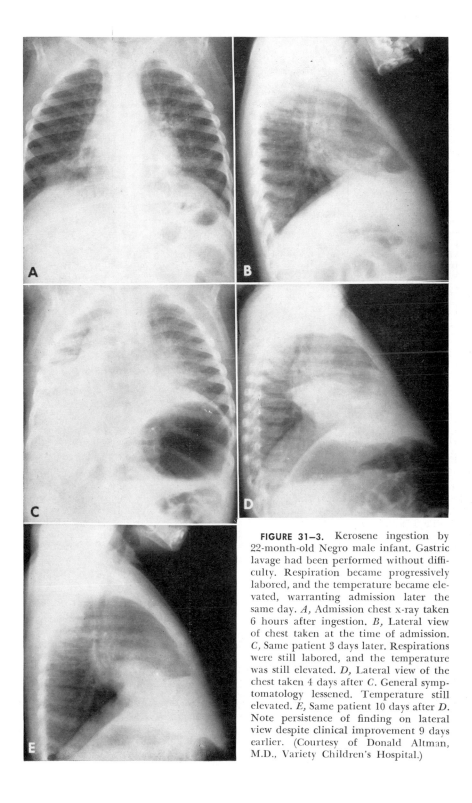

FIGURE 31–3. Kerosene ingestion by 22-month-old Negro male infant. Gastric lavage had been performed without difficulty. Respiration became progressively labored, and the temperature became elevated, warranting admission later the same day. *A*, Admission chest x-ray taken 6 hours after ingestion. *B*, Lateral view of chest taken at the time of admission. *C*, Same patient 3 days later. Respirations were still labored, and the temperature was still elevated. *D*, Lateral view of the chest taken 4 days after *C*. General symptomatology lessened. Temperature still elevated. *E*, Same patient 10 days after *D*. Note persistence of finding on lateral view despite clinical improvement 9 days earlier. (Courtesy of Donald Altman, M.D., Variety Children's Hospital.)

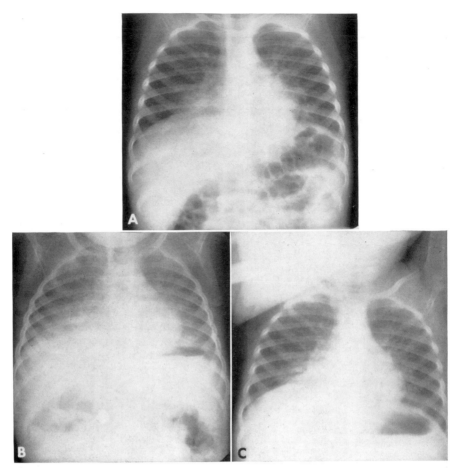

FIGURE 31–4. A 17-month-old white female infant had vomited 1½ hours after ingesting a half-bottle of furniture polish containing mineral seal oil. She was relatively asymptomatic. Twenty-four hours later she became drowsy and was unable to walk, and had a temperature elevation. *A,* Admission film taken 48 hours after ingestion. The child was drowsy and cyanotic with tachypnea. *B,* Twelve days later. The patient was treated with oxygen, moisture and antimicrobial therapy. Five days after admission the temperature remained under 100°. Seven days after admission she had clinical improvement and was removed from oxygen and moisture without recurrence of respiratory difficulty. *C,* The patient was discharged home 24 hours after *B* was taken. She has been completely asymptomatic, but findings persist 11 days later. (Courtesy of Donald Altman, M.D., Variety Children's Hospital.)

FIGURE 31–5. A 15-month-old female infant had ingested kerosene. Gastric lavage was performed immediately. The child was placed in oxygen for 48 hours. The temperature climbed steadily, and on the fifth day the child became lethargic and by the seventh day was dehydrated and transferred to Variety Children's Hospital for further definitive care. *A,* The cyst in the left lung is evident in this figure. *B,* The patient remained seriously ill. Progression was noted in size of the cyst. *C,* Clinical improvement 24 hours after *B.* The child continues to improve, although a fluid level is evident in one or more cysts 4 days after *B.* *D,* Three days after *C.* Fluid levels have disappeared. The child remains clinically improved. Anemia was treated with transfusion. Suggestion of multiple cysts persists. *E,* Fifteen days after *D.* The child has remained well, and the pulmonary cysts are not apparent. (Courtesy of Donald Altman, M.D., Variety Children's Hospital.)

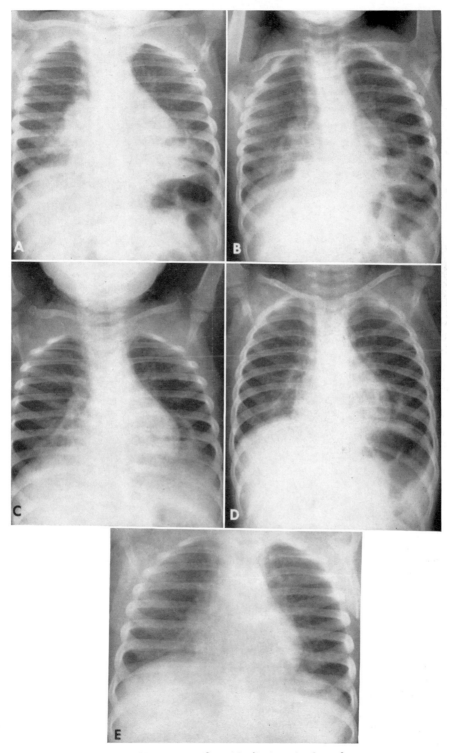

FIGURE 31–5. *See opposite page for legend.*

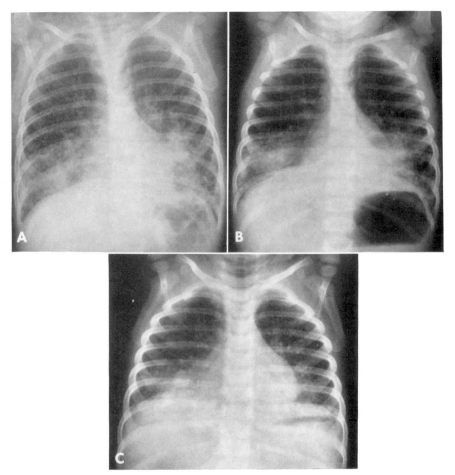

FIGURE 31–6. A 14-month-old male infant had ingested furniture polish 6 days prior to this illustration. Gastric lavage was performed. The child was treated with oxygen, but, owing to increasing severity of symptoms, was transferred to Variety Children's Hospital. *A*, Film taken on admission. The bilateral pulmonary involvement was evident. *B*, Five days after *A* the patient was clinically improved. Transfusion was given for anemia. The patient had been digitalized and treated with oxygen and mist. Effusion of the right pleural cavity is evident. *C*, Fifteen days after *B*. The patient is clinically well. He had no temperature elevation or respiratory difficulty or any symptoms in the past 12 days. Roentgenographic evidence of involvement of right and left hemithorax persists. (Courtesy of Donald Altman, M.D., Variety Children's Hospital.)

verity of symptoms and the degree of aspiration pneumonia following inhalation. As a rule, vegetable oils are less toxic than oils of animal origin; however, chaulmoogra oil (of vegetable origin) is very dangerous. Similarly, the hydrocarbons differ in the reactivity which they elicit. The constitution of kerosene appears to vary according to the temperature at which the cracking process was carried out. Such differences may help explain some of the vagaries of the reaction to aspiration. Petrolatum, another hydrocarbon, is chemically less irritating.

Any of these substances in large enough quantity can theoretically cause suffocation by mechanical blockage. Drowning is an example of aspiration of water accompanied by suffocation. If the victim survives the initial suffocation aspect, pulmonary edema may occur and may be difficult to differentiate from aspiration pneumonia and the superimposed infection which frequently follows.

Bronchitis and asthmatic attacks have been observed to follow the inhalation of dust. Finely powdered clays are particular offenders, but dusts of any appropriate particle size and of any origin are potential pathogens.

In some cases the dust may be infective and result in an actual aspiration pneumonia usually considered under a different classification. Histoplasmosis from the inhalation of dried, infected dung dust from chickens and bats is an excellent example of such an infection. (See the chapter on Histoplasmosis.)

The technicological developments of products, vehicles and packaging methods will lead to the identification of many other causes of aspiration pneumonia in the future. Thesaurosis, due to hair spray inhalation, is one example already cited. (See the chapter on Thesaurosis.) Similar problems can be expected with the continued use of spray packages both from the primary substances contained and from the propellants used, e.g. kerosene as a propellant for insect sprays. Possibly as many or more of the reactions will be hypersensitivity reactions as will be inflammatory or directly obstructive.

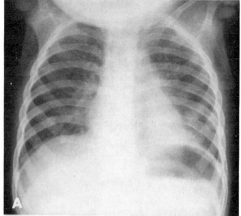
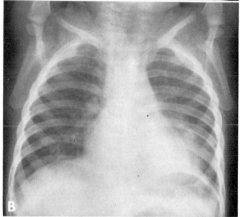

FIGURE 31–7. A 20-month-old male infant had ingested insecticide with petroleum distillate vehicle 14 hours before this x-ray. Choking and coughing developed immediately. Subsequently gastric lavage was performed. *A*, Within 4 hours an increase in respiratory rate with progression of cough and vomiting and the development of fever was noted. Child was brought to Variety Children's Hospital for admission. *B*, Four days after *A*. The patient has been treated with antimicrobial therapy and humidification of inspired air. Within 24 hours of admission the respirations had returned to normal, although the temperature remained elevated for 72 hours after this film was taken. Persistent involvement of the left lung is noted. (Courtesy of Donald Altman, M.D., Variety Children's Hospital.)

An anticipatory diagnosis of aspiration pneumonia, accompanied by considerable morbidity, can be made whenever a history of the ingestion of kerosene or turpentine is obtained.

Similar anticipatory diagnoses with the likelihood of a lesser morbidity may be made with the history of ingestion of large doses of animal oils, and the like. Aspiration pneumonia as an acute process is obvious when there are sudden respiratory symptoms accompanying the known inhalation or ingestion of a substance such as those listed above. A retrospective diagnosis may be made when incidental chest x-rays suggest an aspiration pneumonia and additional history or chemical findings corroborate the impression.

Treatment

The best therapy of aspiration pneumonia is prophylaxis. The process of making the public aware of aspiration pneumonia is the primary prophylactic approach. Through community education the problems of the use of zinc stearate powders, oily nose drops, the accidental and inappropriate ingestion of kerosene, and the use of aerosol house and cosmetic sprays under improper conditions may be eliminated.

Once respiratory symptoms are present, the administration of humidified oxygen frequently becomes necessary. Mechanical assistance or actual mechanical replacement of the respiratory effort with or without tracheostomy may be required. Bronchoscopic drainage of aspirated material may be of benefit in carefully selected patients. Postural drainage (and the coincidental enhancement of the cough) seems warranted for most of the patients who can tolerate the necessary positioning.

Cough medication (expectorants, suppressants and drying agents) may be prescribed for specific indications.

When the aspirated material is infectious or if a superimposed infection occurs, appropriate antimicrobial therapy is indicated. The efficacy of the steroids in the treatment of lipid and hydrocarbon pneumonia has not yet been established.

Poison control centers throughout the country find the ingestion of kerosene and other hydrocarbons to be a great problem in both incidence and morbidity. The pulmonary complications are responsible for much of the morbidity. The controversy

over the pathogenesis of pulmonary complications has been discussed. Most of those who are particularly interested in the investigation and treatment of accidental poisoning agree that vomiting is to be avoided after kerosene, mineral oil, fuel oil, and so on, have been ingested. Careful gastric lavage is indicated, especially if the amount ingested has been large or if decided central nervous system depression occurs early. The smaller the amount of kerosene or hydrocarbon ingested, the less is the danger of pneumonia.

Saline catharsis is indicated in either instance. Mineral oil has been advocated to retard the absorption of kerosene, but Gerade has presented a serious argument favoring olive over mineral oil for this purpose.

REFERENCES

Adams, W. C.: Poison Control Centers: Their Purpose and Operation. *Clin. Pharm. & Therap.,* 4:293, 1963.

Ashkenazi, A. E., and Berman, S. E.: Experimental Kerosene Poisoning in Rats, "Use of C14 Labeled Hendecane as Indicator of Absorption." *Pediatrics,* 28:642, 1961.

Baldachin, B. J., and Melmed, R. N.: Clinical and Therapeutic Aspects of Kerosene Poisoning: A Series of 200 Cases. *Brit. M.J.,* 2:28, 1964.

Balogna, N. A., and Woody, N. C.: Kerosene Poisoning. *N. Orleans Med. Surg. J.,* 101:256, 1948.

Brimblecombe, F. S. W., Crome, M. L., and Tizard, J. P. M.: Oil Aspiration Pneumonia in Infancy. *Arch. Dis. Childhood,* 26:141, 1951.

Foley, J. C., Dryer, N. B., Soule, A. J., and Wall, E.: Kerosene Poisoning in Young Children. *Radiology,* 62:817, 1954.

Graham, J. R.: Pneumonitis Following Aspiration of Crude Oil and Its Treatment by Steroid Hormone. *Tr. Am. Clin. Climatological Ann.,* 67:104, 1955-56.

Gerarde, H. W.: Toxocological Studies on Hydrocarbons. V. Kerosene. *Toxicol. Appl. Pharm.,* 1:462, 1959.

Haggerty, R. J.: Furniture Polish. *New England J. Med.,* 260:835, 1959.

Moran, T. J.: Milk Aspiration Pneumonia in Human and Animal Subjects. *Arch. Path.,* 55:286, 1953.

Nassau, E.: Ueber die Behandlung der Aspiration

von Petroleum mit Cortison. *Ann. paediat.*, 178:181, 1952.

Nelson, W. E.: *Textbook of Pediatrics.* 8th ed. Philadelphia, W. B. Saunders Company, 1964, p. 855.

Olstad, R. B., and Lord, R. M.: Kerosene Intoxication. A.M.A. *J. Dis. Child.,* 83:446, 1952.

Press, E.: Cooperative Kerosene Poisoning Study, Evaluation of Gastric Lavage and Other Factors in Treatment of Accidental Ingestion of Petrolatum Distillate Products. *Pediatrics,* 29: 1962.

Reed, E. S., Leiken, S., and Kerman, H. D.: Kerosene Intoxication. *Am. J. Dis. Child.,* 79:623, 1950.

Soule, A. B., Jr., and Foley, J. C.: Poisoning from Petroleum Distillates—The Hazards of Kerosene and Furniture Polish. *J. Maine Med. Assoc.,* 48:103, 1957.

Taylor, E. E., and Adams, W. C.: Factors Associated with Accidental Poisoning in Childhood: A Progress Report from the Louisville Poisoning Control Program. *South. M.J.,* 50:447, 1957.

Thatcher, E. W.: *Postural Drainage and Respiratory Control.* 2nd ed. London, Lloyd-Luke (Medical Books), Ltd., 1963.

Verhulst, H. L., and Page, L. A.: Adrenal Cortico Steroids in the Treatment of Kerosene Poisoning. *J. New Drugs,* 1:147, 1961.

CHAPTER THIRTY-TWO

Hypostatic Pneumonia

WILLIAM CURTIS ADAMS, M.D.

Hypostatic pneumonia is a natural complication of those conditions predisposing to prolonged maintenance of a prone position. Severe scleroderma, dermatomyositis, tetanus and poliomyelitis are examples of debilitating conditions that may be complicated by hypostatic pneumonia. The early classic symptoms of pneumonia are characteristically absent, and the physical signs of dullness and rales must be carefully looked for in the dependent lung fields. X-ray evidence of consolidation in the dependent areas will confirm the diagnosis in questionable cases.

Prevention by frequent change of position and maintenance of good pulmonary function is the primary therapeutic approach. Postural drainage and physiotherapy are cornerstones of both prophylaxis and active therapy. If the underlying condition prohibits normal pulmonary activity, appropriate partial or full mechanical respiratory support, humidification, and the like, should be selected. If superimposed infection occurs, appropriate antimicrobial therapy should be instituted.

If hypostatic pneumonia has been permitted to develop, therapy should be directed toward the re-establishment of normal function in the involved lung.

CHAPTER THIRTY-THREE

Idiopathic Diffuse Interstitial Fibrosis of the Lung (Hamman-Rich Syndrome)

WILLIAM A. HOWARD, M.D.

Idiopathic diffuse interstitial fibrosis of the lung is a chronic, progressive, usually fatal pulmonary disorder of unknown origin and diverse clinical manifestations. The syndrome, originally described by Hamman and Rich in 1935, has been enlarged to include a number of entities with similar physiologic and pathologic findings, and characterized by a variable response to treatment and a poor prognosis. Over 130 cases have been reported, largely in adults, and the disease appears to be rare under the age of ten years.

Etiology

Although no etiologic agents have been proved, interest has centered around the possibility of tissue hypersensitivity as a factor because of similar findings in certain known collagen disorders such as scleroderma. The response of certain patients to corticosteroid therapy, the presence of tissue eosinophilia, and the experimental production of a similar condition in rats who were given rabbit antirat lung serum intratracheally, all suggest a hypersensitivity phenomenon. Other etiologic agents which have been suggested include viral diseases such as atypical pneumonia, influenza and pleuropneumonia infections, chemical irritants, bacterial infections and chronic pulmonary lymphedema. Silverman and Talbot suggest that idiopathic interstitial pulmonary fibrosis is a syndrome probably produced or initiated by a variety of agents.

Clinical Manifestations

The disease is apparently more common in males and is relatively rare in infants and children. The onset is insidious, and dyspnea is usually the earliest symptom, first appearing on exertion, but later present at rest, and unaffected by position. Cough may be troublesome, and there may be hemoptysis and chest pain. Fever, when present, is usually due to superimposed infection, which may be an unrelated but serious problem. Anorexia, weight loss, fatigability and weakness accompany the progressive course, while cyanosis and clubbing appear only late in the disease. The appearance of peripheral edema, hepatomegaly, accentuation of the pulmonic second sound and elevated venous pressure indicate the presence of right ventricular heart failure, which is common in the later stages of the disease.

X-ray findings, though not diagnostic, are initially suggestive of diffuse reticular infiltration; later the involvement may consist of finely nodular densities, most prominent in the middle and lower lung fields (Fig. 1). Cardiac enlargement may be present, and pleural effusion may appear during episodes of congestive failure. Compensatory emphysema may be seen, and occasionally pneumothorax will occur.

There are no pathognomonic laboratory findings except those associated with intercurrent infections. Secondary polycythemia may appear after prolonged reduction in arterial oxygen saturation, and the electrocardiogram may be indicative of right ventricular hypertrophy.

Pathology

There is extensive and diffuse proliferation of fibrous tissue throughout all the lobes of the lungs, associated with organization of intra-alveolar exudate. The alveolar lining cells are enlarged, with necrosis of alveolar and bronchial epithelium, and with interstitial eosinophilia. There are few leukocytes or bacteria.

Lung biopsy early in the disease may show a cellular appearance with infiltration of lymphocytes, plasma cells and occasional eosinophils, located within the walls of the alveoli, alveolar ducts and peribronchial tissues. Fibrosis is difficult to discern in the early stages.

Diagnosis

The primary problem in patients with diffuse interstitial fibrosis of the lung is reduction in the diffusion capacity of the lung, without obstructive ventilatory dis-

ease, the so-called alveolar-capillary block. These patients have markedly reduced lung compliance, sometimes less than 50 per cent of the expected value; ventilation must be accomplished by a relatively rapid respiratory rate with a small tidal volume. Maximum midexpiratory flow rates and maximum voluntary ventilation values are usually normal, but lung capacities (vital capacity, total lung capacity) are reduced. At rest the arterial oxygen saturation is near normal, but is sharply reduced during exercise. Pulmonary function studies, therefore, are an excellent means for identifying the patient with restrictive lung disease due to pulmonary fibrosis. A more definitive delineation of the type of fibrosis can be made only by tissue study, and this is accomplished with relative ease by lung biopsy.

Differential diagnosis should include collagen diseases, sarcoidosis and other granulomatous processes, and malignancy. In some instances the disease appears to be familial, and the term "familial fibrocystic pulmonary dysplasia" has been suggested to distinguish those cases with a

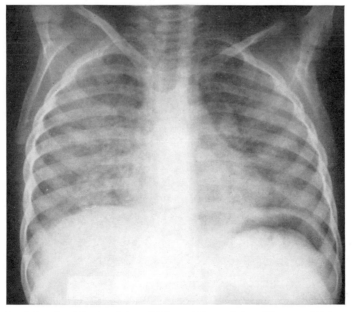

FIGURE 33–1. Nodular densities in right middle and lower lobes. Hamman-Rich syndrome. (Courtesy of W. W. Waring, M.D., Tulane University School of Medicine, New Orleans.)

possible genetic background from other examples of the Hamman-Rich syndrome.

Course and Complications

The development of clinical signs and symptoms in interstitial pulmonary fibrosis depends upon the extent to which pulmonary reserve has been compromised by the underlying disease process. A superimposed acute inflammatory process will produce exacerbation of all symptoms and may precipitate cardiac decompensation. Progression of the basic pulmonary lesion and repeated infections may lead to cor pulmonale. Death usually occurs as a result of cardiac failure or rapidly progressive respiratory insufficiency. Complete and permanent arrest is unusual.

Treatment

Treatment is generally symptomatic, with emphasis on the prevention and treatment of respiratory infection, correction of the anemia and maintenance of general health. Corticosteroids have been used with apparent symptomatic relief, but with little evidence of improvement in pulmonary function. The dosage must be high, maintained for long periods, and tapered slowly. Maintenance doses may be required for long periods, and these patients may become steroid-dependent. Early inflammatory lesions may respond to corticosteroid therapy, while those that are already fibrotic are likely to be irreversible.

REFERENCES

Diamond, I.: The Hamman-Rich Syndrome in Children. *Pediatrics*, 22:279, 1958.

Donohue, W. L., Laski, B., Uchida, I., and Munn, J. D.: Familial Fibrocystic Pulmonary Dysplasia and Its Relationship to the Hamman-Rich Syndrome. *Pediatrics*, 24:786, 1959.

Gross, P.: The Hamman-Rich Syndrome: A Critique. *Am. Rev. Resp. Dis.*, 85:828, 1962.

Hamman, L., and Rich, A. R.: Fulminating Diffuse Interstitial Fibrosis of the Lungs. *Tr. Am. Clin. Climatol A.*, 51:154, 1935.

Ivemark, B., and Wallgren, G.: Hamman-Rich Syndrome in an Infant. *Acta paediat.*, 51:238, 1962.

Livingston, J. S., Lewis, J. G., Reid, L., and Jefferson, K. E.: Diffuse Interstitial Pulmonary Fibrosis. *Quart. J. Med.*, 23:71, 1964.

Rubin, E. H., and Lunliner, R.: The Hamman-Rich Syndrome: Review of the Literature, and Analysis of 15 Cases. *Medicine*, 36:397, 1957.

Sheridan, L. A., Harrison, E. G., and Divertie, M. B.: The Current Status of Idiopathic Pulmonary Fibrosis (Hamman-Rich Syndrome). *Med. Clin. N. Amer.*, 48:993, 1964.

Silverman, J. J., and Talbot, T. J.: Diffuse Interstitial Pulmonary Fibrosis Camouflaged by Hypermetabolism and Cardiac Failure. *Ann. Int. Med.*, 38:1326, 1953.

CHAPTER THIRTY-FOUR

Pulmonary Alveolar Proteinosis

EDWIN L. KENDIG, JR., M.D.

Pulmonary alveolar proteinosis, a syndrome usually characterized by progressive dyspnea and cough, was first described in 1958 by Rosen, Castleman and Liebow, who reported twenty-seven instances of the disease. Since that time only a few cases have been reported.

On pathologic examination the appear-

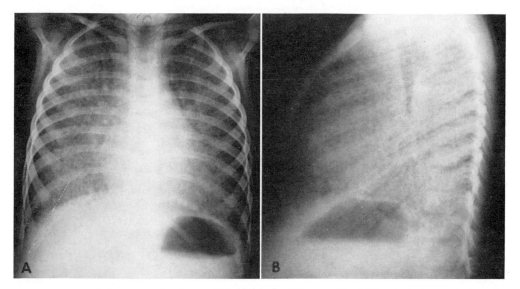

FIGURE 34–1. Pulmonary alveolar proteinosis in a 2½-year-old child. *A,* Anteroposterior view showing punctate and widely distributed densities. *B,* Lateral view showing foci of emphysema interspersed among zones of increased density. (S. H. Rosen, B. Castleman and A. A. Liebow: *New England J. Med.,* 258:1123, 1958.)

ance of the lung is characteristic, although there may be some variation in the extent and distribution of the disease. Multiple yellow-gray or gray nodules, firm to palpation and of varying size, are often present beneath the pleura; consolidation is usually evident in large portions of the lung. The bronchi and bronchioles appear normal, with little evidence of alveolar wall damage or thickening, but the presence of eosinophilic material in some or many of the alveoli is diagnostic. This material is granular and floccular, particularly when stained with PAS; it is also rich in protein and lipid. Suggestion has been made that this material is secreted by the alveolar lining cells, which are swollen and increased in number; these cells may slough into the alveolar lumens, ultimately resulting in rounded or ovoid laminated bodies.

The clinical picture is usually characterized by progressive dyspnea, often accompanied by a cough which may be productive. There is usually increased fatigability and loss of weight. The onset may or may not be heralded by a febrile illness. Physical signs are relatively few.

The roentgen changes as noted by Rosen et al. are "a fine, diffuse, perihilar, radiating, feathery, or vaguely nodular, soft density, resembling in its 'butterfly' distribution the pattern seen in severe pul-

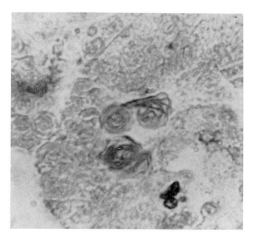

FIGURE 34–2. Laminated bodies, predominating close to alveolar septa, which, despite their cystlike appearance, are thought to represent fragmented residue of cells with deposits of proteinaceous material about them. (S. H. Rosen, B. Castleman and A. A. Liebow: *New England J. Med.,* 258:1123, 1958.)

monary edema." Such shadows may become denser, or there may be a partial or complete resolution.

Death may result from the progressive filling of alveoli, or superimposed fungal or bacterial infection.

There is no specific therapy, and antibiotics appear to be indicated only when there is superimposed bacterial infection. Pulmonary lavage has been shown to be effective in those adults with extreme pulmonary disability with impairment of gaseous exchange.

REFERENCES

Bates, D. V., and Christie, R. V.: *Respiratory Function in Disease*. Philadelphia, W. B. Saunders Company, 1964.

Fraimow, W., Cathcart, R. T., and Taylor, R. C.: Physiologic and Clinical Aspects of Pulmonary Alveolar Proteinosis. *Ann. Int. Med.*, 52:1177, 1960.

Fraimow, W., Cathcart, R. T., Kirshner, J. J., and Taylor, R. C.: Pulmonary Alveolar Proteinosis. A Correlation of Pathological and Physiological Findings in a Patient Followed up with Serial Biopsies of the Lung. *Am. J. Med.*, 28:458, 1960.

Hall, G. F. M.: Pulmonary Alveolar Proteinosis. *Lancet*, 1:1383, 1960.

Jones, C. C.: Pulmonary Alveolar Proteinosis with Unusual Complicating Infections. A Report of Two Cases. *Am. J. Med.*, 29:713, 1960.

Landis, F. B., Rose, H. D., and Sternlieb, R. O.: Pulmonary Alveolar Proteinosis. A Case Report with Unusual Clinical and Laboratory Manifestations. *Am. Rev. Resp. Dis.*, 80:249, 1959.

Lull, G. F., Jr., Beyer, J. C., Maier, J. G., and Morss, D. F., Jr.: Pulmonary Alveolar Proteinosis. Report of Two Cases. *Am. J. Roentgenol.*, 82:76, 1959.

Ray, R. L., and Salm, R.: A Fatal Case of Pulmonary Alveolar Proteinosis. *Thorax*, 17:257, 1962.

Ramirez, R. J., Kieffer, R. G., Jr., and Ball, W. C., Jr.: Bronchopulmonary Lavage in Man. *Ann. Int. Med.*, 63:819, 1965.

Rosen, S. H., Castleman, B., and Liebow, A. A.: Pulmonary Alveolar Proteinosis. *New England J. Med.*, 258:1123, 1958.

Snider, T. H., Wilner, F. M., and Lewis, B. M.: Cardiopulmonary Physiology in a Case of Pulmonary Alveolar Proteinosis. *Ann. Int. Med.*, 52:1318, 1960.

Williams, G. E. G., Medley, D. R. K., and Brown, R.: Pulmonary Alveolar Proteinosis. *Lancet*, 1:1385, 1960.

CHAPTER THIRTY-FIVE

Thesaurosis

WILLIAM CURTIS ADAMS, M.D.

Bergman, Flance and Blumenthal and their co-workers have called attention to the possibility that the repeated inhalation of hair sprays may cause pulmonary infiltration and related findings. All the cases reported to date have been in adults. The National Clearinghouse for Poison Control Centers is unaware of any reported cases in children. Nevertheless both the emphasis on cosmetic and sartorial grooming of teenage girls by the mass advertising media and the employment of female children as actresses or models make hair spray inhalation a potential hazard to children.

Many hair sprays contain macromolecular substances which reportedly cannot be metabolized by the human organism. Draize, Nelson, Neuberger and Kelley have demonstrated that the polyvinyl pyrrolidone type of product (a polymerized vinyl compound) does, however, contain small enough particles to reach the pulmonary aveolar surfaces when the substance is sprayed.

The clinical respiratory symptoms noted in adults have varied from none at all to cough and severe dyspnea. Physical examination of the chest may reveal no abnormality, but rales may be present. Roentgenograms of the chest have demonstrated lung pathology varying from diffuse mottling with stringy densities to extensive bilateral nodular infiltrates with hilar lymph node involvement. By history, the extensive use of hair spray appears to be the most likely potential etiologic factor in these nonspecific roentgenographic findings. Although the causal relationship has not been proved, many of the patients have shown clinical improvement and clearing of the findings when the use of the hair spray has been discontinued.

The primary direct therapeutic action in all cases is discontinuance of the use of hair spray. The signs and symptoms of each case will determine the amount and type of supportive care indicated to provide maximum pulmonary function and drainage. (See the chapter on the Collagen diseases.) In some cases actual respiratory aid and oxygen therapy may be needed. Every effort should be extended to prevent superimposed infection, and appropriate treatment of any such infection should be prompt and adequate. Corticosteroid therapy has been tried, but its efficacy has not been established.

REFERENCES

Bergman, M., Flance, I. J., and Blumenthal, H. T.: Thesaurosis Following Inhalation of Hair Spray; Clinical and Experimental Study. *New England J. Med.*, 258:471, 1958.

Bergman, M., and others: Thesaurosis Due to Inhalation of Hair Spray. *New England J. Med.*, 266:750, 1962.

CHAPTER THIRTY-SIX

Idiopathic Pulmonary Alveolar Microlithiasis

ROBERT H. HIGH, M.D.

This is a rare disease of unknown origin characterized by the formation of tiny stones of calcium carbonate within the pulmonary alveoli. No metabolic aberrations have been recognized in those cases diagnosed before death. In particular, alterations in the metabolism of calcium and phosphorus have not been found. The reported cases have been equally distributed between males and females. A definite familial tendency has been noted, but to date it has not been determined whether a genetic factor is involved in the development of the disease.

The mechanism by which the stones are formed is not known. Their presence in the alveoli eventually leads to interstitial fibrosis and to symptoms and signs of progressive cardiopulmonary failure. Death usually occurs in midadult life.

The onset of the disease is usually insidious, but presumably occurs in childhood. In most instances in which this disease has been recognized in children,

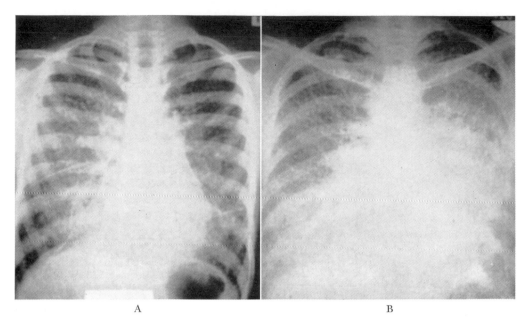

A   B

FIGURE 36–1. *A,* Roentgenogram taken in February 1954, showing minute miliary dissemination except at the apex and peripheral parts of both lungs. Hairline densities were seen from the hilus to peripheral parts. *B,* Roentgenogram taken in April 1964. Minute miliary dissemination became confluent at the hilus and striated at the peripheral parts of both lungs. (S. Oka and others: *Am. Rev. Resp. Dis.,* 93:612-16, 1966.)

the diagnosis has been suggested by the roentgenographic abnormalities. Usually the roentgenograms were obtained because of unrelated cardiac or pulmonary disease. In some instances the disease has been noted on roentgenograms made for routine reasons or as part of family surveys after a symptomatic adult has been recognized. Most children have no symptoms and do not show any abnormality by physical examination. A few children have been studied with a variety of pulmonary function tests and have been found to have normal pulmonary function. Recently impairment in diffusing capacity for carbon monoxide and true membrane diffusing capacity have been demonstrated in two siblings.

Roentgenographic examination of the lungs shows finely granular densities diffusely and relatively uniformly scattered throughout the lungs. The apices and bases of the lungs may appear to be un-

involved. At times the densities may be so numerous that the cardiac outline is indistinct. According to Clark and Johnson, "the appearance somewhat resembles the granular alveolar density of an overfilled normal bronchogram."

The diagnosis can be confirmed by microscopic examination of the pulmonary tissue obtained by percutaneous or open biopsy of the lung.

There is no known effective treatment, and management is entirely symptomatic.

REFERENCES

Clark, R. B., and Johnson, F. C.: Idiopathic Pulmonary Alveolar Microlithiasis. *Pediatrics,* 28:650, 1961.

Oka, S., and others: Pulmonary Alveolar Microlithiasis. *Am. Rev. Resp. Dis.,* 93:612, 1966.

Sosman, M. C., Dodd, G. D., Jones, W. D., and Pillmore, G. U.: Familial Occurrence of Pulmonary Microlithiasis. *Am. J. Roentgenology,* 77:947, 1957.

CHAPTER THIRTY-SEVEN

Pulmonary Hemosiderosis

DOUGLAS C. HEINER, M.D.

The term "pulmonary hemosiderosis" indicates an abnormal accumulation of iron as hemosiderin in the lungs. It results from bleeding into the lungs and is much more likely to follow diffuse alveolar hemorrhage than bleeding from large arteries or arterioles. It may be primary in the lungs or secondary to cardiac or systemic disease. In most instances in which it is primary the cause is unknown, but a significant percentage of cases occurring in infants appear to be related to the ingestion of cow's milk. Pulmonary hemosiderosis in adults is commonly secondary to cardiac disease involving left ventricular failure or pulmonary venous hypertension such as occurs in mitral stenosis. This elevation of venous pressure may result in recurrent or chronic capillary oozing of blood into the alveoli with resultant hemosiderosis (brown induration) of the lungs. In children, on the other hand, primary pulmonary hemosiderosis is more frequent than the secondary varieties. The majority of all primary cases occur during childhood.

Although the first description of the pathologic features of brown induration of the lungs was by Virchow in 1864, the clinical picture of idiopathic pulmonary hemosiderosis was not reported until Ceelen's description in 1931. The first antemortem diagnosis was recorded by Waldenstrom in 1940, and knowledge of the disease has since been amplified by many authors. In Europe the idiopathic form is frequently referred to as "Ceelen's disease," or "Ceelen-Gellerstedt's disease."

As with most diseases, there is a wide variation in clinical manifestations, and many years have been required to delineate several distinct subgroups. It now seems likely that several disease processes may lead to primary as well as to secondary pulmonary hemosiderosis, and as time progresses the diagnosis of idiopathic pulmonary hemosiderosis should apply to a smaller and smaller proportion of patients. At present it is convenient to classify and describe pulmonary hemosiderosis as follows:

I. Primary pulmonary hemosiderosis
   A. Isolated
   B. With myocarditis
   C. With glomerulonephritis (Goodpasture's syndrome)
   D. With sensitivity to cow's milk
II. Secondary pulmonary hemosiderosis
   A. With primary cardiac disease
   B. With primary collagen vascular or purpuric disease

ISOLATED PRIMARY PULMONARY HEMOSIDEROSIS

This diagnosis refers to those instances in which no cause and no significant associated disease are apparent. It may occur at any age, but is most common in children and young adults. It is commonly referred to as idiopathic pulmonary hemosiderosis.

Symptoms and Physical Findings

The most helpful clinical signs are iron deficiency anemia which is sometimes resistant to iron therapy, recurrent or chronic pulmonary symptoms including cough, hemoptysis, dyspnea, wheezing, and often cyanosis, and characteristic abnormalities on chest roentgenograms. Hemoptysis in children is an especially helpful clue to the diagnosis, although one must be aware that sometimes it is difficult to determine the origin of blood

365

when there is both coughing and vomiting. In some infants swallowed blood from the lungs is vomited without coughing, so that the possibility of a pulmonary source of bleeding should be kept in mind in children with unexplained hematemesis, particularly when there are roentgenographic abnormalities in the lungs. Any of the features noted above may be the first manifestation of the disease. For example, subjects have been recorded in whom there was apparently an asymptomatic iron deficiency anemia as an initial single abnormal finding. Others have had hemoptysis, persistent cough or another pulmonary symptom before anemia was apparent. Pulmonary symptoms may occur with or without detectable roentgenographic abnormalities, or there may be striking roentgenographic changes before pulmonary symptoms or other features are clearly manifest. The clinical picture is usually characterized by recurrent episodes of pulmonary bleeding during which there is fever, tachycardia, tachypnea, leukocytosis, an elevated sedimentation rate, abdominal pain and often other findings suggesting a bacterial pneumonia. Occasionally pneumonia appears to be confirmed by positive sputum or throat cultures, and only long-term follow-up combined with an awareness of the possibility of pulmonary hemosiderosis leads to the correct diagnosis. Poor weight gain and easy fatigue are common in subjects with moderate to severe disease. Physical findings vary, depending on the status of the patient at the time of examination. There may be pallor, dyspnea, bronchial or suppressed breath sounds, rales, rhonchi, wheezing and an emphysematous chest. Liver or spleen enlargement is sometimes found and may be transient.

Laboratory and Roentgenologic Findings

The anemia is typically microcytic and hypochromic, and the serum iron concentration is low in spite of an excessive accumulation of iron in the lungs. Trace labeling of red blood cells with radioisotopes has shown that large volumes of blood may exude into the lungs, the iron subsequently becoming largely sequestered and relatively unavailable for use in the formation of new red blood cells. Animal experiments suggest, however, that there may be slow utilization of hemosiderin iron from the lungs for hematopoiesis, and it is possible that in human pulmonary hemosiderosis the rate of deposition of iron in the lungs in most instances merely exceeds the rate of utilization. The fact that symptoms, chest roentgenograms and anemia sometimes clear completely indicates that in remission there may be significant net removal of iron from the lungs.

There is a variable hematologic response to oral or intramuscular iron. Some patients have a good reticulocyte and hemoglobin response, but others appear to have defective hematopoiesis while the disease process is active. Many have reticulocytosis during periods of active pulmonary bleeding whether or not iron therapy is administered, and this, along with mild jaundice and an elevated urobilinogen excretion, may lead to an erroneous diagnosis of hemolytic anemia. This diagnosis seems even more credible in the few subjects who have a positive direct Coombs test result suggesting that anti-red blood cell antibodies are adherent to the erythrocyte surfaces. Circulating cold agglutinins may also be found, and like a positive Coombs test result, suggest the presence of an unusual immune response.

Eosinophilia has been present in one fifth to one eighth of the reported cases, but experience suggests that eosinophile counts fluctuate markedly in this disease and that the likelihood of finding eosinophilia is proportional to the number of times it is looked for in a given case. If frequent differential leukocyte or absolute eosinophile counts are obtained, more than this proportion of subjects will be found to have eosinophilia.

Stool guaiac test results are frequently positive, and the presumption is that this is due to swallowed blood from the tracheobronchial tree. Reasonable evidence for this presumption comes from the fact that most patients with pulmonary hemosiderosis produce bloody sputum, some of which is obviously swallowed. In addition, the gastric juice usually contains iron-laden macrophages (siderophages) from the lungs even when there is no obvious hemoptysis. It is possible, however, that direct bleeding into the gastrointestinal tract may occur in some subjects.

The finding of siderophages in the stomach in the presence of otherwise unexplained pulmonary disease is good presumptive evidence of pulmonary hemosiderosis (Fig. 1). It is the simplest reliable diagnostic laboratory test in infants and young children. The Prussian-blue reaction with potassium ferrocyanide and hydrochloric acid provides a good stain, the hemosiderin granules within macrophages acquiring an easily recognized deep blue color. Siderophages may also

be found in the sputum or in washings of the tracheobronchial tree, or within the alveoli of biopsy specimens obtained by needle aspiration or open operation. Most workers accept siderophages in gastric or bronchial secretions as diagnostic if typical clinical features are present and are not accompanied by evidence of extrapulmonary disease.

A biopsy diagnosis is considered necessary by some workers. The pathologic findings on biopsy have been summarized in detail by Soergel and Sommers. They include alveolar epithelial hyperplasia and degeneration with excessive shedding of cells, large numbers of siderocytes, varying amounts of interstitial fibrosis and mast-cell accumulation, elastic fiber degeneration, and sclerotic vascular changes. Most of these features were present in the specimen shown in Figure 2. Vasculitis is usually absent, but, if found, suggests that the disorder may not be primary, but rather secondary to a systemic colla-

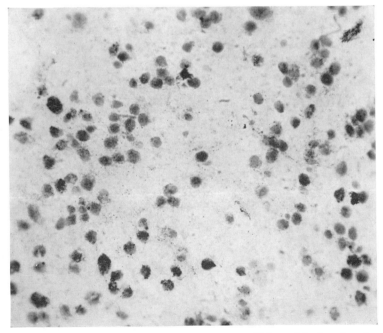

FIGURE 37–1. Siderophages in gastric washings of a 15-year-old boy with chronic pulmonary disease, recurrent hemoptysis and iron deficiency anemia. Bronchial washings showed similar iron-laden macrophages. There was no evidence of cardiovascular, renal, collagen or purpuric disease, but multiple precipitins to cow's milk were present in high titer. Chronic cough and hemoptysis ceased coincidentally with removal of milk from the diet. Prussian blue stain × 150.

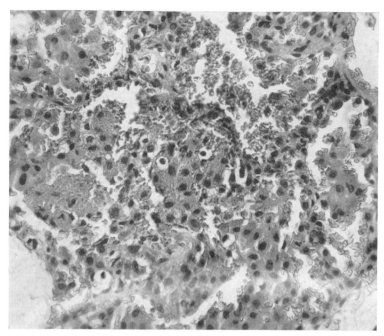

FIGURE 37–2. Microscopic section of lung from 1-year-old infant with primary pulmonary hemosiderosis. The alveoli are filled with macrophages, many of which contained hemosiderin granules demonstrated by an iron stain. Fresh intra-alveolar hemorrhage is also evident, and there is proliferation and shedding of alveolar epithelial cells. H & E stain × 150.

gen vascular disease. Biopsies would seem justified in those subjects in whom clinical findings are atypical or if the diagnosis is still in doubt after all simpler procedures have been done, including a careful search for siderophages in several specimens of gastric juice, sputum or bronchial washings. Needle aspiration biopsy may be as risky as open biopsy under anesthesia, or more risky. The author has had an experience with one subject in whom the clinical picture suggested primary pulmonary hemosiderosis with active pulmonary lesions and in whom needle biopsy was attempted under local anesthesia. The procedure was considered benign when it was done, but seemed to be the turning point to deterioration with a rapidly progressive downhill course, massive pulmonary hemorrhage and a fatal termination several hours later. Postmortem examination confirmed the clinical diagnosis. Other authors have suggested that needle biopsy is not without danger in this disease.

Roentgenographic abnormalities vary from minimal transient infiltrates to massive parenchymal involvement with secondary atelectasis, emphysema and hilar lymphadenopathy. The findings are somewhat variable from patient to patient and may change in a given subject with each new bleeding or with clinical remission. Diffuse, soft perihilar infiltrates are common. In some subjects the appearance is similar to that of pulmonary edema. In others it is more like bronchial or lobar pneumonia, and in still others it may resemble the findings in miliary tuberculosis, Gaucher's disease or Wegener's granulomatosis. Thus there frequently is thickening of interlobar septa with horizontal lines and fine nodulations suggesting interstitial fibrosis. The resulting reticular or reticulonodular pattern may be widespread, but is often present chiefly in the lower lobes and is likely to persist for months or years after acute infiltrative lesions have cleared in those who survive. Illustrative roentgenograms are shown in Figures 3 and 4.

Pulmonary function tests have not been reported in detail, but the vital capacity, maximal breathing capacity and arterial oxygen saturation have each been reduced in individual subjects. Cardiac catheterization has revealed variable findings, some patients showing no abnormalities, others having pulmonary arterial hypertension and even right ventricular failure as an end-result of cor pulmonale.

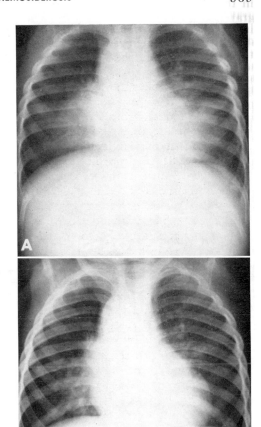

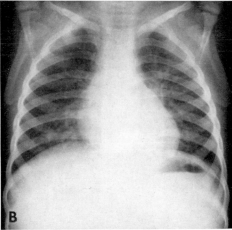
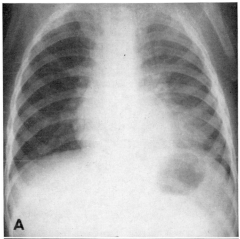

FIGURE 37–4. *A,* Roentgenogram of a boy with primary pulmonary hemosiderosis at 2 years of age, showing diffuse, soft perihilar infiltrates, somewhat suggestive of pulmonary edema. *B,* Same subject 6 months later, showing less pronounced soft infiltrates in right middle lobe and left hilar regions, and some horizontal septal lines suggesting fibrosis.

FIGURE 37–3. *A,* Roentgenogram of a boy with primary pulmonary hemosiderosis of 2 years' duration during an exacerbation at 27 months of age. Note soft perihilar infiltrates, most evident along the left cardiac border. *B,* Same subject 4 months later when asymptomatic. Note decrease in soft infiltrates, but prominent bilateral reticulonodular pattern suggesting interstitial fibrosis.

Significant abnormalities in pulmonary function and demonstrated pulmonary hypertension indicate a more guarded prognosis than if these physiologic parameters are normal, although most deaths are due to active bleeding rather than to pulmonary or cardiac insufficiency.

Treatment

When possible, treatment should be preceded by vigorous attempts to rule out known factors which might be important in the causation of, or which might aggravate, idiopathic hemosiderosis. These include appropriate studies to detect heart disease, diffuse collagen vascular disease, thrombocytopenic purpura, and attempts to uncover sensitivity to drugs, inhaled substances, and foods. Acute crises should be treated with oxygen. Severely dyspneic patients may benefit from its administration by intermittent positive pressure. Blood transfusions are indicated to correct severe anemia or shock. The blood should be obtained from a healthy nonallergic donor and carefully cross-matched. It should be given under close supervision, since several acutely ill patients have been thought to do less well during and immediately after transfusions. ACTH, 10 to 25 units daily, or hydrocortisone, 4 mg. per kilogram of body weight per day, by intravenous infusion is recommended. Critically ill subjects are probably best kept on intravenous fluid therapy with nothing by mouth for twenty-four to forty-eight hours. After this foods may be introduced, and prednisone, 2 mg. per kilogram may be given orally instead of ACTH or hydrocortisone. After a clinical remission has been well established the corticosteroid level can be gradually decreased until the drug is discontinued or until pulmonary symptoms recur. If maintenance corticosteroid therapy seems necessary, attempt should be made to establish the minimum dose which will suppress symptoms, but not produce undesirable side effects. This should be continued for three months before again trying to discontinue it. Growth retardation and other steroid side effects may be minimized in some patients by administering the corticosteroid on three consecutive days of each week, or by giving the calculated amount for two days as a single dose. If pulmonary disease recurs at any time, corticosteroids should be reinstituted, or the dosage temporarily increased, in an attempt to suppress the process. Control of the disease should be judged by symptoms, hematologic studies and roentgenographic findings. Subjects

with idiopathic pulmonary hemosiderosis are in constant danger of relapse and even death; hence careful, long-term medical supervision is indicated.

Three additional approaches to therapy are worth consideration. The first is a trial on a milk-free diet. It is the author's belief that all subjects with idiopathic pulmonary hemosiderosis should be placed on a milk-free diet for six months or until it is shown that there is persistent active or recurrent disease in spite of this measure (see section on Pulmonary Hemosiderosis with Sensitivity to Cow's Milk). A milk-free diet is innocuous, and although little is known about its value in the group of patients who do not have unusual precipitins or obvious evidences of milk sensitivity, it has appeared to help substantially several such subjects.

Another measure which may be worthy of trial in subjects who respond poorly to other measures or who have chronic pulmonary symptoms or persistent roentgenologic findings is the use of the iron-chelating drug deferoxamine (Desferrioxamine). This agent has been found to be useful in removing excessive accumulations of tissue iron from subjects with transfusion hemosiderosis, acute iron toxicity, idiopathic hemochromatosis in whom repeated phlebotomies are not feasible, and other conditions. Although as yet experience has been insufficient to prove its value in the majority of patients with pulmonary hemosiderosis, its demonstrated margin of safety would suggest that further trials are warranted. The results in one subject reported by Cavalieri were particularly encouraging. Present evidence indicates that urinary iron excretion in subjects with excessive iron accumulation is directly proportional to the number of grams of deferoxamine administered up to 1.6 Gm. daily or about 25 mg. per kilogram per day. The drug seems to be most effective when given intramuscularly in divided doses eight hours apart. Levels of 24-hour urinary iron excretion should be studied for several days before and after institution of chelate therapy. If the daily urinary iron excretion is increased by more than 4 or 5 mg. per gram of administered chelate, there is good evidence of the removal of excessively accumulated iron. An increase in serum iron levels should also occur, and if iron deficiency anemia is present, it may improve. Periodic checks of 24-hour urinary iron excretion should be made with any long-term chelate therapy in order to indicate its continued value.

Nonspecific suppression of the immune response by splenectomy has been recommended by several authors (particularly Steiner). Its value has been questioned by others. The rationale for its use lies in the circumstantial evidence that primary pulmonary hemosiderosis is an immunohematologic disorder and in the theory that removal of splenic antibody-producing capacity will help suppress the production of antibodies contributing to the pathogenesis of the disease. In the present state of knowledge other measures should be tried initially and splenectomy recommended only for those who fail to respond. Even then, an immunosuppressant drug such as azathioprine (Imuran), in combination with high-dose prednisone therapy, is likely to be of more help than splenectomy.

PRIMARY PULMONARY HEMOSIDEROSIS WITH MYOCARDITIS

Some subjects with idiopathic pulmonary hemosiderosis have been found at postmortem examination to have inflammatory infiltrates in the myocardium. These have varied from minimal scattered lesions to extensive myocardial disease. If significant myocardial disease is present when the pulmonary disease is discovered, it may be difficult or impossible to decide whether the pulmonary hemosiderosis is a primary or secondary phenomenon. According to Soergel and Sommers, there may be distinctive alterations demonstrable on lung biopsy which may help in the differential diagnosis.

From a clinical point of view, when myocarditis is the primary disorder, the heart should be large and other evidences of congestive failure should be present early in the course of the disease; whereas if the heart is normal in size at the time pulmonary hemosiderosis is recognized and then enlarges, one can assume that the lung disease is primary rather than secondary to myocarditis.

The treatment of idiopathic pulmonary hemosiderosis is the same whether or not myocarditis is present with one exception. If congestive failure is detected, it should be treated appropriately with digitalis, diuretics, and other measures of recognized value.

PRIMARY PULMONARY HEMOSIDEROSIS WITH GLOMERULONEPHRITIS (GOODPASTURE'S SYNDROME)

In 1918 Goodpasture described a patient with pulmonary bleeding and glomerulonephritis. Although it is not certain that his patient had primary pulmonary hemosiderosis, the eponym "Goodpasture's syndrome" has been applied to the association of primary pulmonary hemosiderosis and proliferative or membranous glomerulonephritis. There is some debate as to whether Goodpasture's syndrome is different from, or related to, isolated pulmonary hemosiderosis. Several authors have pointed out possible differences in the clinical picture and in pathologic findings in the lung to support the contention that they are distinct entities. Thus it is known that Goodpasture's syndrome usually occurs in young adult males and is rare or nonexistent in infants. It is more likely to be fatal than is isolated pulmonary hemosiderosis, although neither disease has a generally good prognosis. Examination of lung tissue in Goodpasture's syndrome has been reported to show necrotizing alveolitis with degenerative changes of the alveolar capillary basement membranes, occasional arteritis, and relatively little alveolar epithelial proliferation or hemosiderosis, all of which are somewhat in contrast with the findings in isolated pulmonary disease. In spite of these apparent differences, however, the clinical disease usually is characterized by initial pulmonary involvement with hemoptysis, iron deficiency anemia and typical siderophages. Thus in the early stages before evidences of renal disease appear, the disease may be clinically indistinguishable from isolated pulmonary hemosiderosis. Death may result either from the renal disease or from pulmonary hemorrhage. In a few subjects renal disease becomes apparent before, or concomitantly with, the pulmonary disease.

Treatment is the same as that described for isolated pulmonary hemosiderosis, corticosteroids being the most helpful single therapeutic agent. Results of therapy are much better when kidney lesions have not progressed to the point of renal insufficiency. If a remission occurs, careful follow-up is mandatory, and attempts should be made to suppress recurrent pulmonary or renal disease as soon as either appears. It is possible that use of a prednisone-azathioprine combination may be helpful in this disorder, since the simultaneous administration of these drugs has been useful in suppressing immune responses in experimental animals and has been beneficial in subjects with advanced membranous glomerulonephritis not associated with pulmonary hemosiderosis.

PRIMARY PULMONARY HEMOSIDEROSIS WITH SENSITIVITY TO COW'S MILK

In 1962 four patients were described who fulfilled the criteria for primary pulmonary hemosiderosis in that each had recurrent pulmonary disease, hemoptysis, iron deficiency anemia, and iron-laden macrophages in gastric or bronchial washings or at lung biopsy. Additional distinctive features included unusually high titers of precipitins to multiple constituents of cow's milk, positive intradermal skin tests to various cow's milk proteins, chronic rhinitis, recurrent otitis media, and growth retardation. The symptoms of each patient improved when cow's milk was removed from the diet and returned with reintroduction of milk. Since this report the author has attended an additional subject with proved pulmonary hemosiderosis and multiple precipitins to cow's milk in high titer who improved after removal of milk from his diet. Serums from three other patients with an established diagnosis have been sent to the author and have been found to have multiple precipitins to cow's milk. Each of these was felt by his physician to have much less hemoptysis or none at all and to show general improvement when cow's milk was removed from his diet. An almost immediate clearing of chronic rhinitis and cough in several subjects who were placed on a milk-free diet seems to have provided an early clue that a lasting improvement would result in the pulmonary status. Most of the subjects having an important element of sensitivity to cow's milk were small infants, although one was fifteen years of age. A possible role of milk aspiration has been suggested in some subjects with pulmonary disease related to milk ingestion, but it has not been proved.

It should be emphasized that not all subjects with primary pulmonary hemosiderosis have unusual precipitins to cow's milk, and some without this finding do not change dramatically when on a milk-free diet. Nevertheless two subjects with proved diagnoses, but without multiple precipitins, have been felt by competent pediatricians to clearly improve on a milk-free diet, and the one who was challenged with milk reintroduction had an immediate recurrence of symptoms. This suggests that in at least some subjects with pulmonary hemosiderosis and clinical sensitivity to milk, precipitins may not play an etiologic role in the disorder. When present, they may simply indicate a vigorous immune response and may be unrelated to the direct pathogenesis of the hypersensitive state, although the point is unsettled.

There are several similarities between subjects having pulmonary hemosiderosis with sensitivity to cow's milk and infants who have milk-induced gastrointestinal bleeding and iron deficiency anemia. Both are likely to have multiple precipitins to cow's milk in high titer, and both are usually recognized between the ages of six months and two years. Symptoms and abnormal bleeding can be repeatedly induced in each by the ingestion of cow's milk, and symptom-free intervals without bleeding occur on a milk-free diet. There seems to be a direct relation between the amount of milk ingested and the severity of symptoms and bleeding in both groups. Some in each category become less sensitive to cow's milk as they grow older. One observable difference is that most patients with milk-induced gastrointestinal bleeding and iron deficiency anemia do not have positive intradermal skin test results to milk proteins, whereas those with milk-related pulmonary hemosiderosis do. Neither group commonly has reaginic antibodies to milk demonstrable by Prausnitz-Küstner reactions.

The treatment of subjects with milk-related pulmonary hemosiderosis is identical to that described above under idiopathic pulmonary hemosiderosis. Cow's milk and milk products should be removed from the diet until a complete remission has been attained. Subsequent challenge with cow's milk in moderate amounts (16 to 32 ounces daily) for several weeks is probably justified in a patient who is not critically ill in an effort to confirm a relation of milk ingestion to symptoms. If obvious pulmonary disease recurs when milk is reintroduced and clears when it is again eliminated, a milk-free diet should be maintained indefinitely. Some subjects are able to tolerate milk with minimal symptoms after a milk-free diet for six months to a year. Nevertheless persistent and recurrent pulmonary infiltrates have been found in several such subjects. suggesting that a milk-free diet should have been continued.

The possibility that foods other than cow's milk may play a role in some instances of pulmonary hemosiderosis should be considered, and if a food comes under suspicion as a result of history, skin tests or immunologic studies, temporary elimination of, and diagnostic challenge with, the food is warranted. A suggested technique to help identify other offending dietary constituents is that of placing the subject on a diet restricted to well cooked meats, vegetables and fruits as soon as the diagnosis is made and oral ingestion of foods allowed. Then new foods such as cereals, eggs, fish, raw fruits and vegetables, chocolate and nuts soon are added one at a time at weekly intervals and in relatively large quantities. If it is possible to demonstrate a consistent relation between the ingestion of a specific food and the occurrence of respiratory tract symptoms, that food is eliminated from the diet.

PULMONARY HEMOSIDEROSIS SECONDARY TO HEART DISEASE

Any form of heart disease which results in a chronic increase in pulmonary venous and capillary pressure may theoretically lead to diapedesis of red cells into the alveoli and secondary pulmonary hemosiderosis. The most common defect causing this sequence of events is mitral stenosis, but it has occurred in chronic left ventricular failure of several varieties. If significant heart disease is present, therefore, one must consider this in the interpretation of iron-laden macrophages in gastric and bronchial washings, sputum and even in lung biopsies. In these instances the burden of proof is on the person who suggests an origin other than cardiac. According to some authors, even the pathologic findings in biopsy sections may look enough like those of idiopathic pulmonary hemosiderosis to be difficult to distinguish. Others, however, report distinctive features in hemosiderosis secondary to heart disease and list concentric hypertrophy of pulmonary arterioles, thickened alveolar capillary basement membranes, and an interstitial diapedesis of red blood cells as findings which are not seen in the primary pulmonary forms of the disease.

If mitral stenosis, cor triatriatum or infradiaphragmatic drainage of the pulmonary veins is present in association with pulmonary hemosiderosis, a vigorous program of medical therapy followed by surgical repair of the obstructive lesion is mandatory, since reversal of the disease process is otherwise unlikely. Special diagnostic procedures, including cardiac catheterization with measurement of the gradient across the mitral valve or other sites of obstruction, and selective angiocardiograms to define precisely the pathologic anatomy, may be necessary to establish an accurate diagnosis.

If chronic myocardial disease or another cause of left ventricular failure is primarily at fault, every effort must be made to determine the cause of the disorder and to provide appropriate medical and surgical therapy.

PULMONARY HEMOSIDEROSIS AS A MANIFESTATION OF DIFFUSE COLLAGEN-VASCULAR OR PURPURIC DISEASE

A number of instances have been recorded in which the lesions of polyarteritis nodosa have been limited to a few organs, including pulmonary involvement with hemosiderosis. In such instances it may initially be impossible to distinguish this disease from primary pulmonary hemosiderosis except by biopsy. Nevertheless, with or without therapy, the passage of time may result in involvement of other organs, and this may lead to a suspicion of polyarteritis and also provide more accessible material for biopsy. Sometimes pulmonary hemosiderosis occurs as part of Wegener's granuloma, which is considered by some to be a variant of polyarteritis nodosa involving

chiefly the nasal septum, lungs, spleen, liver and kidney. Other collagen diseases, including lupus erythematosus, rheumatic fever and rheumatoid arthritis, have occasionally resulted in pulmonary hemosiderosis, usually in association with a diffuse vasculitis. Treatment in those instances of diffuse collagen-vascular disease with pulmonary hemosiderosis is much the same as that outlined for idiopathic pulmonary hemosiderosis. It should also include any measures or precautions indicated for the management of the collagen disease itself.

Several subjects have been reported to have pulmonary hemosiderosis in association with anaphylactoid purpura, and others in association with thrombocytopenic purpura. When either occurs, treatment must be directed at the basic disease as well as at the pulmonary complication. Splenectomy is likely to be particularly helpful in thrombocytopenic purpura with pulmonary hemosiderosis, if an early and lasting remission does not occur with steroid therapy alone.

REFERENCES

Anspach, W. E.: Pulmonary Hemosiderosis. *Am. J. Roentgenol.*, 41:592-6, 1939.

Apt, L., Pollycove, M., and Ross, J. F.: Idiopathic Pulmonary Hemosiderosis: A study of the Anemia and Iron Distribution Using Radioiron and Radiochromium. *J. Clin. Invest.*, 36:1150-59, 1957.

Azen, E. A., and Clatanoff, D. V.: Prolonged Survival in Goodpasture's Syndrome. *Arch. Int. Med.*, 114:453-60, 1964.

Bronson, S. M.: Idiopathic Pulmonary Hemosiderosis in Adults: Report of a Case and Review of the Literature. *Am. J. Roentgenol.*, 83:269-73, 1960.

Browning, J. R., and Houghton, J. D.: Idiopathic Pulmonary Hemosiderosis. *Am. J. Med.*, 20:374-82, 1956.

Bruwer, A. J., Kennedy, R. L. J., and Edwards, J. E.: Recurrent Pulmonary Hemorrhage with Hemosiderosis: So-Called Idiopathic Pulmonary Hemosiderosis. *Am. J. Roentgenol.*, 76:98-107, 1956.

Cameron, A. H.: Pulmonary Haemosiderosis in Association with Bronchiectasis. *Thorax*, 11:105-12, 1956.

Campbell, S.: Pulmonary Haemosiderosis and Myocarditis. *Arch. Dis. Childhood*, 34:218-22, 1959.

Canfield, C. J., Davis, T. E., and Herman, R. H.: Hemorrhagic Pulmonary-Renal Syndrome. *New England J. Med.*, 268:230-34, 1963.

Cavalieri, S.: Desferrioxamine with Corticosteroids in a Case of Idiopathic Pulmonary Hemosiderosis. *Fracastoro*, 56:389-403, 1963.

Cavalieri, S., and others: Study of Two Cases of Idiopathic Pulmonary Hemosiderosis. *Minerva Pediat.*, 15:683-94, 1963.

Ceelen, W.: Die Kreislaufstörungen der Lungen; in F. Henke and O. Lubarsch (Eds.): *Handbuch der speziellen pathologischen Anatomie und Histologie*. Berlin, J. Springer, 1931, Vol. 3, pp. 1-163.

Cook, C. D., and Hart, M. C.: cited by L. W. Hill: Some Advances in Pediatric Allergy in the Last Ten Years. *Pediat. Clin. N. Amer.*, 11:17-30, 1964.

Cooper, A. S.: Idiopathic Pulmonary Hemosiderosis: Report of a Case in an Adult Treated with Triamcinolone. *New England J. Med.*, 263:1100-1103, 1960.

Cruickshank, J. G., and Parker, R. A.: Pulmonary Haemosiderosis with Severe Renal Lesions (Goodpasture's syndrome). *Thorax*, 16:22-9, 1961.

DeCastro-Freire, L., and Cordeiro, M.: Hemoptysie sub-aigüe recidivante par diathese hemorragique thrombocytopenique: Splenectomieguerlson. *Helvet, paediat. Acta*, 3:255-63, 1948.

DeGowin, R. L., Oda, Y., and Evans, R. H.: Nephritis and Lung Hemorrhage. Goodpasture's Syndrome. *Arch. Int. Med.*, 111:16-22, 1963.

Denson, H. B.: Idiopathic Pulmonary Hemosiderosis: An Adult Case with Acute Onset, Short Course, and Sudden Fatal Outcome. *Ann. Int. Med.*, 53:579-85, 1960.

Editorial: Idiopathic Pulmonary Haemosiderosis. *Lancet*, 1:979-80, 1963.

Elgenmark, O., and Kjellberg, S. R.: Hemosiderosis of the Lungs—Typical Roentgenological Findings. *Acta Radiol.*, 29:32-6, 1948.

Emparaza, E., Hasbun, J., Vildosola, J., and Olcese, A.: Idiopathic Pulmonary Hemosiderosis. *Rev. Chile Paediat.*, 34:607-13, 1963.

Fleischner, F. G., and Berenberg, A. L.: Idiopathic Pulmonary Hemosiderosis. *Radiology*, 62:522-6, 1954.

Gellerstedt, N.: Ueber die essentielle anamisierende Form der braunen lungeninduration. *Acta Path. et Microbiol. Scandinav.*, 16:386-400, 1939.

Gellis, S. S., Reinhold, P. L. D., and Green, S.: Use of Aspiration Lung Puncture in Diagnosis of Idiopathic Pulmonary Hemosiderosis. *A.M.A. J. Dis. Child.*, 85:303-307, 1953.

Glanzmann, E., and Walthard, B.: Idiopathische progressive braune Lungeninduration im Kindesalter mit hereditärer Hämoptyse, intermittierender sekundärer Anämie und Eosinophile und embolischer Herdenephritis. *Mschr. Kinderheilk.*, 88:1-45, 1941.

Goodpasture, E. W.: Significance of Certain Pulmonary Lesions in Relation to the Etiology of Influenza. *Am. J.M. Sc.*, 158:863, 1919.

Gurewich, V., and Thomas, M. A.: Idiopathic Pulmonary Hemorrhage in Pregnancy. Report of a Case Suggesting Early Pulmonary Hemosiderosis with Clinical Recovery After Steroid Therapy. *New England J. Med.*, 261:1154-9, 1959.

Halvorsen, S.: Cortisone Treatment of Idiopathic Pulmonary Hemosiderosis. *Acta paediat.*, 45:139-46, 1956.

Hammond, D., and Crane, J.: Sequestration of Iron in the Lungs in Idiopathic Pulmonary Hemosiderosis. *A.M.A. J. Dis. Child.*, 96:503, 1958. (Abstract.)

Hanssen, P.: Haemosiderosis Pulmonum. *Acta paediat.*, 34:103-11, 1947.

Heiner, D. C.: Pulmonary Hemosiderosis; in S. Gellis and B. M. Kagan (Eds.): *Current Pediatric Therapy, 1966-1697*. Philadelphia, W. B. Saunders Company, 1966, pp. 147-8.

Heiner, D. C., Sears, J. W., and Kniker, W. T.: Multiple Precipitins to Cow's Milk in Chronic Respiratory Disease. A Syndrome Including Poor Growth, Gastrointestinal Symptoms, Evidence of Allergy, Iron Deficiency Anemia, and Pulmonary Hemosiderosis. *Am. J. Dis. Child.*, 103:634-54, 1962.

Heptinstall, R. H., and Salmon, M. J.: Pulmonary Hemorrhage with Extensive Glomerular Disease of the Kidney. *J. Clin. Path.*, 12:272, 1959.

Holland, N. H., Hong, R., Davis, N. C., and West, C. D.: Significance of Precipitating Antibodies to Milk Proteins in the Serum of Infants and Children. *J. Pediat.*, 61:181-95, 1962.

Hukill, P. B.: Experimental Pulmonary Hemosiderosis. The Liability of Pulmonary Iron Deposits. *Lab. Invest.*, 12:577-85, 1963.

Hwang, Y-F., and Brown, E. B.: Evaluation of Deferoxamine in Iron Overload. *Arch. Int. Med.*, 114:741-53, 1964.

Irvin, J. M., and Snowden, P. W.: Idiopathic Pulmonary Hemosiderosis: Report of Case with Apparent Remission from Cortisone. *J. Dis. Child.*, 93:182-7, 1957.

Johnson, J. R., and McGovern, V. J.: Goodpasture's Syndrome and Wegener's Granulomatosis. *Australasian Ann. Med.*, 11:250-59, 1962.

Launay, C., and others: Idiopathic Pulmonary Hemosiderosis. *Ann. Pediat.* (Paris), 10:379-85, 1963.

Lexow, P., and Sigstad, H.: Glomerulonephritis with Initial Lung Purpura. *Acta Med. Scand.*, 168:405-11, 1960.

Loftus, L. R., Rooney, P. A., and Webster, C. M.: Idiopathic Pulmonary Hemosiderosis and

Glomerulonephritis. Report of a Case. *Dis. of Chest*, 45:93-8, 1964.

McCanghey, W. T., and Thomas, B. J.: Pulmonary Hemorrhage and Glomerulonephritis. The Relation of Pulmonary Hemorrhage to Certain Types of Glomerular Lesions. *Am. J. Clin. Path.*, 38:577-89, 1962.

MacGregor, C. S., Johnson, R. S., and Turk, K. A. D.: Fatal Nephritis Complicating Idiopathic Pulmonary Haemosiderosis in Young Adults. *Thorax*, 15:198-203, 1960.

MacMahon, H. E., Derow, H. A., and Patterson, J. F.: Clinicopathologic Conference. *Bull. New England Med. Center*, 15:161, 1953.

Montaldo, G.: Sopra un Caso di Anemia emolitica con Emosiderosi Pulmonare. *Hematologica*, 19:353-9, 1938.

Negoita, C., and others: Idiopathic Pulmonary Hemosiderosis. An Immuno-allergic Disease. *Med. Intern.* (Bucur), 15:1085-9, 1963.

Nitschke, A.: Das klinische Bild der Eisenlunge. *Klin. Wschr.*, 23:348, 1944.

Ognibene, A. J., and Johnson, D. E.: Idiopathic Pulmonary Hemosiderosis in Adults. Report of a Case and Review of Literature. *Arch. Int. Med.*, 111:503-10, 1963.

Parkin, T. W., Rusted, I. E., Burchell, H. B., and Edwards, J. E.: Hemorrhagic and Interstitial Pneumonitis with Nephritis. *Am. J. Med.*, 18:220-36, 1955.

Pilcher, J. D., and Eitzen, O.: Pulmonary Hemosiderosis in a Six Year Old Boy. A Clinical and Pathological Report. *Am. J. Dis. Child.*, 67:387-92, 1944.

Pinals, R. S., and Clark, W. H.: Case Records of Massachusetts General Hospital. Case 9-1964. *New England J. Med.*, 270:414-21, 1964.

Powell, A. H., and Bettez, P. H.: Goodpasture's Syndrome: Pulmonary Hemosiderosis with Glomerulonephritis. *Canad. M.A.J.*, 90:5, 1964.

Propst, A.: Morphologie und Pathogenase der essentiellen Lungenhämosiderose. *Arch. Path. Anat.*, 326:633-63, 1955.

Reye, D.: Pulmonary Hemosiderosis. *Med. J. Aust.*, 1:35-7, 1945.

Rose, G. A., and Spencer, H.: Polyarteritis Nodosa. *Quart. J. Med.*, 26:43-81, 1957.

Rudnick, P. A., and Takamura, T.: Idiopathic Pulmonary Hemosiderosis: Report of a Case from Japan. *Am. Rev. Resp. Dis.*, 84:256-62, 1961.

Rusby, N. L., and Wilson, C.: Lung Purpura with Nephritis. *Quart. J. Med.*, 29:501-11, 1960.

Saltzman, P. W., West, M., and Chomet, B.: Pulmonary Hemosiderosis and Glomerulonephritis. *Ann. Int. Med.*, 56:409-21, 1962.

Schaar, F. E., and Rigler, L. G.: Idiopathic Pulmonary Hemosiderosis: Essential Brown Induration of the Lungs; Report of a Case and Review of Literature. *J. Lancet*, 76:126-34, 1956.

Scheidegger, S., and Dreyfus, A.: Braune Lungeninduration des Kindes mit seckundärer Anämie. *Ann. Pediat.*, 165:2-11, 1945.

Schmide, H. W.: Lung Purpura and Pulmonary Hemosiderosis. *Med. Clin. N. Amer.*, 48:1011-14, 1964.

Schuler, D.: Essential Pulmonary Hemosiderosis. *Ann. Paediat.*, 192:107-25, 1959.

Selander, P.: Idiopathische Lungenhämosiderose. Essentielle braune Lungeninduration. *Acta paediat.*, 31:286, 1944.

Sinapius, D.: Essentielle Lungenhämosiderose mit extrapulmonalen Gefassveränderungen. *Frankfurt Z. Path.*, 70:389 97, 1960.

Smith, W. E., and Feinberg, R.: Early Nonrecurrent Idiopathic Pulmonary Hemosiderosis in an Adult; Report of a Case. *New England J. Med.*, 259:808-11, 1958.

Soergel, K. H.: Idiopathic Pulmonary Hemosiderosis: Review and Report of Two Cases. *Pediatrics*, 19:1101-1108, 1957.

Soergel, K. H., and Sommers, S. C.: Idiopathic Pulmonary Hemosiderosis and Related Syndromes. *Am. J. Med.*, 32:499-511, 1962.

Idem: The Alveolar Epithelial Lesions of Idiopathic Pulmonary Hemosiderosis. *Am. Rev. Resp. Dis.*, 85:540-52, 1962.

Sprecace, G. A.: Idiopathic Pulmonary Hemosiderosis. Personal Experience with Six Adults Treated Within a Ten-Month Period, and a Review of the Literature. *Am. Rev. Resp. Dis.*, 88:830-41, 1963.

Steiner, B.: Essential Pulmonary Hemosiderosis as an Immunohematological Problem. *Arch. Dis. Childhood*, 29:391-7, 1954.

Idem: Immunoallergic Pulmonary Hemorrhage. *Acta paediat.*, Acad. Sci. Hung., 3:253-69, 1962.

Swierenga, J.: Idiopathic Hemosiderosis of the Lung in Adults. *J. Franc. Med. Chir. Thorac.*, 18:5-17, 1964.

Thomas, A. M.: A Case of Wegener's Granulomatosis. *J. Clin. Path.*, 11:146-54, 1958.

Torin, D. E., and Gregoratos, G.: Goodpasture's Syndrome. Report of a Case with Renal Biopsy and Autopsy Finding. *Military Med.*, 128:628-34, 1963.

Virchow, R.: *Die Krankhaften Geschwulste.* Bd. 2, S. 470. Berlin, 1864.

Waldenstrom, J.: Anemia and Iron Deficiency. Blodbust och jarubrist. *Nord. Med.*, 6:940-46, 1940.

Idem: Relapsing, Diffuse, Pulmonary Bleeding or Hemosiderosis Pulmonum—New Clinical Diagnosis. *Acta Radiol.*, 25:149-62, 1944.

Walker, J. M., and Joekes, A. M.: Survival After Haemophysis and Nephritis. *Lancet*, 2:1198, 1963.

Walsh, J. R., Mass, R. E., Smith, F. W., and

Lange, V.: Desferrioxamine Effect on Iron Excretion in Hemachromatosis. *Arch. Int. Med.*, 113:435-41 1964.

Weismann, W., Wolvins, D., and Verbop, M. C.: Idiopathic Pulmonary Hemosiderosis. *Acta Med. Scandinav.*, 146:341-5, 1953.

Wigod, M.: Idiopathic Pulmonary Hemosiderosis. *New England J. Med.*, 253:413, 1955.

Wilson, J. F., Heiner, D. C., and Lahey, M. E.: Studies on Iron Metabolism. IV. Milk-Induced Gastrointestinal Bleeding in Infants with Hypochromic Microcytic Anemia. *J.A.M.A.*, 189:568-72, 1964.

Wyllie, W. G., Sheldon, W., Bodian, M., and

Barlow, A.: Idiopathic Pulmonary Hemosiderosis, Essential Brown Induration of the Lungs. *Quart. J. Med.*, 17:25-48, 1948.

Wynn-Williams, N., and Young, R. D.: Idiopathic Pulmonary Hemosiderosis in an Adult. *Thorax*, 11:101-104, 1956.

Yettra, M., Goldenberg, E., and Weiner, H.: Idiopathic Pulmonary Hemosiderosis. *Calif. Med.*, 93:330-36, 1960.

Zollinger, H. W., and Hegglin, R.: Die idiopathische Lungen-Haemosiderose als pulmonale Form der Purpura Schönlein-Henoch. *Schweiz. med. Wschr.*, 88:439-43, 1958.

CHAPTER THIRTY-EIGHT

Atelectasis

ROSA LEE NEMIR, M.D.

For some years the term "atelectasis," meaning imperfect expansion, has been a subject for discussion, but the clinical concept of nonaerated lung has been known for more than a century. It was described in 1819 by Laennec from necropsy findings, and was produced experimentally in 1845 by Traube. This chapter deals with *acquired* atelectasis and refers to postnatal collapse of a segment, lobe or lobes of the lung.

Causes

Acquired atelectasis may arise under a variety of circumstances: (1) *Bronchial obstruction*, due to causes in the bronchial lumen, such as mucous plugs, foreign bodies; in the wall of the bronchus, such as mucosal edema and inflammation; tumors, smooth muscle spasm; or from peribronchial factors such as pressure from tumors, or from lymph nodes enlarged by infections or lymphomas. (2) *Abnormal alveolar surface tension* following altera-

tion of the alveolar lining layer. (3) Direct local *pressure on parenchymal tissue* from contiguous masses, or from misplaced viscera, such as diaphragmatic hernia or eventration of the diaphragm. (4) *Increased intrapleural pressure*, resulting from exudate, blood, pus or air in the pleural space. (5) *Neuromuscular pathology*, such as paralysis of the diaphragm in poliomyelitis and diphtheria and in congenital anomalies, such as amyotonia congenita. Contraction of the "myoelastic fibers" in the terminal pulmonary alveolar passages under the control of the autonomic nervous system has also been implicated as a cause of atelectasis, especially massive collapse.

Pathophysiology

When a bronchus becomes occluded, air is trapped in the part of the parenchyma ventilated by the affected bronchus, and the trapped gases are absorbed into the blood perfusing that part of the lung. The rate at which absorption occurs depends on the solubility of the constituent gases: atmospheric air, nitrogen and helium are absorbed in two to three hours; oxygen is absorbed in a few minutes, leading to rapid collapse. Rahn, in a study of a dog breathing oxygen, has reported experimental collapse of a lung within six minutes. This observation has serious implications when applied to operative procedures utilizing oxygen.

The rate and extent of collapse are further modified by collateral ventilation through interalveolar pores and through bronchiole-alveolar communications. The presence of interalveolar pores described by Kohn has been confirmed in several studies. The experimental work of Van Allen and Lindskog in dogs and human specimens first called attention to this collateral ventilation.

More recently a different and even more significant collateral ventilating mechanism has been described by Lambert, who found short epithelium-lined communications, approximately 30 microns in diameter, between the distal bronchioles and neighboring alveoli. These tubules are about three times the diameter of most interalveolar pores, and can aerate hundreds of alveoli adjacent to a peripheral bronchiole.

After the collapse of a segment or lobe, ventilation of the affected parenchyma becomes minimal, while perfusion of the area may be only slightly decreased, resulting in abnormality of ventilation-perfusion relations in the involved area of the lung. Yet shunting of blood from the collapsed portion of the lung to normally ventilated areas results in a circulatory adjustment. If the obstructed area is large enough, cyanosis may result.

Another important change which occurs after obstruction of a bronchus is the accumulation and stasis of secretions; these furnish a favorable site for the growth of microorganisms. As the secretions accumulate, they may distend a collapsed segment to more than its normal size ("drowned lung"). Later, with the absorption of fluids, the affected portion contracts.

The internal surface of mammalian lungs is lined by a film containing a surface-acting factor which reduces alveolar tension. Von Neergard first called attention to the importance of this factor in maintaining alveolar patency. This lining layer, surfactant, has the unusual property of varying surface tension with changes in area, thereby preventing collapse and the emptying of the smaller alveoli into the larger lung units. By histochemical techniques this film has been identified as a lipoprotein with a high phospholipid content. The unusual property of variable surface tension is probably attributable to the phospholipid component. The lining layer appears to be synthesized in the mitochondria of the epithelial cells. The normal lining layer may be damaged or inactivated under a variety of pathologic conditions, promoting collapse of the affected alveoli. Extracts of abnormal lungs have been found to have high surface tensions in a variety of conditions: immature newborns, respiratory distresss syndrome, following pulmonary artery ligation and pulmonary edema; and in adults with pneumonia and collapse. The high surface tensions found in these conditions imply that increased retractive forces are operating on the involved alveoli, promoting collapse of the smaller units.

The mechanical effect of the decreased volume of the collapsed segment is to distend the adjacent parenchyma. This compensatory effect may be so great that small collapsed areas are not noticed clinically or on roentgenogram. This is especially true for those areas or segments adjacent to the heart where the small triangular paracardiac shadow may go unnoticed. The heart and the mediastinum may also take part in the adjustment of intrathoracic pressures, and may be displaced toward the atelectatic lung to fill the space previously occupied by expanded lung. The diaphragm on the affected side is often elevated.

Nonobstructive pulmonary collapse has

provoked extensive study and analysis. In addition to the surface tension factor (surfactant), and the neurogenic factor, such as paralysis of the diaphragm and intercostal muscles, another concept for nonobstructive atelectasis is based on the altered normal pulmonary physiology affecting the neuromuscular structure of the terminal air passage. Much evidence has accumulated to support the belief that the lung contains smooth muscle fibers which in the most distally located portion of the air passages, including the alveolar sacs, are interwoven with elastic fibers. This "myoelastic" element is responsible for maintaining a state of contraction of pulmonary tissue similar to the continuous tonus provided by smooth muscle elsewhere—such as the stomach, intestines, bladder, arteries and veins. The precipitating factor may be severe pain, as in broken ribs, thoracic surgery, abdominal surgery or the stimulation of bronchi as in bronchography. Corssen described photomicrographs of diseased and apparently normal lung tissue obtained from twenty-six patients during various surgical procedures. Muscular tissue was found extending beyond the terminal bronchioles.

Similarly, abnormal alterations in the depth of breathing have been suggested as a basis for atelectasis. In an experimental study conducted on the influence of morphine on dogs, Egbert and Bendixen showed a decrease in the depth of breathing; they suggest a causal relation of this drug effect to atelectasis.

Segmental atelectasis is commonly seen in young infants with respiratory infections and less frequently in older children. The larger bronchial lumen and the stiffer cartilaginous structure of bronchi in the older child make atelectasis less likely than in the infant. In addition, the more rigid thoracic walls favor the clearing of obstructed bronchi in the older child.

Incidence

The incidence of postnatal or acquired atelectasis in childhood depends on several factors: the age of the patient, the kind of population sampled, the awareness and interest of the physician in the discovery of atelectasis, and the utilization of different views in chest roentgenograms.

A report by an anesthesiologist may feature postoperative atelectasis, although improved anesthesiology has rendered this complication infrequent; in a report by a physician who sees many children with infectious diseases, measles and pertussis (the latter disease now infrequently encountered in communities with adequate health services) may predominate; a bronchoscopist may emphasize aspiration of a foreign body, or vomitus, or obstruction by mucous plugs during infections and, less commonly, bronchial obstruction by extrinsic masses from lymph nodes in the hilar or mediastinal areas.

In an effort to avoid the error of bias from a study of selected material, James and others analyzed every known case (854 patients) of pulmonary collapse seen on x-ray study in a London hospital during the period 1945 to 1952. Pertussis was the leading cause of "pulmonary collapse," occurring in 18.9 per cent; upper and lower respiratory tract infections, sinobronchitis and pneumonia accounted for 58.2 per cent, all four in approximately equal proportion. The remainder of the group was associated with asthma, tuberculosis (6 per cent each), measles, miscellaneous, and postoperative causes, 3.6 to 2.3 per cent. Since 1954, the time of termination for this study, several changes have occurred. Pertussis pneumonia is rarely seen now because of the wide use of prophylactic pertussis vaccine in infancy. In the United States sinusitis, although still present and often overlooked, is becoming uncommon; this is probably due in large measure to the successful use of appropriate antimicrobial therapy for respiratory infection, especially against such microorganisms as the streptococcus and the pneumococcus.

On the pediatric service of New York University-Bellevue Medical Center the most common causes of atelectasis in the first two years of life are respiratory infections, especially bronchiolitis, broncho-

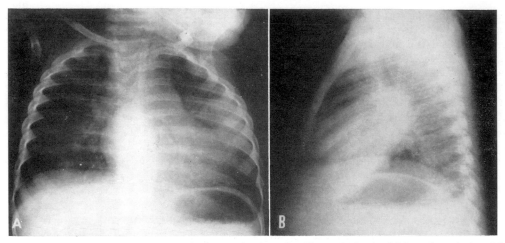

FIGURE 38–1. A homogeneous density is seen in the left midlung field (*A*) which on lateral view (*B*) is apparently segmental, involving the entire lingula. This corresponds to the bronchoscopic findings as reported. These roentgenographic findings remained unchanged for many months.

pneumonia, tuberculosis and measles. In the school-age child, pneumonia and asthma are more frequent and tuberculosis is less common. Aspiration of lipids was seen in the period 1930 to 1940, but with the intensified prophylactic measures, including parent and physician education, this form of pulmonary disease is now rare.

Aspiration of vomitus is an uncommon but often serious cause of atelectasis, especially in the young, debilitated or physically handicapped infant. Organized preventive efforts to prevent foreign body aspiration are constantly being made by many medical and lay groups, including the American Academy of Pediatrics, local and national health organizations, voluntary agencies, the toy and drug industries, and insurance companies. Much educational material is available and distributed widely to parents and other groups, with special emphasis on the preschool ages, one through four years.

Atelectasis Due to Bronchial Obstruction

The most common cause of *extrabronchial obstruction* leading to atelectasis is compression of the adjacent bronchi by hilar and mediastinal lymph nodes. Such

nodal enlargement may be due to infection of the lungs and pleura or, rarely, from descending drainage into the bronchi from an infection in the upper respiratory tract. The most common agents are tubercle bacilli, respiratory viruses (especially measles), and bronchiolitis and pertussis in infants. Other causes are lymphomas, Hodgkin's disease, leukemias, and metastasis from malignancy in other organs, such as Wilms's tumor, adrenal neuroblastoma, retinoblastoma, osteogenic sarcoma and teratoma of the testes. Tuberculous lymph node bronchial compression resulting in obstruction is described elsewhere (see Chap. 53). Two patients are shown in Figures 1 and 2, one illustrating atelectasis due to tuberculous nodal compression of the bronchus, and the second demonstrating atelectasis due to caseous material filling the bronchus after rupture of the infected gland into the bronchus.

Primary malignant tumors of the lung are rare in childhood. Dargeon in his wide experience at Memorial Hospital, New York, has reported only one case, a leiomyosarcoma in a four-year-old boy in whom atelectasis of the right middle and lower lobes was demonstrated on x-ray film.

Congenital anomalies of the diaphragm

(eventration, hiatus hernia) may permit sufficient pressure on the bronchi by *displaced viscera* to produce atelectasis of the parenchyma supplied by the bronchus. Certainly this is a rare cause of pulmonary collapse in our experience. Presenting symptoms of the atelectasis are minimal or absent; those of the hernia may be unnoticed for years and consist of fleeting pain and discomfort. Occasionally bleeding or intestinal obstruction may lead to the diagnosis. Sweet, in an analysis of 130 patients with hiatus hernia, found only ten instances of pulmonary complications; six of these had transitory atelectasis, and four had pulmonary emboli from which they recovered.

The cause of *intrabronchial obstruction* may be endogenous or exogenous; an example of the latter is aspiration of a foreign body; the former may originate within the bronchus as a part of disease

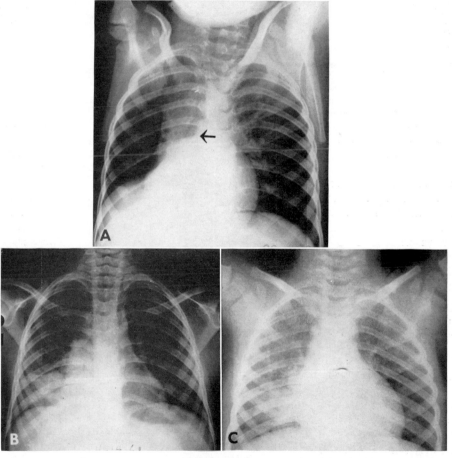

FIGURE 38–2. *A,* There is a homogeneous dense shadow above the right diaphragm extending from the periphery to the heart border, bounded superiorly by a straight edge at the level of the fifth rib anteriorly, consistent with atelectasis. There is hypoaeration in the right lung above this area. There is also displacement of the heart and mediastinum to the right (even discounting the effect of some torsion to the right). The bronchi to the right middle and lower lobes were obstructed as determined by bronchoscopy. *B,* Four days later after bronchoscopy and suction of caseous material from the right middle and lower lobes, there is partial expansion of the atelectatic segment. The costophrenic angle is clear. The shadow is less dense in the right base, but there is still displacement of the heart and mediastinum. Note the large dense shadow in the right hilar area. *C,* One month later after a second bronchoscopy and suction of large amounts of cloudy fluid material, there is almost complete clearing of the atelectasis and return of the mediastinal structures to normal position.

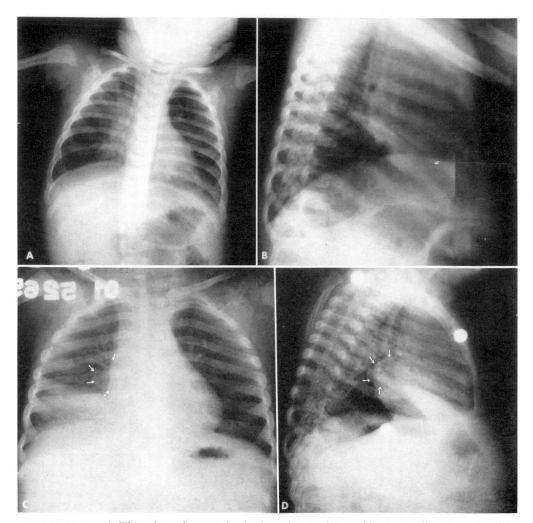

FIGURE 38-3. *A,* There is an increase in the bronchovascular markings extending from the right root, and some patchy infiltration is seen in the hilar area along the heart border and extending upwards into the right upper lobe. *B,* In the lateral view there is a mottled density in the medial aspect of the lung extending from the bronchial bifurcation and overlying the heart shadow, but this is not definitely segmental in distribution. *C,* There is some displacement of trachea, heart and mediastinum to the right. A rounded fairly dense area in the right hilar area suggests nodal enlargement. There is a homogeneous shadow above the diaphragm extending as a wedge-shaped shadow to the periphery. The costophrenic angle is clear. *D,* A shrunken right middle density may be seen, suggesting atelectasis of the entire right middle lobe with questionable hilar density surrounding the apex of the lobe. These films were taken during 2 months of recurrent pneumonia which failed to respond to antibiotics. Bronchoscopy was negative. Atelectasis may be due to disturbed respiration from pathology of the central nervous system in this hydrocephalic infant.

or infection, such as granulomatous tissues, chiefly tuberculous in origin, or mucous material frequently secondary to cystic fibrosis or asthma.

The course and duration of such atelectasis in children depend on many factors, most important of which is the physiologic state of the obstructed bronchus. In asthmatic patients the smooth muscle spasm promotes narrowing of the lumen and facilitates obstruction. Effective medication quickly restores the lumen to almost normal diameter. On the other hand, in bronchopneumonia, bronchiolitis and cystic fibrosis the inherent disease of the bronchi manifested by both edema and swelling within the bronchi, peribronchial exudate, and the mucoid material filling the bronchus favor obstruction at various areas which, even when relieved in one area, may appear in another as long as the infection thrives.

The special qualities of the material producing obstruction affect the outcome and also influence the kind of therapy. (For foreign body aspiration, see below.) The viscid quality of the mucus in cystic fibrosis (mucoviscidosis) favors atelectasis and makes ordinary medication ineffective; mucolytic agents are frequently required.

The chronicity of the infection, which results in damage to bronchi, and the sort of material obstructing the lumen of the bronchus also determine the outcome of the atelectasis. Frequently these intra-

bronchial plugs cannot be removed by bronchoscopy. Shaw described mucus plugs in ten asthmatic patients, eight of whom required surgical resection. These plugs were greenish gray, and had a thick, tenacious consistency; on cut section there was lamination, and they varied in size from 2.5 to 3.5 cm. in length and from 0.9 to 2.3 cm. in diameter.

Foreign bodies aspirated into the lung usually enter a noninfected lung with healthy bronchi. The sequence of events in this circumstance will depend on the patient, his age, state of consciousness and health, the nature of aspirated material, the promptness of correct diagnosis, and the speed and success of appropriate therapy. The younger the patient, the more rapidly atelectasis occurs when the bronchi are occluded. In the young in-

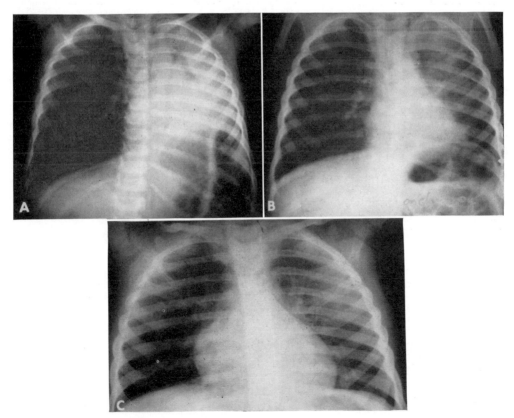

FIGURE 38–4. *A,* Complete shift of heart and mediastinal structures into the left hemithorax, where there is a homogeneous density filling the chest. Signs are suggestive of massive atelectasis of the left lung. A peanut was removed from the left main stem bronchus by bronchoscopy, immediately clearing the obstruction (*B*). Within a few days the patient completely recovered (*C*).

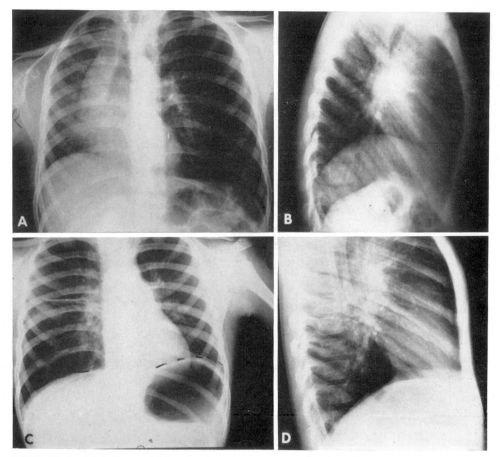

FIGURE 38–5. This 7-year-old boy has been known as an allergic child for 4 years and treated for asthmatic attacks from time to time. *A, B,* Roentgenograms taken a few hours after an acute, severe asthmatic attack. There is obvious massive displacement of mediastinal structure to the right with elevation of the right diaphragm. Extensive distention of the left hemithorax, widening of the interspaces and flattening of the diaphragm. In the lateral film (*B*) the increased anteroposterior diameter of the chest, the elevated diaphragm, and the hyperaeration anteriorly and posteriorly are apparent. *C, D,* Roentgenograms taken the following day after the patient has spent the night in an oxygen tent. Return of structures to relatively normal position may be seen. Horizontal fissures on the right are visualized, and widened intercostal spaces are present bilaterally.

This patient is shown to illustrate sudden massive (partial) obstruction to the left main bronchus which clears spontaneously within 24 hours. The cause of the obstruction is not definitely known. It is plausible to suggest a mucous plug as the etiologic factor.

fant it can develop within a few hours, while in the older child a longer period is usually required. Metallic aspirants may produce obstruction because of their size, and injury because of their shape, but vegetal aspirants have a particularly irritating quality, resulting in prompt mucosal swelling and obstruction. Some of these, such as peanuts, beans, maize, peas and watermelon seed, swell to many times their size and constitute a most serious problem; diagnosis is often obscure, too, because nonopaque aspirant is not visible on roentgenogram and the history is incomplete. The right lung is involved more often than the left, probably because of the sharper angulation of the left main bronchus.

Signs and Symptoms of Bronchial Obstruction

Obviously these vary, depending on the cause of the pulmonary collapse. In general, atelectasis which occurs during the course of tuberculosis, lymphoma, neoplasm, asthma or infections such as bronchiolitis, bronchitis, bronchopneumonia and sinobronchitis produces no change in the clinical picture unless the obstructed area is a main bronchus. This is rare in the course of these pulmonary infections. The patients are already sick, with considerable cough and some fever. Because of the diminished aeration of lung associated with obstruction, the symptoms of tachypnea, dyspnea, cough and stridor, when present, may be increased.

Occasionally a localized constant wheeze, diminished breath sounds and impaired resonance may suggest atelectasis; diagnosis is confirmed by chest roentgenogram. Careful observation may reveal a difference in respiratory expansion; there may be diminished expansion and contraction of the ribs over the atelectatic area and fullness and widened intercostal spaces over the adjacent, compensating, overdistended portion of the lung. Displacement of the heart and the mediastinum and elevation of the diaphragm

are detectable only if the atelectasis involves a large area.

In young infants the mobility of the mediastinum makes evaluation of the tracheal position important; examination should be carried out for epigastric pulsations.

When a previously well child has aspirated a foreign body, there is usually a definite history of respiratory disturbance. The signs may go unnoticed until secondary signs of infection and obstruction become prominent. Coughing, choking and gagging occur at the time of aspiration. If a large bronchus is involved, cyanosis or asphyxia may occur. A wheeze is heard, sometimes without the use of a stethoscope. If the obstruction is at the site of the main bronchus, bilateral wheezing will be evident; otherwise the wheeze is localized to the area obstructed. In many instances, and especially if the obstructed area is limited to a segment or a subsegment, the incident of choking may be followed by a symptomless period of many days; then infection in the area of atelectasis results in fever, cough and malaise. If the infection has involved other parts of the lung, there may be an increased respiratory rate. At this point the clinical picture is that of pneumonitis with atelectasis; the severity of the pneumonitis is related to the virulence of the infecting organism and the nature of the aspirated foreign body.

Diagnosis

When there is lobar atelectasis, the differential diagnosis includes pneumonia and, in the case of the swollen, wet, atelectic lung, pleural effusion. Embolism is a rare complication in childhood. In differential diagnosis the position of the heart, mediastinum and diaphragm, and the nature of both tactile and vocal fremitus are most helpful. Egophony or nasal voice sounds suggest the presence of fluid. Rales are usually present in patients with pneumonia, especially in bronchopneumonia when crackling rales are often heard. Rales are usually absent in the atelectatic lung, especially after clearing of the "wet" stage. The etiologic agent of the pleural fluid may be the determining factor in the production of rales. In an effusion caused by the staphylococcus rales are often heard over the lung. They are usually absent when there is a pneumococcus effusion, and in tuberculosis. With effusion the heart and the mediastinum are displaced toward the normal side, unless there is an underlying collapse of lung; there is no displacement in patients with pneumonia, and the displacement is toward the affected side in atelectasis. The position of the diaphragm is best established by x-ray film, but occasionally physical examination may be helpful in determining free movement of the diaphragm. Other clinical features commonly associated with pneumonia are fever, cough, tachypnea or dyspnea, and evidence of infection.

Laboratory aids in determining the presence of infection, such as blood cell counts, sedimentation rates, and cultures from the nose and throat, the blood and other sources, are valuable guides both in understanding the clinical picture and in treating the patient. The tuberculin skin test, as well as other skin tests when indicated, may be necessary to establish the diagnosis.

The most valuable diagnostic tool is the roentgenogram of the chest. The earliest roentgenographic evidence of atelectasis may be a swollen lung with fissure lines extending beyond its normal areas, thus indicating a swollen or larger segment or lobe; there are often convex curves instead of the usual straight pleural line. Shortly afterwards, as the lung becomes truly atelectatic or airless, the fissure lines become concave and the segment or lobe contracts to a much smaller size. This progression of change is best exemplified in atelectasis of the right middle lobe, especially if the atelectasis has been present over a period of time; the lobe may become so small that on x-ray film it is seen as a dense band suggesting pleural thickening rather than a completely atelectatic lobe.

Understanding of these roentgenographic findings can best be obtained by a review of Spain's experimental production of "acute nonaeration of the lung" in dogs. The earliest pathologic change consisted in congestion and edema. Within thirty-six hours, however, there was some reduction in the size of the lung, and inflammatory cells appeared. The correlation with serial roentgenograms in patients with obstructed bronchi is obvious.

Robbins and Hale have pointed out that there is x-ray evidence of elevation of the hilus on the atelectatic side, but in such interpretation it must be remembered that the left hilus is normally higher than the right. The position of the septa and the hilus should therefore be recorded in the study of the chest x-rays. Elevation of the diaphragm and an elevated position of the hilus on the affected side reflect the smaller volume of the lung containing an atelectatic area or areas. The position of the diaphragm may be of diagnostic aid; it is usually unaffected in lobar pneumonia, and is displaced downward and often flattened on the side of pleural effusion; it sometimes cannot be visualized if fluid overlies it. For proper interpretation and diagnosis of atelectasis, roentgenograms should be obtained in both lateral and posteroanterior views. Films taken during inspiratory and expiratory phases of respiration are also helpful, especially when aspiration of a nonopaque foreign body is the cause of atelectasis.

Atelectasis may occur in any lobe or segment of the lung. The least frequently affected is the left upper lobe. When all causes for obstruction of the airway are considered, the right lower and left lower lobes are most frequently collapsed. The age of the patient and the cause of the atelectasis determine the frequency of lobe obstruction. In lower respiratory tract infections the left lower and right middle lobes are most frequently involved. The right middle lobe is most vulnerable when there is enlargement of the hilar lymph nodes. In childhood tuberculosis the right upper and middle lobes are more frequently obstructed than any other lobes. Aspirated material in young infants more often produces right upper lobe obstruction; this probably results because of the recumbent position of the baby and because of the sharp angulation of the right upper lobe bronchus which tends to trap aspirated material rather than permit expulsion into the main bronchus.

Treatment

Atelectasis associated with acute infections of the lower respiratory tract is usually short-lived and clears with or before the acute infection. This is especially true in acute bronchitis, bronchiolitis and pneumonia in infants. In such instances, therefore, it is pointless to treat the atelectasis; therapy should be directed toward the respiratory infection. Change in the position of the patient, maintenance of moisture in the air, and sometimes bronchodilators are indicated. Bronchoscopy is not advisable during the early stages of an acute infection.

When atelectasis occurs in a patient who has had chronic or recurrent pulmonary disease, the bronchi may be damaged, and the secretions in such areas may be retained or expelled more slowly. These children require careful investigation of the underlying cause of recurrent or chronic infection, including special studies if they are asthmatic or have cystic fibrosis. Cultures for the etiologic agent should be carried out; postural drainage should be used, and the administration of a bronchodilator is often helpful. In those with recurrent episodes of pulmonary obstruction, positive-pressure breathing exercises may be of value. Adequate medical treatment must always be given proper trial before bronchoscopy is done.

On the other hand, if there is a history of aspiration, or a serious coughing or choking spell followed by a wheeze, or an unexplained *unilateral* wheeze, bronchoscopy should immediately be considered. Only about 2 to 4 per cent (Jackson and Jackson) spontaneously cough up the aspirated material. Delay in removal of the foreign body seriously alters the prognosis. The foreign body not only becomes embedded, injures the bronchus and generates infection, but may also descend deeper into the smaller bronchi, thereby making removal by bronchoscopy more difficult.

In general, the object of therapy in obstructive atelectasis is to locate the cause of bronchial obstruction, to remove it as soon as possible by appropriate methods, and to maintain good pulmonary ventilation at all times. Infection, when the cause of obstruction, should be suitably treated. If it is not, secondary infection usually develops. Removal of secretions or similar intrabronchial material, the use of antispasmodics and bronchodilators in an effort to increase the lumen of the obstructed bronchi, the liquefaction of secretions (aerosols), and the use of postural drainage should be utilized as needed. If these measures are ineffectual, mechanical suction or bronchoscopy is indicated. Proper administration of oxygen to maintain healthy pulmonary ventilation may be necessary.

When atelectasis persists for many months, damage to the lung is likely (fibrosis) and renders this portion of the lung parenchyma functionless. If medical treatment and bronchoscopy have been ineffectual in reaerating the lung, surgical removal of the lobe or segment should be considered. Bronchograms and pulmonary function studies are necessary to arrive at such a decision. James and others suggest a waiting period of two years before final decision because they observed fifteen patients whose lungs re-expanded between one and two years. Many factors will influence the ultimate choice of surgical removal of the diseased portion of the lung: the age of the patient, the location of the diseased lobe or segments, the extent of damage to the lung, the result of pulmonary functional studies, the underlying cause of the atelectasis, the presence of infection, and the general health of the child. (See the chapter on Bronchiectasis.) Successful medical management of respiratory infections with antibiotics and skillful and effective thoracic surgery offer an optimistic outlook in either choice for many children. Fortunately, persistent collapse is uncommon.

Preventive therapy, especially in obstructive atelectasis, should succeed in decreasing the incidence of this pulmonary complication. Attention has been directed toward the efforts to educate all those responsible for small children as to the common causes of aspiration of foreign bodies and their prevention. Antibiotics, mucolytic agents, detergents as inhalants, and postural drainage on a prophylactic basis may greatly reduce the incidence of pulmonary collapse associated with bronchial obstruction by secretions. Occasionally liquefaction of secretions by expectorants is also indicated.

Complications

Permanent damage to the proximal bronchi occluded often follows prolonged atelectasis. Fibrosis and bronchiectasis frequently follow atelectasis. (See pages 358 and 377 for a discussion of these conditions.)

Emphysematous areas may exist simultaneously with atelectactic areas and result from the same etiologic factors. In the former instance the occlusion is partial; in the latter the occlusion may be complete, resulting in an airless lung. Prolonged emphysema also causes damage to the lung. In children this is a rare complication.

Prognosis

Many factors are involved in the prognosis of the patient with atelectasis; among these are the cause of the collapse, the duration of the atelectasis, the extent of the concomitant infection, the age of the patient, and the effectiveness of therapy in preventing superimposed infection and in clearing the airways. The two aspects for consideration are prognosis for recovery or fatality, and prognosis in terms of permanent damage to the lung as a result of the airlessness of the lung parenchyma.

A fatal outcome is likely only (1) when the underlying cause for the atelectasis is life-threatening, or (2) when extensive loss of the ventilating function follows a massive lung area involvement which is unresponsive to treatment. Foreign body aspiration unrecognized or untreated may fall in the first category, because of acute secondary pneumonia. Hence diagnostic acumen in such cases is vital, and suspicion should be aroused when pneumonia follows collapse, when the disease progresses despite apparently proper therapy, when constant, localized wheezing is heard, or when the clinical picture is atypical. Bronchoscopy in such cases may be a lifesaving measure. To illustrate further, in patients who have atelectasis during the course of cystic fibrosis or extensive heart disease, the ultimate prognosis is not favorable, not because of the pulmonary collapse, but because of the advanced pathologic stage of the two disease processes.

Permanent damage to the lung following atelectasis is not uncommon, the damage being to the architecture of the bronchial tree. A decade ago pertussis, measles and bronchopneumonia were among the most common offenders in producing bronchiectasis. Today these diseases are increasingly rare as forerunners of severe pulmonary complications. Long-standing bronchial obstruction in childhood tuberculosis is associated with a high incidence of bronchopulmonary damage. (See the chapter on Bronchiectasis.)

In general, pulmonary collapse during the course of acute infections has a good immediate and long-range prognosis.

Careful medical follow-up care to ensure proper pulmonary hygiene is valuable and essential to continued good health.

NONOBSTRUCTIVE ATELECTASIS

There is growing evidence that this etiologic category for the airless lung is more common than was previously suspected. The surface tension factor (surfactant), sometimes called the "antiatelectasis" factor, seems most important during infancy, but it may apply at any time. The contraction of the smooth muscles in the terminal air passages, the "myoelastic" factor, has been reported as responsible for atelectasis at all ages.

Burbank and others have suggested that the lung is an actively contractile organ and that, under the stimulus of unusual pain, a reflex mechanism is responsible for the terminal alveolar muscular spasm which, together with the resultant changes in surface tension and intraluminal air pressure, results in collapse. This may occur in pneumonia and nonobstructive atelectasis, fracture of ribs and during the course of bronchography.

The importance of the neurogenic factor affecting the muscles of respiration was described by Pasteur. Churchill has also called attention to this factor in the nonobstructive cause of atelectasis as a weakened force in respiratory muscle action.

Atelectatic episodes have been described following thoracotomy, during extensive poliomyelitis, during diphtheria, and in patients with neuromuscular anomalies, such as amyotonia congenita or injuries to the spinal cord. Berry and Sanislow have described "acute respiratory insufficiency" which they called atelectasis, and defined as characterized by an "unobstructive, nontransudative alveolar collapse and intense interstitial pulmonary capillary congestion," following intensive parenteral fluid therapy.

The clinical features and diagnostic aspects of nonobstructive atelectasis are dependent on the underlying cause and on the extent of the atelectasis. Some patients are symptomless or show little difference in the symptoms already existing with the illness; others are acutely ill with respiratory symptoms resulting from the disturbed pulmonary physiology. The roentgenograms are similar to those described for obstructive atelectasis. Attention should be given to the position of the diaphragm in various positions and phases of respiration, to the intercostal spaces and to the vertebral bodies. Absence of opaque foreign bodies and of mediastinal or hilar masses is a differential feature between obstructive and nonobstructive atelectasis.

Treatment

Analysis of the underlying cause of the atelectasis and evaluation of the presenting symptoms are essential to intelligent therapy.

When the etiologic agent appears to be related to surfactant, attempt may be made to repair the defective alveolar lining layer by inhalations of aerosols of substances with similar physical properties. In contrast to the natural surfactant, most synthetic surface-active agents have fixed surface tensions which are not altered with changes in the alveolar area. Such agents are the detergents, the "Tweens" (hydrophilic nonionic surfactants) and the "Spans" (lipophilic surfactants); if administered in an aerosol, these tend to replace the normal lining by a film of fixed surface tension, increasing the retractive forces in the lung. Experimental study of excised lung lined with synthetic surfactant demonstrates the beneficial effect on inflation and deflation pressure-volume curves. Radigan and King have demonstrated the value of detergents in preventing postoperative atelectasis. The object of this therapy is to stimulate involuntary and forceful coughing. In pediatrics a similar objective may be achieved by inhalation in nonsurgical patients when coughing is desired.

An ingenious therapeutic device for massive atelectasis of the right lung due to amyotonia congenita in a three-year-old child was used by Townsend and Squire. A jacket encircling the chest attached to a 3-pound weight designed to concentrate traction along the midaxillary line was successful in relieving the collapse within a few days. The patient remained clear for months and, in subsequent bouts of atelectasis, responded to similar treatment without the use of bronchoscopy.

In other respects the treatment of obstructive and nonobstructive atelectasis does not differ. Massive postoperative atelectasis may also be nonobstructive; the additional aspect of treatment for these postoperative patients is given in the succeeding section.

MASSIVE PULMONARY COLLAPSE

Acute massive pulmonary collapse may occur under a variety of circumstances, but most commonly follows upper abdominal or thoracic surgery or bronchial obstruction, resulting from foreign body aspiration or more frequently from mucoid material or the aspiration of vomitus. It is also seen after chest trauma. In the last instance the collapse is usually on the injured side, but may occur on the opposite side, possibly owing to aspiration of blood. Although diaphragmatic paralysis or paresis is also associated with massive atelectasis, it is rarely seen now, because the two most frequent offenders, diphtheria and poliomyelitis, are rapidly disappearing. This section will be devoted to a discussion of massive postoperative collapse.

Incidence

From our own experience at Bellevue Hospital and from the recent literature, it is clear that this massive atelectasis in children is uncommon, especially as a postoperative complication. A comprehensive study by two large city hospitals for the period 1931 to 1941 reported only twenty-one cases. A later study in a Philadelphia hospital, covering 1941 to 1945, analyzed 1240 patients with upper abdominal surgery and reported massive atelectasis in twenty-two children.

Pathogenesis

Massive postoperative atelectasis of the lung may be due to obstructive or nonobstructive factors, although it is thought that the latter, such as hypoventilation or ineffectual respirations, are much more frequent. The same etiologic mechanisms described under both obstructive and nonobstructive atelectasis apply here. In addition, there are other factors directly related to the surgical procedures. These are preoperative and postoperative medications, increased bronchial secretions associated with the operation, excessive pain (especially in thoracic and abdominal surgery), effects on respiration of injury to abdominal muscles, direct effects of anesthetics on the respiratory tract, absence of cough reflex, and inactivity of the patient from both positioning and surgical bandages.

The importance of deep breathing and occasional sighing in normal respirations has been demonstrated. Severe abdominal pain affects the kind and depth of respiration, and morphine has been shown to affect the breathing pattern by causing respiratory depression and eliminating the occasional normal spontaneous deep breaths.

The experimental work of de Takats and associates has led them to conclude that the essential basis for postoperative atelectasis is a combination of increased bronchial secretion associated with reflex bronchoconstriction and bronchial obstruction. Bronchial secretions may be increased in intra-abdominal manipulation during operation, by blunt injury to the chest wall or by pulmonary embolism. Lindskog has postulated the release of a histamine-like substance from the sites of operation; theoretically, this provokes the secretions and bronchiolar constriction. This is found less frequently in newborn and very young infants.

Anesthesia resulting in hypoxia may also be a mechanism leading to atelectasis. The early experimental work of Briscoe pointed out the importance of position of the patient with regard to the development of atelectasis. Long periods in a supine position with constricting abdominal bandages affect the diaphragmatic movements, leading to inadequate ventilation and collapse.

Clinical Features

Symptoms of massive collapse usually appear on the first postoperative day. They consist of fever, respiratory distress, dyspnea, cyanosis and anxiety. The diagnosis is easily made by physical examination and roentgenograms. The heart and the mediastinum are displaced toward the affected side, and there is dullness and markedly diminished to absent breath sounds, and tactile and vocal fremitus; tachypnea and tachycardia are present. There may be a lag in respiration and narrowing of the interspaces on the affected side. By roentgenogram, the diaphragm is elevated.

The diagnosis may be verified by various tests to determine the perfusion of the nonventilated parenchyma, such as arterial blood desaturation, a useful and relatively accurate test using the technique of earpiece oximetry. Such tests may also be a guide to impending atelectasis. Pulmonary function studies are more tedious, but more accurate. These tests may be valuable in determining postoperative pulmonary complications.

The differential diagnosis includes pneumonia, pulmonary embolism, pleural effusion and pneumothorax. The last two may be distinguished by the shift of the heart and mediastinal structures to the opposite side. Pneumonia may coexist with or follow atelectasis; the degree of fever, presence of rales, and other clinical signs and laboratory tests such as bacterial cultures are diagnostic aids. Pulmonary embolism occurs rarely in childhood. It is accompanied by symptoms of shock and often hemoptysis.

Prognosis

The prognosis in this alarming picture is good unless there is an underlying complication such as pneumonia or embolism. Most patients recover spontaneously with the use of simple mechanical measures such as coughing and positioning.

Treatment

Active treatment consists in the removal of the obstruction to airways: by coughing, often accompanied by forceful blows to the thorax or supplemented by tracheal suction, by oxygen inhalation, by medications directed toward liquefying secretions, by mucolytic solutions, and the inhalation of bronchodilators. If voluntary coughing cannot be relied on, positive-pressure breathing may be used after careful evaluation of the airway obstruction and estimation of the probable pressure in the pleural spaces. The use of appropriate antibiotics and the application of the preventive measures, with special attention to the exclusion of medications which depress cough and respiration, are indicated. It is important to remember that atelectasis may clear spontaneously and that good general care of the patient and encouragement of deep inspiration are desirable for a short time before extensive therapeutic measures are used.

Bronchoscopy for postoperative atelectasis has long been recognized as a lifesaving measure, and the techniques and methods are fully described. The experienced, well equipped endoscopist has no difficulty with children, even the very young.

The best results with intermittent positive-pressure breathing are obtained when the treatment is begun on the first postoperative day and used three or four times daily for fifteen minutes each time; 40 per cent oxygen and 60 per cent helium or air under 10 to 12 cm. of water pressure, at a rate of eight to ten respirations per minute, are utilized. Medication consisting of bronchodilators, antibiotics, expectorants or detergents may be added as indicated.

Preventive Therapy

Cooperative efforts by the team of physicians involved in the care of the surgical patient are most important in the prevention of atelectasis. The absence of respiratory infection preoperatively, the choice of the site for abdominal surgical incision to minimize muscular injury, economy of time during the operation, care in the choice of the anesthetic, depth of anesthesia, together with postoperative supervision encouraging cough, changes of position, and elimination of secretions or vomitus, or blood, are all essential elements of good prophylactic care. Some patients can be encouraged to use intermittent positive-pressure breathing the day before operation.

The science of anesthesiology and the growth of this specialty by excellent teaching have made massive atelectasis of the lung a rare occurrence. The many research contributions by physiologists, surgeons, internists, pediatricians and other physicians have been helpful in understanding the causes and in developing effective preventive measures.

REFERENCES

Auspach, W. E.: Atelectasis and Bronchiectasis in Children. *Am. J. Dis. Child.*, 47:1011, 1934.

Avery, M. E.: The Alveolar Lining Layer. A Review of Studies on Its Role in Pulmonary Mechanics and in the Pathogenesis of Atelectasis. *Pediatrics*, 30:324, 1962.

Barino, C.: Brief Clinical Consideration of the Pathogenesis of "Functional" Atelectasis. *Riv. Ital. Radiol. Clin.*, 6:41, 1956.

Becker, A., Barak, S., Braun, E., and Meyers, M. P.: The Treatment of Postoperative and Pulmonary Atelectasis with Intermittent Positive Pressure Breathing. *Surg. Gynec. & Obst.*, 111:517, 1960.

Bendixen, H. H., Smith, G. M., and Mead, J.: Pattern of Ventilation in Young Adults. *J. Appl. Physiol.*, 19:195, 1964.

Berry, R. E. L., and Sanislow, C. A.: Clinical Manifestations and Treatment of Congestive Atelectasis. *Arch. Surg.*, 87:153, 1963.

Briscoe, J. C.: The Mechanism of Postoperative Massive Collapse of the Lungs. *Quart. J. Med.*, 13:293, 1919-1920.

Idem: The Muscular Mechanism of Respiration and Its Disorders. *Lancet*, 1:637, 749, 857, 1927.

Brock, R. C.: *The Anatomy of the Bronchial Tree*. London, Oxford Medical Publications, 1954.

Brown, E. S., Johnson, R. P., and Clements, J. A.: Pulmonary Surface Tension. *J. Appl. Physiol.*, 14:717, 1959

Burbank, B., Cutler, S. S., and Sbar, S.: Nonobstructive Atelectasis: Its Occurrence with Pneumonitis. *J. Thoracic & Cardiovasc. Surg.*, 41:701, 1961.

Caffey, J.: *Pediatric X-ray Diagnosis*. 4th ed. Chicago, Year Book Publishers, Inc., 1961.

Churchill, F. D.: Pulmonary Atelectasis, with Special Reference to Massive Collapse of the Lung. *Arch. Surg.*, 11:489, 1925.

Idem: The Segmental and Lobular Physiology and Pathology of the Lung. *J. Thor. Surg.*, 18:279, 1949.

Idem: The Architectural Basis of Pulmonary Ventilation. *Ann. Surg.*, 137:1, 1953.

Corssen, G.: Changing Concepts of the Mechanism of Pulmonary Atelectasis, A Study of Smooth Muscle Elements in the Human Lung. *J.A.M.A.*, 188:485, 1964.

Coryllos, P. N., and Birnbaum, G. L.: The Circulation in the Compressed Atelectatic, and Pneumonic Lung. *Arch. Surg.*, 19:1346, 1929.

Culiner, M. M.: Personal communication, 1965.

Culiner, M. M., Reich, S. B., and Abouav, J.: Nonobstructive Consolidation-Atelectasis Following Thoracotomy. *J. Thor. Surg.*, 37:371, 1959.

Dargeon, H. W.: *Tumors of Childhood*. New York, Paul B. Hoeber, Inc., 1960.

Dawson, J.: Valvular Bronchial Obstruction. A Report of Three Cases. *Brit. J. Radiol.*, 25:557, 1952.

DeTakats, G., Beck, W. C., and Fenn, G. K.: Pulmonary Embolism. *Surgery*, 6:339, 1939.

DeTakats, G., Fenn, G. K., and Jenkinson, E. L.: Reflex Pulmonary Atelectasis. *J.A.M.A.*, 120:686, 1942.

Dripps, R. D., and Deming, Van M.: Postoperative Atelectasis and Pneumonia. *Am. Surg.*, 124:94, 1946.

Egbert, L. D., and Bendixen, H. H.: Effect of Morphine on Breathing Pattern. A Possible Factor in Atelectasis. *J.A.M.A.*, 188:485, 1964.

Ferris, B. J., Jr., and Pollard, D. S.: Effect of Deep and Quiet Breathing on Pulmonary Compliance in Man. *J. Clin. Invest.*, 39:143, 1960.

Goodwin, T. C.: Lipoid Cell Pneumonia. *Am. J. Dis. Child.*, 48:309, 1934.

Gordon, R. A.: Bronchoscopy in the Treatment of Pulmonary Atelectasis. *Canad. M.A.J.*, 54:6, 1946.

Hamilton, W. K.: Atelectasis, Pneumothorax and Aspiration as Postoperative Complications. *Anesthesiology*, 22:708, 1961.

Hamilton, W. K., McDonald, J. S., Fischer, H. W., and Bethards, R.: Postoperative Respiratory

Complications: A Comparison of Arterial Gas Tensions, Radiographs and Physical Examination. *Anesthesiology*, 25:607, 1964.

Hoffstaedt, E. G. W.: Modern Concept of Pulmonary Collapse: Study in Functional Pathology. *Tubercle*, 34:234, 1953.

Huppler, E. G., Clagett, O. T., and Grindlay, J. H.: Elimination and Transport of Mucus in the Lung. *J. Thor. Surg.*, 32:661, 1956.

Jackson, C., and Jackson, C. L.: *Diseases of the Nose, Throat and Ear*. Philadelphia, W. B. Saunders Company, 1959, pp. 842-55.

Jacobaeus, H. C.: A Study of Acute Massive Atelectatic Collapse of the Lung. *Brit. J. Radiol.*, 3:50, 1930.

Idem: Spontaneous Collapse of the Lung. *Med. Klin.*, 38:673, 1932.

James, U., Brumblecombe, F. S. W., and Wells, J. W.: The Natural History of Pulmonary Collapse in Childhood. *Quart. J. Med.*, 25:121-36, 1956.

Johanssen, L., and William-Olsson, G.: Foreign Bodies in the Bronchi. *Acta Chirurgica Scandinavia*, Suppl. 283, 1961, p. 153.

Klaus, M., Reiss, O. K., Tolley, W. N., Piel, C., and Clements, J. A.: Alveolar Epithelial Cell Mitochondria as Source of the Surface-Active Lung Lining. *Science*, 137:750, 1962.

Kohn, H. H.: Zur Histologie des indurirenden fibrinosen Pneumonie. *Muench. med. Wchschr.*, 40:42, 1893.

Krahl, V. E.: Microscopic Anatomy of the Lungs. *Am. Rev. Resp. Dis.*, Suppl., 80:24, 1959.

Laennec, R. T. H.: *Diseases of the Chest* (1819). 4th ed. Translated by John Forbes in 1834. London.

Lambert, M. W.: Accessory Bronchiole-Alveolar Communications. *J. Path. Bact.*, 70:311, 1955.

Idem: Accessory Bronchiolo-alveolar Channels. *Anat. Rec.*, 127:472, 1957.

Lance, J. S., and Latta, H.: Hypoxia, Atelectasis and Pulmonary Edema. *Arch. Path.*, 75:373, 1963.

Liebow, A. A.: The Genesis and Functional Implications of Collateral Circulation of the Lungs. *Yale J. Biol. Med.*, 22:637, 1950.

Lindskog, G. E.: Studies on the Etiology of Postoperative Pulmonary Complications. *J. Thoracic Surg.*, 10:635, 1941.

Macklin, C. C.: The Musculature of the Bronchi and Lungs. *Physiol. Rev.*, 9:1, 1929.

Mead, J., Whittenberger, J. L., and Radford, E. P., Jr.: Surface Tension as a Factor in Pulmonary Volume Pressure Hysteresis. *J. Appl. Physiol.*, 10:191, 1957.

Michael, P.: *Tumors of Infancy and Childhood*. Philadelphia, J. B. Lippincott Company, 1964, p. 251.

Moersch, H. J.: Bronchoscopy in Treatment of Postoperative Atelectasis. *Surg., Gynec. & Obst.*, 77:435, 1943.

Molonoy, C. J.: Postoperative Pulmonary Collapse in Childhood. *Am. J. Dis. Child.*, 66:280, 1943.

O'Brien, E.: Vegetal Bronchitis. A Summation of Thoughts on Its Etiology. Presentation of Twenty-Three Cases. *Laryngoscope*, 58:1013, 1948.

Palley, A.: Factors Leading to Production of Bronchiectasis in Childhood and Its Prevention. *South African M. J.*, 22:169, 1948.

Pasteur, W.: Respiratory Paralysis After Diphtheria as a Cause of Pulmonary Complications, with Suggestions as to Treatment. *Am. J.M. Sc.*, 100:242, 1890.

Idem: Massive Collapse of the Lung. *Lancet*, 2:1351, 1908.

Idem: Active Lobar Collapse of the Lung After Abdominal Operations. *Lancet*, 2:1080, 1910.

Pattle, R. E.: Properties, Function and Origin of the Alveolar Lining Layer. *Proc. Roy. Soc.* (Biol.) London, Series B, 148:217, 1958.

Pattle, R. E., and Thomas, L. C.: Lipoprotein Composition of the Film Lining the Lung. *Nature*, 189:844, 1961.

Pinck, R. L., Burbank, R., Cutler, S. S., Sbar, S., and Mangieri, M.: Nonobstructive Atelectasis. *Am. Rev. Resp. Dis.*, 91:909, 1965.

Radford, E. P., Jr.: Method for Estimating Respiratory Surface Area of Mammalian Lungs from Their Physical Characteristics. *Proc. Soc. Exper. Biol. & Med.*, 87:58, 1954.

Idem: Recent Studies of Mechanical Properties of Mammalian Lungs; in J. W. Remington (Ed.): *Tissue Elasticity*. Washington, D.C., American Physiological Society, 1957, pp. 177-90.

Radigan, L. R., and King, R. D.: A Technique for the Prevention of Postoperative Atelectasis. *Surgery*, 47:184, 1960.

Rahn, H.: The Role of N_2 Gas in Various Biological Processes, with Particular Reference to the Lung. *Harvey Lectures*, Series 55, 1959-60, p. 173.

Reinhardt, K.: Total Left Pulmonary Atelectasis Following Bronchography. *J. Radiol. Electr.*, 32:470, 1951.

Robbins, L. L., and Hale, C. H.: Roentgen Appearance of Lobar and Segmental Collapse of Lung. Technic of Examination. *Radiology*, 44:107, 1945.

Ross Conference on Pediatric Research #37. Normal and Abnormal Respiration in Children. 1960, pp. 36-45.

Rudy, N. E., and Crepeau, J.: Role of Intermittent Positive Pressure Breathing Postoperatively. *J.A.M.A.*, 167:1093, 1958.

Shaw, R. R.: Mucoid Impaction of the Bronchi. *J. Thor. Surg.*, 22:149, 1951.

Siebecker, K. L., Sadler, P. E., and Mendenhall, J. T.: Postoperative Ear Oximeter Studies in Patients Who Have Undergone Pulmonary Resection. *J. Thor. Surg.*, 36:88, 1958.

Singer, J. J., and Graham, E. A.: Roentgen-Ray Study of Bronchiectasis. *Am. J. Roentgenol.*, 15:54, 1926.

Smith, T. C., and Siebecker, K. L.: Postoperative Ear Oximeter Studies in Thoracotomy Patients. II. Variations with Operative Procedures and with the Stir-up Regime. *J. Thor. Cardiov. Surg.,* 39:478, 1960.

Smith, T. C., Cook, F. D., De Kornfield, T. J., and Siebecker, K. L.: Pulmonary Function in the Immediate Postoperative Period. *J. Thor. Cardiov. Surg.,* 39:788, 1960.

Spain, D. M.: Acute Nonaeration of Lung: Pulmonary Edema Versus Atelectasis. *Dis. of Chest,* 25:550, 1954.

Stein, M., Koota, G. M., Simon, M., and Frank, H. A.: Pulmonary Evaluation of Surgical Patients. *J.A.M.A.,* 181:765, 1962.

Strum, A.: Der Lungenkrampf: Kontraktionatektase durch pulmonalen Spasmus. *Deutsch med. Wchnschr.,* 71:201, 1946.

Idem: Ist die Lunge kontraktil? *Schweiz med. Wchnschr.,* 81:859, 1951.

Sutnick, A. I., and Soloff, L. A.: Pulmonary Surfactant and Atelectasis. *Anesthesiology,* 25: 676-81, 1964.

Sweet, R. H.: Analysis of 130 Cases of Hiatus Hernia Treated Surgically. *J.A.M.A.,* 151:367, 1953.

Tannenberg, O., and Pinner, M.: Atelectasis and Bronchiectasis. *J. Thor. Surg.,* 11:571, 1942.

Tooley, W., Gardner, R., Thung, N., and Finley, T.: Factors Affecting the Surface Tension of Lung Extracts. *Federation Proc.,* 20:428, 1961.

Townsend, E. H., Jr., and Squire, L.: Treatment of Atelectasis by Thoracic Traction. *Pediatrics,* 17:250, 1956.

Traube, L.: Die Usrsachen und die Beschaffenheit der jenigen Veranderungen, welche das Lungenparenchym nach Durchschneidung der Nn. Vagi erleidet. Kritisch-experimenteller Beitrag zur Lehre von der Pneumonie und Atelektase. *Beitr. z. exper. Path. u. Physiol.,* 1:65, 1846.

Van Allen, C. M., and Lindskog, G. E.: Collateral Respiration in the Lung. *Surg., Gynec. & Obst.,* 53:16, 1931.

Von Neergaard, K.: Neue Auffassungen über einen Grundbegriff der Atemmechanik. Die Retraktions Kraft der Lunge, abhangig von der Oberflachenspannung in den Alveolen. *Ztachr. ges. exper. Med.,* 66:373, 1929.

Xalabarder, C.: What Is Atelectasis? *Tubercle,* 30:266, 1949.

CHAPTER THIRTY-NINE

Pulmonary Edema

ROBERT H. HIGH, M.D.

Pulmonary edema occurs when serous fluid passes from the pulmonary capillaries into the alveolar spaces and the bronchioles.

Pulmonary edema is most commonly secondary to severe cardiovascular anomalies, such as aortic stenosis or coarctation of the aorta, or to myocarditis caused by rheumatic fever, Coxsackie infections, and so forth. Edema of the lung is also common in a variety of acute or chronic renal diseases, especially those in which hypertension or hypoproteinemia is present. Pulmonary edema may be noted with certain acute infections or with poisoning by morphine, alcohol, barbiturates and other substances. The inhalation of toxic gases, such as household illuminating gas, ammonia, nitrogen dioxide, can produce acute pulmonary edema, as can the inhalation of smoke. Pulmonary edema often occurs as one of the terminal events in patients with acute fulminating infections or chronic debilitating diseases.

The manifestations of pulmonary edema develop rapidly in most instances, but occasionally, as in chronic cardiac failure, may have an insidious onset. Tachypnea is often the first manifestation. Other common symptoms are cough —sometimes associated with the production of frothy, pinkish sputum—chest pain and increasing respiratory distress. Physical examination reveals the presence of many, scattered fine rales which are often most prominent in the dependent portions of the lungs. Percussion may reveal some dullness, especially at the lung bases. Cyanosis is commonly noted. The cardiac sounds are faint, and the peripheral pulses are often weak. The symptoms and signs of the primary disease are also present.

Although the diagnosis of pulmonary edema is often readily apparent from the clinical manifestations, roentgenographic examination of the chest is recommended to exclude the presence of pneumonia. Roentgenographic changes are those of a diffusely overfilled pulmonary vascular tree, often showing a diffuse, rather uniform haziness of the lungs; sometimes there is evidence of freely movable pleural fluid. The fluid is best demonstrated in roentgenograms taken in the erect or lateral decubitus position.

Treatment is directed at the primary disease causing pulmonary edema. The administration of oxygen is often useful in relieving some of the chest pain and tachypnea. Bubbling oxygen through 50 per cent ethyl alcohol to reduce the surface tension of the foamy secretions has been advocated, but the efficacy of this procedure has been questioned. Oxygen may be administered by tent, mask or a mechanical respirator using intermittent positive pressure. The tent method is most generally applicable. Dyspnea is often severe, and relief usually follows the administration of morphine sulfate subcutaneously or intravenously in a dosage of 0.1 to 0.2 mg. per kilogram of body weight. Many patients are more comfortable when placed in a semierect position. If cardiac failure is present, rapid digitalization is indicated. When pulmonary edema is secondary to hypertension of renal origin, the parenteral administration of reserpine and Apresoline is recommended. Those instances of pulmonary edema secondary to poisoning should be treated with specific antidotes when such are available, e.g. the administration of

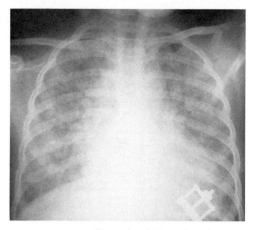

FIGURE 39–1. Extensive bilateral pulmonary edema secondary to acute renal failure.

nalorphine hydrochloride (Nalline) to combat the effect of morphine poisoning. If pulmonary edema is secondary to excessive parenteral administration of fluids or blood or to the twin transfusion syndrome of the newborn, phlebotomy may be life saving. The application of tourniquets or inflated blood pressure cuffs ("bloodless phlebotomy") to the extremities or the withdrawal of blood from a vein may be performed. In those instances in which pulmonary edema is part of the terminal events in patients suffering from incurable diseases, heroic therapeutic efforts do not seem to be indicated.

REFERENCES

Gootnick, A., Lipson, H. J., and Turbin, J.: Inhalation of Ethyl Alcohol for Pulmonary Edema. *New England J. Med.*, 245:842, 1951.

Haddy, T. B., and others: The Effect of Acute Pulmonary Edema upon Lung Compliance. *Pediatrics*, 33:55-62, 1964.

Masson, I.: Pulmonary Edema During or After Surgery. *Anesth. Analg.*, 43:440-45, 1964.

Nelson, W. E.: Pulmonary Edema; in W. E. Nelson (Ed.): *Textbook of Pediatrics*. 8th ed. Philadelphia, W. B. Saunders Company, 1964, p. 865.

Robbins, J. J., and others: Pulmonary Edema from Teflon Fumes; Report of a Case. *New England J. Med.*, 271:360-61, 1964.

CHAPTER FORTY

Emphysema

ROBERT H. HIGH, M.D.

Emphysema, or overaeration of the lung, produces distention and sometimes rupture of the alveoli. In most instances emphysema in children can be corrected by appropriate medical or surgical treatment. Irreversible emphysema is seldom seen in childhood except as a manifestation of cystic fibrosis of the pancreas, severe and intractable asthma, extensive bronchiectasis, or the like. Idiopathic pulmonary emphysema as noted in adults, possibly from excessive smoking or chronic bronchitis, is almost never observed in childhood.

Emphysema is usually associated with some pulmonary disease such as anomalies of the lungs or major blood vessels (see p. 493), bronchiolitis (see p. 272), aspiration (see p. 125), bronchial asthma (see p. 449), cystic fibrosis (see p. 541) and certain other specific diseases. The causes of emphysema in newborn infants are often different from those observed in older infants and children and are discussed in Chapter 4. The physiologic alterations produced by emphysema and the methods for measuring the functional impairment in emphysema are presented in Section I.

Emphysema may be *localized* to a portion of one lung or may be *generalized,* involving all of one or both lungs. Emphysema usually implies some degree of obstruction in the airway, so that the ingress of air to the involved area(s) occurs freely, but the egress is impaired by some cause such as an increase of secretions, foreign body, bronchospasm, bronchial narrowing, extraluminal bronchial compression, bronchostenosis, endobronchial granulations, and the like.

Compensatory emphysema may occur when a major area of the lung is collapsed, as with lobar or massive pulmonary atelectasis. Compensatory emphysema is also noted in the normal lung in the presence of agenesis of the contralateral lung or following pneumonectomy.

Localized emphysema is usually secondary to narrowing of the bronchial lumen and may involve the entire lung, a lobe or a portion of a lobe, depending upon the site of the obstruction. Most instances of localized obstructive emphysema are acquired. They are often secondary to aspirated foreign objects, retained secretions, mucous plugs, or endobronchial granulomas secondary to tuberculosis or other infectious diseases. Less frequently, localized emphysema is produced by narrowing of the bronchial lumen from extraluminal compression by enlarged hilar and mediastinal lymph nodes, as may be noted with tuberculosis (see p. 656), the pulmonary mycoses (see p. 568) or malignancies involving the lymph nodes.

Localized emphysema of a congenital nature may be noted in congenital lobar emphysema, congenital narrowing of the bronchus, extraluminal compression of a bronchus by a large anomalous vessel, and the like.

The symptoms and abnormalities noted on physical examination vary according to the extent of the emphysema. At times no abnormalities are noted and localized emphysema is demonstrable only by roentgenographic examination. When severe localized emphysema is present, cough, dyspnea, tachypnea and cyanosis are noted. Percussion over the involved area produces a hyperresonant note, and the heart and the trachea may be shifted to the opposite side. Auscultation often reveals high-pitched, whistling inspiratory sounds, and expiratory wheezes are often heard over the involved area. The expira-

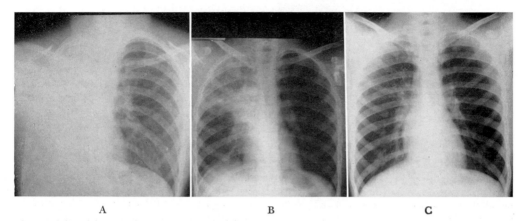

A B C

FIGURE 40–1. *A,* Compensatory emphysema of left lung secondary to massive collapse of entire right lung during asthmatic attack. *B,* Same day, showing improvement following bronchoscopic aspiration of thick secretions. *C,* Three weeks later lung is normal.

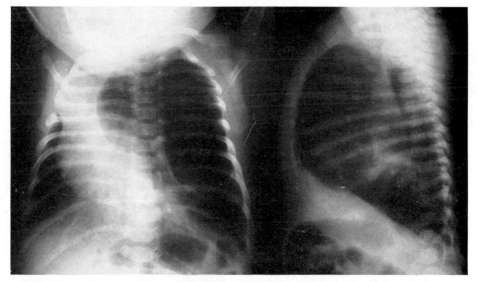

FIGURE 40–2. Congenital lobar emphysema of left upper lobe. Recovery followed lobectomy.

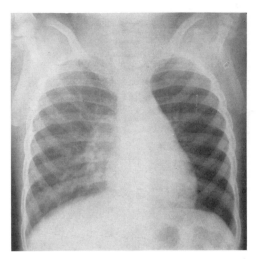

FIGURE 40–3. "Apparent" emphysema of left lung secondary to coarctation of the left main pulmonary artery. Note the reduced vascular markings on the left and absence of shift of the mediastinum.

tory phase of respiration is often prolonged, and sometimes it is difficult to perceive any movement of air with expiration. The involved hemithorax is often overexpanded and does not change with expiration.

Roentgenographic study and fluoroscopic examination are most helpful in confirming the presence of localized emphysema and often indicate the area where the obstruction is present. Films should be exposed in inspiration and expiration; fluoroscopic examination and cinefluorographic movies are also useful diagnostic studies. Opaque foreign bodies may be demonstrated. Examination during inspiration shows the emphysematous area, and the heart and mediastinal structures may be shifted to the opposite side. During expiration the uninvolved areas of the lung empty normally, but the involved area does not. The heart and mediastinal structures show a greater shift toward the normal side. In the presence of severe localized emphysema, e.g. with congenital lobar emphysema, the emphysematous areas may herniate across the mediastinum.

Bronchoscopic examination is usually

indicated, and bronchography may be required to demonstrate the area and extent of bronchial abnormality. In those instances in which extraluminal compression is caused by vascular abnormalities, contrast studies of the esophagus and angiocardiographic examination are often necessary diagnostic studies.

Treatment varies according to the cause of the obstructing mechanisms. Appropriate antimicrobial treatment is indicated in the presence of infectious processes. Bronchoscopic manipulations are needed to remove secretions, mucous plugs, foreign bodies, endobronchial granulations, and the like. Surgical treatment such as lobectomy or correction of vascular anomalies may be indicated.

Attention is directed to the pulmonary findings in certain cardiovascular anomalies such as coarctation of the pulmonary artery or in some instances of patent ductus arteriosus. Because of greatly reduced blood flow to one lung, that lung will have some superficial radiographic resemblance to an emphysematous one. The involved lung will appear darker, as if it contained an increased amount of air, because of the decreased vascular flow. If any shift of the heart and mediastinal structures occurs with respiration, the shift is toward the involved side. These

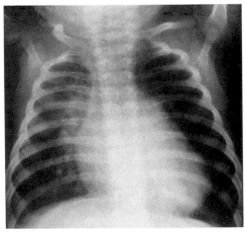

lung secondary to a large patent ductus arteriosus
FIGURE 40–4. "Apparent" emphysema of left shunting most of the blood to the right lung.

characteristic findings readily permit differentiation from localized emphysema of one lung. Cardiac catheterization and angiocardiography will delineate the nature of the vascular anomaly and will indicate whether remediable surgery can be undertaken.

Generalized obstructive emphysema occurs in the presence of widespread inflammatory disease or bronchospasm, so that both lungs are diffusely and usually uniformly overaerated.

It should be noted that some degree of overaeration of both lungs is often present during the acute phase of many pulmonary infections even when the area of involvement is localized, e.g. in lobar pneumonia. Under these circumstances the generalized emphysema is not extensive and is best appreciated by comparing roentgenograms obtained during the acute phase of the infection with those obtained after recovery has occurred.

Generalized obstructive emphysema is noted in bronchial asthma, cystic fibrosis, acute bronchiolitis, after the aspiration of secretions or liquids, after the inhalation of irritant substances, and the like. (See appropriate sections for details.)

Bullous emphysema (pneumatoceles) may follow overdistention of the alveoli with rupture of a number of them. They may be observed in newborn infants who had difficulty in initiating respiration and

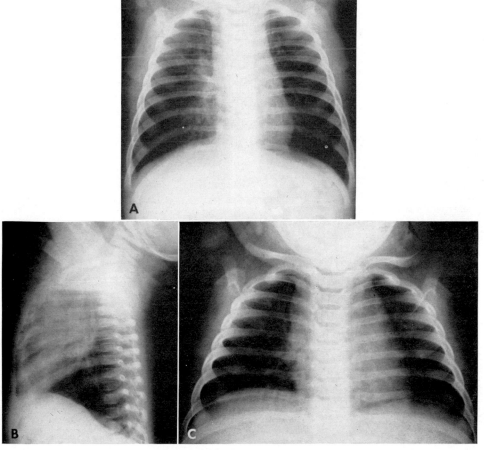

FIGURE 40–5. *A, B* (4/7/64), Acute generalized obstructive emphysema secondary to acute bronchiolitis. *C* (4/14/64), Normal chest after recovery.

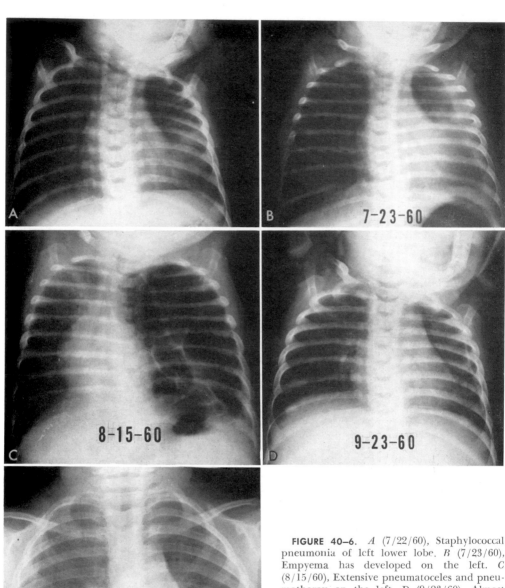

FIGURE 40–6. *A* (7/22/60), Staphylococcal pneumonia of left lower lobe. *B* (7/23/60), Empyema has developed on the left. *C* (8/15/60), Extensive pneumatoceles and pneumothorax on the left. *D* (9/23/60), Almost complete resolution of the preceding disease. *E* (11/1/62), Complete resolution.

often in those infants who required some active measures of rescuscitation (see p. 143). Pneumatoceles most commonly occur during the course of pneumonia caused by staphylococci (see p. 289), but can follow infections caused by pneumococci, Friedlaender's bacilli, *M. tuberculosis,* and others.

Pneumatoceles vary in number and size and often do not cause any symptoms. Very large or numerous pneumatoceles may cause respiratory distress which occasionally is severe. In rare instances a pneumatocele may rupture, causing a tension pneumothorax. Sometimes fluid accumulates in a pneumatocele, and air-fluid levels will be noted in the roentgenogram. Such lesions can usually be distinguished from lung abscesses (see p. 334). When fluid accumulates in a pneumatocele, there is no deterioration in the patient's general response; e.g. fever does not recur, leukocytosis does not worsen. Roentgenographic examination does not reveal an increase in parenchymal density adjacent to the pneumatocele.

Almost all pneumatoceles ultimately resolve completely, often within a few weeks, but an occasional one will persist for months before it finally disappears.

Attempts at surgical manipulation, such as needle aspiration, should be strongly discouraged. In the rare instance in which tension pneumothorax develops, surgical aspiration is obviously urgently needed. Since the expected events are those of spontaneous resolution without residual functional defects, conservative treatment of the underlying process is recommended.

Subcutaneous emphysema, though not a disturbance of the respiratory tract, may originate from abnormalities of it. Subcutaneous emphysema may originate from disease, injury or surgery in the respiratory tract from the nose to the lungs. In most instances subcutaneous emphysema is secondary to tracheostomy, especially one performed without a bronchoscope in the trachea, or to diseases of the lungs which cause obstructive emphysema. In the former instance, air enters through the surgical wound and dissects into the subcutaneous tissues along the fascial planes. Subcutaneous emphysema occurring from this source is usually not extensive. In the case of subcutaneous emphysema originating from pulmonary disease, it is thought, according to the studies of Macklin and Macklin, that alveolar rupture occurs, permitting air to dissect back toward the

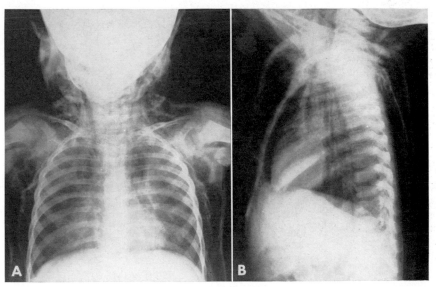

FIGURE 40–7. Severe subcutaneous emphysema and pneumomediastinum secondary to cystic fibrosis of the pancreas.

mediastinum in the perivascular and peribronchial spaces. Free air enters the mediastinum and from there may break out into the pleural cavity, causing a pneumothorax (see p. 487), or the air may remain in the mediastinum, producing pneumomediastinum (see p. 487). Sometimes air from the mediastinum passes upwards along the perivascular, fascial planes and other structures to the supraclavicular area, where it spreads subcutaneously. It may also extend downward along the aorta or the substernal structures to enter the abdomen or the subcutaneous areas of the abdominal wall. When subcutaneous emphysema is secondary to pulmonary obstruction, it may become widespread, extending over almost the entire body.

Subcutaneous emphysema may be seen in association with cystic fibrosis of the pancreas, pertussis, bronchial asthma, bronchiolitis, aspiration of foreign bodies, after violent coughing efforts as occasionally occur with bronchoscopy, and the like.

Treatment is largely symptomatic. The primary disease requires appropriate treatment. Should tension pneumothorax or tension pneumomediastinum develop, aspiration or suction drainage may be indicated. The subcutaneous emphysema is usually associated with surprisingly few symptoms in children and is usually absorbed in a few days or so.

Subcutaneous emphysema may also be secondary to the growth of anaerobic, gasforming clostridial species which enter the tissues through penetrating wounds.

REFERENCES

Binet, J. P., Nezelof, C., and Fredet, J.: Five Cases of Lobar Tension Emphysema in Infancy; Importance of Bronchial Malformation and Value of Postoperative Steroid Therapy. *Dis. of Chest,* 4:126, 1962.

Kress, M. B., and Finklestein, A. H.: Giant Bullous Emphysema Occurring in Tuberculosis in Childhood. *Pediatrics,* 30:269, 1962.

Leape, L., and Longino, L.: Infantile Lobar Emphysema. *Pediatrics,* 34:346, 1962.

Nelson, W. E.: Emphysema; in W. E. Nelson (Ed.): *Textbook of Pediatrics.* 8th ed. Philadelphia, W. B. Saunders Company, 1964, pp. 862-5.

Nelson, W. E., and Smith, L. W.: Generalized Obstructive Emphysema in Infants. *J. Pediat.,* 26:36, 1945.

CHAPTER FORTY-ONE

Tumors of the Chest

JAMES W. BROOKS, M.D.

Neoplasms of the chest in children may be divided into the following categories:

1. Pulmonary
   a. Benign
   b. Malignant
   c. Metastatic
2. Mediastinal
   a. Cysts
   b. Solid tumors
   c. Lymphatic
   d. Vascular
3. Cardiac
4. Diaphragmatic
5. Chest wall

PULMONARY TUMORS

In the pediatric age group all forms of primary pulmonary tumors are unusual.

Benign Pulmonary Tumors

Hamartoma

The term "hamartoma" was coined in 1904 by Albrecht, who defined it as a tumor-like malformation formed by an abnormal mixing of the normal components of the organ. Hamartomas of the lung consist largely of cartilage and also include variable quantities of epithelium, fat and muscle (Fig. 1). They are usually located in the periphery of the lung, but involvement of intermediate and primary bronchi has been reported. Developmental derangement is apparently responsible for their occurrence.

The incidence of hamartoma in all patients is 0.25 per cent (Lindskog and Liebow), but only six have been reported in the pediatric age group; four of these were discovered at autopsy, and two were successfully removed.

Although fifty-three cases of endobronchial hamartoma have been reported in adults, none have been seen in children.

Unlike hamartomas in adults, which are usually asymptomatic and small, the rare case found in infancy has been large and symptomatic and has contributed to the death of the infant (prematurity combined with respiratory inadequacy). At least four of the six reported hamartomas had obvious progressive intrauterine development and had attained considerable size at the time of birth.

Recognition and prompt removal of such large intrapulmonic tumors is necessary for survival. Difficult resuscitation or early demise, however, makes this difficult.

Although solid masses seen on chest x-rays in infants may cause one to suspect hamartoma, the diagnosis cannot be substantiated without thoracotomy. Surgical removal is the treatment of choice.

Holder and Christy have collected from the literature thirty-two cases of cystic adenomatoid malformation of the lung in newborn infants. These authors suggest that the entity be designated "adenomatoid hamartoma"; although this is a form

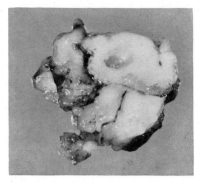

FIGURE 41–1. Hamartoma removed from right upper lobe of an adult. Note predominance of cartilage.

of congenital cystic disease of the lung resulting from abnormal growth of normal lung components, it is not a true hamartoma.

Polypoid Intrabronchial Mesodermal Tumors

As far as can be determined, chondromas, granular cell myoblastomas and mesenchymomas have not been reported in the pediatric age group.

Benign Parenchymal Tumors of Mesodermal Origin

A benign plasma cell granuloma of the lung in a seven-year-old girl has been reported by Liebow and Lindskog.

Study of the literature has revealed no case of sclerosing hemangioma in the pediatric age group.

Bronchial Adenoma

Bronchial adenoma is a neoplasm arising from either the cells of the mucous glands of the bronchi or the cells lining the excretory ducts of these glands.

Two histologic types are defined.

The *carcinoid type* (90 per cent) has histologic resemblance to carcinoid tumors of the small bowel; it is composed of somewhat oval cells filled almost entirely by nucleus. The cells, which have barely detectable lumens, are arranged in

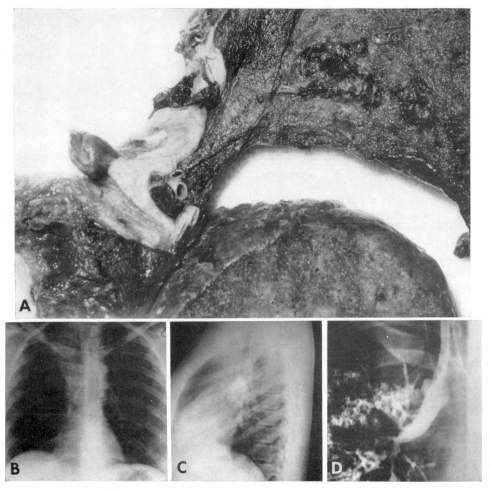

FIGURE 41–2. Bronchial adenoma (carcinoid type) (*A*) with total obstruction of the right upper lobe bronchus and distal atelectasis (*B* and *C*). Recurrent pneumonitis, cough and hemoptysis had occurred. Diagnosis by biopsy at the time of bronchoscopy. *D,* Obstruction of right upper lobe bronchus demonstrated with bronchograms. Treated by right upper lobectomy.

a quasi-acinar fashion and are piled up in several layers. The tumor is very vascular and is surrounded by a thin capsule of fibrous tissue which is not invaded by the tumor cells. Metaplastic epithelium of the bronchial mucosa covers the intrabronchial component. The tumor is frequently shaped like a dumbbell, with the smaller component intrabronchial and the larger one intrapulmonic. Though considered a benign tumor, bronchial adenomas have a definite malignant potential; lymph node metastasis (15 per cent) is more frequent than distant blood-borne metastasis.

The *cylindromatous type* (10 per cent) is made up of cuboidal or flattened epithelial cells, arranged in two layers, which form corelike structures of the cylinders. Histologically, it closely resembles mixed tumors of the salivary glands and basal cell carcinoma of the skin. There is a 40 per cent chance of malignancy.

Ten cases of bronchial adenoma, all apparently of the carcinoid type, have been reported in the pediatric age group. There were no metastases, and the carcinoid syndrome was not described.

The most prominent symptoms and signs are recurrent and refractory pneumonitis, elevated temperature, cough and chest pain due to bronchial obstruction with associated distal infection. Hemoptysis and wheeze are not as common in children as in adults. The right main bronchus is most commonly involved, and the diagnosis can usually be made by biopsy obtained at bronchoscopy. The tumor occurs five times more commonly in males. Although the youngest recorded patient was a ten-month-old infant, all the others were seen in children at least eight years of age (Fig. 2).

No case of peripheral bronchial adenoma has come to our attention.

Thoracotomy and resection of a segment, lobe or total lung according to the degree of involvement is indicated. Treatment by bronchoscopy is not effective, since complete removal of the tumor cannot be thus carried out. Rarely, a bronchial adenoma can be removed by bronchial resection.

Papilloma of the Trachea and Bronchi

Twenty-three cases of papilloma of the trachea and bronchi have been recorded in children (Fishman). These lesions, the cause of which is not known, may be single, but are more frequently multiple. The tendency for these tumors to disappear spontaneously at puberty has suggested a hormonal relationship.

Symptoms depend on the location and size of the tumor. The lesion may be attached by a pedicle and oscillate in and out of orifices during inspiration and expiration (flutter valve). Single, slow-growing, high lesions within the trachea may be asymptomatic for years. Dyspnea and stridor are the most common symptoms, occurring in 63 per cent of the cases. Cough, at first dry and later productive, is another frequent symptom.

Wheeze, audible at the open mouth, is the earliest sign of papilloma of the trachea. This eventually develops into stridor and is associated with slowly increasing dyspnea. Such secondary changes as obstructive emphysema, atelectasis, pneu-

monia, lung abscess and bronchiectasis may result in the distal parts of the tracheobronchial tree; empyema may also occur. Unless diverted, the usual course is one of increasing dyspnea which terminates in asphyxia.

These tumors should be removed because of their tendency to obstruction. Distal pulmonary infection or death from asphyxia may result. Ogilvie has reported two instances of malignancy arising from tracheobronchial papillomas.

Excision is the treatment of choice. Owing to the frequent multiplicity of the papillomas, treatment may be difficult and tedious, requiring numerous endoscopic procedures. Electrocoagulation can be used, and x-ray therapy has been most beneficial when there are multiple papillomas. The prognosis is good, but there is a tendency to recurrence, and constant vigilance with repeat bronchoscopic follow-up is indicated.

Fibroma of the Trachea

Nine cases of fibroma of the trachea have been recorded in infants (Gilbert).

Angioma of the Trachea

Six children with benign angioma have been reported by Gilbert. Congenital hemangioma of the trachea may cause death by the compromise of a vital structure, bleeding complications, intractable cardiac failure from atrioventricular shunting of blood within the tumor, or malignant change. In infants and children these tumors are usually below the vocal cords, sessile, flat, and associated with dyspnea. Ninety per cent of the recorded patients have been six months of age at the time of the onset of symptoms, and females predominate over males 2 to 1. Fifty per cent of the infants have hemangiomas elsewhere.

The onset is insidious with symptoms of respiratory obstruction, such as stridor, retraction, dyspnea, wheezing, and sometimes cyanosis and cough. The symptoms tend to be intermittent and labile. Usually fever and leukocytosis are absent, but superimposed infection may produce fever and an elevated white blood cell count. The best diagnostic tools are x-ray and endoscopy. Biopsy is not advisable at the time of endoscopy, since bleeding may cause asphyxia or an exsanguinating hemorrhage. Tracheostomy with x-ray therapy is probably the best form of therapy.

Leiomyoma of the Lung

Grossly, these tumors cannot be differentiated from other benign tumors of the lung. Leiomyomas of the lung are usually asymptomatic unless there is partial or complete bronchial obstruction. In a review of the world literature, Guida found only one case in a child. This six-year-old had a tumor in the right lower lobe, successfully treated by lobectomy.

Lipoma

Review of the literature reveals no case of lipoma of the bronchus or lung in the pediatric age group.

Neurogenic Tumors

Primary intrapulmonic neurogenic tumors have been recorded in three children out of thirty-two proved cases in the world literature. One was a neurofibroma, and the other two were neurilemmomas.

Malignant Pulmonary Tumors

Bronchogenic Carcinoma

Only sixteen cases of primary bronchogenic carcinoma of the lung in children have been reported. In three of these, congenital malformations of the lung were present; two had cystic disease and one had congenital atelectasis. The cases were equally distributed between males and females. The youngest patient was a five-month-old female infant with cystic lung disease and malignancy in the left lung reported by Schwyter in 1928. Every cell type except alveolar cell carcinoma, giant cell carcinoma, mucoepidermoid and carcinosarcoma has been seen in the pediatric age group.

1. Carcinoma 4
2. Adenocarcinoma 4
3. Squamous cell epithelioma 5
4. Oat cell carcinoma 2
5. Undifferentiated carcinoma 1

All patients have had widespread disease at the time when diagnosis was made. None has been resected. The longest recorded survival was seven years in a case treated by irradiation (Wasch). At the time of death there were widespread metastases.

Fibrosarcoma of the Bronchus

Review of the literature reveals only five cases of primary fibrosarcoma of the bronchus in the pediatric age group. Three were in girls and two in boys.

Fever, probably due to bronchial obstruction and distal infection, is the most common symptom; hemoptysis is relatively uncommon. Diagnosis in these cases should be established by bronchoscopy. Resection is the treatment of choice, since recurrence is frequent when any other mode of therapy is used. As a rule, metatastasis occurs by way of the blood stream, but lymph node involvement is possible.

Leiomyosarcoma

There have been three cases of primary leiomyosarcoma and four cases of nonspecific primary sarcoma of the lung reported in children. Cough, dyspnea and signs of obstructive pneumonitis are usually present. Surgery is indicated.

Multiple Myeloma

Multiple myeloma is usually limited to the medullary space. Extramedullary plasma cell tumors are relatively uncommon (myeloma or solitary plasmacytoma of the lung parenchyma). In a review of the literature Sekulich found only nineteen cases since 1911; one of these was a plasmacytoma in a three-year-old girl. Sputum cytology may be diagnostic.

Chorioepithelioma

A case of chorioepithelioma of the lung in a seven-month-old, white, female infant has been reported by Kay and Reed. The presenting symptoms were fever, dyspnea and anorexia; massive hemoptysis then occurred. X-ray film showed almost complete opacity of the right side of the chest. Pneumonectomy was performed, but the child died several hours postoperatively.

Systemic Neoplasms Affecting the Lung

Myeloid and lymphatic leukemia may have a pulmonary component, but isolated pulmonary disease has not been recorded. Similarly, Hodgkin's disease and lymphosarcoma may involve the lung during the course of the disease, but neither occurs as an isolated pulmonary lesion.

Metastatic Pulmonary Tumors

Primary sarcomas occur much more frequently in children than do primary carcinomas. The literature does not contain a report of a primary carcinoma in an infant with metastases to the lung; however, there are a number of references to primary sarcomas with pulmonary involvement by metastases. Primary sarcoma of the kidney (Wilms's), primary malignant skeletal tumors (chondrosarcoma and osteogenic sarcoma), Ewing's tumor, reticulum cell sarcoma, and soft tissue sarcomas (fibrosarcoma, rhabdomyosarcoma, liposarcoma, malignant neurilemmoma and synovioma) may metastasize to the lung. In general, the indications for resection of metastatic pulmonary disease should be based on the following criteria: (1) unilateral pulmonary involvement, (2) evidence of local control of the primary

malignancy for a period of one year before pulmonary resection.

If the lesion is thought to be unilateral, planigrams of the opposite lung should be obtained before resection is carried out. Pneumonectomy may be necessary for the removal of multiple unilateral lesions.

Bilateral pulmonary resections for metastatic disease are seldom indicated.

Discussion

Children who have symptoms of pulmonary involvement which do not disappear promptly when treated in the usual manner by expectorants and antibiotics must be suspected of having a space-occupying lesion. Posteroanterior and lateral chest x-rays are mandatory whenever respiratory symptoms persist.

Indeed, it would seem logical that all children should have a routine chest x-ray within the first six months of life. Certainly a physical examination in the adult patient is no longer considered complete without a chest x-ray. Why should the child be excluded from this advanced form of diagnosis? Without such refinement, how can we expect to help those with potentially curable lesions? Only by such techniques can obstructive emphysema (Fig. 3), atelectasis (Fig. 4) or actual solid masses be seen at a stage of development when active resectional surgery may have some hope of cure (Figs. 5, 6, 7, 8, 9).

In addition to a probing history and complete physical examination, children with respiratory symptoms should have other studies.

SPUTUM. It is impossible to obtain sputum voluntarily from the infant, but swabs from the posterior portion of the pharynx may be studied. In older children, however, sputum can be collected. A small catheter placed through the nose and adjusted into the trachea, thereby producing cough, will allow one to collect sputum through the catheter (Fig. 10). Any sputum thus collected should be

(Text continued on page 413.)

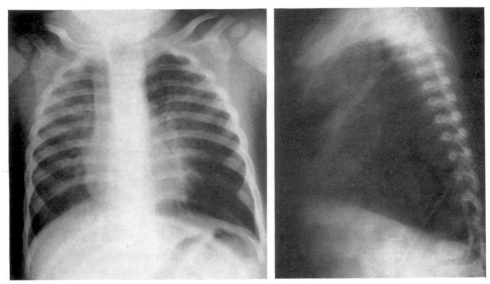

FIGURE 41–3. Obstructive emphysema of left lower lobe bronchus caused by partial occlusion of lumen. Left diaphragm is flattened, mediastinal and cardiac shadows are displaced toward right, left upper lobe is compressed, and there is increased radiolucency of left lower lobe.

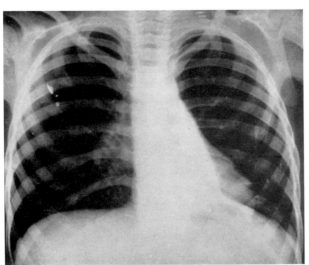

FIGURE 41–4. Total atelectasis of left lower lobe secondary to inflammatory stricture of left lower lobe bronchus. Retrocardiac position tends to confuse diagnosis in some cases.

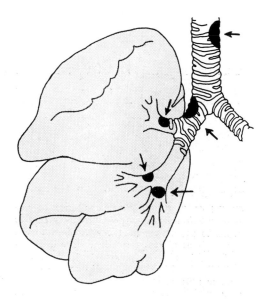

FIGURE 41–5. Diagram illustrating locations of lesions within the lumen of major bronchi. Location of such lesions will dictate area of pulmonary involvement, unilateral or bilateral, and extent of signs and symptoms.

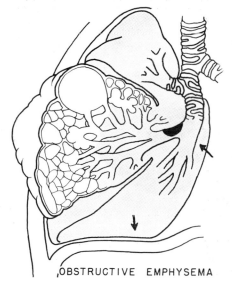

OBSTRUCTIVE EMPHYSEMA

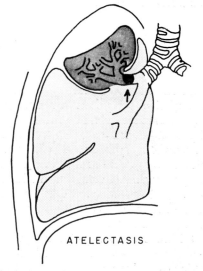

ATELECTASIS

FIGURE 41–6. Partial obstruction leads to retention of air in pulmonary parenchyma distal to obstructed bronchus. This will cause ipsilateral compression of adjacent normally aerated lung tissue, widening of intercostal spaces, descent of diaphragm, shift of mediastinum away from lung with partially obstructing lesion, and wheeze accompanied by decreased breath sounds over affected pulmonary tissue.

FIGURE 41–7. Persistence of the lesion with ultimate total obstruction gives rise to atelectasis, absent breath sounds over affected lung tissue, overexpansion of surrounding lung tissue, and shift of diaphragm to more normal position, with return of mediastinum to midline. Bronchial secretions may actually decrease in amount.

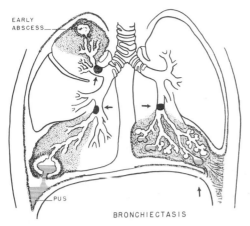

FIGURE 41–8. Continuing persistence of obstructing lesion leads to permanent destructive changes in pulmonary parenchyma distal to the lesion such as abscess formation, chronic pneumonitis with fibrosis, pleursy, empyema, and bronchiectasis with parenchymal contracture secondary to fibrosis.

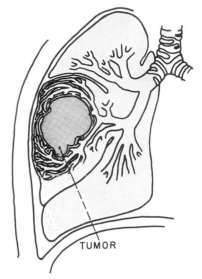

FIGURE 41–9. If tumor is within pulmonary parenchyma, pressure on adjacent lung and bronchi will give surrounding zone of pneumonitis that may actually show incomplete, temporary improvement on conservative management.

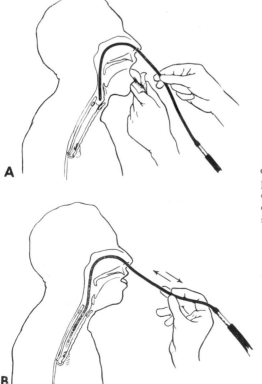

FIGURE 41–10. Diagram illustrating placement of rubber catheter through nose into posterior pharynx (*A*), followed by insertion into the trachea (*B*) through opened epiglottis at time of deep inspiration or cough to obtain bronchial secretions.

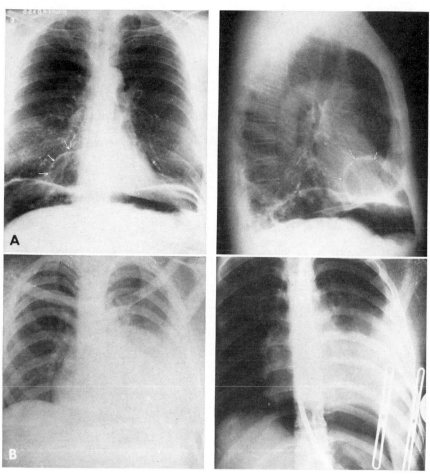

FIGURE 41–11. *A*, Diagnostic pneumoperitoneum showing congenital diaphragmatic hernia of Morgagni; and (*B*) outlining normal diaphragm with intrapleural or pneumonic density above.

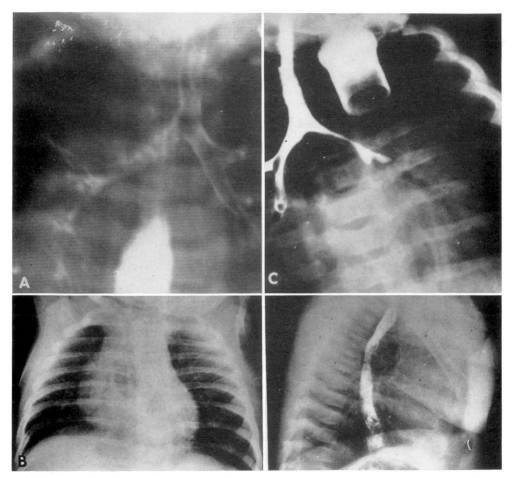

FIGURE 41–15. Adequate lung biopsy with specimens to bacteriology and pathology laboratories are anterior and lateral chest x-rays in infant with congenital bronchogenic cyst at carina and clinical respiratory distress. *C,* Contrast tracheobronchogram delineates narrowing of left main bronchus and displacement of right main bronchus.

studied by smear and culture for routine bacteria, acid-fast bacilli and fungi; bacteria should be tested for *antibiotic* sensitivity. Cytologic analysis for tumor cells should be carried out.

SKIN TESTS. The tuberculin, coccidioidin, blastomycin and histoplasmin skin tests should be applied.

BLOOD TESTS. Protein electrophoresis may show hypogammaglobulinemia to be a primary or secondary etiologic factor in recurrent pulmonary infectious processes. Complement fixation studies for fungal infections are generally more reliable than the skin tests. Pulmonary complications of hematologic disorders such as leukemia, Hodgkin's disease or lymphosarcoma may be properly identified by examination of the peripheral blood smear.

BONE MARROW. Examination of the bone marrow may give diagnostic evidence of blood dyscrasias such as leukemia or myeloma, or even metastatic malignancy.

SWEAT CHLORIDES. Cystic fibrosis as a cause of chronic recurrent pulmonary inflammatory disease may be suggested or ruled out by sweat chloride determination. (See the chapter on Cystic Fibrosis, p. 541.)

ROENTGENOLOGIC EXAMINATION of the chest with fluoroscopy and cinefluoroscopy, special views such as apical lordotic, right and left oblique, and planigrams may be necessary for final definition. Cinefluoroscopy allows repeated examination of the thoracic organs in motion (function) without subjecting the infant to excessive radiation exposure. During this examination and at the time of fluoroscopy, studies with barium in the esophagus will aid in determining any displacement of the posterior mediastinum.

PNEUMOPERITONEUM. The introduction of air into the peritoneal cavity, outlining the diaphragm, may aid in the diagnosis of abnormalities adjacent to the diaphragm; congenital diaphragmatic hernias may also be visualized (Fig. 11).

ANGIOGRAPHY. Angiocardiograms, outlining the cardiac chambers, will point up any displacement due to masses in the lung, mediastinum or pericardium. Certain lesions may be studied better by venous angiography outlining the major veins of the mediastinum. The use of aortograms will assist in ruling out such vascular causes for symptoms as vascular ring, congenital aneurysm, or congenital vascular malformations of the pulmonary tree.

BRONCHOGRAMS. Bronchograms are ex-

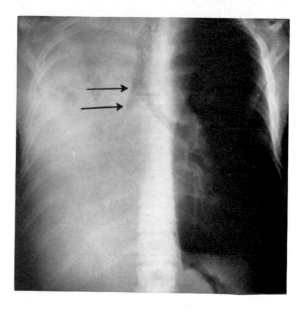

FIGURE 41–13. Air bronchogram showing complete block of right main bronchus in patient with total right lung atelectasis.

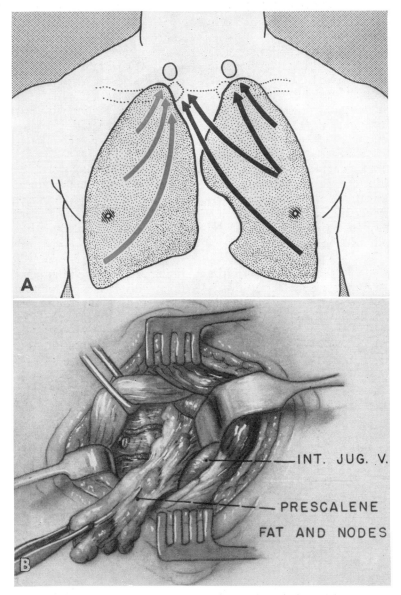

INT. JUG. V.

PRESCALENE

FAT AND NODES

FIGURE 41–14. *A,* Disease within the right lung usually drains into the right scalene lymph node group, while that in the left lung may drain to either scalene node group in a pattern similar to that indicated on the illustration. Generally, left lung disease requires bilateral scalene node biopsy, while right lung disease requires only right scalene node biopsy. Regardless of the side of lung disease, all palpable nodes in the scalene node area should be biopsied. *B,* The scalene group of nodes are contained in the fat pad bounded medially by the internal jugular vein, inferiorly by the subclavian vein and superiorly by the posterior belly of the omohyoid muscle. The base of the triangle is formed by the anterior scalene muscle. Retraction of the internal jugular vein is essential in order to get all nodes in this group.

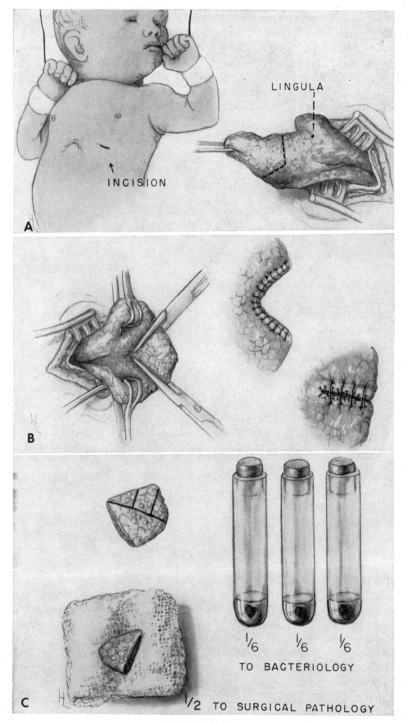

FIGURE 41–15. Adequate lung biopsy with specimens to bacteriology and pathology laboratories are essential. In general a small open thoracotomy has many advantages over the blind needle biopsy technique.

tremely useful in study of the trachea, major bronchi, and lobar and segmental bronchi. Intraluminal lesions, obstructive lesions and those causing displacement of bronchial segments may be identified (Fig. 12). Air bronchograms may give detail sufficient to dispense with contrast liquid materials (Fig. 13).

BRONCHOSCOPY. Bronchoscopy is the best available procedure for the study of tracheobronchial and pulmonary disease. This procedure enables visual study of the vocal cords, larynx, trachea, major bronchi and their important segmental orifices. Congenital anatomic abnormalities may be visualized; lesions within the lumen can be biopsied for a definitive diagnosis; prognosis in extensive lesions is evaluated by study of the carina and trachea. Aspiration of secretions is an important therapeutic contribution. Study of secretions and washings must include cytologic studies for malignant cells, routine bacterial smear, culture, and sensitivity studies, acid-fast smear and cultures, and fungal smear and cultures.

LYMPH NODE BIOPSY. Biopsy of palpable lymph nodes may be of aid in the diagnosis of abnormal processes in the lung. Most important are the scalene lymph nodes which drain the pulmonary parenchyma. Regardless of palpability, these nodes should be biopsied in those cases of pulmonary disease in which the diagnosis is uncertain and thoracotomy is contemplated. Scalene lymph node biopsy is of great help in the diagnosis of sarcoidosis, lymphatic malignancy such as Hodgkin's disease and lymphosarcoma, and in primary neoplasms of the lung and mediastinum. Lymph nodes obtained at the time of biopsy should be subjected to histologic study, and a portion sent to the bacteriology laboratory for routine bacterial smear, culture, studies for sensitivity of organism to antibiotics, acid-fast smear and culture and fungal smear and culture (Fig. 14).

LUNG BIOPSY AND THORACOTOMY. When all other methods have failed to produce a definitive diagnosis, thoracotomy should be considered. A limited incision may first be made, and biopsy of the lung obtained. If the situation appears to be an inoperable problem, biopsy may afford useful information (Fig. 15). Thoracotomy should not be unnecessarily delayed when definitive diagnosis has not been made.

MEDIASTINAL TUMORS

The mediastinum, the portion of the body which lies between both lungs, is bounded anteriorly by the sternum and posteriorly by the vertebrae. Superiorly, it extends from the suprasternal notch and terminates inferiorly at the diaphragm. Cysts or tumors which arise within the mediastinum may originate from any of the structures contained therein, or may be the result of developmental abnormalities. The mediastinum is lined on both sides by parietal pleura, and contains all structures of the thoracic cavities except the lungs. At times the lungs may herniate into the mediastinum. For ease of definition of sites of disease the mediastinum may be divided into four arbitrary compartments (Fig. 16): (1) the superior mediastinum—that portion of the mediastinum above a hypothetical line drawn from the junction of the manubrium and gladiolus of the sternum (angle) to the intervertebral disk between the fourth and fifth thoracic vertebrae; (2) the anterior mediastinum—that portion of the mediastinum which lies anterior to the anterior plane of the trachea; (3) the middle mediastinum—that portion containing the heart and pericardium, the ascending aorta, the lower segment of the superior vena cava, bifurcation of the pulmonary artery, the trachea, the two main bronchi, and bronchial lymph nodes; (4) the posterior mediastinum—that portion which lies posterior to the anterior plane of the trachea.

A great number of lesions (even very large ones) in the mediastinum will remain asymptomatic for a considerable period of time and will be discovered only through the use of routine chest x-rays.

The patient becomes aware of lesions within the mediastinum only when pressure is exerted upon sensitive structures of the mediastinum or the structures are displaced; therefore the severity of symptoms depends upon the size and location of the tumor, the rapidity of growth, and the presence or absence of the actual invasion of organs. Symptoms resulting from mediastinal lesions may become manifest according to the disturbance of function of the various organs in the mediastinum.

RESPIRATORY SYMPTOMS. In mediastinal lesions of children respiratory symptoms are the most important. These symptoms are the result of direct pressure on some portion of the respiratory tract.

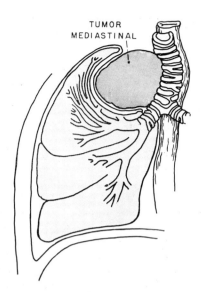

FIGURE 41–17. Diagram illustrating large mediastinal tumor or cyst with pressure on tracheobronchial tree as well as pulmonary parenchyma, thus possibly giving rise to pulmonary symptoms.

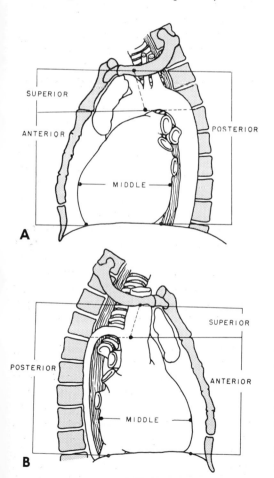

FIGURE 41–16. A, Mediastinal compartments as seen from left hemithorax. B, Mediastinal compartments as seen from right hemithorax.

This pressure causes narrowing of the trachea or the bronchi, or compression of the lung parenchyma (Fig. 17). Dry cough may be present; stridor or wheeze may occur at the same time or may precede it. The compression may be sufficient to produce enough occlusion so that there is distal obstructive emphysema or atelectasis, pneumonitis or chronic recurrent lower respiratory tract infections with associated fever and leukocytosis. The dry cough may be replaced by a productive one with mucoid sputum; if infection occurs, the secretion will become purulent. The unilateral nature of the wheezing and respiratory complaints serves to rule out asthma, bronchiolitis or chronic recurrent infections secondary to cystic fibrosis or hypogammaglobulinemia, but will not eliminate the possibility of endobronchial or endotracheal lesions; nor can the possibility of a foreign body in the tracheobronchial tree be discarded. Bronchoscopy is necessary in order to make this differentiation.

If the lesion in the mediastinum exerts pressure on the recurrent laryngeal nerve, hoarseness and a brassy cough will result.

Dyspnea, which may be progressive, is a common symptom of mediastinal tumors. Acute episodes of dyspnea with associated pneumonitis may occur when there is tracheal or bronchial obstruction leading to distal infection. Hemoptysis occurs in less than 10 per cent of mediastinal tumors in children.

GASTROINTESTINAL SYMPTOMS. Symptoms referable to the gastrointestinal tract result primarily from pressure on the esophagus. Regurgitation of food, and dysphagia with a slight sensation of sticking in the lower esophagus, are common. Displacement of the esophagus usually does not cause dysphagia; however, if there is fixation of the mass secondary to infection, hemorrhage or malignant degeneration, thereby causing interference with the peristaltic activity of the esophagus, dysphagia will occur. Vomiting is rare when the tumor is benign, but may occur when it is malignant; this is the result of the systemic effects of the malignancy.

NEUROLOGIC SYMPTOMS. In older children there is often a feeling of vague intrathoracic discomfort, fullness or ache caused by pressure on the sensitive intercostal nerves. Such pain may be mild or severe and is common in tumors of neurogenic origin. The appearance of herpes zoster indicates involvement of an intercostal nerve, but this is not common in the pediatric age group. When lesions impinge on the pleura, the pain may be of pleuritic nature. Erosion of vertebrae causes a boring pain located in the interscapular area. A malignant lesion which invades the brachial plexus causes severe pain in the upper extremities; Horner's syndrome indicates involvement of the cervical sympathetics. Inflammation, intracystic hemorrhage, or malignant degeneration of the phrenic nerve may result in hiccups. Certain dumbbell tumors of the spinal cord and mediastinum may exhibit symptoms referable to spinal cord pressure.

VASCULAR SYMPTOMS. Benign lesions of the mediastinum rarely cause obstruction of the great vessels in the mediastinum; however, obstruction is a common finding in malignant mediastinal tumors and carries a poor prognosis. Superior vena caval involvement gives rise to a dilatation of veins in the upper extremity, head and neck. As the obstruction progresses there is cyanosis of the head and neck area associated with bounding headaches and tinnitus. Either innominate vein may be involved, causing unilateral venous distention and edema of the upper extremity, head and neck (ipsilateral). Pressure on the inferior vena cava is less common, but when present there may be associated edema of the lower extremities.

MISCELLANEOUS SYMPTOMS. Fever is uncommon in mediastinal lesions unless there is secondary infection in the tracheobronchial tree; it may also be present with Hodgkin's disease, lymphosarcoma, or breakdown of malignant disease. Weight loss, malaise, anemia and anorexia are uncommon unless there is malignancy.

PHYSICAL FINDINGS. Physical findings are frequently absent; wheeze, rhonchi or rales may be present. There may be dullness to percussion over the area of mediastinal enlargement; this extends laterally from each sternal border or posteriorly between the scapulae and above the diaphragm. Occasionally there is tenderness over the chest wall when a mediastinal tumor exerts pressure on the parietal pleura in that area.

DIAGNOSTIC PROCEDURES. The same diagnostic procedures apply in cases of lung lesions and mediastinal tumors. Certain situations unique to mediastinal tumors will be mentioned.

A tumor or lesion of the mediastinum should never be aspirated pre-operatively when operation is clearly indicated. If a neoplasm is present, such needle aspiration will cause spread of the tumor cells. Needle aspiration of lesions of the mediastinum should be reserved for the inoperable tumor, or the acute emergency when tremendous cystic enlargement may jeopardize the child's life or may interfere with a good course of induction at the time of anesthesia.

The use of trial x-ray therapy for un-diagnosed mediastinal lesions is not war-ranted. Deep x-ray therapy can be ad-ministered in dosage sufficient to produce shrinkage of hyperplasia of the thymus, mediastinal nodes in Hodgkin's disease and lymphosarcoma. The danger of ra-diation-induced thyroid carcinoma makes the use of deep x-ray therapy for the shrinkage of hyperplasia of the thymus inadvisable. Peripheral node biopsy is preferable in suspected cases of Hodg-kin's disease or lymphosarcoma. If such nodes are not diagnostic, thoracotomy is then indicated.

Hydatid disease is not common in the United States, and only when it is present in the lung adjacent to the mediastinum can mediastinal tumor be simulated. The precipitin and skin test results are posi-tive in hydatid disease with an active hydatid cyst. Often hooklets may be found in the sputum of patients so affected.

Mediastinal abscess will rarely be con-fused with a neoplasm of the mediasti-num. Usually there is a history of trauma, foreign body in the esophagus, or instru-mentation. High fever, tachycardia, dysp-nea, extreme weakness, and prostration usually come on rapidly; thus the signs and symptoms of acute infection are paramount. The development of a fluid level in the mediastinum is diagnostic of mediastinal abscess if the above-men-tioned physical findings are also present. Intensive antibiotic therapy and prompt surgical drainage are indicated. There may be masses in the neck secondary to extension from lesions within the medias-tinum.

Primary Mediastinal Cysts

Lesions occurring within the mediasti-num may be predominantly cystic or predominantly solid. Those in the cystic group are usually benign, while the solid group has a more malignant potential.

Primary mediastinal cysts probably rep-resent abnormalities in embryologic devel-opment at the site of the foregut just

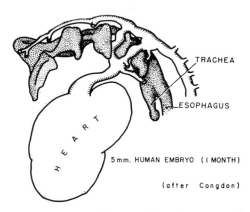

FIGURE 41–18. Foregut lying between tra-cheal and esophageal buds is probable site of em-bryologic maldevelopment which gives rise to foregut cyst development.

when separation of esophageal and lung buds occurs (Fig. 18).

Structures which arise from the foregut are the pharynx, thyroid, parathyroid, thymus, respiratory tract, esophagus, stomach, upper part of the duodenum, liver and pancreas; thus abnormal de-velopment at this stage may give rise to (1) bronchogenic cysts, (2) esophageal du-plication cysts, and (3) gastroenteric cysts.

Bronchogenic Cysts

Maier has classified bronchogenic cysts according to location (Fig. 19) as (a) tra-cheal, (b) hilar (Fig. 20), (c) carinal (Fig. 21), (d) esophageal, (e) miscellaneous.

Bronchogenic cysts are usually located in the midmediastinum, but have been described in all mediastinal subdivisions. Microscopically, bronchogenic cysts may contain any or all of the tissues normally present in the trachea and bronchi (fi-brous connective tissue, mucous glands, cartilage, smooth muscle, and a lining formed by ciliated pseudostratified co-lumnar epithelium or stratified squamous epithelium). The fluid inside the cyst is either clear, water-like liquid, or vis-cous, gelatinous material.

Bronchogenic cysts are usually asymp-tomatic. There may, however, be frequent upper respiratory tract infections, vague feelings of substernal discomfort, and re-

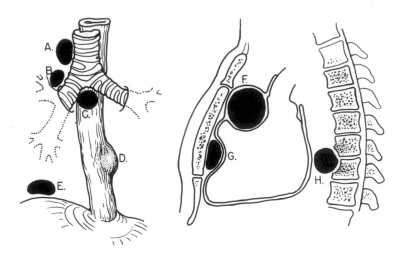

FIGURE 41–19. Diagrammatic illustration of location of bronchogenic cysts as suggested by Maier; *B* and *C* are the most common sites recorded.

spiratory difficulty (cough, noisy breathing, dyspnea, and possibly cyanosis). Bronchogenic cysts may communicate with the tracheobronchial tree and show varying air-fluid levels accompanied by the expectoration of purulent material. If communication with the tracheobronchial tree is present, this may be visualized by bronchoscopy and by bronchograms. Hemoptysis may occur when there is infection and communication of the cyst with the tracheobronchial tree.

On x-ray examination the bronchogenic cyst is usually a single, smooth-bordered, spherical mass (Fig. 23). It has a uniform density similar to the cardiac shadow. Calcification is unusual. Fluoroscopic examination of the cyst may demonstrate that it moves with respiration, since it is attached to the tracheobronchial tree; its shape may be altered during the cycles of respiration. Evidence of bone erosion with bronchogenic cysts is not recorded.

When the bronchogenic cyst is located at the carina, it may cause severe respiratory distress due to compression of either one or both major bronchi (Fig. 24). Early diagnosis and prompt removal are necessary.

The recorded incidence of bronchogenic cysts varies greatly. For example,

Gross found one bronchogenic cyst out of a total of thirty-three cysts and tumors of the mediastinum, while Heimburger and Battersby found seven cases (20 per cent) in their series of thirty-six cysts and tumors. When the latter combined five series from the literature, bronchogenic cysts were found in 10 per cent of the cases.

In a review of the literature by Dabbs and Berg there were ten cases of intrapericardial bronchogenic cysts.

Bronchogenic cysts should be treated by surgical removal. Their exact diagnosis can rarely be confirmed prior to thoracotomy. Removal is indicated because the lesion represents an undiagnosed thoracic mass; inflammation and intracystic hemorrhage may cause symptoms of severe respiratory distress and complicate removal; and finally, continued growth will embarrass surrounding vital structures.

Esophageal Cysts (Duplication)

Esophageal cysts are located in the posterior mediastinum; they are usually on the right side, and are intimately associated in the wall of the esophagus (Fig. 25). They occur more frequently in males than in females.

There are two types of esophageal
(*Text continued on page 426.*)

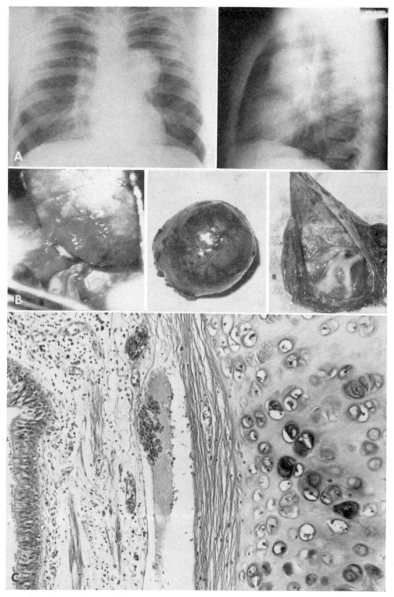

FIGURE 41–20. *A,* Typical left hilar bronchogenic cyst, with rounded, smooth border, and density similar to cardiac density. *B,* At the time of thoracotomy solid stalk was found attached to left main bronchus. Cyst was unilocular, containing thick, yellowish mucoid material. The wall was thin with typical trabeculations. *C,* Microscopic study revealed cartilage, smooth muscle and pseudostratified, ciliated, columnar epithelium.

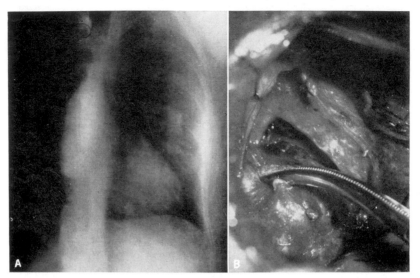

FIGURE 41–21. *A,* Overexposed posteroanterior chest film showing a carinal bronchogenic cyst. *B,* At operation the location is clearly seen at the carina with a solid fibrous stalk attached at the carina and separated just beneath the instrument dissector.

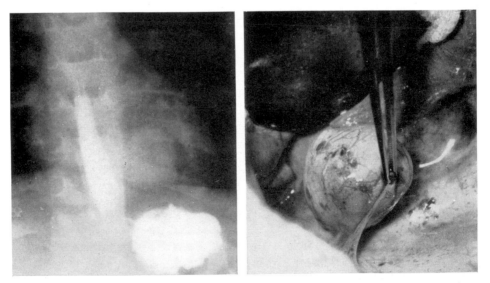

FIGURE 41–22. Bronchogenic cyst in child located retropleurally, overlying the distal thoracic aorta and not attached to the respiratory tract or esophagus.

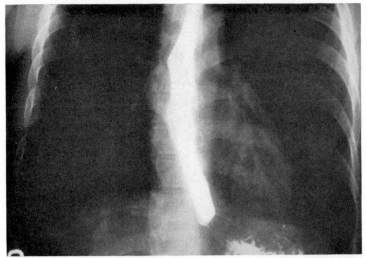

FIGURE 41–23. Hilar bronchogenic cyst with esophageal indentation seen on esophagogram.

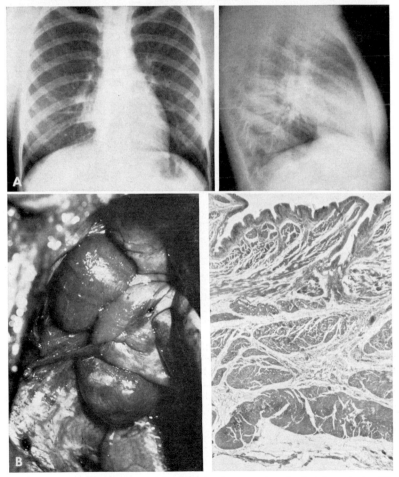

FIGURE 41–24. *A,* Bronchogenic cyst in a child whose mother had tuberculosis. The child was treated with antituberculous drugs for one year without change. *B,* At operation a dumbbell-shaped bronchogenic cyst was found is the region of the inferior pulmonary vein. Microscopic section shows a wall with ciliated epithelium, but no cartilage, and smooth muscle wall of 2 layers.

423

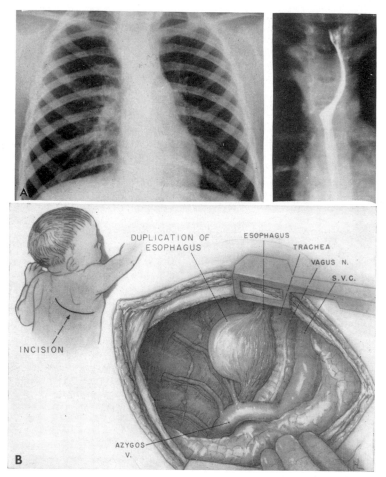

FIGURE 41–25. *A*, Posteroanterior chest x-ray taken in a child with an upper respiratory tract infection. A mass is seen in the posterior, superior mediastinum and presenting into the right hemithorax. At the time of an esophagogram the esophagus is seen displaced toward the left by a smooth mass. *B, C, D*, Artist's drawings of findings at operation. Note the plane of separation from the mucosa of the esophagus and lack of communication with the esophageal lumen. *E*, Opened operative specimen, cavity of which was filled with mucoid fluid. Lining of duplication was typical squamous cell.

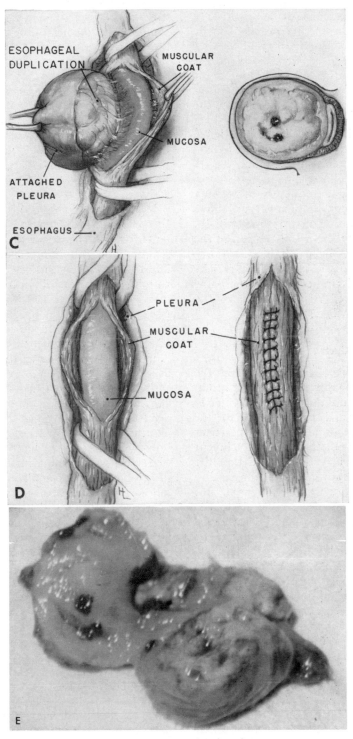

FIGURE 41–25. *Continued.*

cysts; the more characteristic type resembles adult esophagus with the cyst lined by noncornified, stratified squamous epithelium having a well defined muscularis mucosae and striated muscle in the wall. Intimate association in the muscular wall of the esophagus is not accompanied by communication with the lumen of the esophagus.

The second type is lined by ciliated mucosa, thus resembling that of the fetal esophagus. Esophageal cysts may be associated with mild dysphagia and regurgitation, but most frequently are asymptomatic. Barium esophagogram shows smooth indentation of the esophagus. On esophagoscopy there is indentation of the normal mucosa by a pliable, movable, soft, extramucosal mass. Removal by thoracotomy is indicated for the same reasons as noted in discussion of the therapy of bronchogenic cysts.

Gastroenteric Cysts

The third type of cyst arising from the foregut is the gastroenteric. This group of cysts lies against the vertebrae, posterior or lateral to and usually free of the esophagus, and usually in the posterior mediastinum with the main attachment posteriorly. It may be recalled that the early esophagus is lined by columnar epithelium, much of which is ciliated, and this is only gradually converted to the stratified epithelium of the definitive organ. The change is generally complete or almost complete at birth (Arey). Thus if a cyst arises from the embryonic esophagus, the ciliated lining is expected.

The enteric nature of a posterior mediastinal cyst is presumably certain if microscopic examination reveals a frank gastric or intestinal type of epithelium, but in general a better index of the nature and origin of such a cyst is the presence of well developed muscularis mucosae, tela submucosa, and two or even three main muscle coats. Gastric glands are most frequent, but esophageal, duodenal or small intestinal glands may be found. At operation the cyst sometimes seems grossly

"stomach-like" or "bowel-like." The significant fact is that cysts encountered in the posterior mediastinum show a highly developed mesodermal wall, and even the presence of Meissner's and Auerbach's plexuses, whereas the lining epithelium from case to case may range from columnar ciliated epithelium to a typical small intestinal type.

Two types of gastroenteric cysts have been described: (1) acid-secreting cysts which are functionally active; (2) cysts in which the mucosa has no functional activity.

Males predominate in this abnormality. In contrast with other foregut cysts, the posterior gastroenteric cyst is usually symptomatic. The symptoms are usually due to pressure on thoracic structures or rupture into bronchi with massive hemoptysis and death. Calcification also is frequent. Ossification has been reported by Steele and Schmitz in a cyst from a fifteen-year-old girl.

If the lining is gastric, dyspnea is the usual presenting symptom and occurs early; of the eighteen cases collected by Christoffersen (1947), all patients were under four with an average age of sixteen months. Actual peptic perforation of the lung with hemorrhage has been recorded.

Hemoptysis in young infants is difficult to distinguish from hematemesis; it may follow ulceration of a gastroenteric cyst (with gastric lining) of the mediastinum, with subsequent erosion into the lung. Gastric epithelium associated with intestinal or respiratory epithelium is apparently less secretory. Many functional cysts may lose their functional activity when the secretive areas of the mucosa are destroyed. Rennin, pepsin, chlorides and free hydrochloric acid have been demonstrated in the contents of some of the cysts.

Posterior gastroenteric foregut cysts of the mediastinum are frequently associated with two other types of congenital anomalies; (1) mesenteric and (2) vertebral abnormalities. Both types may occur in the same case. In the embryo the notocord and the entoderm are at one time in intimate contact; thus this combined developmental anomaly may result from abnormal embryonic development.

Penetration of the diaphragm by a cyst arising primarily from the thorax may occur; conversely, penetration of the diaphragm by the free end of an intramesenteric intestinal duplication is also possible.

A survey of the literature on mediastinal cysts combined with vertebral anomalies reveals that hemivertebra, spinal bifida anterior or infantile scoliosis has been reported in 61 per cent of eighteen cases. Most of these vertebral lesions involve the upper thoracic and lower cervical vertebrae, and the cyst tends to be caudad to the vertebral lesion. Planigrams may be necessary for diagnosis.

The presence of spina bifida anterior, congenital scoliosis, Klippel-Feil syndrome or similar but less defined lesions in the cervical or dorsal vertebra suggests the possibility that enteric cysts may be present in the mediastinum or in the abdomen.

In a survey by Abell four such gastroenteric cysts (3 per cent) were present in a series of 133 tumors of the mediastinum; they comprised 10 per cent of the mediastinal cysts in this series. All produced symptoms, were present in patients whose ages ranged from seven months to five years, were located in the posterior mediastinum, had abnormalities of the cervical or dorsal spine, and were resected succesfully.

Pericardial Celomic Cysts

These mesothelial cysts are developmental in origin, and formal genesis is related to the pericardial celom. The primitive pericardial cavity forms by the fusion of celomic spaces on each side of the embryo. During the process, dorsal and ventral parietal recesses are formed. Dorsal recesses communicate with the pleuroperitoneal celom, while the ventral recesses end blindly at the septum transversum. Persistence of segments of the ventral parietal recess accounts for most pericardial celomic cysts.

The cysts are usually located anteriorly in the cardiophrenic angles, more frequently on the right, and occasionally on or in the diaphragm (Fig. 26). They are usually asymptomatic and are discovered by routine chest x-ray. Rarely do they reach sufficient size to cause displacement of the heart or produce pressure upon the pulmonary tissue. Infection is unusual.

Pericardial cysts are usually unilocular. The walls are thin and the intersurfaces smooth and glistening, lined by a single layer of flat mesothelial cells. The mesothelium is supported by fibrous tissue with attached adipose tissue.

These cysts are usually not diagnosed in the pediatric age group. There are no recorded cases of symptomatic pericardial celomic cysts in children.

Intrathoracic Meningoceles

Intrathoracic meningoceles are not true mediastinal tumors or cysts; they are diverticuli of the spinal meninges which protrude through the neuroforamen adjacent to an intercostal nerve and present beneath the pleura in the posterior medial thoracic gutter. The wall represents an extension of the leptomeninges, and the content is cerebrospinal fluid. Enlargement of the intervertebral foramen is common; vertebral or rib anomalies adjacent to the meningocele are also frequent. The most commonly associated anomalies are kyphosis, scoliosis, and bone erosion or destruction. The wall of these cysts is formed by two distinct components; these are the dura mater and the arachnoidea spinalis, with small nerve trunks and ganglia occasionally incorporated in the wall.

Of the forty-six reported cases of intrathoracic meningocele, four were in the pediatric age group.

A threefold syndrome with generalized neurofibromatosis (von Recklinghausen's disease), kyphoscoliosis and intrathoracic meningocele may occur, but thoracic meningocele as an isolated defect is much less frequent. This lesion is usually asymp-

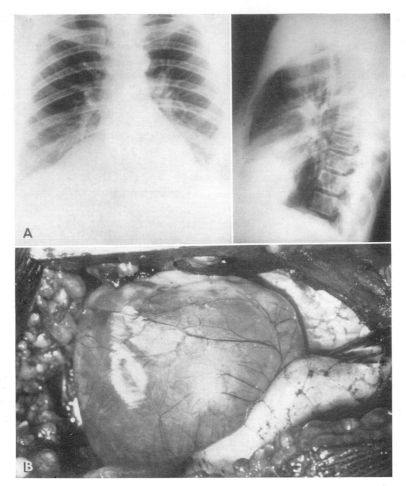

FIGURE 41–26. *A,* Typical location of pericardial cyst in posteroanterior and lateral chest films at the right cardiophrenic angle. *B,* Large cyst seen at the time of thoracotomy.

tomatic; it occurs on the right side approximately three times as often as on the left. Rarely the lesion may be bilateral. In patients with neurofibromatosis posterior sulcus tumors are more likely to be meningoceles and are rarely neurofibromas.

On x-ray examination the lesion is a regular, well demarcated, intrathoracic density located in the posterior sulcus; there are associated congenital anomalies of the spine and thorax. On fluoroscopy, pulsations may be noted in the sac. Diagnosis may be confirmed by myelograms.

When diagnosis is established, no therapy is indicated unless the lesion is symptomatic.

Operative complications such as empyema, meningitis and spinal fluid fistula have been greatly reduced since the advent of the antibiotics.

Thymus

Normally the thymus is located in the anterior superior mediastinum, but abnormalities of the thymus have been reported in all areas of the mediastinum. Abnormalities of the thymus in children are (1) hyperplasia of the thymus, (2) thymic neoplasms, (3) benign thymomas, (4) thymic cysts, (5) teratoma in the thymus, (6) tuberculosis of the thymus.

Hyperplasia of the Thymus

Thymic masses are the most common of the mediastinal masses in children; of these, hyperplasia of the thymus is most frequent.

The function of the thymus is still not clear, but recent studies suggest that it may in some way be involved in the determination of immunologic individuality. The thymus varies greatly in size. Steroids, infection, androgens and irradiation may make the thymus smaller; those stimuli which cause it to increase in size are not understood. Local variations in size are, as in other ductless glands, probably related to chance.

In a review of normal chest x-rays, Ellis found that there was almost always a recognizable thymic shadow present during the first month of life; there was great variation in the size and shape. The mediastinal shadow in this age group seemed to be proportionally wider than in older children and adults because of the proportionally larger heart and thymic shadow. In the age group from one to twelve months the thymic shadow was still present, if it had been seen earlier. Between one year and three years very little of the thymic shadow remained. Two per cent of children over four years of age still have a recognizable thymus on x-ray examination. It does not contain calcium, and there are transmitted pulsations on fluoroscopy. Noback, in a study of the thymus in both live and still-born infants, found a cervical extension of the thymus gland in 80 per cent of the cases. If located in the superior thoracic inlet, enlargement of the thymus may cause tracheal compression (Fig. 27).

The diagnosis of obstruction from an enlarged gland is established by good x-ray films, made in full inspiration with the child's head in a neutral position when the lateral film is made. Both esophageal and angiographic studies can be used to exclude a vascular ring. In cases of vascular ring obstruction, most patients find that their distress is relieved by hyperextension of the head.

Treatment of an enlarged thymus causing respiratory obstruction may be carried out in one of three ways.

First, the thymus responds rapidly to small doses (70 to 150 r) of irradiation; however, the danger of carcinogenic effect has caused this method of treatment to be abandoned.

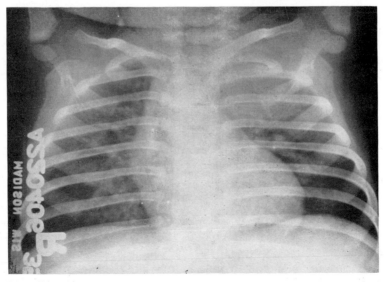

FIGURE 41–27. Mild respiratory distress in an infant with an enlarged thymus. Gradual improvement with age and no specific therapy.

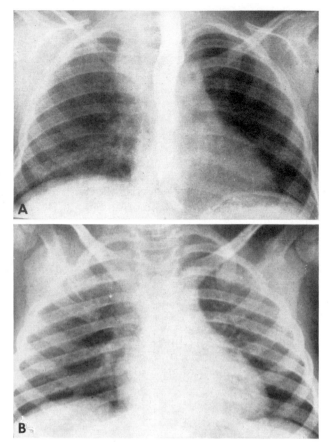

FIGURE 41–28. *A*, Enlarged thymus in an infant with (*B*) reduction in size after 7 days of steroid therapy.

Second, corticosteroids cause a rapid decrease in the size of the thymus, usually within a period of five to seven days. After cessation of corticosteroid therapy the gland may reach a size greater than that before treatment was instituted. Such a response may also be used in distinguishing between a physiologic enlargement of the thymus and a neoplasm (Fig. 28).

Third, surgery may be indicated both for the treatment of respiratory obstruction and for diagnosis.

Neoplasm of the Thymus

In a review of the literature in 1948 Neal found forty-seven malignant thymic tumors in children. Of this group, there were forty-four cases of lymphosarcoma, two of carcinoma, and one of primary Hodgkin's disease of the thymus. In none of these cases was there an associated myasthenia gravis.

Benign Thymoma

Only six benign thymic tumors have been reported in children (Fig. 29).

Thymic Cysts

Multiple small cysts of the thymus are frequently observed in necropsy material, but large thymic cysts are rare (Fig. 30). Fridjon described a large cyst in the thymus of a one-day-old infant. Thymic cysts have been resected from the neck (Fig. 31).

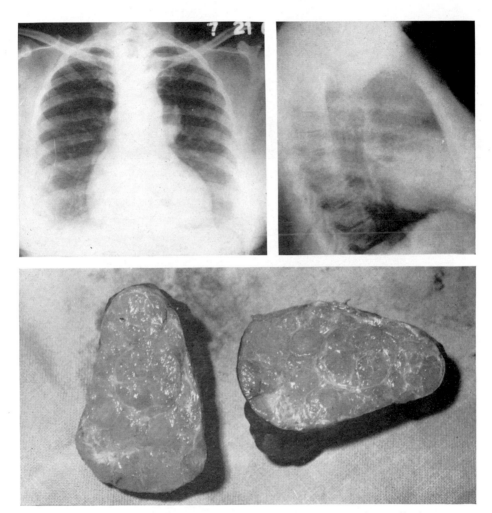

FIGURE 41–29. Benign thymoma located in the anterior superior mediastinum.

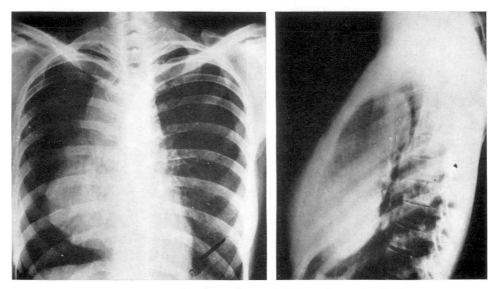

FIGURE 41–30.   Large thymic cyst in an adult located near the diaphragm.

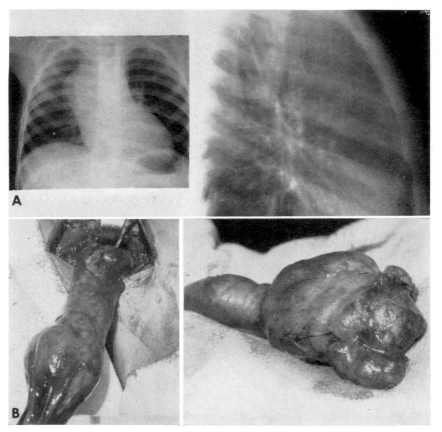

FIGURE 41–31.   *A,* Large thymic cyst in 4-year-old boy which presented in the right side of the neck as well as by chest x-ray. Removal required thoracotomy and supraclavicular incision. *B,* Thymic cyst as seen after thoracotomy and at time of removal through neck incision.

Teratoma of the Thymus

Teratoma of the thymus in a two-day-old white female infant has been described by Sealy; there was progressive respiratory distress, and she underwent operation at seven weeks of age.

Tuberculosis of the Thymus Gland

A single case of tuberculosis involving only the thymus gland has been described in a stillborn infant.

Teratoid Tumors

Teratoid tumors of the mediastinum may be classified as (1) benign cystic teratomas, (2) benign teratoids (solid), (3) teratoids (carcinoma).

Benign Cystic Teratoma

Teratoma of the anterior mediastinum probably results from faulty embryogenesis of the thymus or from local dislocation of tissue during embryogenesis.

Benign cystic teratoma (mediastinal dermoid cyst) contains such elements of ectodermal tissue as hair, sweat glands, sebaceous cysts and teeth. Other elements, including mesodermal and entodermal tissue, may also be found when benign cystic teratoid lesions are subjected to comprehensive examination; thus such tumors are more properly classified as teratoid than dermoid cysts.

Cystic teratomas are more common than solid ones. These lesions are predominantly located in the anterior mediastinum and may project into either hemithorax, more commonly the right. In children, females are affected more often than males. Malignant degeneration is less common than in the solid form of teratoid tumor.

It seems reasonable to assume that most if not all mediastinal teratomas are present at birth; however, Edge and Glennie have reported two adult patients from whom large teratoid tumors were re-moved two and four years after a routine chest x-ray was normal.

These cystic masses usually cause symptoms because of pressure on or erosion into the adjacent respiratory system. Symptoms are usually those of vague chest discomfort associated with cough, dyspnea and pneumonitis. Infection may cause a sudden exacerbation of symptoms, and rupture into the lung may occur with expectoration of hair; rupture into the pleura or pericardium may also occur.

The lesion is usually in the anterior mediastinum. On x-ray film the lesion is well outlined with sharp borders; definite diagnosis is not possible unless teeth can be demonstrated in the mass. Calcification is not unusual, and appears as scattered masses rather than diffuse, small densities. Cystic swelling in the suprasternal notch may occur.

Benign cystic teratomas should be removed. In cases in which infection, perforation, intracystic hemorrhage or malignant degeneration has occurred, complete removal may be difficult or impossible, owing to adherence to surrounding vital structures.

Benign Solid and Malignant Teratoid Tumors

Teratoma is the most common tumor occurring in the anterior mediastinum of infants and children (Fig. 32). The solid tumors in the teratoid group are much more complex and have a greater propensity for malignant change (Fig. 33). The incidence of malignancy is about 20 per cent.

In the benign solid teratoid tumors there are well differentiated structures which are rarely observed in the malignant group. Whereas the connective tissue stroma of malignant teratoma is usually poorly arranged, that of benign teratoma is dense and of the adult type. In the benign type, nerve tissue, skin and teeth may be found. Skin and its appendages are usually present and remarkably well formed. Hair follicles preserve their normal slightly oblique position relative to

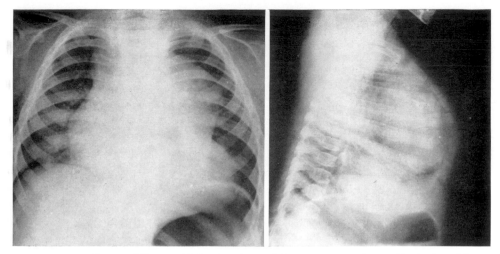

FIGURE 41–32. Large solid teratoid, benign, in an infant. Note anterior mediastinal position and forward displacement of the sternum.

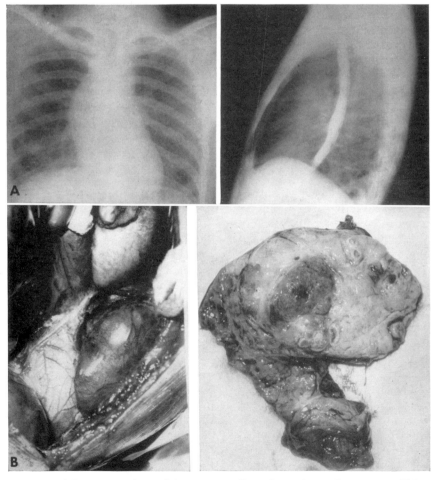

FIGURE 41–33. *A,* Posteroanterior and lateral x-ray films of anterior malignant teratoid in an older child. *B,* Note the anterior mediastinal position with teratoid wedged between the heart and sternum.

434

the free surface and are always accompanied by well developed sebaceous glands. Sweat glands, often of the apocrine type, are frequently located near the sebaceous glands. Smooth muscle, closely resembling arrectores pilorum, is occasionally encountered.

Mesodermal derivatives such as connective tissue, bone, cartilage and muscle arranged in organoid pattern are frequently found. When present, hematopoietic tissue is found only in association with cancellous bone. Smooth muscle is most often observed as longitudinal or circular bundles in organoid alimentary structures. Occasionally it is also seen in bronchial walls.

Entodermal derivatives representing such structures as intestine, and respiratory and pancreatic tissue are also present.

In a review of mediastinal tumors Ellis and DuShane found 27.6 per cent teratomatous tumors in infants. Of this group of sixteen teratomatous tumors, eight were benign teratomas, five were teratoid cysts, and three were teratoid carcinoma.

The symptoms, signs and x-ray findings in these cases are identical to those found in teratoid cysts unless malignant spread has occurred.

The final decision as to malignancy can be determined only after removal and histologic study of the tumor. Malignant degeneration usually involves only one of the cellular components.

Heuer and Andres reviewed 217 cases of teratoid tumors and found that only 5.5 per cent were discovered under the age of twelve years. Both benign and malignant teratoid tumors may occur within the pericardial sac.

Neurogenic Tumors

Neurogenic tumors, by far the most common of posterior mediastinal origin, may be classified as follows:

1. Neurofibromas and neurilemmoma
   a. Malignant schwannomas
2. Tumors of sympathetic origin
   a. Neuroblastomas
   b. Ganglioneuroma
   c. Ganglioneuroblastoma
   d. Pheochromocytomas
3. Chemodectoma

Benign neurofibromas, neurilemmoma and malignant schwannomas are extremely unusual in the pediatric age group and when present are most often asymptomatic (Fig. 34).

The neuroblastoma is a malignant tumor arising from the adrenal medulla and occasionally from ganglia of the sympathetic nervous system; it consists of uniform cell layers with or without pseudorosettes. The cells have a dark nucleus and scant cytoplasm, and are separated by an eosinophilic fibrillar stroma. Cellular differentiation is sometimes very poor. Although the primary neuroblastoma may cause the first clinical signs or symptoms, metastases in the bone, skin or lymph nodes may be the first indication of its presence.

The ganglioneuroma is a benign tumor made up of mature ganglion cells, few or many in number, in a stroma of nerve fibers.

Ganglioneuroblastoma is a tumor composed of various proportions of neuroblastoma and ganglioneuroma.

Ganglioneuroma and ganglioneuroblastoma are more likely to occur after the age of two years. The more malignant forms such as neuroblastoma frequently occur before the age of two years. Ganglioneuroma is more common in children than in adults; respiratory symptoms are rare (Fig. 35).

Tumors of nerve origin usually occur in the upper two thirds of the hemithorax and tend to extend locally. They may grow into the lower part of the neck, across the midline through the posterior mediastinum to the opposite hemithorax, descend through the diaphragm into the upper part of the abdomen, or into the intercostal spaces posteriorly and involve one or several of the vertebral foramina. Ganglioneuroblastoma rarely metastasizes to lymph nodes.

A large number of neurogenic tumors, more often the benign type, may be

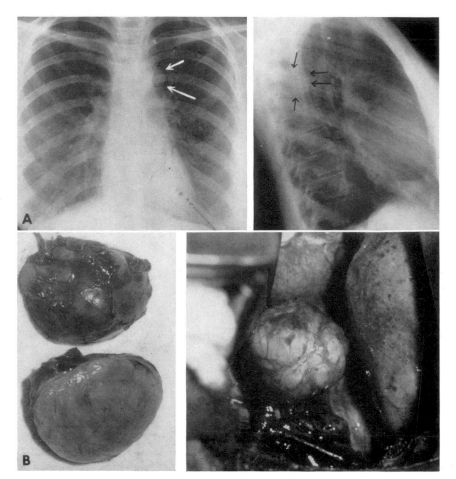

FIGURE 41–34. *A,* Neurofibroma seen posteriorly located in posteroanterior and lateral films. *B,* Note solid nature of lesion, round, smooth outline and attachment to intercostal nerve.

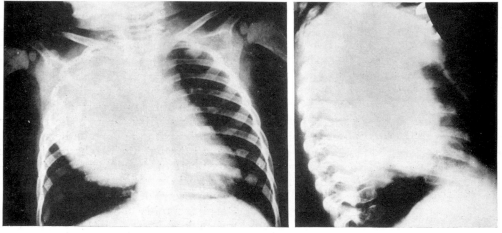

FIGURE 41–35. Large ganglioneuroma in infant. Benign lesion was removed with good follow-up result.

asymptomatic. Symptoms such as radicular pain, paraplegia, motor disturbances or Horner's syndrome may occur.

Upper respiratory tract infections, dyspnea, elevated temperature, weight loss and asthenia may occur. Neurogenic tumors of the neuroblastoma group usually occur in younger children, and respiratory symptoms, thoracic pain and fever are more common (Fig. 36).

On x-ray examination neurogenic tumors are round, oval or spindle-shaped, and are characteristically located posteriorly in the paravertebral gutter. On thoracic x-rays the ganglioneuroma appears as an elongated lesion and may extend over a distance of several vertebrae. Typically, a neurofibroma tends to be more rounded in outline. Calcifications within the tumor may be seen, more commonly in the malignant forms. Even though not demonstrated on x-ray examination, calcification may be found at the time of histologic examination. Bone lesions such as intercostal space widening, costal deformation, vertebral involvement and metastatic bone disease are not unusual with neurogenic tumors.

The therapy for neurogenic tumors of the thoracic cavity is surgery. Every case of ganglioneuroma reported in a study by Schweisguth was amenable to resection. In malignant neurogenic tumor all possible tumor growth should be excised and postoperative irradiation therapy instituted. X-ray therapy must be given judiciously, since growth disturbances, pulmonary fibrosis and other sequelae may develop. In the hourglass type of tumor, laminectomy must precede thoracotomy.

Mediastinal chemodectomas are usually located anteriorly; they are likely to be associated with similar tumors in the carotid body and elsewhere. There is a tendency for these tumors to be multiple.

Mediastinal pheochromocytomas are extremely rare and have not been recorded in the pediatric age group.

In Heimburger and Battersby's series of mediastinal tumors in childhood, 25 per cent of thirty-six tumors were of the neurogenic type. Ellis and DuShane reported 32 per cent neurogenic tumors in a review of primary mediastinal cysts and neoplasms in infants.

Lymph Nodes

Abnormalities of the lymph nodes in the mediastinum may be classified as follows:

1. Leukemia
2. Hodgkin's disease
3. Lymphosarcoma
4. Sarcoidosis

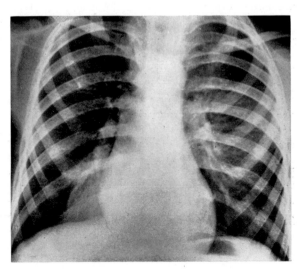

FIGURE 41–36. Neuroblastoma in a 6-year-old boy.

5. Inflammatory
   a. Tuberculosis
   b. Fungus
   c. Nonspecific

Any lymph node enlargement in a child should be viewed with suspicion. Lymphatic tumors are one of the more frequently observed malignant growths in childhood. The diagnosis is made by biopsy. Tumors of the Hodgkin's lymphosarcoma and reticulum cell sarcoma group are found primarily in children over three years of age with a peak incidence from eight to fourteen years. Over 95 per cent of children with primary lymphatic malignancy will have lymph node enlargment as the presenting sign. Tonsillar hypertrophy and adenoidal hyperplasia, pulmonary hilar enlargement, splenomegaly, bone pain, unexplained fever, anemia, infiltrative skin lesions, and rarely central nervous system symptoms may also be present. The diagnosis should be sought through the study of peripheral blood smears, lymph node biopsy or bone marrow examination.

Surgery has limited value in lymphosarcoma, since the disease is usually widespread. When, however, the lesions are apparently isolated in the neck, axilla, mediastinum or gastrointestinal tract, surgery may be of great benefit. With few exceptions, all the tumors in this group are radio-sensitive; however, they are not curable by x-ray.

In most cases of mediastinal malignancy bilateral hilar enlargement, as well as bilateral mediastinal enlargement, will be present. The lymph node enlargement may rarely be unilateral and relatively localized. In such cases routine study of the blood smear, scalene lymph node biopsy and bone marrow studies may not provide the diagnosis, and open thoracotomy may be necessary. In such cases complete lymph node removal should be carried out if technically feasible.

Inflammatory

Lymph node enlargement in the hilus of the lung or mediastinum may be secondary to tuberculous, fungal or bacterial lung disease. Diagnosis is usually confirmed by means of sputum culture, washings from the tracheobronchial tree at the time of bronchoscopy, scalene node biopsy, and skin tests correlated with the general clinical picture. The same is true in sarcoidosis. In sarcoidosis there may be involvement of the eye, skin, peripheral lymph nodes, mediastinal or hilar lymph nodes, and the lung parenchyma. It is possible to establish the diagnosis with this clinical picture and scalene node biopsy in approximately 80 to 85 per cent of the cases of sarcoidosis.

Although nonspecific symptomatic or asymptomatic enlargement of the mediastinal lymph nodes may occur, a cause can usually be found. For example, histoplasmosis may produce the clinical picture outlined.

Venezilae et al. have described angiofloccular hyperplasia of the mediastinal lymph nodes. Although this rare, benign localized lymph node enlargement may occur in extrathoracic locations, it most often occurs as an isolated asymptomatic mediastinal or pulmonary hilar tumor. Grossly, the tumors are moderately firm and usually well encapsulated. Calcification may occur, but is unusual. Microscopically, the two main features of these lymphoid masses are a diffuse follicular replacement of the lymph node architecture and much follicular and interfollicular vascular proliferation. Sixty per cent of patients with this entity are asymptomatic. When symptoms occur, they may include cough, colds, fatigue, chest pain and fever. Surgical excision is the treatment of choice and is usually successful.

Vascular and Lymphatic Abnormalities

Vascular and lymphatic abnormalities of the mediastinum may be classified as (1) cavernous hemangioma, (2) hemangiopericytoma, (3) angiosarcoma, (4) cystic hygroma.

Vascular tumors of the mediastinum in

children are rare, and preoperative diagnosis is unusual. Vascular tumors may occur at any level in the mediastinum, but are more frequently seen in the upper portion of the thorax and in the anterior mediastinum. They are uniformly rounded in appearance and are moderately dense. Calcification within the tumor is unusual. They are usually asymptomatic.

Cystic hygromas are relatively rare, but occur more often in infants and children than in adults. These tumors consist of masses of dilated lymphatic channels containing clear, watery fluid; they are lined with flat endothelium and are usually multilocular. They may appear to be isolated in the mediastinum (Fig. 37), but more often have an associated continuation into the neck. They may be rather large and unilateral with lateral masses in the superior mediastinum. In 1948 Gross and Hurwitt reported twenty-one cases of cervical mediastinal hygromas and only eight cases of isolated mediastinal hygromas.

Diagnosis of a cervico-mediastinal hygroma is made by physical examination of the cervical swelling and x-ray examination of the chest. Periodic fluctuation in size frequently occurs in cervical hygromas. This is even more characteristic of the combined cervico-mediastinal lesions; in these the cervical component may increase in size during inspiratory movements. X-ray films and fluoroscopic examination may show descent of the mass into the mediastinum on inspiration with a prominence in the neck during expiration.

Cystic hygromas confined to the mediastinum are usually discovered at autopsy or as an unanticipated finding on x-ray examination. The soft and yielding nature of the cysts allows them to attain considerable size without producing symptoms. On x-ray film there is a somewhat lobulated, smoothly outlined mass; however, it is usually not possible to distinguish hygromas from other benign tumors or cysts of the mediastinum by this method.

When respiratory infections occur, hygromas often become infected. Such infec-

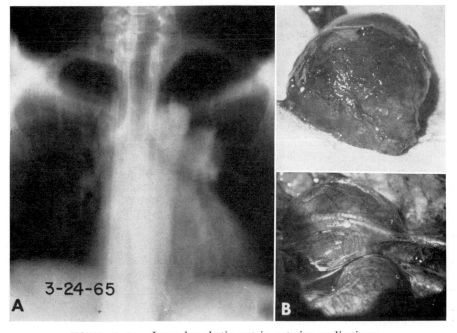

3-24-65

A

B

FIGURE 41–37. Large lymphatic cyst in anterior mediastinum.

tions are usually controlled by chemotherapy or by incision and drainage. A mediastinal or blood stream infection may result, however, or infection may be followed by local fibrosis and the disappearance of the mass. Spontaneous or post-traumatic hemorrhage into a cyst may result in extension of the cyst; this may cause sudden tracheal compression, a surgical emergency. Malignant change in hygroma has not been reported.

Surgical excision is the treatment of choice. Mediastinal hygromas can usually be excised with little difficulty because tissue planes around the cysts are well developed.

Chylothorax may result when there is cervical hygroma with involvement of the thoracic duct.

Mediastinal Lipoma and Liposarcoma

Intrathoracic lipoma is rare in children. Lipomas of the mediastinum have been divided into three groups according to their location and form: (1) tumors confined within the thoracic cage; (2) intrathoracic lipomas which extend upward into the neck; (3) intrathoracic lipomas with an extrathoracic extension, forming a dumbbell configuration.

Of the eighty cases of lipoma reported in the world literature, sixty-one were intrathoracic, eight cervico-mediastinal, and eleven of the dumbbell type. Only two occurred in the pediatric age group, and these were intrathoracic. There have been three cases of liposarcoma of the mediastinum in children. Although these tumors usually do not metastasize, their invasiveness and tendency to recur place them in the malignant group.

In general, lipomas of the subcutaneous tissue are benign, while those of the retroperitoneal area and deep somatic soft tissue are usually malignant. The tumors of the mediastinum seem to have an incidence and behavior similar to those of lipomas in the peritoneal region.

Radical surgical excision is the procedure of choice. Repeated surgical attacks may serve as a method of extended control, and x-ray therapy may be added for palliative use.

Thyroid and Parathyroid

Substernal thyroid is a common anterior superior mediastinal tumor in the adult age group, but apparently does not occur before puberty. Ectopic thyroid in the mediastinum does occur in children, and in such cases blood supply is derived from a mediastinal vessel.

Parathyroid adenoma with a typical syndrome of hyperparathyroidism does not occur before puberty.

PRIMARY CARDIAC AND PERICARDIAL TUMORS

Primary tumors of the heart in infants may cause cardiac enlargement or enlargement of the cardiac silhouette, giving rise to symptoms in the lungs or esophagus. Most frequently the signs and symptoms of congestive heart failure are much more prominent than those of the respiratory system or esophagus.

Rhabdomyoma appears to be the only cardiac tumor showing a definite predilection for the younger age groups. This is particularly true in children with tuberous sclerosis, in whom rhabdomyoma of the heart is prone to occur. Such tumors are not considered true neoplasms, but probably represent an area of developmental arrest in the fetal myocardium. It is not unusual for rhabdomyoma to regress spontaneously without causing any appreciable impairment of cardiac function.

Myxoma is by far the most frequent primary tumor of the heart; this accounts for slightly more than 50 per cent of all primary cardiac tumors. It may be encountered at almost any age. The signs and symptoms vary widely, but ultimately lead to cardiac failure which does not respond to the usual medical management. Most myxomas are located in the atria, more frequently on the left than on the right. They tend to proliferate and project into the chambers of the heart, preventing normal cardiac filling by obstruction to the mitral or tricuspid valve. The origin appears to be in the atrial septa.

Primary sarcoma of the heart is less common than myxoma, but may occur at any age. It does not, as a rule, proliferate into the lumens of the heart; it infiltrates the wall of the myocardium and frequently extends into the pericardial cavity.

Other primary tumors of the heart are angioma, fibroma, lipoma and hamartoma. All are rare and usually produce prominent circulatory symptoms.

Primary neoplasms of the pericardium are rare. Histologically, the predominant tumors are mesotheliomas (endothelioma) and sarcomas, but occasionally leiomyomas, hemangiomas and lipomas may occur.

A single instance of a large cavernous hemangioma of the pericardium has been described; this occurred in an eight-year-old girl and was successfully removed.

TUMORS OF THE DIAPHRAGM

Tumors involving the diaphragm may cause chest pain and discomfort or pulmonary compression; thus they may simulate mediastinal or primary pulmonary neoplasms. Primary tumors of the diaphragm are extremely rare in the pediatric age group.

Benign tumors of the diaphragm which have been reported, though not necessarily in children, are lipoma, fibroma, chondroma, angiofibroma, lymphangioma, neurofibroma, rhabdomyofibroma, fibromyoma and primary diaphragmatic cysts.

Malignant tumors of the diaphragm which have been reported are fibrosar-coma, rhabdomyosarcoma, myosarcoma, leiomyosarcoma and fibromyosarcoma. None of these tumors appears to have been reported in children.

PRIMARY TUMORS OF THE CHEST WALL

Lipoma of the chest wall is frequent in adults, but rare in the pediatric age group. As noted previously, these may be dumbbell in shape, presenting on the chest wall with a large component intra-thoracically. Chest x-ray will aid in its definition.

Extensive cavernous hemangiomas of the thoracic wall are seen in infancy or childhood. They may be isolated or associated with similar lesions in other tissues, including the lung. In these cases the diagnosis of Osler-Weber-Rendu syndrome is suggested. Intrathoracic extension of these lesions may occur.

In von Recklinghausen's disease multiple cutaneous and subcutaneous nodules are present. These patients should be carefully studied for the possible coexistence of mediastinal neurofibromas or intrathoracic meningocele.

Chondroma and chondrosarcoma are the principal bony tumors of the chest wall; 80 per cent of these occur in the ribs or sternum, usually in the anterior extremity of a rib near the costochondral junction. They may also occur in the sternum, scapula, clavicle or vertebral bodies. There may be few if any symptoms. X-ray examination reveals a discrete expansion of the bone with an intact, thinned-out cortex.

Chondrosarcoma of the rib occurs more frequently in males; it is usually seen in the posterior half and paravertebral portion of the rib, but sometimes involves the transverse process and the vertebral body either primarily or secondarily. Occasionally the direction of growth appears to be entirely internal, thus simulating the radiologic appearance of a primary pleural or mediastinal tumor. Usually, how-

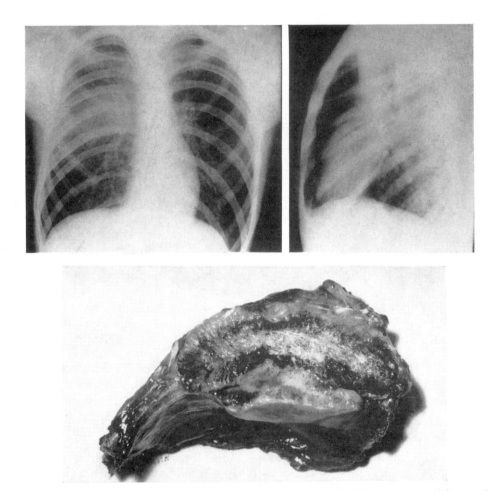

FIGURE 41–38.   Reticulum cell sarcoma in chest wall of 8-year-old white boy. Survival longer than 18 months.

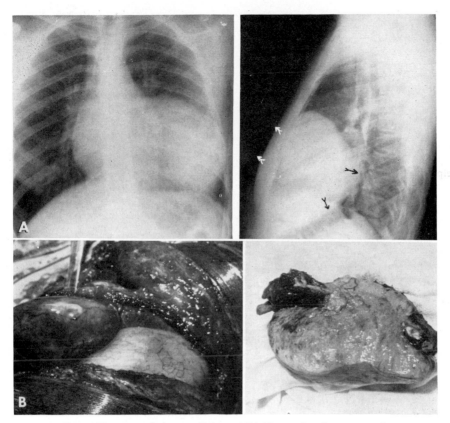

FIGURE 41-39. Desmoid tumor of chest wall in a child 18 months after patent ductus surgery. The desmoid was in the line of the posterior lateral incision.

ever, there is an externally visible and palpable tumefaction. This usually occurs during the middle decades of life.

Solitary plasmacytoma, a lesion histologically similar to multiple myeloma, but localized to a single bone, may involve any part of the thoracic cage; it may involve the vertebrae, rarely attacks the ribs, and may involve the lung itself. In solitary plasmacytoma the bone is thinned and can be greatly expanded.

Ewing's tumor is sometimes primary in a rib, and is unusual before the second decade of life.

REFERENCES

General

Ackerman, L. V., and del Regato, J. A.: *Cancer: Diagnosis, Treatment and Prognosis*. 2nd ed. St. Louis, C. V. Mosby Company, 1954.

Arey, L. B.: *Developmental Anatomy*. 7th ed. Philadelphia, W. B. Saunders Company, 1965.

Ariel, I. M., and Pack, G. T.: *Cancer and Allied Diseases of Infancy and Childhood*. Boston, Little, Brown and Co., 1960.

Banyai, A. L.: *Nontuberculous Diseases of the Chest*. Springfield, Ill., Charles C Thomas, 1954.

Benedict, E. B., and Nardi, G. L.: *The Esophagus: Medical and Surgical Management*. Boston, Little, Brown and Co., 1958.

Benson, C. D., Mustard, W. T., Ravitch, M. M., Snyder, W. H., Jr., and Welch, K. J.: *Pediatric Surgery*. Chicago, Year Book Publishers, Inc., 1962, Vol. I.

Blades, B.: *Surgical Diseases of the Chest*. St. Louis, C. V. Mosby Company, 1961.

Clinical Pathologic Conference, Children's Medical Center, Boston, Mass. *J. Pediat.*, 54:529, 1959.

Felson, B.: *Fundamentals of Chest Roentgenology*. Philadelphia, W. B. Saunders Company, 1960.

Flavell, G.: *The Oesophagus*. London, Butterworth, 1963.

Fried, B. M.: *Tumors of the Lungs and Mediastinum*. Philadelphia, Lea & Febiger, 1958.

Gibbon, J. H., Jr.: *Surgery of the Chest*. Philadelphia, W. B. Saunders Company, 1962.

Gilbert, J. G., Mazzarella, L. A., and Feit, L. J.: Primary Tracheal Tumors in the Infant and Adult. A.M.A. *Arch. Otolaryngology*, 58:1, 1953.

Gross, R. E.: *The Surgery of Infancy and Childhood*. Philadelphia, W. B. Saunders Company, 1953.

Hinshaw, H. C., and Garland, L. H.: *Diseases of the Chest*. 2nd ed. Philadelphia, W. B. Saunders Company, 1963.

Hollinger, P. H., Slaughter, D. P., and Novak, F. J., III: Unusual Tumors Obstructing the Lower Respiratory Tract of Infants and Children. *Tr. Am. Academy Ophthal. & Otol.*, 54th Session: 223, 1949.

Keith, A.: *Human Embryology and Morphology*. 6th ed. Baltimore, Williams & Wilkins Company, 1948.

Leigh, T. F., and Weens, H. S.: *The Mediastinum*. Springfield, Ill., Charles C Thomas, 1959.

Lindskog, G. E., Liebow, A. A., and Glenn, W. W. L.: *Thoracic and Cardiovascular Surgery with Related Pathology*. Des Moines, Iowa, Meredith Publishing Comapny, 1962.

Myers, J. A.: *Diseases of the Chest—Including the Heart*. Springfield, Ill., Charles C Thomas, 1959.

Naclerio, E. A.: *Bronchopulmonary Diseases, Basic Aspects, Diagnosis and Treatment*. New York, Paul B. Hoeber, Inc., 1957.

Pack, G. T., and Ariel, I. M.: *Treatment of Cancer and Allied Diseases*. 2nd ed. Vol. IV, Tumors of the Breast, Chest and Esophagus. New York, Paul B. Hoeber, Inc., 1960.

Perry, K. M. A., and Sellors, T. H.: *Chest Diseases*. London, Butterworth, 1963, Vol. 2.

Postlethwait, R. W., and Scaly, W. C.: *Surgery of the Esophagus*. Springfield, Ill., Charles C Thomas, 1961.

Potts, W. J.: *The Surgeon and the Child*. Philadelphia, W. B. Saunders Company, 1959.

Rubin, E. H.: *The Lung as a Mirror of Systemic Disease*. Springfield, Ill., Charles C Thomas, 1956.

Rubin, E. H., and Rubin, M.: *Thoracic Diseases, Emphasizing Cardiopulmonary Relationships*. Philadelphia, W. B. Saunders Company, 1961.

Schaffer, A. J.: *Diseases of the Newborn*. 2nd ed. Philadelphia, W. B. Saunders Company, 1965.

Shaw, R. R., and Paulson, D. L.: *The Treatment of Bronchial Neoplasms*. Springfield, Ill., Charles C Thomas, 1959.

Smithers, S. W., and Bignall, J. R.: *Neoplastic Diseases at Various Sites*. Vol. I, Carcinoma of the Lung. London, E. & S. Livingstone, Ltd., 1958.

Spain, D. M.: *Diagnosis and Treatment of Tumors of the Chest*. New York, Grune & Stratton, Inc., 1960.

Stout, A. P.: Tumors of the Peripheral Nervous System; in *Atlas of Tumor Pathology*. Washington, D.C., 1949.

Sweet, R. H.: *Thoracic Surgery*. 2nd ed. Philadelphia, W. B. Saunders Company, 1954.

Symposium on Certain Tumors of the Bronchi and on Tumors of the Trachea. *Proc. Staff Meet. Mayo Clin.*, 21:409, 1946.

Terracol, J., and Sweet, R. H.: *Diseases of the Esophagus*. Philadelphia, W. B. Saunders Company, 1958.

Unin, J.: *Neoplastic Diseases*. 4th ed. Philadelphia, W. B. Saunders Company, 1940.

Benign Pulmonary Tumors

Albrecht, E. E.: *Verhandl. d. deutsch. Path. Gesellsch.*, 7:153, 1904.

Archer, F. L., Harrison, R. W., and Moulder, P. V.: Granular Cell Myoblastoma of the Trachea and Carina Treated by Resection and Reconstruction. *J. Thor. Surg.*, 45:539, 1963.

Baker, D. C., and Pemington, C. L.: Congenital Hemangioma of the Larynx. *Tr. Am. Laryng., Rhinol., Otol. Soc.*, 60th Meeting: 84, 1956.

Barrett, N. R., and Barnard, W. G.: Some Usual Thoracic Tumors. *Brit. J. Surg.*, 32:447, 1945.

Blackman, J., Cantril, S. T., Lund, T. K., and Sparkman, D.: Tracheobronchial Papillomatosis, Treated by Roentgen Irradiation. *Radiology*, 73:598, 1959.

Campbell, J. S., Wiglesworth, F. W., Latarroca, R., and Wilde, H.: Congenital Subglottic Hemangiomas of the Larynx and Trachea in Infants. *Pediatrics*, 22:727, 1958.

Cavin, E., Masters, J. H., and Moody, J.: Hamartoma of the Lung. *J. Thor. Surg.*, 35: 816, 1958.

Doermann, P., Lunseth, J., and Segnitz, R. H.: Obstructing Subglottic Hemanigoma of the Larynx in Infancy, Review of the Literature and Report of a Deceptive Case. *New England J. Med.*, 258:68, 1958.

Ferguson, C. F., and Flake, C. G.: Subglottic Hemangioma as a Cause of Respiratory Obstruction in Infants. *Tr. Am. Bronchoesoph. A.*, 41:27, 1961.

Fishman, L.: Papilloma of the Trachea. *J. Thor. & Cardiov. Surg.*, 44:264, 1962.

Graham, G. G., and Singleton, J. W.: Diffuse Hamartoma of the Upper Lobe in an Infant: Report of a Successful Surgical Removal. A.M.A. *J. Dis. Child.*, 89:609, 1955.

Guida, P. N., Fultcher, T., and Moore, S. W.: Leiomyoma of the Lung, *J. Thor. Surg.*, 49: 1058, 1965.

Holder, T. M., and Christy, M. G.: Cystic Adenomatoid Malformation of the Lung. *J. Thor. Surg.*, 47:590, 1964.

Jackson, C. L., Konzelmann, F. W., and Norris,

C. M.: Bronchial Adenoma. *J. Thor. Surg.*, 14:98, 1945.

Jones, C. J.: Unusual Hamartoma of the Lung in the Newborn Infant. *Arch. Path.*, 48: 150, 1949.

Jones, H., MacKenzie, K. W., and Biddle, E.: Bronchial Adenoma, A Case Report. *Brit. J. Tubercul.*, 37:113, 1943.

Kramer, R., and Som, M. L.: Further Study of Adenoma of the Bronchus. *Ann. Otol., Rhin. & Laryng.*, 44:861, 1935.

Kumis, F. D., and Conn, J. H.: Endobronchial Hamartoma. *J. Thor. Surg.*, 50:138, 1965.

Littler, E. R.: Asphyxia Due to Hemangioma in the Trachea. *J. Thor. & Cardiov. Surg.*, 45: 552, 1963.

Lukens, R. M.: Papilloma of the Trachea. *Ann. Otol., Rhin. & Laryng.*, 45:872, 1936.

Ogilvie, O. E.: Multiple Papillomas of the Trachea with Malignant Degeneration. A.M.A. *Arch. Otolaryngology*, 58:10, 1953.

Peterson, H. O.: Benign Adenoma of the Bronchus. *Am. J. Roentgenol.*, 36:836, 1936.

Rosenblum, P., and Klein, R. I.: Adenomatous Polyp of the Right Main Bronchus Producing Atelectasis. *J. Pediat.*, 7:791, 1935.

Smoller, S., and Maynard, A. DeL.: Adenoma of the Bronchus in a Nine Year Old Child. *Am. J. Dis. Child.*, 82:587, 1951.

Som, M. L.: Adenoma of the Bronchus: Endoscopic Treatment in Selected Cases. *J. Thor. Surg.*, 18:462, 1949.

Souders, C. R., and Kingsley, J. W.: Bronchial Adenoma. *New England J. Med.*, 239:459, 1948.

Stein, A. S., and Volk, B. M.: Papillomatosis of the Trachea and Lung. A.M.A. *Arch. Path.*, 124:127, 1959.

Thomas, M. R.: Cystic Hamartoma of the Lung in a Newborn Infant. *J. Path. & Bact.*, 61:599, 1949.

Walcott, C. C.: Bronchial Adenoma. *Laryngoscope*, 72:1952.

Ward, D. E., Jr., Bradshaw, H. H., and Prince, T. C.: Bronchial Adenoma in Children. *J. Thor. Surg.*, 27:295, 1954.

Wilkins, E. W., Darling, R. C., Soutter, L., and Sniffen, R. C.: A Continuing Clinical Survey of Adenomas of the Trachea and Bronchus in a General Hospital. *J. Thor. & Cardiov. Surg.*, 46:279, 1963.

Womack, N., and Graham, E. A.: Mixed Tumors of the Lung. *Arch. Path.*, 26:165, 1938.

Primary and Metastatic Malignant Pulmonary Tumors

Bartley, J. D., and Arean, V. M.: Intrapulmonic Neurogenic Tumors. *J. Thor. Surg.*, 50:114, 1965.

Beardsley, J. M.: Primary Carcinoma of the Lung in a Child. *Canadian M.A.J.*, 29:257, 1933.

Berman, L.: Extragenital Chorionepithelioma

with Report of a Case. *Am. J. Cancer*, 38:23, 1940.

Bogardus, G. M., Knudston, K. P., and Mills, W. H.: Pleural Mesothelioma. *Am. Rev. Tuberc.*, 71:280, 1955.

Breton, A., Gaudier, R., and Ponte, C.: Tumeurs bronchiques chez l'enfant. *Pediatrie* (Lyon), 13:43, 1958.

Breton, A., Gaudier, B., Delacroiz, R., Dupont, A., and Poingt, O.: Neurinomes intrapulmonaires primitives. *Arch. Franç. Pediat.*, 18:26, 1961.

Cayley, C. K., Mersheimer, W., and Caez, H. J.: Primary Bronchogenic Carcinoma of the Lung in Children. A.M.A. *J. Dis. Child.*, 82:49, 1951.

Curry, J. J., and Fuchs, J.: Expectoration of a Fibrosarcoma. *J. Thor. Surg.*, 19:135, 1950.

Doesel, H.: Intrabronchioles psammöses Neurofibroma. *Thoraxchirurgie*, 8:657, 1961.

Donahue, F. E., Anderson, H. A., and McDonald, J. B.: Unusual Bronchial Tumor. *Ann. Otol., Rhinol. & Laryngol.*, 65:820, 1956.

Drews, G. A., and Willman, K. H.: Das primare Lungensarkon. *Langenbecks Arch. klin. Chir.*, 274:95, 1953.

Dyson, B. C., and Trentalance, A. E.: Resection of Primary Pulmonary Sarcoma. *J. Thor. Surg.*, 17:577, 1961.

Feldman, P. A.: Sarcoma of the Lungs, A Report of Three Cases. *Brit. J. Tuberculosis & Chest Dis.*, 51:331, 1957.

Gerber, I. E.: Ectopic Chorioepithelioma. *J. Mt. Sinai Hosp.*, 2:135, 1935.

Gray, F. W., and Tom, B. C. K.: Diffuse Pleural Mesothelioma: A Survival of One Year Following Nitrogen Mustard Therapy. *J. Thor. & Cardiov. Surg.*, 44:73, 1962.

Harris, W. H., and Schattenberg, H. H.: Anlagen and Rest Tumors of the Lung. *Am. J. Path.*, 18:955, 1942.

Herring, N., Templeton, J. Y., III, Haup, G. J., and Theodos, P. A.: Primary Sarcoma of the Lung. *Dis. of Chest*, 42:315, 1962.

Hill, L. D., and White, M. L., Jr.: Plasmacytoma of the Lung. *J. Thor. Surg.*, 25:187, 1953.

Hirsch, E. F.: Extragenital Choriocarcinoma, with Comments on the Male Origin of Trophoblastic Tissues. *Arch. Path.*, 48:516, 1949.

Hochberg, L. A.: Endothelioma of the Pleura. *Am. Rev. Tuberc.*, 63:150, 1951.

Hollinger, P. H., Johnston, K. C., Gosswiller, N., and Hirsch, E. C.: Primary Fibrosarcoma of the Bronchus. *Dis. of Chest*, 37:137, 1960.

Kay, S., and Reed, W. G.: Chorioepithelioma of the Lung in a Female Infant Seven Months Old. *Am. J. Path.*, 29:555, 1953.

Killingsworth, W. P., McReynolds, G. S., and Harrison, A. W.: Pulmonary Leiomyosarcomas in a Child. *J. Pediat.*, 42:466, 1963.

Lewis, J.: Sarcoma of the Bronchus. *Proc. Roy. Soc. Med.*, 40:119, 1947.

Mallory, T. B.: Cabot Case, N. R. 20202. *New England J. Med.*, 218:843, 1938.

Idem: Case Record 24202, Mass. Gen. Hosp. *New England J. Med.*, 218:845, 1938.

Merrit, J. W., and Parker, K. R.: Intrathoracic Leiomyosarcoma. *Canad. M.A.J.*, 77:1031, 1957.

Noehren, T. H., and McKee, F. W.: Sarcoma of the Lung. *Dis. of Chest*, 25:633, 1954.

Ochsner, S., and Ochsner, A.: Primary Sarcoma of the Lung. *Ochsner Clinic Reports*, 3:105, 1957.

Randell, W. S., and Blades, B.: Primary Bronchogenic Leiomysarcoma. *Arch. Path.*, 42:543, 1946.

Sekulich, M., Pandola, G., and Simon, T.: A Solitary Pulmonary Mass in Multiple Myeloma: Report of a Case. *Dis. of Chest*, 48:100, 1965.

Shaw, R. R., Paulson, D. L., Kee, J. L., and Lovett, V. F.: Primary Pulmonary Leiomyosarcomas. *J. Thor. & Cardiov. Surg.*, 41:430, 1961.

Sherman, R. S., and Malone, B. H.: A Study of Muscle Tumors Primary in the Lung. *Radiology*, 54:507, 1950.

Stout, A. P., and Himidi, G. M.: Solitary (Localized) Mesothelioma of the Pleura. *Ann. Surg.*, 133:50, 1951.

Wasch, M. G., Lederer, M., and Epstein, B. S.: Bronchogenic Carcinoma of Seven Years' Duration in an 11-Year-Old Boy. *J. Pediat.*, 17:521, 1940.

Watson, W. L., and Anlyan, A. J.: Primary Leiomyosarcoma of the Lung. *Cancer*, 7:250, 1954.

Mediastinal Tumors

Abell, M. R.: Mediastinal Cysts. A.M.A. *Arch. Path.*, 61:360, 1956.

Ackerman, L. R., and Taylor, F. H.: Neurogenic Tumors Within the Thorax. *Cancer*, 4:669, 1951.

Adams, F. H.: Unusual Case for Bronchogenic Lung Cyst Simulating Dextrocardia. *J. Pediat.*, 39:483, 1951.

Adams, W. E., and Thornton, T. F., Jr.: Bronchogenic Cysts of the Mediastinum: With Report of Three Cases. *J. Thor. Surg.*, 12:503, 1943.

Adler, R. H., Taheri, S. A., and Waintraub, D. G.: Mediastinal Teratoma in Infancy. *J. Thor. Surg.*, 39:394, 1960.

Andrus, W. D. W., and Foote, N. C.: Report of a Large Thymic Tumor Successfully Removed by Operation. *J. Thor. Surg.*, 6:648, 1937.

Archer, O., Pierce, J. C., and Good, R. A.: Role of the Thymus in the Development of the Immune Response. *Fed. Proc.*, 20:26, 1961.

Arnason, B. G., Jankovic, B. D., and Wadsman, B. H.: A Survey of the Thymus and Its Relation to Lymphocytes and Immune Reactions. *Blood*, 20:617, 1962.

Arnheim, E. E.: Cervicomediastinal Lymphangioma (Cystic Hygroma). *J. Mt. Sinai Hosp.*, 10:404, 1943.

Arnheim, E. E., and Gemson, B. L.: Persistent Cervical Thymus Gland: Thymectomy. *Surg.*, 27:603, 1950.

Bednav, B.: Malignant Intrapericardial Tumor of Heart. (Translation.) *Casopis Lekaro*, 48:1355, 1950.

Bernard, E. D., and James, L. S.: The Newborn Cardiac Silhouette in Newborn Infants: A Cinematographic Study of the Normal Range. *Pediatrics*, 27:713, 1961.

Bernatz, P. E., Harrison, E. G., and Clagett, O. T.: Thymoma: A Clinicopathologic Study. *J. Thor. & Cardiov. Surg.*, 42:424, 1961.

Bill, A. H., Jr., Sentrill, S. T., and Creighton, S. A.: The Spectrum of Malignancy in Childhood Compared with That Seen in Adults. Personal communication.

Bill, A. H., Jr., and others: Common Malignant Tumors of Infancy and Childhood. *Pediat. Clin. N. Amer.*, 6:1197, 1959.

Bjorn, T., and Hayes, L. L.: Duplication of the Stomach. *Surg.*, 44:585, 1958.

Blades, B.: Mediastinal Tumors: Report of Cases Treated at Army Thoracic Surgery Centers in the U.S. *Ann. Surg.*, 123:749, 1946.

Bremmer, J. L.: Diverticuli and Duplications of the Intestinal Tract. *Arch. Path.*, 38:132, 1944.

Brescis, M. A.: Chylothorax, Report of a Case in an Infant. *Arch. Ped.*, 58:345, 1941.

Brewer, L. A., III, and Dolley, F. S.: Tumors of the Mediastinum: A Discussion of Diagnostic Procedure and Surgical Treatment Based on Experience with 44 Operated Cases. *Am. Rev. Tubercul.*, 60:419, 1949.

Burnett, W. E., Rosemond, G. P., and Bucher, R. M.: The Diagnosis of Mediastinal Tumors. *Surg. Clin. N. Amer.*, 32:1673, 1952.

Caffey, J., and Silbey, R.: Regrowth and Overgrowth of the Thymus After Atrophy Induced by Oral Administration of Adrenocorticosteroids to Human Infants. *Pediatrics*, 26:762, 1960.

Cicciarelli, E. H., Soule, E. H., and McGoon, D. C.: Lipoma and Liposarcoma of the Mediastinum, a Report of Fourteen Tumors Including One Lipoma of the Thymus. *J. Thor. Surg.*, 47:411, 1964.

Claireaux, A. E., An Intrapericardial Teratoma in a Newborn Infant. *J. Path. & Bact.*, 63:743, 1951.

Clark, D. E.: Association of Irradiation with Cancer of the Thyroid in Children in Adolescence. *J.A.M.A.*, 157:107, 1955.

Conklin, W. S.: Tumors and Cysts of the Mediastinum. *Dis. of Chest*, 17:715, 1950.

Conti, E. A., Patton, G. D., Conti, J. E., and Hempelmann, L. H.: The Present Health of Children Given X-Ray Treatment to the

Anterior Mediastinum in Infancy. *Radiol.*, 74:386, 1960.

Cruickshank, D. B.: Primary Intrathoracic Neurogenic Tumors. *J. Fac. Radiol.*, 8:369, 1957.

Curreri, A. R., and Gale, J. W.: Mediastinal Tumors. *Arch. Surg.*, 58:797, 1949.

Dameshek, W.: The Thymus and Lymphoid Proliferation. (Editorial.) *Blood*, 20:629, 1962.

Davidson, L. R., and Brown, L.: Gastrogenous Mediastinal Cyst. *J. Thor. Surg.*, 16:458, 1947.

Dobbs, C. H., Berg, R., Jr., and Pierce, E. C., II: Intrapericardial Bronchogenic Cysts. *J. Thor. Surg.*, 34:718, 1957.

Dowd, C. N.: Hygroma Cysticum Colli, Its Structure and Etiology. *Ann. Surg.*, 58:112, 1913.

Drash, E. C., and Hyer, H. J.: Mesothelial Mediastinal Cysts: Pericardial Celomic Cysts of Lambert. *J. Thor. Surg.*, 19:755, 1950.

Duffy, B. J., Jr., and Fitzgerald, P. J.: Thyroid Cancer in Childhood and Adolescence: Report of 28 Cases. *Cancer*, 3:1018, 1950.

Duprez, A., Corlier, R., and Schmidt, P.: Tuberculoma of the Thymus. *J. Thor. & Cardiov. Surg.*, 44:115, 1962.

Edge, J. R., and Glennie, J. S.: Teratoid Tumors of the Mediastinum Found Despite Previous Normal Chest Radiography. *J. Thor. & Cardiov. Surg.*, 40:172, 1960.

Ellis, F. H., Jr., and DuShane, J. W.: Primary Mediastinal Cysts and Neoplasms in Infants and Children. *Am. Rev. Tubercul. & Pulmonary Dis.*, 74:940, 1956.

Ellis, F. H., Jr., Kirklin, J. W., and Woolner, L. B.: Hemangioma of the Mediastinum: Review of Literature and Report of Case. *J. Thor. Surg.*, 30:181, 1955.

Ellis, F. H., Jr., Kirklin, J. W., Hodgson, J. R., Woolner, L. B., and DuShane, J. W.: Surgical Implications of the Mediastinal Shadow in Thoracic Roentgenograms of Infants and Children. *Surg., Gynec. & Obst.*, 100:532, 1955.

Emerson, G. L.: Supradiaphragmatic Thoracic Duct Cysts. *New England J. Med.*, 242:575, 1950.

Evans, A.: Developmental Enterogenous Cysts and Diverticula. *Brit. J. Surg.*, 17:34, 1929.

Fallon, M., Gordon, A. R. G., and Lendrum, A. C.: Mediastinal Cysts of Fore-Gut Origin Associated with Vertebral Abnormalities. *Brit. J. Surg.*, 41:520, 1954.

Ferguson, J. O., Clagett, O. T., and McDonald, J. R.: Hemangiopericytoma (Glomus Tumor) of the Mediastinum: Review of the Literature and Report of Case. *Surg.*, 36:320, 1954.

Forsee, J. H., and Blake, H. A.: Pericardial Celomic Cyst. *Surg.*, 31:753, 1952.

Fridjohn, M. H.: Cyst of the Thymus in a Newborn Baby. *Brit. M.J.*, 2:553, 1943.

Garland, H. L.: Cancer of the Thyroid and Previous Radiation. *Surg., Gynec. & Obst.*, 112:564, 1961.

Gebauer, P. W.: Case of Intrapericardial Teratoma. *J. Thor. Surg.*, 12:458, 1953.

Gledhill, E. Y., and Marrow, A. G.: Ciliated Epithelial Cyst of the Esophagus: Report of Case. *J. Thor. Surg.*, 20:923, 1950.

Godwin, J. T., Watson, W. L., Pool, J. L., Cahan, W. G., and Nardiello, V. A.: Primary Intrathoracic Neurogenic Tumors. *J. Thor. Surg.*, 20:169, 1950.

Gondos, B., and Reingold, I. M.: Mediastinal Ganglioneuroblastoma. *J. Thor. Surg.*, 47:430, 1964.

Greenfield, E., Steinberg, I., and Touroff, A. S. W.: "Spring Water" Cyst of the Mediastinum: Case Report. *J. Thor. Surg.*, 12:495, 1943.

Griffiths, S. P., Levine, O. R., Baker, D. H., and Blumenthal, S.: Evaluation of an Enlarged Cardiothymic Image in Infancy: Thymolytic Effect of Steroid Administration. *Am. J. Cardiol.*, 8:311, 1961.

Gross, R. E.: Thoracic Surgery for Infants. *J. Thor. Surg.*, 48:152, 1964.

Gross, R. E., Holcomb, G. W., and Farber, S.: Duplications of the Alimentary Tract. *Pediatrics*, 9:449, 1952.

Gross, R. E., and Hurwitt, E. S.: Cervical Mediastinal Cystic Hygromas. *Surg., Gynec. & Obst.*, 87:599, 1948.

Grutezner, P.: *Ein Fall von mediastinal Tumor durch ein lymphosarcom Bedingt.* Berlin, G. Lang, 1869.

Guinn, H.: Mediastinal Teratoma. *Radiology*, 8:438, 1927.

Hardy, L. M.: Bronchogenic Cysts of the Mediastinum. *Pediatrics*, 4:108, 1949.

Hedblom, C. A.: Intrathoracic Dermoid Cysts and Teratomata, with Report of Six Personal Cases and 185 Cases Collected from the Literature. *J. Thor. Surg.*, 3:22, 1933.

Herlitzka, H. A., and Gayle, J. W.: Tumor and Cysts of the Mediastinum. *A.M.A. Arch. Surg.*, 76:697, 1958.

Heuer, G. J.: The Thoracic Lipomas. *Ann. Surg.*, 98:801, 1933.

Heuer, J., and Andrus, W.: The Surgery of Mediastinal Tumors. *Am. J. Surg.*, 50:146, 1940.

Hollingsworth, R. K.: Intrathoracic Tumors of the Sympathetic Nervous System. *Surg., Gynec. & Obst.*, 82:682, 1946.

Hopkins, S. M., and Freitas, E. L.: Bilateral Osteochondroma of the Ribs in an Infant, an Unusual Cause of Cyanosis. *J. Thor. Surg.*, 49:247, 1965.

Jackson, C.: Thymic Tracheostenosis, Tracheoscopy, Thymectomy, Cure. *J.A.M.A.*, 48:1753, 1907.

Jellen, J., and Fisher, W. B.: Intrapericardial Teratoma. *Am. J. Dis. Child.*, 51:1397, 1936.

Joel, J.: Ein Teratom auf der artena pulmonalio Innerhalb des Herzbeutals. *Arch. Path. Anat.*, 122:381, 1890.

Jones, J. C.: Esophageal Duplications or Mediastinal Cysts of Enteric Origin. *West. J. Surg.,* 55:610, 1947.

Kauffman, S. L., and Stout, A. P.: Lipoblastic Tumors of Children. *Cancer,* 12:912, 1959.

Kennedy, R. L. J., and New, G. B.: Chronic Stridor in Children Sometimes Erroneously Attributed to Enlargement of the Thymus Gland. *J.A.M.A.,* 96:1286, 1931.

Kent, E. M., Blades, B., Valle, A. R., and Graham, E. A.: Intrathoracic Neurogenic Tumors. *J. Thor. Surg.,* 13:116, 1944.

Kessel, A. W. L.: Intrathoracic Meningocele, Spinal Deformity and Multiple Neurofibromatosis. *J. Bone & Joint Surg.,* 33B:87, 1951.

Key, J. A.: Mediastinal Tumors. *Surg. Clin. N. Amer.,* 34:959, 1954.

Koop, C. P., Kiesewetter, W. B., and Horn, R. C.: Neuroblastoma in Childhood: An Evaluation of Surgical Management. *Pediatrics,* 16:652, 1955.

Kuipers, F., and Wieberdink, J.: An Intrathoracic Cyst of Enterogenic Origin in a Young Infant. *J. Pediat.,* 42:603, 1953.

Ladd, W. E., and Scott, H. W., Jr.: Esophageal Duplications or Mediastinal Cysts of Enteric Origin. *Surg.,* 6:815, 1944.

Laipply, T. C.: Cysts and Cystic Tumors of the Mediastinum. *Arch. Path.,* 39:153, 1945.

Lambert, A. V.: Etiology of Thin-Walled Thoracic Cysts. *J. Thor. Surg.,* 10:1, 1940.

Lillie, W. E., McDonald, J. R., and Clagett, O. T.: Pericardial Celomic Cysts and Pericardial Diverticula: Concept of Etiology and Report of Cases. *J. Thor. Surg.,* 20:494, 1950.

Longino, L. A., and Meeker, E., Jr.: Primary Cardiac Tumors in Infancy. *J. Pediat.,* 43:724, 1953.

McLetchie, N. G. B., Purves, J. K., and Saunders, R. L.: Genesis of Gastric and Certain Intestinal Diverticula. *Surg., Gynec. & Obst.,* 99:135, 1954.

Maksim, G., Henthorne, J. C., and Allebach, H. K.: Neurofibromatosis with Malignant Thoracic Tumor and Metastasis in a Child. *Am. J. Dis. Child.,* 57:381, 1939.

Maier, H. C.: Bronchogenic Cysts of the Mediastinum. *Ann. Surg.,* 127:476, 1948.

Mason, C. B.: Intrathoracic Lymph Nodes. *J. Thor. Surg.,* 37:251, 1959.

Mayo, P.: Intrathoracic Neuroblastoma in a Newborn Infant. *J. Thor. Surg.,* 45:720, 1963.

Meltzer, J.: Tumorformige Nebenlunge in Herzbeutal. *Virchows Arch. f. path. anat.,* 308:199, 1941.

Miscall, L.: Cited by H. P. Goldberg and I. Steinberg: Primary Tumors of the Heart. *Circulation,* 11:936, 1955.

Mixter, C. G., and Clifford, S. H.: Congenital Mediastinal Cysts of Gastrogenic and Bronchogenic Origin. *Ann. Surg.,* 90:714, 1929.

Myers, R. T., and Bradshaw, H. H.: Benign Intramural Tumors and Cysts of the Esophagus. *J. Thor. Surg.,* 21:470, 1951.

Nanson, E. M.: Thoracic Meningocele Associ-

ated with Neurofibromatosis. *J. Thor. Surg.,* 33:650, 1957.

Neal, A. E., and Menten, M. L.: Tumors of the Thymus in Children. *Am. J. Dis. Child.,* 76:102, 1948.

Nicholls, M. F.: Intrathoracic Cyst of Intestinal Structure. *Brit. J. Surg.,* 28:137, 1940.

Olken, H. G.: Congenital Gastroenteric Cysts of the Mediastinum, Review and Report of a Case. *Am. J. Path.,* 20:997, 1944.

Patcher, M. R.: Mediastinal Non-chromaffin Para Ganglioma. *J. Thor. Surg.,* 45:152, 1963.

Perry, T. M., and Smith, W. A.: Rhabdomyosarcoma of the Diaphragm, A Case Report. *Am. J. Cancer,* 35:416, 1939.

Pickardt, O. C.: Pleuro-diaphragmatic Cyst. *Ann. Surg.,* 99:814, 1934.

Pohl, R.: Meningokele im Brustraum unter dem Bilde eines intrathorakalen Rundschattens. *Röntgenpraxis,* 5:747, 1933.

Raeburn, C.: Columnar Ciliated Epithelium in the Adult Oesophagus. *J. Path. & Bact.,* 63:157, 1951.

Ranström, S.: Congenital Cysts of the Esophagus. *Acta oto-laryng.,* 33:486, 1945.

Reiquam, C. W., Beatty, E. C., and Allen, R. P.: Neuroblastoma in Infancy and Childhood. *Am. J. Dis. Child.,* 91:588, 1956.

Reuben, S., and Stratemeier, E. H.: Intrathoracic Meningocele, A Case Report. *Radiology,* 58:552, 1952.

Richards, G. E., Jr., and Reaves, R. E.: Mediastinal Tumors and Cysts in Children. *J. Dis. Child.,* 95:284, 1958.

Sabiston, D. C., and Scott, H. W.: Primary Neoplasms and Cysts of the Mediastinum. *Ann. Surg.,* 135:777, 1952.

Saini, V. K., and Wahi, P. L.: Hour Glass Transmural Type of Intrathoracic Lipoma. *J. Thor. Surg.,* 47:600, 1964.

Schwarz, H., II, and Williams, C. S.: Thoracic Gastric Cysts, Report of Two Cases with Review of the Literature. *J. Thor. Surg.,* 12:117, 1942.

Schweisguth, O., Mathey, J., Renault, P., and Binet, J. P.: Intrathoracic Neurogenic Tumors in Infants and Children: A Study of Forty Cases. *Ann. Surg.,* 150:29, 1959.

Scott, O. B., and Morton, D. R.: Primary Cystic Tumor of the Diaphragm. *Arch. Path.,* 41:645, 1946.

Sealy, W. C., Weaver, W. L., and Young, W. G., Jr.: Severe Airway Obstruction in Infancy Due to the Thymus Gland. *Ann. Thor. Surg.,* 1:389, 1965.

Seybold, W. D., McDonald, J. R., Clagget, O. T., and Harrington, S. W.: Mediastinal Tumors of Blood Vascular Origin. *J. Thor. Surg.,* 18:503, 1949.

Seydel, G. N., Valle, E. R., and White, M. L., Jr.: Thoracic Gastric Cysts. *Ann. Surg.,* 123:377, 1946.

Skinner, G. E., and Hobbs, M. E.: Intrathoracic

Cystic Lymphangioma, Report of Two Cases in Infants. *J. Thor. Surg.*, 6:98, 1936.

Singleton, A. O.: Congenital Lymphatic Disease —Lymphangiomata. *Ann. Surg.*, 105:952, 1937.

Smid, A. D., Ellis, F. H., Logan, G. B., and Olson, A. M.: Partial Respiratory Obstruction in an Infant Due to a Bronchogenic Cyst, Report of a Case. *Proc. Staff Meet., Mayo Clin.*, 30:282, 1955.

Smith, R. E.: Case of Mediastinal Dermoid Cyst in an Infant. *Guy's Hosp. Rep.*, 80:466, 1930.

Sochberg, L. A., and Robinson, A. L.: Primary Tumor of the Pericardium Involving the Myocardium, Surgical Removal. *J. Circulation*, 1:805, 1950.

Soloman, R. D.: Malignant Teratoma of the Heart: Report of a Case with Necropsy. *A.M.A. Arch. Path.*, 52:561, 1951.

Soto, M. V.: Un Caso de Lipoma de la Cara Toracica del Diafragma. *J. Internat. Coll. Surgeons*, 6:146, 1943.

Starer, F.: Successful Removal of an Anterior Mediastinal Teratoma from an Infant. *Arch. Dis. Childhood*, 27:371, 1952.

Steele, J. D., and Schmitz, J.: Mediastinal Cyst of Gastric Origin. *J. Thor. Surg.*, 14:403, 1945.

Stich, M. H., Rubinstein, J., Freidman, A. B., and Morrison, M.: Mediastinal Lymphosarcoma in an Infant. *J. Pediat.*, 42:235, 1953.

Stout, A. P.: Ganglioneuroma of the Sympathetic Nervous System. *Surg., Gynec. & Obst.*, 84: 101, 1947.

Stowens, D.: Neuroblastomas and Related Tumors. *A.M.A. Arch. Path.*, 63:451, 1957.

Svien, H. J., Seybold, W. D., and Thelen, E. P.: Intraspinal and Intrathoracic Tumor with Paraplegia in a Child: Report of Case. *Proc. Staff Meet., Mayo Clin.*, 25:715, 1950.

Swift, E. A., and Neuhof, H.: Cervicomediastinal Lymph Angioma with Chylothorax. *J. Thor. Surg.*, 15:173, 1946.

Touroff, A. S. W., and Sealey, H. P.: Chronic Chylothorax Associated with Hygroma of the Mediastinum. *J. Thor. Surg.*, 26:318, 1953.

Veneziale, C. M., Sheridan, L. A., Payne, W. S., and Harrison, E. G., Jr.: Angiofollicular Lymph Node Hyperplasia of the Mediastinum. *J. Thor. Surg.*, 47:111, 1964.

Ware, G. W.: Thoracic Neuroblastoma. *J. Pediat.*, 49:765, 1956.

Welch, C. S., Ettinger, A., and Hecht, P. L.: Recklinghausen's Neurofibromatosis Associated with Intrathoracic Meningocele: Report of Case. *New England J. Med.*, 238:622, 1948.

Weimann, R. B., Hallman, G. L., Bahar, D., and Greenberg, S. D.: Intrathoracic Meningocele. *J. Thor. Surg.*, 46:40, 1963.

Weinstein, E. C., Payne, W. S., and Soule, E. H.: Surgical Treatment of Desmoid Tumor of the Chest Wall. *J. Thor. Surg.*, 46:242, 1963.

Williams, K. R., and Burgord, T. H.: Surgical Treatment of Granulomatous Paratracheal Lymphadenopathy. *J. Thor. Surg.*, 48:13, 1964.

Williams, M. H., and Johnson, J. F.: Mediastinal Gastric Cysts, Successful Excision in an Eight Week Old Infant. *A.M.A. Arch. Surg.*, 64: 138, 1952.

Willis, R. A.: In Intrapericardial Teratoma in an Infant. *J. Path. & Bact.*, 58:284, 1946.

Wilson, J. R., and Bartley, T. D.: Liposarcoma of the Mediastinum. *J. Thor. Surg.*, 48:486, 1964.

Wilson, J. R., Wheat, M. W., Jr., and Arean, V. M.: Pericardial Teratoma. *J. Thor. Surg.*, 45:670, 1963.

Wyllie, W. G.: Myasthenia Gravis. *Proc. Roy. Soc. Med.*, 39:591, 1946.

Ya Deau, R. E., Clagett, O. T., and Divertie, M. B.: Intrathoracic Meningocele. *J. Thor. Surg.*, 49:202, 1965.

Yater, W. M.: Cyst of the Pericardium. *Am. Heart J.*, 6:710, 1931.

CHAPTER FORTY-TWO

Asthma

SUSAN C. DEES, M.D.

Bronchial asthma is a common, capricious disorder of respiration affecting persons of all ages with repeated attacks of difficulty in breathing; this may develop into continuous respiratory embarrassment. Its characteristic features are wheezing, labored breathing, an irritative tight cough and tenacious sputum.

The symptoms range from the mildest cough and wheeze to the most severe respiratory distress which may result in prostration and fatal asphyxia. A combination of edema of the bronchial mucosa and bronchospasm decreases the caliber of bronchioles and bronchi and produces bilateral obstructive emphysema.

The usual cause for this sequence of events is an allergic reaction in the bronchi. In some instances no allergic or immunologic process can be recognized, however, and the assumption is then made that some degree of bronchial obstruction is produced by factors other than those resulting from antigen-antibody union. This has led to the classification of asthma into *allergic* and *nonallergic* types. Although most asthma in children is of the allergic type, there may occasionally be nonallergic causes for wheezing, such as compression or compromise of the bronchi by external pressure, by foreign body in the airway, or by a diffuse endobronchial inflammatory reaction, as in bronchiolitis. Rackeman suggested separating asthma into *extrinsic asthma,* caused by allergens or external factors, and *intrinsic asthma,* caused by nonallergic factors. Intrinsic asthma has been used to designate asthma due to bacterial infection, which in the strict sense is not of intrinsic origin. This term has also been applied to asthma attacks provoked by emotional stimuli, and to a different type of asthma, usually seen in elderly patients, which is associated with pulmonary fibrosis. Asthma is further described as *spasmodic,* if isolated attacks occur with long symptom-free intervals; *continuous,* when some daily wheezing is present; *intractable,* when symptoms are constant and unrelieved by bronchodilators; and as *status asthmaticus,* when little or no response is obtained to bronchodilators such as epinephrine, and the patient's respiratory metabolism is greatly unbalanced. Kraepelien et al. developed a helpful classification for asthma according to severity: grade I, consisting of less than five attacks per year, grade II of five to ten attacks per year, and grade III of ten or more attacks per year or the presence of continuous symptoms.

Incidence

Asthma is accepted as such a common condition in both children and adults, by the public as well as by the medical profession, that familiarity has blinded everyone to its true significance as a health hazard. Furthermore, since asthma ranges widely in its severity, frequency and duration, mild forms are frequently confused with the so-called common respiratory infections which everyone is resigned to endure periodically. On the other hand, severe forms of asthma often masquerade as other incapacitating and recurring pulmonary conditions, such as pneumonitis. Thus its ability to produce serious damage is not adequately appreciated, and recognition of its potential gravity is further suppressed by the comforting but misleading belief that children "outgrow" asthma.

It comes as a surprise to many people to learn that in the most recent United States National Health Survey by the United States Public Health Service (1959-1961) asthma, hay fever and other allergies accounted for one third of all chronic conditions occurring annually in children under seventeen years of age (Fig. 1). In a summary based on this survey, "Illness Among Children" (Schiffer and Hunt) prepared by the Children's Bureau, Department of Health, Education, and Welfare, it was reported that the rate of prevalence of asthma, hay fever and other allergies was 74.3 per 1000 children, being divided equally among asthma (25.8), hay fever without asthma (24.5), and other allergies (24.0). The rate for chronic sinusitis, bronchitis and other respiratory diseases for this age group was 34.2 per 1000 children. These two groups of conditions, the allergic and the sinobronchial, accounted for almost half of all the chronic conditions reported for children. The survey further found that nearly one child in five, practically 14 million children, had some kind of chronic condition. This means that at least 4.6 million children have chronic allergic problems, and more than 1.5 million have asthma. The distribution of chronic conditions by age is shown in Figure 2, in which it will be seen that even at fifteen to sixteen years of age, allergies account for one quarter of the chronic medical problems of childhood. This information is summarized for asthma and other chronic illnesses in Table 1, which shows the average annual number of conditions, the percentage distribution, and the rate per 1000 children based on data from the 1959-61 United States National Health Survey.

For purposes of the United States Public Health Survey, asthma, hay fever and rheumatic fever were classified as chronic conditions even though their onset occurred within a three-month period, which was the upper limit of onset period for acute conditions. Because of this definition and the selection of three months as a dividing point for the duration of illness between acute and chronic conditions, it is possible that some incapaci-

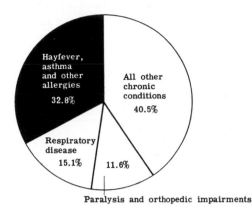

FIGURE 42–1. Incidence of asthma among chronic diseases of children under 17 years of age. Based on United States National Health Survey data as reported in interviews during period July 1959-June 1961. (From C. G. Schiffer and E. P. Hunt: Illness Among Children. Children's Bureau Publ. No. 405, Washington, D.C., United States Department of Health, Education, and Welfare, 1963, p. 14.)

tating, recurrent, yet purely seasonal cases of asthma and hay fever lasting only three months were excluded from the tabula-

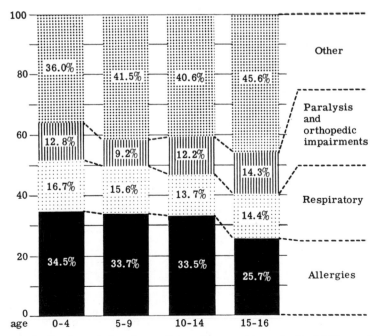

FIGURE 42–2. Distribution of chronic conditions by age. (From C. G. Schiffer and E. P. Hunt: Illness Among Children. Children's Bureau Publ. No. 405, Washington, D.C., United States Department of Health, Education, and Welfare, 1963.)

Table 1. *Chronic Conditions in Children Under 17 Years of Age*

Condition	No. in 1000's	% Distribution	Rate/1000 Children
All chronic conditions	13,996	100	226.1
Infective parasitic*	154	1.1	2.5
Hay fever	1,518	10.8	24.5
Asthma	1,595	11.4	25.8
Other allergies	1,485	10.6	24.0
Total allergy	4,598		73.3

Condensed from Table 13, Illness Among Children. Children's Bureau Publication No. 405, United States Department of Health, Education, and Welfare, Washington, D.C., 1963, p. 72.
* Excludes tuberculosis.

tion of either chronic or acute illness. This would make the reported incidence of allergy lower than the actual incidence. That these and other factors are recognized as minimizing is evident in the statement, "It is believed that the National Health Survey data is on the side of under-reporting," from The Children's Bureau Publication No. 405 (1963) "Illness Among Children," from which these statistics have been quoted.

Other surveys with slightly different design, but still based on household interview technique, made in Connecticut and metropolitan New York, found that one in five children of school age suffered from allergy (Rapaport, Appel and Szanton). A study of allergic diseases in adolescents, done in Denver, Colorado, showed asthma to be present in twenty-eight per 1000, the same prevalence given in the National Health Survey (Freeman et al.).

The incidence of asthma found in various pediatric practices, with the diagnosis made by examination, was 6.6 to 9 per cent or higher (London; Dees, 1957). Asthma ranked fifth as a cause for medical appointments in children under fourteen years in a survey made in Washington (Standish). These statistics could be amplified by many similar ones from other parts of the world, the more recent ones showing a trend toward higher rates for asthma and all allergy.

Morbidity

Translating these statistics into terms of the amount of handicapping illness

produced in these millions of children by asthma gives them an even more impressive and unexpected significance. The United States National Health Survey of 1959-61 reports that "the single chronic condition causing the highest percentage of days lost from school was asthma; 22.9 per cent of all days lost from school because of chronic conditions was due to asthma." Allergic diseases which were the chief cause of restricted activity, along with respiratory disease, caused 55.2 per cent of days lost from school (Fig. 3). The survey found that nearly 33 million school days were lost because of chronic conditions or three days for each child with at least one chronic condition. When one analyzes these days of illness by condition, the large part asthma contributed

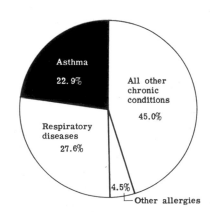

FIGURE 42–3. School days lost because of chronic conditions. (From C. G. Schiffer and E. P. Hunt: Illness Among Children. Children's Bureau Publ. No. 405, Washington, D.C., United States Department of Health, Education, and Welfare, 1963.)

Table 2. *Days of Illness Due to Chronic Conditions*

	Age 0-16 yrs.		*6-16 yrs.*
	(*Days Expressed in 1000's*)		
	Activity Restricted	*Bed Days*	*School Days Lost*
All chronic conditions	136,660	54,633	32,927
Hay fever without asthma	2,517	725	566
Asthma with or without hay fever	24,163	11,656	7,524
Other allergies	7,095	822	967
Heart disease	3,507	1,200	859
Paralysis	2,587	1,681	743
Impairment of extremities:			
Upper extremities	1,009	234	76
Lower extremities and hip	6,482	818	303

Condensed from Table 21, Illness Among Children. Children's Bureau Publication No. 405, United States Department of Health, Education, and Welfare, Washington, D.C., 1963, p. 80.

to the over-all averages of disability can be seen more clearly. Table 2, which outlines the days of illness caused by chronic conditions, shows 24,163,000 restricted activity days, 11,656,000 bed days, and 7,524,-000 school days lost because of asthma. This is more than twice the combined total restricted activity days for heart disease, paralysis and orthopedic impairment; it is three times the bed days, and nearly four times the lost school days for these other, more obviously disabling conditions.

Mortality

Fortunately, the high frequency of asthma in childhood is largely offset by a low death rate, the mortality rate being much lower than in the later years of life. Death from asthma occurs so rarely in any one physician's experience, in fact, that it is always a shocking and unexpected outcome. Yet because of the large number of asthmatics, asthma still ranks among the sixty leading causes of death in the United States (Vital Statistics of the United States, 1963). To evaluate properly the meaning of the mortality from asthma, it must be considered against the background of general mortality rates for this country and must also be compared with rates for other leading causes of death. The rates for those conditions which have special importance in

childhood, either as preventable, hereditary or major causes of illness, offer the best perspective on the significance of asthma mortality, as shown in Table 3. In 1963 the United States total average death rate at all ages for both sexes was 961.9 per 100,000 population, exclusive of fetal deaths. There is a wide range by age as seen in rates of 25.4 per 1000 under one year, 1 per 1000 for one to four years and 0.4 per 1000 for five to fourteen years. There has been a slight rise in total death rate for all causes from 9.2 to 9.6 per 1000 from 1954 to 1963. For several decades the death rate for asthma was stationary, but from 1954 to 1963 the total rate for asthma declined from the level of 3.8 to 2.7 per 100,000 (rates for specific diseases are given per 100,000 population). During this same ten-year period, however, death rates from other diseases fell much more impressively: rates for tuberculosis, for example, fell from 10.2 to 4.9; rates for rheumatic fever and chronic rheumatic heart disease went from 12.1 to 8.8; the total death rate for acute poliomyelitis fell from 0.8 to 0.0; and death rates from diphtheria, pertussis, measles, dysentery and meningococcal infections dropped from 0.6 to 0.0 per 100,000.

The low rates for the infectious diseases which once decimated our child population are the result of widespread, active prophylaxis, greater availability of medical care and facilities and the de-

Table 3. *Death Rates by Age Groups—Rate per 100,000 Population**

	Total	Years			
		0-1	1-4	5-9	10-14
All causes	961.9	2537.2	99.5	45.2	41.5
Tuberculosis, all forms	4.9	0.8	0.5	0.1	0.1
Diphtheria	0.0	0.1	0.1	0.1	—
Whooping cough	0.1	2.2	0.2	—	—
Meningococcal infection	0.4	5.0	1.6	0.3	0.1
Acute poliomyelitis	0.0	0.1	0.0	0.0	—
Measles	0.2	1.9	1.0	0.4	0.1
Other infective and parasitic diseases ...	3.2	19.4	2.7	1.1	0.7
Asthma	*2.7*	*0.6*	*0.4*	*0.2*	*0.3*
Diabetes	17.2	0.4	0.2	0.2	0.4
Pneumonia**	33.8	210.0	13.4	2.4	1.8
Bronchitis	2.9	13.4	1.4	0.3	0.1
Other bronchopulmonary diseases	12.3	33.6	1.1	0.1	0.1
Congenital malformations	11.0	357.8	10.8	3.2	2.4
Rheumatic fever†	8.8	0.1	0.2	0.3	0.7
Accidents:	53.4	86.3	31.0	18.6	17.9
Motor	23.1	7.9	10.0	8.8	7.2
Nonmotor	30.3	78.4	21.0	9.9	10.7

From "Vital Statistics of the United States," Vol. IIA, Table 1-26, Death rate for 60 selected causes by 5 years, pp. 1-248 through 1-261, 1963.
  * Excludes fetal deaths.
  ** Excludes newborn.
  † Includes other chronic rheumatic diseases.

velopment of new, specific therapeutic measures, some of which are applicable to asthma. In terms of actual numbers, from a United States population of 58,-734,000 children under fifteen years (1963 census), 135,485 deaths were reported. Five conditions accounted for more than half of these deaths: accidents, malformations, pneumonias, respiratory diseases and neoplasms. The remainder were distributed through the other 280 reportable

causes of death. (The conditions which are compared with asthma as a cause of childhood deaths are listed in Table 4.)

These mortality statistics, along with the morbidity rates, indicate that asthma is neither a completely benign condition nor an inconsequential health problem in childhood. On the contrary, it looms as one of the biggest hazards of childhood.

Pathogenesis

Allergic asthma is the most important form of spontaneously occurring human hypersensitivity. Asthma, hay fever, infantile eczema, urticaria and angioedema are the diseases for which the term "atopy" (strange disease) was coined by Coca and Cooke in 1923. They are characterized by a heritable tendency (Cooke and Vander Veer; Spain and Cooke) and by the presence of a unique sort of circulating antibody. Initially, it was believed that this sort of sensitivity occurred only in human beings, but in recent years atopic conditions have been found in

Table 4. *Number of Deaths in Children Under 15 Years of Age, United States, 1963, Due to Selected Conditions*

Condition	Total
Asthma	182
Rheumatic fever with heart disease ..	203
Tuberculosis	142
Measles	345
Cystic fibrosis	654
Poliomyelitis	21
Diphtheria	37

From "Vital Statistics of the United States," Vol. IIA, Table 1-23, pp. 1-86 to 1-147, 1963.

dogs, horses, walruses and other animals. Furthermore, patients with these disorders have been found in whom neither the circulating antibodies nor the hereditary features are present. Despite these exceptions and some new light which recent, sophisticated techniques have shed upon our concepts of the nature and behavior of the atopic antibody, the original criteria of Coca and Cooke and others remain valid in their essential outline.

The current definition of atopic antibody (reagin) (Raffel) is an antibody which (1) is skin-sensitizing in the subject and has an affinity for the mucous membranes of the respiratory and gastrointestinal tracts and the conjunctiva of the sensitized person, (2) can be passively transferred to a normal person's skin (Prausnitz-Küstner reaction) and to nonhuman primates, but not to guinea pigs, (3) is heat-labile, becoming inactivated at 56°C. after two hours, (4) cannot be measured by any of the conventional invitro serologic techniques, (5) can be detected by in-vitro histamine release in monkey ileum and by PCA (passive cutaneous anaphylaxis) in monkey, and (6) does not usually cross the placenta from mother to fetus.

The atopic antibodies appear after sensitization to environmental substances, which are often poor but complete antigens or are haptens which combine with serum protein to form a sensitizing antigen. Pollen, dust, animal dander, foods, fungi, bacteria, insect stings and certain drugs (such as penicillin, aspirin and iodides) which are not noxious agents are examples of allergens which sensitize and are incriminated in asthma. Injections of animal serums may produce both atopic and precipitating antibodies.

The nature of the antibodies present in human allergy is currently the subject of active investigation, and since data are constantly being added and concepts modified, the reader should consult current reviews on the subjects of allergy and immunology, published annually, for up-to-date information. Antibody activity has been associated with serum fractions containing the immunoglobulin IgA (formerly referred to as γ_{1A} or β_{2A}) as the only detectable immunoglobulin, and the Prausnitz-Küstner reaction has been blocked by prior or concomitant injections of similar fractions from nonallergic serums in the area being sensitized. This fraction (IgA) has been estimated to have a molecular weight of 160,000 (plus polymers), has a sedimentation coefficient of 7 to 18S, is found in serum at an average concentration of 2.5 to 3 mg. per milliliter, and occurs as the sole or principal detectable type of antibody in tears, saliva, tracheal and bronchial mucous and other external secretions, and in colostrum. It is attractive to associate reagin with this antibody fraction, since it is found in such high concentration in the areas of the body frequently involved in atopic hypersensitivity. Nevertheless the sporadic finding that persons who completely lack this immunoglobulin in their serum or external secretions may have skin-sensitizing antibody casts some doubt on the constancy of this association. It is entirely possible that reagin exists in an as yet unidentified immunoglobulin fraction which migrates with, and is separated from, serum by many of the same procedures used to isolate IgA.*

In spite of the many large gaps in the knowledge of the nature and properties of atopic antibody, the earliest investigators made a practical application of their observations on skin and mucous membrane sensitization, passive transfer and heat lability in developing the clinical diagnostic tests for specific sensitization in allergic patients. These observations form the basis on which modern clinical allergy rests; current immunologic investigation should ultimately produce additional aids which will elucidate the basic pathophysiology of the allergic diseases.

---

* Ishizaka proposes IgE to designate an immunoglobulin different from IgA and IgG, which he has recently identified as the fraction which contains the principal reaginic activity in several serums (*J. Allergy*, 23:169, 336, 1966).

let cell glands of the bronchial and bronchiolar mucosa. Droplets of mucus are extruded into the bronchial lumen and coalesce to form mucous plugs, which often occlude the lumen. When it occurs in lesser degree, this is a normal process, as shown in sections of normal bronchus (Fig. 4). In the mucus from an asthmatic patient, desquamated bronchial epithelial cells and eosinophils are seen. Eosinophils also may be seen infiltrating the mucosa and bronchial wall. There may be a loss of cilia in patches or apparently in large areas. The mucosa may become redundant, with strong infoldings which may become almost polypoid. In some patients, especially very young children, the lymph nodes are greatly enlarged, and clumps of lymphocytes are present along the bronchial wall. Structural changes in bronchial smooth muscle are difficult to detect, so that it is difficult, if not impossible, to demonstrate contraction or spasm of this muscle in pathologic sections, and for this reason some investigators have questioned

whether muscle spasm is actually a feature of asthma. Their objection is at variance, however, with the well known relief from asthma produced by the bronchodilating drugs.

The alveolar walls usually appear to be normal in younger patients (Fig. 5). In older persons dying of asthma, emphysema of variable degree is seen, with the characteristic thinning, fibrosis and rupture of the alveolar walls. Thickening of the adventitia and the muscular layers of blood vessels is much less frequently seen in young children than in adults.

The majority of pathologic studies have utilized autopsy material. The sections from asthmatic lung illustrated in Figure 6, however, were taken from surgical specimens obtained at lobectomy. They do not differ in any essential features from the autopsy material, except that the cilia seem to be more intact.

No characteristic gross or microscopic pathologic changes have been reported in other organs in autopsy material, al-

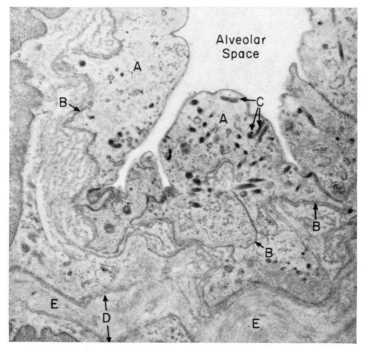

FIGURE 42–5. Alveolar wall from young asthmatic, showing (*A*) alveolar epithelial cells, (*B*) basal membrane, (*C*) lysosomes, (*D*) septal membrane, (*E*) collagen fibrils in septal membrane. The capillary endothelium is at lower margin of section. × 23,000.

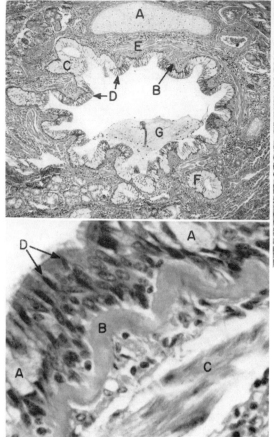

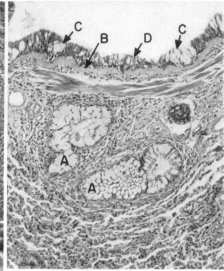

FIGURE 42–6. Sections of asthmatic lung. *Top left,* Cross section of bronchus (× 66) showing (*A*) cartilage, (*B*) basement membrane which is thickened, (*C*) epithelium containing many goblet cells, (*D*) area of many ciliated epithelial cells, (*F*) mucous gland, (*G*) mucous plug. *Top right,* Bronchial epithelium (× 136) showing (*A*) mucous glands, (*B*) hyaline basement membrane, (*C*) goblet cells, (*D*) ciliated cells. *Bottom left,* Bronchial epithelium (× 700) showing (*A*) goblet cell, (*B*) basement membrane, (*C*) connective tissue, (*D*) ciliated respiratory epithelial cells.

though right-sided cardiac hypertrophy has been present in some patients. In one child who suffered a fatal paroxysm of asthma, we noted considerable eosinophilic infiltration of tissues and cerebral edema, with eosinophils clustered around the cerebral blood vessels.

Since most severe asthmatics who die in acute asthmatic attacks have usually undergone extensive, long-term corticosteroid treatment, some of the pathologic changes encountered have been attributed to prolonged steroid therapy (Keeney).

Pathophysiology

The concept that allergic antibodies are fixed to lung tissue and mucous membranes and that the antigen-antibody interaction releases enzymes or substances which can produce tissue damage has evolved over the years as the explanation for the pathophysiology of asthma and allergic reactions. The substances which are thought to act as mediators of immediate hypersensitivity in man are histamine (H-substance), acetylcholine, and slow-reacting substance (SRS-A) (reviews of subject by Logan, 1959, 1960). Various animals have, in addition to these three, serotonin (5-hydroxytryptamine), bradykinin, other kinins, and heparin released in anaphylaxis; thus far these latter substances have not been demonstrated to be active mediators in human beings. The histamine present during an immediate hypersensitivity reaction in man is thought both to come from the actual union of antigen and antibody protein and to originate from mast cells. The granules of mast cells contain large amounts of histamine which is liberated with their disruption; this occurs as the mast cells "degranulate" when damaged, e.g. during the allergic reaction. Histamine produces capillary dilatation which increases the permeability of blood vessel walls, contracts smooth muscle and stimulates mucous gland secretions. The lungs and bronchi of allergic persons hyperreact to a smaller amount of histamine and acetylcholine aerosol than do those of normal persons.

Acetylcholine can duplicate many of the effects of histamine. It has been shown in sensitized guinea pigs that acetylcholine concentration rises after injection of specific antigens. In man the use of atropine and anticholinergic agents has exhibited some effect in decreasing asthma and other allergic reactions. It has been suggested that these two substances, histamine and acetylcholine, act as mediators by way of the autonomic nervous system, and that the autonomic state of the end-organ at the time of their release determines the clinical picture of asthma. Experience has shown that nonspecific factors often heighten asthma and allergic reactions. These are trauma, chilling, emotional stresses, fatigue, and the administration of certain drugs such as codeine and morphine, all of which release histamine and also evoke a parasympathetic response. Stimulation of the parasympathetic nervous system may magnify the direct effect of histamine on tissue; it also may evoke symptoms by means of acetylcholine. The various pieces of evidence of the asthmagenic interrelation of histamine and acetylcholine are not yet fully integrated, and many of the theories in this area are subject to constant revision (Voorhorst). The recent development of several new techniques for rapid assay of small amounts of histamine should advance our understanding of this complex relation.

SRS-A (slow-reacting substance A of Brocklehurst) was first identified in 1956 as causing contraction of bronchial smooth muscle in human and guinea pig lung at antigen-antibody union. Since SRS-A is a relative newcomer, less is known about its properties than about those of the other mediators, but it is antagonized by atropine, epinephrine and theophylline, and increases in Ca^{++} ion concentration minimize its effect in vitro on guinea pig ileum. These intriguing observations suggest its potential significance in some, if not all, cases of human asthma.

Clinical Features

SYMPTOMS. The symptoms of asthma reflect the major component of bronchial and bronchiolar obstruction and are directly due to interference in air exchange. Hacking and paroxysmal, irritative, nonproductive cough marks the *first stage*, i.e. bronchial edema. The tenacious mucus which accumulates may also act somewhat like a foreign body in stimulating cough.

As secretion becomes more profuse in the *second stage* of asthma, the cough becomes more rattling and productive of frothy, clear, gelatinous sputum. At this stage the patient begins to feel slightly short of breath, he attempts to breathe more deeply, his expiration becomes prolonged, and exhalation produces a high-pitched musical wheeze. He is seen to have retraction of the soft tissue of the neck and retraction of the intercostal spaces, and his facial expression is anxious. He speaks in short, panting, broken phrases, and he sits in a hunched-over position, hands on the edge of the bed or chair, his braced arms supporting his chest to facilitate the use of accessory muscles of respiration. He is often pale, although some children have a rosy malar flush and bright red ears. The lips assume a deep, dark red hue, but later they may become cyanotic, as may the nailbeds and the skin, especially about the mouth. The chest becomes overdistended and rounded and moves relatively little with each breath. The younger children revert to abdominal breathing, with suprasternal and intercostal retraction and flaring of the rib margins at each breath. Young infants and children become very restless during this second stage and cannot be made comfortable in any position in bed, often resting only briefly upright in an attendant's arms. The cough becomes less effective, the respiratory rate increases, breathing becomes shallow, panting or grunting, and cyanosis rapidly increases.

The *third stage* is that of severe bronchial obstruction or spasm, when so little air is moved per breath that breath sounds and rales become almost inaudible. This is a dangerous stage of asthma, and one which is often misinterpreted as improvement by those unfamiliar with the disorder. The absence of rales is taken to represent clearing, whereas in actuality no sound is being made because no air is moving; even cough seems to be suppressed at this point. Shallow or irregular respirations and sudden rise in respiratory rate are ominous signs indicating that asphyxia may be imminent.

In some children the order of these groups of symptoms is reversed and the attack may be initiated by a sudden acute, severe, generalized bronchospasm which may follow one or two harsh, sharp coughs. Some instances of sudden death from asthma have occurred with this sequence of events, and the bronchospasm has been so severe and generalized that an adequate airway could not be established rapidly enough to maintain life. Fortunately, in most instances the bronchospasm is neither so rapid in onset nor so extensive, and even though respiration is seriously embarrassed, there is sufficient time for the child to effect some adjustment to this and for relief measures to be instituted.

It has been suggested that this sudden bronchospasm is an anaphylactic-like reaction, the challenging agent reaching all the bronchi simultaneously by way of the blood stream and not by inhalation. The validity of this hypothesis in spontane-ously occurring asthma cannot easily be tested in human patients because the emergency situation is not suitable for such direct study. By inference from data involving penicillin and other drug reactions, serum reactions after insect stings and anaphylactic accidents during skin testing, however, this challenge by blood stream appears to occur occasionally. In addition, a few instances of anaphylactic-like reactions to foods suggesting blood stream challenge have been reported in children (Crawford et al.).

PHYSICAL SIGNS. The principal physical findings in asthma are rapid, labored respiration, paroxysmal cough and prolonged expiration. It has already been noted that the chest is emphysematous or overdistended, the shoulders tend to be held high, the sternocleidomastoid and upper chest muscles are taut, and the ribs are widely spaced with the rib margins flared. The anteroposterior diameter of the chest is increased. The supraclavicular and suprasternal areas retract with inspiration, and the intercostal spaces may also retract. The angle made by the margin of the rib cage and the sternum becomes obtuse.

Percussion is hyperresonant over the entire chest, especially over the lower posterior part of the chest. The excursion of the diaphragms may be decreased to 1 to 2 cm. The cardiac borders are difficult to outline because of the overlying inflated lungs. Tactile fremitus is usually normal, although it may be decreased.

Breath sounds are distant, with a prolongation of expiration. There are musical rales of inconstant nature over the entire chest, changing in intensity after cough or deep breathing. In latent asthma, compression of the chest wall between the stethoscope and the examiner's hand may elicit wheezing rales (Glaser). In addition, sibilant and coarse, moist, sonorous rales may be present over the larger bronchi. Spoken voice sounds are normal or increased.

The pulse rate is accelerated, and the volume may become weak and thready.

Paradoxical pulse and slowing and diminution of pulse volume with inspiration may be present. The heart may show signs of right-sided failure in acute episodes of asthma which are severe and protracted. This condition should be suspected when the pulse rate increases without good cause, the basilar rales take on a moist or wet nature, the liver enlarges or becomes tender, and the eyelids have a puffy appearance.

In young infants and toddlers the prolongation of expiration is not as apparent as in older children because of the more pliable chest and more rapid respiratory rate. Unfortunately, the distinction between expiratory and inspiratory dyspnea is less clear at this age when it would be most helpful in differentiating the non-asthmatic causes of dyspnea.

Many asthmatics have the so-called adenoidal or allergic facies, with narrow maxilla and nose, high palate and mal-occlusion, but there seems to be no particular type seen in asthma, nor is there necessarily any alteration in growth pattern. Spock has recently reviewed the growth patterns in 200 asthmatic children from our clinic and reports that they have a tendency to be a little below the mean in both height and weight. A few children are chronically ill and show the decreased height and weight expected for their degree of illness. Others are short because of steroid therapy. Clubbing of fingers and toes is not characteristic even for severe chronic asthma, unless it is complicated by some other chronic lung or heart disease; even then it may be absent.

Generalized slight enlargement of superficial lymph nodes is common in asthmatic children, tonsils often appear large and cryptic, and adenoids may be palpated or seen extending into the nasopharynx. When removed surgically, adenoids tend to recur rapidly as bits or clusters of lymphoid tissue over the posterior pharyngeal wall. The soft palate ordinarily has a peculiar "goose flesh" appearance due to the prominence of minute lymphoid follicles.

Clinical Types

Classification of asthma by clinical type (Table 5) has obvious limitations and exceptions, but it does serve one significant and useful purpose: it directs the physician to the most likely causes and therefore to the most suitable treatment programs. At the same time it emphasizes that asthma has many origins and, like headache, cannot be expected to run the same course in all patients.

ALLERGIC (ATOPIC) ASTHMA. *Dermal-Respiratory Syndrome.* "Dermal-respiratory syndrome" (Ratner) or "eczema-prurigo-asthma syndrome" (Bray) describes the truly "allergic child" who has atopic eczema in infancy with respiratory symptoms or coryza (allergic rhinitis) and who later suffers asthma with persistent neurodermatitis continuing into childhood and adult life. The classic findings of atopy are present here: vasomotor lability with white dermographism, strong sensitivities with positive immediate skin test results to protein allergens, and blood and tissue eosinophilia. Other family members are likely to have allergic disorders, and many nonspecific factors may precipitate symptoms.

The infant's asthmatic breathing may be first noted with respiratory infections which last longer and seem more prostrating than expected. Attacks are often recurrent with only a few days of normal breathing before a second episode begins.

Table 5. *Clinical Types of Asthma in Children*

A. Allergic (atopic)
    1. Dermal-respiratory syndrome (Ratner)
       Eczema-asthma-prurigo (Bray)
       Spasmodic
       Continuous
       Intractable
    2. Allergic rhinitis-asthma
       Seasonal (hay fever)
       Nonseasonal (inhalant)
B. Nonallergic (nonatopic)
    1. Infectious—lung damage
    2. Mechanical obstruction
C. Status asthmaticus

Asthma follows eczema in about one half to two thirds of true atopic eczema patients, regardless of the severity of the eczema (Dees, 1957). The respiratory symptoms become more prominent by about two years of age. These babies are likely to have a strongly positive immediate skin test results to egg, although egg may not be a major or primary cause of symptoms. Buffum feels that this positive reaction is significant in that it indicates that allergic sensitization is present, and it may herald the persistence of asthma beyond ten years of age.

In this group of patients one sees the emergence of a stereotyped set of symptoms. As the child reaches three to five years of age, definite "attacks" of asthma occur. They frequently come on abruptly at night, with little or no warning, or they may be preceded by a few hours or a whole day of coryza, nasal obstruction and hacking cough. Dyspnea and cough of increasing severity finally culminate in hard wheezing and labored breathing. The cough may be so severe that vomiting results, and this in turn is often followed by improvement in dyspnea.

If untreated, such an attack will last several hours or days, until the child appears completely exhausted. Then there may be sudden, rapid improvement, all symptoms quickly subsiding, and the child returns to his normal state in a relatively short time. During the attack he often loses 5 to 10 pounds in weight, which is rapidly regained thereafter. If treated with an adequate bronchodilator, the attack is shorter and milder. The eczema usually improves when asthma begins, but small patches may "flare up" just before the asthma attack and may serve as a warning of impending trouble. In other children whose eczema has remained active there may be a remission during asthma with prompt recurrence on recovery from asthma. Each child tends to follow a repetitive pattern of the same antecedent symptoms, exhibiting these each time he has asthma. In some children mild to severe cramping mid-abdominal pain is the premonitory complaint. Other children may have one or more of the following: constipation or diarrhea, abnormal appetite, darkening of the periocular skin (aptly termed "allergic shiners" by Marks), a glassy-eyed appearance, and allergic tension-fatigue (Crook) consisting of a change in disposition usually associated with irritability, whining, listlessness or hyperactivity. Occasionally the hyperactivity extends to insomnia and nightmares. Some mothers report that the child sweats excessively at night or has enuresis in this prodromal stage. Others may have a peculiar type of throat-clearing or itching of the throat.

Between attacks these children are apt to wheeze briefly if they laugh suddenly or overexert themselves. They are also very susceptible to weather and temperature changes, and they frequently sneeze, cough and wheeze when exposed to a draft or sudden chilling. Many other nonspecific irritants and stresses also appear to act as immediate causes of symptoms.

A variety of factors may determine whether the asthma occurs intermittently in attacks, with symptom-free intervals gradually decreasing in duration until finally the wheezing is mild, constant and punctuated by more severe symptoms. Variation in the individual asthmatic pattern is partly related to the nature of the specific causes and to the degree of sensitivity of the particular child, as well as to the amount of exposure he has to his particular allergens. In some children whose asthma becomes intractable despite apparently complete and efficient removal of noxious agents from the environment, the reason for worsening is obscure. In these cases one usually finds considerably decreased pulmonary function, abnormal bronchi (when tissue is available for study), and the nonspecific factors of emotional tension, fatigue, and hyperreaction to temperature change, all operating in an important way. These are the children who are destined to become pulmonary cripples, and every effort should be made to detect them early and to institute vigorous antiallergic treatment with the hope of arresting or reversing the process. Unfortunately, much still remains to be explained about the various causes of intractable asthma.

ALLERGIC RHINITIS-ASTHMA. Another clinical type of allergic asthma is that associated with hay fever or perennial allergic rhinitis. Asthma may appear after several years of upper respiratory allergic symptoms, or both may develop about the same time. Specific causes are usually airborne allergens, either pollen, dusts or animal danders. Sensitization can be regularly demonstrated by direct and indirect skin tests or other conventional allergy tests and can be confirmed by provocative tests. If hay fever is the antecedent, patients are usually five to six years of age or older at the onset of asthma. If perennial allergic rhinitis is present, the age at onset is usually much younger, even as early as one to two years.

The severity of symptoms in the upper and lower airways varies directly with the level of the patient's sensitivities and with the frequency, duration and amount of exposure to the inciting allergen(s). Nonspecific factors which aggravate symptoms are the presence of vasomotor rhinitis or intercurrent infection, anatomic malconfiguration of the upper airway, inclement weather, and other provocative environmental conditions. These factors all contribute to produce a variable clinical picture, ranging from the mildest infrequent attack to intractable asthma and, rarely, to status asthmaticus. This allergic rhinitis-asthma group of patients consists of those in whom response to specific etiologic treatment and improvement after medication are the most clear-cut. Allergic rhinitis, both seasonal and perennial, may persist after asthma has been controlled. From the foregoing it is obvious that the ultimate prognosis for both the improvement and control of asthma symptoms can be better in this group than in the preceding dermal-respiratory type, or in the lung-damage type to be described below.

NONALLERGIC (NONATOPIC) ASTHMA. *Infectious or Lung-Damage Asthma.* Lung-damage type of asthma, as it has been designated by Bray and others, is a type of asthma in which hereditary features are lacking or are minor and which may have originated so soon after an attack of measles, bronchiolitis, influenza or some other viral disease which affects the lung that this appears to have been the initial insult. From then on an infection of any kind seems to precipitate an asthmatic attack. There is fever with the attack, leukocytosis is higher than with other types of asthma, and pathogenic bacteria are often cultured from the sputum, paranasal sinuses or nasopharynx. Although elimination of these bacteria does not completely prevent attacks, the symptoms always seem worse when they are present. There is much fibrosis and more emphysema of an irreversible type in these children than in those of the atopic group; the skin tests to allergens are likely to yield unimpressive results, but they may show strong immediate and delayed reactions to bacterial vaccines and extracts.

Some of these children will suffer sufficient pulmonary insult from the initial illness that they are never well thereafter, becoming pulmonary cripples with a poor prognosis for both health and life and exhibiting a course comparable to that in adults with the "vanishing lung syndrome."

STATUS ASTHMATICUS. Many of the children who suffer status asthmaticus, or completely unresponsive asthma, come from the "infectious asthma" group. They present with signs of severe asthma within a short time after the initial onset of an apparently minor respiratory infection. The asthma does not improve until the infection is controlled. Clinical evidence suggests that these children often have immunologic deficiencies, and they usually suffer more frequent complications of asthma than children with the strong atopic trait.

In some instances of uncomplicated

"infectious asthma" the outlook becomes less gloomy as the child grows older and he seems to handle the respiratory infections better and with decreasing bronchospasm. If extensive damage has not occurred within the first few years of the disease, the prospects brighten as the child improves and eventually remains well except for rare sporadic asthma with respiratory infection. Asthma of this type is then considered to have been "outgrown." Children with this form of asthma present diagnostic problems and are difficult to classify; certainly, some have bronchial obstruction due to inflammatory reaction of a particular infection, and hence perhaps more properly should be considered to have bronchiolitis or "asthmatic bronchitis," although the latter term has fallen into disfavor. As refinements in both viral isolation and immunologic methods become available for general clinical use, and as the techniques of bronchial and lung biopsy become less formidable, some of this confusion in differentiation may disappear.

Laboratory Findings

SPUTUM.   The sputum in asthma is a peculiar clear to whitish, gelatinous, glairy material, very tenacious and sticky, which is coughed up in stringy casts or molds of the bronchioles (Curschmann spirals). Sometimes small, firm, pellet-like matter is present; these are similar rolled-up casts which are twisted and convoluted and often contain air bubbles. The chemical composition has not been completely established, but mucopolysaccharides, serum albumin and globulins (IgA) are present, the last in higher concentration than is found in serum or saliva. The sputum lacks a proteolytic enzyme found in nonasthmatic, purulent sputum (Mendes et al.; Dennis et al.).

The sputum consists largely of an amorphous eosinophilic-staining mucus, eosinophils and polymorphonuclear cells, with few bacteria (Kim et al.). The Charcot-Leyden crystals are also a unique feature of asthmatic sputum and are seen in specimens several hours old. *The unmistakable appearance of asthmatic sputum is a useful and neglected diagnostic aid in recognizing asthma.* Even when there is some degree of complicating infection, the casts retain their shape, although they may become an opaque yellow. In more extensive infections this may be overshadowed by an excess of purulent secretion, but asthmatic sputum rarely has the homogeneous appearance seen in other pulmonary conditions. In children too young to cough on command, tracheal aspirate will yield the same characteristic secretion.

NASAL SECRETION.   Nasal secretion has been the object of much interest in asthma, particularly in nasal allergy, since Hansel popularized the use of staining for eosinophils as a diagnostic test. He describes the secretion as alkaline and nonirritating to nasal mucosa and skin, in contrast to infectious exudate, which is acid and irritating. IgA globulin has been isolated from the nasal secretion, as from other body fluids.

BLOOD.   Most asthmatic children tend to have hematocrit values and hemoglobin concentrations above average, findings which are related directly to the degree of hypoxia and its duration. In very young children during an attack of asthma it is not uncommon to see values of 14 to 15 gm. per 100 ml. or higher, which then fall 2 to 3 gm. (to 12 to 13 gm. per 100 ml.) when the dyspnea is relieved. Dehydration may contribute to this, as the white blood cell count may rise without demonstrable infection. Eosinophils are frequently present in concentrations over 5 per cent, and values may reach 30 to 40 per cent in severe, long-standing asthma or in drug or parasite-induced asthma. Although Cooke (1947) believed that infectious asthma was characterized by a higher eosinophilia than that seen in asthma due to allergens, this opinion is not universally shared. During the peak of an asthmatic attack eosinophils may virtually disappear from the blood smear and then reappear with improvement. Recently, interest has centered on the basophil, which may be found in either increased or decreased concentration in chronic or acute allergic states (Shelley). This has been related to the mast cell degranulation of anaphylaxis (Selye). In some children neutropenia and decrease in platelets occur during an asthmatic attack. Various theories as to their transient disappearance have been offered, among them one hypothesis that sequestration in the lung or other shock organ is responsible, and another that their dissolution is brought about by the products of antigen-antibody union.

Much has been written about the gamma globulin levels in asthmatic children, but no conclusive proof has been presented that there is any constant quantitative or qualitative alteration in gamma globulin (Abernathy; Dees and Grunt). There appears, however, to be a small percentage of young children and an almost minute percentage of older children in whom gamma globulin level is low and features of both allergic disorders and collagen diseases are present. In addition, these children have a high family incidence of arthritis and collagen diseases and are found to have a dysgammaglobulinemia, often with reduction or absence of one portion of the gamma globulin component, commonly the IgA or IgM globulin. This condition may be suspected on clinical grounds if the skin test results are negative or weakly positive and if the isoagglutinins are reduced. Only if immunoelectrophoretic or quantitative analysis shows a reduction in IgG globulin, which is the fraction present in commercial gamma globulin, is there any reason to give gamma globulin injections to these patients. The development of sensitization to gamma globulin after repeated injections makes it imperative to restrict its therapeutic use to unequivocal necessity (Allen and Kunkel).

The Weltmann reaction, a simple test for qualitative changes in the serum protein, gives a normal value of 6 in uncomplicated asthma, less than 6 in infected cases, and more than 6 in patients with pulmonary fibrosis (Dees, 1941). Deviations from this value have been shown to closely parallel changes in the amounts and proportion of the globulins in asthmatics (Dees and Grunt). This test can be used as a screening device to detect abnormal serums, which should be studied with more precise measurements of serum protein in order to detect children whose asthma is attended by immunologic abnormalities and by infection.

The sedimentation rate is slow in allergic diseases, including asthma; 0 to 2 mm. per hour, Wintrobe, uncorrected, is a usual range. When infection supervenes, more rapid rates are found, but they are frequently slower than in nonallergic patients with comparable active infections.

There are no specific changes or trends seen in asthma in the various other blood tests used for detecting the presence of infection, such as C-reactive protein, latex fixation, antistreptolysin O, cold and heterophile agglutinins. Also, the various chemical constituents of the blood do not show any characteristic changes or trends in asthma.

SWEAT. In our experience sweat chloride levels are normal or low in asthmatics, and Gharib et al. reached the same conclusion. This contrasts with an early report by Hsia, who found some elevated levels in asthmatics. Values above 30 to 40 mEq. per liter are present in cystic fibrosis, whereas normal and allergic children do not reach this concentration if sweating is normal. Thus the sweat test for chlorides is an aid in differentiating the two conditions.

GASTRIC SECRETION. Gastric secretion tends to have a low hydrochloric acid content in allergic children. It has been suggested that this condition may be a predisposition to food sensitization, since protein is not subjected to normal amounts of the acid for digestion and thus may reach the absorption areas of the small bowel in an incompletely degraded state, with antigenic potential. This possible mechanism needs re-examination with current methods for studying intestinal physiologic processes before it can be accepted as the explanation for food sensitization, however.

Dynamics of Respiration

The dynamics of respiration are discussed in detail by Comroe (1962) and by Bates and Christie, and in various other studies of special aspects of lung physiology. (See also the section on The Functional Basis of Respiratory Pathology, page 3.) The consensus of these investigators regarding the abnormalities in asthma is that bilateral obstructive emphysema is produced by a decrease in the caliber of the bronchi and bronchioles. The extra effort required to inhale and expel air through a narrowed airway, in order to accommodate to increased resistance to outflow, produces an abnormal breathing pattern with prolonged expiration. As this abnormal pattern continues, the rate increases, the fatigue which results from inefficient respiratory movements deepens, expiration becomes more prolonged, and inspiration becomes shallow and panting until finally the chest is almost fixed in an overdistended inspiratory position. This, in turn, results in the distention of alveoli, inadequate and uneven alveolar ventilation, pulmonary hypertension, and loss of lung elasticity and compliance.

The ventilating capacity for static lung volumes and forced vital capacity in twenty-one asthmatic children from attack to symptom-free status has been studied by Engström by means of a closed-circuit helium-dilution technique. The mechanics of breathing, tidal volume, flow rate and changes in intraesophageal pressure were measured simultaneously to calculate lung compliance and pulmonary flow resistance. A reverse body plethysmograph was used for measuring tidal volume.

During an asthmatic attack, Engström found increased inspiratory and expiratory pulmonary flow resistance to be the characteristic expression of bronchial obpage 3.) The consensus of these investistruction:

$$\frac{E}{I} = 1.6$$

where E represents expiratory and I in-

Table 6. *Summary of Trends in Ventilatory Capacity in 21 Asthmatic Children*

	Attack	Symptom-free Interval
Pulmonary flow resistance (R)	↑	N* or ↑
Functional residual capacity (V_{FRC})	↑	↓
Residual volume (V_R)	↑	↓
Dynamic compliance (C)	↓	↑ or N
Vital capacity (V_{VC})	↓	↑
Forced expiratory 1-second volume ($FEV_{1.0}$)	↓	↑
Total lung capacity (V_{TLC})	↓	↑

Modified from I. Engström (1964).
* N = normal.

spiratory resistance; vital capacity and dynamic compliance were low. Five days after the asthma attack all parameters had reverted toward normal, but hyperinflation and reduced ventilatory ability persisted. In the symptom-free interval, forced expiratory 1-second volume ($FEV_{1.0}$) was always lower than would have been expected for the amount of pulmonary resistance found (Table 6).

Previous study (Kraepelien, Engström and Karlberg) suggested that accelerated growth of the lung occurred in those asthmatic children in whom vital capacity (VC) was greater than normal at symptom-free status. Normal growth of the lung is consistent with widening of the alveoli and airways. During an asthmatic attack, expansion of alveoli also occurs; this is reversed when bronchial obstruction is removed. Engström's recent study suggests that after repeated attacks the expansion no longer reverses completely, and airways seem to expand in proportion to alveoli. By assuming an inspiratory position in the thorax, the lungs may be aided in maintaining a hyperventilated state without bronchial obstruction, thus hampering expiratory movement. This, in turn, implies that there may be increased distensibility of the lung, with air-trapping in addition to bronchial obstruction, to explain hyperinflation at normal pulmonary flow resistance in symptom-free periods. Pecora and Bernstein reported that pulmonary diffusing capacity in eight children with intractable asthma without hyperinflation was slightly lower than the normal range, whereas it was normal in seventeen others with hyperinflation.

In addition to the measurement of various parameters in asthma, the changes in vital capacity (V_{VC}), forced expiratory 1-second volume ($FEV_{1.0}$), maximum voluntary ventilation (MVV) and pulmonary resistance (R) after the inhalation of a bronchodilator (such as isoproterenol) provide a good estimate of the degree of bronchospasm in asthma and aid in the detection of emphysema and air trapping.

Status asthmaticus is the term used to designate the extreme stage of refractory asthma when so little air is exchanged with each breath that carbon dioxide retention, respiratory acidosis, loss of chloride and constantly deepening hypoxia result. The disturbed acid-base balance may then become compensated by respiratory alkalosis, so that carbon dioxide narcosis develops as the final stage of respiratory failure. Examples of the change in pH, pCO_2, base excess and oxygen saturation, ranging from those seen in respiratory acidosis, which develops first as the result of various combinations of partial decompensation, through those due to respiratory alkalosis are shown in Table 7.

The measurement of plasma bicarbonate and blood pH is crucial in determining the amount of carbon dioxide retention. This information is essential for correction of the metabolic derangement in severe status asthmaticus, particularly in the very young child, in whom fatigue may develop so rapidly that his appearance may not accurately reflect the seriousness of his condition. When facilities for the direct measurement of pCO_2, pO_2, oxygen saturation and total base in plasma are not available, but when blood pH value can be obtained, a recently conceived formula for deriving an estimated pCO_2 can be applied (Kassirer and Bleich). This now makes it possible for any physician who can obtain blood pH and total carbon dioxide content to follow this crucial parameter of his patient's metabolism. Kassirer and Bleich described their method as follows:

Estimation of Blood [H+] from pH

Hydrogen ion concentration in nanomoles (10^{-9} moles) per liter can readily be estimated from blood pH over a wide range of pH values. Two fortuitous relations form the basis of this empirical conversion . . .

The two digits that follow the decimal point in the normal blood pH of 7.40 and the normal value for blood hydrogen ion concentration of 40 nanomoles per liter are numerically identical.

Over a wide range of values, each deviation in pH of 0.01 unit from the normal value corresponds to a deviation in [H+] of 1 nanomole per liter.

Table 7. *Summary of Metabolic Derangements in Severe Asthma*

	pH	pCO_2	Base Excess	O_2 Saturation
Respiratory acidosis, plain	7.22	79	+ 2.5	80.5%
Chronic respiratory acidosis:				
Partially compensated	7.25	87.2	+ 7.2	< Rx IPPB* Before Rx
Overcompensated with metabolic alkalosis	7.52	38.0	+ 9.8	< After Rx
Respiratory acidosis-metabolic alkalosis:				
Due to decreased K+**	7.49	45	+ 11.6	
After treatment with K+**	7.43	40	+ 3.0	
Respiratory alkalosis-metabolic acidosis	7.39	33	− 3.3	61%
Respiratory alkalosis	7.45	34.7	+ 3.0	87%

  * IPPB = intermittent positive-pressure breathing.
  ** K+ = potassium ion.

Estimation of Plasma pCO_2 from $[H^+]$ and Total Carbon Dioxide Content

The blood pH of 7.16 is 0.24 unit more acid than normal, and thus

blood $[H^+] \approx 40 + 24$, or 64 nanomoles per liter;

$$\text{blood } pCO_2 \approx [H^+] \times \frac{\text{total } CO_2 \text{ content}}{25}$$

$$= 64 \times \frac{[20]}{25}, \text{ or 51 mm. Hg.}$$

The actual value for pCO_2, calculated from the Henderson-Hasselbalch equation with the aid of a table of logarithms, is 53 mm. of mercury (Kassirer and Bleich).

Differential Diagnosis

Each of the characteristic features of asthma—the tight cough, rapid respiration, dyspnea, obstructive emphysema and wheezing—may be found to some degree in a wide variety of different chest conditions and general systemic diseases. Furthermore, many very young asthmatic children, under four years of age, do not respond typically to skin tests or exhibit other characteristic features of atopic asthma, thus making it essential for the physician to be informed enough to rule out the nonallergic causes of wheezing and cough (Table 8). Most frequent among these are croup, asthmatic bronchitis, acute respiratory disease, frequently due to rhinovirus or respiratory syncytial virus, and bronchiolitis. Croup is characterized by the sudden onset of a harsh, barking cough, but differs from asthma in its inspiratory stridor. All the rest diffusely involve the bronchioles in inflammatory edema and bronchospasm and are characterized by some fever, wheezing and dyspnea. Emphysema and prostration are especially marked in bronchiolitis occurring in young infants, and are much more severe than in asthma. Since most cases of bronchiolitis are due to viral infections, and since tests for antiviral antibodies and direct viral cultures as yet are too time-consuming to make them diagnostically feasible, one must rely on finding evidence of infection and on observing the response to bronchodilating drugs. This response will be much less impressive, if detectable, in bronchiolitis than in asthma.

The presence of a foreign body in either

Table 8. *Differential Diagnosis of Asthma in Infants and Young Children**

1. *Foreign body,* any part of airway
2. Upper airway
    - Nose: enlarged adenoids, choanal atresia, polyps
    - Throat: retropharyngeal or peritonsillar abscess, *flaccid epiglottis, short neck*
    - Larynx: *croup, infection,* structural anomalies, paralysis of vocal cord, polyps, allergic edema, tetany
3. Lower airway
    - Trachea: *tracheomalacia, infection,* external compression by nodes, tumor, vascular ring, or foreign body in esophagus
    - Bronchus: infection, such as *asthmatic bronchitis, bronchiolitis, bronchitis* or bronchiectasis; obstruction due to endobronchial disease, stenosis or *external compression*
    - Lungs: *pneumonias, cystic fibrosis,* tuberculosis, histoplasmosis, pertussis, aspiration pneumonia, pneumothorax, Pneumocystis carinii, *atelectasis,* compression from lung or enteric cysts, intralobar emphysema, sequestration of lung, anomalies of lung such as agenesis of a lobe, etc., Loeffler's syndrome
4. Extrarespiratory disorders
    - Cardiovascular: congenital heart disease of various types, vascular ring, anomalies of great vessels
    - Central nervous system: hyperventilation, encephalitis, hysteria, cerebral palsy, palate paralysis, myasthenia gravis, drug intoxication (e.g. salicylism)

Modified from S. C. Dees: *J.A.M.A.,* 175:365, 1961.
* Italicized conditions are most common.

the trachea or esophagus must be considered in *every* child who shows difficulty in breathing. Removal of this cause for wheezing requires prompt and often emergency treatment. Small children, of course, present with this condition much more often than older children, and the parents characteristically report that symptoms began abruptly (often the exact moment can be recalled long afterward), describing some degree of respiratory difficulty or dysphagia, usually accompanied by harsh, barking, irritative cough and varying amounts of persistent wheezing. If the foreign body is lodged in one or the other main stem bronchus, unilateral wheezing is often heard. If the object is freely movable, one may hear a "click" or "slap" as it moves up and down the airway with breathing. If the object nearly but not completely obstructs the bronchus, a ball-valve effect results with emphysema occurring in the lung distal to the foreign body. With complete obstruction of a bronchus, atelectasis of the lobe supplied by that bronchus results. It is important to bear in mind that a foreign body may produce reflex bronchospasm with generalized signs which may easily obscure localizing ones.

Other important causes of wheezing and cough frequently mistaken for asthma are pertussis and cystic fibrosis of the pancreas (mucoviscidosis). In pertussis a markedly elevated white blood cell count with lymphocytosis is a helpful diagnostic sign. In cystic fibrosis the sweat test is diagnostic. Atelectasis, usually of the right middle lobe, may be associated with a wheezing, irritative cough, and may be suspected from the clinical signs of respiratory infection and the nature of the sputum. Roentgenographically, it can be recognized by a characteristic wedge-shaped area of increased density on lateral view or by blurring of the right cardiac border and obliteration of the right cardiophrenic angle. Other frequent causes of wheezy cough are flaccid epiglottis, tracheomalacia and laryngeal stridor. These abnormalities occur in early infancy, are primarily heard in inspiration,

and the signs of respiratory difficulty can be corrected or greatly decreased by change of position and by other maneuvers such as advancing the mandible; they diminish with age.

Less common but not less important and correctable causes of cough and wheeze are vascular rings and other anomalies of blood vessels which compromise tracheal or bronchial function. Also, hilar lymph nodes enlarged from any cause, but especially from tuberculosis, may compress the trachea or bronchus and cause wheezing.

Clinical Course and Complications

The clinical course of asthma assumes many variations in different patients; many different factors influence it. In addition to the degree of allergic sensitivity and the amount, duration and frequency of exposure to allergens, a number of nonspecific factors are influential; among these are infections, chilling, fatigue, emotional stress, physical debility, and predisposition by age and sex. Allowing for these many variables, the natural history of a representative (hypothetical) case of asthma may be described as follows:

A four-year-old boy with a feeding problem, mild transient facial eczema in infancy, and frequent "colds" accompanied by much mucus in the postpharynx and trachea all his life suddenly has acute, moderately severe nocturnal wheezing two days after the onset of his first fall "cold." The attack improves after treatment with steam, cough medicine and an antibiotic. Two weeks later there is a recurrence, more severe than the first, which is refractory to the previous treatment and progresses to severe respiratory distress with accompanying cyanosis; this improves promptly after treatment with a bronchodilator such as epinephrine or aminophylline. During the next year he appears to have less trouble when milk and peanuts are removed from his diet.

In the two ensuing years, wheezing of varying severity accompanies every respiratory infection. At seven years of age he has asthma attacks without infection, and although by nine years of age foods no longer seem to disagree with him, his respiratory difficulties are obviously worse at particular seasons of the year. He also finds that he cannot ride horseback without wheezing, nor can he handle his dog without mild symptoms. His health remains about the same until he is fourteen years old, when he begins to improve, and by seventeen years of age he no longer has asthma attacks, except for mild wheezing with strenuous exertion. He continues to have hay fever and perennial nasal obstruction made bearable by an occasional dose of antihistamine. For the next two decades he has so little trouble that he forgets he ever had any allergy. At thirty-five years of age, however, he has become an avid gardener and golfer, and while he is engaged in these hobbies his hay fever recurs. Several months later, on a cool damp evening in the fall, he has an attack of asthma. From then on he notices increasing dyspnea on exertion; there is

also coughing and wheezing. Asthma attacks become more and more frequent, so that by the time he is fifty years old he is emphysematous and has almost continuous mild asthma with severe attacks associated with respiratory infection.

Contrary to the usual pattern described above, asthma may begin abruptly in some children; in these cases food sensitivity seldom appears to play a significant role in producing symptoms. Asthma attacks may merely show a gradual increase in severity and frequency. These children are almost invariably sensitive to airborne allergens and have some associated nasal symptoms, with either perennial allergic rhinitis or hay fever. Also, many of them react to changes in temperature and humidity, worsening with every spell of cold, damp weather; sometimes their parents can even predict inclement weather by the child's heightened symptoms. These are children whose chronic nasal obstruction leads to changes in the structure of the mouth and nasal

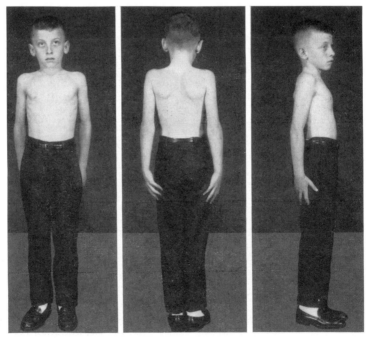

FIGURE 42–7. Asthmatic habitus, showing typical posture of 12-year-old boy with chronic grade III asthma. Note flattened malar bones, circles beneath eyes, narrow nose, protruding upper teeth. Shoulders are squared, supraclavicular area retracted, neck muscles tense, scapulae prominent and anteroposterior chest diameter increased.

passages, producing malocclusion of the jaws and a detrimental cosmetic effect, often improperly termed the "adenoid facies." The narrowing of the upper jaw, with high palate, causes the upper teeth to protrude, and the nasal passage becomes narrow and elongated. The tendency to mouth-breathe directs the flow of air upward against the hard palate. This constant mild pressure on the hard palate may further aggravate the tendency toward elevation in the central part, which, in turn, decreases the size of the nasal passage above. In bypassing the normal cleaning and warming function of the nose, the air which reaches the lungs is also prevented from being in the more or less "steady state" provided by constant humidification. Children with asthma previously associated with perennial allergic rhinitis are more likely to have sinus complications in later years. They also are more apt to have serous otitis media than are the children with the dermal-respiratory syndrome. It appears, however, that serous otitis media is seen less often in the children who have asthma combined with perennial allergic rhinitis than with allergic rhinitis alone.

Although there seems to be no demonstrable reason for it, the asthmatic girl has only half as good a chance of "outgrowing" her ailment around puberty as has the asthmatic boy. The dermal-respiratory syndrome may occur a little more frequently in boys than in girls, and in our series more girls had persistent eczema or neurodermatitis at puberty than did the boys, but the severity and persistence of asthma appeared to be the same in both sexes. Among a very small group of patients (thirty) with right middle lobe syndrome and complicated asthma, the girls outnumbered the boys two to one. This group is too small to permit conclusions, but the incidence in girls appeared to be predominant only in this instance.

The various complications seen in asthma could be woven into the hypothetical asthmatic story, but for brevity they are listed as follows:

1. Other allergic disorders—hay fever, perennial allergic rhinitis, eczema, urticaria, serous otitis media, gastrointestinal allergy, etc.
2. Infection—sinusitis, bronchitis, bronchiolitis, pneumonias (all types), otitis media, tuberculosis, early rubeola
3. Atelectasis—partial, recurrent or chronic with bronchiectasis involving one or more lobes (usually the right middle lobe)
4. Massive collapse of the entire lung
5. Pneumothorax — pneumomediastinum, subcutaneous emphysema
6. Status asthmaticus
7. Emphysema
8. Right-sided cardiac failure
9. Emotional and behavior problems
10. "Adenoid" or "allergic" facies—malformation of the nose and dental arches due to chronic mouth-breathing caused by associated chronic nasal allergy
11. Immunologic disorders, dysgammaglobulinemia.

Certain of these complications deserve special emphasis, but all warrant the same warning—that it is a grave mistake to attribute all respiratory symptoms to asthma and not constantly bear in mind that other lung conditions may be marked by overt wheezing.

Hyperinflation, ultimately culminating in the emphysematous chest with depressed diaphragms and increased anteroposterior chest diameter, is illustrated radiographically in Figure 8. Atelectasis, complete or partial, and usually involving the right middle lobe (Fig. 9), is often the cause of persistent and severe refractory wheezing; this may arise in connection with pneumonia and last long after the pneumonia has cleared. It may also arise from other causes of compression of the right middle lobe (or other) bronchus, or it may be due to endobronchial obstruction by a foreign body, accumulated secretion (mucous plug) or bronchostenosis, sometimes congenital. Endobronchial masses are rarely found in children, although one boy with atelectasis recently had a polypoid fold of mucosa extensively infiltrated with lymphocytic cells obstructing the bronchus. To date no endobron-

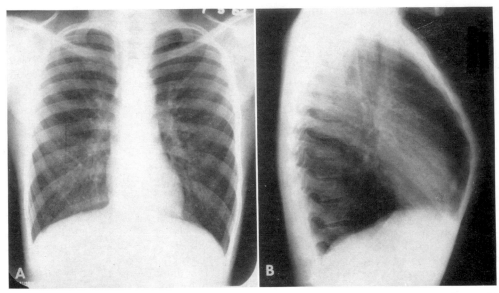

FIGURE 42–8. Roentgenogram of asthmatic chest. *A,* Posteroanterior projection showing radiolucent lungs, low diaphragm, wide interspaces between ribs, and small, centrally placed heart. *B,* Lateral projection. Note the increased radiolucent lung anterior to the heart.

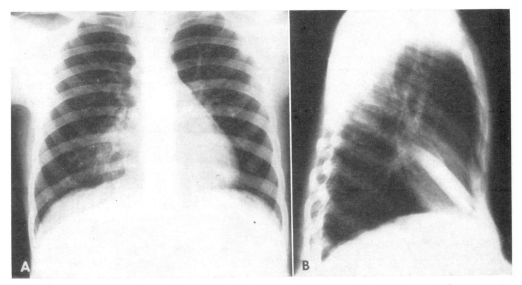

FIGURE 42–9. Atelectasis of right middle lobe during asthma attack. *A,* Posteroanterior roentenogram shows only an indistinctly outlined infiltration along the right cardiac border. *B,* Lateral projection shows a dense area of infiltration representing complete atelectasis of the right middle lobe.

chial malignancies in children have been seen in our clinic, but obviously this a main cause of wheezing and atelectasis in older persons.

Massive collapse rarely occurs in asthma, but is a critical emergency when it does occur. When complete obstruction of a main bronchus is responsible, good intrapulmonary circulation will cause the air to be rapidly absorbed so that the lung becomes atelectatic (Fig. 10). On the other hand, a tiny rupture of an alveolar wall may result in the slow accumulation of air in the extrapleural space, producing pneumothorax and lung collapse. Incessant cough, shift of the mediastinum and its contents, rapid, shallow respirations with no movement of the affected side, deviation of the trachea away from the affected side, hyperresonance and absence of breath sounds are the most frequent findings in pneumothorax. If the process is gradual in the older child whose mediastinum is a little more stable, respiratory embarrassment will be present, but may not be severe. Often the alveolar rupture will close spontaneously, and the intra-

pleural air already present will be slowly resorbed with consequent spontaneous re-expansion of the lung. The air may dissect along the fascial planes into the mediastinum, causing varying degrees of cardiac embarrassment. Other common pathways for extrapleural air are the cervical fascial planes leading to subcutaneous emphysema in the neck and over the chest.

The most dangerous kind of massive collapse is that associated with tension pneumothorax which occurs when a large amount of air enters the pleural space at one time and continues to be drawn into the thorax with each breath. (See the chapter on pneumothorax, page 487.) Such collapse often occurs as a complication of staphylococcal pneumonia, and we have seen it three times in asthmatic children who were receiving treatment with intermittent positive-pressure breathing apparatus (IPPB). It may also occur in asthmatics during the height of a paroxysm of coughing. Prompt thoracotomy with continuous drainage of the pneumothorax is necessary to permit re-expansion

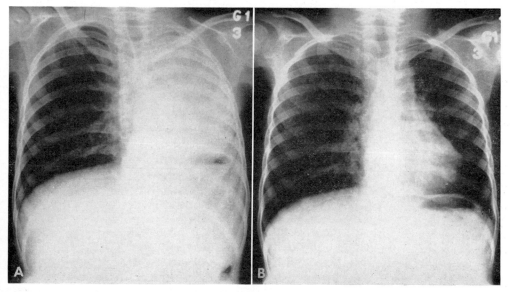

FIGURE 42–10. Massive collapse of the left lung during an asthmatic attack. A, Posteroanterior projection roentgenogram showing trachea deviated to the affected left side, with the heart and mediastinum shifted to the left. Note the elevated left diaphragm as shown by air in the stomach. B, Resolution of density in the left lung, with re-expansion. Note that the trachea is nearer the midline.

of the lung and relieve the respiratory embarrassment.

Status asthmaticus has been described previously in respect to the deranged respiratory metabolism, and treatment will be discussed later. Its frequency in asthmatic children is difficult to estimate. Children who have once suffered status asthmaticus tend to become repeaters; these children almost invariably react in this way to apparently minor respiratory infections. To date no one has offered an entirely satisfactory explanation for the development of status asthmaticus and atelectasis. Although Kravis and Lecks have suggested lack of surfactant or an abnormality in the substance as the causative factor, this attractive hypothesis has not been proved. Although this condition is fortunately infrequent, it accounts for many of the hospital admissions for asthma. A basic emergency routine for such patients should be established in each hospital so that prompt treatment can be instituted and properly monitored by the blood gas and pH determinations to correct metabolic derangements and to prevent irreversible changes.

Prognosis

The various reports on the prognosis of asthma are generally characterized by confusion and discrepancies due largely to the lack of uniformity of methods of sampling, the use of divergent classifications, and the inconsistencies in data inherent in retrospective studies. It is obvious from the preceding discussion of the variables in asthma that the prognosis for either control of symptoms or the eventual disappearance of symptoms ("cure") will differ among children with rare infrequent attacks, those with constant wheezing, and those who are subject to episodes of status asthmaticus. Thus it is inaccurate to base the prognosis on sex, age, duration of disease, or prior treatment. Furthermore, none of the reported studies use uniform criteria for the selection of patients; nor do they separate like kinds of asthma in every respect. Ryssing and Flensborg attempted this, but did not clearly differentiate the types of therapy. Also, in almost all reports some sort of therapy is superimposed on the entire group, thereby coloring the prognosis for the natural course of the illness.

Although recognizing these problems and the capricious nature of asthma, one can nevertheless conclude that an impressive number of asthmatic children lose their symptoms at puberty. This is borne out by the well established observation that boys with asthma outnumber girls two to one under the age of fifteen years, while after that age the sex ratio is nearly equal, and in early and later adulthood

Table 9. *Prognosis in Asthma**

Author	Date	Place	Number of Patients	Cured	Percentage Improved	Unchanged**
Ryssing and Flensborg	1963	Copenhagen	442	37	9	54
Aas	1963	Oslo	174	44	17	39
Wilken-Jensen	1963	Copenhagen	625	65	29	6
Kraepelien	1963	Stockholm	528	29	65	6
Freeman et al.	1964	Colorado	608	57	—	—***
Dees	1957	North Carolina	236	44	36	20
Rackemann	1952	Massachusetts	449<13 yrs.†	31	56	13
			239>13 yrs.	22	26	52

* Based on evaluation of asthmatic patients, both treated and untreated, between adolescence and young adulthood (see text).
** Includes mortalities from asthma or other causes.
*** Not stated.
† Asthma began before 13 years (< 13 yrs.), after 13 years (> 13 yrs.).

Table 10. *Correlation Between Severity and Prognosis in Asthma*

Grade of Disease Attacks/Year		Percentage		Author
		Cured	Improved	
Grade I 0- 5		73	82	Aas
Grade II 5-10		30	30	
Grade III ....10 or more		Less than 30		
Grade I		—	—	Ryssing and Flensborg
Grade II		0	49	
Grade III		0	27	
Grade I		—	—	Wilken-Jensen
Grade II		—	33	
Grade III		—	37	

women asthmatics slightly outnumber men.

The data from the Scandinavian countries, reported in *Acta paediatrica* (1963), probably represent the largest and most nearly comparable series of asthmatics to date, but even here significant differences exist in the selection and grouping of patients, making it impossible to summarize the results and compare them in all respects (Table 9). Nevertheless in each series (Ryssing and Flensborg; Aas; Kraepelien) the percentage of untreated or minimally treated patients reported as asthma-free ("cured") at puberty or after a ten-year follow-up ranged from 30 to 44 per cent. Wilken-Jensen analyzed a series of 625 treated patients and reported 65 per cent to be asthma-free. Investigators concur that prognosis for "cure" or improvement depends on the severity of the asthma (Table 10), multiplicity of allergic diseases, multiple sensitivity, positive family history of allergy, and the duration of disease before the onset of treatment. The more severe and numerous the symptoms, the longer they have been present, and the more allergic the family, the poorer is the prognosis for improvement. Wilken-Jensen, however, found a slightly higher rate of improvement among his treated patients with a positive family history. He suggests that the increased enlightenment in the patient's family regarding allergy may be a possible explanation.

However comforting it may be for the parents of young asthmatic boys to hear that asthma is largely a preadolescent phenomenon, the statistics do not reveal which particular child may "outgrow" asthma, nor do they tell which boy may merely enjoy a free interval between adolescence and early adulthood, only to relapse into wheezing and chronic emphysema in later years (Freeman et al.). In fact, when the evaluation of "cure" is based on examination and pulmonary function studies and not merely on the patient's statement, one finds a far higher number of adolescent boys with asthma than predicted by the alleged "outgrowing" phenomenon which is supposed to occur at puberty. One also finds that upper respiratory and other forms of allergy do not decline in these so-called cured patients and may indeed become more severe at this age. It would appear, then, that there may be a shift in the major shock organ at this age (from bronchi to nose), rather than true loss of allergy—just as a shift from skin to bronchi is often seen at the end of infancy.

The attempts to separate those children who will "outgrow" their sensitivity from those who will not have not been successful.

Treatment

LONG-RANGE TREATMENT. The foregoing discussion of the prognosis in asthma has already alluded to the long-range treatment of asthma. The keystone of this kind of "allergy program" is an evaluation of the patient's general health combined with an accurate assessment of both the specific allergic factors and the nonspecific factors which precipitate symptoms. Specific allergens may be detected by skin, conjunctival or other mucous membrane tests with protein allergy extracts; direct skin tests by scratch or intradermal technique are most frequently used. Indirect skin tests by Prausnitz-Küstner reaction are performed by injection of the serum of the patient's blood into the recipient's skin and the testing of these sites with allergens. Sensitivities can also be detected by inhalation testing or by controlled exposure (such as diet trial).

After the identification of significant allergens and the confirmation by provocative tests, the first step in therapy is the avoidance of the noxious substances. If avoidance is impossible (as in allergies to airborne pollen), a hyposensitization program may be initiated. A series of injections of allergens of gradually increasing potency are administered at intervals to cause the increasing production of antibodies in the allergic patients; sensitivity to the particular antigen is thereby minimized.

Although this form of treatment (hyposensitization) has been used for more than fifty years, the mechanism invoked in the process is incompletely understood (Noon) and is now the subject of active reinvestigation in many laboratories and clinics. It is thought that such injections stimulate the production of an antibody different from the spontaneously occurring skin-sensitive "reagin" (called a "blocking" antibody since it blocks skin tests); this antibody selectively shows greater affinity for the allergen than does the reagin present in the sensitized shock organ or cell. It has therefore been postulated that antigen-antibody union is consummated by the "blocking" antibody, thereby protecting cells from the damage caused by the mediators of an allergic reaction which would otherwise have taken place in some vulnerable tissue such as the bronchial tree or the lungs. There are,

however, many experimental and clinical observations which cannot be reconciled with this oversimplified explanation. For details of these controversial points, as well as the relative merits of aqueous, oil emulsion repository (Loveless) and alum-precipitated pyridine (Allpyral) (Fuchs and Strauss) extracts, of bacterial and fungal vaccines and of various treatment schedules—preseasonal, coseasonal, perennial—the reader is referred to the various texts and specialty journals of allergy.

In some instances the removal of environmental factors will suffice as a preventive measure, as evidenced by the improvement noted when a child who is dog- or cat-sensitive no longer has exposure to the animal, or when egg is removed from the diet of an egg-sensitive child. Since most allergic persons are sensitive to house dust (a substance produced by the aging of cotton linters and other household furnishings), use of precautions to decrease household dust exposure, particularly by setting up a "dust-free" bedroom,* is one of the most common treatment measures. This is accomplished by removing excess room appointments and bric-a-brac, encasing pillows, mattresses, box springs and similar furnishings in airtight plastic covers, or the substitution of synthetic or rubber foam products for these furnishings. These rearrangements and modifications, plus frequent scrupulous cleaning, often supply immediate and significant relief to dust-sensitive children.

Treatment directed toward the nonspecific factors which often trigger allergic symptoms is also important. This includes provision for adequate humidity in the house (especially in winter), protection of the child from temperature extremes, with simultaneous and systematic exposure of the child to temperature differences so that he will develop greater tolerance, and the decrease of exposure to airborne irritants such as dust, pollens and chemicals by the installation of an air conditioner equipped with a special activated-charcoal

---

* Specific instructions for preparing a dust-free bedroom for the patient can be obtained from manufacturers of nonallergic bedding.

filter or an electronic air cleaner. For special problems in which emotional stress plays a leading role, psychotherapy, change of environment, and separation from the family with temporary residence in a foster home or special asthma residence are often utilized with much benefit.

Aerosol therapy is frequently used as a prelude to a breathing exercise program. Any one of several bronchodilator drugs (e.g. epinephrine and isoproterenol, alone or diluted with physiologic saline or with any anionic detergent as Alevaire or Tergemist) is inhaled as an aerosol, ideally of particles 3 to 9 microns in size. Among the several brands of nebulizers which will produce aerosol particles of this size are the DeVilbiss #40 and #640. If this nebulizer is attached to a small compressor (DeVilbiss #501) or to a bicycle pump as a source of pressure, with a gallon jug interposed, an even flow of aerosol is produced which can easily be inhaled (Halpern).

Another technique is the use of an intermittent positive-pressure breathing (IPPB) apparatus to propel the aerosol into the lungs with more force. This method has particular effectiveness in the treatment of acute bronchospasm. Several different manufacturers have efficient IPPB machines, but for technical reasons the Bird seems particularly well suited for use with children. Micronefrin is recommended by the manufacturer as a bronchodilator for use with the Bird machine.

Still other devices for aerosol therapy are the hand-operated bulb or "bomb" type dispensers with the active drug packaged under pressure and propelled by inert gas (Mercer et al.). Epinephrine, isoproterenol and steroids are marketed for nebulization in this aerosol form. Unfortunately, all share the disadvantage of requiring perfect timing and coordination between the peak of inhalation and the full force of aerosol spray to be maximally effective; such coordination and timing are usually impossible to accomplish with small children. Often brief relief is so attractive to patients that they quickly

become "spray addicts" and are unable to be separated from the nebulizer. The danger of repeated constant use of concentrated aerosols lies in chemical irritation of the airway in which a vicious cycle of cough, spray, cough, wheeze is set up.

Corrective breathing and posture exercises, plus general physical fitness programs, are helpful in improving the asthmatic child's exercise tolerance. Certain children can be taught so to control their breathing that they can use exercises designed to relieve shortness of breath and thereby abort the kind of asthmatic attack triggered by a sudden laugh or overexertion. Postural drainage for all or certain lung areas is frequently helpful for the "wet" asthmatic child who has excessive bronchial secretions, and for the patient with copious secretion and cough in the phase of asthma after bronchospasm has been relieved. The child with asthma and concomitant bronchitis, bronchiectasis or atelectasis also benefits from postural drainage. The aid of a physical therapist for instruction and assistance is invaluable, but, lacking this, one may obtain an instructive pamphlet by Livingstone and Reed, Asthma Research Council, London, which illustrates and describes various helpful exercises.* (See chapter on Diagnostic and Therapeutic Procedures, page 80.)

The use of bacterial vaccines in treating asthmatic patients is a controversial subject and may be both a specific and a nonspecific treatment measure. When it is established that a child has a true bacterial sensitivity, treatment with appropriate stock or autogenous bacterial vaccines or extracts may be followed by improvement, or, if tolerance is exceeded, it may provoke actual attacks. Sometimes respiratory bacterial vaccines and extracts are also used for nonspecific protein effect, as were typhoid and pertussis vaccines, sterile milk, snake venom and autohemotherapy injections some years ago. The efficacy of these agents has never been con-

---

* Available through Chicago Medical Book Publishers, Chicago, Ill.

clusively proved by controlled studies, however. The same is true for injections of precipitated sulfur, of extracts of *Rhus quercifolia* (Anergex), bacterial pyrogens (Piromen) and ethylene disulfonate. Other forms of therapy not generally accepted, but still with enthusiastic advocates, are hypnosis, glomectomy (surgical removal of the carotid body), sympathectomy, the Gay treatment (potassium iodide and Fowler's solution), ultraviolet light treatment, inhalation of negative ionized air, ozone, and fumes of "asthma powders," and even sleeping with a chihuahua dog to "take" the asthma, or the wearing of amber beads.

Other conventional and widely applied forms of treatment of respiratory infection in asthmatic children involve the use of antibiotics. Some physicians avoid the use of penicillin in allergic or asthmatic children for fear of aggravating present sensitization or initiating future sensitization; although this practice is certainly defensible in theory, a useful drug should not be denied asthmatic children when it is the drug of choice for significant infection unless there is reason to suspect intolerance to it.

When antibiotics are to be used in an asthmatic child, they should be administered in therapeutic doses for a full therapeutic course, or not at all. It is our impression that microbial drug sensitization and resistance most often arise in the child who receives frequent short courses of an antibiotic which are inadequate to eradicate the infection. Admittedly, viral and bacterial infection may be difficult to differentiate clinically even though it may be presumed that the majority of respiratory illnesses in young children are viral and not amenable to antibiotic therapy. Moreover, it is often impossible to establish immediately whether respiratory symptoms are all due to allergy, to infection or to a combination. The physician is thus led into using antibiotics on occasions when subsequent events may cast doubt on the wisdom of his decision.

There is no easy answer to this dilemma, but some help may be derived from using the policy outlined by Glaser. He recommends treating dubious respiratory symptoms in an allergic child at their earliest onset with immediate bed rest and the administration of antiallergic drugs. The child is then observed for a period of one to several hours; unless definite signs of infection (fever and so forth) develop during this interval, antibiotics are withheld. His response and the developments thereafter then determine whether antiallergic medications are to be repeated or given in more potent form, or whether antibiotics are in order. Since the mother is instructed in this sort of home treatment, there is no delay in commencing therapy; it is well known that allergic symptoms can be most easily aborted or overcome in the earliest stages.

Tonsillectomy and adenoidectomy were once almost routine procedures for asthmatics before falling into disfavor in some quarters because of an alleged increase in the incidence and severity of asthma after surgery. The present consensus among many pediatricians and allergists and some nose and throat surgeons is that indications for tonsillectomy and adenoidectomy should be the same for allergic as for nonallergic children. It also is recommended that operation involving the nasopharynx should not be performed during a pollen season on an asthmatic sensitive to pollen, but should be deferred until allergic symptoms are brought under the best possible control. This policy has been followed in our clinic for many years, and asthma has never apparently worsened after operation in any child in whom these precautions were taken. The children on whom tonsillectomy and adenoidectomy were performed derived the same expected amount of benefit from improved ventilation of the upper airway after operation as nonallergic children with the same operation. We also have a few asthmatic patients in whom these precautions were apparently not taken; they appeared to have a subsequent increase in asthma which may have been coincidental or related to the timing of the operation.

We have been so impressed with the high incidence of family epidemics of infection and with family carriers of pathogens, usually either beta hemolytic streptococci or coagulase-positive staphylococci, among the infection-prone allergic and asthmatic children (Dees), that we now consider a search for such carriers an integral part of the child's treatment. If it were practical to do similar samplings for respiratory viruses among family members, one would undoubtedly find an even higher incidence of infection, and possibly of carriers. Until such testing is possible, however, and until a satisfactory vaccine is generally available for unusually susceptible children, this very important aspect of respiratory illness will continue to be undocumented and without specific treatment.

Much has been written about the gamma globulin levels in allergic children and about the therapeutic use of gamma globulin in large intramuscular or small intradermal doses for the treatment of childhood asthma (Scherr). At this time no clear-cut evidence has been produced to justify the administration of gamma globulin to asthmatics, unless they have one of the accepted conditions indicating its use. These indications, it will be recalled, are measles and infectious hepatitis which gamma globulin may prevent or modify, agammaglobulinemia (as yet unreported in asthma), or hypogammaglobulinemia with low IgG. Recent studies have shown the existence of various hereditary serologic types of gamma globulin to which children who have had multiple transfusions produce antibodies. It therefore seems completely unwarranted to subject a child to the added hazard of gamma globulin sensitivity and the possibility of inducing autoimmune disorders without better indication than is now available.

ACUTE TREATMENT. Acute attacks of asthma should be treated as a medical emergency. It is imperative for physicians, nurses and parents to learn the dictum that the more promptly bronchospasm is relieved, the less medication will be required, the less heroic will treatment need

to be, and the greater likelihood that relief will be complete. It is almost impossible for one who has not experienced acute severe air hunger to appreciate the anxiety and panic this produces. When this physiologic reaction is recognized and appreciated, asthmatics receive better care, and some of their demanding, anxious, clinging behavior is more easily understood and dispelled.

The objectives in treating acute asthma are the relief of bronchial obstruction (a) by bronchodilation, (b) by reduction of the edema of the mucous membranes, and (c) by the removal of excess bronchial secretions, and to prevent and relieve fatigue. The drugs which serve these objectives—bronchodilators, expectorants and sedatives—are listed individually with 24-hour dosage instruction in Table 11.

Rapidly acting bronchodilators are the sympathicomimetic drugs epinephrine (Adrenalin), ephedrine and isoproterenol. These drugs are often supplemented or used in conjunction with xanthines, theophylline and theophylline ethylenediamine (aminophylline) because the latter are equally potent and have a longer-lasting bronchodilating effect. Table 12 lists the most commonly used individual compounds with their trade names. (It is not feasible to list the prescription or over-the-counter antiasthmatic combinations of these drugs, since *Physician's Desk Reference* lists more than 250 now on the market.)

Subcutaneous doses of 0.1 ml. of epinephrine 1:1000 in aqueous solution will rapidly relieve most uncomplicated severe acute asthma; aminophylline (3 mg. per pound) given orally, rectally or intravenously as a single dose is equally effective. Isoproterenol either in solution (1:100 or 1:200) or as a dry powder is used by inhalation, and is also effective when absorbed sublingually. Oral administration of ephedrine or one of its derivatives will usually relieve an attack of asthma at its onset or will control one which is moderate or mild. These drugs are also useful to maintain the brief relaxation effected by more potent and rapidly active bron-

Table 11. *Dosages of Drugs Commonly Used for Allergic Children*[1, 2]

Drug	Dose	Warning
Bronchodilators		
Epinephrine hydrochloride (Adrenalin Chloride) USP	1:1000 aq. 0.01 ml./kg./*DOSE* (Max. 0.5 ml.) Repeat q. 4 h. prn. 1:100 aq. nebulizer prn. 0.1 ml./dose/4 hrs. 1:200 aq. suspension 0.1-0.25 ml./dose/12 hrs. 1:500 oil 0.01-0.02 ml./kg. Daily or every 12 h. im	*Vasopressor*
Ephedrine sulfate USP NF	3 mg./kg./24 hrs. (max. 30 mg./dose) Divide in 4-6 doses (o, sq, iv) Syrup—4 mg./ml.	*Excitation*
Isoproterenol USP, NNR	1:100 0.3 ml.; 1:200 0.5 ml.; 10%, 25% powder for inhalation, 3 × day 0.4 mg./kg./24 hrs. (o), divide in 3 doses	*Palpitation*
Aminophylline USP (Theophylline ethylenediamine)	15 mg./kg./24 hrs. Divide in 4 doses (iv, im, o) Rectal 2 × above	*Poisoning overdose*
Expectorants		
Iodides (saturated solution potassium iodide) USP	1 drop/yr. of age (up to 15 yrs.)** 3 × day in milk or water	*Nausea*
Glyceryl guaiacolate (Robitussin Syrup,* Glycotuss)	10/mg./kg./24 hrs. (o) divide in 3-4 doses 20 mg./ml.	
Ipecac syrup USP	5 drops first year of age** 1 drop per year thereafter per dose May repeat in 2 hrs. (max. 0.5-2 ml.)	*Vomiting Poisoning*
Ammonium chloride USP	75 mg./kg./24 hrs. Divide in 4 doses (o) Give 1 glass water per dose	*Acidosis*
Sedatives		
Phenobarbital USP	6 mg./kg./24 hrs. Divide in 3 doses (o, iv or im)	*Habituation Poisoning*
Chloral hydrate USP (Noctec)*	50 mg./kg./24 hrs. (max. 1 Gm./ dose) Divide 3-4 doses (o or r)	*Liver*
Acetylsalicylic acid USP (Aspirin)	65 mg./kg./24 hrs. Divide in 4-6 doses (o) *Max.* 3.6 Gm./24 hrs.	*Poisoning Acidosis*

* From *Physician's Desk Reference*, Oradel, N. J., Medical Economics, Inc., 1966.
** Spear, Fred: *The Allergic Child*. New York, Hoeber, 1963.
[1] W. Nelson: *Textbook of Pediatrics*. 8th ed., pp. 210-27.
[2] L. S. Goodman and A. Gilman: *Pharmacalogic Basis of Therapeutics*. 2nd ed. New York, Macmillan, 1955.

Key   o = oral.
        sq = subcutaneous.
        im = intramuscular.
        iv = intravenous.
         r = rectal.

Table 12. *Drugs Used as Bronchodilators*

Generic Name	Trade Name
Sympathicomimetic amines	
Epinephrine hydrochloride USP	Adrenalin
	Sus-Phrine
Ethyl-norepinephrine hydrochloride	Bronkephrine
Isoproterenol hydrochloride USP (14)*	Isuprel
	Aludrin (Aerolone)
	Proterenol
Isoproterenol sulfate NNR	Medihaler-iso
	Norisodrine
Ephedrine hydrochloride NF	Ephedrine hydrochloride
Ephedrine sulfate USP (36)*	Isofedrol
	Ephedresol
Racephedrine hydrochloride NF	Ephetonin
Phenylephrine hydrochloride USP (73)*	Neo-Synephrine
	Isophrine
Phenylpropanolamine NNR (42)*	Propadrine
Methoxyphenamine hydrochloride NNR	Orthoxine hydrochloride
Xanthines	
Theophylline USP (34)	
Theophylline-ethylenediamine USP (14)	Aminophylline, Elixophyllin
Choline theophyllinate (oxtriphylline)	Choledyl
Theophylline monoethanolamine	Fleet-Theophylline
Theophylline sodium glycinate NF	Synophylate
Theophylline glyceryl	Iphyllin

*( ) = Number of commercial preparations containing this drug as listed in *Physician's Desk Reference,* Oradell, N. J., Medical Economics, Inc., 1966.

chodilators such as epinephrine, aminophylline or isoproterenol. To counteract the stimulation and excitation they may produce, they are usually combined with a sedative. One should never give morphine for a severe asthmatic attack, however, since this suppresses the respiratory center and has apparently supplied the *coup de grâce* in many reported fatal attacks of asthma. For the same reason and because of the ease of addiction, meperidine (Demerol) and the repeated use of other opiates, such as codeine, should be avoided.

The side effects of all these bronchodilating compounds are excitation, nervousness, wakefulness, headache, tremor and tachycardia. Epinephrine and ephedrine raise blood pressure, and isoproterenol tends to produce flushing, palpitation and dizziness. The xanthines act as diuretics and gastric irritants, and they may cause vomiting and diarrhea. As their effect is cumulative, intoxication from overdose may result in convulsions, coma and sometimes in fatality (White and Daeschner). When given too rapidly by the intravenous route, aminophylline may cause an alarming drop in systolic blood pressure. It should always be given in a sufficient volume of fluid (5 per cent dextrose solution) to require at least one-half hour for administration, and preferably should be given as a slow intravenous drip of 2 to 2.5 mg. per pound every eight to twelve hours. When rectal suppositories (Dees, 1943) or instillation is used, care must be taken that the rectum is empty in order for the drug to be absorbed promptly. Rectal doses of 3 mg. per pound every eight hours in children over four years of age are recommended; this usually affords effective and long-lasting relief. Rarely, a child will complain of local burning or pain in the legs after the use of suppositories.

Aminophylline should be utilized with care. Side effects include nausea and vomiting and convulsions. Aminophylline intoxication may be fatal.

Water, as steam and by mouth, is the most effective means of liquefying secretions. This must be constantly kept in mind, especially when the child is ill with acute, severe asthma, or when there has been a severe attack of asthma of several days' duration and he has become dehydrated. Expectorants are the usual type of drug used in both acute and chronic asthma to assist in the liquefying of secretions; the patient is thus more readily able to rid himself of these secretions by coughing them up. Those most useful are potassium iodide or other iodides, glyceryl guaiacolate and syrup of ipecac.

The variation and combination of proprietary antiasthmatic preparations is bewildering in number and complexity. Many pharmaceutical companies have added sedatives (chiefly barbiturates), antihistamines, and occasionally salicylates and corticosteroids. None of these offers any real, basic advantage over the simple drugs used alone or compounded to order, however, except possibly a minor economic one. Furthermore, they invite the hazard of prescribing by "name" and the danger of ordering an inflexible combination with possible excess of certain ingredients. If combined therapy is used, one should thoroughly familiarize himself with one or two combinations and use these whenever practical.

Relief of the symptoms of severe asthma was one of the first recognized clinical applications for the adrenal corticosteroid compounds. After the first flush of en-

thusiasm, however, there has been increased recognition of the occurrence of steroid dependency and undesirable side effects; these include cushingoid changes, increased susceptibility to infection, arrest or retardation in growth, and rarely pseudotumor cerebri—all features which seriously detract from the general usefulness and safety of steroids for children.

When first introduced, ACTH given intravenously in a 10- to 20-mg. dose over a twelve-hour period was often used for treating status asthmaticus. This is still good treatment for this purpose, provided the child's adrenal cortex is capable of maximal stimulation. The possibility of encountering unresponsive or suppressed adrenal function, or more rarely anaphylaxis to ACTH, has made this mode of treatment less popular than formerly. ACTH gel (injected intramuscularly) is similarly used for less severe allergic symptoms when a longer action depot effect is desired (Table 13); the same potential hazard of sensitivity exists with the gel as with the aqueous preparation.

The corticosteroids, of which there have been many synthetic derivatives since Compound E was identified, are in more general use at present. These are listed with equivalent biologically active doses, trade names and manufacturers in Table 14. These drugs are preferable to ACTH in that they are effective when given by mouth, they replace or supplement and do not require an active adrenal response, and they have not been observed to cause sensitization. The dose of 25 to 37.5 mg. of cortisone or hydrocortisone is appar-

Table 13. *Adrenocorticotropic Hormone Preparations Used in Asthma**

Trade Name	Manufacturer	Dose (for All Preparations)
H-P Acthar Gel	Armour	Infants, 20-40 units/24 hrs.
H-P Acthar Sol		Children, 1-2 units/kg./24 hrs.
ACTH Gel	National	Aqueous, divide in 4 doses IM.
ACTH Sol		Gel, daily or in 2 doses IM.
Cortrophin-Zinc	Organon	
Depo ACTH Sol	Upjohn	
Duracton	Nordic	
El Acorte Gel	Breon	

* From *Physician's Desk Reference.* Oradell, N. J., Medical Economics, Inc., 1966.

Table 14.   *Equivalent Doses of Corticosteroids Used in Asthma**

Generic Name	Trade Name	Manufacturer
Cortisone acetate	Cortisone Acetate	Upjohn
25 mg.	Cortone Acetate	Merck Sharp & Dohme
	Cortogen	Schering
Hydrocortisone	Hydrocortone	Merck Sharp & Dohme
20 mg.	Cortef	Upjohn
	Cortril	Pfizer
Prednisone	Meticorten	Schering
5 mg.	Deltasone	Upjohn
	Deltra	Merck Sharp & Dohme
	Delta-Dome	Dome Chemical
	Paracort	Parke Davis
	Prednisone	West-ward
Prednisolone	Meticortelone	Schering
5 mg.	Delta-Cortef	Upjohn
	Sterane	Pfizer
	Hydeltra	Merck Sharp & Dohme
	Predne-Dome	Dome Chemical
	Prednisolone	West-ward
	Paracortol	Parke Davis
	Prednis-C.V.P.	U. S. Vitamin
	Sterolone	Rowell
	Prednisolone	Rexall
Methyl prednisolone	Medrol	Upjohn
4 mg.	Wyacort	Wyeth
Triamcinolone	Aristocort	Lederle
4 mg.	Kenacort	Squibb
Betamethasone	Celestone	Schering
0.6 mg.		
Dexamethasone	Decadron	Merck Sharp & Dohme
0.75 mg.	Deronil	Schering
	Dexameth	U. S. Vitamin
	Gammacorten	Ciba
	Hexadrol	Organon
Paramethasone acetate	Haldrone	Lilly
2 mg.		

* From *Physician's Desk Reference.* Oradell, N. J., Medical Economics, Inc., 1966.

ently the basic daily amount equivalent to the amount of hormone required for the survival of an adrenalectomized person or one with suppressed adrenals. The biologic activity of 25 mg. of cortisone is equal to 5 mg. of prednisone. Cortisone, hydrocortisone and prednisone appear to slow growth less than the other corticosteroids, although there is less sodium retention and possibly less hypertension with the newer drugs. The advantage of the smaller dosage (in milligrams) of the latest synthetic variations is highly questionable. The dose of corticosteroids for asthma cannot be based on age or weight, but must be determined by pharmacologic need. In status asthmaticus we have sometimes used 400 to 600 mg. of hydrocortisone per day for several days, and in less severe asthma a five- to seven-day course has been commenced with 100 mg. of cortisone or the equivalent, decreased as tolerated thereafter (Dees and McKay).

We agree with many others who find it difficult to refrain from using steroids when other drugs seem ineffective, even though the more often steroids are used in a patient, the more difficult it may be to forego them the next time. Eventually, continuous use may develop insidiously because of decreasing symptom-free intervals without the drug. In such instances the problems imposed on the patient by intractable or poorly controlled asthma must be weighed against those attending the long-term use of steroids.

STATUS ASTHMATICUS. The treatment of status asthmaticus must be individualized, since there will be some patients with complicating conditions or some who are more ill and refractory than others. By definition, status asthmaticus is a continuous state of severe asthma resistant for more than twenty-four hours to vigorous therapeutic measures, particularly to epinephrine injections. The general principles which serve as a therapeutic guide (to be modified, of course, as necessary) are outlined in Table 15.

As the attack subsides, one may change to oral administration of fluids and medication, utilize postural drainage and breathing exercises to help remove secretion, and discontinue steroids and other heroic treatment as rapidly as feasible. No attempt should be made to perform diagnostic allergy tests immediately after an episode of status asthmaticus, since the results will probably be unreliable, owing to unreactive skin. There seems to be a tendency for certain children to have repeated attacks of status asthmaticus; in some no obvious irritating cause can be found, and in others localized lung disease is discovered after careful investigation.

At the earliest opportune time these

Table 15.   *Treatment of Status Asthmaticus*

1. Immediate hospitalization
2. Immediate intravenous administration of fluids to correct dehydration, liquefy secretion, and provide route for medication
3. Sedatives: mild for rest and relaxation—choral hydrate, small doses of barbiturates (e.g. phenobarbital), paraldehyde, Librium (chlordiazepoxide), ether and olive oil in equal parts given per rectum (1 to 2 ounces)
4. Bronchodilators: aminophylline intravenously or per rectum, isoproterenol or epinephrine, Micronephrine per aerosol or by IPPB (aminophylline may restore the effectiveness of epinephrine by injection)
5. Expectorants: steam, sodium iodide intravenously, potassium iodide, glyceryl guaiacolate or syrup of ipecac, orally
6. Corticosteroids: intravenous doses of 100 mg. of Solu-Cortef or equivalent of other steroids repeated as needed every 4 to 8 hours, and later given orally; in selected cases, ACTH, 10 to 20 mg. given intravenously over 12-hour period
7. Antibiotics: full therapeutic dose
8. Oxygen and steam: as indicated
9. Digitalis: if cardiac strain is present (follow with electrocardiogram)
10. Correct metabolic imbalance with sodium lactate, sodium bicarbonate electrolytes, or THAM buffer
11. Other treatment, occasionally indicated:
    a. Tracheal suction
    b. Bronchoscopy
    c. Tracheostomy
    d. Assisted respiration (by respirator)
12. Procedures for diagnosis and monitoring of the patient's condition:
    a. Chest x-ray—posteroanterior and lateral (portable if necessary)
    b. Cultures of nasopharynx, sputum and tracheal aspirate
    c. Blood gas and pH determination at frequent intervals as indicated
    d. Blood electrolytes, as above
    e. Blood cell count and urinalysis
    f. Stool specimen for blood if steroids are used
    g. Blood pressure one or more times daily
    h. Eye grounds examination daily for papilledema in comatose patients

children should undergo a thorough allergic study and be started on appropriate treatment to prevent recurrence. There is no more alarming situation than status asthmaticus, nor one which calls for more prompt, persistent, coordinated treatment or constant vigilance from medical personnel, who must conceal their own anxiety from the frightened child and family in order to be effective. Respiratory failure and death do occur in status asthmaticus, though rarely. Because a child may have a dangerous degree of carbon dioxide retention in a matter of a few minutes, and one or two coughs may be the only prelude to asphyxia, the acutely ill child should *never* be left unattended.

Summary

It should be apparent at this point that asthma embraces more than one disease and that the gamut of the clinical syndrome—its pathophysiology, etiology and immunology—embraces many different disciplines. The various approaches to comprehensive treatment and management, about which we know a great deal without fully understanding the fundamental causes of allergy, are complex. The physician dealing with asthma must be a "jack-of-all-trades," able to change tempo in a moment from the considered atmosphere of the consultation room to the supercharged tension of emergency surgery.

Fresh approaches in research into the nature of asthma must be found. Parents must be encouraged to take a middle course in their attitudes between overprotection and freedom. The severely involved child must be treated supportively with relief from his anxiety, while he is simultaneously being taught to care for himself within his limitations. Finally, the general public, educators and public health officials must be educated about asthma and its problems and informed of the heavy toll which illness from asthma takes from school children and young adults in their most productive years.

REFERENCES

Aas, K.: Prognosis for Allergic Children. *Acta paediat.* (Stockholm) (Suppl. 140), 87:81, 1963; *Pediatrics*, 21:980, 1958.

Abernathy, R. S., and others: Chronic Asthma in Childhood. Double Blind Study of Treatment with Gamma Globulin. *Pediatrics*, 21: 980, 1958.

Allen, J. C., and Kunkel, H. G.: Antibodies to Genetic Types of Gamma Globulin After Multiple Transfusions. *Science*, 139:419, 1963.

Bates, D. V., and Christie, R. V.: *Respiratory Function in Disease*. Philadelphia, W. B. Saunders Company, 1964, p. 131.

Bray, G. W.: *Recent Advances in Allergy*. 3rd ed. Philadelphia, Blakiston, 1937.

Brocklehurst, W. E.: Histamine and Other Mediators in Hypersensitivity Reactions; in B. N. Halpern, and A. Holtzer (Eds.): *Reports of the Third International Congress of Allergology*. Paris, Flammarion, 1958.

Idem: A Slow-Reacting Substance in Anaphylaxis—"SRS-A"; in G. E. W. Wolstenholme, and C. A. O'Connor (Eds.): *Ciba Foundation Symposium*: Jointly with the Physiological Society and the British Pharmacological Society on Histamine: Honouring Sir Henry Dale. Boston, Little, Brown and Co., 1956.

Buffum, W. P.: The Prognosis of Asthma in Infancy. *Pediatrics*, 32:453, 1963.

Coca, A. F., and Cooke, R. A.: On the Classification of the Phenomena of Hypersensitiveness. *J. Immunol.*, 8:163, 1923.

Cohen, S., and Porter, R. R.: Structure and Biological Activity of Immunoglobulins; in *Advances in Immunology*. New York, Academic Press, Inc., 1964, vol. 4, pp. 287-342.

Comroe, J. H.: *Physiology of Respiration*. Chicago, Year Book Publishers, Inc., 1965.

Comroe, J. H., and others: *The Lung*. 2nd ed. Chicago, Year Book Publishers, Inc., 1962.

Cooke, R. A.: *Allergy in Theory and Practice*. Philadelphia, W. B. Saunders Company, 1947, p. 139.

Cooke, R. A., and Vander Veer, A.: Human Sensitization. *J. Immunol.*, 1:201, 1916.

Crawford, J. D., and others: Observations of a Metabolic Lesion in Cow's Milk Allergy. *Pediatrics*, 22:122, 1958.

Crook, W. G.: The Allergic Tension-Fatigue Syndrome; in F. Speer (Ed.): *The Allergic Child*. New York, Paul B. Hoeber, Inc., 1963, Chap. 21.

Dees, S. C.: The Value of the Weltmann Serum Coagulation Reaction in Allergic Disease. *South. Med. J.*, 34:586, 1941.

Idem: The Use of Aminophylline Rectal Suppositories in Treatment of Bronchial Asthma. *J. Allergy*, 14:492, 1943.

Idem: Development and Course of Asthma in Children. *Am. J. Dis. Child.*, 93:228, 1957.

Idem: Infection and the Allergic Child. *Virginia Med. Monthly*, 87:607, 1960.

Idem: Asthma in Infants and Young Children. *J.A.M.A.*, 175:362, 1961.

Dees, S. C., and Grunt, J. A.: A Survey of the Serum Protein Electrophoresis Pattern in Allergic Children. *Ann. Allergy*, 18:50, 1960.

Dees, S. C., and McKay, H. W.: Occurrence of Pseudotumor Cerebri (Benign Intracranial Hypertension) During Treatment of Children with Asthma by Adrenal Steroids. *Pediatrics*, 23:1143, 1959.

Dennis, E. V., Hornbrook, M. M., and Ishizaka, K.: Serum Proteins in Sputum of Patients with Asthma. *J. Allergy*, 35:464, 1964.

Engström, I.: Respiratory Studies in Children. XI. Mechanics of Breathing, Lung Volumes and Ventilatory Capacity in Asthmatic Children from Attack to Symptom-Free Status. *Acta paediat.*, Suppl. 155, 1964.

Idem: Respiratory Studies in Children. XII. Serial Studies of Mechanics, Breathing, Lung Volumes and Ventilatory Capacity in Provoked Asthmatic Attacks. *Acta paediat.*, 53: 345, 1964.

Falliers, C. J.: Corticosteroids and Anabolic Hormones for Childhood Asthma. *Clin. Pediat.*, 4:441, 1965.

Freeman, G. L., and others: Allergic Diseases in Adolescents. I. Description of Survey; Prevalence of Allergy. *Am. J. Dis. Child.*, 107:549, 1964.

Freeman, G. L., and others: Allergic Diseases in Adolescents. II. Changes in Allergic Manifestations During Adolescence. *Am. J. Dis. Child.*, 107:560, 1964.

Fuchs, A. M., and Strauss, M. B.: The Clinical Evaluation and the Preparation and Standardization of Suspension of a New Water-Insoluble Whole Ragweed Pollen Complex. *J. Allergy*, 30:66, 1959.

Gharib, R., and others: Sweat Chloride Concentration. A Comparative Study in Children with Bronchial Asthma and with Cystic Fibrosis. *Am. J. Dis. Child.*, 109:66, 1965.

Glaser, J.: *Allergy in Childhood.* Springfield, Ill., Charles C Thomas, 1956.

Halpern, S., and others: Practical Tips on Aerosol Therapy in Asthma. *Am. J. Dis. Child.*, 107:280, 1964.

Hansel, F. K.: *Allergy of the Nose and Paranasal Sinuses.* St. Louis, C. V. Mosby Company, 1936.

Hsia, D. Y.-Y., and others: Abnormal Sweat Electrolytes in Patients with Allergies. *Am. J. Dis. Child.*, 96:685, 1959.

Kallós, P., and Waksman, B. H. (Eds.): *Progress in Allergy.* Basel and New York, S. Karger, 1965, Vols. I-IX.

Kassirer, J. P., and Bleich, H. L.: Rapid Estimation of Plasma Carbon Dioxide Tension from pH and Total Carbon Dioxide Content. *New England J. Med.*, 272:1067, 1965.

Keeney, E. L.: The Pathology of Corticosteroid-Treated Asthma. *J. Allergy*, 36:97, 1965.

Kim, C.-J., and others: Ciliocytophoria (CCP) in Asthmatic Children. *J. Allergy*, 35:159, 1964.

Kraepelien, S.: Prognosis of Asthma in Childhood, with Special Reference to Pulmonary Function and the Value of Specific Hyposensitization. *Acta paediat.*, (Suppl. 140), 87:92, 1963.

Kraepelien, S., Engström, I., and Karlberg, P.: Respiratory Studies in Children. II. Lung Volumes in Symptom-Free Asthmatic Children, 6-14 Years of Age. *Acta paediat.*, 47: 399, 1958.

Kravis, L. P., and Lecks, H. I.: Therapeutic Aerosols in Childhood Asthma. A Review with Clinical Observations on Two New Preparations. *Clin. Pediat.*, 4:193, 1965.

Livingstone, J. L., and Reed, J. M.: *Exercises for Asthma and Emphysema.* 9th ed. Asthma Research Council, King's College, Strand, London, 1957.

Logan, G. B.: Mechanism of the Immediate Allergic Reaction and Some Therapeutic Implications. *Am. J. Dis. Child.*, 97:163, 1959.

Idem: Steps Toward a Better Understanding of the Acute Allergic Reaction. *Ann. Allergy*, 18:17, 1960.

London, A. H., Jr.: The Composition of an Average Pediatric Practice. *J. Pediat.*, 10:762, 1937.

Loveless, M. H.: Repository Injections in Pollen Allergy. *J. Immunol.*, 79:68, 1957.

Marks, M. B.: Significance of Discoloration in the Lower Orbitopalpebral Grooves in Allergic Children (Allergic Shiners). *Ann. Allergy*, 21:26, 1963.

Mendes, E., and others: Immunochemical Studies of the Asthmatic Sputum. *Acta allerg.*, 18:17, 1963.

Mercer, T. T., and others: Output Characteristics of Several Commercial Nebulizers. *Ann. Allergy*, 23:314, 1965.

Miller, F. F.: Eosinophilia in the Allergic Population. *Ann. Allergy*, 23:177, 1965.

Noon, L.: Prophylactic Inoculation Against Hay-Fever. *Lancet*, 1:1572, 1911.

Pecora, L. J., and Bernstein, I. L.: Pulmonary Diffusing Capacity in Children with Intractable Asthma with and Without Chronic Hyperinflation of the Lung. *J. Allergy*, 35: 479, 1964.

Rackemann, F. M.: Intrinsic asthma. *J. Allergy*, 11:147, 1940.

Raffel, S.: *Immunity.* 2nd ed. New York, Appleton-Century-Crofts, Inc., 1961, pp. 300-302.

Rapaport, H. G., Appel, S. J., and Szanton, V. L.: Incidence of Allergy in a Pediatric Population. Pilot Survey of 2,169 Children. *Ann. Allergy*, 18:45, 1960.

Ratner, B., Crawford, L. V., and Flynn, J. A.: Allergy in the Infant and Preschool Child. *Am. J. Dis. Child.*, 91:593, 1956.

Ryssing, E., and Flensborg, E. W.: Prognosis After Puberty for 442 Asthmatic Children Examined and Treated on Specific Allergologic Principles. *Acta paediat.*, 52:97, 1963.

Scherr, M. S.: The Intradermal Use of Human Immune Globulin in Allergic Conditions. A Double Blind Study. *Rev. Allergy & Appl. Immunology*, 19:289, 1965.

Schiffer, C. G., and Hunt, E. P.: Illness Among Children (Data from U.S. National Health Survey). Children's Bureau Publ. No. 405. Washington, D.C., U.S. Dept. of Health, Education, and Welfare, 1963.

Selye, H.: *The Mast Cells.* London, Butterworth, 1965.

Shelley, W. B.: The Circulating Basophile as an Indicator of Hypersensitivity in Man. *Arch. Derm. Syph.*, 88:759, 1963.

Spain, W. C., and Cooke, R. A.: Studies in Specific Hypersensitiveness. II. The Familial Occurrence of Hay Fever and Bronchial Asthma. *J. Immunol.*, 9:521, 1924.

Spock, A.: Growth Patterns in 200 Asthmatic Children. *Ann. Allergy,* 23:608, 1965.

Standish, E., and others: *Why Patients See Doctors.* Seattle, University of Washington Press, 1955, p. 35.

Stiehm, E. R., and Fudenberg, H. H.: Antibodies to Gamma Globulin in Infants and Children Exposed to Isologous Gamma Globulin. *Pediatrics*, 35:229, 1965.

U.S. Dept. of Health, Education, and Welfare: Vital Statistics of the United States. Washington, D.C., 1963, Vol. IIA.

Van Metre, T. E., and Pinkerton, H. L., Jr.: Growth Suppression in Asthmatic Children Receiving Prolonged Therapy with Prednisone or Methylprednisone. *J. Allergy*, 30: 103, 1959.

Voorhorst, R.: *Basic Facts of Allergy.* Leiden, H. E. Stenfert, Kroese N. V., 1962.

Wilken-Jensen, K.: Prognosis of Asthma in Childhood. *Acta paediat.* (Suppl. 140), 87:90, 1963.

White, B. H., and Daeschner, C. W.: Aminophylline poisoning in Children. *J. Pediat.,* 49: 262, 1956.

CHAPTER FORTY-THREE

Pneumothorax and Pneumomediastinum

ROBERT H. HIGH, M.D.

Pneumothorax and pneumomediastinum may occur alone or may be associated with each other. The mechanisms by which these develop have been described elsewhere (see the Chapter on Emphysema, p. 396). Pneumothorax and pneumomediastinum may occur in the newborn infant (see Chap. 5) and are most commonly noted in those infants who had difficulty in initiating respiration. They seem to be more frequent in infants who were resuscitated with some mechanical respirator or in those who were assisted in breathing by insufflation such as mouth-to-mouth resuscitation. The impression should not be left, however, that the method of resuscitation was solely responsible for the development of pneumothorax or pneumomediastinum, since the infant may well have had some abnormality in its lungs. In older infants and children, pneumothorax and pneumomediastinum are usually secondary to diseases producing obstructive emphysema or to surgical procedures in the cervical region. Pneumothorax is usually unilateral, but may be bilateral. Serous fluid may develop in the pleural cavity, leading to the occurrence of hydropneumothorax. When the pneumothorax is secondary to an infectious process, the pleural cavity may rapidly become infected, leading to a pyopneumothorax. These latter developments are common with staphylococcal pneumonia (see Chap. 21). Pneumothorax occasionally occurs without known cause (spontaneous pneumothorax), but this is uncommon until adolescence or early adult life. Those persons who have repeated episodes of spontaneous pneumothorax are often ultimately found to have some abnormality of the lung. Subcutaneous emphysema (see p. 401) may be associated with either disturbance.

The symptoms of pneumothorax are chiefly secondary to compression of the lung, sometimes the great vessels, and to the irritative effects of air in the pleural cavity. The symptoms of the underlying disease, such as pneumonia or lung abscess, are also present. The onset of pneumothorax is usually manifested by the sudden appearance of chest pain, dyspnea and tachypnea. Cyanosis may be noted. When pneumothorax occurs bilaterally, the symptoms are severe, and occasionally death occurs before treatment can be undertaken. Minimal accumulations of pleural air may produce few symptoms, and the pneumothorax may be a coincidental roentgenographic finding.

The physical examination (see Chap. 2) reveals changes dependent upon the extent of the pneumothorax. In those of minimal extent, no abnormality may be apparent. A large pneumothorax is associated with a hyperresonant percussion note, and auscultation reveals the breath sounds to be diminished or absent. The trachea and the heart may be shifted to the opposite side. When fluid is present, a sharp delineation of its extent can often be made because of the hyperresonant percussion note over the collection of air associated with a dull to flat note over the area where the serous fluid or purulent exudate is present.

The symptoms of pneumomediastinum are chiefly those of respiratory and circulatory distress secondary to compression of the trachea and great vessels. Dyspnea, tachypnea and chest pain, chiefly substernal, are common.

Physical examination may reveal an anterior bulge of the thorax; this finding is most often seen in newborn and young infants. The area beneath the sternum is more resonant to percussion because of the collection of air in the mediastinum. Auscultation over the mediastinal area reveals a peculiar sound, the mediastinal crunch, produced by the cardiovascular and respiratory movements. Cyanosis may be present and, because of compression of the blood vessels, may be more evident in the upper part of the body.

Roentgenographic examination of the chest is useful to demonstrate the extent of either of these disturbances. In pneumomediastinum, air may outline the thymus, producing an angular area lateral to the cardiac border. This has been likened to the sail of a boat. Air may also be detected in the neck or abdomen when pneumomediastinum is present.

Pneumomediastinum and pneumothorax may follow perforation of the esophagus. These circumstances, though uncommon, are serious because of the likely complication of suppurative mediastinitis.

Treatment of the underlying disease, when such is present, must continue. Patients with pneumothorax of minimal extent may require no treatment other than the relief of pain, but they must be observed closely for increasing respiratory distress. When the pneumothorax is large, symptoms can usually be relieved by performing a thoracentesis and aspirating as much air as possible. Often one aspiration of the pneumothorax is sufficient, and residual air is absorbed. Such is often the case if the cause is corrected or improves spontaneously, as in diseases such as asthma or bronchiolitis. If the pneumothorax reaccumulates and produces respiratory distress after the initial aspiration, continuous closed intrapleural drainage is recommended as in empyema (see p. 343). This procedure is recommended initially in the presence of extensive bilateral pneumothorax. If pneumothorax persists, the presence of a bronchopleural fistula is likely, and surgical exploration may be indicated.

Roentgenographic examination will help in the diagnosis of some disturbances which may simulate pneumothorax, including congenital lobar emphysema (see p. 530), congenital cystic adenomatoid malformation of the lung (see p. 536), congenital diaphragmatic hernia (see p. 505), postpneumonic pneumatoceles, and the like.

Pneumothorax which follows the rupture of a postpneumonic pneumatocele deserves special mention. Such pneumatoceles seldom rupture, but when they do, they are best treated by continuous closed intrapleural drainage, since most resolve rather quickly. Surgical treatment of pneumatoceles is rarely necessary.

Pneumomediastinum is often of small extent and does not require treatment, since the air is absorbed rapidly. These circumstances are usual when the air has entered the mediastinum after tracheostomy or other surgical manipulations in the neck. Also, the minimal degree of pneumomediastinum which occurs in pneumothorax in which the site of air leakage is from ruptured pulmonary alveoli usually requires no specific treatment. Massive pneumomediastinum which produces pulmonary or circulatory distress is an emergency situation requiring immediate relief. Aspiration of the mediastinum by needle and suction is usually helpful. This procedure may be performed under fluoroscopic guidance. Occasionally surgical drainage with continuous suction is necessary.

When pneumomediastinum is secondary to rupture of the esophagus, prompt surgical drainage of the mediastinum is indicated. Intensive antimicrobial treatment, as in the treatment of putrid empyema (see p. 344) or putrid lung abscess (see p. 337), should be initiated immediately.

The routine administration of antibiotic agents is not indicated for prophylactic purposes in patients with uncomplicated pneumothorax or pneumomediastinum.

REFERENCES

Becker, A. H., and others: Mediastinal Emphysema. *Clin. Pediatrics,* 3:335-8, 1964.

Chasler, C. N.: Pneumothorax and Pneumomediastinum in the Newborn. *Amer. J. Roentgen.,* 91:550-59, 1964.

High, R. H.: Pneumothorax and Pneumomediastinum; in S. S. Gellis and B. M. Kagan (Eds.): *Current Pediatric Therapy* 1966-1967. Philadelphia, W. B. Saunders Company, 1966, pp. 154-5.

Jan, S. Y., Rudolph, A. J., and Teng, C. T.: Pneumomediastinum in Infancy. *J. Pediat.,* 62:754-61, 1963.

Lodan, W. D., Jr., Pausa, S. G., and Crispin, R. H.: Spontaneous Pneumothorax of the Newborn. *Dis. of Chest,* 42:611-14, 1962.

Reams, G. B.: Simplified Treatment of Pneumothorax. *J.A.M.A.,* 183:901, 1963.

Vines, R.: Suction Drainage for Pneumothorax in Neonates. *M.J. Australia,* 50:202-203, 1963.

Welch, K. J.: Pneumothorax; in S. S. Gellis and B. M. Kagan (Eds.): *Current Pediatric Therapy* 1966-1967. Philadelphia, W. B. Saunders Company, 1966, pp. 133-4.

SECTION X

Other Diseases
with a Prominent
Respiratory Component

CHAPTER FORTY-FOUR

Congenital Malformations of the Lower Respiratory Tract

ARNOLD M. SALZBERG, M.D.

STERNAL CLEFTS

A partial or total midline vertical split in the sternum represents a persistence of the embryonic separation of the two sternal cartilage bars which have failed to unite (Hansen). This can be associated with an ectopic but otherwise normal heart or ectopia cordis with intrinsic congenital cardiac disease. Sternal clefts may also accompany a more complex abnormality with pathologic apertures in the abdominal wall, diaphragm and pericardium and a herniated, malformed heart.

The midline defect is appreciated on physical examination. The paradoxical movements of the anterior chest wall and the subcutaneous cardiac dance are specific findings.

The unfused sternal bars of the flexible chest wall can be surgically apposed in the neonatal period. Sabiston has described a sound method of repair in the older infant by oblique mobilization of the costal cartilages. Autogenous cartilage has also been advocated in this situation.

PECTUS CARINATUM

This is an uncommon structural deformity of the sternum in which segmental or total sternal protrusion occurs with or without unilateral or bilateral costal cartilage recession.

The surgical indications are cosmetic and psychic.

The operative procedure consists of variously placed sternal osteotomes and chondrectomy of offending cartilages.

Mortality and morbidity are very low, and the immediate and long-term results are satisfactory.

PECTUS EXCAVATUM (FUNNEL CHEST)

There are characteristic morphologic deformities in pectus excavatum which have been known since antiquity and make the diagnosis fairly obvious on inspection. Physiologic implications and therapy are not quite so standardized, however; these are under current scrutiny and debate and have not been unanimously resolved.

The three anatomic segments of the sternum are not equally involved in pectus excavation. The superior manubrium is normal. The sharp slope inward, toward the vertebral column, begins at the manubrio-gladiolar junction, and the depression is deepest at the gladiolar-xiphoid articulation. The depth of this concavity varies widely from a shallow excavation to near contact with the vertebral column. The xiphoid or ensiform may then proceed outward, deviate laterally, or become rotated. Deformities of the lower costal cartilages form an essential part of the malformation. From the costochondral junctions, the cartilages proceed away from the chest wall, then angulate sharply

493

inward toward their sternal attachments and thus become abnormal in length and direction.

Etiologic concepts are legion, but can be distilled into a workable number. Both Brodkin and Chin have implicated a functional deficiency of the anterior diaphragm which, by default, allows the unopposed remaining diaphragm to distort a pliable sternum and costal cartilages. Respiratory obstruction cannot be a frequent causative factor, but may aggravate an existing deformity. Bowers has emphasized defective pectoral muscles, while Brown described a short central tendon running between the diaphragm and the sternum. These two factors are not consistently present. An arresting etiologic possibility is that of a primary, misdirected, excessive growth of cartilage which eventually drives the lower part of the sternum backward. Of course, simultaneous or sequential diaphragmatic weakness with cartilage overgrowth is also a possibility.

The degree of structural deformity at birth may be minimal or extensive and remain stationary, progress or regress. With age, growth of the thorax in an anteroposterior direction is restricted, but lateral development is uninhibited, and the disparity in the different diameters becomes obvious. Functionally, in the newborn and the infant, the labile breast bone may move paradoxically, but this relents with fixation and rigidity, and a deeply concave pectus may move normally with respiration as the child becomes older.

The depth of the gladiolar-ensiform excavation influences the position and volume of the intrathoracic viscera. There is cardiac compression between the sternum and vertebrae or dislocation of the heart into the left hemithorax with encroachment on the space occupied by the left lung. The basis for pulmonary and cardiac dysfunction exists, and the right side of the heart appears especially vulnerable, but it is difficult to document physiologic aberrations precisely. Bates and Christy conclude that no consistent data have been accumulated which would incriminate pectus excavation as an etiologic factor in the production of chronic pulmonary disease.

Clinically, the deformity is apparent at or shortly after birth, but is not associated with symptoms at this time except for the occasional occurrence of paradoxical movement of the lower part of the sternum which rarely produces respiratory distress. In the older infant or child there may be decreased exercise tolerance, chest pain, palpitations, repeated upper respiratory tract infections, wheezing, stridor and

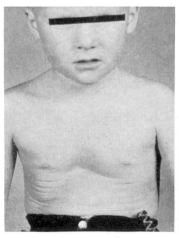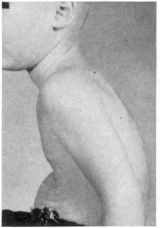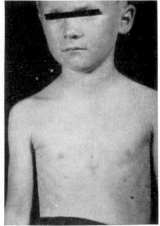

FIGURE 44–1. A moderate pectus excavatum in a 4-year-old boy with rounded shoulders, kyphosis and protuberant abdomen. There is a reasonable cosmetic result one year after surgical correction.

cough. The deformity is frequently cosmetically objectionable and embarrassing to the child and the parents. This may be the only or chief complaint. On physical examination the inward angle of the gladiolar-xiphoid junction in the infant may be exaggerated with inspiration, documenting the paradoxical movement. Obliteration of the deformity should occur with expiration, and Chin felt that failure to do so was a sign of irreversibility. On further inspection, the anteroposterior diameter of the elongated chest is narrow compared to the lateral diameter. The round shoulders accentuate a dorsal kyphosis or kyphoscoliosis and a protuberant abdomen (Fig. 1). The apical cardiac impulse is often shifted to the left and may be accompanied by a systolic murmur.

X-ray examination of the chest quantitatively confirms the clinical diagnosis. The mediastinum and the heart are squeezed to the left of the vertebral column. The chest is wide on the posteroanterior view and narrow on lateral films (Fig. 2). Barium paste on the skin of the sternal depression nicely delineates the curvature and the restricted area between the posterior breast bone and the anterior vertebral column. Bronchograms have shown left lower lobe bronchiectasis.

The electrocardiogram may record a complex variety of changes, including right axis deviation, which probably represents displacement and not intrinsic or concomitant heart disease. An increased venous pressure has been noted occasionally as a reflection of cor pulmonale and may be associated with a slight increase in right atrial pressure on cardiac catheterization. Pulmonary function studies have not demonstrated a consistent pattern. Often, vital capacity, maximal breathing capacity and functional, residual and total lung capacities are within the normal range. Welch, however, found a reduction in the vital and maximal breathing capacities in the lung volume in three of nine children so tested.

The clinical and laboratory information, then, in the majority of patients is likely to exhibit a cosmetic deformity with variable psychologic implications, vague

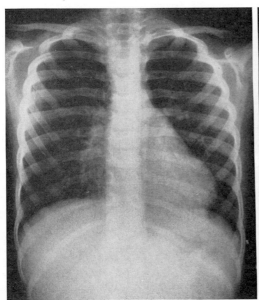
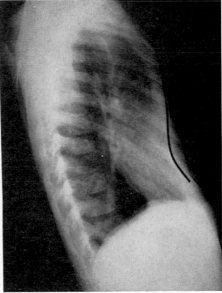

FIGURE 44–2. Typical x-ray findings in a 5-year-old boy with a pectus excavation, demonstrating an absent right cardiac border and minimal deviation of the cardiac mass into the left hemithorax with angulation of the anterior ends of the middle and lower ribs. The chest is wide in the anteroposterior view and narrow in the lateral film. The lung fields are normal.

cardiorespiratory symptoms and minimal objective evidence of heart-lung dysfunction. Later in life a few patients with severe pectus excavation and chronic pulmonary sepsis whose chest wall becomes rigidly fixed are said to have an insidious decrease in pulmonary function and perhaps emphysema. For this small group, operative correction has been advised as a prophylactic measure. Certainly, however, the selection of patients on the basis of future invalidism is most difficult.

Additional indications for the surgical treatment of pectus excavation might include children whose seriously depressed funnel chest is associated with measurable evidence of cardiopulmonary disease, and a cosmetic deformity which is psychologically oppressive and cannot be otherwise handled. This approach would exclude the newborn and the infant from surgery except for the rare neonate with uncontrollable paradoxical movement, whose diaphragm might be separated from the sternum as suggested by Phillips.

The contemporary surgical treatment for funnel chest was instigated by Brown, who proposed the limited procedure of detaching or removing the xiphoid from the substernal ligament and diaphragm. Unfortunately, recurrence was frequent and stimulated the development of a host of more extensive thoracic wall operations. Basically, the deformity must be freed from all attachments, overcorrected and splinted. The technique popularized by Ravitch is preferred by many because it fulfills the technical principles simply and without cumbersome external appliances or internal foreign body support.

Postoperatively, exercise tolerance may increase and growth and development may accelerate. Other associated symptoms have been relieved. In a few instances improvement in cardiac and pulmonary function studies has been noted. The immediate results, cosmetically, are usually acceptable, and tend to remain so for the first three years, especially if the correction is performed before five years of age. Long-term follow-up studies are not quite so encouraging. Chin's clinic reported a 40 per cent recurrence after ten years.

REFERENCES

Adkins, P. C.: Pectus Excavatum. *Amer. Surg.,* 24:571, 1958.

Adkins, P. C., and Gwathmey, O.: Pectus Excavatum: An Appraisal of Surgical Treatment. *J. Thorac. Surg.,* 36:714, 1958.

Ashmore, P. G.: Management of Some Deformities of the Thoracic Cage in Children. *Canad. J. Surg.,* 6:430, 1963.

Avery, M. E.: *The Lung and Its Disorders in the Newborn Infant.* Philadelphia, W. B. Saunders Company, 1964, p. 95.

Ballinger, W. F., II: The Thoracic Wall, in J. H. Gibbon, Jr. (Ed.): *Surgery of the Chest.* Philadelphia, W. B. Saunders Company, 1962, pp. 193, 195, 201.

Bates, D. V., and Christie, R. V.: *Respiratory Function in Disease, An Introduction to the Integrated Study of the Lung.* Philadelphia, W. B. Saunders Company, 1964, p. 261.

Becker, J. M., and Schneider, K. M.: Indications for the Surgical Treatment of Pectus Excavatum. *J.A.M.A.,* 180:22, 1962.

Bigger, I. A.: The Treatment of Pectus Excavatum or Funnel Chest. *Amer. Surg.,* 18:1071, 1952.

Brodkin. A. H., Jr.: Pectus Excavatum: Surgical Indications and Time of Operation. *Pediatrics,* 11:582, 1953.

Brodkin, H. A.: Pigeon Breast—Congenital Chondrosternal Prominence. *A.M.A. Arch. Surg.,* 77:261, 1958.

Brown, A. L.: Pectus Excavatum (Funnel Chest). *J. Thorac. Surg.,* 9:164, 1939.

Brown, A. L., and Cook, O.: Cardio-respiratory Studies in Pre and Post Operative Funnel Chest (Pectus Excavatum). *Dis. of Chest,* 20:378, 1951.

Brown, J. J. M.: The Thoracic Wall; in J. J. M. Brown (Ed.): *Surgery of Childhood.* Baltimore, Williams & Wilkins Company, 1963, p. 790.

Cantrell, J. R., Haller, J. A., and Ravitch, M. M.: The Syndrome of Congenital Defects Involving the Abdominal Wall, Sternum, Diaphragm, Pericardium, and Heart. *Surg., Gynec. & Obst.,* 107:602, 1958.

Chin, E. F.: Surgery of Funnel Chest and Congenital Sternal Prominence. *Brit. J. Surg.,* 44:360, 1957.

Chin, E. F., and Adler, R. H.: Surgical Treatment of Pectus Excavatum (Funnel Chest). *Brit. M.J.,* 1:1064, 1954.

Fink, A., Rivin, A., and Murray, J. F.: Cardiopulmonary Effects of Funnel Chest. *Arch. Int. Med.,* 108:427, 1961.

Flavell, G.: *An Introduction to Chest Surgery.*

London, Oxford University Press, 1957, p. 66.

Gross, R. E.: *The Surgery of Infancy and Childhood, Its Principles and Techniques*. Philadelphia, W. B. Saunders Company, 1953, p. 57.

Groves, L. K.: Deformities of the Anterior Chest Wall. *Cleveland Clin. Quart.*, 30:55, 1963.

Hanlon, C. R.: Surgical Treatment of Funnel Chest (Pectus Excavatum). *Amer. Surg.*, 22:408, 1956.

Hansen, F. N.: The Ontogeny and Phylogeny of the Sternum. *Am. J. Anat.*, 26:41, 1919.

Hansen, J. L., and Jacoby, O.: Pulmonary Function in Pectus Excavatum Deformity. *Acta Chir. Scand.*, 111:25, 1956.

Hay, W., and Dodsley, J.: *Deformity*. London, 1754, pp. 4, 20.

Howard, R.: Funnel Chest: Its Effect on Cardiac Function. *Arch. Dis. Childhood*, 34:5, 1959.

Howard, R. N.: Funnel Chest: Report of a Series of One Hundred Cases. *Med. J. Aust.*, 2:1092, 1955.

Humphreys, G. H., and Connolly, J. E.: The Surgical Technique for the Correction of Pectus Excavatum. *J. Thorac. Cardiov. Surg.*, 40:194, 1960.

Jackson, J. L., and others: Pectus Excavatum. *Am. J. Surg.*, 98:664, 1959.

Jensen, N. K., Schmidt, W. R., and Garamella, J. J.: Funnel Chest: A New Corrective Operation. *J. Thorac. Cardiov. Surg.*, 43:731, 1962.

Jewett, T. C., Butsch, W. L., and Hug, H. R.: Congenital Bifid Sternum. *Pediat. Surg.*, 52:932, 1962.

Kondraisin, N. I.: Congenital Funnel Chest in Children. *Pediatrica*, 42:56, 1963.

Koop, E. C.: The Management of Pectus Excavatum. *Surg. Clin. N. Amer.*, 36:1627, 1956.

Lam, C. R., and Brinkman, G. L.: Indications and Results in the Surgical Treatment of Pectus Excavatum. A.M.A. *Arch. Surg.*, 78:322, 1959.

Lester, C. W.: Funnel Chest and Allied Deformities of Thoracic Cage. *J. Thorac. Surg.*, 19:507, 1950.

Idem: Funnel Chest: Its Cause, Effects, and Treatment. *J. Pediat.*, 37:224, 1950.

Idem: Pigeon Breast. *Ann. Surg.*, 137:482, 1953.

Idem: Pigeon Breast, Funnel Chest, and Other Congenital Deformities of Chest. *J.A.M.A.*, 156:1063, 1954.

Idem: The Etiology and Pathogenesis of Funnel Chest, Pigeon Breast, and Related Deformities of the Anterior Chest Wall. *J. Thorac. Surg.*, 34:1, 1957.

Idem: Funnel Chest, The Status 360 Years After Its First Description. *Arch. Pediat.*, 75:493, 1958.

Idem: Pectus Carinatum, Pigeon Breast and Related Deformities of the Sternum and Costal Cartilages. *Arch. Pediat.*, Oct. 1960, p. 399.

Idem: Surgical Treatment of Protrusion Deformities of the Sternum and Costal Cartilages (Pectus Carinatum, Pigeon Breast). *Ann. Surg.*, 153:441, 1961.

Lindskog, G. E., and Felton, W. L., II: Considerations in the Surgical Treatment of Pectus Excavatum. *Ann. Surg.*, 142:654, 1955.

Lindskog, G. E., Liebow, A. A., and Glenn, W. W. L.: *Thoracic and Cardiovascular Surgery with Related Pathology*. New York, Appleton-Century-Crofts, Inc., 1962, p. 31.

Logan, W. D., Jr., and others: Ectopia Cordis: Report of a Case and Discussion of Surgical Management. *Surgery*, 57:898, 1965.

Moghissi, K.: Long-Term Results of Surgical Correction of Pectus Excavatum and Sternal Prominence. *Thorax*, 19:350, 1964.

Paltia, V., Parkkulainen, K. V., and Sulamaa, M.: Indications for Surgery in Funnel Chest. *Ann. Pediat. Fenniae*, 5:183, 1959.

Peters, R. M., and Johnson, G., Jr.: Stabilization of Pectus Deformity with Wire Strut. *J. Thorac. Cardiov. Surg.*, 47:814, 1964.

Phillips, W. L.: Pectus Excavatum. *South Afr. M.J.*, 34:6, 1960.

Pilcher, R. S.: Trachea, Bronchi, Lungs and Pleura; in J. J. M. Brown (Ed.): *Surgery of Childhood*. Baltimore, Williams & Wilkins Company, 1963, p. 664.

Polgar, G., and Koop, C. E.: Pulmonary Function in Pectus Excavatum. *Pediatrics*, 32:209, 1963.

Potts, W. J.: *The Surgeon and the Child*. Philadelphia, W. B. Saunders Company, 1964, p. 79.

Ramsay, B. H.: Transplantation of the Rectus Abdominis Muscle in the Surgical Correction of a Pectus Carinatum Deformity with Associated Parasternal Depressions. *Surg. Gynec. & Obst.*, 116:507, 1963.

Ravitch, M. M.: Operative Treatment of Pectus Excavatum. *Ann. Surg.*, 129:429, 1949.

Idem: Pectus Excavatum and Heart Failure. *Surgery*, 30:178, 1951.

Idem: Operation for Correction of Pectus Excavatum. *Surg., Gynec. & Obst.*, 106:618, 1958.

Idem: Operative Correction of Pectus Carinatum (Pigeon Breast). *Ann. Surg.*, 151:705, 1960.

Idem: Operative Treatment of Congenital Deformities of the Chest. *Am. J. Surg.*, 101:588, 1961.

Idem: Congenital Deformities of the Chest Wall; in C. D. Benson and others (Eds.): *Pediatic Surgery*. Chicago, Year Book Medical Publishers, Inc., 1962, Vol. 1, p. 235.

Idem: Technical Problems in the Operative Correction of Pectus Excavatum. *Ann. Surg.*, 162:29, 1965.

Rehbein, F., and Wernicke, H.-H.: The Operative Treatment of the Funnel Chest. *Arch. Dis. Childhood*, 32:5, 1957.

Robicsek, F., and others: The Surgical Treatment of Chondrosternal Prominence (Pectus Carinatum). *J. Thorac. Cardiov. Surg.*, 45:691, 1963.

Roccaforte, D. S., Mehnert, J. H., and Peniche, A.: Repair of Bifid Sternum with Autogenous Cartilage. *Ann. Surg.*, 149:448, 1959.

Sabiston, D. C.: The Surgical Management of Congenital Bifid Sternum with Partial Ectopia Cordis. *J. Thorac. Surg.*, 23:118, 1958.

Sanger, P. W., Robicsek, F., and Taylor, F. H.: Surgical Management of Anterior Chest Deformities: A New Technique and Report of 153 Operations Without a Death. *Surg.*, 48:510, 1960.

Sanger, P. W., Taylor, F. H., and Robicsek, F.: Deformities of the Anterior Wall of the Chest. *Surg. Gynec. & Obst.*, 116:515, 1963.

Schaub, F., and Wegmann, T.: Elektrokardiographische Veränderungen bei Trichterbrust. *Cardiologia*, 24:39, 1954.

Swenson, O.: *Pediatric Surgery.* 2nd ed. New York, Appleton-Century-Crofts, Inc., 1962, p. 119.

Van Buchem, F. S. P., and Nieveen, J.: Findings with Funnel Chest. *Acta Med. Scand.*, 174:657, 1963.

Wachtel, F. W., Ravitch, M. M., and Grishman, A.: Relation of Pectus Excavatum to Heart Disease. *Am. Heart J.*, 52:121, 1956.

Welch, K. J.: Satisfactory Surgical Correction of Pectus Excavatum Deformity in Childhood. *J. Thorac. Surg.*, 36:697, 1958.

Wichern, W. A., Jr., and Lester, C. W.: Funnel Chest. *Arch. Surg.*, 84:170, 1962.

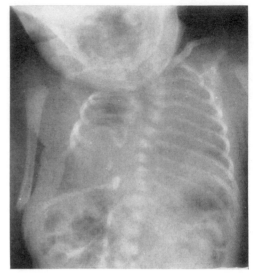

FIGURE 44–3. Anteroposterior x-ray film of the thorax demonstrates absent and deformed ribs on the right. Soft tissue changes, consistent with the loss of supporting structures, are also present. There is scoliosis with convexity to the left, and the heart is dislocated into the left hemithorax. Segmentation anomalies of the dorsal spine are also noted.

CONGENITAL ABSENCE OF RIBS

This is an unusual bony deformity of the thoracic cage, usually associated with other muscular and orthopedic anomalies (Fig. 3). The defect frequently involves the highest and lowest ribs, and clinical repercussions are minimal. Conversely, when ribs in the midthoracic region are absent, lung function may be altered.

In 1895 Thompson suggested that perhaps the hand of the fetus, applying pressure on the chest wall, produced the defect, which may be unilateral or bilateral and usually extends from the sternum anteriorly to the posterior axillary line. Involvement of the second, third, fourth and fifth ribs would remove part of the origin of the pectoralis major muscle, and therefore absence of this muscle is a common associated defect; less common is breast agenesis on the same side. Hemivertebrae and kyphoscoliosis may be present.

Often the defect produces no physio-logic disturbance if the anomaly is single, small, and so localized that a lung hernia is not produced. If the second through the fifth ribs are absent anteriorly, a large lung hernia may occur, and lack of chest wall support here can lead to dramatic paradoxical respirations. Kyphoscoliotic heart disease, with cor pulmonale and congestive heart failure, may complicate congenitally absent ribs.

Symptoms may vary from none to severe dyspnea secondary to paradoxical respiratory movements and mediastinal flutter. Relatively few infants, however, present with advanced respiratory distress, and less serious difficulties will gradually disappear as the lung protrusion diminishes with growth.

Therapy is based on the contribution of the rib defect to the clinical picture and is seldom required. When symptoms are severe enough to produce respiratory embarrassment, local pressure may stabilize the chest, although Rickham feels that an inappropriate bandage may worsen the distress. Certainly, if critical symptoms persist in spite of conservative chest wall support, homologous rib grafting should be done.

REFERENCES

Aschner, B. B., Kaizer, M. N., and Small, A. R.: Flaring of Ribs Associated with Other Skeletal Anomalies. *Conn. M.J.*, 19:383, 1955.

Ballinger, W. F., II: The Thoracic Wall; in J. H. Gibbon, Jr. (Ed.): *Surgery of the Chest.* Philadelphia, W. B. Saunders Company, 1962, p. 192.

Brown, J. J. M.: The Thoracic Wall; in J. J. M. Brown (Ed.): *Surgery of Childhood.* Baltimore, Williams & Wilkins Company, 1964, p. 789.

Fishmann, A. P., Turino, G. M., and Bergofsky, E. H.: Disorders of Respiration and Circulation in Subjects with Deformities of Thorax. *Mod. Conc. Cardiov. Dis.*, 27:449, 1958.

Flavell, G.: *An Introduction to Chest Surgery.* London, Oxford University Press, 1957, p. 65.

Goodman, H. I.: Hernia of Lung. *J. Thorac. Surg.*, 2:368, 1933.

Ravitch, M. M.: The Operative Treatment of Congenital Deformities of the Chest. *Am. J. Surg.*, 101:588, 1961.

Idem: The Chest Wall; in C. D. Benson and others (Eds.): *Pediatric Surgery.* Chicago, Year Book Medical Publishers, Inc., 1962, Vol. 1, p. 245.

Rickham, P. P.: Lung Hernia Secondary to Congenital Absence of Ribs. *Arch. Dis. Childhood*, 34:14, 1959.

Swenson, O.: *Pediatric Surgery.* 2nd ed. New York, Appleton-Century-Crofts, Inc., 1962, p. 118.

Thomson, J.: *Teratologia.* Edinburgh, W. Green and Sons, 1895, Vol. 2, p. 1.

CONGENITAL ANTERIOR DIAPHRAGMATIC HERNIA (MORGAGNI)

Morgagni hernias occur behind the sternum through a defect in the diaphragm. Although these hernias may be the most frequent tumor in the anterior inferior mediastinum in the pediatric age, they are the rarest type of congenital diaphragmatic hernia. More than half have a sac containing omentum or transverse colon.

Many infants and children with an anterior diaphragmatic defect are asymptomatic. Others may have abdominal complaints simulating gallbladder or peptic ulcer disease or constipation. A third group presents with chest symptoms of retroxiphoid pain, dyspnea and cough. Finally, acute findings with strangulation are said to occur in 10 per cent. Here a succussion sound synchronous with the cardiac impulse may be diagnostic.

The diagnosis may be ultimately supported by roentgenograms showing a moderately dense tumor at the cardiophrenic angle. A barium enema may delineate a thoracic transverse colon and also demonstrate an elevated transverse colon if omentum is incarcerated. An omental hernia may also be suggested by changes in angulation of the transverse colon with inspiration and expiration. Pneumoperitoneum has been used for diagnosis.

Abdominal herniorrhaphy is advised for most Morgagni hernias.

CONGENITAL DIAPHRAGMATIC HERNIA OF BOCHDALEK

Posterolateral diaphragmatic hernia through the pleuroperitoneal sinus is perhaps the most urgent of all neonatal thoracoabdominal emergencies. If the diagnosis is not immediate, many neonates with no other abnormalities will expire. The same fate may await those whose diagnosis is prompt, but operation delayed.

The maldevelopment has been catalogued as frequently as one in 2200 to one in 3500 births, or about 8 per cent of major congenital anomalies, and occurs on the left side in 80 per cent of the cases. At present it may be outnumbered by hiatal hernia, but requires operative intervention as a lifesaving measure much more often. Concomitant defects that occur with some regularity are midgut malrotation, extralobar sequestration and congenital heart disease.

The common channel between the chest and the abdomen results from a failure of development or fusion of diaphragmatic muscle. The diaphragm is largely formed from the septum transversum and dorsal mesentery, which, at first, separates the thoracic systems from the abdominal organs. The defect in the posterolateral areas of the diaphragm is the last to close and is eventually bridged at the sixth to eighth week of fetal development by pleural and peritoneal membranes. Body wall mesoderm eventually insinuates between these membranes and becomes the diaphragmatic muscle. Early, arrested development in the region of the foramen of Bochdalek, prior to the presence of pleura and peritoneum, produces a hernia without a sac, and this is the most frequent anatomic situation. The left side is favored because diaphragmatic closure normally occurs here later than on the right. If the pleuroperitoneal membranes are formed without muscular development, a hernial sac for the Bochdalek defect has been created. Finally, aborted muscle ingrowth between the properly fashioned pleura and peritoneum may lead to a thin, fibrous tissue layer rather than substantial contractile muscle, and eventration results. Baffes has emphasized the role of an early return of the midgut from its umbilical domicile to the peritoneal cavity in the creation and maintenance of Bochdalek hernias.

The aperture in the posterolateral leaf of the diaphragm may vary in size from a small defect to absence or agenesis of the entire muscle, and this may occur bilaterally. Small and large bowel, stomach and spleen on the left and liver on the right have been found in the appropriate pleural cavity. In less than 10 per cent of the cases a constricting hernia sac is present. Without this peritoneal or pleural investment the herniated viscera may extend to the apex of the thorax. This migration of intraperitoneal structures is possible because of their insecure posterior peritoneal attachments, and is reflected in the reported 20 per cent incidence of simultaneous malrotation. As in omphalocele, the peritoneal cavity shrinks down to accommodate the remaining viscera.

Since the Bochdalek hernia has been present since the eighth week of intrauterine life, compression atelectasis of the ipsilateral lung is predictable. In spite of this time interval, remarkably few adhesions occur between the abdominal organs and the parietal or visceral pleura. Development of the compressed lung has excited a great deal of curiosity and over-enthusiastic application of the term "pulmonary hypoplasia" to a chronic compression syndrome. Actually, after proper operation, lung expansion does occur, and the microscopic picture demonstrates a normal, mature alveolar pattern.

The pathogenesis of symptoms is based on usurpation of pleural space from the ipsilateral lung with atelectasis, mediastinal shift and contralateral lung compression, aggravated by gastrointestinal distention from swallowed air. This chain of events is likely to occur in the immediate neonatal period with a large diaphragmatic orifice and no restraining sac and is rapidly worsened by labored respiratory efforts which draw more abdominal viscera into the crowded pleural space by negative intrathoracic pressure. A smaller hole in the posterolateral diaphragm may restrict the degree of herniation, but strangulation becomes easier.

On examination of the newborn, immediate cardiorespiratory distress is striking and does not clear with pharyngotracheal toilet. Cyanosis, dyspnea, tachypnea and tachycardia are fairly constant. The involved hemithorax, usually the left, is relatively protuberant, and chest expansion is bilaterally uneven. Breath sounds are absent on the left, and percussion may be resonant. It is unusual to hear thoracic peristalsis. The apical cardiac impulse is dislocated to the right, and the abdomen is scaphoid. Feedings, face mask resuscitation without an endotracheal tube and delayed surgical intervention aggravate a precarious situation.

The majority of patients with Bochdalek hernia have critical symptoms within the first month of life. After this, survival is likely to be marred by chronic respiratory and gastrointestinal ailments, and strangulation may occur.

Plain films of the chest in conventional views are almost always diagnostic, and the use of contrast material gives little constructive aid to the work-up and introduces the danger of aspiration. The mediastinum is markedly displaced, and very little lung tissue on either side aerates properly. The diaphragmatic line on the affected side is difficult or impossible to visualize. Signet ring radiolucencies in the thorax suggestive of air-filled loops of bowel are contrasted with a distinct loss of the normal gastrointestinal pattern within the abdomen (Fig. 4). If the hernia is right-sided, the liver alone may encroach on intrathoracic space, and pneumoperitoneum may be necessary for diagnosis. An intravenous pyelogram will often show upward displacement of the ipsilateral kidney, especially when the defect is on the right side.

In preparing for the differential diagnosis, Moore has emphasized the triad of dyspnea, cyanosis and apparent dextrocar-

dia. On x-ray film the lesions simulate diffuse congenital pulmonary cysts and pneumatoceles. Neither is particularly frequent in the immediate neonatal period, and an infectious background is often lacking. Moreover, with both, the abdominal gastrointestinal configuration is normal. Other entities which can be separated with minimal difficulty are laryngotracheal obstruction, atelectasis, pneumothorax, true dextrocardia, congenital heart and cerebral disease and lobar emphysema. It may be impossible, but is unnecessary, to separate Bochdalek hernia, eventration and phrenic nerve paralysis. The treatment in the presence of catastrophic symptoms is surgical in each instance.

Since a significant number of neonates with congenital posterolateral diaphragmatic hernias expire shortly after birth even with a correct, prompt diagnosis, proper emergency attention may enable the infant to survive the short preopera-

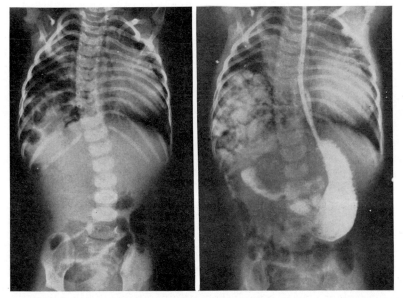

FIGURE 44–4. The plain anteroposterior thoracoabdominal radiograph shows a scoliosis of the spine and asymmetry of the chest with the left side larger. The heart and trachea are dislocated to the left. The dome of the left diaphragm is intact; the right cannot be seen. Multiple signet ring radiolucencies and mottled densities are noted in the lower half of the right hemithorax. The right lung is confined to the upper half of the hemithorax, and the peripheral left lung is hyperaerated. The normal gastrointestinal air pattern within the abdomen is absent.

Through the nasogastric tube, contrast material has been instilled and superfluously documents the findings apparent in the plain film.

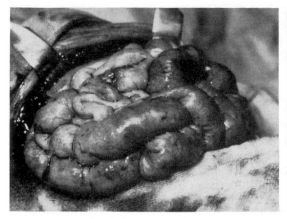
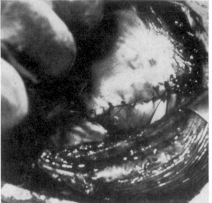

FIGURE 44–5. Small bowel extrudes through a low posterolateral right thoracotomy incision, relieving the pulmonary and mediastinal tamponade. After the hernial contents have been replaced within the abdomen, the diaphragmatic defect is closed in 2 layers.

tive interval. In this regard, effective, constant nasogastric suction may relieve or prevent the devastating intrathoracic gastrointestinal distention. Gentle positive-pressure resuscitation must be done through an endotracheal tube to avoid forcing oxygen down the esophagus and further dilating the gastrointestinal tract. Overenthusiastic inflation of the lungs may produce unilateral or bilateral pneumothorax.

Hedblom, in 1925, encouraged the emergency surgical approach for Bochdalek hernia by reporting a neonatal mortality rate of 75 per cent without operation. Today the prompt use of surgery has reduced neonatal mortality to a range of 15 to 25 per cent. After one month of age the operative mortality rate drops to 6 per cent with a 2 per cent recurrence rate.

It has been emphasized that operation should be done when the diagnosis is made, preceded by the shortest possible period of correct preoperative resuscitation, because a patient who is apparently well may become moribund within minutes and fail to respond. The surgical incision may be made transthoracically or transperitoneally, and there are advocates for each (Fig. 5). We favor the abdominal route for neonatal hernias on the left side and the transpleural approach for hernias of the right side and all those repaired later than six months of age. If reduction of the viscera into the abdomen and a layered abdominal wall closure create prohibitive intra-abdominal pressures, additional space may be obtained by just approximating the skin. A further extension of this concept has been proposed by Meeker and Snyder, who suggest the construction of a gastrostomy and an intentional ventral hernia when the operation is done in the newborn. Ventral herniorrhaphy may be accomplished after one year of age.

Closure of the posterolateral defect is usually uncomplicated, although the absence of a hemidiaphragm may pose serious technical problems which have been ingeniously handled by Teflon, Marlex and Ivalon grafts, pedicled abdominal or thoracic wall flaps, and liver.

During the operation the anesthesiologist cannot forcibly expand the atelectatic lung and, accordingly, must exert restraint in breathing for the patient in order to avoid pneumothorax, pneumomediastinum and a bronchopleural fistula. Postoperatively, chest drainage is used without excessive negative pressure, and the lung will expand within a few days to several weeks.

REFERENCES

Avery, M. E.: *The Lung and Its Disorders in the Newborn Infant*. Philadelphia, W. B. Saunders Company, 1964, p. 93.

Baffes, T. G.: Diaphragmatic Hernia; in C. D. Benson and others (Eds.): *Pediatric Surgery*. Chicago, Year Book Medical Publishers, Inc., 1962, Vol. 1, p. 251.

Belsey, R.: The Surgery of the Diaphragm; in J. J. M. Brown (Ed.): *Surgery of Childhood*. Baltimore, Williams & Wilkins Company, 1963, pp. 758, 780.

Benjamin, H. B.: Agenesis of the Left Hemidiaphragm. *J. Thorac. Surg.*, 46:265, 1963.

Bentley, G., and Lister, J.: Retrosternal Hernia. *Surgery*, 57:567, 1965.

Bowers, V. M., Jr., McElin, T. W., and Dorsey, J. M.: Diaphragmatic Hernia in the Newborn: Diagnostic Responsibility of the Obstetrician. *Obst. & Gynec.*, 6:262, 1955.

Butler, N., and Claireaux, A. E.: Congenital Diaphragmatic Hernia as a Cause of Perinatal Mortality. *Lancet*, 1:659, 1962.

Campanale, R. P., and Rowland, R. H.: Hypoplasia of the Lung Associated with Congenital Diaphragmatic Hernia. *Ann. Surg.*, 142:176, 1955.

Carter, R. E. B., Waterson, D. J., and Aberdeen, E.: Diaphragmatic Hernia in Infancy. *Lancet*, 1:656, 1962.

Cerilli, G. J.: Foramen of Bochdalek Hernia. *Ann. Surg.*, 159:385, 1964.

Filler, R. M., Randolph, J. G., and Gross, R. E.: Esophageal Hiatus Hernia in Infants and Children. *J. Thorac. Surg.*, 47:551, 1964.

Flavell, G.: *An Introduction to Chest Surgery*. London, Oxford University Press, 1957, p. 231.

Fitchett, C. W., and Tavarex, V.: Bilateral Congenital Diaphragmatic Herniation. *Surg.*, 57:305, 1965.

Gans, S. L., and Hackworth, L. E.: Respiratory Obstructions of Surgical Import. *Pediat. Clin. N. Amer.*, 6:1023, 1959.

Gross, R. E.: *The Surgery of Infancy and Childhood, Its Principles and Techniques*. Philadelphia, W. B. Saunders Company, 1953, p. 428.

Hajdu, N. H., and Sidhva, J. N.: Parasternal Diaphragmatic Hernia Through the Foramen of Morgagni. *Brit. J. Radiol.*, July 1955, p. 355.

Harrington, S. W.: Various Types of Diaphragmatic Hernia Treated Surgically; Report of 430 Cases. *Surg. Gynec. & Obst.*, 86:735, 1948.

Haupt, G. L., and Myers, R. N.: Polyvinyl Formalized (Ivalon) Sponge in the Repair of Diaphragmatic Hernia. *A.M.A. Arch. Surg.*, 80:103, 613, 1960.

Hedblom, C. A.: Diaphragmatic Hernia. *J.A.M.A.*, 85:947, 1925.

Hermann, R. E., and Barber, D. H.: Congenital Diaphragmatic Hernia in the Child Beyond Infancy. *Cleveland Clin. Quart.*, 30:73, 1963.

Holcomb, G. W., Jr.: A New Technique for Repair of Congenital Diaphragmatic Hernia with Absence of the Left Hemidiaphragm. *Surgery*, 51:534, 1962.

Hope, J. W., and Koop, C. E.: Differential Diagnosis of Mediastinal Masses. *Pediat. Clin. N. Amer.*, 6:379, 1959.

Jemerin, E. E.: Diaphragmatic Hernia Through Foramen of Morgagni. *J. Mount Sinai Hosp.* (N.Y.), 30:415, 1963.

Keith, A.: *Human Embryology and Morphology*. London, Edward Arnold, 1948.

Kelly, K. A., and Bassett, D. L.: An Anatomic Reappraisal of the Hernia of Morgagni. *Surgery*, 55:495, 1964.

Kenigsberg, K., and Gwinn, J. L.: The Retained Sac in Repair of Posterolateral Diaphragmatic Hernia in the Newborn. *Surgery*, 57:894, 1965.

Kiesewetter, W. B., Gutierrez, I. Z., and Sieber, W. K.: Diaphragmatic Hernia in Infants Under One Year of Age. *Arch. Surg.* 83:561, 1961.

Kinsbourne, M.: Hiatus Hernia with Contortions of the Neck. *Lancet*, 1:1058, 1964.

Ladd, W. E., and Gross, R. E.: *Abdominal Surgery of Infancy and Childhood*. Philadelphia, W. B. Saunders Company, 1941.

Meeker, I. A., Jr., and Snyder, W. H., Jr.: Surgical Management of Diaphragmatic Defects in the Newborn, A Report of Twenty Infants Each Less than One Week Old. *Am. J. Surg.*, 104:196, 1962.

Moore, T. C., and others: Congenital Posterolateral Diaphragmatic Hernia in the Newborn. *Surg., Gynec. & Obst.*, 104:675, 1957.

Murphy, D. R., and Owen, H. F.: Respiratory Emergencies in the Newborn. *Am. J. Surg.*, 101:58, 1961.

Neville, W. E., and Clowes, G. H. A., Jr.: Congenital Absence of Hemidiaphragm and Use of a Lobe of Liver in Its Surgical Correction. *A.M.A. Arch. Surg.*, 69:282, 1954.

Nixon, H. H., and O'Donnell, B.: *The Essentials of Pediatric Surgery*. London, William Heinemann, Ltd., 1961, p. 36.

Polk, H. C., and Burford, T. H.: Hiatal Hernia in Infancy and Childhood. *Surgery*, 54:521, 1963.

Potts, W. J.: *The Surgeon and the Child*. Philadelphia, W. B. Saunders Company, 1959, p. 64.

Richardson, W. R.: Thoracic Emergencies in the Newborn Infant. *Am. J. Surg.*, 105:524, 1963.

Riker, W. L.: Congenital Diaphragmatic Hernia. *A.M.A. Arch. Surg.*, 69:291, 1954.

Rosenkrantz, J. G., and Cotton, E. K.: Replacement of Left Hemidiaphragm by a Pedicled Abdominal Muscular Flap. *J. Thorac. Cardiov. Surg.*, 48:912, 1964.

Sabga, G. A., Neville, W. E., and Del Guercio, L. R. M.: Anomalies of the Lung Associated with Congenital Diaphragmatic Hernia. Surgery, 50:547, 1961.

Schuster, S. R.: The Recognition and Management of Diaphragmatic Hernias in Infancy and Childhood. *Quart. Rev. Pediat.,* 15:171, 1960.

Shaffer, J. O.: Prothesis for Agenesis of the Diaphragm. *J.A.M.A.,* June 15, 1964, p. 168.

Snyder, W. H., and Greany, E. M.: Congenital Diaphragmatic Hernia; 77 Consecutive Cases. *Surgery,* 57:576, 1965.

Sulamaa, M., and Viitanen, I.: Congenital Diaphragmatic Hernia and Relaxation. *Acta Chir. Scand.,* 124:288, 1962.

Thomsen, G.: Diaphragmatic Hernia in the Newborn, Incidence of Neonatal Fatalities. *Acta Chir. Scand.,* Suppl., 283:267, 1961.

White, M., and Dennison, W. M.: *Surgery in Infancy and Childhood, A Handbook for Medical Students and General Practitioners.* Edinburgh, E. & S. Livingstone, Ltd., 1958, p. 300.

CONGENITAL EVENTRATION OF THE DIAPHRAGM

Congenital eventration of all or part of one diaphragm follows the maldevelopment of diaphragmatic muscle and is commoner than acquired eventration secondary to phrenic nerve paralysis.

Embryologically, there is a complete or partial absence of muscular development in the septum transversum in the presence of normal pleura above and peritoneum below. These two membranes may be in direct juxtaposition or separated only by a thin fibrous sheath; usually a small rim of muscle lies anteriorly between the pleuroperitoneal folds. Total eventration is said to be more frequent on the left, while a more localized or partial eventration is likely to be on the right side. The lesion has been found in the fetus, along with other local congenital anomalies, such as high renal ectopia and extralobar pulmonary sequestration.

Gross pathologic analysis demonstrates an absence or diminution of the diaphragmatic muscle, which becomes fibrous, thin and abnormally elevated. The phrenic nerve is smaller than normal; microscopically, there is degeneration of the muscle, but not of the nerve.

Symptoms are produced by an ex-tremely elevated diaphragm with minimal or no function, but usually without paradoxical movements compressing the ipsilateral lung. The resultant mediastinal shift and rotation then encroaches on the opposite lung. Respiratory findings are compounded by elevation and angulation of the stomach.

The clinical picture may vary from an asymptomatic, elderly patient to an early neonatal death. It is not unusual to have respiratory distress of the order seen with a Bochdalek hernia, with dyspnea, tachypnea and cyanosis. Physical examination may demonstrate tracheal and cardiac shift, with dullness and absent breath sounds over the involved thorax. Gastrointestinal complaints of vomiting, flatulence and indigestion or cough with bronchitis, and repeated pneumonia may predominate in the older child

Fluoroscopy and chest x-rays are essential to the diagnosis. The degree of diaphragmatic elevation is precisely documented by visualization of a definite, thin, unbroken arc above the abdominal viscera (Fig. 6). At first diaphragmatic excursions may be properly synchronous, but minimal; later, perhaps, the diaphragm may move paradoxically and create mediastinal flutter. Atelectasis and mediastinal shift are seen.

The differential diagnosis includes congenital posterolateral diaphragmatic hernia and phrenic nerve paralysis. If the congenital eventration moves paradoxically, it cannot be clinically separated from a hernia with a sac or a diaphragm elevated from nerve injury. In the usual Bochdalek hernia without a sac, however, the remaining diaphragm is difficult to see and when seen is located normally and not elevated. Other diagnoses that should be entertained are various tumors and cysts, Morgagni hernia and perhaps pleural effusion. Barium studies and pneumoperitoneum separately or combined can help in the differential diagnosis.

The course with congenital eventration is as unpredictable as the symptomology. Deaths have been reported in the untreated patient, and survival may be com-

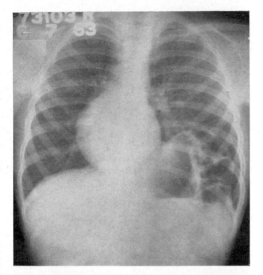

FIGURE 44–6. This is a 6-year-old boy with a modest, asymptomatic eventration of the diaphragm whose x-ray film was taken during an infrequent respiratory infection. The heart is shifted to the right, and the right diaphragm is intact and at the proper level. The arc of the left diaphragm is elevated 2 interspaces above the right and surrounds gas-containing abdominal viscera.

plicated by chronic pulmonary suppuration, diaphragmatic rupture and ulcer and volvulus of the stomach. Usually, however, supportive treatment will suffice in the barely symptomatic infant. With dyspnea and cyanosis in the newborn, eventration should be handled by thoracotomy as urgently as is a Bochdalek hernia. With plication, which lowers the diaphragm, mortality is low, respiratory distress is promptly abolished, and the immediate and long-term results are eminently satisfactory. The ipsilateral lung function may eventually approach normality. Goulston has demonstrated the efficacy of operation in older children with chronic gastric and respiratory complaints.

REFERENCES

Allison, P. R.: The Diaphragm; in J. H. Gibbon, Jr., (Ed.): *Surgery of the Chest.* Philadelphia, W. B. Saunders Company, 1962, p. 280.

Arnheim, E. E.: Congenital Eventration of the Diaphragm in Infancy. *Surgery,* 35:809, 1954.

Avery, M. E.: *The Lung and Its Disorders in the Newborn Infant.* Philadelphia, W. B. Saunders Company, 1964, p. 91.

Baffes, T. C.: Diaphragmatic Hernia; in C. D. Benson and others (Eds.): *Pediatric Surgery.* Chicago, Year Book Medical Publishers, Inc., 1962, Vol. 1, p. 259.

Belsey, R.: The Surgery of the Diaphragm; in J. J. M. Brown (Ed.): *Surgery of Childhood.* Baltimore, Williams & Wilkins Company, 1963, p. 786.

Bisgard, J. D.: Congenital Eventration of Diaphragm. *J. Thorac. Surg.,* 16:484, 1947.

Chin, E. F., and Lynn, R. B.: Surgery of Eventration of the Diaphragm. *J. Thorac. Surg.,* 32:6, 1956.

Flavell, G: *An Introduction to Chest Surgery,* London, Oxford University Press, p. 233.

Gans, S. L., and Hackworth, L. E.: Respiratory Obstructions of Surgical Import. *Pediat. Clin. N. Amer.,* 6:1023, 1959.

Goulston, E.: Eventration of the Diaphragm. *Arch. Dis. Childhood,* 32:9, 1957.

Laxdal, O. E., McDougall, H., and Mellin, G. W.: Congenital Eventration of the Diaphragm. *New England J. Med.,* 250:401, 1954.

Lindskog, G. E., Liebow, A. A., and Glenn, W. W. L.: *Thoracic and Cardiovascular Surgery with Related Pathology.* New York, Appleton-Century-Crofts, Inc., 1962, p. 546.

Michelson, E.: Eventration of the Diaphragm. *Surgery,* 49:410, 1961.

Schaffer, A. J.: *Diseases of the Newborn.* Philadelphia, W. B. Saunders Company, 1960, p. 145.

CONGENITAL HIATAL DIAPHRAGMATIC HERNIA

According to Belsey, and Filler, Randolph and Gross, hiatal hernias are common in the pediatric age group, especially during the first year. The extension of the stomach into the lower part of the chest occurs through an exaggerated crural defect which is usually congenital, but may be acquired by gastric expansion in an upward direction during excessive vomiting. This may explain some of the hiatal hernias associated with pyloric stenosis.

The majority of hiatal protrusions in infancy and childhood are sliding hernias in which the esophagogastric junction is above the crural level of the diaphragm. This particular anatomic configuration

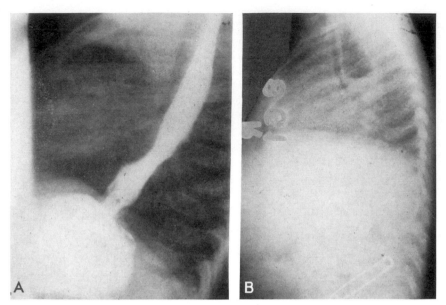

FIGURE 44–7. A 7-month-old male infant with persistent bile-free vomiting, recurrent episodes of aspiration pneumonia and poor weight gain. *A,* The lateral esophagogram reveals minimal dilatation in the region of the middle third with tapering and irritability of the distal portion of the esophagus. The presence of gastric mucosa above the diaphragm in a hiatal hernia is demonstrated. *B,* One month later an air-fluid level is seen in the posterior mediastinum at the level of the carina with considerable dilatation of the proximal part of the esophagus, documenting the progression of the stricture secondary to the hiatal hernia. A transthoracic approach to this sliding hiatal hernia with repair and dilatation resulted in complete rehabilitation.

abolishes the acute esophagogastric angle and, with a wide crural ring, allows free gastric reflux which produces the symptoms of the disease. The rarer paraesophageal hiatal hernia has a normal esophagogastric junction and crural aperture, the stomach herniating into the chest parallel to, but separated from, the esophagus by strands of diaphragmatic muscle. Incarceration may occur with this arrangement, but reflux is less likely.

Persistent bile-free vomiting, projectile or regurgitant, is found consistently. This may begin soon after birth or start at the third or fourth month and simulate a late pyloric stenosis. The incessant vomiting may occur at night with aspiration and repeated bouts of pneumonia. Slow growth and development are often systemic manifestations of malnutrition, dehydration and chronic infection. Hematemesis is not unusual. Later, dysphagia from esophageal stricture and chronic pneumonitis with pulmonary fibrosis are

seen. A peculiar contortion of the neck with hiatal hernia has been described.

Both hematemesis and melena can be confirmed by the clinical laboratory and are reflected in a blood loss anemia. The barium swallow corroborates the diagnosis and the stricture formation, and plain chest films document the aspiration pneumonia (Fig. 7). Burford has emphasized the role of esophagoscopy in detailing the esophagitis and stenosis.

The differential diagnosis in the newborn and the infant involves other entities which produce chronic, relentless vomiting with failure to thrive, repeated pneumonias, upper gastrointestinal bleeding, anemia and dysphagia.

In the majority of patients the hernia is small and symptoms are not critical, although there is no correlation between size and symptoms. In this sizable group, conservative therapy consisting of the continuous upright position, antacids and antispasmodics will suffice. If the symptoms are severe, regardless of the size of the hernia, conservative therapy should be exhausted before operative intervention and the lesion may respond. Surgical repair, either thoracic or abdominal, is reserved for patients who fail to grow and develop normally, continue with bleeding, are developing a stricture and accordingly are considered medical failures. Hiatal herniorrhaphy can reverse this sequence of events by obliterating the hernial sac and reconstructing the normal esophagogastric junction and angle. The addition of a pyloroplasty permits prompt gastric drainage. The results following a technically satisfactory procedure are gratifying.

CHYLOTHORAX

Pleural chylous effusion is a rare but important reason for neonatal respiratory distress because the prognosis is fairly optimistic with conservative therapy.

Chylothorax (see also p. 345) which occurs later in infancy or childhood follows accidental trauma or left thoracotomy, usually for congenital cardiovascular anomalies. In the newborn the etiologic factors are less precise The basic defect probably involves a malformation of the mediastinal and pulmonary lymphatics with failure of orderly fusion and the production of multiple lymphatic fistulas. This may explain the generalized sources of chylous fluid found at postmortem examination. The remainder of the lymphatic system is normal.

A newborn may present with the usual stigma of respiratory distress—dyspnea, tachypnea and cyanosis without evidence of sepsis. On physical examination the mediastinum is displaced with unilateral dullness and diminished breath sounds, although bilaterality has been reported at least once. Chest x-rays demonstrate opacification, usually on the right with verification of the mediastinal shift.

The respiratory problem, which is secondary to compression atelectasis and mediastinal shift, is promptly relieved by aspiration of clear pleural fluid which turns opalescent only after milk has been digested. The withdrawal of pleural chyle, of course, establishes the diagnosis, and thoracenteses are continued until the pleural cavity remains dry. Varying numbers of thoracenteses have been used to control the effusion, which has a considerable protein content. Ancillary help is provided by a low fat, high protein, high caloric diet.

In a few instances the chylothorax has persisted in spite of multiple aspirations, and thoracotomy was performed. In one patient, operated on by Gross and Randolph, ligation of the thoracic duct controlled the lymphatic extravasation. Pleurodesis with iodized talc may have a place.

Although the over-all prognosis is favorable, death may occur from infection and malnutrition.

REFERENCES

Avery, M. E.: The Lung and Its Disorders in the Newborn Infant. Philadelphia, W. B. Saunders Company, 1964, p. 157.
Boles, E. T., and Izant, R. J., Jr.: Spontaneous Chylothorax in the Neonatal Period. Am. J. Surg., 99:870, 1960.
Forbes, G. B.: Chylothorax in Infancy. J. Pediat., 25:191, 1944.
Gingell, J. C.: Treatment of Chylothorax by Producing Pleurodesis Using Iodized Talc. Thorax, 20:261, 1965.
Maier, H. C.: The Pleura; in J. H. Gibbon, Jr. (Ed.): Surgery of The Chest. Philadelphia, W. B. Saunders Company, 1962, p. 244.
Nelson, W. E.: Chylothorax; in W. E. Nelson (Ed.): Textbook of Pediatrics. 8th ed. Philadelphia, W. B. Saunders Company, 1964, p. 875.
Perry, R. E., Hodgman, J., and Cass, A. B.: Pleural Effusion in the Neonatal Period. J. Pediat., 62:838, 1963.
Randolph, J. G., and Gross, R. E.: Congenital Chylothorax. A.M.A. Arch. Surg., 74:405, 1957.
Ravitch, M. M.: Chylothorax; in C. D. Benson and others (Eds.): Pediatric Surgery, Chicago, Year Book Medical Publishers, Inc., 1962, Vol. 1, p. 353.
Schaffer, A. J.: Diseases of the Newborn. Philadelphia, W. B. Saunders Company, 1960. p. 177.
Williams, K. R., and Burford, T. H.: The Management of Chylothorax. Ann. Surg., 160:131, 1964.

TRACHEAL AGENESIS AND STENOSIS

Aplasia, atresia or agenesis of the trachea is a rare congenital anomaly which to date seems incompatible with life.

Basically, the defect most often consists of a partial or complete absence of the trachea below the larynx or cricoid, main stem bronchi which join in the midline, and a bronchoesophageal fistula.

In at least one instance the diagnosis was suspected and confirmed and recon structive surgery ingeniously performed with survival for six weeks. Intragastric oxygen at birth may prolong life and permit emergency surgical treatment, which in Fonkalsrud's case consisted in division of the cervical esophagus with utilization of the proximal end as a salivary fistula and the distal stoma for the airway, division of the esophagus below the congenital esophagobronchial fistula and gastrostomy.

Additional corrective surgery would be necessary for long-term survival and may depend eventually on progress in transplantation.

Stenosis of the trachea has been reported by Holinger as a fibrous stricture in the form of webs. Respiratory difficulty is characterized by continuous stridor. The diagnosis may be suspected on lateral x-ray films of the neck and chest, and the stenosis may be treated bronchoscopically. Tracheostomy may be necessary. Successful transthoracic repair has been reported by Cantrell and Guild.

REFERENCES

Bigler, J. A., and others: Tracheotomy in Infancy. *Pediatrics*, 13:476, 1954.

Cantrell, J. R., and Guild, H. G.: Congenital Stenosis of the Trachea. *Am. J. Surg.*, 108:297, 1964.

Fonkalsrud, E. W., Martelle, R. R., and Maloney, J. V.: Surgical Treatment of Tracheal Agenesis. *J. Thorac. Cardiov. Surg.*, 45:520, 1963.

Holinger, P. H.: The Infant with Respiratory Stridor. *Pediat. Clin. N. Amer.*, 2:403, 1955.

Holinger, P. H., and Johnston, K. C.: Clinical Aspects of Congenital Anomalies of the Trachea and Bronchi. *Dis. of Chest*, 31:613, 1957.

Holinger, P. H., and others: Congenital Malformations of the Trachea, Bronchi and Lung. *Ann. Otol.*, 61:1159, 1952.

Ochsner, J. L., and LeJeune, F. E., Jr.: Tracheal and Esophageal Obstructions in Infants. *South. M.J.*, 57:1340, 1964.

Oliver, P., and others: Tracheotomy in Children. *New England J. Med.*, 267:631, 1962.

Rubin, L. R., and others: Elective Tracheostomy in Infants and Children. *Am. J. Surg.*, 98:880, 1959.

Witzleben, C. L.: Aplasia of the Trachea. *Pediatrics*, 32:31, 1963.

TRACHEOMALACIA

In infancy the tracheal lumen is largely maintained by tracheal cartilages. If cartilaginous rings are congenitally absent, small, malformed or too pliable, essential support is lacking, and such lack may lead to a functional tracheal stenosis and obstruction. This primary tracheomalacia is an unusual, but usually benign, form of respiratory distress in the newborn and the young infant and must be distinguished from the secondary type, produced by extrinsic compression from a vascular ring or mediastinal tumor.

Tracheal expansion and contraction occur with inspiration and expiration respectively; these variations in airway size are minimized during sleep and shallow respiration and exaggerated by forceful breathing, as with crying. With incomplete structural support of the trachea, the normal luminal narrowing during expiration becomes exaggerated, and in severe instances the lumen may be small for inspiration.

Clinically, there may be wheezing, cough, stridor, dyspnea, tachypnea and cyanosis, and these are made worse by pulmonary sepsis and secretions. On physical examination, expiration is prolonged, and there may be emphysema, but there is no localization by auscultation except with secondary infection. Opisthotonos has been reported. The neck, the mouth and the pharynx are normal; ear cartilage may be absent. Chest roentgenograms are almost invariably done in inspiration, and the lungs may be exceptionally well aerated. Tracheal narrowing may be visible on lateral films.

The esophagogram is normal, but a contrast tracheogram done with cinefluorography in the lateral view may demonstrate the abnormal tracheal wall mobility. Laryngoscopy is normal down to the vocal cords, which, too, may be excessively soft; the combination of laryngotracheomalacia is not unusual. Careful bronchoscopy under local anesthesia with inspection of the entire trachea may show close approximation of the anterior and posterior tracheal walls near the carina at any phase of respiration, but most often during expiration. Passage of the bronchoscope to the carina is followed by less respiratory distress, since the flaccid area is splinted.

The differential diagnosis involves a vascular ring, mediastinal tumor, tracheal web, foreign body, and obstructive lesions of the upper airway. Unfortunately, the ultimate diagnosis of tracheomalacia must often be established by exclusion. The positive findings of excessive tracheal wall mobility and airway relief with the passage of the bronchoscope are at times arbitrary and inconclusive.

Treatment involves the control of infection and secretions by specific antibiotics and humidification. Conservative therapy should be persistent, since cartilaginous development will eventually support the airway, and this may be correlated with concomitant stiffening of the aural cartilages. Clinical improvement is definite in the majority of cases by six months of age, and spontaneous recovery in the remainder may be anticipated at one year. Tracheostomy has been used, but is rarely indicated.

REFERENCES

Cox, W. L., and Shaw, R. R.: Congenital Chondromalacia of the Trachea. *J. Thorac. Cardiov. Surg.*, 49:1033, 1965.

Burford, T. H., and Ferguson, T. B.: Congenital Lesions of the Lungs and Emphysema; in J. H. Gibbon (Ed.): *Surgery of the Chest.* Philadelphia, W. B. Saunders Company, 1962, p. 332.

Holinger, P. H., and Johnston, K. C.: The Infant with Respiratory Stridor. *Pediat. Clin. N. Amer.*, 2:403, 1955.

Holinger, P. H., and others: Congenital Malformations of the Trachea, Bronchi, and Lung. *Ann. Otol.*, 61:1159, 1952.

Levin, S. J., Scherer, R. A., and Adler, P.: Cause of Wheezing in Infancy. *Ann. Allerg.*, 22:20, 1964.

Ochsner, J. L., and LeJeune, F. E., Jr.: Tracheal and Esophageal Obstruction in Infants. *South. M.J.*, 57:1333, 1964.

VASCULAR RING

In 1945 Gross inaugurated the current surgical management of vascular ring anomalies, over 200 years after their morphologic description. Since then, documentation of this early contribution to cardiovascular surgery has been profuse.

Although numerous variations from the normal aortic arch development have been reported, only a few distinct patterns can produce extrinsic tracheal obstruction, and even these may be incidental findings without clinical correlation. The most likely types that compromise the trachea or esophagus, single or together, are (1) right aortic arch with left ligamentum arteriosum or patent ductus arteriosus; (2) double aortic arch; (3) anomalous innominate or left carotid artery; (4) aberrant right subclavian artery.

A right aortic arch represents a persistent right fourth brachial vessel which normally disappears. If this artery, in front of the trachea, is combined with a ductus or a ligamentum arteriosum which runs behind the esophagus, circular incarceration of the trachea and esophagus has taken place, and symptoms may follow.

With double aortic arch, the ascending aorta bifurcates and sends one branch to the right of the trachea and esophagus and then posterior to the esophagus to help form the descending aorta after joining the second branch of the arch which proceeded in front and to the left of the

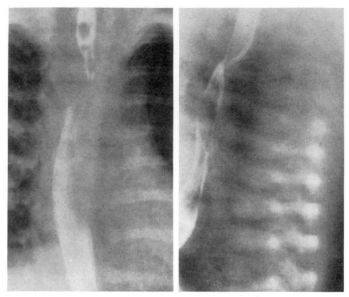

FIGURE 44–8. A posteroanterior and lateral barium swallow demonstrates encirclement of the esophagus at the level of the aortic arch in a 2-month-old infant with dyspnea and noisy respirations. There is narrowing of the lumen from extrinsic pressure with forward displacement, noted best in the lateral projection. The posteroanterior film shows minimal deviation to the left with tapering of the esophagus proximal to a horizontal area of constriction.

trachea. Again, a ring is fashioned and there may be respiratory distress.

Anomalous innominate or left carotid arteries may produce direct anterior pressure on the tracheal wall because of delayed or premature take-off from the arch. Thus the innominate origin from the arch is to the left of its normal source, while the left carotid arises to the right of its usual site. Both vessels must then run over the tracheal cartilages to reach their eventual destination and in so doing may produce a pressure phenomenon.

The aberrant right subclavian artery is most often asymptomatic, but may constrict the posterior esophageal wall and produce dysphagia as it courses from the descending aorta toward the right and behind the esophagus. It is not likely to produce respiratory symptoms.

The common denominator in these arch anomalies is compression and narrowing of the tracheo-esophageal complex. Air exchange is impeded, especially expiration. There is interference with deglutition, and esophageal distention proximal to the area of obstruction may further

constrict the narrowed trachea. Respiratory tract secretions are usually increased and badly handled. Aspiration almost becomes inevitable.

The clinical findings usually begin earlier and are most acute with a double aortic arch; they usually begin later and are less acute with a right aortic arch associated with an encircling ligamentum or ductus, and still less with anomalies that only produce pressure anteriorly, such as aberrant left carotid and innominate arteries.

Signs and symptoms frequently start in the nursery with raucous respirations, dyspnea and tachypnea. There is an invariable exacerbation of the respiratory problem with feedings, and cyanosis with coughing is likely at this time. On examination the chest may be slightly emphysematous, expiration is prolonged, and stridor apparent. Auscultation may demonstrate expiratory wheezing and rhonchi which are diffuse and sometimes transmitted. Opisthotonos has been emphasized, and neck flexion is not tolerated.

Plain x-ray films in the conventional

views may show unusually well aerated lungs, migratory atelectasis, pneumonia, and sometimes a right aortic arch. Chest x-rays may fail, however, to explain the respiratory difficulty. On good lateral films the trachea may be narrowed just above the carina, and contrast material in the esophagus will document various combinations of posterior or lateral indentations at the same level as the tracheal constriction (Fig. 8). Endoscopy will confirm these findings. If respiratory distress is not critical, contrast material in the trachea will delineate the anterior tracheal wall compression. In the infant this can be done without general anesthesia by direct tracheal instillation or by overflow from the hypopharynx.

The presence of a vascular ring can be proved by angiocardiography, either through the venous system or by way of the brachial artery (Fig. 9). This demonstration in the presence of clinical symptoms and x-ray or endoscopic evidence of tracheo-esophageal compression secures the diagnosis. In addition, contrast studies may facilitate the dissection and uncover other cardiovascular anomalies that were clinically unsuspected.

The differential diagnosis involves the clinical picture of respiratory distress, stridor and dysphagia. Cervical and hypopharyngeal obstruction can be ruled out by physical examination of the neck and the mouth and laryngoscopy. Mediastinal tumors and most foreign bodies are excluded by the radiographs. This restricts the diagnostic possibilities to a vascular ring, tracheal stenosis, tracheo-esophageal fistula without atresia, and tracheomalacia. The esophagogram is the next step in the orderly establishment of the diagnosis and begins to limit the possibilities.

After the diagnosis has been established a short period of observation is useful, since only those patients with severe symptoms should be considered for surgery (Mustard). With prolonged hospitaliza-

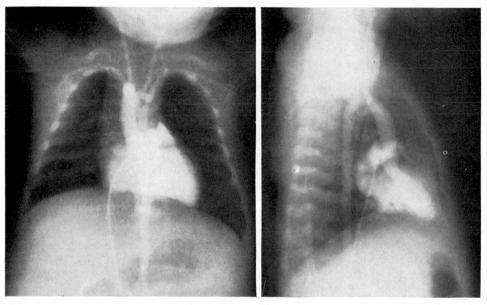

FIGURE 44–9. Selected posteroanterior and lateral films from a venous angiocardiogram, done by Dr. Page Mauck, through the right atrium, foramen ovale and left atrium demonstrates 2 separate, contrast-filled channels originating at the superior aspect of the ascending aorta. On the lateral view the larger superior posterior arch and smaller inferior anterior limb fuse posteriorly at the origin of the descending aorta. In the 2 composite films the innominate artery arises prior to the formation of the double arch, while the left-sided branches arise from the smaller anterior limb. In the frontal projection the posterior arch has a short diagonal course to the left and downward before merging to form the descending aorta.

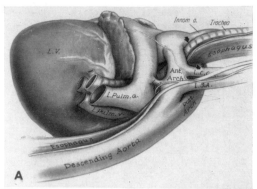

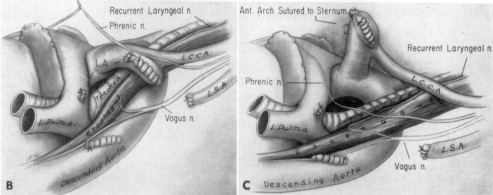

FIGURE 44–10. *A,* The operative findings through a left posterolateral fourth interspace incision confirm the presence of a double aortic arch. *B,* The left subclavian artery and ligamentum arteriosum were divided and the smaller anterior arch transected well to the left of the origin of the left common carotid artery. *C,* The anterior arch was then sutured to the under surface of the sternum.

tion, however, a considerable mortality arises from the natural course of the disease, especially with a double aortic arch or right arch-left ligamentum arteriosum. Death may be sudden and due to compression or septic and secondary to pneumonia. In the severely symptomatic infant, tube feeding, frequent pharyngeal suction, specific antibiotic therapy, high humidity and controlled oxygen and temperature are indispensable in the preoperative period. Careful, direct tracheal aspiration may be appropriate at this time.

The surgical treatment for an offensive vascular ring is now fairly standard. With right aortic arch and a ligamentum arteriosum, division of the latter provides relief. A double aortic arch will require division of the smaller arch, usually the

anterior one. The ligamentum or ductus should also be interrupted and the remnant of the anterior arch separated gently from the trachea and sutured to the under surface of the sternum (Fig. 10). Inspection of the trachea may reveal a cartilaginous deformity which might alter the postoperative course.

Surgical intervention for an aberrant innominate or left carotid artery is rarely required. When indicated, it consists in displacement of the vessel rather than division.

The immediate postoperative period may be precarious because operative and anesthetic trauma may compromise the airway. Fortunately, tracheostomy is rarely required. The stridor usually disappears, and feedings are taken without choking or aspiration. Respirations are not affected by flexion or extension of the head, but the loud nature persists for a few months.

Operative results are uniformly good, and relief from the respiratory distress is predictable. Surgical mortality and morbidity rates are low.

REFERENCES

Abreu, A. L., Surgery of the Heart and Great Vessels; in J. J. M. Brown (Ed.): *Surgery of Childhood.* Baltimore, Williams & Wilkins Company, 1963, p. 705.

Avery, M. E.: *The Lung and Its Disorders in the Newborn Infant.* Philadelphia, W. B. Saunders Company, 1964, p. 66.

Bahnson, H. T.: The Aortic Arch and the Thoracic Aorta; in J. H. Gibbon, Jr. (Ed.): *Surgery of the Chest.* Philadelphia, W. B. Saunders Company, 1962, p. 550.

Bernatz, P. E., Lewis, D. R., and Edwards, J. E.: Division of the Posterior Arch of a Double Aortic Arch for Relief of Tracheal and Esophageal Obstruction. *Proc. Staff Meet., Mayo Clin.,* 34:173, 1959.

Blumenthal, S., and Ravitch, M. M.: Seminar on Aortic Vascular Rings and Other Anomalies of the Aortic Arch. *Pediatrics,* 20:896, 1957.

Boyle, W. F., and Shaw, C. C.: Right-Sided Aortic Arch. *New England J. Med.,* 256:392, 1957.

Cartwright, R. S., and Bauersfield, S. R.: Thoracic Aortography in Infants and Children. *Ann. Surg.,* 150:266, 1959.

De Bord, R. A.: Double Aortic Arch in Infancy. *Ann. Surg.,* 161:479, 1965.

Fineberg, C., and Stofman, H. C.: Tracheal Compression Caused by an Anomalous Innominate Artery Arising from a Brachiocephalic Trunk. *J. Thorac. Surg.,* 37:214, 1959.

Gans, S. L., and Hackworth, L. E.: Respiratory Obstructions of Surgical Import. *Pediat. Clin. N. Amer.,* 6:1023, 1959.

Griswold, H. E., and Young, M. D.: Double Aortic Arch: Report of 2 Cases and Review of the Literature. *Pediatrics,* 4:751, 1949.

Gross, R. E.: *The Surgery of Infancy and Childhood, Its Principles and Techniques.* Philadelphia, W. B. Saunders Company, 1953, pp. 806, 913.

Idem: Thoracic Surgery for Infants. *J. Thorac. Cardiov. Surg.,* 48:152, 1964.

Gross, R. E., and Neuhauser, E. B. D.: Compression of the Trachea or Esophagus by Vascular Anomalies; Surgical Therapy in 40 Cases. *Pediatrics,* 7:69, 1951.

Gross, R. E., and Ware, P. F.: The Surgical Significance of Aortic Arch Anomalies. *Surg., Gynec. & Obst.,* 83:435, 1946.

Holinger, P. H., and Johnston, K. C.: The Infant

with Respiratory Stridor. *Pediat. Clin. N. Amer.,* 2:403, 1955.

Holinger, P. H., and others: Congenital Malformations of the Trachea, Bronchi and Lung. *Ann. Otol.,* 61:1159, 1952.

Lasher, E. P.: Types of Tracheal and Esophageal Constriction Due to Arterial Anomalies of the Aortic Arch, with Suggestions as to Treatment. *Am. J. Surg.,* 96:228, 1958.

Lindskog, G. E., Liebow, A. A., and Glenn, W. W. L.: *Thoracic and Cardiovascular Surgery, with Related Pathology.* New York, Appleton-Century-Crofts, Inc., 1962, p. 750.

Mahoney, E. B., and Manning, J. A.: Aortic Arch; Congenital Abnormalities. *Pediat. Digest,* March 1965.

Mustard, W. T.: Vascular Rings Compressing the Esophagus and Trachea; in C. D. Benson and others (Eds.): *Pediatric Surgery.* Chicago, Year Book Medical Publishers, Inc., 1962, Vol. 1, p. 427.

Nelson, W. E. (Ed.): *Textbook of Pediatrics.* 8th ed. Philadelphia, W. B. Saunders Company, 1964, p. 950.

Nixon, H. H., and O'Donnell, B.: *The Essentials of Paediatric Surgery.* London, William Heinemann, Ltd., 1961, p. 40.

Ochsner, J. L., and LeJeune, F. E., Jr.: Tracheal and Esophageal Obstruction in Infants. *South. M.J.,* 57:1333, 1964.

Richardson, D. W.: Thoracic Emergencies in the Newborn Infant. *Am. J. Surg.,* 105:524, 1963.

Riker, W. L., and Potts, W. J.: Cardiac Lesions Amendable to Surgery: Current Status. *Pediat. Clin. N. Amer.,* 6:1055, 1959.

Schaffer, A. J.: *Diseases of the Newborn.* Philadelphia, W. B. Saunders Company, 1960, p. 63.

Swenson, O.: *Pediatric Surgery.* 2nd ed. New York, Appleton-Century-Crofts, Inc., 1962, p. 202.

TRACHEO-ESOPHAGEAL FISTULA WITHOUT ESOPHAGEAL ATRESIA

Instances of communication between the trachea and the esophagus with an otherwise normal esophagus occur in about 3 per cent of tracheo-esophageal fistulas, and, according to Schneider and Becker, approximately twenty-eight such infants are born each year in the United States. Although symptoms from this congenital abnormality are fairly gross, the diagnosis is usually delayed, and a considerable amount of respiratory morbidity is likely to result (Fig. 11).

The tracheo-esophageal connection is

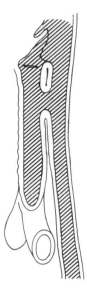

FIGURE 44–11. Diagram of tracheo-esophageal fistula without esophageal atresia. The actual communication is much smaller than depicted.

almost always small, and the majority are found in the neck, from below the larynx to the thoracic inlet. With this arrangement the lungs become, in essence, a diverticulum of the esophagus, and continuous and relentless pulmonary soiling is the basis for extensive pulmonary infection.

The diagnosis should be considered in the presence of recurrent pneumonitis without clear cause or when bouts of coughing, choking or cyanosis follow the ingestion of fluids. There is no dysphagia, and solids may be swallowed and gavage feedings given without difficulty. On physical examination, gastric distention is prominent, especially after crying and coughing, as air is fed through the fistula into the esophagus and the stomach. The lung fields are noisy after liquid feedings, but clear before such feedings. The severity of symptoms may parallel the size of the fistula.

Plain chest x-rays often demonstrate the stigma of chronic pulmonary sepsis, especially in the right upper lobe. In addition, attempts should be made to visualize the fistula by x-ray or endoscopy. Esophagograms in the various prone positions may be fruitful, especially if cinefluoroscopy is used. With continuous recording of the contrast swallow, filling of the trachea through a fistula can be distinguished from overflow aspiration. Esophagoscopy and bronchoscopy may demonstrate the specific orifices, and dyes, such as methylene blue inserted into one lumen, may be recovered in the other lumen, especially if the esophagus distal to the fistula is occluded with a Foley catheter.

The differential diagnosis of this variant of tracheo-esophageal fistula should include chronic bacterial pulmonary disease, chalasia, achalasia, hiatal hernia, cystic fibrosis, neurogenic dysphagia, vascular ring and agammaglobulinemia.

Operative division and suture of the fistula through a transcervical approach are satisfactory in most instances. Very few must be handled transthoracically. The operative mortality rate is reasonable, and deaths are largely due to the crippling nature of the chronic pulmonary disease in patients whose diagnosis has not been prompt.

ESOPHAGEAL ATRESIA

The various types of esophageal atresia comprise an important segment of those congenital abnormalities that produce respiratory distress in the newborn.

The commonest anatomic configuration of this primitive foregut anomaly, with an incidence of 85 per cent, is esophageal atresia with distal tracheo-esophageal fistula. In perhaps 5 to 10 per cent of the cases of esophageal atresia there is no fistula between the distal esophagus and the trachea (Fig. 12). Atresia with proximal tracheo-esophageal fistula and tracheal fistula from both upper and lower esophageal pouches present infrequently.

The incidence of this anomaly has been variously recorded, but one in 3500 births is a reasonable census, and males predominate. At least 25 per cent are premature, and the same percentage have additional critical malformations such as congenital heart disease, mongolism, hydronephrosis, imperforate anus, duodenal atresia and tracheomalacia.

Aberrations in the development of the primary, common respiratory-digestive anlage form the basis for this anomaly. Separation into the anterior pulmonary and posterior gut components by fusion of internal septa is incomplete and may explain the presence of communications or fistulas. A complete lack of septal ingrowth is associated with the more serious, related deformity of laryngotracheo-esophageal cleft. The intrauterine interruption of the vascular supply to the esophagus, vascular anomalies with constriction, or the failure of intraluminal esophageal vacuolization may explain the atresia.

Gross pathologic information is useful in the diagnosis and management of this lesion. With the usual proximal atresia and distal fistula arrangement, the upper blind pouch is large and substantial and usually ends about 10 cm. from the superior alveolar ridge in the region of the azygous vein. The arterial supply from the inferior thyroid artery is rich, runs in a vertical manner, and is difficult to interrupt. Conversely, the lower segment is small and flimsy and originates from the region of the distal posterior membranous trachea, carina or right mainstem bronchus. Its arteries are distributed radially from the intercostals, and a small tracheal vessel may nourish the esophageal end of the tracheo-esophageal fistula. Accordingly, ischemia and necrosis of the distal esophagus are constant hazards of the operative dissection. Congenital stenosis and a diaphragm-like atresia below the tracheo-esophageal fistula in the distal esophagus have been reported.

The attachment of the lower part of the esophagus to the region of the bifurcation of the trachea places this segment in some juxtaposition to the upper pouch. Fortunately, in a third of such cases the two muscle walls are in actual contact and anastomosis is relatively simple; in the remaining two thirds the anastomosis is more difficult because the segments are separated by a gap varying from 1 mm. to several centimeters. In the 5 to 10 per

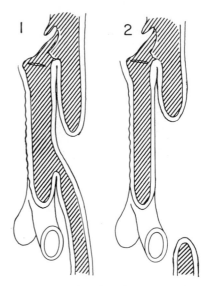

FIGURE 44–12. By far the commonest morphologic variation of esophageal atresia is proximal atresia with distal tracheo-esophageal fistula (1). Much less frequent is proximal atresia without a tracheo-esophageal fistula in which the distal part of the esophagus, seen diagrammatically, actually ends blindly just above the crura of the diaphragm (2).

cent of atresias without fistula, the proximal esophagus is similar to its counterpart in the more usual variance, but the distal esophagus is actually a small gastric diverticulum which barely extends above the diaphragmatic crura and, of course, ends blindly. The two segments are widely separated and cannot be joined surgically.

The respiratory distress sustained by newborns with proximal atresia and distal fistula is instigated by three factors. Obviously, secretions which collect in the upper pouch may overflow into the trachea. Secondly, gastric juice refluxes through the tracheo-esophageal fistula and floods the lungs. And finally the fistula provides a convenient route for gastric distention, upward displacement of the diaphragm and critical interference with pulmonary function.

The clinical picture begins with a history of hydramnios in 25 per cent of the mothers. Profuse, bubbly, oral mucus appears early and almost continuously covers

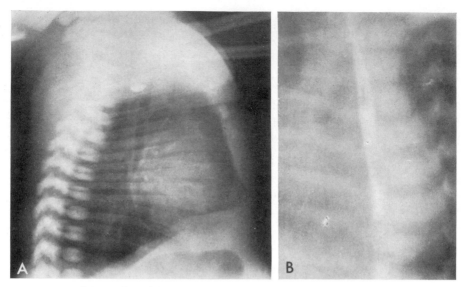

FIGURE 44–13. *A,* Lateral upright chest x-ray after instillation of 0.5 ml. of contrast material into the esophagus defines the atresia at the level of the fourth thoracic vertebra. There is gas in the stomach. *B,* A spot film 3 weeks after surgical repair demonstrates an adequate, undistorted lumen.

the baby's chin in spite of persistent oropharyngeal aspiration. Tachypnea and dyspnea soon follow with intermittent episodes of choking and cyanosis. Regurgitation promptly occurs after the initial and subsequent feedings, and the aspiration explosively exacerbates the respiratory distress. This latter finding is exaggerated in the rare atresia with a proximal fistula, since the ingested liquid reaches the lungs directly through the fistula as well as by overflow of the proximal pouch. On further examination the abdomen is protuberant, flatus is quickly and incessantly passed, and consolidation may be demonstrated in the region of the right upper lobe. If the abnormality is an atresia without a fistula, the incidence of maternal hydramnios may be higher, pulmonary consolidation lower, and the abdomen is scaphoid. Otherwise, the findings in these two groups are similar.

Thoracoabdominal roentgenograms in conventional views may show consolidation of the right upper lobe or more diffuse pneumonitis. Air in the gastrointestinal tract is seen with the usual atresia and distal fistula, although it is said that small fistulas may prevent air

from leaking into the stomach. Conversely, large amounts of gastric air may suggest a large fistula, and therapy becomes more urgent because of the exaggerated respiratory distress. An airless abdomen is presumptive evidence of atresia without a distal fistula. On lateral thoracic x-ray films the proximal atretic pouch may be delineated by air, but this is made clearer by the insertion of a small radiopaque urethral catheter under fluoroscopy. Coiling of a fairly stiff catheter at a level between the second and fourth thoracic vertebrae or demonstration of the blind pouch by 0.5 ml. of contrast material will conclude the regional diagnostic exercise. The contrast material should be aspirated at the conclusion of the examination (Fig. 13).

These and other diagnostic studies are utilized to establish the presence of additional anomalies which may affect therapy. Thus the mediastinal dissection can be done with more alacrity if a right-sided aortic arch has been noted preoperatively. Congenital heart, cerebral, gastrointestinal and neurologic anomalies must be considered and uncovered with some dispatch before the correct operative approach can be planned. Associated cardiovascular anomalies are particularly lethal.

The diagnosis, then, of atresia with fistula should be strongly suspected on the basis of maternal hydramnios, excessive mucus, respiratory distress, and regurgitation. The suspicion is strengthened by the passage of a catheter into the esophagus which stops 8 to 12 cm. from the gums. The final confirmation is obtained by fluoroscopic examination.

Preoperatively, the upper pouch is aspirated through an indwelling catheter. A semi-upright position should be maintained during transportation or in the nursery Isolette to prevent or minimize gastric reflux through the fistula. High humidity and antibiotics are used to control pneumonia. Constant nursing of a high order should be started on admission and continued until the issue is no longer in doubt.

The operative management of isolated atresia without a fistula will eventually require a reversed gastric tube or colon transplant, since the two ends of the esophagus are widely separated and cannot be anastomosed. The operation immediately after diagnosis is gastrostomy under local anesthesia. Contrast study through the stomach with the infant in sharp Trendelenburg position will outline the short, blind, distal esophageal stump. Since an anastomosis is technically impossible, a cervical esophagostomy is created to drain saliva, and esophageal replacement is anticipated at two years of age. The same steps can be followed when a large gap prevents anastomosis in the usual variety of atresia (Fig. 14).

Several operative approaches are available for atresia with distal fistula. The ultimate decision is based on the degree of prematurity, presence of other anomalies, time of diagnosis, presence or absence of pneumonia, exact anatomic configuration of the lesion, and the preference of the surgeon. Transpleural or extrapleural ligation of the fistula and esophago-esophagostomy with or without gastrostomy in one stage is ideal and is the accepted

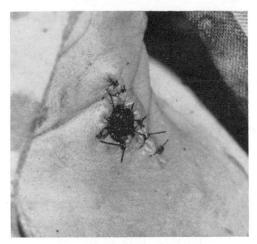

FIGURE 44–14. Proximal esophagostomy, or salivary fistula, in the right side of the neck of a newborn with esophageal atresia without fistula.

approach in the full-term newborn with no serious anomalies or pneumonia. Varying degrees of prematurity, pneumonitis and concomitant abnormalities drastically alter mortality, so that staged procedures have assumed some popularity in certain clinics. Gastrostomy then becomes the primary, emergency step to decompress the fistula and control the pneumonia. Later, ligation of the fistula and fixation of the oversewn distal esophagus to the endothoracic fascia permits feeding while the upper pouch remains on continuous or intermittent suction. With good nursing care this arrangement is compatible with growth and development and the esophageal anastomosis may be accomplished at a time of election in a better-risk infant. If such nursing cannot be provided, aspiration pneumonia from the upper pouch is almost inevitable, and in these circumstances the very premature infant had best be committed to a salivary fistula and esophageal substitute. This is less than ideal, but the mortality is a distinct improvement over that of primary repair in this group.

The acute postoperative period is critical and deserves maximum attention. All the advantages of an Isolette are utilized. The pharynx must be carefully aspirated,

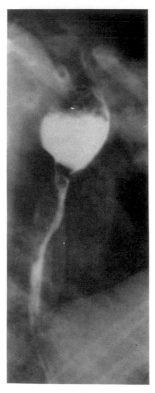

FIGURE 44–15. A barium swallow in a one-year-old male infant with dysphagia who was born with proximal esophageal atresia and distal tracheo-esophageal fistula managed by ligation of the fistula and esophago-esophagostomy in one stage. This single film shows gross saccular dilatation of the proximal esophagus above an area of stricture at the level of the anastomosis. Several dilatations over a string provided an adequate lumen.

without injury to the fresh anastomosis, to prevent aspiration and stimulate coughing. Postoperative feeding should be started with homeopathic amounts of glucose water and formula, initially administered by slow drip through a small nasogastric or gastrostomy tube. Oral feedings are started with a 0.6-cc. medicine dropper; this minimal volume can be handled by the proximal esophagus and its anastomosis without overflow (Potts).

Complications are legion, but the most catastrophic is disruption of the suture line and resultant empyema. The mortality from this can be lessened by an extrapleural operative approach which would confine the contamination to an extrapleural plane. The brassy postoperative cough is usually temporary and not related to a recurrence of the fistula, which, fortunately, is rare. Anastomotic strictures occur within three months in one third of the survivors and are heralded by dysphagia, regurgitation, cough and recurrent pneumonia (Fig. 15). Treatment at first consists in dilatation, started on the basis of dysphagia correlated with x-ray changes. Holinger, however, prefers to treat postoperative strictures early because of the danger of aspiration pneumonia. Resection has been advised for recalcitrant strictures. Postoperative pneumonia can also be instigated by faulty motility of the distal esophagus with reflux following operative vagus nerve damage.

The over-all rate of survivors with primary definitive operations from a generous aliquot of children's and general hospitals approaches 60 per cent; this is elevated to 70 per cent of full-term newborns and perhaps 80 per cent full-term neonates who are otherwise normal. Primary anastomosis in prematures carries a 60 to 70 per cent mortality rate, but this can be reversed with operative staging.

REFERENCES

Avery, M. E.: *The Lung and Its Disorders in the Newborn Infant.* Philadelphia, W. B. Saunders Company, 1964, p. 89.

Baker, D. C., Flood, C. A., and Ferrer, J. M., Jr.: Postoperative Esophageal Stenosis. *Ann. Otol.,* 63:1082, 1954.

Blumberg, J. B.: Laryngotracheoesophageal Cleft, the Embryologic Implications: Review of the Literature. *Surgery,* 57:559, 1965.

Burford, T. H., and Ferguson, T. B.: Congenital Lesions of the Lungs and Emphysema; in J. H. Gibbon, Jr. (Ed.): *Surgery of the Chest.* Philadelphia, W. B. Saunders Company, 1962, p. 331.

Cohen, S. J.: Unusual Types of Esophageal Atresia and Tracheoesophageal Fistulae. *Clin. Pediat.,* 4:271, 1965.

DeBoar, A., and Potts, W. J.: Congenital Atresia of the Esophagus with Tracheo-esophageal Fistula. *Surg. Gynec. & Obst.,* 104:475, 1957.

Desjardins, J. G., Stephens, C. A., and Moes, C. A. F.: Results of Surgical Treatment of

Congenital Tracheo-esophageal Fistula, with a Note on Cine-fluorographic Findings. *Ann. Surg.*, 100:14, 1964.

Falletta, G. P.: Recommunication on Repair of Congenital Tracheoesophageal Fistula. *Arch. Surg.*, 88:779, 1964.

Flavell, G.: *The Oesophagus.* London, Butterworth, 1963, pp. 20, 24.

Franklin, R. H.: The Oesophagus; in J. J. M. Brown (Ed.): *Surgery of Childhood*, Baltimore, Williams & Wilkins Company, 1963, pp. 747, 754.

Gans, S. L., and Hackworth, L. E.: Respiratory Obstructions of Surgical Import. *Pediat. Clin. N. Amer.*, 6:1023, 1959.

Goldenberg, I. S.: An Unusual Variation of Congenital Tracheoesophageal Fistula. *J. Thorac. Cardiov. Surg.*, 40:114, 1960.

Gross, R. E.: *The Surgery of Infancy and Childhood, Its Principles and Techniques.* Philadelphia, W. B. Saunders Company, 1953, p. 77.

Groves, L. K.: Surgical Treatment of Esophageal Atresia and Tracheo-esophageal Fistula in the Infant. *Cleveland Clin. Quart.*, 25:227, 1958.

Haight, C.: Congenital Tracheo-esophageal Fistula Without Esophageal Atresia. *J. Thorac. Surg.*, 17:600, 1948.

Idem; The Management of Congenital Esophageal Atresia and Tracheo-esophageal Fistula. *Surg. Clin. N. Amer.*, 41:1281, 1961.

Idem: The Esophagus; in C. D. Benson and others (Eds.): *Pediatric Surgery.* Chicago, Year Book Medical Publishers, Inc., 1962, Vol. 1, p. 266.

Hays, D. M.: An Analysis of the Mortality in Esophageal Atresia. *Am. J. Dis. Child.*, 103:765, 1962.

Idem: Esophageal Atresia: Current Management. *Pediat. Digest*, April 1965.

Hays, D. M., and Snyder, W. H.: Results of Conventional Operative Procedures for Esophageal Atresia in Premature Infants. *Am. J. Surg.*, 106:19, 1963.

Heimlich, H. J.: Peptic Esophagitis with Stricture Treated by Reconstruction of the Esophagus with a Reversed Gastric Tube. *Surg., Gynec. & Obst.*, 114:673, 1962.

Helmsworth, J. A., and Pryles, C. V.: Congenital Tracheoesophageal Fistula Without Esophageal Atresia. *J. Pediat.*, 38:610, 1951.

Herwig, J., and Ogura, J.: Congenital Tracheoesophageal Fistula Without Esophageal Atresia. *J. Pediat.*, 47:298, 1955.

Holder, T. M.: Problems Peculiar to Infants; in J. H. Gibbon, Jr. (Ed.): *Surgery of the Chest.* Philadelphia, W. B. Saunders Company, 1962, p. 107.

Idem: Transpleural Versus Retropleural Approach for Repair of Tracheoesophageal Fistula. *Surg. Clin. N. Amer.*, 44:1433, 1964.

Holder, T. M., and Gross, R. E.: Temporary Gastrostomy in Pediatric Surgery. *Pediatrics*, 26:37, 1960.

Holder, T. M., McDonald, V. G., and Woolley, M. W.: The Premature or Critically Ill Infant with Esophageal Atresia: Increased Success with a Staged Approach. *J. Thorac. Cardiov. Surg.*, 44:344, 1962.

Holder, T. M., and others: Esophageal Atresia and Tracheoesophageal Fistula. *Pediatrics*, 34:542, 1964.

Holinger, P. H., Brown, W. T., and Maurizi. D. G.: Endoscopic Aspects of Post-surgical Management of Congenital Esophageal Atresia and Tracheoesophageal Fistula. *J. Thorac. Cardiov. Surg.*, 49:22, 1965.

Holinger, P. H., and others: Congenital Malformations of the Trachea, Bronchi and Lung. *Ann. Otol.*, 61:1159, 1952.

Humphreys, G. H., Hogg, B. M., and Ferrer, J.: Congenital Atresia of Esophagus. *J. Thorac. Surg.*, 32:332, 1956.

Karlan, M., Thompson, J., and Clatworthy, H. W.: Congenital Atresia of the Esophagus with Tracheoesophageal Fistula and Duodenal Atresia. *Surgery*, 41:544, 1957.

Killen, D. A., and Greenlee, H. B.: Transcervical Repair of H-Type Congenital Tracheoesophageal Fistula: Review of the Literature. *Ann. Surg.*, 162:145, 1965.

Koop, C. E.: Atresia of the Esophagus: Technical Considerations in Surgical Management. *Surg. Clin. N. Amer.*, 42:1387, 1962.

Koop, C. E., Kiesewetter, W. B., and Johnson, J.: Treatment of Atresia of the Esophagus by the Transpleural Approach. *Surg., Gynec. & Obst.*, 98:687, 1954.

Lindskog, G. E., Liebow, A. A., and Glenn, W. W. L.: *Thoracic and Cardiovascular Surgery with Related Pathology.* New York, Appleton-Century-Crofts, Inc., 1962, p. 481.

Lloyd, J. R., and Clatworthy, H. W.: Hydramnios as an Aid to Early Diagnosis of Congenital Obstruction of the Alimentary Tract: A Study of the Maternal and Fetal Factors. *Pediatrics*, 21:903, 1958.

Lynn, H. B., and Davis, L. A.: Tracheo-esophageal Fistula Without Atresia of the Esophagus. *Surg. Clin. N. Amer.*, 41:871, 1961.

Martin, L. W., and Hogg, S. P.: Esophageal Atresia and Tracheoesophageal Fistula. *A.M.A. J. Dis. Child.*, 99:828, 1960.

Mellins, R. B., and Blumenthal, S.: Cardiovascular Anomalies and Esophageal Atresia. *Am. J. Dis. Child.*, 107:160, 1964.

Morse, G. W., Anderson, E. V., and Arenson, N.: Congenital Tracheo-esophageal Fistula Without Esophageal Atresia: An Improved Method of Demonstration. *Am. Surg.*, 24:112, 1958.

Murphy, D. R., and Owen, H. F.: Respiratory Emergencies in the Newborn. *Am. J. Surg.*, 101:581, 1961.

Nixon, H. H., and O'Donnell, B.: *The Essen-*

tials of Pediatric Surgery. London, William Heinemann, Ltd., 1961, p. 32.

Rehbein, F., and Yanagiswa, F.: Complications After Operation for Oesophageal Atresia. *Arch. Dis. Childhood,* Feb. 1959, p. 24.

Reploge, R. L.: Esophageal Atresia: Plastic Sump Catheter for Drainage of the Proximal Pouch. *Surgery,* 54:296, 1963.

Richardson, W. R.: Thoracic Emergencies in the Newborn Infant. *Am. J. Surg.,* 105:524, 1963.

Sandegard, E.: The Treatment of Oesophageal Atresia. *Arch. Dis. Childhood,* 32:475, 1957.

Schaffer, A. J.: *Diseases of the Newborn.* Philadelphia, W. B. Saunders Company, 1960, pp. 149, 155.

Schneider, K. M., and Becker, J. M.: The "H-Type" Tracheoesophageal Fistula in Infants and Children. *Surgery,* 51:677, 1962.

Schultz, L. R., and Clatworthy, H. W.: Esophageal Strictures After Anastomosis in Esophageal Atresia. *Arch. Surg.,* 87:136, 1963.

Schwartz, S. I., and Dale, W. A.: Unusual Tracheo-esophageal Fistula with Membranous Obstruction of the Esophagus and Postoperative Hypertrophic Pyloric Stenosis. *Ann. Surg.,* 142:1002, 1955.

Shaw, R. R., Paulson, D. L., and Siebel, E. K.: Congenital Atresia of the Esophagus with Tracheo-esophageal Fistula, Treatment of Surgical Complications. *Ann. Surg.,* 142:204, 1955.

Stephens, C. A., Mustard, W. T., and Simpson, J. S.: Congenital Atresia of the Esophagus with Tracheo-esophageal Fistula. *Surg. Clin. N. Amer.,* 36:1465, 1956.

Swenson, O., and others: Repair and Complications of Esophageal Atresia and Tracheoesophageal Fistula. *New England J. Med.,* 267:960, 1962.

Swenson, O.: *Pediatric Surgery.* 2nd ed. New York, Appleton-Century-Crofts, Inc., 1962, p. 155.

Tuqan, N. A.: Annular Stricture of the Esophagus Distal to Congenital Tracheoesophageal Fistula. *Surgery,* 52:394, 1962.

Waterston, D. J., Bonham-Carter, R. E., and Aberdeen, E.: Congenital Tracheo-esophageal Atresia. *Lancet,* 2:55, 1963.

Yahr, W. Z., Azzoni, A. A., and Santulli, T. V.: Congenital Atresia of the Esophagus with Tracheoesophageal Fistula: An Unusual Variant. *Surgery,* 52:937, 1962.

Zachary, R. B., and Emery, J. L.: Failure of Separation of Larynx and Trachea from the Esophagus: Persistent Esophagotrachea. *Surgery,* 49: 525, 1961.

CONGENITAL BRONCHIAL STENOSIS

Congenital stricture of the bronchus occurs predominantly in a main stem or middle lobe bronchus and can produce acute and chronic pulmonary infection (Swenson). Inflammatory scarring of the congenitally stenosed bronchus provides an ideal environment for distal suppuration, atelectasis and bronchiectasis.

Chest x-rays will demonstrate various stages of pneumonitis, atelectasis and perhaps compensatory emphysema.

Bronchoscopy and bronchography confirm the diagnosis.

Treatment will eventually consist of varying degres of lung resection, although plastic reconstruction of a main stem bronchus may have a place.

REFERENCES

Holinger, P. H., and others: Congenital Malformations of the Trachea, Bronchi and Lung. *Ann. Otol.,* 61:1159, 1952.

Swenson, O.: *Pediatric Surgery.* 2nd ed. New York, Appleton-Century-Crofts, Inc., 1962, p. 123.

BRONCHOGENIC CYST

Congenital intrathoracic tumors of bronchogenic origin are found in the posterior or midmediastinum, behind or close to the tracheobronchial tree and often attached to it by an obliterated or patent stalk. These malformations are usually single, more frequent on the right, and associated with local bronchovascular anomalies, including a systemic pulmonary blood suply. A few bronchogenic cysts have been reported within the esophagus, pericardium and pulmonary parenchyma.

Embryologically, respiratory tissue, at various stages of development, becomes pinched off and separated, and the eventual location and histology of the bronchogenic cyst depend partly on the time of this dislocation from the main respiratory body. Early partition from the foregut may produce a cyst with some similarity to esophageal and gastroenteric duplications. Later cystic development from distal bronchoalveolar structures may simulate congenital pulmonary cysts.

The majority of bronchogenic cysts will be paratracheal, carinal, hilar or para-esophageal in location (Maier), between 2 and 10 cm. in diameter, unilocular, have a substantial wall and contain mucus, pus or blood. Microscopically, there is a lining of ciliated columnar respiratory epithelium surrounded by disorganized muscle, cartilage and fibrous tissue.

There may be some difficulty, pathologically and clinically, in separating congenital bronchogenic cysts from acquired cysts and abscesses, especially in the older infant and the child. The presence of respiratory epithelium lining a cyst in embryos and newborns is considered evidence of a congenital abnormality. Unfortunately, secondary infection can obliterate this characteristic lining, and subsequent healing may occur with bronchial mucosa; the final histologic picture, then, is similar to an epithelialized, chronic lung abscess.

Clinical findings are based on (1) proximal tracheobronchial obstruction with respiratory distress, (2) moderate obstruction with distal pulmonary sepsis, (3) suppuration of the cyst by contamination through a tracheobronchial communica-tion. This may be followed by slough of the respiratory epithelium and replacement by granulation tissue with chronic infection. (4) Finally, some cysts are asymptomatic and are diagnosed only by routine x-ray examination or x-ray films taken for some other reason.

Carinal cysts usually produce dramatic symptoms of respiratory obstruction in infancy, and the distress parallels the size of the cyst to the point of sudden death (Fig. 16). Cysts in other locations are more likely to become infected or lead to repeated pulmonary parenchymal infection in the older infant and the child. The clinical picture may mimic a lung abscess with fever, chest pain, wheezing, cough, dysphagia, hemoptysis, purulent sputum, and plain or push-up stridor.

The diagnosis may be suspected after x-ray examination of the chest by various techniques (Fig. 17). Fluoroscopic or cineradiographic visualization of ascent with swallowing is possible if a firm tracheal attachment is present. Displacement, separation and compression of the trachea and esophagus and elevation of the carina with flattening of the bronchial angle can also be seen at the same examination. Chest x-rays will document these findings and demonstrate a solitary, smooth-

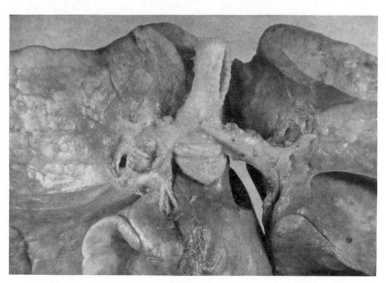

FIGURE 44–16. Autopsy specimen of a carinal bronchogenic cyst.

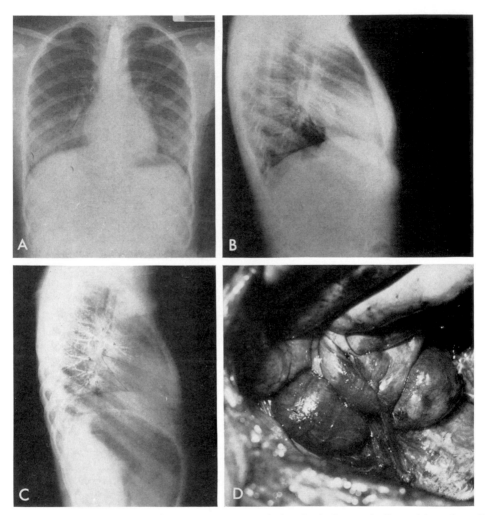

FIGURE 44–17. A 10 year-old girl, exposed to tuberculosis, who had a markedly positive tuberculin skin test reaction. A mediastinal mass did not regress after 6 months of therapy in a sanatorium. *A, B,* The posteroanterior and lateral chest films show a normal cardiovascular silhouette. There is a mass posterior to the border of the right side of the heart with smooth margins, which covers almost 2 interspaces. The lateral film localizes the density to the area beneath the right hilus. The mass is denser than surrounding lung, but more radiolucent than the heart. The lung fields are otherwise not remarkable. *C,* A lateral bronchogram shows no filling of the middle lobe, with adequate filling elsewhere. *D,* At thoracotomy a bilobed bronchogenic cyst, in the region of the inferior pulmonary vein and ligament, was resected.

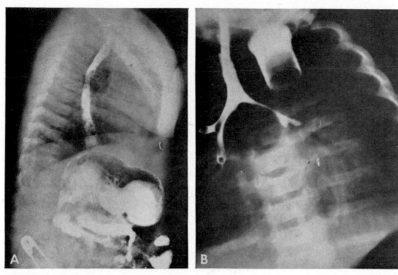

FIGURE 44—18. A 2-month-old infant with intermittent, severe respiratory distresss. *A*, A lateral film with a barium-filled esophagus demonstrates an irregular, smoothly marginated radiolucency in the midmediastinum at the level of the carina with slight narrowing of the esophagus at this level. *B*, The anteroposterior tracheobronchogram reveals widening of the tracheal bifurcation and narrowing of the left main stem bronchus by extrinsic pressure. Within the limbs on the 2 main stem bronchi is an area of radiolucency with smooth borders, compatible with an air-filled cyst under tension. A bronchogenic cyst attached to the left main stem bronchus was removed.

walled, noncalcified tumor widening the mediastinum on one side or both sides and sometimes associated with pneumonia, atelectasis or emphysema. With a tracheobronchial communication a fluid level in a thick-walled cyst shouud arouse suspicion. Planigrams and bronchograms are occasionally helpful (Fig. 18).

Low-lying mediastinal cysts or even those centrally located may be difficult to separate from a host of other mediastinal tumors. The differential diagnosis includes diaphragmatic hernia, tuberculosis, pyogenic lung abscess, sarcoidosis, emphysema, lymphoma, teratoma, hamartoma, mediastinal granuloma and metastatic lung tumors.

Since a bronchogenic cyst may rupture into a bronchus or pleura, bleed profusely, become badly infected, undergo tumorous degeneration and produce sudden death, surgical intervention should be utilized unless there is some serious contraindication, in order to establish a diagnosis and to avoid annoying or catastrophic sequelae. The actual surgical exercise involves resection of the cyst alone or with various amounts of pulmonary tissue surrounding the cyst. Aberrant systematic arteries and bronchial anomalies can be troublesome.

REFERENCES

Ackerman, L. V.: Personal communication cited in J. H. Gibbon, Jr. (Ed.): *Surgery of the Chest.* Philadelphia, W. B. Saunders Company, 1962, p. 339.

Bressler, S., and Wiener, D.: Bronchogenic Cyst Associated with an Anomalous Pulmonary Artery Arising from the Thoracic Aorta. *Surgery,* 35:815, 1954.

Bruwer, A., Clagett, O. T., and McDonald, J. R.: Anomalous Arteries to the Lung Associated with Congenital Pulmonary Abnormality. *J. Thorac. Surg.,* 19:957, 1950.

Culiner, M. M., and Grimes, O. F.: Localized Emphysema in Association with Bronchial Cysts or Mucoceles. *J. Thorac. Cardiov. Surg.,* 41:306, 1961.

Burford, T. H., and Ferguson, T. B.: Congenital Lesions of the Lungs and Emphysema; in J. H. Gibbon, Jr. (Ed.): *Surgery of the Chest.* Philadelphia, W. B. Saunders Company, 1962, p. 338.

Dabbs, C. H., Peirce, E. C., and Rawson, F. L.: Intrapericardial Interatrial Tertoma (Bronchogenic Cyst). *New England J. Med.*, 256: 541, 1957.

Flavell, G.: *An Introduction to Chest Surgery.* London, Oxford University Press, 1957, p. 126.

Gans, S. L., and Hackworth, L. E.: Respiratory Obstructions of Surgical Import. *Pediat. Clin. N. Amer.*, 6:1023, 1959.

Greenfield, L. J., and Howe, J. S.: Bronchial Adenoma Within the Wall of a Bronchogenic Cyst. *J. Thorac. Cardiov. Surg.*, 49:398, 1965.

Gross, R. E.: *The Surgery of Infancy and Childhood, Its Principles and Techniques.* Philadelphia, W. B. Saunders Company, 1962, p. 780.

Hope, J. W., and Koop, C. E.: Differential Diagnosis of Mediastinal Masses. *Pediat. Clin. N. Amer.*, 6:379, 1959.

Jones, P.: Developmental Defects in Lungs. *Thorax*, 10:205, 1955.

Leigh, T. F., and Weens, H. S.: *The Mediastinum.* Springfield, Ill., Charles C Thomas, 1959, p. 136.

Lindskog, G. E., Liebow, A. A., and Glenn, W. W. L.: *Thoracic and Cardiovascular Surgery, with Related Pathology.* New York, Appleton-Century-Crofts, Inc., 1962, p. 452.

Maier, H. C.: Bronchogenic Cysts of the Mediastinum. *Ann. Surg.*, 127:476, 1948.

Moersch, H. J., and Clagett, O. T.: Pulmonary Cysts. *J. Thorac. Surg.*, 16:179, 1947.

Opsahl, T., and Berman, E. J.: Bronchogenic Mediastinal Cysts in Infants: Case Report and Review of Literature. *Pediatrics, 30:372*, 1962.

Pilcher, R. S.: Trachea, Bronchi, Lungs and Pleura; in J. J. M. Brown (Ed.): *Surgery of Childhood,* Baltimore, Williams & Wilkins Company, 1963, p. 667.

Pontius, R. G.: Bronchial Obstruction of Congenital Origin. *Am. J. Surg.*, 106:8, 1963.

Potts, W. J.: *The Surgeon and the Child.* Philadelphia, W. B. Saunders Company, 1964, p. 71.

Schaffer, A. J.: *Diseases of the Newborn.* Philadelphia, W. B. Saunders Company, 1960, p. 168.

Schlumberger, H. G.: Tumors of the Mediastinum; in *Atlas of Tumor Pathology.* Fascicle 18. Washington, D.C., Armed Forces Institue of Pathology, 1951.

Swenson, O.: *Pediatric Surgery.* 2nd ed. New York, Appleton-Century-Crofts, Inc., 1962, p. 124.

Trossman, C. M.: Push-Up Stridor Caused by a Bronchogenic Cyst. *J. Dis. Child.*, 107:293, 1964.

Webb, W. R., and Burford, T. H.: Studies of the Re-expanded Lung After Prolonged Atelectasis. *Arch. Surg.*, 66:801, 1953.

Weisel, W., Claudon, D. B., and Darin, J. C.: Tracheal Adenoma in Juxtaposition with a Mediastinal Bronchogenic Cyst. *J. Thorac. Surg.*, 37:687, 1959.

PULMONARY AGENESIS, APLASIA AND HYPOPLASIA

Varying degrees of absence of pulmonary tissue have been recorded in a number of instances. Bilateral pulmonary agenesis is a rare malformation and may occur with acephalic monsters (Potter). Slightly more frequent is unilateral pulmonary agenesis, in which the trachea runs directly into the sole bronchus, with an absent carina. Pulmonary aplasia is the commonest variant and consists of a carina and mainstem bronchial stump with an absent distal lung. Functionally, unilateral lung agenesis and aplasia are similar. Lobar agenesis and aplasia are rarer than complete absence of one lung and usually occur as a combination of the right upper and middle lobes. Finally, pulmonary hypoplasia has been described as a mass of poorly differentiated lung parenchyma connected to a malformed bronchus.

Embryologically, these malformations correspond to a failure of development of the respiratory system from the foregut. Arrest at the stage of the primitive lung bud produces bilateral pulmonary agenesis. The respiratory anlage at a later stage may develop only unilaterally and lead to lung agenesis. Lobar agenesis then becomes developmental arrest on one side in an older embryo. Lastly, pulmonary hypoplasia may occur during the last trimester of pregnancy with failure of final alveolar differentiation. The high incidence of associated cardiac, gastrointestinal and skeletal malformations, as well as frequent variations in the bronchopulmonary vasculature, lends support to generalized teratogenic factors.

Pathologically, the sole lung is larger than normal in pulmonary agenesis, and this enlargement is true hypertrophy and not emphysema. In addition, Lukas has reported vascular changes, secondary to hypertension, in the residual lung.

The wide variation in clinical findings is only partially explained by the amount of involved pulmonary tissue, although obviously this is an important factor. About 50 per cent of the patients with unilateral pulmonary agenesis survive. This segment is probably devoid of other serious anomalies, except for an occasional instance of retarded development.

The history may include harsh breathing, dyspnea, tachypnea, repeated upper respiratory tract infections and respiratory distress, with cyanosis, on exertion. Inspection of the chest does not suggest an absent lung, since the external appearance is normal. Herniation of the sole lung and massive mediastinal shift and rotation fill the empty hemithorax. In addition, there is flat percussion over a dislocated heart, which may suggest dextrocardia in the presence of a right-sided agenesis. Breath sounds from the herniated, hypertrophied lung are heard on the side of the agenesis except in the axilla and the base. With lobar agenesis, respiratory symptoms and mediastinal displacement occur, but are more subtle.

X-ray films of the chest show a homogeneous density on the involved, agenetic side, with mediastinal rotation and shift. Lung herniation can be seen beneath the sternum on lateral films. X-ray films of lobar agenesis may simply exhibit mediastinal shift.

The diagnosis should be suspected when respiratory difficulty occurs with tracheal deviation in the presence of a symmetrical chest and the chest roentgenogram is suggestive of massive atelectasis and mediastinal shift. Body section roentgenograms may strengthen the possibility of pulmonary agenesis. The diagnosis is confirmed by bronchoscopy which fails to demonstrate one major bronchus and bronchography which documents this finding. With lobar aplasia, bronchograms are indispensable, since the pathologic changes may not be visible to the bronchoscopist. Angiography may demonstrate suspected cardiac anomalies and aberrant pulmonary vessels.

It is difficult to separate atelectasis from pulmonary or lobar agenesis on clinical grounds. In the differential diagnosis, Schaffer suggests that bilateral peripheral aerated lung rules out the diagnosis of unilateral pulmonary agenesis. Endoscopy and bronchography can settle the issue.

In reviewing the mortality from pulmonary agenesis, it is apparent that chronic dyspnea with cough and repeated respiratory infections are ominous prognostic signs; so indeed is a right-sided agenesis. A tracheobronchial foreign body may produce the initial symptoms, and at least three fatalities have been reported during attempts at endoscopic removal.

Pulmonary resection may be indicated in lobar agenesis if the lung parenchyma on the side of the agenesis is supplied by abnormal bronchi or arteries to which incapacitating symptoms can be ascribed (Adler, Herman and Jewett). For pulmonary agenesis, acute infections are treated conventionally; repeated infections may deserve continuous antibiotic therapy.

REFERENCES

Adler, R. H., Herrmann, J. W., and Jewett, T. C.: Lobar Agenesis of the Lung. *Ann. Surg.*, 147:267, 1958.

Avery, M. E.: *The Lung and Its Disorders in the Newborn Infant.* Philadelphia, W. B. Saunders Company, 1964, pp. 83, 84.

Brunner, S., and Nissen, E.: Agenesis of the Lung. *Am. Rev. Resp. Dis.*, 87:103, 1963.

Burford, T. H., and Ferguson, T. B.: Congenital Lesions of the Lungs and Emphysema; in J. H. Gibbon, Jr. (Ed.): *Surgery of the Chest.* Philadelphia, W. B. Saunders Company, 1962, p. 332.

Claireaux, A. E., and Ferreira, H. P.: Bilateral Pulmonary Agenesis. *Arch. Dis. Childhood*, 33:364, 1958.

Harris, G. B. C.: The Newborn with Respiratory Distress: Some Roentgenographic Features. *Radiol. Clin. N. Amer.*, 1:499, 1963.

Holinger, P. H., and others: Congenital Malformations of the Trachea, Bronchi, and Lung. *Ann. Otol.*, 61:1159, 1952.

Landing, B. H.: Anomalies of the Respiratory Tract. *Pediat. Clin. N. Amer.* 4:73, 1957.

Lindskog, G. E., Liebow, A. A., and Glenn, W. W. L.: *Thoracic Cardiovascular Surgery, with Related Pathology*. New York, Appleton-Century-Crofts, Inc., 1962, p. 103.

Lukas, D. S., Dotter, C. T., and Steinberg, I.: Agenesis of the Lung and Patent Ductus Arteriosus with Reversal of Flow. *New England J. Med.*, 249:107, 1953.

Martinez-Jimenez, M., and others: Agenesis of the Lung with Patent Ductus Arteriosus Treated Surgically. *J. Thorac. Cardiov. Surg.*, 50:59, 1965.

Minetto, E., Galli, E., and Boglione, G.: Agenesia, Aplasia, Hypoplasia Pulmonare. *Minerva Med.*, 49:4635, 1958.

Morison, J. E., *Foetal and Neonatal Pathology*. London, Butterworth & Co., 1952.

Morton, D. R., Klassen, K. P., and Baxter, E. H.: Lobar Agenesis of the Lung. *J. Thorac. Surg.*, 20:665, 1950.

Oyamada, A., Gasul, B. M., and Holinger, P. H.: Agenesis of the Lung. Report of a Case with Review of All Previously Reported Cases. *Am. J. Dis. Child.*, 85:182, 1953.

Pilcher, R. S.: Trachea, Bronchi, Lungs, and Pleura; in J. J. M. Brown (Ed.): *Surgery of Childhood*. Baltimore, Williams & Wilkins Company, 1963, p. 665.

Potter, E. L.: *Pathology of the Fetus and the Newborn*. Chicago, Year Book Publishers, Inc., 1952, p. 261.

Ravitch, M. M.: Agenesis of the Lung; in C. D. Benson and others (Eds.): *Pediatric Surgery*, Chicago, Year Book Medical Publishers, Inc., 1962, Vol. 1, p. 346.

Schaffer, A. J.: *Diseases of the Newborn*. Philadelphia, W. B. Saunders Company, 1960, p. 133.

Spencer, H.: *Pathology of the Lung*. New York, Macmillan Company, 1962, p. 27.

Tuynman, P. E., and Gardner, L. W.: Bilateral Aplasia of Lung. *Arch. Path.*, 54:306, 1952.

Waddell, J. A., Simon, G., and Reid, L.: Bronchial Atresia of the Left Upper Lobe. *Thorax*, 20:214, 1965.

CONGENITAL PNEUMONOCELE (PULMONARY HERNIA)

The presence of lung tissue outside the usual confines of an intact bony thorax is a most infrequent finding in the neonatal period. About 20 per cent of all lung hernias are congenital; the remainder follow trauma.

The usual site of a congenital pulmonary hernia is the cervical region because of the absence of the endothoracic fascia in this area. Hernias in the region of the axilla have also been reported. Conversely, acquired post-traumatic hernias will occur in the midthoracic region.

The infant is usually asymptomatic, although local tenderness and slight dyspnea have been observed. Examination may demonstrate a supraclavicular mass which will increase in size with crying.

Treatment is usually superfluous.

REFERENCES

Ballinger, W. F., II: The Thoracic Wall; in J. H. Gibbon, Jr. (Ed.): *Surgery of the Chest*. Philadelphia, W. B. Saunders Company, 1962, p. 206.

Goodman, H. I.: Hernia of Lung. *J. Thorac. Surg.*, 2:368, 1933.

Lindskog, G. E., Liebow, A. A., and Glenn, W. W. L.: *Thoracic and Cardiovascular Surgery, with Related Pathology*. New York, Appleton-Century-Crofts, Inc., 1962, p. 51.

Rickham, P. P.: Lung Hernia Secondary to Congenital Absence of Ribs. *Arch. Dis. Childhood*, 34:14, 1959.

CONGENITAL PULMONARY CYSTS

Cooke and Blades have classified congenital cystic disease of the lung into (1) bronchogenic, (2) alveolar, and (3) a combination of these types. The entire group is probably outnumbered by acquired cysts; nevertheless it includes a substantial segment of salvageable infants and children with respiratory distress and suppuration. There is a relative absence of other anomalies; cystic disease elsewhere is rare, and the pulmonary cystic problem, whether single or multiple, is usually limited to one lobe.

Since cysts have been recorded in late embryos and newborns, an anomalous development of the bronchopulmonary system has been postulated at the stage of terminal bronchiolar or early alveolar formation. This may evolve by intrapulmonary alveolar dissociation or partial bronchiolar recanalization with stenosis. The distal alveolated pulmonary cyst is then formed on the basis of expiratory obstruction through an area of bronchiolar narrowing. These essential postuterine respiratory dynamics might explain the paucity of these cysts in embryos.

The usual gross pathologic specimen exhibits a single, multiloculated, unilobar, peripheral air-filled cyst with a tracheobronchial communication. Common variants include multiplicity of cysts, bilateral lung or segmental distribution and absence of bronchial communication. Pus may be present. On microscopic examination the thin congenital cyst wall contains bits of smooth muscle and perhaps cartilage and is lined by columnar epithelium. With the exception of acute staphyloccocal pneumatocele, which has an obvious acute infectious background, most acquired cysts have an inner lining of squamous epithelium and can be separated histologically from the congenital cyst. Unfortunately, contamination and inflammation may destroy these helpful criteria, so that an infected congenital cyst, acquired cyst and lung abscess may be indistinguishable, pathologically and clinically.

The clinical pathogenesis derives from a cyst-airway connection, either directly or through the pores of Kohn, with free access on inspiration and obstruction during expiration. Under these circumstances there is an acute or chronic distention of the cyst leading to progressive increase in intrathoracic tension, frequently in the neonatal period. Compression of the unilateral lung and of the diaphragm, mediastinal shift and contralateral atelectasis are the usual sequence of events. If cyst drainage is poor, suppuration develops.

In the newborn and the infant, clinical findings are usually due to progressive tension as the congenital pulmonary cyst gradually distends with air. Respiratory and circulatory embarrassment is manifested by tachypnea, tachycardia, dyspnea, stridor, cyanosis, hyperresonance, absence of breath sounds, and displaced trachea and heart without history or signs of infection. By late infancy and childhood, infection is almost invariably present, and cough, fever and hemoptysis with repeated, localized episodes of pulmonary sepsis become more prominent as the cyst evolves into a lung abscess.

Although at times there is a startling lack of correlation between symptoms and roentgen findings, plain roentgenograms of the chest will corroborate the diagnosis and help in the differential diagnosis. The congenital pulmonary alveolar cyst may occupy the entire hemithorax and appear as a circular or oval, thin-walled, air-filled cavity containing faint strands of lung. Normally aerated or atel-

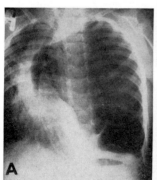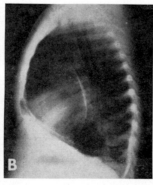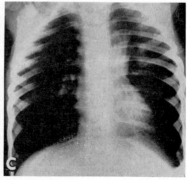

FIGURE 44–19. A 13-month-old infant with minimal respiratory distress. Posteroanterior and lateral chest films demonstrate gross hyperlucency of the left hemithorax. Frontal projection shows mediastinal displacement to the right. Pulmonary septal markings are noted within the area of hyperinflation. There is herniation of the left lung across the anterior mediastinum with flattening of the left diaphragm and widening of the left intercostal spaces. The right lung is compressed. C, After left upper lobe lobectomy an overexposed x-ray film reveals good aeration bilaterally with return of the mediastinum toward the midline.

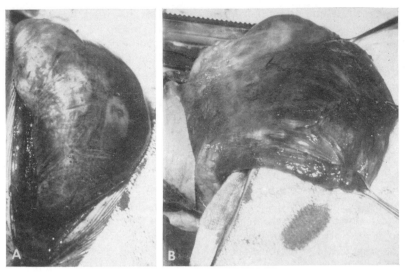

FIGURE 44–20. *A,* Extrusion of a left upper lobe pulmonary cyst, under tension, through an intercostal incision, with relief of respiratory distress which had become accentuated during the induction of anesthesia. *B,* The multiloculated cyst after deflation.

ectatic lung may be present at the apex and the base, but not at the hilus. There is a mediastinal shift, the diaphragm is depressed, pneumonia is absent, the pleura is not thickened, and other areas of translucency may be seen (Fig. 19). A fluid level with the cyst is unusual. Bronchography may be useful.

It is difficult, perhaps impossible, to separate pulmonary cysts from lobar emphysema. Emphysematous respiratory distress may be more explosive, but this is not a substantial differential factor in the face of common x-ray findings. The treatment is similar. The pulmonary cysts of cystic fibrosis and Letterer-Siwe disease should be excluded by the absence of other manifestations of the disease. Diaphragmatic hernia may simulate multiple lung cysts, but the immediate neonatal appearance of the hernia is very suggestive and makes the use of barium contrast x-ray studies academic. A staphylococcal pneumatocele may complicate a virulent pneumonia, and the changes in size and configuration of this type of acquired cyst may be volatile. Since spontaneous resolution here is expected, it would be a great error to confuse pneumatoceles with congenital cysts. An infected congenital

cyst and encapsulated empyema may look alike; many cysts have been drained with a diagnosis of empyema, but characteristically, unlike empyema, obliteration of the infected cyst does not occur in the presence of adequate dependent drainage. The respiratory distress will suggest pneumothorax, but there are no linear strands in or around the area of translucency, and a hilar shadow representing compressed lung is likely with pneumothorax.

The fate of congenital pulmonary cystic disease is rarely spontaneous regression. Instead, pleural rupture with tension pneumothorax, infection with abscess, recurrent disabling bronchopneumonia and expansion with suffocation may be encountered. Accordingly, thoracotomy is advised in order to avoid these complications and the exceedingly poor prognosis associated with large, moderately symptomatic cysts. Elective lobectomy is the usual planned procedure, and every attempt should be made to conserve functioning pulmonary tissue (Fig. 20). Pneumonectomy for more generalized disease has been reported. At times emergency resection must be done for the acute respiratory distress which threatens life. In this situation, needle aspiration and decompression of the tension cyst may be a worth-while preparatory step on the way to the operative suite. Thoracentesis cannot be used definitively because pneumothorax and pleural soiling will follow.

The repeatedly infected lung cyst deserves systemic antibiotic therapy in the preoperative period, and resection should be done without prior drainage. At operation, Clatworthy suggests aspiration of a fluid-filled cyst in order to provide exposure and to prevent bronchotracheal spillage. Aberrant systemic arteries must be considered, especially for lower lobe cysts. Postoperative nursing should be carried out in an intensive care unit with appropriate equipment and must be of the highest order.

REFERENCES

Avery, M. E.: The Lung and Its Disorders in the Newborn Infant. Philadelphia, W. B. Saunders Company, 1964, p. 69.

Bowden, K. M.: Congenital Cystic Disease of Lung. Med. J. Aust., 2:311, 1948.

Boyden, E. A.: Bronchogenic Cysts and the Theory of Intralobar Sequestration: New Embryologic Data. J. Thoracic Surg., 35:604, 1958.

Burford, T. H., and Ferguson, T. B.: Congenital Lesions of the Lungs and Emphysema; in J. H. Gibbon, Jr. (Ed.): Surgery of the Chest. Philadelphia, W. B. Saunders Company, 1962, p. 334.

Caffey, J.: On the Natural Regression of Pulmonary Cysts During Early Infancy. Pediatrics, 11:48, 1953.

Clatworthy, H. W., Jr.: Intrathoracic Tumors and Cysts; in I. M. Ariel, and G. T. Pack (Eds.): Cancer and Allied Diseases of Infancy and Childhood. Boston, Little, Brown and Company, 1960, p. 143.

Cooke, F. N., and Blades, B.: Cystic Disease of the Lungs. J. Thorac. Surg., 23:546, 1952.

Dickson, J. A., Clagett, O. T., and McDonald, J. R.: Cystic Disease of the Lung and Its Relation to Bronchiectatic Cavities: A Study of 22 Cases. J. Thorac. Surg., 15:196, 1946.

Donald, J. G., and Donald, J. W.: Congenital Cysts of the Lung. Ann. Surg., 141:944, 1955.

Egan, R. W., Jewett, T. C., and Macmanus, J. E.: Congenital Lesions of the Thorax in Infancy Demanding Early Surgical Treatment. A.M.A. Arch. Surg., 77:584, 1958.

Gans, S. L., and Hackworth, L. E.: Respiratory Obstructions of Surgical Import. Pediat. Clin. N. Amer., 6:1023, 1959.

Gilbert, J. W., and Myers, R. T.: Intrathoracic Tension Phenomena in the Neonatal Period and Infancy. A.M.A. Arch. Surg., 76:402, 1958.

Grimes, O. F., and Farber, S. M.: Air Cysts of the Lung. Surg., Gynec. & Obst., 113:720, 1961.

Gross, R.: Congenital Cystic Disease: Successful Pneumonectomy in a Three Week Old Baby. Ann. Surg., 123:229, 1946.

Guest, J. L., and others: Pulmonary Parenchymal Air Space Abnormalities. Ann. Thorac. Surg., 1:102, 1965.

Herrmann, J. W., Jewett, T. C., and Galletti, G.: Bronchogenic Cysts in Infants and Children. J. Thorac. Surg., 37:242, 1957.

Holinger, P. H., and others: Congenital Malformations of Trachea, Bronchi, and Lung. Ann. Otol., 61:1159, 1952.

Landing, B. H.: Anomalies of the Respiratory Tract. Pediat. Clin. N. Amer., 4:73, 1957.

Lichtenstein, H.: Congenital Multiple Cysts of the Lung. Dis. of Chest, 24:646, 1953.

Lindskog, G. E., Liebow, A. A., and Glenn, W. W. L.: Thoracic and Cardiovascular Surgery, with Related Pathology. New York, Appleton-Century Crofts, Inc., 1962, p. 104.

Maier, H. C.: The Pleura; in J. H. Gibbon, Jr. (Ed.). Surgery of the Chest. Philadelphia, W. B. Saunders Company, 1962, p. 243.

Minnis, J. F., Jr.: Congenital Cystic Disease of the Lung in Infancy. J. Thorac. Cardiov. Surg., 43:262, 1962.

Murphy, D. R., and Owen, H. F.: Respiratory Emergencies in the Newborn. Am. J. Surg., May, 1961, p. 581.

Nixon, H. H., and O'Donnell, B.: The Essentials of Pediatric Surgery. London, William Heinemann, Ltd., 1961, p. 38.

Opsahl, T., and Berman, E. J.: Bronchogenic Mediastinal Cysts in Infants. Pediatrics, 30: 372, 1962.

Potts, W. J., and Riker, W. L.: Differentiation of Congenital Cysts of Lung and Those Following Staphylococcal Pneumonia. Arch. Surg., 61:684, 1950.

Potts, W. J.: The Surgeon and the Child. Philadelphia, W. B. Saunders Company, 1964, p. 68.

Pryce, D. M.: Lining of Healed but Persistant Abscess Cavities in Lung with Epithelium of Ciliated Columnar Type. J. Path. Bact., 60: 259, 1948.

Ravitch, M. M.: Congenital Cystic Disease of the Lung; in C. D. Benson and others (Eds.): Pediatric Surgery. Chicago, Year Book Medical Publishers, Inc., 1962, Vol. 1, p. 355.

Ravitch, M. M., and Hardy, J. B.: Congenital Cystic Disease of Lung in Infants and Children. Arch. Surg., 59:1, 1949.

Riker, W. L.: Lung Cysts and Pneumothorax in Infants and Children. Surg. Clin. N. Amer., 36:1613, 1956.

Schaffer, A. J.: Diseases of the Newborn. Philadelphia, W. B. Saunders Company, 1960, p. 158.

Slim, M. S., and Melhem, R. E.: Congenital Pulmonary Air Cysts. *Arch. Surg.,* 88:923, 1964.

Spandler, B. P.: Pathogenesis and Treatment of Pulmonary Tension Cavities. *Am. Rev. Tuber. Pul. Dis.,* 76:370, 1957.

Spencer, H.: *Pathology of the Lung (Excluding Pulmonary Tuberculosis).* New York, Macmillan Company, 1962, pp. 40, 45.

Swan, H., and Aragon, G. E.: Surgical Treatment of Pulmonary Cysts in Infancy. *Pediatrics,* 14:651, 1954.

Swenson, O.: *Pediatric Surgery* 2nd ed. New York, Macmillan Company, 1962, p. 120.

Szots, I., and Jakab, T.: Indications for Urgent Operation in Pulmonary Tension Disorders in Childhood. *Arch. Dis. Childhood,* 39:172, 1964.

Woods, F. M.: Cystic Diseases of the Lung. *J. Internat. Coll. Surgeons,* 19:568, 1953.

LOBAR EMPHYSEMA

Abnormal lobar distention can produce subtle or gross respiratory distress in an otherwise normal newborn or infant. Recognition of this entity is rewarding, since excisional therapy is fairly specific and the results are satisfactory.

The disease is usually unilobar and often confined to either an upper or middle lobe, but may be segmental, bilobar or bilateral or involve an entire lung. Ten per cent of the patients have congenital heart disease; chondroectodermal dysplasia has been reported as a rare associated anomaly.

Etiologic factors are profuse and, at times, specifically applicable; more often the underlying mechanism is vague and escapes pathologic confirmation. Certainly the emphysema secondary to a foreign body, tuberculosis, ECHO virus infection, mediastinal tumor, bronchial adenoma and stenosis is well established, but does not often produce the distinctive pattern of infantile lobar emphysema. The current favorite explanation for this form of lobar hyperaeration involves partial bronchial obstruction or intrinsic alveolar disease. The bronchial obstruction can be engendered by complete absence of cartilage, bronchomalacia, exuberant muco-

sal folds, extrinsic vascular and lymph node compression, bronchial distortion from an anterior mediastinal lung hernia and retained secretions. The common denominator hinders expiration by organic bronchial narrowing compounded by functional expiratory bronchial collapse. This valvular arrangement leads to a hugely overdistended, noncollapsible lobe with widespread alveolar emphysema and rupture and small subpleural blebs. The pulmonary arteries are normal in contradistinction to unilateral pseudoemphysema, in which small pulmonary arteries supply a normal or small emphysematous lobe. The report of the surgical pathologist, although confirming the emphysematous nature of the distal parenchymatous disease, is often disappointing in its etiologic parameters. Perhaps the majority of surgical specimens are resected distal to intrinsic intrabronchial disease, or extrinsic causative factors such as anomalous vessels are left undisturbed. Finally, Bolande and co-workers have suggested that alveolar fibrosis cannot handle normal expiration without the development of emphysema. Leape and Longino, in a substantial clinical contribution, postulate the etiologic combination of alveolar disease with bronchial obstruction.

The clinical profile is formed by a space-occupying emphysematous lobe producing ipsilateral lobar atelectasis and diaphragmatic compression, mediastinal shift and contralateral lung atelectasis. Decompression of the overdistended lobe into the atelectatic lobe is prevented by the immaturity and distortion of the pores of Kohn.

Progressive respiratory distress from birth to four months of age, but especially in the first month, will parallel the degree of emphysema. Cough, wheezing, dyspnea, tachypnea, tachycardia, expiratory stridor and intermittent cyanosis are aggravated with feeding. To this may be added retraction and bulging of the thorax, tracheal and cardiac shift, hyperresonant percussion and diminished breath sounds. There is no history of infection.

Thoracic roentgenograms, in various

positions, especially during expiration, must be obtained. On lateral view a translucent anterior mediastinum is suggestive of lung herniation. Anteroposterior films will show a large hyperlucent area containing vague lung and bronchovascular markings. Adjacent lobes are compressed, the diaphragm is pushed downward, rib interspaces are wide, and the mediastinum is shifted into the opposite hemithorax with compression of the lung (Fig. 21). On fluoroscopy the emphysematous segment remains constant in area, regardless of the phase of respiration. Bronchograms demonstrate incomplete distal filling of the affected bronchi.

The differential diagnosis must exclude those lesions producing respiratory distress, but for which thoracotomy may not be indicated. Bronchoscopy can be utilized if foreign body is a possibility. Postpneumonic pneumatocele and bronchiolitis both have a septic background. Pulmonary cystic disease may be similar, but usually begins a little later in life. Fortunately, excision is proper for both. A tension pneumothorax will not have

lung markings in the area of radiolucence, and the nubbin of compressed lung in this condition is likely to be hilar rather than supradiaphragmatic or apical. Atelectasis with compensatory emphysema is not characterized by such pronounced respiratory distress. Pulmonary agenesis can be ruled out by bronchoscopy and bronchograms. Diaphragmatic hernia should not pose a problem, but can be separated by the use of contrast material.

Rarely, symptomatic infantile lobar emphysema will resolve spontaneously. The usual course is relentlessly progressive toward tension emphysema. The prognosis then, without treatment, is exceedingly poor, and the mortality rate high. Accordingly, excisional therapy, almost always lobectomy, should be done when the diagnosis is accompanied by symptoms. Only when the diagnosis is purely on a radiologic basis can thoracotomy be deferred.

Early age or severe respiratory symptoms should not contraindicate operation. Lobectomy has been done successfully within the first day of life. If the newborn

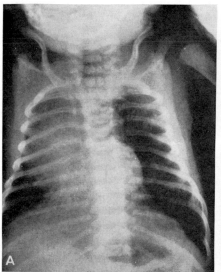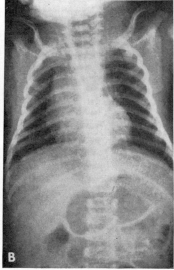

FIGURE 44–21. *A,* The anteroposterior chest x-ray of this newborn with respiratory distress demonstrates a shift of the mediastinum to the right with overinflation of the left lower lobe. There is depression of the left diaphragm, and the volume of the right lung is restricted. *B,* After left lower lobe lobectomy for lobar emphysema the mediastinum has returned toward the midline, and the diaphragm is normally located. There is better aeration of the right lung and slight radiolucency of the upper lobe, which has expanded and filled the left hemithorax.

is *in extremis*, thoracentesis can provide time for thoracotomy at the expense of a tension pneumothorax. This is its only role, and aspiration should not be used definitely. During the induction of anesthesia vigorous inflation of the emphysematous lobe may produce an extension of the respiratory distress. The emergency is over when the distended lobe herniates through the posterolateral thoracotomy incision with decompression of the thorax. There is no peculiar postoperative morbidity, and relief is immediate.

The operative mortality rate today is less than 5 per cent. Long-term follow-up shows normal growth and development, marred in rare instances by similar or less severe emphysema of other lobes.

REFERENCES

Avery, M. E.: *The Lung and Its Disorders in the Newborn Infant*. Philadelphia, W. B. Saunders Company, 1964, p. 78.

Baker, D.: Chronic Pulmonary Disease in Infants and Children. *Rad. Clin. N. Amer.*, 1:519, 1963.

Backman, A., Parkkulaimen, K. V., and Sulammaa, M.: Pulmonary Tension Emergencies in Infants. *Ann. Paediat. Fenn.*, 5:172, 1959.

Bates, D. V., and Christie, R. V.: *Respiratory Function in Disease, an Introduction to the Integrated Study of the Lung*. Philadelphia, W. B. Saunders Company, 1964, p. 227.

Binet, J. P., Nezelof, C., and Fredet, J.: Five Cases of Lobar Emphysema in Infancy; Importance of Bronchial Malformation and Value of Postoperative Steroid Therapy. *Dis. Chest*, 41:126, 1962.

Bolande, R. B., Schneider, A. F., and Boggs, J. D.: Infantile Lobar Emphysema, an Etiological Concept. *Arch. Path.*, 61:289, 1956.

Burford, T. H., and Ferguson, T. B.: Congenital Lesions of the Lung and Emphysema; in J. H. Gibbon, Jr. (Ed.): *Surgery of the Chest*. Philadelphia, W. B. Saunders Company, 1962, p. 346.

Burman, S. O., and Kent, E. M.: Bronchiolar Emphysema (Cirrhosis of the Lung). *J. Thorac. Cardiov. Surg.*, 43:253, 1962.

Butterfield, J., and others: Cystic Emphysema in Premature Infants, Report of an Outbreak with the Isolation of Type 19 ECHO Virus in One Case. *New England J. Med.*, 268:18, 1963.

Campbell, D., Bauer, A. J., and Hewlett, T. H.: Congenital Localized Emphysema. *J. Thorac. Cardiov. Surg.*, 41:575, 1961.

Ehrenhaft, J. L., and Taber, R. E.: Progressive Infantile Emphysema, a Surgical Emergency. *Surgery*, 34:412, 1953.

Egan, R. W., Jewett, T. C., and Macmanus, J. E.: Congenital Lesions of the Thorax in Infancy Demanding Early Surgical Treatment. *A.M.A. Arch. Surg.*, 77:584, 1958.

Fischer, H. W., Potts, W. J., and Holinger, P. H.: Lobar Emphysema in Infants and Children. *J. Pediat.*, 41:403, 1952.

Fischer, H. W., Lucido, J. L., and Lynxwiler, C. P.: Lobar Emphysema. *J.A.M.A.*, 166:340, 1958.

Floyd, F. W., and others: Bilateral Congenital Lobar Emphysema Surgically Corrected. *Pediatrics*, 31:87, 1963.

Gans, S. L., and Hackworth, L. E.: Respiratory Obstructions of Surgical Import. *Pediat. Clin. N. Amer.*, 6:1023, 1959.

Henry, W.: Localized Pulmonary Hypertrophic Emphysema. *J. Thorac. Surg.*, 27:197, 1954.

Jewett, T. C., Jr., and Adler, R. H.: Localized Pulmonary Emphysema of Infancy. *Surgery*, 43:926, 1958.

Jones, J. C., and others: Lobar Emphysema and Congenital Heart Disease in Infancy. *J. Thorac. Cardiov. Surg.*, 49:1, 1965.

Kanphuys, E. H. M.: Congenital Lobar Emphysema. *Arch. Chir. Neerl.*, 14:93, 1962.

Korngold, H. W., and Baker, J. M.: Non-surgical Treatment of Unilobar Obstructive Emphysema of the Newborn. *Pediatrics*, 14:296, 1954.

Kress, M. B., and Finkelstein, A. H.: Giant Bullous Emphysema Occurring in Tuberculosis in Childhood. *Pediatrics*, 30:269, 1962.

Landing, B. H.: Anomalies of the Respiratory Tract. *Pediat. Clin. N. Amer.*, 4:73, 1957.

Leape, L. L., and Longino, L. A.: Infantile Lobar Emphysema. *Pediatrics*, 34:246, 1964.

Lewis, J. E., and Potts, W. J.: Obstructive Emphysema with a Defect of the Anterior Mediastinum. *J. Thorac. Surg.*, 21:438, 1959.

Lindskog, G. E., Liebow, A. A., and Glenn, W. W. L.: *Thoracic and Cardiovascular Surgery, with Related Pathology*. New York, Appleton-Century-Crofts, Inc., 1962, p. 357.

May, R. L., Meese, E. H., and Timmes, J. J.: Congenital Lobar Emphysema: Case Report of Bilateral Involvement. *J. Thorac. Cardiov. Surg.*, 48:850, 1964.

Mercer, R. D., Hawk, W. A., and Darakjian, G.: Massive Lobar Emphysema in Infants: Diagnosis and Treatment. *Cleveland Clin. Quart.*, 28:270, 1961.

Moore, T. C.: Chondroectodermal Dysplasia (Ellis-Van Creveld Syndrome) with Bronchial Malformation and Neonatal Tension Lobar Emphysema. *J. Thorac. Cardiov. Surg.*, 46:1, 1963.

Murphy, D. R., and Owen, H. F.: Respiratory

Emergencies in the Newborn. *Am. J. Surg.*, 101:581, 1961.

Myers, N. A.: Congenital Lobar Emphysema. *Aust. New Zeal. J. Surg.*, 30:32, 1960.

Nelson, T. Y.: Tension Emphysema in Infants. *Arch. Dis. Childhood*, 32:38, 1957.

Nelson, W. E. (Ed.): *Textbook of Pediatrics*. 8th ed. Philadelphia, W. B. Saunders Company, 1964, p. 862.

Nelson, T. Y., and Reye, D.: Tension Emphysema: A Surgical Emergency in Infants. *Med. J. Aust.*, Aug. 28, 1954, p. 342.

Nixon, H. H., and O'Donnell, B.: *The Essentials of Pediatric Surgery*. London, William Heinemann, Ltd., 1961, p. 40.

Overstreet, R. M.: Emphysema of a Portion of the Lung in the Early Months of Life. *A.M.A. J. Dis. Child.*, 57:861, 1939.

Potts, W. J.: *The Surgeon and the Child*. Philadelphia, W. B. Saunders Company, 1959, p. 70.

Riker, W. L.: Neonatal Respiratory Distress; in C. D. Benson and others (Eds.): *Pediatric Surgery*. Chicago, Year Book Medical Publishers, Inc., 1962, Vol. 1, p. 352.

Robertson, R., and James, E. S.: Congenital Lobar Emphysema. *Pediatrics*, 8:795, 1951.

Schaffer, A. J.: *Diseases of the Newborn*. Philadelphia, W. B. Saunders Company, 1960, p. 97.

Spencer, H.: *Pathology of the Lung (Excluding Pulmonary Tuberculosis)*. New York, Macmillan Company, 1962, p. 408.

Thomson, J., and Forfar, J. O.: Regional Obstructive Emphysema in Infancy. *Arch. Dis. Childhood*, 33:97, 1958.

White, M., and Dennison, W. M.: *Surgery in Infancy and Childhood, a Handbook for Medical Students and General Practitioners*. Edinburgh, E. & S. Livingston, Ltd., 1958, p. 304.

Williams, H., and Campbell, P.: Generalized Bronchiectasis Associated with Deficiency of Cartilage in the Bronchial Tree. *Arch. Dis. Childhood*, 35:182, 1960.

Wiseman, D. H.: Unilateral Pseudoemphysema— A Case Report. *Pediatrics*, 35:300, 1965.

Zatzkin, H. R., Cole, P. M., and Bronsther, B.: Congenital Hypertrophic Lobar Emphysema. *Surgery*, 52:505, 1962.

PULMONARY SEQUESTRATION

Pulmonary tissue that is embryonic and cystic, does not function, is isolated from normal functioning lung and is nourished by systemic arteries has been aptly called pulmonary sequestration. The intrapulmonary variant is contained within otherwise normal lung parenchyma. The less common extralobar sequestration is divorced from and accessory to the ipsilateral lung.

Fundamentally, pulmonary sequestration represents a malformation of the primitive respiratory and vascular systems in which fetal lung tissue is segregated from the main tracheobronchial apparatus and ultimately has its own systemic artery. The sequence and time of these embryologic events have aroused a great deal of curiosity. Pryce feels that persistent aberrant fetal pulmonary blood vessels exert traction on a segment of an equally primitive lung bud which then splits off from the parent lung. The arterial trauma during and after the actual detachment is thought to lead to cystic degeneration. Others propose a primary pulmonary separation soon after the foregut stage with subsequent acquisition of a blood supply from the nearest and most convenient source, which happens to be the aorta. Smith, in 1956, suggested that sequestration was secondary to pulmonary artery deficiency and that the cysts followed systemic blood pressure flow after birth. Boyden concludes from the available data that the respiratory and vascular anomalies are unexplained, may not be related as to cause and occur coincidentally. Finally, Halasz, Lindskog and Liebow postulate the presence of an additional, low, anterior foregut respiratory duplication with subsequent sequestration, but retention of the original aortic blood supply. The occasional association of esophagobronchial fistula with sequestration supports this contention.

Both types of sequestration have certain similar pathologic characteristics as well as clear-cut differences. The pathologic tissue is largely fetal and profusely cystic, and contains disorganized, airless and nonpigmented alveoli, bronchi, cartilage, respiratory epithelium and a systemic artery. It is often secondarily infected, bronchiectatic, or atelectatic, and is usually located in the region of the lower lobes (Fig. 22). The aberrant arteries may arise from the thoracic or abdominal aorta and, in the latter instance, pierce the dia-

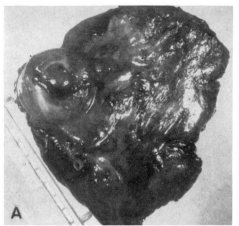
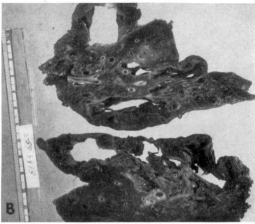

FIGURE 44–22. *A,* Gross external appearance of intralobar sequestration, left lower lobe, in an older child. Note aberrant systemic artery in lower left corner of specimen. *B,* Cross section of inflated, formalin-fixed specimen with multiple cysts, surrounded by compressed parenchyma. (Courtesy of Drs. James W. Brooks and Saul Kay, Medical College of Virginia.)

phragm and run through the pulmonary ligament before reaching the sequestration. The elastic vessel walls may become atherosclerotic, and the lumen varies considerably in size.

The intralobar sequestration is encircled by visceral pleura, usually of the lower lobes, although Clagett has reported the lesion in the upper lobes. The remainder of the affected lobe and lung is normal except that a small communication with the sequestration may have been maintained, reopened, or created by infection. A communication with the gastrointestinal tract is rare, and so are other anomalies. The systemic arteries are likely to be large, and the veins drain into the pulmonary system.

Extralobar sequestration can occur from the thoracic inlet to the upper part of the abdomen, but characteristically is a left-sided, ball-like, pliable mass between the diaphragm and the lower lobe and outside of the visceral pleura. Communications with the trachea, bronchi, esophagus, stomach and small bowel have been reported, but are rare. The systemic arteries are small, the venous drainage is likewise systemic through the azygous system, and other anomalies, principally congenital pleuroperitoneal hernias, are frequently concurrent.

The basis for symptoms is infection through a fistula between the sequestration and either the airway or digestive tract. The congenital, pathologic tissue may be contaminated by contiguous pneumonitis or hematogenous localization with the formation of the primary or additional fistulas. Accordingly, the arresting clinical feature, especially with intralobar sequestration, is recurrent, persistent, progressive pulmonary sepsis in the form of pneumonitis or lung abscess, or both. This is manifested by weight loss, chills, fever, cough, hemoptysis and pyoptysis. Physical examination may elicit pathologic findings at the bases paravertebrally. With extralobar sequestration, infection is less frequent and the child may be asymptomatic.

Plain chest films will show a triangulated density in the region of the medial basal segment of a lower lobe with displacement of the bronchovascular markings. Sometimes there is a dense linear projection toward the aorta. Body section radiography may amplify these findings. With abscess, of course, a fluid level may be present along with surrounding pneumonitis. The diagnosis is suggested by the restriction and localization of x-ray findings to the same area associated with repeated clinical episodes.

Bronchography is extremely helpful, since the sequestration will not fill with dye, but its periphery is outlined by bronchi that are filled. Aortography through the descending aorta will delineate the anomalous arterial supply and thus confirm the nature of the pulmonary density. At bronchoscopy purulent secretions are absent from the main stem bronchi, even with pulmonary suppuration.

Extirpation is the only reasonable approach after the diagnosis has been established. Antibiotics must be used for the acute infection and should be given before and after operation. Intralobar sequestration is handled by lobectomy; segmental resection will not suffice, since the sequestration is not clearly demarcated. An extralobar sequestration can be removed without disturbing the remaining lobes and the Bochdalek hernia repaired, if present. The only technical problem with either form of sequestration is the anomalous systemic artery, and exsanguination has followed its inadvertent division. The frequency of this vascular anomaly should be appreciated in all lower lobe lesions in infants and children exposed to thoracotomy.

Morbidity and mortality rates are exceedingly low if resection precedes repeated infections. Postoperative results are uniformly good.

REFERENCES

Asp, K., and others: Sequestrations in Children. *Ann. Paediat. Fenn.*, 9:270, 1963.

Avery, M. E.: *The Lung and Its Disorders in the Newborn Infant*. Philadelphia, W. B. Saunders Company, 1964, p. 86.

Boyden, E. A.: *Segmental Anatomy of the Lungs*. New York, McGraw-Hill Book Company, Inc., 1955.

Boyden, E. A.: Bronchogenic Cysts and the Theory of Intralobar Sequestration: New Embryologic Data. *J. Thorac. Surg.*, 35:604, 1958.

Breton, A., and others: Pulmonary Sequestration: Aortographic Diagnosis and Pathogenic Discussion. *Arch. Franç. Pediat.*, 16:751, 1959.

Britton, R. C., Weston, J. T., and Landing, B. H.: Plastic Injection Techniques in Pediatric Pathology, with Particular Reference to Roentgenographic Analysis of Injected Specimens. *Bull. Int. A.M. Mus.*, 31:124, 1950.

Bruwer, A., Clagett, O. T., and McDonald, J. R.: Anomalous Arteries to the Lung Associated with Congenital Pulmonary Abnormality. *J. Thorac. Surg.*, 19:957, 1950.

Burford, T. H., and Ferguson, T. B.: Congenital Lesions of the Lungs and Emphysema; in J. H. Gibbon, Jr. (Ed.): *Surgery of the Chest*. Philadelphia, W. B. Saunders Company, 1962, p. 341.

Byron, N. D., Campbell, D. C., and Hood, R. H.: Lower Accessory Lung. *J. Thorac. Cardiov. Surg.*, 47:605, 1964.

Claman, M. A., and Ehrenhaft, J. L.: Bronchopulmonary Sequestration. *J. Thorac. Cardiov. Surg.*, 39:531, 1960.

DeBakey, M., Arey, J. B., and Brunazzi, R.: Successful Removal of Lower Accessory Lung. *J. Thorac. Surg.*, 19:304, 1950.

Elliott, G. B., and others: Thoracic Sequestration Cysts of Fetal Bronchogenic and Esophageal Origin. *Canad. J. Surg.*, 4:522, 1961.

Ellis, F. H., McGoon, D. C., and Kincaid, O. W.: Congenital Vascular Malformations of the Lungs. *Med. Clin. N. Amer.*, 48:1069, 1964.

Flavell, G.: *An Introduction to Chest Surgery*. London, Oxford University Press, 1957, p. 129.

Gallagher, P. G., Lynch, J. P., and Christian, H. J.: Intralobar Bronchopulmonary Sequestration of the Lung. *New England J. Med.*, 257:643, 1957.

Gans, S. L., and Potts, W. J.: Anomalous Lobe of Lung Arising from the Esophagus. *J. Thorac. Surg.*, 21:313, 1951.

Gerard, F. P., and Lyons, H. A., Anomalous Artery in Intralobar Bronchopulmonary Sequestration. *New England J. Med.*, 259:662, 1958.

Halasz, N. A., Lindskog, G. E., and Liebow, A. A.: Esophagobronchial Fistula and Bronchopulmonary Sequestration. *Ann. Surg.*, 155:215, 1961.

Kafka, V., and Beco, V.: Simultaneous Intra- and Extrapulmonary Sequestration. *Arch. Dis. Childhood*, 35:51, 1960.

Kergin, F. G.: Congenital Cystic Disease of Lung Associated with Anomalous Arteries. *J. Thorac. Surg.*, 23:55, 1952.

Kilman, J. W., and others: Pulmonary Sequestration. *Arch. Surg.*, 90:648, 1965.

Landing, B. H.: Anomalies of the Respiratory Tract. *Pediat. Clin. N. Amer.*, 4:73, 1957.

Lindskog, G. E., Liebow, A. A., and Glenn, W. W. L.: *Thoracic and Cardiovascular Surgery, with Related Pathology*. New York, Appleton-Century-Crofts, Inc., 1962, p. 105.

Mannix, E. P., and Haight, C.: Anomalous Pulmonary Arteries and Cystic Disease of the Lung. *Medicine*, 34:193, 1955.

Muller, H.: Inaugural Dissertation, University of Halle; quoted by J. N. Ramsey and D. L. Reiman; Bronchial Adenomas Arising in

Mucous Glands. *Am. J. Path.*, 29:339, 1953.

Pryce, D. M.: Lower Accessory Pulmonary Artery with Intralobar Sequestration of Lung. *J. Path. Bact.*, 58:457, 1946.

Pryce, D. M., Sellors, T. H., and Blair, L. G.: Intralobar Sequestration of Lung Associated with an Abnormal Pulmonary Artery. *Brit. J. Surg.*, 35:18, 1947.

Quinlan, J. J., Schaffer, V. D., and Hiltz, J. E.: Intralobar Pulmonary Sequestration. *Canad. J. Surg.*, 6:418, 1963.

Ravitch, M. M.: Congenital Cystic Disease of the Lung; in C. D. Benson and others (Eds.): *Pediatric Surgery*. Chicago, Year Book Medical Publishers, Inc., 1962, Vol. 1, p. 360.

Simopoulos, A. P.: Intralobar Bronchopulmonary Sequestration in Children: Diagnosis by Intrathoracic Aortography. A.M.A. *J. Dis. Child.*, 97:796, 1959.

Smith, R. A.: A Theory of the Origin of Intralobar Sequestration of Lung. *Thorax*, 11:10, 1956.

Idem: Some Controversial Aspects of Intralobar Sequestration of the Lung. *Surg., Gynec. & Obst.*, 114:57, 1962.

Solit, R. W.: The Effect of Intralobar Pulmonary Sequestration on Cardiac Output. *J. Thorac. Cardiov. Surg.*, 49:844, 1965.

Song, Y. S.: Lower Pulmonary Aberrant Lobe. *South. M. J.*, 49:1137, 1956.

Spencer, H.: *Pathology of the Lung (Excluding Pulmonary Tuberculosis)*. New York, Macmillan Company, 1962, p. 32.

Talalak, P.: Pulmonary Sequestration. *Arch. Dis. Childhood*, 35:57, 1960.

Turk, L. N., III, and Lindskog, G. E.: The Importance of Angiographic Diagnosis in Intralobar Pulmonary Sequestration. *J. Thorac. Cardiov. Surg.*, 41:299, 1961.

Van Rens, T. J. G.: Intralobar Sequestration of Lung: Review of Its Possible Origin and Report on Five Cases. *Arch. Chir. Neerl.*, 14:63, 1962.

Waddell, W. R.: Organoid Differentiation of Fetal Lung; Histologic Study of Differentiation of Mammalian Fetal Lung in Utero and in Transplants. *Arch. Path.* 47:227, 1949.

Witten, D. M., Clagett, O. T., and Hiltz, J. E.: Intralobar Pulmonary Sequestration Involving the Upper Lobes, *J. Thorac. Cardiov. Surg.*, 43:523, 1962.

CONGENITAL CYSTIC ADENOMATOID MALFORMATION OF THE LUNG

Cystic adenomatoid pulmonary hamartoma, first described by Chin and Tang in 1949, is a rare variant of congenital cystic disease and, like it, can produce respiratory difficulty by tension and infection.

Careful investigation of postmortem material by Kwittken and Reiner would seem to implicate a developmental overgrowth of pulmonary tissue in the region of the end bronchioles and alveolar ducts. Grossly, this presents as a massive and fleshy unilobar enlargement, although bilobar and bilateral involvement has been described. Microscopically, cystic degeneration, excessive terminal bronchiolar tissue and areas of premature alveolar differentiation are interspersed with the normal lung.

The basis for symptoms is the pulmonary replacement by the malformation and compression of normal lung and mediastinum by the bulky size of the hamartoma and its enlarging cysts. Premature infants with hydramnios and anasarca are frequently afflicted, and the presenting picture is respiratory distress soon after birth. Examination demonstrates mediastinal shift toward the opposite side in a newborn with associated dyspnea, tachypnea and perhaps cyanosis. Fairly specific radiologic findings, described by Craig, Kirkpatrick and Neuhauser, include a pulmonary density with radiolucent areas and mediastinal shift to the opposite side.

The differential diagnosis is essentially a radiologic one and includes the more usual forms of congenital and acquired cystic disease, lobar emphysema, and Bochdalek hernia.

The urgency for operation in the newborn parallels that for obstructive emphysema, and indeed the tension phenomenon in both is remarkably similar. Lobectomy has been curative in a number of instances, some of which have been reported in small prematures, soon after birth. Later in life, secondary infection, which is almost inevitable, constitutes an indication for thoracotomy.

REFERENCES

Avery, M. E.: *The Lung and Its Disorders in the Newborn Infant*. Philadelphia, W. B. Saunders Company, 1964, p. 74.

Bain, G. O., Congenital Adenomatoid Malformation of the Lung. *Dis. of Chest,* 36:430, 1959.

Belanger, R., Lafleche, L. R., and Picard, J. L.: Congenital Cystic Adenomatoid Malformation of the Lung. *Thorax,* 19:1, 1964.

Chin, K. Y., and Tang, M. Y.: Congenital Adenomatoid Malformation of One Lobe of a Lung with General Anasarca. *Arch. Path.,* 48:311, 1949.

Craig, J. M., Kirkpatrick, J., and Neuhauser, E. B. D.: Congenital Cystic Adenomatoid Malformation of the Lung in Infants. *Am. J. Roentgen.,* 76:516, 1956.

Holder, T. M., and Christy, M. G.: Cystic Adenomatoid Malformation of the Lung. *J. Thorac. Cardiov. Surg.,* 47:590, 1964.

Kwittken, J., and Reiner, L.: Congenital Cystic Adenomatoid Malformation of the Lung. *Pediatrics,* 30:759, 1962.

Landing, B. H.: Anomalies of the Respiratory Tract. *Pediat. Clin. N. Amer.,* 4:73, 1957.

CONGENITAL PULMONARY LYMPHANGIECTASIS

This unusual congenital dilatation of the pulmonary lymphatics produces severe respiratory distress in the newborn and is often associated with other crippling anomalies, such as congenital heart disease.

Pathologically, according to Laurence, there is diffuse overgrowth of the entire lymphatic system of both lungs, which become heavy, bulky and inelastic, with grossly prominent subpleural cystic lymphatics. It is quite unlike a localized lymphangioma and is not associated with chylothorax.

Symptomatically, there is immediate respiratory distress with dyspnea and cyanosis. X-ray films of the chest may show a diffuse, generalized mottling similar to hyaline membrane disease, along with emphysema in the remaining functioning lung (Carter and Vaughn).

Treatment is nonspecific, and the prognosis with diffuse involvement is hopeless.

REFERENCES

Avery, M. E.: *The Lung and Its Disorders in the Newborn Infant.* Philadelphia, W. B. Saunders Company, 1964, p. 76.

Carter, R. W., and Vaughn, H. M.: Congenital Pulmonary Lymphangiectasis. *Am. J. Roent.,* 86:576, 1961.

Javett, S. N., Webster, I., and Braudo, J. L.: Congenital Dilatation of the Pulmonary Lymphatics. *Pediatrics,* 31:416, 1963.

Landing, B. H.: Anomalies of the Respiratory Tract. *Pediat. Clin. N. Amer.,* 4:73, 1957.

Laurence, K. M.: Congenital Pulmonary Cystic Lymphangiectasis. *J. Path. Bact.,* 70:325, 1955.

Idem: Congenital Pulmonary Lymphangiectasis. *J. Clin. Path.,* 12:62, 1959.

Idem: Personal Communication; cited in H. Spencer: *Pathology of the Lung.* New York, Macmillan Company, 1962, p. 58.

Spencer, H.: *Pathology of the Lung (Excluding Pulmonary Tuberculosis).* New York, Macmillan Company, 1962, p. 58.

PULMONARY ARTERIOVENOUS FISTULA

A congenital pulmonary arteriovenous fistula represents a direct intrapulmonary connection between pulmonary artery and vein without an intervening capillary bed. This cavernous arteriovenous aneurysm is the basis, then, for a right-to-left shunt and an uncommon cause of symptoms, including cyanosis, in the pediatric age group. Accordingly, the diagnosis is not often made in children in spite of its congenital nature. Bosher, in an exhaustive review in 1959, reported seventeen patients below ten years, and Shumaker, in 1963, recorded thirty-one patients who were treated surgically between five months and sixteen years of age. From this material it is apparent that the fistula occurs in the lower lobes in about 60 per cent of the instances, is single in 65 per cent and unilateral in 75 per cent. Bilateral multiplicity is found in the remainder.

Etiologically, the pulmonary vascular malformation represents a failure of maturation of the fetal splanchnic bed in which arteriovenous communications may normally exclude the pulmonary capillaries. There may, however, be a widespread basic blood vessel abnormality, since familial hemorrhagic telangiectasis of the Osler-Weber-Rendu variety often occurs simultaneously.

On gross pathologic examination the actual arteriovenous fistula is subpleural or hilar and may simulate a saccular, cavernous hemangioma because of its aneurysmal swelling. The fistula is fed by at least one afferent artery, usually pulmonic, less often bronchial, and drained by several veins, almost always pulmonary. There are numerous communications between artery and vein in this tortuous, dilated wormlike vessel mass. Microscopically, the arteriovenous fistula is lined with vascular endothelium. Carcinomatous degeneration has been recorded by Hall and Wollstein.

The clinical picture of this anomaly is created by an intrapulmonic right-to-left shunt in which unoxygenated pulmonary artery blood flows directly into the pulmonary veins and thence into the systemic circulation without gas exchange in the pulmonary capillaries. Although 50 per cent of the blood volume can be so rerouted in massive fistulization, Ellis has estimated that a 25 per cent shunt will produce diagnostic clinical findings.

Generalized telangiectasis, noted especially on the skin and mucous membranes, has been described in half of the patients with pulmonary arteriovenous fistula. Dyspnea, rubor, cyanosis, clubbing of the fingers and toes, hemoptysis, epistaxis, exercise intolerance and hemorrhagic conjunctiva are common complaints. On physical examination a thrill may be felt, and a systolic or continuous murmur and bruit may be heard over the shunt, especially during inspiration. The heart is normal to auscultation. The blood pressure, pulse, venous pressure, electrocardiogram and cardiac output are within normal variations.

Clinical pathologic and radiologic studies are essential for the final diagnosis. Polycythemia in the range of 7 to 10 million red blood cells and 18 to 25 gm. of hemoglobin is fairly standard. This is reflected by an increase in the red blood cell and total blood volume and a hematocrit level of 60 to 80 per cent. The arterial oxygen saturation is consistently low, drops lower with exercise and will rise, but not to normal, with 100 per cent oxygen.

Routine chest films in various views demonstrate one or more homogeneous, noncalcified pulmonary densities with irregular, fairly sharp peripheral margins, and confluent with the ipsilateral hilus. Body section roentgenograms may bring out the vascular nature of the tissue between the peripheral lesion and the hilus. At fluoroscopy the tumor may pulsate, decrease in size during the Valsalva maneuver, and become larger with the Muller test. Venous cine-angiography with full chest films can accurately delineate the offending fistula and uncover smaller fistulas which were not hitherto suspected (Fig. 23). Pressure studies may record a normal systolic but low diastolic pulmonary artery pressure.

Cyanotic cardiac anomalies are excluded in the differential diagnosis by the presence of a lung tumor and the absence of various murmurs and aberrations in pulse, blood pressure, venous pressure, cardiac output, heart size configuration and electrocardiogram, all of which are normal in pulmonary arteriovenous fistula.

Complications during the natural history of the untreated disease are formidable. Exsanguination from a massive spontaneous hemothorax or hemoptysis can occur. Subacute bacterial endarteritis may initiate septicemia and brain abscess, and polycythemia can lead to embolic and thrombotic phenomena. The prognosis is obviously more serious and less manageable with widespread bilateral shunts or diffuse hereditary telangiectasis.

Excisional therapy should be done in symptomatic infants and children with localized disease. In thirty-one pediatric patients there has been one operative death, and the morbidity rate is equally low. The results have been eminently satisfactory and have stimulated a more aggressive surgical approach toward the isolated pulmonary arteriovenous aneurysm with minimal or no symptoms and the more widely distributed fistulas with gross symptoms. Several experienced ob-

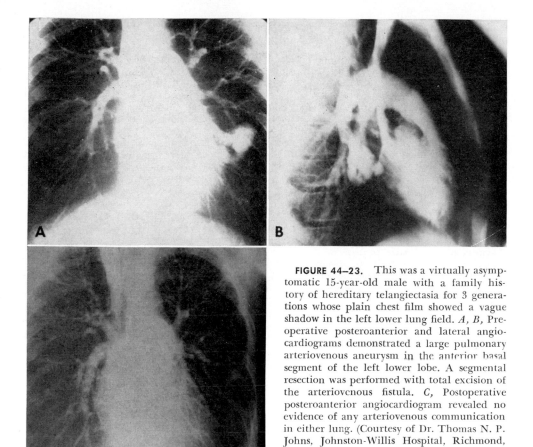

FIGURE 44–23. This was a virtually asymptomatic 15-year-old male with a family history of hereditary telangiectasia for 3 generations whose plain chest film showed a vague shadow in the left lower lung field. *A, B,* Preoperative posteroanterior and lateral angiocardiograms demonstrated a large pulmonary arteriovenous aneurysm in the anterior basal segment of the left lower lobe. A segmental resection was performed with total excision of the arteriovenous fistula. *C,* Postoperative posteroanterior angiocardiogram revealed no evidence of any arteriovenous communication in either lung. (Courtesy of Dr. Thomas N. P. Johns, Johnston-Willis Hospital, Richmond, Virginia.)

servers have commented on the clinical improvement following excision of the major dominant pulmonary fistula even though smaller diffuse fistulas remain unmolested.

Lobectomy has been the procedure of choice in the majority of children. Unfortunately, normal pulmonary parenchyma was sacrificed because the dissection was not limited to the actual borders of the pathologic tissue. Since multiple shunts are often of paramount importance, postoperative results parallel the conservation of functioning lung. Accordingly, Bosher and then Murdock have described the technique and practicality of local excision in a bloodless field in preference to segmental resection or lobectomy.

REFERENCES

Bosher, L. H., Jr., Blake, D. A., and Byrd, B. R.: An Analysis of the Pathologic Anatomy of Pulmonary Arteriovenous Aneurysms, with Particular Reference to the Applicability of Local Excision. *Surgery,* 45:91, 1959.

Burford, T. H., and Ferguson, T. B.: Congenital Lesions of the Lung and Emphysema; in J. H. Gibbon, Jr. (Ed.): *Surgery of the Chest.* Philadelphia, W. B. Saunders Company, 1962, p. 348.

Charbon, B. C., Adams, W. F., and Carlson R. F.: Surgical Treatment of Multiple Arteriovenous Fistulas in the Right Lung in a Patient Having Undergone a Left Pneumonectomy Seven Years Earlier for the Same Disease. *J. Thorac. Surg.,* 23:188, 1952.

Clatworthy, H. W., Jr.: Intrathoracic Tumors and Cysts; in I. M. Ariel and G. T. Pack (Eds.): *Cancer and Allied Diseases of Infancy and Childhood.* Boston, Little, Brown, and Company, 1960, p. 149.

Dargeon, H. W.: *Tumors of Childhood, a Clinical Disease.* New York, Paul B. Hoeber, Inc., 1964.

Goldman, A.: Pulmonary Arteriovenous Fistula with Secondary Polycythemia Occurring in Two Brothers. *J. Lab. & Clin. Med.,* 32:330, 1947.

Idem: Arteriovenous Fistula of the Lung: Its Hereditary and Clinical Aspects. *Am. Rev. Tuber.,* 57:266, 1948.

Hall, E. M.: Malignant Hemangioma of the Lung with Multiple Metastasis. *Am. J. Path.,* 11:343, 1935.

Hodgson, C. H., and Kaye, R. L.: Pulmonary Arteriovenous Fistula and Hereditary Hemorrhagic Telangiectasia. *Dis. of Chest,* 43:-449, 1963.

Hope, J. W., and Koop, C. E.: Differential Diagnosis of Mediastinal Masses. *Pediat. Clin. N. Amer.,* 6:379, 1959.

Husson, G. S., and Wyatt, T. C.: Primary Pulmonary Obliterative Vascular Disease in Infants and Young Children. *Pediatrics,* 23:-493, 1959.

Klassen, K.: Personal communication to H. W. Clatworthy, Jr., in I. M. Ariel and G. T. Pack (Eds.): *Cancer and Allied Diseases of Infancy and Childhood.* Boston, Little, Brown and Company, 1960, p. 149.

Landing, B. H.: Anomalies of the Respiratory Tract. *Pediat. Clin. N. Amer.,* 4:73, 1957.

Lansdowne, M.: Discussion of Paper by A. Goldman: *J. Lab. & Clin. Med.* (v. s.).

Lindgren, E.: Roentgen Diagnosis of Arteriovenous Aneurysm of the Lung. *Acta Radiol.,* 27:586, 1946.

Lindskog, G. E., Liebow, A. A., and Glenn, W. W. L.: *Thoracic and Cardiovascular Surgery, with Related Pathology.* New York, Appleton-Century-Crafts, Inc., 1962, p. 110.

Maier, H. C., and others: Arteriovenous Fistula of the Lung. *J. Thorac. Surg.,* 17:13, 1948.

Michael, P.: *Tumors of Infancy and Childhood.* Philadelphia, J. B. Lippincott Company, 1964, p. 252.

Mitchell, F. N.: Pulmonary Arteriovenous Telangiectasis, *South. M.J.,* 47:1157, 1954.

Moyer, J. H., and Ackerman, A. J.: Hereditary Hemorrhagic Telangiectasis Associated with Pulmonary Arteriovenous Fistula in Two Members of a Family. *Ann. Int. Med.,* 29:775, 1948.

Murdock, C. E.: Pulmonary Arteriovenous Fistulectomy *Arch. Surg.,* 86:44, 1962.

Muri, J.: Arterio-Venous Aneurysm of the Lung. *Dis. of Chest,* 24:49, 1953.

Nelson, W. E. (Ed.): *Textbook of Pediatrics.* 8th ed. Philadelphia, W. B. Saunders Company, 1964, p. 1515.

Ravitch, M. M.: Anomalies of the Pulmonary Vessels; in C. D. Benson and others (Eds): *Pediatric Surgery.* Chicago, Year Book Medical Publishers, Inc., 1962, Vol. 1, pp. 361, 363.

Seaman, W. B., and Goldman, A.: Roentgen Aspects of Pulmonary Arteriovenous Fistula. *Arch. Int. Med.,* 89:70, 1952.

Shefts, L.: Discussion of Paper by H. C. Maier, et al.

Shumaker, H. B., Jr., and Waldhausen, J. A.: Pulmonary Arteriovenous Fistulas in Children. *Ann. Surg.,* 158:713, 1963.

Sweet, R. H.: Discussion of Paper by H. C. Maier, et al.

Taber, R. E., and Ehrenhaft, J. L.: Arteriovenous Fistulae and Arterial Aneurysms of the Pulmonary Arterial Tree. A.M.A. *Arch. Surg.,* 73:567, 1965.

Weiss, D. L. and Czeredarczuk, O.: Rupture of an Angiomatous Malformation of the Pleura in a Newborn Infant. A.M.A. *J. Dis. Child.,* 96:370, 1958.

Wollstein, M.: Malignant Hemangioma of the Lung with Multiple Visceral Foci. *Arch. Path.,* 12:562, 1931.

GENERAL REFERENCES

Arey, L. B.: *Developmental Anatomy, a Textbook and Laboratory Manual of Embryology.* 7th ed. Philadelphia, W. B. Saunders Company, 1965.

Avery, M. E.: *The Lung and Its Disorders in the Newborn Infant.* Philadelphia, W. B. Saunders Company, 1964.

Bates, D. V., and Christie, R. V.: *Respiratory Function in Disease, an Introduction to the Integrated Study of the Lung.* Philadelphia, W. B. Saunders Company, 1964.

Benson, C. D., and others (Eds.): *Pediatric Surgery.* Chicago, Year Book Medical Publishers, Inc., 1962, Vol. 1.

Brown, J. J. M. (Ed.): *Surgery of Childhood.* Baltimore, William & Wilkins Company, 1963.

Comroe, J. H., Jr., and others: *The Lung, Clinical Physiology and Pulmonary Function Tests.* 2nd ed. Chicago, Year Book Medical Publishers, Inc., 1962.

Flavell, G.: *An Introduction to Chest Surgery.* London, Oxford University Press, 1957.

Flavell, G.: *The Oesophagus.* London, Butterworth, 1963.

Gibbon, J. H., Jr., (Ed.): *Surgery of the Chest.* Philadelphia, W. B. Saunders Company, 1962.

Gross, R. E.: *Surgery of Infancy and Childhood, Its Principles and Techniques.* Philadelphia, W. B. Saunders Company, 1953.

Hamilton, W. J., Boyd, J. D., and Mossman, H. W.: *Human Embryology (Prenatal Development of Form and Function).* 2nd ed. Cambridge, W. Heffer & Sons, Ltd., 1952.

Leigh, T. F., and Weens, H. S.: *The Mediastinum.* Springfield, Ill., Charles C Thomas, 1959.

Lindskog, G. E., Liebow, A. A., and Glenn, W. W. L.: *Thoracic and Cardiovascular Surgery, with Related Pathology*. New York, Appleton-Century-Crofts, Inc., 1962.

Nelson, W. E. (Ed.): *Textbook of Pediatrics*, 8th ed. Philadelphia, W. B. Saunders Company, 1964.

Nixon, H. H., and O'Donnell, B.: *The Essentials of Pediatric Surgery*. London, William Heinemann, Ltd., 1961.

Patten, B. M.: *Human Embryology*. 2nd ed. New York, McGraw-Hill Book Publishing Company, Inc., 1953.

Potts, W. J.: *The Surgeon and the Child*. Phila-

delphia, W. B. Saunders Company, 1959.

Schaffer, A. J.: *Diseases of the Newborn*. 2nd ed. Philadelphia, W. B. Saunders Company, 1965.

Spencer, H.: *Pathology of the Lung (Excluding Pulmonary Tuberculosis)*. New York, Macmillan Company, 1962.

Swenson, O.: *Pediatric Surgery*. 2nd ed. New York, Appleton-Century-Crofts, Inc., 1962.

White, M., and Dennison, W. M.: *Surgery in Infancy and Childhood, a Handbook for Medical Students and General Practitioners*. Edinburgh, E. & S. Livingstone, Ltd., 1958.

CHAPTER FORTY-FIVE

Cystic Fibrosis

HARRY SHWACHMAN, M.D.

Cystic fibrosis is a new clinical entity first reported in 1936. In 1938 it was considered a rare pancreatic disorder uniformly fatal and affecting only small infants. Although this disease is not limited to the pancreas, many of the designations refer to the pancreas, such as fibrocystic disease of the pancreas, pancreatic fibrosis, pancreatic infantilism or cystic fibrosis of the pancreas. Farber first pointed out the generalized nature of the disease with involvement of many of the mucous-secreting glands and later suggested the name "mucoviscidosis." Bodian subsequently used the designation "mucosis." Eccrinosis has been suggested by Kagan to indicate a widespread involvement of the exocrine glands. A very early name which did not attain widespread usage for obvious reasons is dysporia entero-broncho-pancreatica congenita familiaris. There is no satisfactory name for this disease.

Numerous advances have been made in the past twenty years which indicate that (1) this is not a disease limited to the pancreas; for that matter, it may occur without evidence of pancreatic insuffi-

ciency; (2) this is no longer a rare disease— it is ten to twenty times as frequent as phenylketonuria; (3) survival into adulthood and even parenthood can be achieved; (4) the diagnosis can be made with ease, even in the neonatal period; (5) it is a hereditary disease transmitted as a mendelian recessive; (6) it is a serious disease affecting the respiratory system in nearly all cases; and (7) the cause of death is most often related to the pulmonary involvement. It is appropriate, therefore, to consider this disease in a text dealing with pulmonary disease in childhood.

Incidence

Accurate incidence figures are not available because reliable diagnostic methods have been in use only a short time. Estimates range from one in 500 to one in 3500 live births. Many patients with mild symptoms escape diagnosis in early childhood because the physician may not be familiar with such a benign course. In a recent study of sixty-five patients over seventeen years of age nearly 50 per cent were first diagnosed after the age of nine years. There is a high incidence of disease in the caucasian race and a low one in the Negro. Until recently it was considered not to exist in the oriental, but in the past few years it has been diagnosed in a number of Japanese and Arab children. We are aware of one case in an American Indian. The clinical and pathologic findings appear the same in cases reported from various racial groups. The disease occurs equally in both sexes and in all levels of social and economic groups. The family background of patients seen in the New England area suggests a wide ethnic source with a predominant Canadian and European origin. The affected families have the following ancestry: French-Canadian, English, Irish, Scottish, Russian, German, Polish, Spanish, Portuguese and Dutch; not unlike the rest of the population in this area. Cystic fibrosis occurs in approximately 3 per cent of the postmortem examinations performed in Children's Hospitals.

Etiology

Cystic fibrosis is a disease of obscure origin. Etiologic considerations include the following: (1) Cystic fibrosis is inherited as a mendelian recessive trait. (2) The disease cannot be reproduced in animals. (3) Theories based on blood incompatibilities, maternal toxicity in pregnancy, failure of secretin formation, vitamin A deficiency and viral infection are most unlikely. (4) Dysautonomia, altered cell membrane permeability, a defective enzyme system involving mucoprotein, "sodium pump" defect, or altered salt crystal structural formation may be responsible for the primary defect resulting in increased viscosity of many body secretions and increased salt content of eccrine and salivary glandular secretions.

Pathogenesis

Cystic fibrosis is a generalized disease involving eccrine and mucous secretory glands. The increase in viscosity of mucus suggested the name "mucoviscidosis." In view of the almost constant abnormality of the sweat glands, this name is no longer in use.

The pathogenetic mechanisms may be depicted as follows:

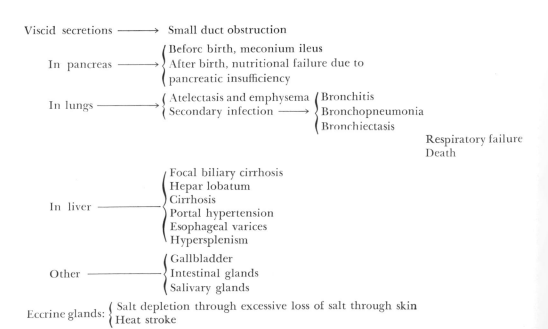

Genetics

Cystic fibrosis is transmitted as a mendelian recessive disorder. The affected patient is the homozygote, and his healthy parents the heterozygotes. His brothers and sisters may appear healthy or may also have the disease in either the same severe form or in a milder degree. Figure 1 illustrates a family of four children, one of whom has cystic fibrosis. Of the three healthy children, one does not carry the gene, and the other two are carriers of the gene or heterozygotes. By definition, all healthy siblings have normal sweat electrolyte levels. In any one family it is impossible to predict the incidence or the outcome of future pregnancies. There is the same chance of cystic fibrosis regardless of the number of previously affected children. We have seen one family with five of six children affected, and another family of eleven children with only one affected child. The parents of our patients do not appear to present abnormal clinical or laboratory findings which would segregate them from the rest of a healthy adult population.

Little progress has been made in identifying the heterozygote. Investigations in which the test individual is subjected to a stress condition prior to collecting sweat have not been successful in detecting the heterozygote. The analysis of certain tissues such as fingernail and toenail clippings for sodium and potassium content may segregate the carrier state in childhood, but not in the adult. Preliminary data indicate that approximately one third of the healthy siblings of children with cystic fibrosis have a distinct elevation of the sodium and potassium content in their nails. The incidence of the heterozygote in the adult population is calculated after the frequency of the disease has been established or estimated. If the incidence of the disease is one in 1600, then the frequency of the gene in the adult population is one in twenty.

Pathology

The name of the disease is derived from the initial description of the changes noted in the pancreas. Farber pointed out that the morphologic changes in this disease are not limited to the pancreas, but occur in many mucus-secreting cells in the body.

The demonstration of altered function of eccrine sweat glands is not reflected in a morphologic or histochemical change in these glands. The changes noted in the pancreas are not fixed; i.e. the lesion may evolve gradually, and the appearance may vary according to the age of the patient or the severity of the disease. The end-stage of the pancreatic lesion which may occur in the older patient is fat replacement and a few clusters of islet cells. When this occurs, the diagnosis of cystic fibrosis cannot be made on a morphologic basis. This progressive change probably explains the increasing incidence of diabetes mellitus in the older patients.

The most characteristic lesion of the pancreas is seen in the first few years and consists in a dilatation of the ducts, a flat-

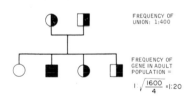

FREQUENCY OF
UNION: 1:400

FREQUENCY OF
GENE IN ADULT
POPULATION =

$$1\sqrt{\frac{1600}{4}} = 1:20$$

IF INCIDENCE OF C.F. IS ASSUMED TO BE 1:1000, FREQUENCY OF THE GENE IN
ADULT POPULATION WILL BE APPROXIMATELY 1:16

○ FEMALE   ☐ MALE   ◐ HETEROZYGOTE   ■ HOMOZYGOTE

A

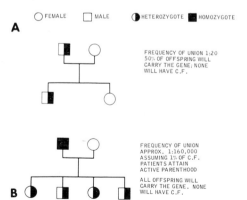

FREQUENCY OF UNION 1:20
50% OF OFFSPRING WILL
CARRY THE GENE; NONE
WILL HAVE C.F.

FREQUENCY OF UNION
APPROX. 1:160,000
ASSUMING 1% OF C.F.
PATIENTS ATTAIN
ACTIVE PARENTHOOD

ALL OFFSPRING WILL
CARRY THE GENE. NONE
WILL HAVE C.F.

B

FIGURE 45–1. Recessive inheritance in cystic fibrosis, based on an estimated incidence of one in 1600 live births.

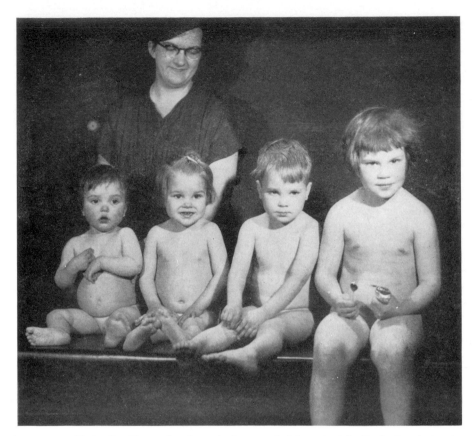

FIGURE 45–2. M. family. The proband case is the second girl on the left. She had typical pulmonary and gastrointestinal symptoms of cystic fibrosis. As soon as the diagnosis was made in November 1953, her 3 siblings were studied. The eldest girl was found to be healthy, and her duodenal fluid showed normal enzymes. The other 2 siblings were found to have the disease, but with milder clinical manifestations. Duodenal intubation on each showed increased viscosity with absent trypsin, lipase and amylase. The sweat test had not yet been discovered, but, when available the following year (1954), confirmed the clinical diagnosis. The mother was pregnant when the photograph was taken, and shortly after delivery her baby was found to be healthy.

The photograph is included to point out (1) the testing of all children in a family as soon as one child is discovered to have cystic fibrosis, and (2) the familial incidence with healthy first and fifth children and 3 affected. There were 3 subsequently healthy children. Two of the 3 children with cystic fibrosis have succumbed, the boy at age 14 years (August 1964) and the proband patient at age 12 years (November 1963).

tening of the epithelium, enlargement of the acini to form cysts, the presence of eosinophilic concretions and a diffuse fibrosis with varying degrees of leukocytic infiltration. Grossly, the pancreas is firm, irregular and shrunken. The lesion need not be uniform in all areas. In such cases functional tests of the pancreas reveal varying degrees of enzyme insufficiencies. In some cases the pancreatic lesion is minimal.

INTESTINE. The earliest lesion and the

one responsible for approximately 10 per cent of all cases of cystic fibrosis occurs in the intestine in the form of meconium ileus. The obstruction is generally in the region of the terminal ileum and is due to the abnormal nature of the meconium. The degree of obstruction may vary, and in a pediatric hospital practice one is more likely to see the severe cases requiring surgical correction. In a small number of patients, however, the meconium obstruction is relieved spontaneously or by means of pancreatin enemas. The meconium is tarry and very sticky, contains a large amount of serum proteins and can readily be liquefied by proteolytic enzymes. In patients with meconium ileus the absence of pancreatic enzymes helps explain the persistence of the large amount of proteins found in the meconium. The intestinal wall in the region of the obstruction is thin, and the lumen may be large. The wall may be hypertrophied proximally and considerably reduced in size distally. The intestinal glands at the site of obstruction are flattened and show evidence of hyperactivity. Complications are frequent and include perforation with meconium peritonitis, volvulus and secondary atresia (see Table 1). On occasion the surgeon may be unable to provide an accurate etiologic diagnosis of intestinal obstruction in the newborn. It is recommended that all newborns with intestinal obstruction be subjected to a sweat test. An attempt to clarify the diagnosis is justified by recent experiences and forms the basis of providing proper therapeutic, prophylactic, prognostic and genetic information to the parents.

Morphologic changes in mucus-secreting glands may be found in various regions of the intestinal tract. Duodenal mucosal biopsy specimens rarely reveal a lesion of diagnostic value, but a biopsy of the rectal mucosa may suggest the disease. The morphologic criteria include the appearance of the surface epithelium, lamina propria and glandular structures. In a typical example the surface epithelium is denuded and disorganized with tortuous disordered glands and a decrease in the number of crypts; these show dilatation with gaping of the crypt mouths. Special stains may reveal an increase in the acid mucopolysaccharides. The appendix may provide a clue, since it may be firm with a thick wall revealing active mucus secretion with inspissation and even extrusion of casts. In older patients intestinal obstruction may result from the inspissation of secretions with the formation of firm intraluminal masses. Intussusception is another complication that is occasionally seen in the older child.

LIVER. The basic changes in the liver include cell atrophy, fatty metamorphosis, periportal fibrosis, and proliferation of the bile ducts, often distended by obstruction. The initial lesion in the liver

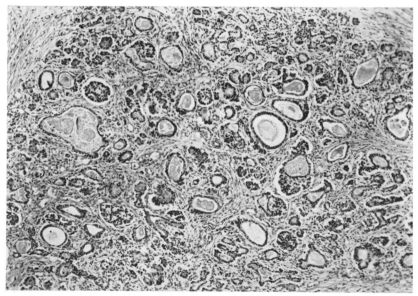

FIGURE 45–3. Microscopic appearance of the pancreas ($\times$ 140). This shows the typical changes with inspissation of secretions, dilatation of ducts and acini, as well as increased fibrosis.

Table 1. *Complications of Meconium Ileus in 127 Infants Requiring Surgery*
(1940 to 1965)

	Total	Surgical Survivals (Beyond 2 Months)	Dead Before Reaching 2 Mo.
Meconium ileus only	68	31	37
Meconium ileus + peritonitis	14	1	13
Meconium ileus + peritonitis + atresia	9	3	6
Meconium ileus + atresia	9	6	3
Meconium ileus + peritonitis + volvulus	12	5	7
Meconium ileus + volvulus	4	..	4
Meconium ileus + peritonitis + volvulus + atresia	3	2	1
Meconium ileus + peritonitis + perforated colon	8	4	4
Birth weight below 5 pounds	10	1	9
Birth trauma	3	..	3
Septicemia	7	1	6
Rh incompatibility	1	1	..
Meningitis	1	..	1
Kernicterus due to prematurity	1	..	1
Convulsion	1	..	1
Subarachnoid hemorrhage	4	1	3
Bleeding ? Hypoprothrombinemia	4		4
Hyaline membrane disease	1	..	1
Epidermolysis bullosa	1	..	1
Acute duodenal ulcer	1	..	1
Congenital abnormalities	9	..	9

Hirschsprung's aganglionic colon and congenital
  short bowel
Herniation of bowel through mesenteric defect—2
  patients
Meckel's diverticulum in 3 patients
Atypical lobulation of left lung
Absent left testis
Polycystic kidneys
Mesenteric pseudocyst

is analogous to the changes noted in the pancreas. Focal obstructive lesions resulting from the bile-containing mucous plugs has suggested the name "focal biliary cirrhosis." This lesion is present in less than one fifth of the cases examined at autopsy. Adjacent to the areas of proliferation of bile ducts with dilated obstructed lumens, the portal areas are broad and fibrosed. When these areas grossly distort the lobule and join one another, the appearance is that of a multilobular cirrhosis or "hepar lobatum." Such advanced changes occur in less than 5 per cent of the cases and may result in the production of clinical symptoms of portal vein obstruction. Hypersplenism,

and hemorrhage from esophageal varices may occur as a result of the increased portal pressure, and shunting procedures with splenectomy may be necessary. Jaundice is rarely noted in spite of extensive liver involvement. Some of the commonly used liver function tests may give normal results, but the prothrombin time may be prolonged and the relative decrease in serum albumin, and the increase in the globulins, especially the gamma globulins, may be striking. The transaminases may also be abnormal.

The fatty changes noted in the liver are common and do not appear to be related to the nutritional status of the patient and are not specific.

The gallbladder is often shrunken and contains a small amount of viscid bile.

RESPIRATORY TRACT. Most deaths are due to chronic pulmonary infection. At autopsy the trachea and bronchi are generally filled with a mucopurulent material. The thorax is rounded, and the lungs are emphysematous. Pleural adhesions, congestion, emphysematous blebs, subpleural hemorrhage and areas of pneumonic consolidation and abscesses may be seen. When dissected, the bronchi may be found dilated and filled with purulent exudate. Lung section reveals areas of bronchopneumonia, emphysema and atelectasis, with widespread dilatation of bronchi which ooze purulent exudate upon pressure. The bronchiectasis is usually tubular and generally involves all lobes. The hilar lymph nodes are enlarged. The bacteria grown from the exudate are generally *Staphylococcus aureus* or *Pseudomonas aeruginosa*.

The initial lesion in the lung is bronchial obstruction, and this is followed by overdistention of the alveoli. Infection supervenes, and a chronic inflammatory process occurs in which the *M. aureus* predominates. The bronchial and tra-

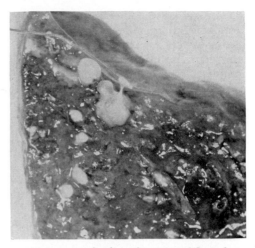

FIGURE 45–4. Section of a resected lung from a child with cystic fibrosis to show the thick, sticky, mucopurulent exudate which oozes from many of the bronchi. A culture revealed mucoid Pseudomonas.

cheal glands appear active and secrete a viscid material. The sticky sputum or mucopurulent secretion is the combined product of the mucus-secreting glands and the infectious process. The infection contributes cellular debris, bacteria and their products and necrotic leukocytes.

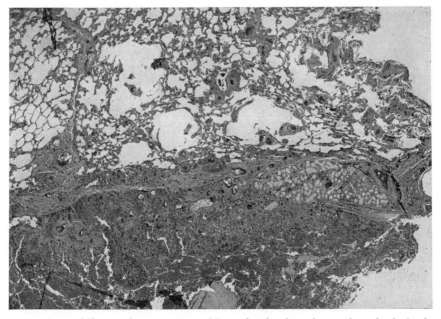

FIGURE 45–5. Microscopic appearance of lung showing bronchus and tracheal glands.

The bronchial walls become thick, and adjacent alveoli are involved in a chronic pneumonia. Focal areas of atelectasis occur when the bronchiolar obstruction is complete. This process is noted more frequently in the smaller infant. Larger segments of the bronchial tree may also obstruct and cause segmental and even lobar collapse. The atelectatic segment may become a seat of abscess cavities. Surgical removal of such areas is feasible, provided the remaining lung tissue is in relatively good condition. The persistence of the chronic bronchial infection results in a cylindrical bronchiectasis. The chest becomes rounded. Digital clubbing occurs. Some of the pulmonary complications include hemoptysis, pneumothorax and cor pulmonale. The chronic infection may result in a granulomatous lesion resembling an actinomycosis and is more properly described as botryomycosis.

The upper respiratory tract is usually affected. Chronic sinus infection is present in the majority of patients with this disease. The mucus-secreting cells may be hyperactive, and the membrane edematous and hypertrophied. The turbinates are often swollen. Nasal polyps may occur as early as three years of age, and there is an incidence of nearly 10 per cent in patients over ten years of age; they may occur at almost any age. Nasal polyps are generally multiple, occur bilaterally and often recur after polypectomy.

OTHER CHANGES. The eccrine sweat glands are histologically normal and produce an abnormal secretion with a high sodium, potassium and chloride concentration. Other serous glands, especially the salivary and parotid glands, likewise may appear normal, yet produce a secretion which may be slightly abnormal. The lacrimal gland secretions are normal.

Lesions secondary to pancreatic insufficiency and malabsorption may occur. Failure to absorb fat and fat-soluble vitamins has led to vitamin A, vitamin E and vitamin K deficiency, hypolipemia and hypocholesterolemia.

Diagnosis

A high degree of clinical suspicion is essential in making a diagnosis of cystic fibrosis. Some years ago physicians commonly remarked that the appearance of the patient was so good that the diagnosis of cystic fibrosis could be discarded. This statement implies that patients with this

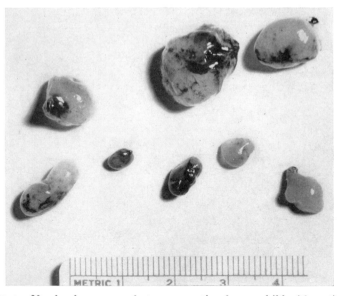

FIGURE 45–6. Nasal polyps removed at one operation from a child with cystic fibrosis.

disease are necessarily severely malnourished and stunted. Perhaps it is for this reason that many cases today are not diagnosed, and only when advanced changes take place does the diagnosis suggest itself.

The disease should be suspected in any child having chronic or recurrent symptoms involving the upper or lower respiratory tract. Some of these symptoms are found in over 90 per cent of the patients at one time or another and may include chronic cough, asthma-like symptoms in infancy, recurrent pneumonitis, bronchitis, or pneumonia, atelectasis, focal or lobar, nasal polyposis (see Fig. 6) and chronic sinusitis, empyema, and bronchiectasis.

The diagnosis should be suspected in any child with symptoms suggesting pancreatic insufficiency or malabsorption. These symptoms are present in approximately 80 per cent of the patients and include slow growth or failure to thrive, a good to huge appetite, frequent large, foul movements, a protuberant abdomen, rectal prolapse (usually recurrent), intestinal obstruction in the newborn, fecal impaction in older children, infants with vitamin K deficiency, infants with hypoproteinemic edema, infants suspected of having milk allergy, and infants suspected of having celiac disease.

The diagnosis should also be suspected in children with cirrhosis of the liver presenting with portal hypertension with or without hypersplenism. A small number of patients may have this complication, and in some cases these symptoms may be the ones for which initial medical attention is sought.

The diagnosis should also be suspected in patients with "heat stroke." The climate as well as diet may influence the occurrence of this complication. In some patients "heat stroke" has been the initial complaint. Conditions causing excess sweating with loss of salt and water result in circulatory collapse.

Whenever the diagnosis is firmly established in any one patient, it is essential to examine and test all siblings. Inquiry should be made about the health of first cousins, noting that the incidence in such persons is approximately ten times as great as in a randomly selected or control group.

The symptoms may vary widely in severity as well as in the age at onset. Some infants have severe manifestations from the first weeks of life and show a rapid downhill course. Others with an early onset of symptoms may respond to therapy and survive to adulthood. Still others have their first symptoms at two years of age or even later. In some cases there is pulmonary disease without any digestive or pancreatic involvement. On the other hand, the gastrointestinal manifestations may predominate for months or years before signs of chronic pulmonary disease appear. By far the largest number of infants and children with this disease have symptoms of pulmonary involvement and pancreatic insufficiency. In recent years most of the newly diagnosed older patients appear to have predomi-

Table 2. *Age at Diagnosis of 85 Patients Seen in 1963*

Age at Diagnosis	No. of Patients	(%)	Accumulated % of Patients
M. I	8	(9)	
1 week–11 months	34	(41)	50
1 year – 3 years	20	(24)	74
4 years– 7 years	15	(18)	91
8 years– 9 years	2	(2)	
10 years–12 years	1	(1)	
13 years–16 years	2	(2)	
17 years–20 years	2	(2)	
Over 21 years	1	(1)	100
Total	85	100	

Table 3. *Differential Diagnosis*

Chronic bronchitis
Recurrent respiratory infection
Bronchopneumonia
Staphylococcal pneumonia
Pertussis
Bronchiectasis
Asthma
Pulmonary tuberculosis
Familial dysautonomia
Agammaglobulinemia
Celiac disease
Milk allergy in early infancy
Protein-losing enteropathy
Intestinal atresia in newborn
Pancreatic insufficiency and bone
  marrow hypoplasia
Cirrhosis—portal hypertension may
  be present
Heat stroke—encephalitis

nantly the respiratory features with no evidence of pancreatic insufficiency.

It may be of interest to show the age at diagnosis of all new patients seen in our clinic in 1963 (Table 2). The total number was eighty-five. Eight had intestinal obstruction at birth, and at the other end of the scale five were first correctly diagnosed after the age of thirteen. It should be noted that approximately 50 per cent of all cases were diagnosed under the age of one year.

MECONIUM ILEUS. The earliest manifestation of cystic fibrosis is intestinal obstruction of the newborn (meconium ileus). This manifestation of cystic fibrosis actually begins in utero and may be associated with a number of complications such as volvulus, perforation of the bowel with meconium peritonitis and secondary atresia. There appears to be a higher incidence of prematurity than in children with cystic fibrosis born without this complication. The mortality rate in this group is high, partly owing to the presence of associated conditions at birth and to the high risk of development of pulmonary symptoms with secondary bronchopneumonia. The majority of infants with meconium obstruction require surgical

correction. A variety of surgical approaches are currently in vogue, and the one favored by Gross is the Mikulicz ileostomy. The over-all mortality rate is in the vicinity of 30 to 40 per cent by two months of age. The survivors of meconium ileus may exhibit the other symptoms of cystic fibrosis, and their subsequent course depends in general on the same factors that determine survival in any other child with the disease. Our oldest patients with this disease are now young adults gainfully employed. We have noted a high incidence of meconium ileus in certain families, and this may suggest the operation of environmental factors in determining the genetic mode of expression of the disease.

The meconium in these infants is usually viscid and contains serum protein. Normal meconium, by contrast, has very little protein. The abnormal meconium can be readily digested by a variety of proteolytic enzymes. The lack of pancreatic function explains the persistence of protein in the meconium. The signs of intestinal obstruction in the newborn do not distinguish this form from many others, although the x-ray appearance may be suggestive of meconium ileus. The appearance of air bubbles entrapped in the meconium provides a clue. One can also perform a pilocarpine iontophoresis sweat test, and if this reveals the characteristic elevation of sodium and chloride, the diagnosis of cystic fibrosis can be made.

PULMONARY MANIFESTATIONS. The earliest pulmonary symptom is usually cough. At first this may attract little attention, but it soon becomes chronic and even paroxysmal, at times suggesting pertussis. Feeding or sudden changes of environmental temperature may induce coughing, and in the older child an emotional response may initiate a paroxysm of coughing. Vomiting associated with coughing is not uncommon in young patients. An observant mother may detect the presence of thick mucus which the baby is unable to expel. In severely affected babies "strings of mucus" can be pulled from the oropharynx. The mother may also note that the respiratory rate is rapid and that the baby breathes noisily. These symptoms may begin as early as two or three weeks of age, but are more common a few months later. The development of frank pneumonia generally ascribed to the *M. aureus* is not uncommon. By two years of age over 75 per cent of children with cystic fibrosis have already had some of the foregoing symptoms.

The auscultatory findings may be normal in the early stages and even with advanced changes may not be striking. Roentgenograms of the chest may reveal the characteristic early changes, namely, evidences of irregular aeration with scattered areas of atelectasis. The lungs are hyperinflated, and the diaphragm may be depressed. The heart size may be small or unaffected. On occasion one may note segmental or lobar atelectasis, a finding more commonly observed on the right side than on the left. On occasion large atelectatic areas may re-expand, but they are more likely to persist and present challenging therapeutic problems. Eventually the peribronchial markings become pronounced, and the diagnosis may be readily suspected from the x-ray appearance of the chest (see Fig. 7). In addition to the cough and elevated respiratory rate, the pulmonary findings in the infant may include intercostal and suprasternal retraction as well as a rounding of the chest. Actual measurements of the lateral and anteroposterior dimensions with calipers will establish this abnormal relationship. Digital clubbing is noted frequently and

Table 4. *Clinical Features of Pulmonary Involvement*

1. Manifestation of widespread bronchial obstruction and infection
2. Often confused with "asthma" in small infants
3. Onset in infancy in majority of patients
4. May present in infancy as lobar or lobular atelectasis or in later childhood as bronchiectasis

Symptoms
    Cough, initially infrequent, later persistent and often paroxysmal. May initiate vomiting and interfere with sleep
    Wheezing is common. The bronchospasm may be secondary to infection, or the patient may also be an atopic individual
    Respiratory rates of over 70 per minute may be noted in small babies
    Easy fatigue and reduced exercise tolerance
    As pulmonary disease progresses
        Cough becomes productive
        Fever may be present
        Poor to fair appetite in a child formerly a good eater
        Weight loss
        Cyanosis

Findings
    Irregular aeration with increased markings noted by x-ray film
    Atelectasis, lobular or lobar. Lobar atelectasis is more common in small infants and occurs more commonly on the right side. It is often transient and responds to vigorous therapy. If persistent, prognosis is worsened
    Rounding of chest, increased AP dimension
    Intercostal and suprasternal retraction
    Stooped shoulders
    Digital clubbing
    Auscultatory changes
    Right-sided failure

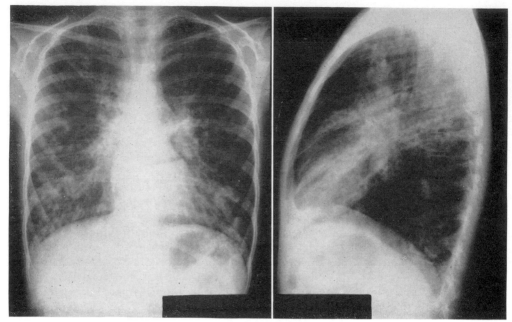

FIGURE 45–7. Chest x-ray of a child with severe pulmonary involvement.

Table 5. Pulmonary Function Studies

These tests confirm in general the impressions gathered from the clinical and roentgeno-graphic examinations. In patients with minimal pulmonary involvement the tidal volume, respiratory rate, lung volumes, lung compliance and resistance are normal. In the severely ill child the changes are striking, as shown in the following data taken from studies of Cook et al. Patient 1 is compared with patient 2. Patient 1 is a 14-year-old girl with minimal pulmonary involvement, and her pulmonary function test results are normal. This patient is well nine years after these studies were carried out. Patient 2 is a severely ill child of 13 years with extensive pulmonary involvement. She had pronounced changes by x-ray and grossly abnormal tests. She died approximately five months after the tests were done.

Respiratory Data in Patients 1 and 2

	Patient 1	Patient 2
Clinical rating	Excellent	Severe
Chest x-ray rating	Excellent	Severe
Respiratory rate/minute	21	30
Tidal volume (ml.)	414	186
Minute ventilation (1)	8.7	5.6
Residual volume*	+ 1	+153
Functional residual capacity	+ 1	+ 59
Vital capacity*	− 9	− 43
Total lung capacity*	− 7	+ 10
Compliance*	−10	− 76
Resistance*	+25	+112
RV/TLC %	25	61
FRC/TLC %	56	72

* Volumes expressed in terms of percent above or below the predicted
value for a normal child of the same height.

The expiratory peak flow can be readily determined with a Wright Peak Flow Meter in the office and is a good indication of pulmonary obstruction. Results are expressed in liters per minute and in per cent of the predicted normal. Serial measurements provide an additional method of assessing progress of the patient.

in our experience is not a very good index of the degree of pulmonary involvement. Fever is usually absent and, when present, signifies frank pulmonary infection. Persistent rales confirm the clinical impression of bronchiectasis. Right-sided cardiac failure may be a terminal event, although extensive bronchiectasis with respiratory failure is more often the cause of death.

Only a small number of patients escape pulmonary involvement in infancy. It is estimated that less than 10 per cent of the recognized patients are free of pulmonary signs or symptoms and have clear lung fields on the roentgenogram.

Clinical Evaluation

A system of clinical evaluation has been devised to aid in determining the severity of the disease and the patient's response to therapy (Table 6). The evaluation is

Table 6. *Clinical Evaluation–System of Rating Severity of Disease*

Grading	Points	General Activity	Physical Examination	Nutrition	X-ray Findings
Excellent (86–100)	25	Full normal activity; plays ball, goes to school regularly, etc.	Normal; no cough; pulse and respirations normal; clear lungs; good posture	Maintains weight and height above 25th percentile; well formed stools, almost normal; fair muscle tone and mass	Clear lung fields
Good (71–85)	20	Lacks endurance and tires at end of day; good school attendance	Resting pulse and respirations normal; rare coughing or clearing of throat; no clubbing; clear lungs; minimal emphysema	Weight and height at approximately 15th to 20th percentile; stools slightly abnormal; fair muscle tone and mass	Minimal accentuation of bronchovascular markings; early emphysema
Mild (56–70)	15	May rest voluntarily during the day; tires easily after exertion; fair school attendance	Occasional cough, perhaps in morning upon rising; respirations slightly elevated; mild emphysema; coarse breath sounds; rarely localized rales; early clubbing	Weight and height above 3rd percentile; stools usually abnormal, large and poorly formed; very little, if any, abdominal distention; poor muscle tone with reduced muscle mass	Mild emphysema with patchy atelectasis; increased bronchovascular markings
Moderate (41–55)	10	Home teacher; dyspneic after short walk; rests a great deal	Frequent cough, usually productive; chest retraction; moderate emphysema; may have chest deformity; rales usually present; clubbing 2 to 3+	Weight and height below 3rd percentile; poorly formed, bulky, fatty, offensive stools; flabby muscles and reduced mass; abdominal distention, mild to moderate	Moderate emphysema; widespread areas of atelectasis with superimposed areas of infection; minimal bronchial ectasia
Severe (40 or below)	5	Orthopneic, confined to bed or chair	Severe coughing spells; tachypnea with tachycardia and extensive pulmonary changes; may show signs of right-sided cardiac failure; clubbing 3 to 4+	Malnutrition marked; large protuberant abdomen; rectal prolapse; large, foul, frequent, fatty movements	Extensive changes with pulmonary obstructive phenomena and infection; lobar atelectasis and bronchiectasis

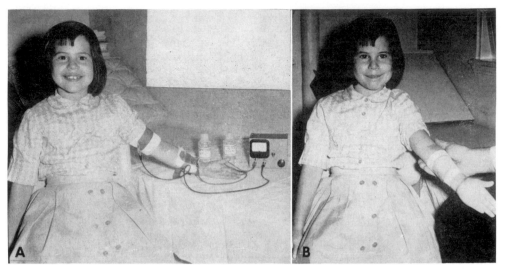

FIGURE 45–8. Pilocarpine iontophoresis. *A,* Stimulation of local sweat glands in the region of the left lower part of the forearm. *B,* Collection of sweat sample.

derived from an appraisal of each of four categories: (1) general activity, (2) physical findings, (3) nutritional status, and (4) findings on chest roentgenograms. Each category is given equal weight, 25 points, 100 points representing a perfect score. The status of the patient is considered excellent when the score is over 85, good when the score is between 71 and 85, mild between 56 and 70, moderate between 41 and 55, and severe when 40 or below. The scoring is made without consideration of the therapeutic regimen in use at the time. This system of scoring, which does not involve complicated laboratory procedures, has been used in assessing the effect of therapeutic programs.

Diagnostic Tests

The most reliable diagnostic test for cystic fibrosis is the quantitative analysis of sweat for both sodium and chloride. In no disease that can be confused with cystic fibrosis is there so great an elevation of electrolyte levels. A positive sweat test result in the absence of symptoms does not establish the diagnosis, however. The only exception to this rule may be made in the study of newborn siblings of patients with cystic fibrosis during the

first weeks of life. The sweat test result may be positive long before clinical symptoms appear.

The sweat test is carried out in three stages: (1) stimulation of sweat glands, (2) collection of the sweat sample, (3) analysis of the sweat. A variety of procedures have been used for each of these steps. To minimize errors it is strongly urged that one person, usually a trained technician, be responsible for the entire procedure. Each laboratory must use a standard procedure which yields reliable and reproducible results and must establish a range of normal in healthy and sick controls. We prefer the painless pilocarpine iontophoresis method of stimulating local sweat production, which takes seven minutes, collection of the sweat produced over a thirty-minute period into a weighed gauze pad, and determination of the chloride concentration by a titration procedure and the sodium and potassium with the flame photometer. A sample of less than 50 mg. is too small for accurate assay by our methods. This test can be performed on babies one day of age, in patients acutely ill and even in patients sleeping in mist tents. The entire procedure can be done in less than an hour. Many factors influence the level of electrolytes in sweat, and a number are listed below (see Table 7).

Elevated values are obtained in patients with adrenal insufficiency, ectodermal dys-

Table 7. *Sweat Test: Factors Influencing Level of Electrolytes*

The Patient
   Nature of the disease
   Genetic stock
   Age
   Sex: no difference noted in childhood; adult females sweat less than males with heat stimulus
   Individual variation: noted on repeated testing; may be of considerable magnitude in some patients
   Condition of patient: dehydration, circulatory failure, respiratory distress, hypothyroidism, malnutrition, edema, adrenal insufficiency, etc.
   Diet, especially salt intake
   Time of day and season of year
   Exhaustion of glands
   Acclimatization
   Activity of patient
   Unknown or unrecognized factors
Sweat Induction and Collection
   Heat vs. drug or combination
   Environmental and body temperature; humidity and effect of evaporation
   Rate of sweating
   Duration of sweat period
   Area of body
   Total body sweat vs. local collection
Drug Used and Application
   Pilocarpine, Furmethide, Mecholyl
   Method of application of drug: I.D. injection or by iontophoresis
Analytical Factors
   Size of sample
   Weight determined in analytical balance by weighing sweat absorbed on gauze pads, cotton, filter paper
   Volume measured directly with volumetric pipet
   Method of determining chloride: semiquantitative, electrometric, titrimetric, polarographic
   Flame-photometric analysis for sodium and potassium
   Dilution factor
   Contamination
   Technical: personal factor

S. Schuster, H. Shwachman and K. T. Khaw. *J. Thoracic & Cardiovasc. Surg.*, 48:5, 1964.

plasia and in some patients with glycogen storage disease. An important factor is age. In the neonatal period the values are higher than after the second week of life. By about sixteen or seventeen years the values for sodium and chloride gradually increase to adult levels, which may be nearly twice the value in childhood.

Figure 9 shows the results of 4231 sweat tests carried out in our laboratory. The end of the bar indicates the mean value, and the numbers in the bar indicate the range of values. Note that in the 745 patients with cystic fibrosis tested, the lowest values recorded are 77 mEq. per liter for chloride and 72 mEq. per liter for sodium. We have omitted seven patients who belong in this category and in whom sweat values varied significantly and generally fell in the borderline zone. The chart also shows the increase with age as noted in the control group; the findings in siblings correspond to the findings in the healthy controls under seventeen years of age, and the results of the sweat test in parents correspond to the results in the older control group. The mean sodium value exceeds the chloride in all groups except the patients with cystic fibrosis, in whom the mean chloride value exceeds the mean sodium. The potassium concentration decreases with increasing age and has no diagnostic value, although the mean value in patients with cystic fibrosis is nearly twice as high as in the control group.

We have not been able to confirm the observation of others that the sweat electrolyte levels are elevated in the heterozygote.

The reliability of the sweat test is close to 98 per cent, indeed a remarkable laboratory finding, since this test reflects on the function of one type of gland which is not known to contribute to the main features of the disease. The level of the salt concentration is not a measure of the severity of the disease. In a small number of patients with cystic fibrosis the values tend to be in the borderline zone or even in the high normal region. The diagnosis is, in such cases, most difficult to establish, and a variety of other pro-

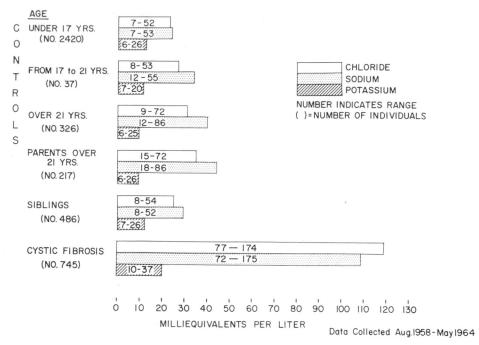

FIGURE 45–9. Concentration of electrolytes in the sweat after pilocarpine stimulation in 4231 patients. The end of the bar in each case represents the mean value. There is little overlapping between the patients with cystic fibrosis and all the others tested except in a small number of subjects over 21 years of age.

cedures are justified. In children the analysis of fingernail and toenail clippings for the sodium and potassium content may help establish the diagnosis in doubtful cases. Repeated sweat tests are indicated when equivocal results are obtained.

Screening tests for sweat chloride levels are helpful, especially when properly done. These tests, of which there are many, should not be regarded as a final diagnostic procedure. We have seen serious errors made with such tests, especially when too much reliance was placed on a single negative result. In our clinic the most reliable procedure is performed on any patient suspected of having cystic fibrosis.

PANCREATIC FUNCTION. The most direct method of studying pancreatic function is to obtain duodenal fluid and determine the activity of pancreatic enzymes. The viscosity measurement of the duodenal aspirate is of considerable value in patients with cystic fibrosis, since this is significantly increased in approximately 90 per cent of patients. The volume of fluid is also reduced, and the pH is lower than in healthy controls. The enzyme assay includes measurement of trypsin, chymotrypsin, lipase and amylase. There is a rough parallelism in enzyme activity in the healthy gland or in the case of complete pancreatic achylia. In the former case all enzyme values are normal, and in the latter all are virtually absent. Under these circumstances assay for trypsin alone is sufficient. In patients with partial involvement of the pancreas, however, a dissociation of enzyme activity may be noted. Complete pancreatic enzyme insufficiency is not indicated by finding low to absent enzyme values in the fasting state, but must include the measurement of enzyme activity following intravenous secretin or intraduodenal stimulation with olive oil.

Indirect tests for pancreatic function are numerous, and one we have developed as a simple test is the gelatin film technique of testing feces. In infants and small children the normal stool contains considerable proteolytic activity; in patients with complete pancreatic insufficiency the stool trypsin is markedly reduced or absent. The measurement of fecal fat by determining the total free fatty acids is a practical one and can be readily performed in most clinical laboratories. Patients with pancreatic insufficiency may excrete as much as 30 gm. or more of fat a day. Nearly all infants and children with pancreatic insufficiency have cystic fibrosis. The small number who do not may have either a congenital anomaly or dysplasia of the pancreas or a syndrome we recently described. Initially the first three patients with this syndrome were regarded as atypical examples of cystic fibrosis because pulmonary manifestations failed to develop, and the patients had normal sweat test results. These cases, which now number ten in our series, include the following clinical and laboratory features: pancreatic insufficiency, failure to thrive, bone marrow hypoplasia, neutropenia, thrombocytopenia or anemia and transient galactosuria.

A variety of oral absorptive tests have been proposed, such as gelatin or casein for measuring protein digestion, vitamin A and Lipiodol for fat absorption, and glucose or xylose for measuring glucose absorption. In patients with pancreatic insufficiency the xylose and glucose absorption test results are normal, whereas protein and fat absorption test results are abnormal.

The clinical response to dietary modifications has often been used to assess pancreatic function. These tests, although helpful, should never be regarded as conclusive evidence unless balance studies are made.

DIAGNOSTIC TESTS IN ADULTS. The sweat test in adults is far less reliable than in children, owing in part to the wide range of values in healthy adults. Some healthy adults may have values well above the diagnostic range, i.e. above 70 mEq. per liter. The presence of diabetes, emphysema, ulcers or other complications seen in cystic fibrosis does not point to the disease when these features are noted in adults. The clinical picture must be consistent with the disease and should include a history of illness beginning in childhood. Roentgenograms of the chest may be helpful, and the family history must also be taken into account.

Treatment

The nature of the basic disorder remains unknown; hence therapy, although effective, must be considered nonspecific or empiric. Treatment is given to relieve the presenting complaints and to prevent complications. Although prophylactic therapy is the most important aspect of managing the child with cystic fibrosis, it is least understood. Three examples of prophylactic therapy each affecting a different system follow: (1) The *eccrine sweat glands*. The use of salt in a warm climate or when the patient sweats excessively even in cold weather may prevent "salt depletion" or "heat stroke." (2) *Respiratory system*. Measles may be a serious disease and may precipitate a downward course; hence measles prophylaxis should be advised in all children with cystic fibrosis. (3) *Gastrointestinal*. Dietary and pancreatic therapy, when given to patients diagnosed in early infancy, will reduce the incidence of rectal prolapse to nearly zero from an incidence of over 20 per cent in untreated patients.

In many communities patients suspected of having cystic fibrosis are hospitalized for study, and if the diagnosis is confirmed, the therapeutic program is instituted and education of parents undertaken. In a center where facilities and personnel are available, hospitalization is reserved for the very sick and in many cases avoided. The amount of time and effort needed to provide parents with an understanding of the disease, the training in methods of physical therapy, the setting up of the mist tent equipment at home, and the evaluation of all siblings is considerable. In our clinic relatively few patients are hospitalized for diagnostic study.

PULMONARY SYSTEM. The chief considerations are the prevention of bronchial obstruction and the accompanying infection. When these already exist, the therapeutic program must be vigorous and include the following measures.

Antibiotic Therapy. Oral therapy is preferred, and the antibiotics may be selected from a fairly large list. The study of sputum or throat cultures and the testing of the microorganisms to a variety of antibiotics may be of help in determining which agent to use. The most common organism recovered in the initial cultures is penicillin-resistant *M. aureus.* Chlortetracycline, oxytetracycline, erythromycin, oxacillin or Lincocin may be used in a dosage of approximately 20 to 50 mg. per kilogram per day, depending on the severity of the disease and the clinical response of the patient. Gram-negative bacteria such as aerogenes, *Klebsiella pneumoniae* and *P. aeruginosa* may be predominant; chloramphenicol may be a clinically effective drug, although the bacteria isolated may be resistant. In patients with persistent infection, continuous antibiotic therapy may be necessary, and when the clinical and radiologic condition deteriorates, the combination of chloramphenicol and oxacillin or erythromycin may be used for long periods. Close observation is essential when chloramphenicol is used, since there may be hematologic, ophthalmologic and neurotoxic complications. In patients with minimal pulmonary disease continuous antibiotic therapy is not necessary. Aerosol antibiotic therapy is a useful adjunct to systematic therapy. Neomycin solution, 50 mg. per milliliter, plus isoproterenol may be used as often as two or three times daily for prolonged periods of time.

Relief of Bronchial Obstruction. The removal of viscid mucus and the exudate produced as a result of infection is the main aim of the following therapeutic measures.

Mist Tent Therapy. The provision of a water-saturated atmosphere makes it easier for the patient to mobilize his secretions. The tent is set up in the home, and the patient sleeps in this tent throughout the night. A variety of effective pieces of equipment are commercially available to provide a mist. A 10 per cent solution of propylene glycol is placed in the nebulizer, and a fine mist with a particle size of less than 3 to 5 microns can be achieved. When first placed in a tent, many patients with moderate pulmonary involvement will report that they slept comfortably for the first time in many a night, that they no longer awoke through the night coughing. They also find it easier to cough up sputum.

Postural Drainage. The use of mechanical means to assist expulsion of pulmonary secretions is advocated. The patient is placed in the appropriate position, i.e. with the bronchus from the area to be drained perpendicular to the ground; by clapping and vibrating the secretions from the affected area are loosened and expelled. Parents are instructed by the physical therapist and may be advised to drain the affected lobes once or more times a day (see Fig. 3-6, *A,* p. 94).

Breathing Exercises. As in most types of obstructive bronchopulmonary disease, the expiratory phase is relatively ineffective and the residual air is increased. Breathing exercises are instituted to remedy this defect.

Other measures include the use of expectorant drugs and mucolytic agents. These drugs may be used for prolonged periods of time and are often beneficial, but in no way affect the basic disorder. Steroid therapy may relieve the bronchospasm in the severely ill infant or may be used in the attempt to prevent the regrowth of nasal polyps.

Pulmonary resection may provide a palliative form of therapy in selected patients who have long-standing areas of persistent atelectasis with underlying abscess formation or bronchiectasis. The areas resected and the results of the twenty-nine resec-

Table 8. *Results of Pulmonary Resections in 29 Patients with Cystic Fibrosis*

Excellent	4 (14%)	Symptom-free and full activity
Good	15 (51.5%)	Definite decrease in symptoms with increased sense of well-being
Fair	4 (14%)	Mild decrease in symptoms with increased sense of well-being
Unsatisfactory	1 (3.5%)	Unchanged
Poor	5 (17%)	Patient either died as result of operation or is worse

Area Resected

Right Side	No. of Patients	Left Side	No. of Patients
Pneumonectomy	1	Pneumonectomy	1
Upper lobe	3	Left upper	2
Middle lobe	4	Lingula	1
Upper and middle lobes	4	Left lower	4
Anterior segment of upper lobe	1	Left lower lobe and lingula	2
Middle and lower lobes	4	Total	10
Lower lobe	1		
Superior segment of lower lobe	1		
Total	19		

tions performed in our hospital are given in Table 8.

DIGESTIVE SYSTEM. No special dietary considerations are needed in patients with good pancreatic function. The majority of patients, however, have either complete or partial insufficiency. The aim of therapy in these patients is to satisfy hunger by providing an adequate diet and vitamin supplementation, and to replace missing pancreatic enzymes. The total caloric intake in untreated patients may be surprisingly high, and as soon as proper dietary therapy is begun, hunger is less intense and the caloric intake diminished to a nearly normal level. The diet consists of food generally consumed by the family with emphasis on restricting the fat and increasing the protein intake. The weight change and the nature and frequency of the stool will in most cases serve as a guide. Many parents are not aware of the stool abnormality, and an inspection by the physician is urged. Commercial pancreatin preparations are effective and are best administered with each meal. We have found the powder suitable for infants and small children and tablets or capsules for older patients. We have had considerable experience with Viokase powder and tablets, and find these products effective. Other available commercial products are Cotazyme and

Pancreatic granules. The effective dose may vary with each child and is determined by the nature of the response. At present nearly all commercially available multivitamin preparations are in water-soluble form. We recommend twice the usual dose and also the addition of vitamin B complex in patients receiving antibiotics orally. Vitamin K is given to all small infants, since they are prone to hypoprothrombinemia.

TREATMENT OF COEXISTING CONDITIONS. Patients with cystic fibrosis are subject to all conditions that appear in the general population. Congenital anomalies that need correction should be dealt with. Associated conditions such as allergies are treated in the accepted manner. The incidence of allergic disorders is no more frequent in patients with cystic fibrosis than in the child population. We have encountered two patients who had an associated lactase deficiency and one who had a gluten-induced celiac disease. These children responded to the appropriate dietary exclusion therapy.

Complications

It is difficult to determine what constitutes a complication or a symptom. When one diagnoses a case in an infant newly born into a family with other cystic

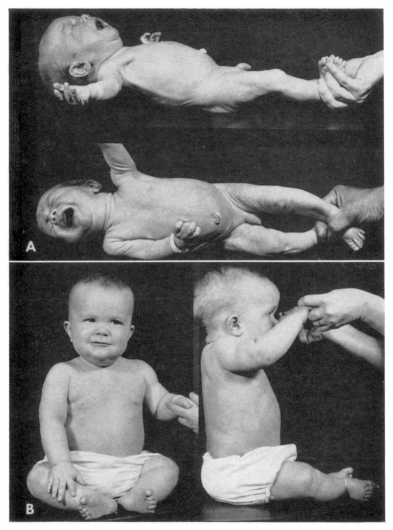

FIGURE 45–10. Patient (*A*) when first seen at 2 months of age and (*B*) after 8 months of therapy.

Table 9. *Complications Versus Features of Disease*

Emphysema	C	Right-sided heart failure	O
Atelectasis	C	Pulmonary hypertension	O
Bronchiectasis	C		
Hemoptysis	O	Botryomycosis	R
Sinusitis	C	Osteomyelitis	R
Nasal polyposis	C	Ocular changes	R
Empyema	R	Salt depletion syndrome	R
Pneumothorax	R	Calcification of pancreas	R

Complications

Growth retardation	C	Intestinal obstruction	C
Delayed sexual development	C	Meconium ileus (see Table 1)	
Gynecomastia	R	Atresia	
Diabetes mellitus	R	Fecal impactions	
Osteoarthropathy	C	Intussusception	R
Parotitis	R	Duodenitis	O
Osteoporosis	O	Duodenal ulcerations	R
Hypoproteinemia*	R	Pancreatitis	R
Edema,* generalized	R	Portal hypertension	O
Anemia secondary to blood loss	R	Hypersplenism	R
Deficient metal-binding globulin*	R	Cirrhosis	C
B_{12} deficiency		Hypergammaglobulinemia	R
Folate deficiency		Ascites	R
Vitamin K deficiency	O	Pneumatosis intestinalis	R
Vitamin A deficiency	O	Rectal prolapse	O
Vitamin E deficiency	O		

Complications—Iatrogenic

Iodides: goiter
          hypothyroidism
Pancreatic replacement: constipation
         Pork allergy: diarrhea
Antibiotics
  Tetracyclines: discoloration of teeth
                deposition in bone
                photosensitivity
                "growth factor"
                bulging fontanel
                vomiting
                diarrhea
  Novobiocin: fever, dermatitis
  Chloramphenicol: ocular changes, loss of vision
                   pancytopenia
                   toxic neuritis
Anabolic agents: androgenic effects
I.P.P.B.: pneumothorax
         extension of infection

* Figure 11 illustrates infant with hypoproteinemia, generalized edema, and anemia.
  R = rare; O = occasional; C = common.

fibrosis children, there are usually no symptoms or complaints. If one observes such an infant carefully, the stools may become abnormal. The baby develops a large appetite and fails to gain, or he may begin to cough or breathe rapidly. Some of these early symptoms can be prevented, and when prophylactic therapy accomplishes this, one is clearly left with a baby symptom-free yet labeled as having cystic

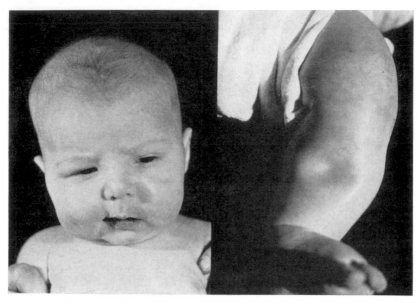

FIGURE 45–11. Patient presenting at 2½ months of age with edema, hypoproteinemia and anemia. The anemia was due to a deficiency in metal-binding globulin. The edema and hypoproteinemia cleared rapidly with changes in formula from a soybean preparation to an evaporated milk formula and the addition of pancreatin. This is an unusual manifestation of cystic fibrosis noted in early infancy.

fibrosis. Our ultimate aim is to establish the diagnosis very early and prevent the complications, many of which are now considered symptoms of the disease. Table 9 lists the complications, and the frequency with which they occur is indicated by the letters *R* for rarely, *O* for occasionally and *C* for commonly. Some of the complications are iatrogenic.

Conclusion

Cystic fibrosis is a frequent cause of chronic pulmonary disease in childhood. Although the cause of the hereditary disorder is unknown, considerable progress has been made in diagnostic methods and in therapeutic management. Early detection and prompt treatment will favorably affect the outcome. The enormous economic and psychologic burden borne by the parents cannot be overemphasized, and successful management cannot be carried out without the cooperation of the parents. Consultation with experts at treatment centers is recommended to assure that the diagnosis is correct, that

proper prophylactic therapy is available, and to provide genetic counseling and financial and other assistance. The knowledge that a small number of patients have reached adulthood, graduated from college, have married and are leading productive lives should encourage us to continue to search for a better understanding of the underlying disorder with the hope of providing a more specific type of therapy.

Prognosis

The outlook for patients with cystic fibrosis has improved a great deal in the past twenty years. Before 1945 most patients diagnosed succumbed to this disease within a few years. At that time the survival of a child beyond ten years of age was unusual. Death was due to the extensive pulmonary involvement, infection playing a large role. With the advent of broad-spectrum antibiotics in 1948 a striking improvement in the course of the disease was noted. As new antibiotics appeared, many were found to be effective in combating the pulmonary infection. Other therapeutic advances included home therapy, aerosols combining antibiotics with bronchodilators or mucolytic agents, mist tent therapy, physical therapy with breathing exercises, and postural drainage. Emphasis on therapy shifted from pancreatic and dietary management to a variety of measures designed to prevent and control pulmonary infection or complications initiated by the process of diffuse bronchiolar plugging. Measles vaccination as well as protection against influenza is widely practiced.

The extent to which we are effective in applying measures to prevent the progress of the pulmonary lesion will in large measure determine the prognosis. Unfortunately, in the past, many patients presented with advanced and irreversible pulmonary lesions. The advent of more reliable and easily performed diagnostic tests plus a greater awareness of the varied clinical manifestations makes it possible to recognize the disease in its earliest stages. Today many cystic fibrosis clinics can boast of a mortality rate of less than 4 per cent per year of all newly diagnosed cases, excluding meconium ileus. In our clinic over 100 patients have reached seventeen years of age, whereas twelve years ago only three patients were over seventeen years. Many have completed college, and at least twelve are married. A current survey of babies born to mothers with documented cystic fibrosis revealed eleven mothers and fourteen deliveries. Two of the babies and three of the mothers succumbed. In our series of older patients the males outnumber females. These observations point to a much better prognosis today than was possible at any previous time.

REFERENCES

Andersen, D. H.: Cystic Fibrosis of the Pancreas and Its Relation to Celiac Disease. *Am. J. Dis. Child.*, 56:344, 1938.

Idem: Pathology of Cystic Fibrosis; in Problems in Cystic Fibrosis. *Ann. New York Acad. Sc.*, 93:500, 1962.

Bodian, M.: *Fibrocystic Disease of the Pancreas: A Congenital Disorder of Mucus Production—Mucosis.* London, Heinemann, 1953.

Cook, C. D., Shwachman, H., and others: Studies of Respiratory Physiology in Children. II. Lung Volumes and Mechanics of Respiration in 64 Patients with Cystic Fibrosis of the Pancreas. *Pediatrics*, 24:2, 1959.

Craig, J. M., Haddad, H., and Shwachman, H.: The Pathological Changes in the Liver in Cystic Fibrosis of the Pancreas. *Am. J. Dis. Child.*, 93:357, 1957.

Doershuk, C. F., Matthews, L. W., Tucker, A. S., and Spector, S.: Prophylactic and Therapeutic Program for Cystic Fibrosis. *Pediatrics*, 36:675, 1965.

Donnison, A. B., Shwachman, H., and Gross, R. E.: A Review of 164 Children with Meconium Ileus. *Pediatrics*, 37:833, 1966.

Fanconi, G., Uehlinger, E., and Knauer, C.: Das Coeliakiesyndrom bei angeborener zystischer Pankreasfibromatose und Bronchiekstasien. *Wien. med. Wchnschr.*, 86:753, 1936.

Farber, S.: Pancreatic Function and Disease in Early Life. V. Pathologic Changes Associated with Pancreatic Insufficiency in Early Life. *Arch. Path.*, 37:238, 1944.

Idem: Some Organic Digestive Disturbances in Early Life. *J. Michigan M. Soc.*, 44:587, 1945.

Glanzmann, E.: Dysporia Entero-bronchopancreatica Congenita Familiaris, Zystische Pankreasfibrose. *Ann. paediat.*, 166:289, 1946.

Grand, R. A., and di Sant'Agnese, P. A.: Personal communication.

Gross, R. E.: *The Surgery of Infancy and Childhood.* Philadelphia, W. B. Saunders Company, 1953, Chap. 13.

Guide to Diagnosis and Management of Cystic Fibrosis. National Cystic Fibrosis Research Foundation, 521 Fifth Ave., N.Y., March 1963.

Kagan, B. M.: Cystic Fibrosis of the Pancreas. Eccrinosis. *Illinois M.J.*, 107:120, 1955.

Katznelson, D., Vawter, G. F., Foley, G. E., and Shwachman, H.: Botryomycosis, a Complication in Cystic Fibrosis. *J. Pediat.*, 65:525, 1964.

Kobayashi, Y.: An Autopsied Case of Cystic Fibrosis of the Pancreas. *Acta Ped. Jap.*, 65:597, 1961.

Kopito, L., Khaw, K. T., Townley, R. R. W., and Shwachman, H.: Studies in Cystic Fibrosis—Analysis of Nail Clippings for Sodium and Potassium. *New England J. Med.*, 272:504, 1965.

Murray, A. B., and Cook, C. D.: Measurement of Peak Expiratory Flow Rates in 220 Normal Children from 4.5 to 18.5 Years of Age. *J. Pediat.*, 62:186, 1963.

Orzalesi, M. M., Kohner, D., Cook, C. D., and Shwachman, H.: Anamnesis, Sweat Electrolyte and Pulmonary Function Studies in

Parents of Patients with Cystic Fibrosis of the Pancreas. *Acta paediat.*, 52:267, 1963.

Rosan, R. C., Shwachman, H., and Kulczycki, L. L.: Diabetes and Cystic Fibrosis of the Pancreas. *Am. J. Dis. Child.*, 104:265, 1962.

Salam, M. Z.: Cystic Fibrosis of the Pancreas in Middle East. *J. Med. Lebanese*, 15:61, 1962.

Schuster, S., Schwachman, H., and Khaw, K. T.: Pulmonary Surgery in Cystic Fibrosis. *J. Thoracic & Cardiovasc. Surg.*, 48:5, 1964.

Shwachman, H., and Kulczycki, L. L.: A Report of 105 Patients with Cystic Fibrosis of the Pancreas Studied over a Five to Fourteen Year Period. *Am. J. Dis. Child.*, 96:6, 1958.

Shwachman, H., Kulczycki, L. L., and Khaw, K. T.: Studies in Cystic Fibrosis. A Report of 65 Patients over 17 Years of Age. *Pediatrics*, 36:689, 1965.

Shwachman, H., Diamond, L. K., Oski, F. A., and Khaw, K. T.: The Syndrome of Pancreatic Insufficiency and Bone Marrow Dysfunction. *J. Pediat.*, 65:645, 1964.

CHAPTER FORTY-SIX

Cytomegalic Inclusion Disease

WILLIAM A. HOWARD, M.D.

Cytomegalic inclusion disease is a systemic infection characterized by the presence of intranuclear and intracytoplasmic inclusions in enlarged cells of many viscera; associated with these inclusions are varying degrees of inflammatory degeneration or necrosis. The disease in the newborn is apparently the result of an infection acquired in utero from an asymptomatically infected mother. If the disease is not fatal, there is usually severe residual damage, especially of the central nervous system. Inapparent postnatally acquired infections are common in children and young adults. Because of the relatively recent development of adequate methods of diagnosis, much is yet to be learned about the frequency of cytomegalic inclusion disease and its clinical patterns in various age groups.

Incidence

Serologic studies, using neutralization and complement fixation techniques, indicate that the virus responsible for the disease is widespread and occurs at all ages, although clinical cases are infrequent. Antibodies may be recognized in 70 per cent or more of newborn infants. This is roughly the same incidence as is found in young adults, indicating passage of the antibody through the placenta, and suggesting the occurrence of inapparent infections in adults. Neither positive serology nor isolation of the virus necessarily warrants a diagnosis of cytomegalic inclusion disease, since the virus has been isolated from a number of fetuses and newborn infants dying from a variety of causes. An interesting finding is that virus isolation occurs approximately twenty times more frequently in institutionalized children and in contacts of children with viruria than in routine examination. Cytomegalic inclusion disease also has been found to occur with greater frequency in debilitated patients, those suffering from chronic illness and those with malignancy.

Etiology

Cytomegalic inclusion disease is caused by one of the group of cytomegaloviruses (CMV) formerly labeled human salivary gland viruses. The cytomegaloviruses are ether-sensitive DNA viruses measuring 120 to 130 microns in diameter, and are heat- and acid-labile. These physical properties, together with the pattern of cellular infection produced, indicate a close relation to the viruses of herpes simplex and varicella, and it is probable that the cytomegaloviruses will be classified with the herpesvirus group.

As a group the human cytomegaloviruses are not antigenically homogeneous. At least three serologic types have been recognized, and it is possible that additional varieties may be isolated as more cases are studied.

Pathogenesis

Despite an apparently large reservoir of subclinical human infection, the mechanism by which the disease is spread from person to person is not readily apparent. The fetus in utero is infected by trans placental passage of the cytomegalovirus from a recently infected mother who herself has an inapparent infection. The mother may continue to excrete virus in spite of the development of a good antibody titer. The presence of antibody apparently does not prevent virus multiplication, but it may prevent the disease from being transmitted in subsequent pregnancies. It is rare to have a succeeding infant afflicted, but this also is possible on the theoretical basis of infection with another serotype of cytomegalovirus.

There is a curious note in the contrasting behavior of the illness in the mother and in her severely affected infant, who may not only have a more severe infection, but may also develop a higher antibody titer, and excrete virus for a longer time (up to three to four years). This makes it appear that the adult host has a greater ability to terminate the infection. Medearis suggests that since endogenous interferon may be responsible for both the limitation and termination of viral infections, and since immature animals (including premature infants) have a deficient interferon-producing capacity,

the presence of interferon produced by cytomegalovirus may play an important role in pathogenesis. This is a notable example of the modifying effect of host maturation on the response of individuals to infectious agents.

At autopsy the widespread disturbance produced by cytomegalic inclusion disease becomes apparent. The virus has been found in salivary glands, lung, kidney, brain, liver, bone marrow and numerous other organs throughout the body. Generally the liver, kidney and lungs are the organs most heavily infected, but the brain is also heavily involved from the viewpoint of functional damage. In almost every instance pulmonary involvement is recognized at autopsy, although clinical evidence may have been mild. The pulmonary changes are diffuse, but are principally those of an interstitial pneumonia, with numerous inclusions found in cells around the terminal air spaces. Occasional instances of placental involvement in cytomegalic inclusion disease have been reported; in Rosenstein and Navarette-Reyna's case approximately 1 per cent of the villi showed focal necrosis, with neutrophils and nuclear debris. A few of the affected villi showed typical intranuclear inclusions.

Clinical Manifestations

Symptoms of the usually congenitally acquired form of cytomegalic inclusion disease appear within a matter of hours to a few days after birth in a prematurely born first child of an apparently healthy mother. Some of these mothers have reported the occurrence of a severe respiratory infection during pregnancy, leading to the supposition that this infection may be the original source of cytomegalovirus infection in the mother and her infant.

The most frequent and severe manifestations of cytomegalic inclusion disease are hepatosplenomegaly, jaundice and petechiae. Hepatosplenomegaly is nearly always present, is considerable, and in survivors may persist into the second or third year of life. Jaundice may appear early, within the first twenty-four hours, and may be intense, persisting for several weeks. Direct bilirubin usually accounts for more than 50 per cent of the bilirubinemia, and the indirect fraction rarely rises above 20 mg. per 100 ml. Petechiae and purpuric areas relatable in part to thrombocytopenia are frequent findings. A hemolytic anemia is often present. Symptoms of nervous system involvement appear early and include twitching, convulsions, motor abnormalities, chorioretinitis and cerebral calcifications in the subependymal region of the lateral ventricles (visible by x-ray film). Microcephaly is present in most infants with the congenital form of the disease, and may become apparent at any time up to one year of age. Spastic paralysis, seizures and blindness may result, and mental retardation is the rule in most survivors. Measured intelligence quotient levels in these retarded infants range from 30 to 50.

Pulmonary manifestations are overshadowed by other striking symptoms, but in many of the severe, eventually fatal cases, pneumonia is diagnosed ante mortem, and is always found post mortem. X-ray examination may be helpful in severe involvement. In some infants in whom the disease appears later in the postnatal period, pneumonitis is the cause of persistent respiratory distress. In the early months of life a pneumonic form with hepatosplenomegaly may be recognized, and cytomegalovirus has been found associated with *Pneumocystis carinii* pneumonia. The frequency of pulmonary involvement increases with increasing age, and in adults it most commonly appears in patients with malignancy. The occurrence of viruria, hepatomegaly and abnormal liver function tests in children without any other underlying disease suggests that cytomegalic inclusion disease is clinically significant, that the process may localize in the liver, and that this may be a possible cause of sporadic cases of chronic hepatitis in childhood.

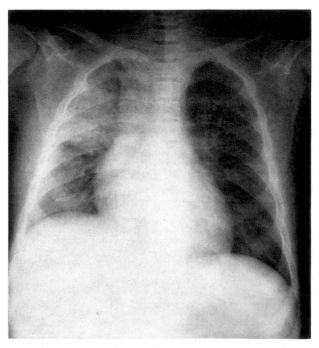

FIGURE 46–1. Cytomegalic inclusion disease following renal transplant. (Courtesy of David Hume, M.D., Medical College of Virginia, Richmond.)

Diagnosis

Initially, the diagnosis could only be suspected during life and confirmed at autopsy by the finding of the typical enlarged inclusion-bearing cells in many tissues and organs of the body. Wyatt, observing that these large cells were almost invariably present in the renal tubules, and often seen lying free in the tubules, suggested that a search of the urinary sediment might aid in diagnosis during life. Fetterman in 1952 reported the first successful identification of these inclusion-bearing cells in urinary sediment, and in 1962 Blanc and Gaetz increased the accuracy of the technique by using millipore filter equipment to collect and concentrate cells in the urine before staining. The characteristically enlarged cells may be as large as 40 microns in diameter, while the intranuclear inclusions range in size from 10 to 15 microns. With hematoxylin-eosin stain the intranuclear inclusion is amphophilic, and is separated from the nuclear membrane by a clear halo (owl's eye cell). Cytoplasmic inclusions are much smaller (4 microns) in size and less characteristic. It has been suggested that the cytologic diagnosis be based only on the finding of intranuclear inclusions, thereby avoiding a good deal of confusion. Cytologic diagnosis is more accurate in infancy, less so in older children and adults. Virus isolation is the most effective method of diagnosis, though viruria does not necessarily mean active disease; cytomegalovirus has been recovered in a high percentage of contacts of patients, and individuals institutionalized for other problems, all without clinical disease. Serologic diagnosis is hampered by lack of reference antiserums in laboratory animals, the diverse strains of the virus, and the equivocal results obtained by complement fixation.

Differential diagnosis runs the gamut of the hemorrhagic and hemolytic processes in the newborn, chiefly sepsis, erythroblastosis fetalis, neonatal thrombocytopenic purpura and congenital leukemia. The neurologic findings may be readily confused with the congenital form of *Toxoplasma gondii* infection. Less commonly, one may consider congenital syphilis and generalized herpes simplex infections.

Prognosis

Though cytomegalic inclusion disease is not necessarily fatal, the problem is a serious one, and almost all patients who recover are left with crippling residual effects. The most significant of these are the neurologic sequelae, including microcephaly, mental retardation, paralysis, blindness and convulsions. It is probable that there are undiagnosed or inapparent infections that might raise the recovery rate, if all instances were recognized. In general the prognosis for future pregnancies is good, since there is only one recorded instance of the infection occurring in a subsequent pregnancy in the same mother.

Treatment

No satisfactory treatment is available. Because of the high proportion of direct bilirubin present, exchange transfusions are seldom required in the management of severe jaundice in these infants. Corticosteroids have been used without apparent success, and it is unlikely that any drug administered postnatally would significantly influence the course of the disease in these infants damaged so severely in utero. Antibiotics may be used when sepsis cannot be ruled out, but have no effect on the underlying pathology. Gamma globulin administration has been without effect.

REFERENCES

Blanc, W. A., and Gaetz, R.: Simplified Millipore Filter Technic for Cytologic Diagnosis of Cytomegalic Inclusion Disease in Examination of the Urine. *Pediatrics*, 29:61, 1962.

Fetterman, G. H.: A New Laboratory Aid in the

Clinical Diagnosis of Inclusion Disease of Infancy. *Am. J. Clin. Path.*, 22:424, 1952.

Hanshaw, J. B.: Clinical Significance of Cytomegalovirus Infection. *Postgrad. Med.*, 35:472, 1964.

Hanshaw, J. B., and Simon, G.: Cytomegaloviruses in the Urine of Children with Generalized Neoplastic Disease. *J. Pediat.*, 58:305, 1961.

Kibrick, S.: Cytomegalic Inclusion Disease, Clinical Clin. Pediat., 3:153, 1964.

Kluge, R. C., Wicksman, R. S., and Weller, T. H.: Cytomegalic Inclusion Disease of the Newborn. Report of a Case with Persistent Viruria. *Pediatrics*, 25:35, 1960.

Kramer, R. I., Cirone, V. C., and Moore, H.: Interstitial Pneumonia Due to Pneumocystis Carinii, Cytomegalic Inclusion Disease, and Hypogammaglobulinemia Occurring Simultaneously in the Same Infant. *Pediatrics*, 29:816, 1962.

McAllister, R. M., Wright, H. T., Jr., and Tasem, W. M.: Cytomegalic Inclusion Disease in Twins. *J. Pediat.*, 64:278, 1964.

Medearis, D. N., Jr.: Observations Concerning Human Cytomegalovirus Infection and Disease. *Bull. Johns Hopkins Hosp.*, 114:181, 1964.

Naib, Z. M.: Cytologic Diagnosis of Cytomegalic Inclusion Body Disease. *Am. J. Dis. Child.*, 105:153, 1963.

Rosenstein, D. L., and Navarette-Reyna, A.: Cytomegalic Inclusion Disease. Observation of the Characteristic Inclusion Bodies in the Placenta. *Am. J. Obst. & Gynec.*, 89:220, 1964.

Rowe, W. P., Hartley, J. W., Cramblett, H. G., and Mastrotta, F.: Detection of Human Salivary Gland Virus in Mouth and Urine of Children. *Am. J. Hyg.*, 67:57, 1958.

Weller, T. H., and Hanshaw, J. B.: Virologic and Clinical Observations on Cytomegalic Inclusion Disease. *New England J. Med.*, 266:1233, 1963.

Weller, T. H., Hanshaw, J. B., and Scott, D. E.: Serologic Differentiation of Viruses Responsible for Cytomegalic Inclusion Disease. *Virology*, 12:132, 1960.

Wyatt, J. P., Saxton, J., Lee, R. S., and Pinkerton, H.: Generalized Cytomegalic Inclusion Disease. *J. Pediat.*, 36:271, 1950.

CHAPTER FORTY-SEVEN

The Mycoses (Excluding Histoplasmosis)

JOHN H. SEABURY, M.D.

The systemic mycoses as a group are believed to occur rarely among pediatric patients. When one considers all the known factors pertinent to systemic fungous infections, this attitude is quite reasonable for infants, but much less so for children and adolescents.

Infants and children with congenital agammaglobulinemia, cystic fibrosis and other constitutional or acquired immunologic or metabolic disturbances may be expected to acquire infection from almost any agent, regardless of its usual pathogenicity. Similarly, the child with leukemia or lymphoma may acquire one or more fungous infections because of alterations produced by the disease or its treatment. This sort of infection, due to serious impairment of host resistance or iatrogenic factors (prolonged use of the same vein for infusions, cutdowns, corticosteroid treatment, or prolonged administration of antibiotics) is best termed "opportunistic." Opportunistic infections in the pediatric age group are not likely to be due to the usual pathogenic fungi, but rather to those saprophytes which are common in nature (e.g. Aspergillus) or in the normal host (e.g. Candida). Since this type of fungous infection usually occurs during management of a primary illness, recognition of mycotic superinfection may be difficult unless one thinks of such complications when the patient's course is unsatisfactory.

The common systemic mycoses, with the exception of actinomycosis, are acquired from exogenous sources in nature which usually require ambulation. Epidemiologic studies of histoplasmosis and coccidioidomycosis indicate a low rate of infection in endemic areas until the child is freely ambulatory outside the home. Rate of infection increases during adolescence and early adult life. The epidemiology of cryptococcosis and North American blastomycosis has not been as clearly established. It appears that both are more intimately associated with restricted "point sources" of infection than is true for either histoplasmosis or coccidioidomycosis in highly endemic areas. Accordingly, the decade of maximum prevalence seems to fall in middle or later adult life. The recognition of purely pulmonary cryptococcosis and "epidemic" North American blastomycosis among pediatric patients may stimulate studies which will necessitate revision of this belief.

Fungous infection as a cause of pulmonary infiltration among pediatric patients is rarely an initial consideration. Acute inhalational histoplasmosis and the thin-walled cavitary residual of coccidioidomycosis are exceptions in areas of high endemicity. The roentgen features of these special manifestations of two mycotic diseases are sufficiently distinct to prompt comment by the experienced radiologist if he is given any clinical information. In other situations the radiologic report should be descriptive, and perhaps suggest a differential diagnosis. The clinician should remember that there are no specific roentgenographic features for any pulmonary infection.

The diagnosis of a pulmonary mycosis, in common with all infectious diseases, depends first of all upon laboratory evidence. Isolation of the agent by culture or animal inoculation is most desirable, but one may have to rely upon microscopy and serology at times. The physician's approach to the diagnosis of pulmonary disease in childhood is likely to involve a too limited differential diagnosis, and a too timid approach to securing adequate specimens for proper diagnosis. Of the two, the latter is the more serious. No one wants to inflict risk and pain, particularly when reasons for the procedure cannot be communicated to the child, but this is scarcely reason for jeopardizing his welfare. Transtracheal aspiration is simple and does not have the hazards of bronchoscopy. Direct needle aspiration of the lung carries no significant risk if pleural symphysis is present over the area of puncture. These procedures should be considered for many children who will not produce sputum. (See the chapter on Diagnostic and Therapeutic Procedures.)

GENERAL METHODS OF LABORATORY DIAGNOSIS

Diagnostic methodology for fungi is grossly inferior to that for bacteria in most hospital laboratories in the United States. The fault is multilateral. There are a few simple things which the clinician can do to improve results.

In the first place, the laboratory must be given suitable material. Swabs, 24-hour sputum collections or sputum contaminated with food or tooth paste are worthless for culture. The collection of specimens should not be left to uninstructed personnel.

If sputum can be obtained, it should be collected in the fasting state after the teeth have been cleaned with plain water only. Whatever sputum can be coughed into a sterile glass container during approximately one-half hour of effort should be taken directly to the laboratory.

When one cannot obtain sputum, transtracheal aspirates or direct needling of pneumonic or cavitary lesions is more likely to give diagnostic materials than are gastric aspirates. All are collected under as aseptic conditions as possible. Lung aspirates or cavitary washings should be transported within the original syringe so that the microbiologist can be responsible for subsequent handling with a minimum of opportunity for contamination.

Biopsy is usually performed by a surgical consultant in the operating room. The specimen should be bisected with sterile instruments; half should be sent for culture and the other half fixed in formalin for histopathology. Preliminary discussion with the surgical consultant or personal attention to the biopsy material by the clinician (or microbiologist) will prevent the common error of fixing the entire specimen in formalin.

Direct communication between clinician and laboratory worker can increase the likelihood of establishing the correct diagnosis. If the microbiologist is approached as a consultant, which he truly should be, not only can he make use of methods which are not routine, but he may also suggest sources for specimens which the clinician has not considered.

Another bonus from the close cooperation of the laboratory and physician is improved interpretation of the results of the laboratory examination. Ultimately, it is the clinician who must decide, but the counsel of a versatile microbiologist or clinical pathologist can often prevent misinterpretation of the results of serologic testing or culture. The isolation of fungi which are usually saprophytic or common laboratory contaminants may prompt additional studies if it is known that the patient has been on antibiotics for some days and an opportunistic fungous infection is being considered.

Aside from serologic methods, the laboratory search for fungi should begin with direct examination unless the amount of material available is so small that blind culture is necessary. Sputum or other exudate is placed in a sterile Petri dish on a black background. Granular material should be handled in a manner different from that applied to grayish or purulent flecks. A single granule may be placed on a slide in sterile saline or water and then crushed beneath the cover glass. If the granule is filamentous, suggesting Actinomyces or Nocardia, the crushed material may be allowed to dry on the slide and stained by the Gram method.

Small flecks of grayish or purulent material are mixed with a small drop of 10 per cent hydroxide on a glass slide and covered for microscopic examination. If yeastlike forms are present, one may be able to make a diagnosis of North or South American blastomycosis, coccidioidomycosis or, rarely, cryptococcosis. Even if morphologically typical forms are not present, a finding of yeast forms is most helpful in guiding the selection of culture media and future efforts. Rarely, intracellular *Histoplasma capsulatum* may be observed in hydroxide-cleared mounts, but their morphologic characteristics are never sufficient for diagnosis. Asteroid clusters or small clumps of narrow hyphae suggest the presence of Nocardia or Actinomyces. The pseudohyphae with attached blastospores of Candida are easily recognized, but blastospores alone may be confusing. Septate hyphae can usually be distinguished from nonseptate ones, but this distinction has no clinical significance.

If the amount of exudate permits, Gram's stain should always be used on a thin smear of a selected fleck. This stain is most useful for the detection of narrow filaments suggestive of Actinomyces or Nocardia. The stain demonstrates the pseudohyphae and blastospores of Candida very well, but is not very useful for the yeastlike fungi.

A Wright's stain of thinly smeared exudate is useful in giving one a good idea of the cellular population present and of the probable source of the exudate (upper or lower respiratory tract). Hyphae and candidal blastospores are usually well delineated. Histoplasma stains well, but cannot be differentiated with certainty from Cryptococcus and other yeastlike fungi. The blastomycetes, Cryptococcus and Coccidioides may appear only as unstained negative images in many preparations. A suspicious smear stained by Wright's method can always be restained by either the periodic acid-Schiff or Gomori methenamine silver nitrate method.

If the study of a hydroxide-cleared preparation suggests the presence of yeast-like fungi, the application of special fungous stains may be indicated. The methenamine-silver method will impregnate a wider variety of fungi than will the periodic acid-Schiff stain. Morphologic detail is better demonstrated by the periodic acid-Schiff method.

The Ziehl-Neelsen stain is useful primarily for the demonstration of *Nocardia asteroides*, *N. brasiliensis* and mycobacteria. For this purpose, destaining with acid alcohol should be shortened to five seconds or be replaced by a 1 per cent aqueous acid solution. Yeastlike fungi will often be demonstrated by the Ziehl-Neelsen stain.

Cultural isolation of pathogenic fungi may be prevented by the earlier growth of bacteria. This problem usually can be controlled by the addition of antibiotics to media at approximately neutral pH. Commercially available media (Mycosel agar, Baltimore Biological Co.; Brain-Heart cc agar, Difco Laboratories) contain chloramphenicol (0.05 mg. per milliliter) and cycloheximide (0.4 mg. per milliliter) to inhibit both bacteria and many nonpathogenic fungi. This type of medium is stable and useful for bacteria-containing specimens. Penicillin (20 units per milliliter) and streptomycin (40 micrograms per milliliter) may be added to solid media during the cooling period immediately prior to tubing, but storage life and bacterial inhibition are relatively brief. Some gram-negative bacilli (e.g. Proteus species) which are not inhibited by chloramphenicol or streptomycin can be controlled by adding polymyxin B (not to exceed 8 micrograms per milliliter), but this is not done routinely because polymyxin frequently inhibits the growth of pathogenic fungi.

Unfortunately, antibacterial substances which are added to media for the isolation of fungi may exert significant fungal inhibition. Streptomycin and chloramphenicol inhibit some strains of *Nocardia asteroides*, and cycloheximide may prevent the growth of Cryptococcus. Actinomyces is completely inhibited by both penicillin and chloramphenicol. Chloramphenicol and cycloheximide have a variable degree of inhibition of Blastomyces and Histoplasma when cultured at 37°C.

The direct examination of unstained or stained preparations may guide the selection of media. Otherwise one must use several containing antibiotics and at least two tubes of plain Sabouraud's glucose agar. It is suggested that at least three different media be inoculated, using two or more slants or plates of each if the volume of the specimen is sufficient. Anaerobic culture for Actinomyces is done in the writer's laboratory only on purulent material from closed infections, biopsies, and those specimens of sputum or sinus tract drainage which appear suspicious during direct examination of wet and stained preparations.

Except when Actinomyces is suspected, all the primary cultures in our laboratory are incubated at room temperature (25 to 27°C.), and most are planted on tube slants. If direct examination has suggested the possibility of a species of Nocardia, both plate and tube cultures are made. Plates are sealed to prevent drying. Only screw-cap tubes 25 by 150 mm. are suitable for routine use in a general laboratory. The media recommended for primary isolation after direct examination are listed in Table 1.

Conversion of the mycelial to the yeast form is a general requirement before making a *final* report of the isolation of the Blastomyces or Histoplasma, and this may apply to Sporotrichum and Coccidioides (if endosporulating spherules have not been seen in the original exudate.) The only practical way of converting *Coccidioides immitis* is by animal inoculation, and sometimes it is the only successful method of obtaining typical yeast forms of Histoplasma or *B. dermatitidis*. Hamsters are

Table 1.   *Media for Primary Isolation of Fungi Producing Pulmonary Disease*

Genus	Medium	Tube Slants (S) or Plates (P)	Temperature (°C)
Actinomyces	BHI	P	37
	BHI + 10% Rabbit blood	P	Anaerobic
	Thio broth	(Tubes)	37
Nocardia	Sab	S	
	Sab P & S	S	
	BHI	P	27
	BHI P & S	P	
Blastomyces, Histoplasma, Coccidioides }	Sab	S	
	BHI P & S	S	
	BHI C & C	S & P	27
	BHI 5% RB C & C	P	
Cryptococcus	BHI P & S	S	
	BHI	S	27
	Sab P & S	S	
Candida, Aspergillus, Sporotrichum, Mucor, Rhizopus }	Sab	S	
	Sab P & S	S	27
	BHI P & S	S	

Key to abbreviations: BHI = Brain-heart infusion agar. P & S = penicillin and streptomycin. C & C = chloramphenicol and cycloheximide.   RB = rabbit blood. Sab = Sabouraud's dextrose agar. Thio broth = Brewer's thioglycollate broth.

the most uniformly susceptible laboratory animal, but some strains of mice are suitable.

Cultural conversion of Histoplasma, Blastomyces and Sporotrichum is achieved by incubation at 37°C. Brain-heart infusion agar with added rabbit blood (10 per cent), brain-heart infusion agar, and Francis's cysteine glucose blood agar are most suitable. Incubation on plates is sometimes successful when tube-slants fail, but moisture should be conserved by sealing the plates. Cultures contaminated by bacteria may fail to convert to the yeast form despite the best cultural conditions. Repeated subculture on an antibiotic-containing medium may "purify" these cultures and permit conversion, but animal inoculation is often faster and simpler.

A microbiological safety hood of the type approved by the Communicable Disease Center is essential equipment for any laboratory processing cultures for fungi. Inoculating from clinical materials is not hazardous, but all cultures should be opened for inspection, subculture, or the making of slide mounts under the hood. Preparation of suspensions of mycelial growth for animal inoculation requires the same precautions.

Slide mounts for microscopic study are made by transferring a small amount of growth to a drop of normal saline on one slide and a drop of lactophenol cotton blue on a second. The selected growth is gently removed from the surface of the medium with one or two teasing needles. Bacteriological loops or nichrome wires are not useful for mycelial sampling.

All cultures should be examined weekly. Unfortunately, cultural identification is rarely possible from young colonies, and slowly growing pathogenic fungi may be overgrown by saprophytes. Therefore, if several different colonies appear, and particularly if one is growing more rapidly than another, subculture of the immature colonies should be made.

Occasionally, direct examination or serologic study will indicate the probability of a fungous infection, but cultural studies will be negative. Repeated culture is certainly indicated, but animal inoculation should be done if possible. Male hamsters are the most useful laboratory animal, both because of their general susceptibility to fungous infection and the ease with which intratesticular and intraperitoneal inoculations can be done. Both routes should be used in the same animal.

REFERENCES

Ajello, L., Georg, L. K., Kaplan, W., and Kaufman, L.: *Laboratory Manual for Medical Mycology*. Public Health Service Pub. No. 994, Washington, D.C., United States Government Printing Office, 1963.

Mowry, R. W.: The Special Value of Methods That Color Both Acidic and Vicinal Hydroxyl Groups in the Histochemical Study of Mucins. With revised directions for the colloidal iron stain, the use of alcian blue 8 GX, and their combinations with the periodic acid-Schiff reaction. *Ann. New York Acad. Sc.*, 106:402, 1963.

Seeliger, H. P. R.: Serology of Fungi and Deep Fungous Infections; in G. Dalldorf (ed.): *Fungi and Fungous Diseases*. Springfield, Ill., Charles C Thomas, 1962, pp. 158-86.

ACTINOMYCOSIS

The Organism

The actinomycetales are relatively primitive organisms whose classification as fungi can be doubted without apology. The obvious morphologic resemblance to the corynebacteria and mycobacteria is reinforced by the similarity of their cell walls in monosaccharide and amino acid patterns and serologic cross-reactivity.

The *Actinomyces* species are all grampositive organisms, 0.5 to 1.0 micron in width, which exhibit some degree of hyphal formation and branching in young

microcolonies. All species grow anaerobically, but some will grow also under microaerophilic and aerobic conditions. Considerable variation in oxygen tolerance can be found among strains of the same species. All species recognized as possibly pathogenic are catalase-negative and produce hydrogen sulfide. Although electron microscopy, serologic and chromatographic analysis of cell wall components, general biochemical reactions, and the usual microscopic and colonial morphologic criteria have been used to establish species differentiation, much more correlative study is necessary to establish the validity of species differentiation because of the rather wide variation between strains of the same species.

Actinomyces bovis, the classic etiologic agent of lumpy jaw of cattle, has taxonomic precedence if species differentiation from *A. israelii* is not valid. Morphologically, microcolonies fragment earlier into diphtheroid forms and show less hyphal development than *A. israelii*. Mature colonies tend to be smooth and soft on agar media and to produce turbidity when thioglycollate cultures are shaken. Except for the absence of catalase, the resemblance to anaerobic or microaerophilic diphtheroids is striking. Rough colonial variants of the same isolate may, according to Georg et al., show morphologic characteristics on solid media and in thioglycollate broth which are typical of *A. israelii*. In addition, their rough variant fails to hydrolyze starch ("characteristic" of *A. bovis*), and both variants fail to reduce nitrate to nitrite (suggestive of *A. bovis*).

A. israelii, supposedly a distinct species, produces actinomycosis in man and at least occasionally in cattle. Its oxygen tolerance overlaps that of *A. bovis*. Classically, young microcolonies show a more definite hyphal configuration with branching, and mature colonies are marginally lobulated ("molar tooth") with peripheral hyphal extension similar to that seen in granules in tissue. Most strains do not hydrolyze starch, whereas most strains of *A. bovis* do. Most strains of *A. israelii* reduce nitrate to nitrite. Production of acid from xylose is variable.

A. propionicus is probably a valid species pathogenic for man. This species is represented by a single reported isolate from human lacrimal canaliculitis. It grows best under anaerobic conditions, but will grow aerobically. It is catalase-negative, reduces nitrate, and produces mycelial microcolonies with branching hyphae. Unlike other known Actinomyces, under anaerobic conditions *A. propionicus* ferments glucose with the formation of carbon dioxide, and acetic and propionic acids. The reported isolate produces dull orange coloration in old colonies.

A. naeslundii grows well aerobically or anaerobically, is catalase-negative, and reduces nitrate to nitrite. Biochemically, it is closer to *A. israelii* than to *A. bovis*. Although it can be isolated frequently from human sources, it has not been proved to be a definite human pathogen.

Georg et al. have characterized an additional species which is probably a human pathogen. Named *A. eriksonii* (X407 and X573), this actinomycete has been found in a lung abscess and in pleural fluid from at least two different patients. Antigenically, it appears to be distinct from, but in many features it resembles, *A. israelii*.

The Clinical Disease

The early pulmonary manifestations of actinomycosis are those of bronchopneumonia or acute lung abscess. In the peribronchial pneumonic type, fever may be minor and remain so until treatment or dissemination. Cough with purulent or sanguinopurulent sputum is rare in children. Aside from weight loss, night sweats and poor tolerance for exercise, there may be little to make one suspect pulmonary disease until it is revealed by auscultation, roentgenography or obvious chest wall involvement. It is felt that lung abscess is usually aspirational and associated with early reactive bronchial occlusion. Fever, leukocytosis and evidence of acute illness are striking. Sputum is usually not produced until the bronchus has opened and a fluid level can be seen within the abscess.

Since it has become customary to prescribe antibiotics for acute pulmonary disease, neither of the two forms above is likely to be recognized unless one is pursuing a special microbiologic study. Instead, one is confronted with either an "unresolved pneumonia" with its possibility of tuberculosis or other granulomatous disease, or a "chronic lung abscess" which may require surgery unless treated properly.

Lung abscesses may be peripheral, and follow the distribution of aspirational abscesses. Pleural involvement is frequent, but may be localized if even suppressive therapy is started early. Empyema is rarely seen now unless the process has been completely neglected.

In recent years the pulmonary actinomycosis seen by the author has consisted almost entirely of unrecognized or neglected undiagnosed pneumonias which have progressed to involvement of the pleurae and chest wall. Chest wall abscesses and sinus tracts have been present, and, as in the patient shown in Figure 1, it has often been unclear whether the initial infection was pulmonary or abdominal. Transdiaphragmatic spread in either direction is different in actinomycosis than in amebiasis. The extension by contiguity in actinomycosis is accompanied by extensive fibrosis; sudden evacuation of purulent material through the bronchi and collections of free pus are not part of the usual clinical course. Neglected pulmonary actinomycosis usually extends to the chest wall, and may result in considerable deformity with or without osteomyelitis of the ribs or vertebrae. Sinus tracts are multiple as a rule, often discharging a rather watery fluid in which the sulfur granules may be found. The degree of fever and rapidity of weight loss are extremely variable, but both usually increase during chest wall involvement. Cerebral metastasis may complicate untreated pulmonary actinomycosis.

From the point of view of help in diagnosis, the description of the roentgenographic spectrum of pulmonary actinomycosis is an utter waste of time. Primary involvement of the lower lobes is more frequent than that of the upper. Pleural involvement is common, particularly in association with loculated empyema. If untreated, actinomycosis tends to produce confluent dense consolidations which suggest a suppurative pneumonitis unless obscured by organizing empyema. Acute hematogenous microabscesses are rare. In the writer's own experience, simultaneous bilateral involvement is rare.

Laboratory Diagnosis

The problem of early diagnosis of actinomycosis in infants and children is particularly difficult. Sputum is rarely available, and the fact that actinomycetes are found in oral secretions of many persons without actinomycosis makes gastric as-

pirates of doubtful value. The x-ray and clinical pictures often suggest the possibility of a foreign body. If bronchoscopy is done, bronchial washings should be obtained for direct study. The saline washings should be placed in a sterile Petri dish and examined with a hand lens against a black background. White or yellow granular material should be examined in the saline material under the microscope. If granules appear to be composed of hyphal elements or coccoidal bodies, the granules may be crushed gently between the cover slip and the slide, and the preparation allowed to dry. The preparation should be placed in alcoholic formalin for at least twenty minutes before attempting to remove the cover slip. The slide and slip are stained by the usual Gram method for study under the oil-immersion objective. Granules of actinomyces usually show definite hyphal elements with branching (Fig. 2) which are rarely as well formed as in tis-

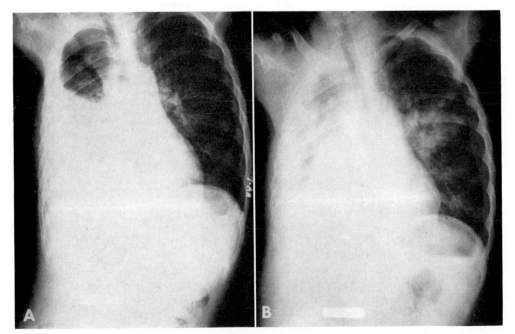

FIGURE 47–1. A ten-year-old child with left hemiparesis and periodic convulsive seizures beginning in the first year of life. *A,* Film taken in the clinic for complaints of epigastric discomfort and constipation. She returned, complaining of an abscess of the lower right hemithorax and fever. *B,* Another film revealed a right bronchopleurocutaneous fistula and pneumonia in the left lung. Empyema fluid was culturally positive for *A. israelii.*

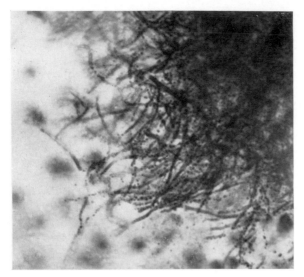

FIGURE 47–2. Gram-stained granule of *A. israelii* in sputum. The oil-immersion objective was used to magnify one margin of the granule to show the fine beading and "coccoidal bodies" which are observed frequently. True hyphal branching can be seen.

sue sections. Inflammatory cells may be present at the periphery of the granule; these and the sheathing or "clubbing" of the hyphae which is so frequent in pus and in tissue section are not frequent in diluted bronchial washings. Small granules may fragment almost completely into clumps and clusters of what appear to be diphtheroids. In addition, Actinomyces may be present in bronchial washings as clusters of diphtheroid-like organisms without granule formation.

Any unresolved pneumonia or lung abscess which has x-ray evidence of definite pleuritis over the area of involvement may be safely needled for aspiration. A portion of the aspirate should be stained by Gram's method prior to utilizing the remainder for culture. Gram-positive filaments in such an aspirate always indicate the necessity of culturing for Actinomyces and Nocardia.

Pus obtained from the lung or from pleural fluid, pleural biopsy, or other surgical materials should be examined directly prior to culture. The exact procedure of culturing is discussed in the section under general laboratory methods. If so-called sulfur granules are present, they should be washed in sterile physiologic saline several times before introducing them into culture media.

Direct examination is particularly im-

portant in actinomycosis because of the necessity of correlating clinical findings with laboratory results. At present few laboratories outside of specialized medical centers appear to be qualified to make the specific identification of an actinomycete. Unless the presence of catalase is determined, it is easy to confuse cultures of anaerobic diphtheroids with Actinomyces. Such misinterpretation has occurred repeatedly. The demonstration of sulfur granules in tissue or exudates is not a *sine qua non* for diagnosis, but it certainly is important in doubtful circumstances.

At present, serologic methods of diagnosis are used only on an experimental basis. Seeliger has found that agglutinins may occur in significant titer in persons without actinomycosis, whereas complement-fixing antibodies are much more specific when present. Since antibodies can be produced in experimental animals, and the method is used for the study of familial and generic relations, it seems reasonable to hope that the Communicable Disease Center will offer assistance in the serodiagnosis of actinomycosis upon consultation.

Epidemiology

A truly free-living form of the anaerobic actinomycetes has never been found.

Their existence in the alimentary tract of man and some other warm-blooded animals is believed to be essentially saprophytic. Noninvasive actinomycetes can be recovered from tonsillar crypts, carious teeth and the adjacent gums. In the absence of a free-living form it is presumed that transmission is from person to person directly or through fomites.

Actinomycosis is worldwide in distribution, and is said to occur more frequently in males than in females. It is an uncommon mycosis in childhood. Better oral hygiene and dental care together with the frequent use of antimicrobials in association with exodontia, tonsillectomy and early undiagnosed bronchopulmonary infections probably account for the lessened incidence in recent years.

Pathogenesis and Pathology

It is known that many people with abnormal oral hygiene, chronic bronchial disease or chronic bronchopulmonary disease have Actinomyces in their mouths or sputum without evidence of actinomycosis. Careful study of early cases of cervicofacial actinomycosis bears out the close association of this form of the disease with significant parodontal disease, extraction or trauma. In this sense, the disease is opportunistic, and by inference a similar pathogenesis has been proposed for primary pulmonary actinomycosis.

It is also known that actinomycosis is seldom, if ever, due to infection with Actinomyces alone. Associated bacteria or the interrelations between the Actinomyces and bacteria are thought to be of primary importance in the initiation of actinomycosis. Primary pulmonary infection presumably takes place after aspiration of an infectious nidus.

Despite the fact that the bacterial flora in pulmonary actinomycosis usually contains anaerobic streptococci which are resistant to penicillin, and often contains gram-negative organisms which are similarly resistant, almost all patients respond as though the disease were due to a penicillin-sensitive organism. The same phe-

nomenon is observed in many aspirational lung abscesses with mixed gram-negative and gram-positive flora.

Actinomycosis is characterized by a mixture of chronic and acute granulation tissue and marginal fibrosis. The Actinomyces usually occur in granules surrounded by an area of suppuration. Small and large abscesses which frequently communicate with one another are common in association with chronic granulation tissue and fibrosis. The reaction around the granules is predominantly polymorphonuclear. At the margin of the granule the individual hyphal tips may be sheathed ("clubbed") by a host material which stains with acidophilic dyes. Multinucleate giant cells are not frequent, but may be present in the chronic granulation tissue adjacent to the area of suppuration.

Actinomycosis tends to spread by contiguity with multiple sinus tracts connecting areas of suppuration and extending through the pleurae into the chest wall or to the surface of the skin.

The individual actinomycotic granule varies greatly in size, but is usually seen easily in routine histologic preparations. The hyphal elements are colored by basophilic stains such as hematoxylin, but are best demonstrated by the Gram method. There are times when the marginal filaments can be demonstrated by either the Gomori methenamine silver method or a periodic acid-Schiff stain with light green counter stain. Although regarded as an inferior procedure for Actinomyces and Nocardia, the latter stain can give excellent structural detail as shown in Figure 3.

A presumptive diagnosis of pulmonary actinomycosis can usually be made from resected tissue even without cultural confirmation. If a pulmonary granule contains definite hyphal filaments of approximately 1 micron in width, one can be sure that either Actinomyces or Nocardia is present. *Nocardia asteroides* is much more commonly present in scattered filaments and loose clumps than in granules. It may, however, produce granules which are indistinguishable from Actino-

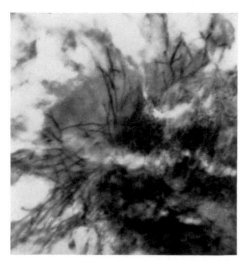

FIGURE 47–3. Actinomycotic granule in lung. The hyphae with their branchings are stained clearly by the periodic acid-Schiff method. The amorphous material surrounding the margin (sheathing) is derived from the host tissue and took the light green counterstain.

myces when stained by Gram's method. Filaments and granules of *Nocardia asteroides* are weakly acid-fast, and this characteristic can be used for differentiating them from Actinomyces.

Treatment and Prevention

Despite the recognized importance of concomitant and mixed bacterial infection in the causation of actinomycosis, combination or broad-spectrum antimicrobial therapy is rarely necessary. The pathogenic Actinomyces are very sensitive to penicillin, erythromycin, chloramphenicol, the tetracyclines and probably most antibacterial antibiotics other than streptomycin. Regardless of the bacterial "associates" which may be found, healing almost always occurs if penicillin is given alone for several months in a daily dosage between 2 and 6 million units. Although it has been shown that the concentration of penicillin needed to suppress the growth of colonies of *A. bovis* exceeds that required to suppress loose filaments, failure of response to penicillin therapy is much more likely to be due to an unrecognized basic pathologic state (e.g.

tuberculosis or penicillin-resistant staphylococcal pneumonia) than to either invasiveness of the usual bacterial "associates" of *A. bovis* or its inherent resistance to penicillin.

Penicillin in dosage sufficient to produce a plasma level between 1 and 2 Oxford units per milliliter should be effective in the treatment of pulmonary actinomycosis if given long enough. The acutely ill patient will respond more rapidly to large intravenous doses. Patients with indolent but extensive involvement may require months of treatment, which can best be given by supplementing oral medication with intermittent intramuscular injections of long-acting penicillins. All our patients are treated with parenteral administration of penicillin, unless contraindicated, until they become asymptomatic and roentgenographic regression is definite. Oral penicillin therapy in equivalent or large dosage is then substituted and continued so long as improvement continues and recovery is evident.

Patients allergic to penicillin may be given erythromycin, tetracycline or chloramphenicol in the usual dosage prescribed for moderate infections. The end-result is probably the same as that achieved with penicillin, but complications of therapy are more common with the broad-spectrum antibiotics.

Unless a free empyema is present, no sort of surgical drainage or exploration is indicated in the immediate treatment of pulmonary actinomycosis. The development of antimicrobial resistance during prolonged treatment for extensive disease has not been a problem. The amount of x-ray and functional improvement which can take place, even in the presence of extensive pleural involvement, is often amazing. Pleural decortication, resection of a destroyed portion of lung, or drainage of a subdiaphragmatic abscess may ultimately be necessary, but one may safely postpone such a decision until after four or more months of continuous and adequate antimicrobial therapy.

There is no indication for preventive measures aimed particularly at actinomycosis. Good oral and dental hygiene is an end in itself. When infected teeth and tonsils must be removed, a few days of postoperative antibiotic therapy is certainly justifiable, and is probably adequate to prevent the development of actinomycosis.

REFERENCES

Buchanan, B. B., and Pine, L.: Characterization of a Propionic Acid Producing Actinomycete, *Actinomyces Propionicus*, Sp. Nov. *J. Gen. Microbiol.*, 28:305, 1962.

Cope, V. Z.: *Actinomycosis*. London, Oxford University Press, 1938.

Georg, L. K., Robertstad, G. W., and Brinkman, S. A.: Identification of Species of *Actinomyces*. *J. Bact.*, 88:477, 1964.

Holm, P.: Studies on the Aetiology of Human Actinomycosis. I. The "Other Microbes" of Actinomycosis and Their Importance. *Acta Path. Microbiol. Scand.*, 27:736, 1950.

Idem. Studies on the Aetiology of Human Actinomycosis. II. Do the "Other Microbes" of Actinomycosis Possess Virulence. *Acta Path. Microbiol. Scand.*, 28:391, 1951.

Kwapinski, J. B.: Antigenic Structure of the Actinomycetales. VII. Chemical and Serological Similarities of Cell Walls from 100 Actinomycetales Strains. *J. Bact.*, 88:1211, 1964.

Nichols, D. R., and Herrell, W. E.: Penicillin in the Treatment of Actinomycosis. *J. Lab. & Clin. Med.*, 33:521, 1948.

Overman, J. R., and Pine, L.: Electron Microscopy of Cytoplasmic Structures in Facultative and Anaerobic *Actinomyces*. *J. Bact.*, 86:656, 1963.

Peabody, J. W., Jr., and Seabury, J. H.: Actinomycosis and Nocardiosis. *J. Chron. Dis.*, 5:374, 1957.

Idem: Actinomycosis and Nocardiosis: A Review of Basic Differences in Therapy. *Am. J. Med.*, 28:99, 1960.

Rosebury, T., Epps, L. J., and Clark, A. R.: Study of the Isolation, Cultivation, and Pathogenicity of *Actinomyces Israelii* Recovered from the Human Mouth and from Actinomycosis in Man. *J. Infect. Dis.*, 74:131, 1944.

Seabury, J. H., and Dascomb, H. E.: Results of the Treatment of Systemic Mycoses. *J.A.M.A.*, 188:509, 1964.

Spilsbury, B. W., Johnstone, F. R. C.: The Clinical Course of Actinomycotic Infections; A Report of 14 Cases. *Canad. J. Surg.*, 5:33, 1962.

Warthin, T. A., and Bushuefe, B.: Pulmonary Actinomycosis. *Arch. Int. Med.*, 101:239, 1958.

Weed, L. A., and Baggenstoss, A. H.: Actinomycosis: Pathologic and Bacteriologic Study of Twenty-One Fatal Cases. *Am. J. Clin. Path.*, 19:201, 1949.

Wright, J. H.: The Biology of the Microorganisms of Actinomycosis. *J. Med. Res.*, 13:349, 1905.

NOCARDIOSIS

The Organism

The genus Nocardia differs from the genus Actinomyces in being aerobic. Members of both are gram-positive and exhibit similar branching of hyphae whose diameter is usually no more than 1 micron. Despite morphologic similarity, it is probable that the genus Nocardia belongs among the fungi and Actinomyces among the bacteria.

Nocardia asteroides has been the causative agent of reported cases of pulmonary nocardiosis in man, but a thoracopulmonary mycetoma due to *Nocardia brasiliensis* has been reported. Both organisms are similar in morphology and may appear identical in colonial characteristics. Of the strains which have been seen, in this laboratory, both species are partially acid-fast and pathogenic for the chick embryo. *N. asteroides*, however, grows poorly or not at all in 0.4 per cent gelatin and does not hydrolyze casein, whereas *N. brasiliensis* grows well in gelatin, forming compact colonies, and hydrolyzes casein.

The hyphal characteristics and branching of Nocardia are best studied in slide cultures, since aerial hyphal production may be slight. Colonies may be white, gray, or various shades of buff through orange.

In pus, sputum or tissues, *N. asteroides* is usually found in small clusters or in open hyphal strands showing various degrees of fragmentation into bacillary or coccobacillary forms. Occasionally one may find asteroid colonies appearing in sputum or pus such as is shown in Figure 4. Grossly, these may resemble tiny gra-

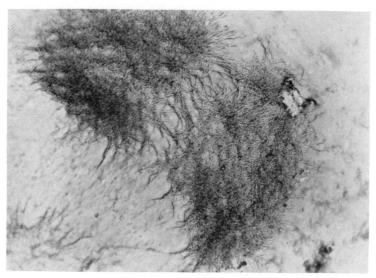

FIGURE 47–4. *Nocardia asteroides* in sputum. These 2 asteroid colonies were seen in a hydroxide-cleared mount of fresh sputum. The mount was fixed in alcoholic formalin before removing the cover slip and staining by a modified Ziehl-Neelsen method. The hyphae were moderately acid-fast.

nules of *A. israelii,* but they are not sheathed, nor is there the same central mycelial mat that one finds in a true actinomycotic granule. The property of acid-fastness of *N. asteroides* is variable, but may be a useful identifying characteristic in fresh exudates and well-fixed tissues. Although 0.5 per cent aqueous sulfuric acid is usually recommended for de-staining smears of sputum and pus after the application of steaming carbol-fuchsin, a three- to five-second de-stain with 3 per cent hydrochloric acid in 95 per cent alcohol appears to be satisfactory, facilitating the use of the standard Ziehl-Neelsen reagents. Acid-fast bacillary forms closely resembling *M. tuberculosis* may be found in abundance, but they are practically always associated with some hyphal elements.

The Clinical Disease

In the adult patient, nocardiosis may present as a subacute or chronic pulmonary illness which closely mimics the course of tuberculosis, or it may present as an acute suppurative pneumonitis which can be rapidly progressive. The number of cases reported in children is too few to establish any special features which would differentiate the childhood disease from that seen in adults.

The x-ray picture may resemble either tuberculosis or suppurative pneumonia (Fig. 5). Occasionally bilateral, patchy pulmonary infiltration may have the appearance of a hematogenous pneumonia. Pleurisy with subsequent empyema occurs in about one fourth of the cases, and chest wall involvement with sinus tract formation may mimic actinomycosis.

Hematogenous dissemination is much more frequent than in actinomycosis. Metastasis is particularly likely to involve the central nervous system, the kidney, and the subcutaneous tissues and bodies of the muscles of the extremities.

There are no particularly helpful symptomatic features of nocardiosis. In general, the symptomatology can be said to simulate either tuberculosis or lung abscess. When sputum is being produced, it is mucopurulent and may be blood-flecked. Leukocytosis with an increase in the polymorphonuclear neutrophils is common.

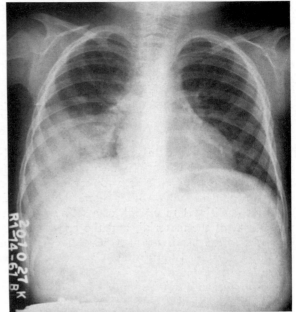

FIGURE 47–5. Pulmonary nocardiosis. This 46-month-old boy failed to improve symptomatically or radiographically during treatment with antibiotics. At thoracotomy the right lower lobe suppurative pneumonitis contained an abscess from which *Nocardia asteroides* was recovered. (Courtesy of C. Harrison Snyder, M.D., Ochsner Clinic.)

Laboratory Diagnosis

When *N. asteroides* occurs in clusters such as shown in Figure 4, it is difficult to overlook the fungus in potassium hydroxide wet mounts of either sputum or pus. Unfortunately, Nocardia may appear in more dispersed filaments which are not recognized in wet mounts of sputum and are overlooked or misinterpreted in wet mounts of pus.

The thin hyphae and bacillary fragments are well seen in thin films of exudates stained by Gram's method, but may be easily overlooked if they are not numerous. If sputum or other exudate contains filaments suggestive of Nocardia, a modified Ziehl-Neelson stain as already discussed should be done before material is planted on culture media.

The genus Nocardia is not fastidious in its growth requirements. Initial isolation may be made on any of the common solid laboratory media. *N. asteroides,* which is the usual cause of pulmonary nocardiosis, grows readily at room temperature or 37°C. The section on general laboratory methods is applicable to the isolation of species of Nocardia with certain qualifications.

The sensitivity in vitro of *N. asteroides* to antibiotics is variable from strain to strain. None of the human isolates of *N. asteroides* studied by the writer has been significantly sensitive to penicillin in vitro, although strains sensitive to penicillin have been reported. Solid media without antibiotics should always be inoculated with materials suspected of containing Nocardia, but unless no other organisms are seen on Gram's staining of the material, the usual antibiotic-containing media recommended in the section on general laboratory methods should also be heavily inoculated. Colonial growth of *N. asteroides* and *N. brasiliensis* usually appears on blood agar or Sabouraud's dextrose agar between seven and ten days after inoculation, but growth may be delayed as long as three weeks. When Sabouraud's dextrose agar containing penicillin and streptomycin is the medium, colony growth is usually slow. The use of a chloramphenicol-cycloheximide-containing medium is a sometimes successful means of purifying bacterially contaminated initial isolates.

Most human isolates of *N. asteroides* are pathogenic to the guinea pig when this animal is inoculated intraperitone-ally with a heavy suspension of the cul-ture, but this property is of doubtful value in species identification.

The yolk sac of the chick embryo is more useful for the study of cultural iso-lates or bacteria-free pus and biopsy materials. Growth in the yolk sac is rapid, the acid-fast property of the hyphae is well developed and the strains of *N. as-teroides* are lethal for the embryo within seven days. *N. brasiliensis* is also lethal for the chick embryo. The yolk sac of seven- to nine-day-old embryos should be inoculated with 0.1 to 0.5 ml. of a saline suspension of the material, and the eggs returned to the incubator at 37°C. They should be candled daily for viability. Upon death, or at the end of a week, smears of the yolk can be stained by the Gram and modified Ziehl-Neelsen meth-ods.

At present there are no serologic meth-ods which have been applied successfully to the diagnosis of nocardiosis in man. The Nocardia appear to be poor stimu-lators of circulating antibody, even under experimental conditions. Serologic study has been of some value in the clarification of taxonomic relations of the Nocardia, but there is, as yet, no direct clinical ap-plication.

Epidemiology

Nocardia asteroides is a normal in-habitant of soil, where it can survive a wide range of temperature. Its distribu-tion is probably worldwide. Nocardiosis is more frequent in males than in females.

The respiratory tract as the ordinary portal of entry is less certain for nocardi-osis than for histoplasmosis, coccidioido-mycosis, cryptococcosis and blastomycosis. Nevertheless, with special effort, *N. as-teroides* can be isolated from the sputum or bronchial washings of a few hospital-ized patients who have no evidence of nocardiosis. Furthermore, there appears to have been an increase in the incidence of opportunistic infections due to *N. as-*

teroides, and most of these have been pul-monary.

The possibility that nocardiosis is a common, self-limited infection has been considered, but no large scale epidemio-logic surveys are available to support this hypothesis.

Pathogenesis and Pathology

The pathogenesis of human nocardiosis is incompletely known. Critical evalua-tion of well documented cases during the last decade suggests that nocardiosis occurs as an opportunistic infection in about 50 per cent of the recognized cases. Whether opportunistic infection takes place from endogenous but inapparent sources or ex-ogenously during the period of increased susceptibility is not known.

The most common expression of pul-monary nocardiosis is that of a suppura-tive pneumonitis. Acute, hematogenous dissemination may appear grossly like miliary tuberculosis. Caseation is not seen, and the predominant cellular response is usually that of polymorphonuclear leukocytes and plasma cells. Multiple, yellow abscesses are frequent in rapidly fatal illness, whereas cavitation and pleu-ral involvement are common in chronic illness.

Filaments, coccobacillary forms and clusters of Nocardia can be demonstrated by the Brown and Brenn modification of the Gram stain in areas of suppuration. Small asteroid colonies may be seen, but there is no sheathing of the peripheral filaments, and no dense granule formation in the lung to suggest actinomycosis. When the filaments are sparse, whether fragmented or not, they are difficult to find and to identify microscopically ex-cept under high magnification. Filaments cannot be seen in ordinary hematoxylin and eosin preparations.

Some patients with chronic nocardiosis have areas of cavitation and of fibrosis and chronic granulomatous reaction not unlike a mixed tuberculous and pyogenic infection. Giant cells may be found in the

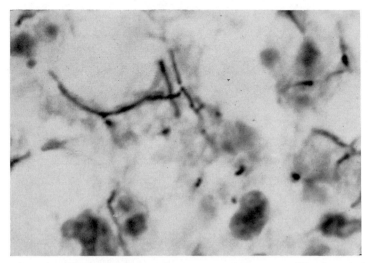

FIGURE 47–6. *N. asteroides* in the lung. The Brown and Brenn modification of the Gram stain shows the slender hyphae, branching, beading and bacillary fragmentation to good advantage. Oil-immersion magnification at the margin of a microabscess.

fibrotic areas of such chronic lesions, and few Nocardia may be found after extensive search with the best staining techniques.

The Gomori methenamine silver stain will demonstrate Nocardia well. Hyphae of Nocardia are stained by the periodic acid-Schiff method. Nevertheless the simpler Brown and Brenn modification of the Gram stain is the method of choice. A Brown and Brenn preparation is shown in Figure 6.

Treatment and Prevention

The fact that clinically recognized nocardiosis is attended by a high mortality rate reflects more upon delay in diagnosis than upon poor therapeutic weapons. The sulfonamides are the most useful drugs. The initial dosage should be calculated to give a blood level between 10 and 15 mg. per 100 ml. if sulfadiazine is used, and this level should be maintained until the disease is symptomatically controlled and shows radiographic improvement.

It is probable that early lesions, corresponding in extent to minimal or even moderately advanced pulmonary tuberculosis, and without evident metastasis, will respond satisfactorily to sulfonamides alone. As a general principle, it seems preferable to resort to two-drug therapy, combining a sulfonamide with either hydroxystilbamidine, streptomycin or cycloserine during the first month or two of treatment. There is experimental and limited clinical evidence to suggest that cycloserine is perhaps the agent of second choice. In children without a history of convulsive manifestations the combination of sulfadiazine and cycloserine may well be the best initial approach to therapy.

Duration of medical therapy in pulmonary nocardiosis can be determined only by judgment based on the clinical and laboratory findings. In general, chemotherapy should be continued for at least two months after all activity of the disease has subsided.

Surgical drainage of closed areas of infection, particularly metastases, should be accomplished soon after chemotherapy has been instituted. Pulmonary infections usually establish drainage transbronchially or through the chest wall, but soft tissue and extrathoracic visceral infections may resist treatment without surgery. If it appears likely that pulmonary resection will be necessary, it should be delayed until the full effects of chemotherapy can be evaluated.

Nocardiosis is not a public health problem, and any discussion of prevention would be meaningless except in relation to opportunistic infections. Children with serious metabolic disease, neoplasia or other disease requiring prolonged antimicrobial or corticosteroid therapy should be carefully monitored with awareness that adverse events may be due to fungal infection, of which nocardiosis is representative. The incidence of nocardiosis among such children is not sufficiently high to justify any specific prophylactic measures.

REFERENCES

Benbow, E. P., Jr., Smith, D. T., and Grimson, K. S.: Sulfonamide Therapy in Actinomycosis; Two Cases Caused by Aerobic Partially Acid-Fast Actinomyces. *Am. Rev. Tuberc.*, 49:395, 1944.

Carlile, W. K., Holley, K. W., and Logan, G. B.: Fatal Acute Disseminated Nocardiosis in a Child. *J.A.M.A.*, 184:477, 1963.

Emmons, C. W.: The Isolation from Soil of Fungi Which Cause Disease in Man. *Tr. New York Acad. Sc.*, 14:51, 1951.

Eppinger, H.: Ueber eine neue Pathogene Cladothrix und eine durch sie hervorgerufene Pseudotuberkulosis (cladothrichica). *Beitr. pathol. Anat. u. allgem. Pathol.*, 9:287, 1891.

Glover, R. P., Herrell, W. E., Heilman, F. R., and Pfeutze, K. H.: Nocardiosis: Nocardia Asteroides Infection Simulating Pulmonary Tuberculosis. *J.A.M.A.*, 136:172, 1948.

Hathaway, B. M., and Mason, K. M.: Nocardiosis; Study of Fourteen Cases. *Am. J. Med.*, 32:903, 1962.

Henrici, A. T., and Gardner, E. L.: The Acid-Fast Actinomycetes. *J. Infect. Dis.*, 28:232, 1921.

Kirby, W. M. M., and McNaught, J. B.: Actinomycosis Due to Nocardia Asteroides; Report of Two Cases, *Arch. Int. Med.*, 78:578, 1946.

Langevin, R. W., and Katz, S.: Fulminating Pulmonary Nocardiosis. *Dis. of Chest.*, 46:310, 1964.

Larsen, M. C., Diamond, H. D., and Collins, H. S.: Nocardia Asteroides Infection: A Report of Seven Cases. *Arch. Int. Med.*, 103:712, 1959.

Murray, J. F., Finegold, S. M., Froman, S., and Will, D. W.: The Changing Spectrum of Nocardiosis; A Review and Presentation of Nine Cases. *Am. Rev. Resp. Dis.*, 83:315, 1961.

Nocard, E.: Note sur la maladie des boeufs de la Guadeloupe connue sous le nom de farcin. *Ann. Inst. Pasteur,* 2:293, 1888.

Peabody, J. W., Jr., and Seabury, J. H.: Actinomycosis and Nocardiosis. *J. Chron. Dis.,* 5:374, 1957.

Idem: Actinomycosis and Nocardiosis: A Review of Basic Differences in Therapy. *Am. J. Med.,* 28:99, 1960.

Raich, R. A., Casey, F., and Hall, W. H.: Pulmonary and Cutaneous Nocardiosis; The Significance of the Laboratory Isolation of Nocardia. *Am. Rev. Resp. Dis.,* 83:505, 1961.

Rhoades, E. R., Riley, H. D., and Muchmore, H. G.: Cycloserine in the Treatment of Human Nocardiosis. *Antimicrob. Agents Chemother.,* 1961, pp. 352-8.

Rivera, J. V., and Perez, J. B.: Pulmonary Nocardiosis Treated with Chloramphenicol. *Arch. Int. Med.,* 100:152, 1957.

Runyon, E. H.: Nocardia Asteroides: Studies on Its Pathogenicity and Drug Sensitivities. *J. Lab. & Clin. Med.,* 37:713, 1951.

Schneidau, J. D., Jr., and Shaffer, M. F.: Studies on *Nocardia* and Other Actinomycetales. I. Cultural Studies. *Am. Rev. Tuberc. Pulm. Dis.,* 76:770, 1957.

Seabury, J. H., and Dascomb, H. E.: Results of the Treatment of Systemic Mycoses. *J.A.M.A.,* 188:509, 1964.

Stadler, H. E., Kraft, B., Weed, L. A., and Keith, H. M.: Chronic Pulmonary Disease Due to *Nocardia. Am. J. Dis. Child.,* 88:485, 1954.

Strauss, R. E., Kligman, A. M., and Pillsbury, D. M.: The Chemotherapy of Actinomycosis and Nocardiosis. *Am. Rev. Tuberc.,* 63:441, 1951.

Tucker, F. C., and Hirsch, E. F.: Nocardiosis, with a Report of Three Cases of Actinomycosis Due to Nocardia Asteroides. *J. Infect. Dis.,* 85:72, 1949.

Webster, B. H.: Pulmonary Nocardiosis: A Review with a Report of Seven Cases. *Am. Rev. Tuberc.,* 73:485, 1956.

Weed, L. A., Andersen, H. A., Good, C. A., and Baggenstoss, A. H.: Nocardiosis: Clinical, Bacteriologic and Pathological Aspects. *New England J. Med.,* 253:1137, 1955.

NORTH AMERICAN BLASTOMYCOSIS

The Organism

Blastomyces dermatitidis is a dimorphic fungus whose free-living form is mycelial. It has been isolated from soils and other organic debris. The parasitic form is yeastlike and thick-walled, and has been found in the tissues of man, dogs and horses.

The characteristics of the parasitic form are more constant in fresh pus or sputum than in wet preparations of cultures at 37°C. Hydroxide-cleared wet mounts of exudates may be supplemented by periodic acid-Schiff stained preparations of the same material in order to study the details of budding and cytology. The yeastlike cells are predominantly spherical to subspherical. Form is preserved as a rule during budding, but some degree of elongation may occur. Resting cells average about 10 to 12 microns in diameter, but may vary from less than 5 to more than 25 microns. The cell wall is thick enough to be distinct, and in phase-contrast or subdued bright-field illumination, the outer and inner limiting optical surfaces may be separated by a central optical membrane producing a "doubly contoured" effect. The cells are multinucleate, whereas those of Histoplasma and Cryptococcus are uninucleate.

Budding is usually single in exudates, but may be multiple, owing to the prolonged period of attachment of the daughter cell. Evagination of the cell wall of the parent is broad, and the protoplasmic bridge is wide. As a general rule, daughter and parent are of approximately equal diameter before separation. In periodic acid-Schiff stained preparations the broad "disjunctive" cell wall margining the protoplasmic bridge is distinct and strikingly unlike that which one may see in similarly stained preparations of cryptocci or Histoplasma (Fig. 7).

B. dermatitidis grows less well at 37°C. than at room temperature, but primary growth of the yeast form can usually be obtained from exudates that contain sufficient organisms to be seen during direct examination. Growth on brain-heart infusion agar or blood agar at 37°C. appears within two weeks after inoculation. The colonies are grayish at first, rapidly become heaped-up and granular, and when mature, vary from light cream to dark brown in color. Pigmentation is greater on blood agar than on brain-heart infusion agar.

Cultures at 37°C. show more variation in cellular morphology than does the study of exudates. Multiple budding, giving rise to clusters or "balls" of yeastlike forms, is much more common, and

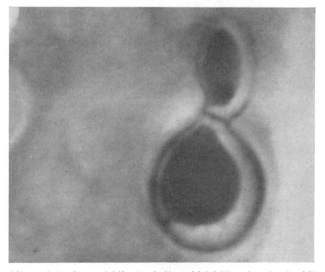

FIGURE 47–7. Budding of *B. dermatitidis.* Periodic acid-Schiff stain of a budding organism under oil-immersion magnification to show the broad attachment and definite cross wall between mother and daughter cells. The cell wall is relatively thick. Compare with Figure 9.

the formation of short germ tubes or abortive hyphae is frequent.

Growth at room temperature is mycelial and more dependable than at 37°C. In the absence of bacterial contamination, growth from clinical specimens may appear within the first week of incubation, but is often delayed until the second. Initial growth may be rapidly spreading as a smooth, membranous, whitish but translucent glaze not unlike the sugar glaze on doughnuts. This growth is generally succeeded by the appearance of bristly aerial hyphae which increase in number and length until the colony is cottony. White, cottony colonies often become tan with age and then resemble colonies of *Histoplasma capsulatum*. Some strains will not give visible growth until the fourth week of incubation, making it necessary to protect cultures against drying. Strains which grow poorly at room temperature may produce small colonies only with little or no typical sporulation. Such strains may not only fail to convert to the yeast phase when subcultured at 37°C., but also may not grow at this temperature. Recognition may be dependent upon heavily inoculating the

mycelial culture intraperitoneally into hamsters and mice. The animals should be sacrificed, cultured, and studied histopathologically three weeks after inoculation.

The mycelial form of *B. dermatitidis* resembles the same form of *H. capsulatum* in many respects. The hyphae of mature colonies are septate and bear a variable number of spherical to ovoid, thin-walled, smooth conidia which range in size from 3 to 6 microns. Some conidia are sessile, but most are borne on slender conidiophores or at the end of hyphae. With aging of the colony, thick-walled chlamydospores may be found on conidiophores or terminally on hyphae. These are similar in diameter (7 to 15 microns) to the chlamydospores of *Histoplasma capsulatum,* but are never tuberculate, whereas those of *H. capsulatum* are usually tuberculate.

The Clinical Disease

It is believed that the respiratory tract is the most common portal of entry for infection with *B. dermatitidis*. Nevertheless there is no recognized clinical picture

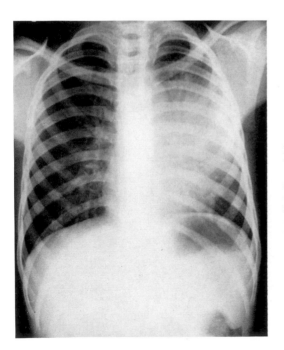

FIGURE 47–8. Pulmonary blastomycosis. A 9-year-old boy with an acute febrile illness and pleuritic chest pain. No sputum was being produced. Fungal skin tests and serology were negative. Needle aspiration of the lung yielded sanguinopurulent material containing numerous *B. dermatitidis.* Despite the suppurative nature of the upper lobe pneumonia, healing occurred without cavitation after treatment with hydroxystilbamidine.

of acute inhalational blastomycosis such as exists for histoplasmosis.

The clinical spectrum of pulmonary blastomycosis is as varied as that of tuberculosis. A segmental pneumonitis is seen sufficiently often to make one believe that this may be a common expression of early disease. This kind of lesion has been seen in children. It may regress spontaneously, apparently stabilize, or progress acutely or subacutely to produce a picture of an acute suppurative pneumonitis (Fig. 8). Circumscribed mass lesions may involve rib and be confused with neoplasm. Fever, chest pain, cough and weight loss have been common symptoms in the pediatric group. Sputum, when produced, is mucopurulent and occasionally blood-streaked. Leukocytosis of mild to moderate degree is the rule in acute disease. Despite the frequency of pleuritic pain, empyema is rare. Rib and subcutaneous chest abscesses may develop without empyema.

Although any sort of radiologic picture may be seen, enlargement of the bronchial or hilar lymph nodes is frequent in all but miliary dissemination. Involvement of anterior segments of the lung is more common than in tuberculosis. The only roentgenographic feature which is particularly helpful, and common to most pulmonary mycoses, is the persistence or slow change of the lesion during treatment with antibacterial antibiotics.

Metastasis to the skin, bones or viscera is frequent during the course of recognized North American blastomycosis. Secondary foci may be more obvious than the pulmonary disease. Nevertheless pulmonary blastomycosis may not only regress without treatment, but also may disappear roentgenographically without evidence of dissemination. It is reasonably certain that primary pulmonary blastomycosis may heal spontaneously, but reliable serologic methods to separate those requiring treatment from those needing observation are not available.

Laboratory Diagnosis

If sputum is being produced, pulmonary blastomycosis can be diagnosed presumptively in most patients by direct examination of sputum. No single laboratory examination is so neglected. Budding yeastlike forms are characteristic to the experienced observer, but many hospital laboratory technologists have a hazy remembrance at best of the diagnostic fea-

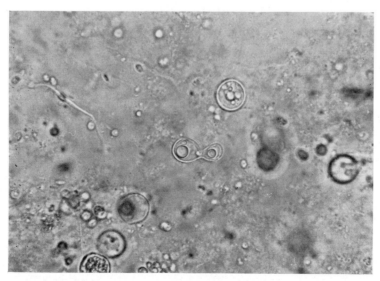

FIGURE 47–9. *B. dermatitidis* in sputum. This is a photograph of a wet preparation of sputum containing numerous blastomycetes. Typical broad-based budding and the "double contour" of the cell wall are illustrated.

tures. Figure 9 is representative of the appearance of B. dermatitidis by direct examination.

The special fungous stains can be applied to fixed smears of sputum, gastric aspirates or other exudates to study morphology. This kind of study is indicated whenever identification by direct examination is uncertain. Although final diagnosis must be made culturally, therapeutic considerations justify rapid methods of making a tentative diagnosis.

Sputum, bronchial washings and gastric aspirates are all suitable for culture, and should be handled according to the methodology outlined in the section on general laboratory methods (p. 569). Pneumonic lesions extending to the pleura may be needled safely and aspirated for culture if insufficient material is obtained for both direct examination and culture. This diagnostic approach is particularly important in children who are not producing sputum. Cultures at 27°C. are much more likely to be positive than those at 37°C. Conversion of the mycelial form to the yeastlike phase by culturing at 37°C. is usually easy, but in healing lesions this may be difficult or even impossible without animal passage. Animal inoculation may not produce macroscopic disease. It is important to sacrifice animals at approximately three weeks after inoculation and to culture homogenates of the liver, spleen, lung, testes and any visible abdominal lymph nodes. Intraperitoneal and intratesticular inoculation of hamsters seems to be as sensitive a method as the intravenous inoculation of mice.

B. dermatitidis is so easily recognized microscopically in sputum, other exudates and tissues that specific aids to diagnosis other than cultures would appear superfluous. There are times, however, when no classic budding forms are seen and cultures, whether because of bacterial contamination or low viability, are negative. In this situation fluorescent microscopy, utilizing specific antiglobulins labeled with fluorescein, may be helpful. Anti-blastomyces rabbit globulin, absorbed with yeast cells of Histoplasma capsulatum and hyphae of Geotrichum candidum and conjugated with fluorescein isothiocyanate, is considered to give specific fluorescence with B. dermatitidis.

Despite the fact that serologic tests for North American blastomycosis lack both sensitivity and specificity, they are useful, when positive, in alerting the physician to the possibility of a yeastlike fungous infection. Agar diffusion-precipitin reactions seem to offer a better serologic potential for diagnosis, but are not as well standardized or as generally available as the complement fixation reaction.

Patients with primary pulmonary histoplasmosis or coccidioidomycosis may give positive complement-fixing reactions with blastomyces antigen to a titer higher than with homologous antigen. Similarly, the patient with North American blastomycosis may give a positive complement fixation reaction with histoplasma antigen and none with homologous antigen. The results of intradermal sensitivity tests and complement fixation tests may be contradictory.

Campbell has demonstrated the frequent occurrence of an increasing titer with homologous antigen and decreasing titer with heterologous ones in serial complement fixation studies during the course of the primary pulmonary infections. This is of considerable immunologic interest, but scarcely helps the diagnostician in his initial contact with the patient. Of my own patients, 53 per cent had positive complement-fixing antibodies and 26 per cent had a positive skin test result with blastomycin.

Epidemiology

North American blastomycosis is a disease of man and some domestic animals in an area extending from Canada through Mexico. Autochthonous cases have been reported from South America and Africa; it seems likely that the increasing interest in medical mycology in all parts of the world will reveal that the characterization of blastomycosis as North American is inappropriate.

The organism has been isolated from soils and other organic debris from old chicken coops, dilapidated houses, and outbuildings. There is a strong possibility that it may occur in association with rotting wood. Recent studies suggest that *B. dermatitidis* has a limited temporal recoverability from soils known to contain the naturally acquired fungus. Ecologic causes for this are not known. It is possible that animal reservoirs are important in bringing about soil inoculation.

Infection of children appears to be relatively infrequent in endemic areas, in contrast to the high incidence noted for other soil-inhabiting fungi such as *Histoplasma capsulatum* and *Coccidioides immitis*. Yet of ten patients with clinical illness due to *B. dermatitidis* during a five-month period in a small community, seven were sixteen years of age or younger, and four of these were under seven. The actual incidence and age distribution of infection in any area must await the development of satisfactory skin test antigens and serologic methods.

Among adults clinical disease is more frequent in males than in females. In my own series the ratio of males to females has been 6:1.

The portal of entry in blastomycosis is almost certainly respiratory in most instances. The clinical characteristics and course of blastomycosis from cutaneous inoculation are different from those seen in the usual cutaneous blastomycosis, which is almost certainly a manifestation of spread from an active or inactive pulmonary focus. The occurrence of self-limited pulmonary blastomycosis lacks the documentation of histoplasmosis and coccidioidomycosis, but has been observed in a few patients.

Pathogenesis and Pathology

Two types of primary pulmonary lesion have been recognized by roentgenographic features, but one can only infer the pathologic changes from older resected specimens and experimental infections in animals.

Bronchopneumonic lesions have been observed to clear spontaneously without cavitation or radiographic evidence of fibrosis, revealing their true nature only by later suppuration of draining lymph nodes or pectoral muscle extension from internal mammary nodes. The histopathology of such lesions has not been documented in man.

The second type of lesion seems to follow the usual evolution of mycotic "coin" granulomas, being well circumscribed and relatively dense from the time of the first roentgenographic recognition. This type of lesion is characterized by a dense fibrotic reaction within and at the margin of the granuloma. Epithelioid tissue and giant cells may predominate, or central caseation may be the outstanding feature. Differentiation from cryptococcal or histoplasmal granulomas may be difficult without culture. Unless typical budding forms and resting forms with definite multiple nuclei are present, histologic differentiation from cryptococcosis may be impossible. The mucicarmine stain does not seem to be as specific for cryptococci as has been stated by some pathologists.

A commonly recognized advanced form of blastomycotic pulmonary disease, a suppurative pneumonitis, is the result of rapid extension of primary bronchopneumonic lesions in a highly susceptible host. Blastomyces are found within areas of suppuration which are more or less circumscribed by epithelioid tissue. They are also present in the fibrinous and polymorphonuclear exudate in the alveoli and terminal bronchioles. Acute suppurative pneumonitis may be followed by cavitation which is often multilocular. Empyema is infrequent even when suppurative pneumonitis and cavitation extend to the pleura. Rib and thoracic soft tissue involvement is not uncommon during the course of acute pulmonary blastomycosis. Extension to the bronchial and hilar lymph nodes is typical.

At the other end of the spectrum of pulmonary response to *B. dermatitidis* are those patients whose x-ray films and tissue sections are suggestive of sarcoidosis. Multiple epithelioid granulomas of varying dimensions with numerous or scanty giant cells and septal fibrosis are scattered throughout the lung. As a general rule, many of the epithelioid granulomas have some degree of central caseation necrosis which alerts the pathologist to the probability of a fungal or mycobacterial origin. Special stains, such as the periodic acid-Schiff, will reveal Blastomyces within giant cells and areas of caseation.

Many adult patients have a subacute or chronic clinical course which is reflected in a mixed suppurative and fibrotic pulmonary pathology. Multiple areas of suppuration may be marginated by epithelioid cell proliferation, plasma cells, fibrosis and a variable number of giant cells. In other areas of the same lung, caseation necrosis may be extensive. In still other areas the histologic picture may be dominated by fibrosis with a lesser element of epithelioid tissue and inflammatory cells. In predominantly fibrotic areas the differentiation of Cryptococcus from Blastomyces by staining methods other than those using fluorescent antibody may be especially difficult.

Treatment

North American blastomycosis responds well to treatment with hydroxystilbamidine as well as with amphotericin B. Patients with involvement of the central nervous system, those whose disease is severely disseminated and those critically ill should be treated with amphotericin B. Otherwise hydroxystilbamidine is preferred, because of its lesser toxicity and fewer side effects.

Although hydroxystilbamidine can be administered intramuscularly, it is best given intravenously in a concentration no greater than 0.5 mg. per milliliter. The infusion can be given within a period of one to two hours. The dosage should be calculated on the basis of 3 to 5 mg. of hydroxystilbamidine per kilogram of body weight per day. The drug is administered daily for twenty-one days and every other day thereafter until the total period of treatment is between eight and twelve weeks. Treatment should not be interrupted, because resistance to hydroxystilbamidine develops more often when treatment is given in courses than when it is given continuously.

If antimicrobial resistance appears, or if the patient relapses, retreatment should be with amphotericin B. This antibiotic can be given according to the recommendations outlined in the section on Treatment of Systemic Mycoses with Amphotericin B (p. 620).

REFERENCES

Abernathy, R. S., and Heiner, D. C.: Precipitation Reactions in Agar in North American Blastomycosis. *J. Lab. & Clin. Med.*, 57:604, 1961.

Acree, P. W., DeCamp, P. T., and Ochsner, A.: Pulmonary Blastomycosis: A Critical Analysis of Medical and Surgical Therapies with a Report of Six Cases. *J. Thoracic Surg.*, 28:175, 1954.

Allison, F., Jr., Lancaster, J. G., Whitehead, A. E., and Woodbridge, H. B.: Simultaneous Infection in Man by Histoplasma Capsulatum and Blastomyces Dermatitidis. *Am. J. Med.*, 32:476, 1962.

Baker, R. D.: Tissue Reaction in Human Blastomycosis: An Analysis of Tissue from 23 Cases. *Am. J. Path.*, 18:479, 1942.

Boswell, W.: Roentgen Aspects of Blastomycosis. *Am. J. Roentgenol.*, 81:224, 1959.

Brandsberg, J. W., Tosh, F. E., and Furcolow, M. L.: Concurrent Infection with Histoplasma Capsulatum and Blastomyces Dermatitidis. *New England J. Med.*, 270:874, 1964.

Buechner, H. A., Anderson, A. E., Strug, L. H., Seabury, J. H., and Peabody, J. W., Jr.: Pulmonary Resection in the Treatment of Blastomycosis. *J. Thoracic Surg.*, 25:468, 1953.

Campbell, C. C.: The Accuracy of Serologic Methods in Diagnosis. *Ann. New York Acad. Sc.*, 89:163, 1960.

Cherniss, E. I., and Waisbren, M. S.: North American Blastomycosis: A Clinical Study of 40 Cases. *Ann. Int. Med.*, 44:105, 1956.

Curtis, A. C., and Bocobo, F. C.: North American Blastomycosis. *J. Chron. Dis.*, 5:404, 1957.

Denton, J. F., and DiSalvo, A. F.: Isolation of Blastomyces Dermatitidis from Natural Sites at Augusta, Georgia. *Am. J. Trop. Med. & Hyg.*, 13:716, 1964.

Denton, J. F., McDonough, E. S., Ajello, L., and Ausherman, R. J.: Isolation of *Blastomyces Dermatitidis* from Soil. *Science*, 133:1126, 1961.

Elson, W. O.: The Antibacterial and Fungistatic Properties of Propamidine. *J. Inf. Dis.*, 76:193, 1945.

Emmons, C. W., and others: North American Blastomycosis: Two Autochthonous Cases from Africa. *Sabouraudia*, 3:306, 1964.

Foshay, L., and Madden, A. G.: The Dog as a Natural Host for *Blastomyces Dermatitidis*. *Am. J. Trop. Med.*, 22:565, 1942.

Furcolow, M. L., Schwartz, J., Hewell, B. A., and Grayston, J. T.: Incidence of Tuberculin, Histoplasmin, and Blastomycin Reactors Among a Group of School Children. *Am. J. Pub. Health*, 43:1523, 1953.

Gilchrist, T. C., and Stokes, W. R.: Further Observations on Blastomycetic Dermatitis in Man. *Bull. Johns Hopkins Hosp.*, 7:129, 1896.

Jones, R. R., and Martin, D. S.: Blastomycosis of Bone: A Review of 63 Collected Cases of Which 6 Recovered. *Surgery*, 10:931, 1941.

Kaplan, W., and Kaufman, L.: Blastomycosis and Histoplasmosis—Specific Fluorescent Antiglobulins for the Detection and Identification of *Blastomyces Dermatitidis* Yeast Phase Cells. *Mycopathol. et Mycol. Appl.*, 19:173, 1963.

Kunkel, W. M., Weed, L. A., McDonald, J. R., and Clagett, O. T.: North American Blastomycosis—Gilchrist's Disease: A Clinicopathologic Study of Ninety Cases. *Surg., Gynec. & Obst.* (Int. Abstr. Surg.), 99:1, 1954.

Lockwood, W. R., Busey, J. F., Batson, B. E., and Allison, F., Jr.: Experiences in the Treatment of North American Blastomycosis with 2-Hydroxystilbamidine. *Ann. Int. Med.*, 57:553, 1962.

Martin, D. S., and Smith, D. T.: Blastomycosis. I. A Review of the Literature. *Am. Rev. Tuberc.*, 39:275, 1939.

Ramsey, F. K., and Carter, G. R.: Canine Blastomycosis in the United States. *J. Am. Vet. Med. A.*, 120:93, 1952.

Seabury, J. H., and Dascomb, H. E.: Results of the Treatment of Systemic Mycoses. *J.A.M.A.*, 188:509, 1964.

Smith, D. T.: Immunologic Types of Blastomycosis: A Report on 40 Cases. *Ann. Int. Med.*, 31:463, 1949.

Smith, J. G., Jr., Harris, J. S., Conant, N. F., and Smith, D. T.: An Epidemic of North American Blastomycosis. *J.A.M.A.*, 158:641, 1955.

Stober, A. M.: Systemic Blastomycosis: A Report of Its Pathological, Bacteriological and Clinical Features. *Arch. Int. Med.*, 13:509, 1914.

SOUTH AMERICAN BLASTOMYCOSIS

The Organism

Paracoccidioides brasiliensis is sometimes termed *Blastomyces brasiliensis*. Unfortunately, both generic names are used, resulting in the confusion of this organism with *B. dermatitidis*.

The free-living form grows slowly and restrictedly on Sabouraud's glucose agar at pH 7 and 27°C. Colonial morphology is variable, occasionally glabrous or cerebriform, but commonly wooly with a short nap. Colonies cannot be considered to be mature until after one month of incubation. Most colonies are pure white, but some may be gray or light brown with aging. Chlamydospores are formed by the septate, branching hyphae.

The parasitic form is diagnostic in either exudates or cultures at 37°C. when the characteristic budding can be seen. The diagnostic cell varies in size from 10 to 60 microns and is seen to have multiple buds extruded through the cell wall. The buds may be elongate, and the budding cell may resemble the wheel of a boat *(roda de leme; rueda del barco)*, or the buds may be relatively large, round to spherical as in Figure 10, and four to five in number. The communication between the mother and daughter cell is narrow and tapering, unlike that seen in *B. dermatitidis*. Budding cells of diagnostic type are more easily found in cultures at 37°C. or in hydroxide-cleared mounts of exudates than in tissue sections.

Growth at 37°C. on blood agar, brainheart infusion agar or Sabouraud's glucose agar (pH 7) appears, as a rule, earlier than at 27°C. Colonies are small, usually cerebriform, translucent to grayish, and produce large numbers of yeastlike cells. Single budding is much more common in cultures, exudates or tissue sections than

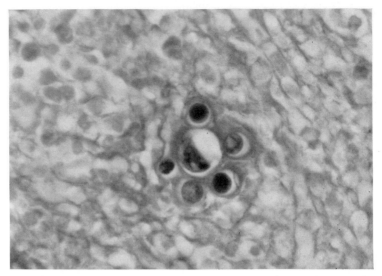

FIGURE 47–10. *Paracoccidioides brasiliensis* in lung. This is a periodic acid-Schiff strain of lung showing a mother cell and 5 daughters. The continuity of cell walls can be seen, but no cytoplasmic communication is evident at this stage.

the typical multiple external budding and is the basis for confusion of *P. brasiliensis* with *B. dermatitidis*. Nevertheless direct examination of cultures at 37°C. or of hydroxide-cleared exudates will reveal the diagnostic budding forms if a diligent search is made. Error is much more likely if microscopic examination of stained tissue sections is the only diagnostic method available.

The Clinical Disease

The South American literature emphasizes the primary disease, in which the portal of entry is usually considered to be the mucous membranes of the mouth or pharynx. Primary inoculation through carious teeth (apical abscesses), nasal mucous membranes, the anus and conjunctivae is considered to be much less frequent. Lacaz has suggested the respiratory tract, however, as one of the most common portals of entry. Perhaps the main fact in favor of primary oropharyngeal infection is the frequency of cervical lymph node involvement.

The most obvious manifestations of South American blastomycosis are ulcerogranulomatous lesions of the skin, mucous membranes and lymph nodes. Involvement of the lymphatic tissue is much greater in South American blastomycosis than in the North American disease. Mucous membrane lesions are similar to those seen in North American blastomycosis, espundia, granuloma inguinale and in some cases of histoplasmosis.

Whether as primary involvement or later dissemination, pulmonary invasion is demonstrable in more than 80 per cent of autopsied cases of South American blastomycosis. Roentgenographic features are nonspecific and differ from those of tuberculosis only in that supposedly "reinfection" disease is more frequent and predominant in the lower lobes. Isolated or multiple granulomas may be seen as in histoplasmosis, cryptococcosis, North American blastomycosis and other pulmonary granulomatous diseases. Small granulomas associated with interstitial fibrosis may simulate sarcoidosis. Cavitary disease is associated with a pneumonic and fibrotic background similar to the usual findings in tuberculosis and histoplasmosis; in this respect South American blastomycosis differs from many cases of progressive primary coccidioidomycosis.

There is a recognized association of

South American blastomycosis with tuberculosis (12 per cent), lymphoma and leishmaniasis; however, this relationship with tuberculosis and neoplasia is no different from that observed for other yeast-like mycoses.

Of 1506 cases tabulated by Lacaz, less than 2 per cent occurred in children of ten years or younger, and less than 13 per cent were under twenty-one years. The patient whose x-ray film is shown in Figure 11 was an adult, but the pulmonary changes are representative of progressive disease in children.

Laboratory Diagnosis

Diagnosis of South American blastomycosis is made regularly on the basis of careful study of hydroxide-cleared mounts of material obtained from granulomatous lesions of the skin or mucous membranes, from sputum or involved lymph nodes. Recognition of typical budding forms is sufficient for clinical diagnosis. Cultural characteristics at 37°C. and the morphology of the organisms present in the exudate when stained by the periodic acid-Schiff method are more useful for

confirmation than information gained from cultures at 27°C.

Filtrates from broth cultures, standardized by Del Negro, yield a paracoccidioidin for skin testing which is comparable in usefulness to commercial histoplasmin. Intradermal reactivity is absent during early infection and in severely disseminated disease, similar to reactivity to coccidioidin in coccidioidomycosis. Cutaneous reactivity is useful for screening, with the usual reservations about negative test results. Cross reactions occur with histoplasmin and blastomycin.

Both complement fixation and precipitin tests have been used in the study of paracoccidioidal infections. A review of Fava Netto's serial studies with a polysaccharide antigen derived from the yeast cells suggests that there is a close parallelism between the serologic fluctuations in coccidioidomycosis and paracoccidioidal infection. The specificity of serologic studies for paracoccidioidomycosis has not been established.

The fluorescent antibody method has been used for the diagnosis of South American blastomycosis. Rabbit antiserums absorbed by the method of Silva and

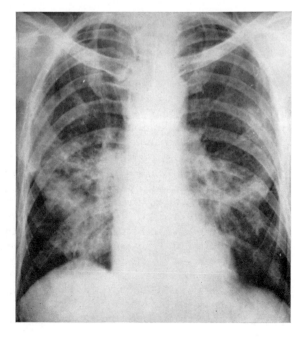

FIGURE 47–11. South American blastomycosis. The bronchopneumonic infiltration and distribution of the disease in the lungs are typical for disseminated South American blastomycosis. The characteristics of primary pulmonary complexes are not yet established. (Courtesy of Prof. Carlos da Silva Lacaz, Faculdade de Medicina da Universidade de São Paulo.)

Kaplan, appear to be specific for the yeast form of *P. brasiliensis.*

Epidemiology

South American blastomycosis is present in Mexico, Central and South America, and Africa (Ghana). *P. brasiliensis* has been isolated from soil in northern Brazil.

The most intensive epidemiologic studies have been in the state of São Paulo, Brazil, a highly endemic region. The disease was distinctly rural until recent years, when it became increasingly frequent in suburban and urban areas, especially in immigrant Japanese, who apparently have great susceptibility to infection by this fungus.

Clinical infection is recognized most frequently during middle life, age distribution being similar to that for North American blastomycosis. Since *P. brasiliensis* is a soil inhabitant, it is anticipated that many pediatric infections will be recognized when minor pulmonary infections are intensively studied in endemic areas and skin testing programs are introduced into the school systems.

Pathogenesis and Pathology

The gross characteristics of the ulcerogranulomatous mucosal and gingival lesions of South American blastomycosis are not distinguishable from those of the North American disease. Suppuration and drainage from the regional lymph nodes are regularly present in South American blastomycosis; lymph nodes are infrequently enlarged in North American blastomycosis. The lymphatic system is more frequently invaded by *P. brasiliensis,* whatever the site of the lesion. Cutaneous lesions are frequent, ulcerogranulomatous or papular, and resemble those produced by *B. dermatitidis* except that central healing is not a prominent feature.

Pulmonary lesions, whether primary or secondary, are not distinctive grossly. The classifications which have been proposed on the basis of gross and microscopic changes are neither helpful in understanding pathogenesis nor useful in differential diagnosis. The pathologic spectrum is like that of North American blastomycosis and tuberculosis.

Microscopically, *P. brasiliensis* may provoke a tissue reaction which is predominantly that of acute, chronic or mixed granulation. The pyogenic reaction is not uncommon in extensive pulmonary disease, but plasma cells are frequent, and there is little difficulty in finding large elements of chronic epithelioid granulation with multinucleate giant cells. Yeast-like cells are visible in most cases after routine hematoxylin and eosin staining, but morphology is demonstrated with greater precision by periodic acid-Schiff and methenamine-silver methods. Although the production of multiple, narrow-necked buds from the periphery of the mother cell is "characteristic" of this fungus, it may require prolonged search of several specially stained sections before they can be found.

In chronic productive tissue reaction, *P. brasiliensis* may not be numerous and may be found predominantly within giant cells of either the Langhans or foreign body type. Such lesions may be confused with Boeck's sarcoid or tuberculosis. Fibrosis of a predominantly interstitial type is common in pulmonary South American blastomycosis which has been treated with either sulfonamides or amphotericin B.

Treatment

Clinically active infections have been treated with sulfonamides since 1940. Some patients have been cured, and many more have had prolonged suppression of the disease. Unfortunately, the development of resistance to sulfonamides is frequent. The diamidines are apparently without value, and this is quite different from their effectiveness in North American blastomycosis.

Amphotericin B is of demonstrated value in the treatment of this disease. It has succeeded in many patients resistant to sulfonamides. Sampaio, who has the largest reported experience, has had excellent results. The recommendations given in the section on treatment with amphotericin B (p. 620) should be followed.

REFERENCES

Azevedo, P. C.: Algumas considerações sôbre a blastomicose Sul-Americana e seu agente etiológico. Tese, Faculdade de Odontologia do Pará, Belém-Pará-Brasil, 1954.

Batista, A. C., Shome, S. K., and Marques dos Santos, F.: Pathogenicity of Paracoccidioides Brasiliensis Isolated from Soil. Publicação No. 373. Insto. de Micologia, Univ. do Recife, Brasil, 1962.

Fava Netto, C.: Estudos quantitatívos sôbre a fixação do complemento no blastomicose Sul-Americana, com antígeno polissacarídico. Arq. Cir. Clin. Exper., 18:197, 1955.

Idem: Contribuição para o estudo immunológico da blastomicose de Lutz (blastomicose Sul-Americana). Rev. Inst. Adolfo Lutz, 21:99, 1961.

Lacaz, C. S.: South American Blastomycosis. An. Fac. Med. Univ. São Paulo, 29:9, 1955.

Lythcott, G. I., and Edgcomb, J. H.: The Occurrence of South American Blastomycosis in Accra, Ghana. Lancet, 1:916, 1964.

Machado Filho, J., and Miranda, J. L.: Considerações relativas a 238 casos consecutivos de blastomicose Sul-Americana. O Hospital, 55:103, 1959.

Mackinnon, J. E., and others: Temperatura ambiental y blastomicosis Sudamericana. An. Fac. Med. Montevideo, 45:310, 1960.

Romero Rivas, O.: El granuloma apical dentario en la blastomicosis Sudamericana. Arch. Peruanos Pat. Clin., 14:203, 1960.

Sampaio, S. de A. P.: Tratamento da blastomicose Sul-Americana com anfotericina B. Tese de concurso para a Cátedra de Dermatologia da Faculdade de Medicina da Universidade de São Paulo, Brasil, 1960.

Silva, M. E., and Kaplan, W.: Specific Fluorescein-Labeled Antiglobulins for the Yeast Form of Paracoccidioides Brasiliensis. Am. J. Trop. Med. & Hyg., 14:290, 1965.

COCCIDIOIDOMYCOSIS

The Organism

Coccidioides immitis is a dimorphic fungus whose free-living form inhabits soils of the Lower Sonoran Life Zone. Mycelial growth gives rise to arthrospores which are easily dislodged and airborne. These arthrospores are the infective units which are inhaled by man or other animals.

When arthrospores encounter a suitable tissue environment, they round up to become relatively small yeastlike spherules (sporangia) which grow to a diameter between 20 and 80 microns before the protoplasm condenses peripherally and undergoes multiple cleavage (endosporulation) to produce many uninucleate endospores (sporangiospores). Growth of the endospores is followed by rupture of the sporangium, liberating the endospores, which perpetuate the cycle by differentiating into sporangia. This process is illustrated in Figure 12. Thus both the endospore and the arthrospore differentiate similarly in susceptible tissue.

Unlike other dimorphic fungi, Coccidioides grows in the form of a mold at 37° C. on ordinary media. Some spherules may be formed rarely, but the mycelial growth predominates except for selected strains which are grown in special media. Mycelial growth is most characteristic at room temperature. Early development is characterized by an adherent, membranous growth like *B. dermatitidis* at a similar stage. Aerial hyphae usually appear, and are white at first. Colonies may remain white, become light to dark gray, or occasionally produce yellow to brown pigment. Fully virulent strains from untreated patients grow luxuriantly as a rule, and produce abundant, loose aerial hyphae which contain arthrospores. The arthrospores are ellipsoidal or rectangular, and are usually from 4 to 6 microns in length. The arthrospores are characteristically separated one from the other by a variable length of clear, empty hypha. An arthrospore-bearing hypha is shown in Figure 13.

The Clinical Disease

In endemic areas of high prevalence most children will acquire primary infection soon after their play activities bring them in contact with contaminated

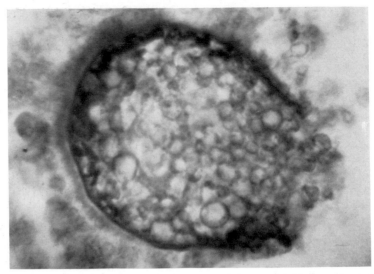

FIGURE 47–12. Mature sporangium of *Coccidioides immitis*. Multiple cleavage of the protoplasm has given rise to many sporangiospores, some of which can be seen leaving the ruptured sporangium. This is a diagnostic tissue form. Periodic acid-Schiff stain.

soils or dusts. Less than half have a recognized or remembered illness which might conceivably have been coccidioidomycosis. In this respect, and in most others, there is a close similarity between coccodioidomycosis, histoplasmosis and tuberculosis. Asymptomatic primary infection can be detected only by serial cutaneous and serologic testing, even though some may show a primary pulmonary complex in later roentgenograms and a very few will experience future activity of the disease.

Primary symptomatic infection may masquerade as a simple respiratory infection, the "flu," "atypical pneumonia," or be severe. In general, there is a parallelism between the severity of the exposure, the duration of the incubation period and the height of the fever. High fever and an incubation period shorter than ten days are associated with heavy infection. The usual incubation period is from ten to twenty-eight days. Constitutional manifestations are those common to any systemic infection. Anorexia and fatigability may persist for days or weeks even if fever has been of low grade and brief duration.

Localizing symptoms may be absent, but pleuritic or other chest pain is common, and more than half the patients have a nonproductive cough. Sputum production, with or without blood-streaking, is uncommon in children with this type of illness.

Erythema nodosum and erythema multiforme occur more frequently than in either histoplasmosis or tuberculosis, but in probably no more than 20 per cent of the symptomatic cases. Arthralgia and arthritis accompany erythema nodosum or erythema multiforme in some patients. If there is an acute febrile stage, a morbilliform exanthem may be present.

Eosinophilia is common among those exhibiting a rash or joint symptoms and is usually associated with some degree of leukocytosis. An elevated erythrocyte sedimentation rate is the most common nonspecific laboratory finding among those with symptomatic primary infection.

Although symptomatic primary disease may be either mild and transient or severe and prolonged over a number of weeks, only about 5 per cent go on to develop chronic pulmonary coccidioidomycosis. Most often extrapulmonary dissemination occurs during the acute stage or during postprimary progression. Dissemination and chronic cavitary disease are less common in children than in adults.

Chronic pulmonary coccidioidomycosis usually manifests itself as a continuation of the symptomatic primary phase. Hemoptysis or blood-streaking of the sputum is more frequent in this type of disease and may be severe. This type of infection is best characterized by the radiologic picture.

The roentgenographic evidence of primary infection may be evanescent and invisible at the time a chest x-ray is taken. The primary lesion is usually similar to that of tuberculosis, North American blastomycosis and some cases of cryptococcosis. Segmental and subsegmental pneumonia are frequent. Bronchial or hilar lymph nodes are enlarged, but may be obscured by the infiltrative density which is frequently in the form of a perihilar wedge. Extensive lesions may develop small areas of cavitation, but most primary lesions resolve completely over a period of several months. The central component of primary infections may extend to the mediastinal lymph nodes or the pericardium. The peripheral component may produce pleural thickening or frank effusion. A mycologically positive pleural fluid should prompt careful, serial serologic studies, since it is frequently part of or forerunner to dissemination.

The primary pulmonary infiltration may fail to resolve completely and may spread. During this sequence of events cavitation is frequent, and the pulmonary coccidioidomycosis becomes chronic. Cavities may persist after clearing of pneumonitis, presenting as the classic cavity without surrounding infiltration, such as is shown in Figure 14. These cavities may remain for years, may close if not too large, or may become filled with inspissated material. Occasionally such cavities may rupture into the pleural space, producing an empyema. If a secondary intrapulmonary spread occurs, the secondary infiltrates may clear completely, remain as fibrotic infiltrates or become nodular.

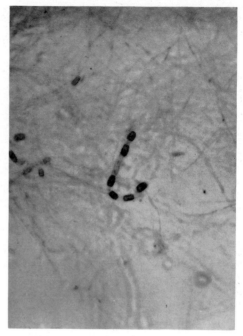

FIGURE 47–13. Arthrospores of *C. immitis.* Developing in the free-living mycelium, these rectangular spores are easily airborne and are highly infectious. Note the empty areas of hypha adjacent to the arthrospores.

Globular peripheral infiltrates, filled cavities and nodular secondary infiltrations may become radiologically dense and constitute "coccidioidomas" which are analogous to other fungal and tuberculous granulomas. Calcium may be deposited in the caseous areas of the granuloma. It may, like a tuberculoma, suddenly liquefy centrally, discharge its content into the bronchus, and become a cavity with or without secondary transbronchial spread.

Some patients with cavitary pulmonary coccidioidomycosis and a stable complement-fixation level remain asymptomatic until surgical resection of the cavitary lung is undertaken. Thereafter new areas of infiltration and cavity formation may develop.

Extrapulmonary dissemination occurs in approximately 0.5 per cent, but will not be discussed in this chapter. High complement-fixing titers, especially with ab-

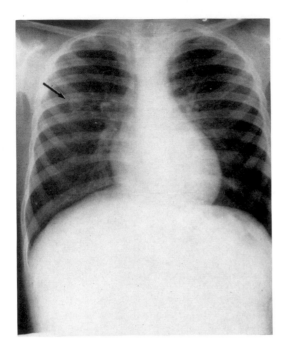

FIGURE 47–14. Cavitary pulmonary coccidi-oidomycosis. Although the right superior hilus is abnormal, there is little infiltration adjacent to the moderately thick-walled cavity in the third anterior intercostal space. A 6-year-old asymptomatic boy whose coccidioidin skin test result was positive. Precipitins were absent, and the complement fixation reaction was 4+ at 1:2 dilution. (Courtesy of Misha Newman, Kern County General Hospital.)

sence of dermal reactivity to coccidioidin in a 1:10 dilution, is pathognomonic of serious dissemination.

Laboratory Diagnosis

Hydroxide-cleared mounts of sputum or pus are usually diagnostic if many spherules are present. Endosporulating sporangia should be identified with certainty, since large yeast forms of Blastomyces may simulate Coccidioides in wet preparations. If in doubt, smears fixed in alcoholic formalin and stained by the periodic acid-Schiff method are frequently conclusive.

Cultures at 27°C. and 37°C. should be made according to the suggestions given in the section on general methods of laboratory diagnosis, but those made at 27° are likely to be more characteristic. If typical sporangia have been observed in fresh clinical materials, the mycelial characteristics will be sufficient for diagnosis. Confirmation by inoculating mice, guinea pigs or hamsters intraperitoneally or intratesticularly with suspensions of the mycelial growth is helpful. Typical tissue forms of Coccidioides can be recovered

from inoculated animals within two or three weeks.

Whether because of the immunologic characteristics of infection with *C. immitis* or the careful and inspired work of C. E. Smith and his colleagues, no other fungous disease is as well understood serologically as coccidioidomycosis. Diagnosis by serologic methods is accurate when serial specimens can be titrated, beginning early after the onset of illness. Furthermore, the course and prognosis of clinical disease and the effects of treatment are reflected, as a rule, in serologic changes.

Primary, truly asymptomatic disease is characterized by the conversion of dermal reactivity to coccidioidin from negative to positive. Precipitins and complement-fixing antibodies in low titer (1:2, 1:4) are found in less than 10 per cent of the recognized asymptomatic infections. Some asymptomatic patients will show evidence of active disease or even dissemination at a later date.

Primary, nondisseminating, symptomatic disease is characterized by the appearance of a dermal reaction to coccidioidin (90 per cent within two weeks), and precipitins against the same antigen. Precipitins are present in 90 per cent of the patients with this form of the disease by the fourth week and have disappeared in 60 per cent by the eighth week. Precipitins are found in no more than 5 per cent of these patients by the twenty-fourth week. Complement-fixing antibodies do not appear in many patients with nondisseminating primary disease, but can be demonstrated in approximately 50 per cent by the fourth week and in about 80 per cent between the eighth and twenty-fourth weeks. These antibodies appear later and persist longer in contrast to precipitins. The titer of complement-fixing antibodies is almost always below 1:32.

The presence of complement-fixing antibodies in a titer of 1:32 or above, and more particularly a serial rise in titers to and beyond this level, is evidence of dissemination and a guarded prognosis. Titers of 1:32 or higher which stabilize for months or years (do not vary by more than one dilution when the test is done in the same laboratory and paired with the previously tested serum specimen) may be found in chronic disseminated disease which can ultimately heal or undergo progressive dissemination to death. Periods of renewed dissemination may be accompanied by the reappearance of precipitins. Both acutely and chronically progressive dissemination are usually associated with a negative skin reaction to coccidioidin. Nevertheless many patients with chronic cavitary pulmonary disease may lose their dermal reactivity to 1:100 coccidioidin, and some of these maintain their low titer of complement-fixing antibodies.

Serologic cross-reactions do occur to some extent between coccidioidomycosis, histoplasmosis and blastomycosis. Serums from patients with coccidioidomycosis rarely give reactions to a significant titer with other fungal antigens, however, and when this does occur, the titer will be higher with coccidioidin if the test is performed correctly.

Epidemiology

Coccidioidomycosis affects all ages and races, but is milder in children than in adults, and more severe in dark-skinned races. It is endemic in portions of southwest Texas, New Mexico, Arizona, small areas of Utah and Nevada, southern California, and parts of Mexico, Guatemala, Honduras, Argentina, Venezuela and Paraguay. Its distribution is limited, apparently, by the features of the Lower Sonoran Life Zone. It is a mistake to think that the environment provided by this zone is associated with widespread culturability of *C. immitis* from the soils.

Although *C. immitis* produces disease in desert rodents and can be isolated from the soil of their burrows, the factors which permit vegetative growth of the fungus in soil and widespread infection are incompletely known. Contrary to popular belief, infected soils are hard to demonstrate and seem to be much more sharply limited than the areas of high prevalence of disease. In this respect coccidioidomycosis is similar to histoplasmosis. Furthermore, it has been established that there is a distinct seasonal variation in the cultural recoverability of *C. immitis* in soils. Culturability may be relatively high shortly after the rainy season and the appearance of warm weather and very low or absent at other times. More disturbing is the fact that a "place" productive of positive cultures for several years may become culturally negative for several years and become positive again without significant variation in climate. Egeberg has suggested that to multiply in number in soil, *C. immitis* requires two allies: (1) the summer sun with its sterilizing effect on the upper layers of soil, and (2) some chemical ally that inhibits the growth of organisms hostile to and competitive with *C. immitis*. Egeberg believes this ally to be one or more of the water-soluble salts found in soil.

Coccidioidomycosis is a disease naturally acquired by the inhalation of arthrospores. It has been stated frequently that contagion does not occur, but this opinion is not biologically sound, although its statistical validity was unquestioned until recently. Arthrospores have been found in many lesions, but especially in chronic pulmonary cavities. Patients with this sort of cavity may have arthrospores in their sputum. Biologically, the possibility of infection from dried sputum of this type must be admitted. Infection of personnel caring for a patient with a plaster cast over coccidioidal involvement of an extremity has been thoroughly documented. A third item of evidence in favor of the possible contagiousness of coccidioidomycosis is the observation of the transmission of disease from an infected female Rhesus monkey to its nursing offspring. One should conclude that arthrospores are capable of producing infection wherever they may be found.

Pathogenesis and Pathology

In the experimental animal inhaled arthrospores of *C. immitis* provoke little immediate tissue response. The development of tissue hypersensitivity is manifested by an acute exudative reaction characterized by infiltration of neutrophils, outpouring of fibrinous fluid about the fungus cells, and a variable degree of simple necrosis. This localized lesion may be resorbed completely or partially fibrosed as immunity develops under favorable host-parasite relations.

If the infection is not quickly contained, the cycle of spherule development and release of endospores provokes a histologic picture which is dependent in large part upon host factors of immunity and hypersensitivity. If complete resolution of the initial infection does not take place early, chronic granulation tissue is produced, particularly about the sporangia. Histiocytic proliferation, epithelioid cells, Langhans's giant cells and caseation necrosis may characterize subacute and chronic pneumonitis as well as coccidioidomas.

Pneumonic lesions are likely to have areas of acute granulomatous reaction about liberated endospores interspersed with the chronic reaction. Coccidioidomas are more adynamic, and show predominantly a hyalinized fibrotic "capsule" with or without calcium deposition surrounding an area of caseation necrosis. Langhan's giant cells occur frequently subjacent to the "capsule," and it is in this region that sporangia in various degrees of degradation are likely to be seen.

The cavitary lesions vary histologically according to their age and the activity of adjacent disease. Chronic cavities are similar to those produced by tuberculosis, including associated bronchiectasis and a pseudomembranous lining of some cavities. Many have a densely fibrotic thin wall surrounded by a few to many caseous nodules.

Lymph node involvement is part of the primary infection. In this respect and in subsequent pathogenetic potentialities, the role of intrathoracic lymph node disease in coccidioidomycosis is the same as in tuberculosis. In progressive, fatal coccidioidomycosis the peribronchial and mediastinal lymph nodes may become greatly enlarged and undergo complete suppuration.

As indicated in the discussion of clinical symptomatology, pleurisy is frequent during the primary infection. This may produce the characteristic signs of fibrinous pleuritis over the area of primary pulmonary involvement. In more severe primary infection, and in progressive pulmonary disease with or without cavitary rupture into the pleural space, a granulomatous pleuritis, sometimes associated with actual empyema, is present.

Active coccidioidomycosis presents no diagnostic problem histologically as a rule. Spherules with endospores can be seen by routine hematoxylin and eosin staining. In subacute and chronic pneumonic lesions and in coccidioidomas the diagnosis may be more difficult to establish unless special stains are utilized. Periodic acid-Schiff or methenamine-silver stains of almost all lesions will give sufficient morphologic detail to be diagnostic. In both chronic cavitary lesions and coccidioidomas hyphal elements of *C. immitis* may be seen.

Culture from active lesions should always be positive if properly done. Growth may be slow and abnormal from some lesions in patients who have been treated with amphotericin B.

Treatment and Prevention

Restriction of activity and increased bed rest are indicated for symptomatic primary and progressive primary infection, especially if complement-fixing antibodies are present and increasing in titer. Activity should be restricted until chest x-rays and serologic studies indicate that the infection is regressing or until it is evident that antimicrobial treatment is desirable. Restriction of activity is not indicated for asymptomatic primary and chronic disease.

The indications for therapy with amphotericin B have not been defined to the point of general acceptance. Under the circumstances, one must give great weight to the opinions and recommendations of those with experience in all manifestations of the disease. Accordingly, the recommendations which follow are those of W. A. Winn, except as otherwise indicated.

Amphotericin B should be administered to patients showing (1) extension or exacerbation of chronic pulmonary disease, (2) impending or actual dissemination, and (3) as coverage before and after any surgical procedure for the disease.

Clinical signs and symptoms are important in deciding when and whom to treat, but the inexperienced therapist may prefer to rely primarily on the results of serial serologic studies. These tests should be done every three or four weeks during symptomatic primary infections until a definite decline in titer is demonstrated. The titer of precipitins has not been accorded any prognostic significance, but persistence or reappearance of precipitins has a serious connotation.

In either threatened or substantiated dissemination, Winn believes that the maximum individual amphotericin B dosage of 1 to 1.5 mg. per kilogram should be given, but the duration of treatment may be tailored to the serologic and clinical responses.

Extrapulmonary coccidioidomycosis is not a concern of this chapter, but in disseminating disease extrapulmonary considerations may determine whether or not amphotericin is to be given. In the presence of continued activity of pulmonary disease, one may not know whether a rising complement fixation titer is due to intrapulmonary or extrapulmonary dissemination or both. In such circumstances treatment with amphotericin B would be favored.

The toxicity of amphotericin B must be weighed against the seriousness of disseminated coccidioidomycosis and the relatively poor results of treatment with amphotericin in widespread or meningeal dissemination. It seems reasonable to administer amphotericin intravenously to all infants and children with severe symptomatic primary or progressive primary disease regardless of the serologic findings at the moment and to all pediatric patients with active pulmonary disease and a complement fixation titer in excess of 1:32, regardless of symptoms. There is some evidence to suggest that although the maximum tolerated individual dose should be administered, the duration of therapy necessary for suppression of acute but nondisseminated disease may be relatively short. The early administration of the antibiotic may be sufficient to permit the host to contain a potentially dangerous infection without resort to a larger or maximal dosage which might produce toxicity, a risk warranted only if the disease should progress. All severely symptomatic primary infections in members of dark-skinned races or those with metabolic diseases which are known to be associated with instability of infectious diseases should also be treated.

The use of amphotericin B has not eliminated the necessity for surgery in selected patients. Progressive cavitary coccidioidomycosis may fail to stabilize after treatment with amphotericin B, but may regress satisfactorily when surgical measures are combined with antibiotic therapy.

Surgical intervention is definitely indicated if a coccidioidal cavity ruptures into the pleural space or if hemoptysis is severe and persistent. Hemoptysis is rarely fatal, and it is probably wise to delay as long as possible unless the cavity is already of the chronic type. Resection of a chronic cavity is less likely to be complicated than resection of progressive primary cavities.

Chronic cavitation and fibrocavitary disease may constitute an indication for surgery, but considerable disagreement exists among physicians writing of their experiences with these problems. Postoperative exacerbation with or without the appearance of new cavities is sufficiently frequent in some series to lead to the recommendations that (1) operation should be preceded and followed by about one month of treatment with amphotericin B, and (2) thoracoplasty should accompany resection in many cases. There is evidence that thoracoplasty is helpful in preventing the postoperative appearance of cavities which were either not present previously or were unrecognized. Thoracoplasty is particularly undesirable in the pediatric age group, and operation should be postponed until after full skeletal growth has been achieved, if possible.

To date, prevention of coccidioidomycosis has been directed toward modifying environmental factors associated with growth and dissemination of the fungus in soils. The application of oils to the surface of infected and agriculturally unworked soils as well as the establishment of grass coverage may be useful in relation to military encampments and village areas. These methods cannot be used to diminish infection among agricultural workers and their children, and these families remain one of the most important sources of new cases.

Experimental work in monkeys and dogs has shown that subcutaneous injection of as few as ten living arthrospores of *C. immitis* will give immunity to subsequent respiratory challenge and will not produce progressive or disseminated disease. A much greater number of arthrospores has been used to immunize dogs which were given amphotericin B orally for twenty-one days after injection of the spores. These dogs became immune while exhibiting no reactions to the vaccine, whereas those animals not receiving amphotericin had significant local and regional reactions, but no dissemination. Since attempts to immunize with nonliving preparations and vaccines have not been fully successful, trials with a living attenuated vaccine among children in highly endemic areas would appear to be very much in order.

REFERENCES

Aronson, J. D., Saylor, R. M., and Carr, E. I.: Relationship of Coccidioidomycosis to Calcified Pulmonary Nodules. *Arch. Path.,* 34: 31, 1942.

Aronstam, E. M., and Hopeman, A. R.: Surgical Experiences with Pulmonary Coccidioidomycosis: A Survey of 112 Operative Cases. *J. Thor. Cardiov. Surg.,* 42:200, 1961.

Birsner, J. W.: Roentgen Aspects of Five Hundred Cases of Pulmonary Coccidioidomycosis. *Am. J. Roentgenol.,* 72:4, 1954.

Carter, R. A.: Coccidioidal Granuloma: Roentgen Diagnosis. *Am. J. Roentgenol.,* 25:715, 1931.

Castleberry, M. W., Converse, J. L., and Del Favero, J. E.: Coccidioidomycosis Transmission to Infant Monkey from Its Mother. *Arch. Path.,* 75:459, 1963.

Cohen, R., Bos, J., and Webb, P. A.: Co-existing Coccidioidomycosis and Tuberculosis in Children. *Arch. Ped.,* 69:267, 1952.

Converse, J. L., Pakes, S. P., Snyder, F. M., and Castleberry, M. W.: Experimental Primary Cutaneous Coccidioidomycosis in the Monkey. *J. Bact.,* 87:81, 1964.

Cotton, B. H., and Birsner J. W.: Surgical Treatment of Pulmonary Coccidioidomycosis. *J. Thor. Cardiov. Surg.,* 38:435, 1959.

Dickson, E. C., and Gifford, M. A.: Coccidioides Infection (Coccidioidomycosis). *Arch. Int. Med.,* 62:853, 1938.

Drips, W., Jr., and Smith, C. E.: Coccidioidomycosis. *J.A.M.A.,* 190:1010, 1964.

Eckmann, B. H., Schaefer, G. L., and Huppert, M.: Bedside Interhuman Transmission of Coccidioidomycosis via Growth on Fomites. An Epidemic Involving Six Persons. *Am. Rev. Resp. Dis.,* 89:175, 1964.

Egeberg, R. O.: Factors Influencing the Distribution of Coccidioides Immitis in Soil. *Recent Progress in Microbiology*, VIII:652-5, U. of Toronto Press (Canada), 1963.

Egeberg, R. O., and Ely, A. F.: Coccidioides Immitis in the Soil of the Southern San Joaquin Valley. *Am. J. Med. Sc.*, 23:151, 1956.

Fiese, M. J.: Coccidioidomycosis. Springfield, Ill., Charles C Thomas, 1958.

Kent, D. C., and Kendall, H. F.: Short Term, Low Dosage Amphotericin B Therapy for Residuals of Coccidioidomycosis. *Dis. Chest*, 47:284, 1965.

Lipschultz, B. M., and Liston, H. E.: Steroid Induced Disseminated Coccidioidomycosis. *Dis. Chest*, 46:355, 1964.

Melick, D. W.: The Surgical Treatment of Pulmonary Coccidioidomycosis, with a Comprehensive Summary of the Complications Following This Type of Therapy. *Am. Rev. Tuberc.*, 77:17, 1958.

Peers, R. A., Holman, E. F., and Smith, C. E.: Pulmonary Coccidioidal Disease. *Am. Rev. Tuberc.*, 45:723, 1942.

Puckett, T. F.: Hyphae of Coccidioides Immitis in Tissues of the Human Host. *Am. Rev. Tuberc.*, 70:320, 1954.

Seabury, J. H., and Dascomb, H. E.: Results of the Treatment of Systemic Mycoses. *J.A.M.A.*, 188:509, 1964.

Sievers, M. L.: Coccidioidomycosis Among Southwestern American Indians. *Am. Rev. Resp. Dis.*, 90:920, 1964.

Smith, C. E.: Diagnosis of Pulmonary Coccidioidal Infections. *California Med.*, 75:385, 1951.

Smith, C. E., Pappagianis, D., Levine, H. B., and Saito, M.: Human Coccidioidomycosis. *Bact. Rev.*, 25:310, 1961.

Smith, C. E., Saito, M. T., Beard, R. R., Rosenberger, H. G., and Whiting, E. G.: Histoplasmin Sensitivity and Coccidioidal Infection. *Am. J. Pub. Health*, 39:722, 1949.

Smith, C. E., Saito, M. T., and Simons, S. A.: Pattern of 39,500 Serologic Tests in Coccidioidomycosis. *J.A.M.A.*, 160:546, 1956.

Winn, W. A.: Recent Advances in the Therapy of Coccidioidomycosis; *in* G. Dalldorf (ed.): *Fungi and Fungous Diseases*. Springfield, Ill., Charles C Thomas, 1962, pp. 315-25.

PULMONARY CRYPTOCOCCOSIS

The Organism

Cryptococcus neoformans, as seen in direct examination of sputum or spinal fluid, is a spherical or oval yeast whose total diameter (including the capsule) is usually between 4 and 10 microns. Smaller forms are seen occasionally, and heavily encapsulated strains may reach a diameter of 20 microns. If the organisms are numerous, budding can be seen in most preparations, but is better studied in India ink or saline mounts from cultures. Budding may be single or multiple from any point on the cell wall. The daughter cell is attached, before separation, by a thin cell wall arising from a small pore in the mother cell wall. Young buds are included within the mother polysaccharide capsule when it is present. During direct examination the mucoid capsules are seen best in India ink mounts. They appear as transparent halos of variable thickness external to the cell wall. In India ink preparations, cryptococci are cleanly separated from the suspension of India ink, whereas exudative cells which may appear to have large "capsules" are encrusted with adherent ink particles around the "cell membrane." Some strains of cryptococci are unencapsulated or have capsules so thin that they cannot be recognized in direct mounts.

Cryptococci grow well on a variety of solid media commonly used in the laboratory. Brain-heart infusion agar, brain-heart infusion rabbit blood agar and Sabouraud's dextrose agar (at pH 7.0) are suitable and generally available. Only *C. neoformans* grows well at 37°C., but other species may show slight growth. Colonial growth usually appears in two to ten days, but occasionally is slower.

The colonies of initial isolation may be either mucoid or pasty. In either case they are white to cream in color and gradually darken to tan or brown. The yeast forms in pasty colonies may not show encapsulation in India ink preparations, although this is usually present after aging of the colony. If capsules cannot be demonstrated after ten days of aging, they almost always appear after subculture. The writer has isolated one strain of *C. neoformans* which did not show encapsulation, except by special mucopolysaccharide stains, until after intracerebral inoculation in mice. Mucoid colonies always contain yeast forms with some degree of encapsulation.

The morphology of the cryptococci from cultural isolates is essentially the same as described for direct mounts. A few elongate cells may remain adherent, producing a short pseudomycelium. No true mycelium is formed, and the cells have the same morphology when grown at 25°C. as at 37°C.

There are seven recognized species of the genus Cryptococcus, none of which ferments any known carbohydrate with the production of gas. All produce extracellular starch on synthetic dextrose-thiamine medium at pH 4.5. The biochemical properties of the cryptococci are used rarely for clinical laboratory diagnosis.

Within the genus Cryptococcus, only *C. neoformans* grows rapidly when subcultured and incubated at 37°C., and only *C. neoformans* is regularly pathogenic for white Swiss mice. There is considerable strain variation in the pathogenicity of *C. neoformans*. If 0.02 or 0.04 ml. of a saline suspension of the organism is injected intracerebrally into white Swiss mice, encapsulated forms can be recovered from the brain and meninges. Most strains of *C. neoformans* kill the mice within two weeks. Intraperitoneal injection should not be relied upon for studies of pathogenicity.

The Clinical Disease

Patients with proved pulmonary cryptococcosis have fallen more or less distinctly into one of two groups. The first group, composed of those who were completely asymptomatic, could recall no significant febrile illness or pulmonary symptoms within the previous several years, and had negative sputum studies for cryptococci. Chest roentgenograms in most revealed one or several nodular lesions similar to that shown in Figure 15. Diagnosis was made after surgical resection. Others in this group were asymptomatic until the onset of central nervous system or cutaneous cryptococcosis. Many of these had negative chest x-rays at the time of diagnosis; the primary pulmonary lesion became evident later in the course of illness or was discovered at autopsy.

The second group of patients, smaller in number, presented with a febrile illness accompanied by cough and sputum production. The sputum was variable in amount, mucoid or mucopurulent, and oc-

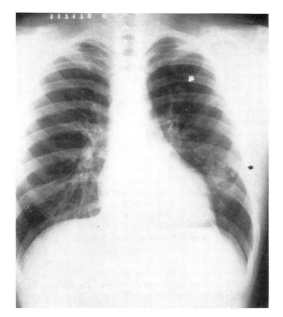

FIGURE 47–15. Asymptomatic pulmonary cryptococcosis. This 17-year-old male could recall no febrile illness or chest symptoms. The x-ray film was a routine preoperative film (pilonidal cyst). Segmental resection was followed by active pulmonary and pleural cryptococcosis.

casionally blood-streaked. Chest pain or discomfort was present in some. The chest x-ray in all patients in this group has shown a pneumonic infiltration of some type, often with nodular lesions as shown in Figure 16. Cryptococci were present in sputum or bronchial washings.

One feature of the clinical history deserves special emphasis. When they were carefully questioned, most of the patients gave a definite history of more than casual contact with pigeons or their droppings. Such a contact history should provoke an intensive search for cryptococci in all patients with a pulmonary disease which does not follow the expected course during treatment.

Physical examination has given no important information as to the cause of the pulmonary disease unless dissemination had occurred. Acneiform or ulcerogranulomatous lesions may be found on the skin, and the peripheral lymph nodes may be enlarged in some patients with disseminated disease.

Fever, when present, varies from a daily maximum of 100°F. to 103°F; in patients without other known disease the fever slowly defervesced over a period of several weeks, often to normal range. The pulmonary infiltration may stabilize or actually regress to a significant degree during hospital observation prior to diagnosis. One such patient had a lobectomy for removal of a residual, irregularly marginated mass lesion. Heavily encapsulated cryptococci were present in large number, but could not be cultured or recovered from young mice inoculated intracerebrally, suggesting that pulmonary cryptococcosis can be a self-limited disease.

Although there are no radiographic features which are specific, globular lesions with fuzzy margins are sufficiently common to invite consideration of cryptococcosis. Mass pneumonic lesions tend to be dense centrally and to have irregular, hazy margins. Some globular lesions develop an air-fluid level and resemble a pyogenic lung abscess. Circumscribed nodular lesions with little or no calcification are often seen in asymptomatic pa-

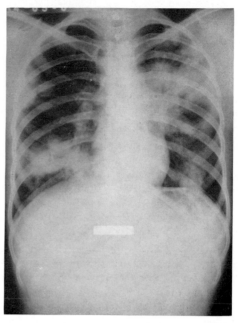

FIGURE 47–16. Active, symptomatic pulmonary cryptococcosis. This 13-year-old girl experienced a sudden onset of left pleuritic pain followed by fever. The sputum contained unencapsulated and thinly encapsulated cryptococci. Note that despite the areas of confluence the basic pattern is globular.

tients. When this type of lesion is found in association with active pneumonic disease, postprimary progression has probably occurred.

The lower lobes, right middle lobe, and lingula are the most common sites of primary lesions, which may be either peripheral or central. The subpleural nodule, so important pathologically, may be invisible in ordinary roentgenograms. These lesions have been observed to enlarge to visibility during corticosteroid therapy for other diseases.

Active lesions may provoke sufficient pleurisy to produce x-ray signs, but frank effusion is uncommon. When it occurs, other causes should be sought unless cryptococci are found in the fluid.

Laboratory Diagnosis

At present no skin test antigen is available commercially; in fact, there is no definite evidence at present that detection of cutaneous hypersensitivity is useful as a diagnostic or epidemiologic tool.

Cryptococcus neoformans has been found to have three basic serologic types: A, B and C. Type specificity is due to the capsular polysaccharides. Although high-titered antiserums can be prepared in rabbits, and specific capsular polysaccharide can be prepared without great difficulty, no serologic method has been generally accepted as suitable for clinical diagnostic purposes. A hemagglutination test which would be technically suitable for hospital laboratories has been reported, but clinical experience with the test is inadequate to date.

Most patients with symptomatic pulmonary cryptococcosis have cryptococci in the sputum or bronchial washings. Unfortunately, children may not cough up sputum even with training, and bronchoscopy is a major procedure in the very young. The saprophytic habitat of cryptococci makes the evaluation of isolates of *C. neoformans* from gastric washings a matter which must be determined by the clinician rather than the laboratorian.

Although the principles for collection and study of materials for laboratory diagnosis have been discussed in the section on General Methods of Laboratory Diagnosis (p. 569), there are some special considerations which apply specifically to cryptococcosis. Direct examination is best accomplished with the aid of India ink. The selected portion of exudate is mixed with a drop of 10 per cent potassium or sodium hydroxide, and then mixed with a drop of India ink. The amount of India ink should be such that there will be adequate transmission of light when a microscope objective with a magnifying power of approximtely 45 times is used. A cover slip large enough to give a thin fluid preparation should be applied carefully to avoid bubble formation. If the suspension of India ink breaks down rapidly into clumps, a second preparation with a drop of weak detergent solution (e.g. Dreft) added to the mixture of alkali and sputum before mixing with India ink

may give a more stable preparation. Wet mounts should be studied promptly to prevent drying and the creation of artefacts. The detection of encapsulated yeast forms is only presumptive evidence of cryptococcosis.

Final diagnosis depends upon the isolation and identification of *Cryptococcus neoformans*. Since sputum and bronchial washings may contain rapidly growing bacteria which obscure or prevent the colonial growth of cryptococci, it is advantageous to use culture media containing antibiotics. Any of the media which have been suggested previously may be used, but cycloheximide should not be incorporated in the medium, since it is a cryptococcostatic agent.

Animal inoculation is occasionally superior to cultural methods for isolation of *C. neoformans*. The intracerebral route should be used in white Swiss mice for final identification of cultural isolates. Direct intracerebral inoculations of bacteria-free fluids (e.g. spinal fluid) may give a diagnosis when cultures are sterile.

Lung biopsies, lymph nodes, or other tissue specimens should be handled as suggested in the section on general methods of laboratory diagnosis. Media without cycloheximide should be used for the culture of the triturated materials.

There are two staining methods which are of great help in the diagnosis of cryptococcosis. Although the mucicarmine method is simple and almost specific, a preferable method entails the use of a colloidal iron-periodic acid-Schiff stain such as that suggested by Mowry for material containing only forms with questionable capsules. These methods are applicable to formalin-fixed smears of sputum or other exudate. In our laboratory these stains have been used on sputum smears on several occasions when the specimen contained so many gram-negative bacteria and saprophytic fungi that there was uncertainty of achieving cultural isolation of the suspected cryptococcus. This difficulty is common in patients who have received several antibiotics for a number of days before a fungous infection is suspected. The organisms shown in Figure 17 were proved to be *C. neoformans*, but no capsules could be seen in hydroxide or India ink mounts.

There are two genera of asporogenous yeasts, closely related to the cryptococci, which may be found in sputum and may cause diagnostic confusion initially. *Torulopsis glabrata* may be found in sputum and can be pathogenic for man. Unlike the cryptococci, *T. glabrata* is an active fermenter of some carbohydrates. It produces gaseous fermentation of glucose and trehalose, but does not assimilate maltose, sucrose or cellobiose. It grows well on ordinary media, producing smooth colonies composed of spherical or ovoid cells. Rhodotorula may also be isolated from sputum. The cells are round to elongate, may produce pseudomycelium, and do not ferment carbohydrates. Pink, red or yellow pigmentation of the colony easily distinguishes it from the cryptococci. At least one species of Rhodotorula (mucilagnosa) has been reported to produce disseminated disease in an infant.

Epidemiology

Although the recognized incidence of cryptococcosis may vary considerably from place to place, it is worldwide in distribution. *Cryptococcus neoformans* exists as a saprophyte in nature, and has been isolated from a variety of sources, including peach juice, normal skin, human gastrointestinal tract, and the milk of cows suffering from cryptococcal mastitis. It is now known that the most important epidemiologic factor is the presence of *C. neoformans* in the excreta of pigeons and starlings, in pigeon nests, and soils which have been contaminated with the excreta.

Animal experimentation and the contact history of patients with acute pulmonary cryptococcosis point to the respiratory tract as the most important portal of entry. Systemic cryptococcosis may be produced in marmosets by feeding large numbers of cryptococci, and it is not unreasonable to suppose that occasional cases of cryptococcosis in association with malignant disease or its treatment may arise from an endogenous source.

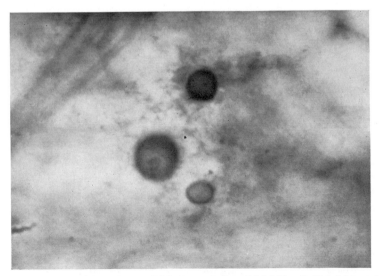

FIGURE 47–17. Cryptococci in sputum. This is periodic acid-Schiff-colloidal iron stain of sputum produced by the patient in Figure 16. The narrow, dark-staining margins of the 3 organisms shown took the colloidal iron and probably represent a thin layer of capsular mucopolysaccharide which could not be seen in India ink preparations. Cultures were positive for pasty colonies. Oil-immersion magnification.

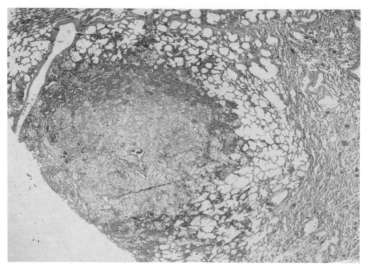

FIGURE 47–18. Subpleural nodule of cryptococcosis. This small nodule was rich in thinly encapsulated cryptococci. Heavily encapsulated forms were present at the periphery of the nodule. The pleural surface is at the right-hand margin.

Because of the lack of a reliable antigen for skin testing and the relatively untested status of serologic studies, there have been no epidemiologic studies of population groups. Nevertheless the increasing frequency of recognition of pulmonary cryptococcosis, the knowledge that pulmonary disease may be present without producing a density in the chest x-ray, the presence of morphologically typical but nonviable organisms in some pulmonary lesions, and the frequency with which airborne exposure must occur in certain areas all suggest that cryptococcosis is much more common and benign than is generally thought.

Pathogenesis and Pathology

Little is known about host-parasite relations in human cryptococcosis. Normal human serum has been shown to have an inhibitory effect upon the growth of cryptococci as well as some other fungi. This inhibitory effect is presumably unrelated to specific antibodies. Vogel et al., utilizing the fluorescent antibody technique, demonstrated the presence of antibody not only in the serums of patients with cryptococcosis, but also in 8 per cent of 339 persons who were considered to be either normal or without fungal disease. Absorption of such positive serums with *Candida albicans* and several other yeasts did not remove the antibody. When factors influencing immunization and subsequent challenge were rigidly controlled, Abrahams and Gilleran were able to demonstrate a significant degree of acquired immunity in mice immunized with formalin-killed vaccine. Both specific and nonspecific immunity may be important in determining the establishment of infection after exposure to *C. neoformans.* The idea that "normal" people do not acquire cryptococcosis is inconsistent with observed data.

So far as is known, there is no systematic study of the histopathology and pathogenesis of experimental pulmonary cryptococcosis in anthropoids. Several different types of lesion are seen in resected and necropsied human lungs. Factors in host and parasite can be correlated with the morphologic expression of infection only by uncertain inference.

The smallest, presumably primary, lesion observed by the writer was immediately subpleural in the costophrenic sinus, 3 mm. in diameter, and had a thin rim of calcium with a semiliquid center containing a few organisms morphologically typical of cryptococci when stained by a modification of the Rhinehart and Abul-Haj method for acid mucopolysaccharides. It was associated with pneumonic cryptococcois extending outward from the hilus of the same lung in a girl being treated with corticosteroids for rheumatic carditis. No other calcific lesion has been seen.

Figure 18 shows a nodule, presumably early and active. Such nodules have no trace of encapsulation, very little fibrosis, and a central mucoid appearance. Microscopically, the central portion of the nodule contained innumerable cryptococci of 2 to 6 microns in diameter with thin capsules. Most of the organisms were apparently free within relatively normal alveolar spaces, but some were within the cytoplasm of greatly distended and distorted histiocytes. No other inflammatory cells were present. Near the periphery of the nodule, single and clustered organisms were present, free or in histiocytes, and had definite and often heavy encapsulation, as shown in Figure 19.

Active, disseminating pulmonary lesions, nodular or pneumonic, are likely to resemble the subpleural nodule shown in Figure 18. "Coin" and mass lesions, more or less stable by roentgenographic criteria, are, in my experience, associated with a rubbery, neoplastic gross appearance and a relatively dense fibrotic reaction microscopically. Judging from the microscopic appearance of the cryptococci in densely fibrotic lesions and the results of a few cultural studies, it may well be that the fibrotic lesion is a manifestation of successful host response to infection.

Large pneumonic lesions may show areas of actively dividing, thinly encapsulated and relatively small cryptococci which are interspersed with larger areas of predominant fibrosis. Haugen and Baker were unable to determine any histologic criteria which they could correlate with the presence or absence of dissemination, but of nine patients with either small or "larger" subpleural nodules, only two had extrapulmonary cryptococcosis.

Multiple, small lesions containing giant cells, lymphocytes, central necrosis and many thinly encapsulated organisms may be found in acutely disseminated pulmonary cryptococcosis and in patients with presumably opportunistic infections associated with diffuse neoplasia, or its treatment. Both these lesions and the densely

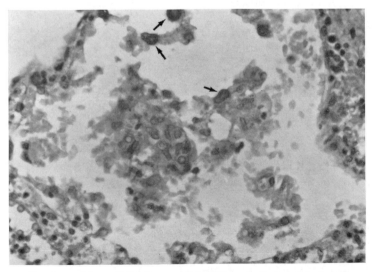

FIGURE 47–19. Cryptococci in a pulmonary nodule. The arrows point to heavily encapsulated organisms, 2 of which are budding. Thinly encapsulated forms are seen intracellularly in the center of the field. Mucicarmine stain.

fibrotic lesions may escape proper recognition unless mucicarmine or, even better, Mowry acid mucopolysaccharide staining is done.

Treatment

The natural history of pulmonary cryptococcosis is not sufficiently well known to permit dogmatism in relation to therapy. Solid cryptococcal granulomas have been resected from a number of adults without postoperative medical treatment and without evidence of active cryptococcosis during several years of follow-up. Occasionally, however, resection of such lesions has been followed by recurrent cryptococcosis. The situation is further complicated by the lack of information about either adequate dosage or the duration of treatment with amphotericin B, the only effective agent available at this time.

On a purely empirical basis the following guide-lines have been established. Regardless of the type of lesion present, if any material obtained for study is positive culturally for *Cryptococcus neoformans*, the patient should receive treatment with amphotericin B. If the diagnosis has been established by lung biopsy and cultures of the biopsy are negative, the patient is observed rather than treated. If cultures have not been made at biopsy, decision is based upon the morphologic appearance of the lesion and the cryptococci unless pleural or parenchymal complications appear in the early postoperative period. All patients with a cultural or histopathologic diagnosis of pulmonary cryptococcosis should have a spinal fluid examination. Asymptomatic involvement of the central nervous system may be present, and if so, the recommendations for treatment would require modification.

For uncomplicated pulmonary cryptococcosis in a patient who appears to be metabolically and immunologically normal, two to three months of treatment with amphotericin at an individual dosage level not exceeding 0.6 mg. per kilogram of body weight is probably adequate. If there is evidence of central nervous system involvement, treatment should be more intensive and extensive. Treatment with amphotericin B is discussed separately (see p. 620).

Prevention

No specific preventive measures have been developed. Although some degree of immunity can be produced experimentally by vaccines, there has been nothing to suggest that immunization would be a useful preventive measure from the public health point of view. It seems probable that children should not be closely associated with the care and raising of pigeons.

REFERENCES

Abrahams, I., and Gilleran, T. G.: Studies on Actively Acquired Resistance to Experimental Cryptococcosis in Mice. *J. Immunol.,* 85:629, 1960.

Anderson, H. W.: Yeast-Like Fungi of the Human Intestinal Tract. *J. Infect. Dis.,* 21: 341, 1917.

Aschner, M., Mager, J., and Leibowitz, J.: Production of Extracellular Starch in Cultures of Capsulated Yeasts. *Nature,* 156:295, 1945.

Baker, R. D., and Haugen, R. K.: Tissue Changes and Tissue Diagnosis in Cryptococcosis; A Study of 26 Cases. *Am. J. Clin. Path.,* 25:14, 1955.

Barron, C. N.: Cryptococcosis in Animals. *J. Am. Vet. M.A.,* 127:125, 1955.

Benham, R. W.: Cryptococci—Their Identification by Morphology and by Serology. *J. Infect. Dis.,* 57:255, 1935.

Idem: The Genus Cryptococcus: The Present Status and Criteria for the Identification of Species. *Tr. New York Acad. Sc.,* 17:418, 1955.

Benham, R. W., and Hopkins, A. M.: Yeastlike Fungi Found on the Skin and in the Intestines of Normal Subjects. *Arch. Derm. & Syph.,* 28:532, 1933.

Berk, M., and Gerstl, B.: Torulosis (Cryptococcosis) Producing a Solitary Pulmonary Lesion; Report of a Four Year Cure with Lobectomy. *J.A.M.A.,* 149:1310, 1952.

Black, R. A., and Fisher, C. V.: Cryptococcic Bronchopneumonia. *Am. J. Dis. Child.,* 54: 81, 1937.

Carter, H. S., and Young, J. L.: Note on the Isolation of *Cryptococcus Neoformans* from a Sample of Milk. *J. Path. & Bact.*, 62:271, 1950.

Cohen, J. R., and Kaufman, W.: Systemic Cryptococcosis; A Report of a Case with Review of the Literature. *Am. J. Clin. Path.*, 22: 1069, 1952.

Collins, V. P., Gelhorn, A., and Trimble, J. R.: The Coincidence of Cryptococcosis and Disease of the Reticulo-endothelial and Lymphatic Systems. *Cancer*, 4:883, 1951.

Cox, L. B., and Tolhurst, J. C.: *Human Torulosis; A Clinical, Pathological, and Microbiological Study with a Report of Thirteen Cases.* Melbourne, Australia, Melbourne University Press, 1946.

Debré, R., and others: Sur la torulose. Etude clinique et expérimentale (à propos d'un cas observé chez un enfant atteint de lymphogranulomatose maligne). *Ann. paediat.*, 168: 1, 1947.

Dezest, G.: Torulose spontanée chez le cobaye. *Ann. Inst. Pasteur*, 85:131, 1953.

Dormer, B. A., Friedlander, J., Wiles, F. J., and Simson, F. W.: Tumor of the Lung Due to Cryptococcus Histolyticus (Blastomycosis). *J. Thoracic Surg.*, 14:322, 1945.

Drouhet, E., and Couteau, M.: Sur les variations sectorielles des colonies de *Torulopsis neoformans. Ann. Inst. Pasteur*, 80:456, 1951.

Durant, J. R., Epifano, L. B., and Eyer, S. W.: Pulmonary Cryptococcosis: Treatment with Amphotericin B. *Ann. Int. Med.*, 58:534, 1960.

Emmons, C. W.: The Isolation from Soil of Fungi which Cause Disease in Man. *Tr. New York Acad. Sc.*, 14:51, 1951.

Idem.: Isolation of Cryptococcus Neoformans from Soil. *J. Bact.*, 62:685, 1951.

Idem: *Cryptococcus Neoformans* Strains from a Severe Outbreak of Bovine Mastitis. *Mycopathol. et Mycol. Appl.*, 6:231, 1952.

Idem: Saprophytic Sources of *Cryptococcus Neoformans* Associated with the Pigeon (*Columbia Livia*). *Am. J. Hyg.*, 62:227, 1955.

Evans, E. E.: The Antigenic Composition of Cryptococcus Neoformans. I. A Serologic Classification by Means of the Capsular and Agglutination Reactions. *J. Immunol.*, 64: 423, 1950.

Evans, E. E., Sorensen, L. J., and Walls, K. W.: The Antigenic Composition of Cryptococcus Neoformans. V. A Survey of Cross-Reactions Among Strains of Cryptococcus and Other Antigens. *J. Bact.*, 66:287, 1953.

Froio, G. F., and Bailey, C. P.: Pulmonary Cryptococcosis; Report of a Case with Surgical Cure. *Dis. Chest*, 16:354, 1949.

Galindo, D. L., and Bohls, S. W.: Combined Pulmonary and Central Nervous System Cryptococcosis; A Case Report. *Mil. Surgeon*, 113:403, 1953.

Gendel, B. R., Ende, M., and Norman, S. L.: Cryptococcosis; A Review with Special Reference to Apparent Association with

Hodgkin's Disease. *Am. J. Med.*, 9:343, 1950.

Greening, R. R., and Menville, L. J.: Roentgen Findings in Torulosis; Report of Four Cases. *Radiology*, 48:381, 1947.

Hamilton, J. B., and Tyler, G. R.: Pulmonary Torulosis. *Radiology*, 47:149, 1946.

Hardaway, R. M., and Crawford, P. M.: Pulmonary Torulosis; A Report of a Case. *Ann. Int. Med.*, 9:334, 1935.

Haugen, R. K., and Baker, R. D.: The Pulmonary Lesions in Cryptococcosis, with Special Reference to Subpleural Nodules. *Am. J. Clin. Path.*, 24:1381, 1954.

Linden, I. H., and Steffen, C. G.: Pulmonary Cryptococcosis. *Am. Rev. Tuberc.*, 69:116, 1954.

Littman, M. L., and Schneierson, S. S.: Cryptococcus Neoformans in Pigeon Excreta in New York City. *Am. J. Hyg.*, 69:49, 1959.

Littman, M. L., and Zimmerman, L. E.: *Cryptococcosis.* New York, Grune & Stratton, Inc., 1956.

Lodder, J., and Kreger-Van Rij, N. J. W.: *The Yeasts, a Taxonomic Study.* New York, Interscience Publishers, 1952.

McConchie, I.: Torula Granuloma of the Lung. *Med. J. Australia*, 38:685, 1951.

McGrath, J. T.: Cryptococcosis of the Central Nervous System in Domestic Animals. *Am. J. Path.*, 30:651, 1954.

Moody, A. M.: Asphyxial Death Due to Pulmonary Cryptococcosis; A Case Report. *California Med.*, 67:105, 1947.

Neuhauser, E. B. D., and Tucker, A.: The Roentgen Changes Produced by Diffuse Torulosis in the Newborn. *Am. J. Roentgenol.*, 59:805, 1948.

Owen, M.: Generalized Cryptococcosis Simulating Hodgkin's Disease. *Texas State J. Med.*, 35:767, 1940.

Peroncini, J., Bence, A. E., Vaccarezza, O. A., and Aguero, J. G.: Torulosis bronquial y meningea. *Medicina Buenos Aires*, 9:363, 1949.

Pollock, A. Q., and Ward, L. M.: A Hemagglutination Test for Cryptococcosis. *Am. J. Med.*, 32:6, 1962.

Poppe, P. K.: Cryptococcosis of the Lung. Report of Two Cases with Successful Treatment by Lobectomy. *J. Thoracic Surg.*, 27:608, 1954.

Potenza, L., Rodriguez, C., and de Feo, M.: Torulopsis neoformans pleural; estudio clinico, patalogico, y micologico del primer caso observado en Venezuela. *Rev. san. y assist. social*, 16:195, 1951.

Procknow, J. J., Benfield, J. R., Rippon, J. W., Diener, C. F., and Archer, F. L.: Cryptococcal Hepatitis Presenting as a Surgical Emergency. *J.A.M.A.*, 191:269, 1965.

Ratcliffe, H. E., and Cook, W. R.: Cryptococcosis; Review of the Literature and Report of a Case with Initial Pulmonary Findings. *U.S. Armed Forces M.J.*, 1:957, 1950.

Reeves, D. L., Butt, E. M., and Hammack, R. W.:

Torula Infection of the Lungs and Central Nervous System; Report of Six Cases with Three Autopsies. *Arch. Int. Med.,* 68:57, 1941.

Rinehart, J. F., and Abul-Haj, S. K.: An Improved Method for Histologic Demonstration of Acid Mucopolysaccharides in Tissues. *A.M.A. Arch. Path.,* 52:189, 1951.

Schepel, J. A. C., and Carsjens, F. W.: Een geval van torulosis met localisatie in de longen. *Nederl. tijdschr. v. geneesk.,* 97:2723, 1953.

Seabury, J. H., and Dascomb, H. E.: Results of the Treatment of Systemic Mycoses. *J.A.M.A.,* 188:509, 1964.

Sheppe, W. M.: Torula Infection in Man. *Am. J.M. Sc.,* 167:91, 1924.

Smith, C. D., Ritter, R., Larsh, H. W., and Furcolow, M. L.: Infection of White Mice with Air Borne Cryptococcus Neoformans. *J. Bact.,* 87:1364, 1964.

Starr, K. W., and Geddes, B.: Pulmonary Torulosis. *Australian & New Zealand J. Surg.,* 18:212, 1949.

Susman, M. P: Torula (Cryptococcus) Infection of the Lung. *Australian & New Zealand J. Surg.,* 23:296, 1954.

Symmers, W. St. C.: Torulosis: A Case Mimicking Hodgkin's Disease and Rodent Ulcer and a Presumed Case of Pulmonary Torulosis with Acute Dissemination. *Lancet,* 265:1068, 1953.

Takos, M. J.: Experimental Cryptococcosis Produced by the Ingestion of Virulent Organisms. *New England J. Med.,* 254:598, 1956.

Takos, M. J., and Elton, N. W.: Spontaneous Cryptococcosis of Marmoset Monkeys in Panama A.M.A. *Arch. Path.,* 55:403, 1953.

Terplan, K.: Pathogenesis of Cryptococcic (Torula) Meningitis. *Am. J. Path.,* 24:712, 1948.

Wickerham, L. J., and Burton, K. A.: Carbon Assimilation Tests for the Classification of Yeasts. *J. Bact.,* 56:363, 1948.

Zimmerman, L. E.: Fatal Fungus Infections Complicating Other Diseases. *Am. J. Clin. Path.,* 25:26, 1955.

Zimmerman, L. E., and Rappaport, H.: Occurrence of Cryptococcosis in Patients with Malignant Disease of Reticuloendothelial System. *Am. J. Clin. Path.,* 24:1050, 1954.

OPPORTUNISTIC AND RARE PULMONARY MYCOSES

The designation "opportunistic fungus infection" has been used for those mycotic infections which develop in the presence of a major host abnormality which either predisposes to infection by fungi rarely pathogenic in normal man or makes possible reactivation of a latent or arrested infection. The basic abnormality may be genetic, acquired or iatrogenic. Commonly recognized factors in opportunism are metabolic and neoplastic diseases; treatment with radiation, antimetabolite, immunodepressive and anti-inflammatory drugs; prolonged or multiple antibiotic therapy; prolonged debilitating illness; burns and surgery; and such nosocomial factors as cutdowns, intravenous catheters and solution contamination.

Classification is related primarily to the host disorder and has broad, statistical implications. For example, diabetes mellitus has been present with North American blastomycosis, histoplasmosis and cryptococcosis in about the same incidence as in patients with tuberculosis. Diabetes is a predisposing factor to such infections, but these have not been considered *usually* opportunistic. Diabetic acidosis has been present in more than 25 per cent of the reported cases of mucormycosis, and this fungous disease is rare in the absence of a major host abnormality.

In the presence of severely impaired defenses the host may be invaded by almost any organism present in the external or internal environment. Unless the laboratory personnel are fully alerted, isolations of common saprophytes or unrecognized organisms may be classified as contaminants and discarded, even when present in blood cultures. The fungi which are considered briefly in this section are those which, although rare in children, have the potential for more frequent recognition.

Aspergillosis

The aspergilli are ubiquitous organisms whose spores are widely airborne. They are a common source of contamination in the laboratory, and may be found on all body surfaces and in the sputum. In culture this genus grows as a mycelium consisting of septate branching hyphae which give rise to aerial conidiophores terminally enlarged to form a vesicle bearing specialized cells (sterigmata) which give rise to chains of small spores (conidia). Some forms are ascosporic. In solid tissue and pus from closed spaces only the hyphae are seen, but the observation of dichotomous branching suggests the presence of this genus. Hyphal elements are usually scanty in ordinary sputum. In plugs of bronchial origin, in the content of pulmonary cavities and in cystic spaces within invaded lung, extensive hyphal elements may be seen together with spores and, occasionally, the vesicle with its sterigmata.

A number of species may be responsible for pulmonary infection, including *A. fumigatus, A. flavus, A. niveus, A. niger* and *A. nidulans*. Species identification is not simple, and undeniably pathogenic human isolates should be submitted for classification to a specialist in the field

Three clinical forms of pulmonary aspergillosis are recognized: the allergic, intracavitary aspergillomatous, and invasive parenchymal varieties. It is not certain whether allergic bronchopulmonary aspergillosis arises as a disease *sui generis* or is always secondary to asthma or bronchitis of other origin. The consensus is that intracavitary aspergilloma is always superimposed upon some anatomic defect. Invasive parenchymal disease, pulmonary or otherwise, occurs both as an opportunistic infection and as an infection unrelated to discernible predisposition.

Allergic bronchopulmonary aspergillosis is classically characterized by episodes of fever, wheezing, transient and often migratory pulmonary infiltration, and eosinophilia in the peripheral blood or sputum, or both. Aspergilli can usually be demonstrated in the sputum, but the immediate skin reactivity to cutaneous prick tests with *A. fumigatus* antigens is more important diagnostically. The explanation for the transient pulmonary infiltrates is, at present, unknown. No definite relation exists between the allergic form of aspergillosis and invasive parenchymal disease. Precipitins may be present in allergic bronchopulmonary aspergillosis, but are not essential for the diagnosis.

Intracavitary aspergilloma occurs as a complication of pulmonary cavitation or infarction due to other diseases in most, if not all, cases. As such, they represent a purely saprophytic adaptation. Immunologic study indicates that these infections are usually accompanied by the presence of species-specific precipitins in the patient's blood and a low incidence of immediate reactivity to skin-inoculated antigen. The frequency of hemoptysis and the high incidence of serum precipitins in patients with intracavitary aspergillomas, together with the demonstration of penetration of the cavitary pseudomembrane by aspergillus hyphae, suggest the possibility that this type of infection may be the precursor of dissemination if host factors are suitable.

The *clinical picture* of intracavitary aspergilloma has only two important features: hemoptysis or blood-streaking of the sputum and the roentgenographic findings. Bloody sputum can be expected from bronchiectatic cavities, but its occurrence and recurrence are not always explainable by assuming a purely saprophytic and inert role for the aspergillus. It is possible that the superficial pericavitary vessels are made to bleed by invasion of hyphae or by the secretory products of the fungus in the cavity.

The radiographic recognition of the fungus ball is well established. The relatively uniform density, separated from the wall of the cavity by a crescentic layer of air which shifts with change of position of the patient, is evidence of a "free-ball" within the cavity. Some aspergillomas are not freely movable within the cavity. Other fungi are capable of producing the same roentgenographic appearance. The development of intracavitary fungus balls may not follow a uniform pattern. The development of the aspergilloma is not always from the dependent portion of the cavity as might be expected. At times the ball may arise on the lateral or superior wall of the cavity and become freely movable only when mature.

Pulmonary aspergillosis which appears suddenly in an apparently normal person is so unusual that some authorities would

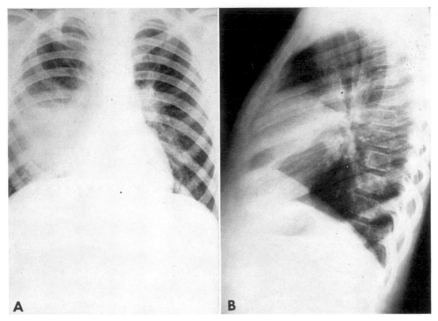

FIGURE 47–20. Invasive pulmonary aspergillosis. A 7½-year-old girl with a 2-week history of right chest pain and low-grade fever presented with a small subcutaneous mass just below the nipple at the time the films were taken. The right middle lobe pneumonia was due to *A. fumigatus,* which metastasized to the brain. The child recovered. *B,* Shows that the initial pneumonia was confined to the middle lobe. (Courtesy of P. E. Conen and *Dis. Chest,* 42:89, 1962.)

give it the special designation "primary aspergillosis." There are, as yet, no defining parameters for this type of infection. Any apparently normal person who has aspergillosis can be said to have "aspergillosis" or "primary aspergillosis," as one chooses. Figure 20 is illustrative of a pediatric patient with this disease.

Invasive aspergillosis is much more common as an opportunistic infection than as a disease in apparently normal children or adults. The most common host abnormality is leukemia, with Hodgkin's disease second in frequency. Of twenty cases of aspergillosis occurring in a cancer hospital, 30 per cent were in children under the age of ten years. It is of some interest that diabetes was also present in 15 per cent of the group. Invasive aspergillosis may be localized to a single organ, particularly as a terminal invader. Since the aspergilli tend to invade blood vessels, dissemination is frequent if the patient lives long enough.

Laboratory diagnosis may be difficult.

The clinical picture, together with cutaneous hypersensitivity, is the usual means of establishing the diagnosis of allergic aspergillosis. Aspergilli may or may not be isolated from the sputum.

Intracavitary aspergilloma is rarely seen in children. Aspergilli may or may not be recoverable from the sputum or bronchial washings. If the cavity is accessible, culture of needle aspirates will confirm the diagnosis if the aspergilli are viable. Serum precipitins are usually present.

Aspergilli are usually present in the sputum of patients with invasive pulmonary aspergillosis. The frequent isolation of aspergilli from the sputum of patients without aspergillosis is the real source of difficulty. Unless the laboratory is aware of the problem, aspergilli may not even be reported, simply being noted as "contaminants.' Whenever possible, it is advisable to isolate aspergilli from tissue, and demonstrate their presence therein by appropriate staining.

Invasive pulmonary aspergillosis is usually characterized by two types of microscopic pathology. The aspergilli tend to occur in colonies which are surrounded by wide zones of hemorrhage and necrosis. Hyphae can often be found within the lumen of blood vessels of all sizes. The walls of such vessels are necrotic, and the lumens are filled with thrombotic material which is frequently eosinophilic, similar to the lesions produced by mucormycosis.

More diffuse lesions or tiny clusters of hyphae may provoke a predominantly pyogenic response. The lesions look like microabscesses, but the tendency for capillary hemorrhage and septal necrosis is usually obvious at the periphery. Large colonies can be seen readily with hematoxylin and eosin staining, but more diffuse lesions, and the rare lesion characterized by a chronic productive reaction with fibrosis and giant cells, may escape detection unless special stains are used.

Treatment of allergic aspergillosis has not been satisfactory. Eradication of the aspergilli from the abnormal bronchial tree is not a simple matter. Treatment with large doses of iodides may be successful, but may produce hypokalemia and hyponatremia. Aerosols of Mycostatin and amphotericin B as well as intrabronchial instillations of these antibiotics have been used with varying success. The poor response to antifungal therapy is regarded by some authors as evidence against the relationship of the aspergilli to the allergic or bronchitic state.

Intracavitary aspergilloma may not require treatment, but if the patient is diabetic or has another major host abnormality, resection of the cavity is desirable. Repeated hemoptysis is also an indication for resection. Medical treatment is not indicated unless operation is impossible or has been complicated by empyema.

Invasive pulmonary aspergillosis probably should be resected whenever possible unless dissemination has already occurred. Medical treatment is not well defined, perhaps because of the variability in sensitivity of aspergilli to therapeutic agents.

There is sufficient evidence to warrant a trial of amphotericin B prior to surgical intervention. Occasionally the therapeutic response will be dramatic, making operation unnecessary. Amphotericin may be instilled directly into empyematous cavities.

Candidiasis

Pulmonary candidiasis, with or without candidemia, is produced more often by *Candida albicans* than by other species of the genus. It is a mistake to believe that all such infections are due to *C. albicans.* Yeast forms (blastospores) may be found intracellularly or extracellularly in exudates or the blood stream. Pseudohyphae or true hyphae are usually demonstrable extracellularly. In culture the Candida give rise to a yeastlike growth of blastospores with varying amounts of hyphae. Species identification on the basis of morphology alone is not reliable. Chlamydospore production is characteristic of *C. albicans* on special media, but chlamydospores may be produced occasionally by *C. stellatoidea* and *C. tropicalis.*

Pulmonary candidiasis is a rarity except as an opportunistic infection. In this form it is most frequently seen in premature or debilitated infants dying in the first year or two of life. Vaginal candidiasis in the mother has been considered an important source of infection in premature and full-term infants experiencing difficult and prolonged delivery. The evidence suggests that this is strictly an aspirational infection.

The most common factors predisposing to infection in children are neoplasia, particularly the leukemia-lymphoma group; administration of multiple antibiotics, or prolonged treatment with one; treatment with adrenocorticotropic hormone or corticosteroids; severe abnormalities of the blood proteins; and prolonged use of the same needle or an intravenous catheter for infusions. Since neither the x-ray nor clinical manifestations of pulmonary candidiasis are in any way specific, they are

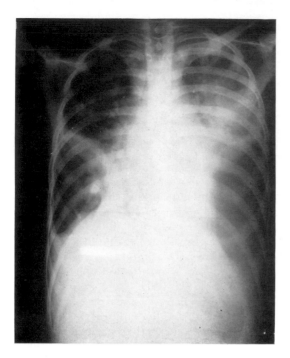

FIGURE 47–21. Opportunistic candidal pneumonia. This 12-year-old girl was being treated with multiple antibiotics for staphylococcal sepsis and pneumonia. Bilateral loculated empyemata had been converted to pyopneumothoraces by needle aspirations. The left upper lung had cleared until one day prior to the x-ray film shown here. Candidemia was present for 5 days. Treatment with amphotericin B controlled the candidemia and induced resolution of the pneumonia.

likely to be obscured by the pre-existing disease.

The signs and symptoms usually suggest either the persistence of bacterial infection or superinfection of a type not etiologically recognizable on clinical grounds. Fever is not always present, even during documented candidemia, but it is the most common sign. The appearance of fever or an increase in fever in a patient receiving antibiotic therapy for bacterial disease should always provoke consideration of opportunistic fungal infection. When pulmonary candidiasis is accompanied by fungemia, some children exhibit mental depression, psychomotor retardation, and toxic manifestations similar to those seen in typhoid fever. Pericarditis is not rare. In severely ill children, oral, cutaneous or urinary tract infection with Candida often precedes pulmonary invasion or fungemia. Such children should have frequent blood cultures so long as antibacterials or adrenocorticosteroids must be given. The pulmonary candidiasis shown in Figure 21 would have escaped proper recognition and treatment had not candidemia been present.

Although Candida are recognized easily by direct examination or staining, species identification from cultures is best done by the methods recommended by Wickerham. Candida are found so commonly in the sputum of patients with bronchopulmonary disease and those receiving antimicrobials, corticosteroids and immunodepressive agents that even repeated isolation of Candida in freshly produced sputum is not acceptable for diagnosis. Isolation from the blood stream, from closed collections of pus or from needle aspiration of pulmonary lesions can be accepted. Circulating antibodies and cutaneous reactivity to candidal antigens are so common among well persons that serologic methods are not helpful in diagnosis.

Candida are distributed throughout the world, and are found particularly in the alimentary tract. They are frequently present on the skin of hospitalized patients. Autopsy studies in patients with cancer suggest that the gastrointestinal tract is a common portal of entry. Candida are present frequently in the vagina in diabetic patients and in pregnant women.

Pathologically, hematogenous pulmonary candidiasis can be recognized by the presence of microabscesses or confluent lobular pneumonitis associated with thrombi containing Candida. As a general rule, the fungus will not be recognized unless periodic acid-Schiff or methenamine-silver stain is used. When the fungus is abundant, both Gram's stain and Giemsa's stain will be satisfactory.

In neonatal pulmonary candidiasis the infection is clearly bronchogenic. Hyphae and pseudohyphae with blastospores can be found within the bronchioles, often in larger bronchi, and growth can be traced out into the air sacs. In some instances there is a definite bronchopneumonia with polymorphonuclear neutrophilic reaction, considerable intra-alveolar fibrinous fluid, and some microabscesses. In other infants there may be practically no parenchymal reaction, indicating that there was aspiration shortly before death with postmortem growth of the fungus.

Although aerosolized nystatin or amphotericin B may be effective in controlling bronchial candidiasis, established pulmonary disease should be treated with intravenous administration of amphotericin B. If infection is recognized early and is secondary to antimicrobial therapy, ten to thirty daily infusions may be adequate. If antibacterial antibiotics or other predisposing drugs can be discontinued, the duration of antifungal therapy is usually less. Blood cultures should be made frequently, utilizing large amounts of broth relative to the size of inoculum; these should not be discarded as negative in less than four weeks. Persistent candidemia may be associated with endocarditis requiring prolonged administration of amphotericin B in maximum tolerated dosage.

Preventive measures are applicable only to infants and children at special risk. It has been suggested that pregnant women harboring Candida in the vagina be treated with topical candicidin near term. This seems unnecessary if normal delivery is anticipated. Infants and children with thrush should be treated orally with nystatin. Diabetic children who must re-

ceive antibacterial antibiotics should be given oral nystatin concomitantly. There are no studies which indicate that prophylaxis with nystatin is of value in children receiving immunodepressive therapy with drugs or x-rays, or those receiving corticosteroids with or without antibacterial antibiotics; the use of nystatin in these circumstances would seem rational.

Phycomycosis (Mucormycosis)

This class contains some fungi which are apparently only opportunistic and others which produce subcutaneous infection in normal persons. The former are the only ones known to involve the lung. All appear in the tissue as broad, nonseptate, irregularly branching hyphae. Although septation may occur among the phycomycetes, its definite presence in tissue sections eliminates the diagnosis without cultural verification.

Too few pulmonary infections have been culturally proved to be dogmatic about the genera involved, but it is probable that most have been in the family Mucoraceae. All grow as molds with coenocytic mycelium and specialized sporangia. A text on mycology should be consulted for generic identification.

The *clinical disease* is most commonly associated with keto-acidosis, leukemia, other neoplasms, and severe burns. Although it may appear first in the lung, primary infection in the paranasal sinuses with subsequent metastasis is relatively common. The clinical course is usually rapid and characterized by fever, cough, hemoptysis, and signs referable to other sites of involvement. Sudden pulmonary, cerebral or orbital signs of infection in any child in acidosis or with disseminated neoplasia should lead to consideration of phycomycosis. There are no helpful roentgenologic signs. In such a clinical setting the finding of a phycomycete in sputum, lung aspirate or other exudate should be sufficient evidence to prompt immediate therapy.

Laboratory diagnosis has been infrequent. The organisms involved are common in the environment, and merit little attention unless the laboratorian knows what is suspected. There is no difficulty in recognizing the phycomycetes in culture, but direct examination of sputum or other exudates is not likely to suggest the diagnosis except in patients with keto-acidosis. Cultural isolation of the Mucoraceae should be reported by the laboratory with the anticipation that the clinician is sufficiently informed to interpret the report.

The phycomycetes are ubiquitous in nature. It is obvious that the opportunity for infection is general. The rarity of infection is evidence of the importance of serious impairment of host resistance in pathogenesis. The portal of entry is not always found. Paranasal sinuses, the lungs and the gastrointestinal tract appear to be the common sites of entry for opportunistic infections.

The *pathology* produced in the lung is similar to aspergillosis. There is often more evidence of vascular invasion with thrombosis and necrosis. Suppuration is usually obvious and extensive, but coagulation necrosis predominates. The hyphae often stain well with hematoxylin and eosin, but the methenamine-silver method is more reliable.

Once the disease is recognized, *treatment* should be started with amphotericin B in maximum tolerated dosage if the underlying host abnormality is correctable. Correction of keto-acidosis may be extremely important, but treatment with amphotericin should not be delayed until after metabolic correction. Superficial infection of burns may be treated with topical amphotericin lotion to prevent deep tissue invasion or phycomycetic septicemia.

Rare Infections

In fungous infections which are known to involve children, but which have been reported rarely as primary pulmonary pathogens, *Sporotrichum schenkii* is the most likely to be found. *Sporotrichosis* of the extremities and face occurs in children, particularly in Central and South America. Dissemination occurs rarely. The fungus is present in soil, wood and many plants. Pulmonary infection in adults may be indolent or spontaneously regressive. The fungus grows well on ordinary laboratory media, being predominantly yeastlike in its growth at 37°C. and mycelial at room temperature. Tissue diagnosis can sometimes be made with periodic acid-Schiff staining, but the fluorescent antibody method is far better. The pulmonary infections are usually asymptomatic; the roentgen findings are those of a persistent patchy bronchopneumonia, and there may be pleural involvement. If treatment with a saturated solution of potassium iodide fails, amphotericin B is effective.

Geotrichosis is reportedly fairly common as a pulmonary or bronchopulmonary disease in certain parts of the world, particularly in Brazil. Geotrichum may be recovered from the sputum of many patients with chronic bronchitis, and it sometimes forms mucosal plaques which are grossly identical with the thrush produced by Candida. Except in Brazil, there is little evidence that Geotrichum is a significant pulmonary pathogen. Lacaz considers the association with bronchopulmonary symptoms to be that of an "associate" or secondary agent. It has been isolated from the blood stream of an infant and also an elderly man. The fungus is usually recognized by direct examination of the sputum if it is present in abundance. The hyphae are septate and narrow, and form arthrospores which are rectangular or elliptical and may resemble those of *Coccidioides immitis*. It grows easily on ordinary media as a rather soft, flat, white to tawny colony which is easily picked from the surface of the agar when grown at room temperature. These colonies will show large numbers of rectangular or elliptical arthrospores together with septate branching hyphae and spherical to subspherical cells which somewhat resemble the yeast form of Blastomyces. Oral potassium iodide therapy has been effective in eliminating the fungus from sputum in many cases. If the fungus were definitely identified in pulmonary biopsies or lung aspirates, the patient should be treated with amphotericin B.

Torulopsis glabrata is a rare cause of fungemia in man; one case of bronchopneumonia associated with this organism has been reported in a ten-year-old boy. Its most common recovery from human sources has been in cultures of urine. *Torulopsis glabrata* grows readily on ordinary media, producing colonies which are smooth and yeastlike in form and white to brownish in color. The cells are ovoid and usually between 3 and 5 microns in dimension. It must be differentiated from Candida and yeasts which might be isolated from human sources. The work of Wickerham should be consulted for the details of identification. In experimental infections in animals, *T. glabrata* grows intracellularly and may be confused with *Histoplasma capsulatum*.

Another asporogenous yeast which has been reported to produce disseminated disease in an infant is *Rhodotorula mucilagnosa*. This yeast may resemble Cryptococcus when seen in body fluids. Cells are round to oval, occasionally elongate, and may produce a scanty amount of pseudomycelium in culture as does Cryptococcus. It reproduces by budding. Cultures may easily be differentiated from Cryptococcus or Torulopsis by means of the red or yellow pigment which colors the colonies.

One would expect that both *T. glabrata* and *R. mucilagnosa* would be sensitive to amphotericin B. At present this antibiotic is the agent of choice in proved pulmonary infections due to either genus.

REFERENCES

Berkel, I., Say, B., and Tinaztepe, B.: Pulmonary Aspergillosis in a Child with Leukemia. Report of a Case and a Brief Review of the Pediatric Literature. *New England J. Med.*, 269:893, 1963.

Baker, R. D.: Leukopenia and Therapy in Leukemia as Factors Predisposing to Fatal My-coses: Mucormycosis, Aspergillosis, and Cryptococcosis. *Am. J. Clin. Path.*, 37:358, 1962.

Baum, G. L.: Significance of Candida Albicans in Human Sputum. *New England J. Med.*, 263:70, 1960.

Borowski, J., Dziedzinszko, A., Mierzejewskki, W., Dubrzynska, T., and Iwanowski, K.: Epidemiology of *Candida Albicans* Infection in Newborn Infants. *Proc. Inter. Symp. Med. Mycol.*, 1963, pp. 133-5.

Burrow, G. N., Salmon, R. B., and Nolan, J. P.: Successful Treatment of Cerebral Mucorcycosis with Amphotericin B. *J.A.M.A.*, 183:370, 1963.

Campbell, M. J., and Clayton, Y. M.: Bronchopulmonary Aspergillosis. Correlation of the Clinical and Laboratory Findings in 272 Patients Investigated for Bronchopulmonary Aspergillosis. *Am. Rev. Resp. Dis.*, 89:186, 1964.

Cawley, E. P.: Aspergillosis and the Aspergilli: Report of a Unique Case of the Disease. *Arch. Int. Med.*, 80:423, 1947.

Conen, P. E., Walker, G. R., Turner, J. A., and Field, P.: Invasive Primary Aspergillosis of the Lung with Cerebral Metastasis and Complete Recovery. *Dis. Chest*, 43:88, 1962.

Crichlow, D. K., Traub, F. B., and Silver, W.: Aspergillosis Due to *Aspergillus Fumigatus* in an Infant. *Bact. Proc.*, 60:138, 1960.

Darja, M., and Davy, M. I.: Pulmonary Mucorcycosis with Cultural Identification. *Canad. M.A.J.*, 89:1235, 1963.

Finegold, S. M., Will, D., and Murray, J. F.: Aspergillosis. *Am. J. Med.*, 27:463, 1959.

Gruhn, J. G., and Sanson, J.: Mycotic Infections in Leukemic Patients at Autopsy. *Cancer*, 16:61, 1963.

Harris, J. S.: Mucormycosis. *Pediatrics*, 16:857, 1955.

Hutter, R. V. P., and Collins, H. S.: The Occurrence of Opportunistic Fungus Infections in a Cancer Hospital. *Lab. Invest.*, 11:1035, 1962.

Kroetz, F. W., Leonard, J. J., and Everett, C. R.: Candida Albicans Endocarditis Successfully Treated with Amphotericin B. *New England J. Med.*, 266:592, 1962.

Louria, D. B., and Dineen, P.: Amphotericin B in Treatment of Disseminated Moniliasis. *J.A.M.A.*, 174:273, 1960.

Louria, D. B., Greenberg, S. M., and Molander, D. W.: Fungemia Caused by Certain Nonpathogenic Strains of the Family Cryptococcaceae. *New England J. Med.*, 263:1281, 1960.

Lupin, A. M., Dascomb, H. E., Seabury, J. H., and McGinn, M.: Experience with *Candida* Recovered from Venous Blood. *Antimicrob. Agents Chemother.*, 1961, pp. 10-19.

Mikkelsen, W. M., Brandt, R. L., and Harrell, E. R.: Sporotrichosis: Report of 12 Cases,

Including Two with Skeletal Involvement. *Ann. Int. Med.,* 47:435, 1957.

Pepys, J., Riddell, R. W., Citron, K. M., Clayton, Y. M., and Short, E. I.: Clinical and Immunologic Significance of Aspergillus Fumigatus in the Sputum. *Am. Rev. Resp. Dis.,* 80:167, 1959.

Ramirez-R., J.: Pulmonary Aspergilloma: Endobronchial Treatment. *New England J. Med.,* 271:1281, 1964.

Ridgeway, N. A., Whitcomb, F. C., Erickson, E. E., and Law, S. W.: Primary Pulmonary Sporotrichosis. *Am. J. Med.,* 32:153, 1962.

Riopedre, R. N., Cesare, I. de, Miatello, E., Caria, M. A., and Zapater, R. C.: Aislamiento de *Rhodotorula mucilagnosa* del l. c. r., heces, orina, exudado faringuo y piel de un lactante de tres meses. *Rev. Assoc. Med. Argent.,* 74:1430, 1960.

Scott, S. M., Peasley, E. D., and Crymes, R. P.: Pulmonary Sporotrichosis: Report of Two Cases with Cavitation. *New England J. Med.,* 265:453, 1961.

Seabury, J. H., and Dascomb, H. E.: Results of the Treatment of Systemic mycoses. *J.A.M.A.,* 188:509, 1964.

Seabury, J. H., and Samuels, M.: Pathogenetic Spectrum of Aspergillosis. *Am. J. Clin. Path.,* 40:1, 1963.

Shelburne, P. F., and Carey, R. J.: Rhodotorula Fungemia Complicating Staphylococcal Endocarditis. *J.A.M.A.,* 180:38, 1962.

Shurtleff, D. B., Peterson, W., and Sherris, J. C.: Systemic *Candida Tropicalis* Infection Treated with Amphotericin. *New England J. Med.,* 269:1112, 1963.

Symmers, W. St. C.: Histopathologic Aspects of the Pathogenesis of Some Opportunistic Fungal Infections, as Exemplified in the Pathology of Aspergillosis and the Phycomycetoses. *Lab. Invest.,* 11:1073, 1962.

Utz, J. P., German, J. L., Louria, D. B., Emmons, C. W., and Bartter, F. C.: Pulmonary Aspergillosis with Cavitation: Iodide Therapy Associated with an Unusual Electrolyte Disturbance. *New England J. Med.,* 260:264, 1959.

Wickerham, L. J.: Apparent Increase in Frequency of Infections Involving *Torulopsis Glabrata.* Procedure for Its Identification. *J.A.M.A.,* 165:47, 1957.

Idem: Taxonomy of Yeasts. U.S. Dept. of Agr. Tech. Bull. 1029, 1961, pp. 1-61.

TREATMENT OF SYSTEMIC MYCOSES WITH AMPHOTERICIN B

Amphotericin B is an antibiotic inhibitory to many fungi and Leishmania, with maximal activity against the yeastlike fungi. Its greatest effectiveness is in the treatment of the blastomycoses, cryptococcosis, histoplasmosis, coccidioidomycosis, candidiasis and disseminated sporotrichosis. It is sometimes useful in infections due to Aspergillus, Mucor and Rhizopus.

Absorption from the gastrointestinal tract is irregular and poor at best. Intramuscular injection is ineffective. The antibiotic can be administered by aerosolization, but there is no acceptable evidence that it is effective when given by this route. Amphotericin B (Fungizone) is used for intravenous administration after dilution with 5 per cent dextrose injection, U.S.P. Each ampule contains 50 mg. of amphotericin B in combination with sodium desoxycholate and phosphate buffers. When reconstituted with 10 ml. of sterile water for injection, U.S.P., a clear colloidal suspension is obtained by shaking, provided the water for injection contains no preservative. A sufficient volume of the reconstituted solution, now diluted to 5 mg. per milliliter, is added to 5 per cent dextrose injection, U.S.P., to give a final concentration of 0.1 mg. of amphotericin B per milliliter.

The diluted solution should be infused over a period of three to four hours. The pediatric scalp vein needle set is satisfactory; *scalp veins should be avoided.* Close observation during the infusion is necessary to detect undesirable reactions and to prevent infiltration of the solution outside of the vein.

By careful regulation of the rate of intravenous infusion, the concentration may be doubled (to 0.2 mg. per milliliter) if the volume of infusate must be restricted.

Dosage and Duration

Neither the optimum total or daily dosage nor the minimal effective duration of treatment has been established for any of the deep mycoses. Dosage is determined primarily by tolerance, and the duration of treatment by clinical judgment.

For disease of average severity an initial infusion of 1 mg. is preferable. If well tolerated, a dose of 0.25 mg. per kilogram is given the following day. The dose is increased by 1 or 2 mg. daily or every other day for infants and small children. The increments of dosage may be doubled for patients weighing more than 30 kg. Whether the dosage is increased daily or every other day is determined entirely by side effects and toxicity. The maintenance dose has been determined primarily by the degree of azotemia and side effects. For patients with coccidioidomycosis, mucormycosis and aspergillosis, the maximum recommended daily dose of 1.5 mg. per kilogram should be administered if possible. A smaller maintenance dose (0.5 and 1.0 mg. per kilogram) is adequate for the treatment of other mycoses of average severity. Once maintenance dosage is achieved, one may elect to administer amphotericin on alternate days or daily, depending upon the judgment of the clinician and the toxicity of the drug to the patient.

Dangerously ill patients may be given 0.33 mg. per kilogram of amphotericin B the first day, 0.66 mg. the second day, and 1 mg. the third day by incorporating either 2 mg. per kilogram of the sodium succinate ester of hydrocortisone or the equivalent of prednisolone sodium hemisuccinate in the infusion. Steroid dosage must be maintained for seven to ten days and then gradually reduced to the level at which mild reactions appear. Rapid achievement of maintenance dosage is accompanied by a prompt rise in the blood urea nitrogen level in most patients.

Except for opportunistic infections, treatment is maintained for several months. Two months is considered to be a minimum period for established pulmonary mycoses. Changes in the chest x-ray are useful as a guide to the duration of therapy only when clearing is progressive. Chronic infections with fibrosis or cavitation often stabilize without much change by x-ray film even after four months of treatment. Culture of bronchial exudate or other available material may indicate the presence of resistant organisms or inadequate dosage, but is not a good guide for the duration of treatment. Cultures usually become negative within two weeks of maintenance of adequate dosage. A significant decrease in titer of complement-fixing antibody also is of help when pretreatment serology has been positive, but, in the last analysis, it is the physician's assessment of the patient's response to treatment which determines when therapy should be stopped. As a general rule, the total dose of amphotericin should be about 50 mg. per kilogram of body weight.

Toxicity and Side Effects

The intravenous administration of amphotericin B is accompanied by a variety of side effects and variable toxicity. Flushing, diaphoresis and general malaise are common during the first week or two of treatment, but are of no consequence.

Chills and fever are usual, particularly in the early phase of treatment or whenever dosage is increased. They may be reduced by premedication with acetylsalicylic acid, and generally diminish or disappear after the maintenance dosage level has been reached. Recrudescence of chills and fever without alteration of dosage has been observed when the production lot number of amphotericin was changed. Fever of some degree usually persists if the interval between infusions is greater than two days.

Anorexia is common during prolonged or high-dosage treatment. It is most intense during and for several hours after infusion. For this reason it is advisable to infuse early in the morning or late in the evening.

Headache and nausea are usually mild and transient. Nausea and vomiting are more common during prolonged or high-dosage therapy. Premedication with intramuscular trimethobenzamide (Tigan) is frequently helpful in the control of vomiting. It may become necessary to reduce the daily dose or give infusions on alternate days. If anorexia, nausea and vomiting are persistent, one should suspect the presence of hypokalemia.

Hypokalemia has appeared in approximately 25 per cent of our patients treated in the past four years. An occasional patient offers no complaints during significant hypokalemia, but the majority complain of anorexia, nausea, vomiting and muscular weakness. Since hypokalemia may produce renal and muscular damage, prevention or prompt replacement of potassium deficit is an important adjunct to amphotericin B therapy. The serum electrolytes should be determined semiweekly. Hypokalemia may occur without nitrogen retention. Once hypokalemia occurs, large amounts of potassium may be required in order to correct it. Potassium supplementation is usually necessary even after hypokalemia has been corrected. Oral potassium medications may be of value in some patients, but they are usually insufficient for the correction of hypokalemia. It has been necessary to give as much as 160 mEq. of potassium chloride intravenously per day to some adult patients for several days before electrolyte balance was restored. The potassium chloride solution is much more irritating to veins than is amphotericin itself, and this may present a serious problem in treatment.

Hyponatremia is an uncommon complication of therapy; it is easily corrected by increasing sodium intake orally or parenterally.

Renal toxicity is a great concern during intravenous therapy with amphotericin. The most serious effect is nephrocalcinosis, which fortunately seldom, if ever, occurs in patients treated with the average dosage. None of our patients has shown clinical evidence of impaired renal function, but several have maintained slight elevation of the blood urea nitrogen level during several years of post-treatment observation. The usual changes in renal morphology are similar to the tubular changes seen in hypokalemic nephropathy; some observers have emphasized the importance of glomerular involvement.

Nitrogen retention is a common manifestation of renal toxicity. Rapid achievement of maintenance dosage is almost always accompanied by an abrupt rise in the blood urea nitrogen level. For unknown reasons, the incidence of nitrogen retention among our patients increased when the colloidal suspension of amphotericin B replaced the insoluble suspension, and there has been a further increase in incidence since 1961. The administration of amphotericin is continued without reduction of dosage unless the blood urea nitrogen level exceeds 40 mg. per 100 ml. A reduction of the daily dose by approximately 30 per cent generally results in significant lowering of the blood urea nitrogen level. If reduction in dosage does not decrease nitrogen retention satisfactorily, it may be necesary to interrupt treatment for as long as two or three weeks. Whenever dosage is interrupted for more than a week, it is advisable to resume therapy at a level of 0.25 mg. per kilogram of body weight. The blood urea nitrogen or nonprotein nitrogen level should be determined semiweekly.

If intravenous treatment must be interrupted for several weeks, or if relapse dictates retreatment, therapy should be approached with caution. Initial reactions to amphotericin during retreatment have frequently been more severe than during the first course.

Cramping abdominal pain, usually epigastric, has accompanied or followed intravenous infusion of amphotericin during a part of the therapeutic course in approximately 25 per cent of our patients. Feces may contain occult blood, and frank melena and hematemesis have been observed. Hemorrhagic gastroenteritis may occur, as is reported in dogs. If melena or hematemesis occurs, treatment should be interrupted.

Normochromic, normocytic anemia occurs routinely during the course of treatment. It usually stabilizes at a level which does not require transfusion (hematocrit level approximately 26 to 28 per cent), but an occasional patient will benefit from blood. This toxic manifestation seems to be of little clinical importance, and no patient has had persistent or progressive anemia after treatment was terminated.

Phlebitis is considered to be a frequent side effect of intravenous infusion with amphotericin. The low incidence in our own series may be due in part to the relatively short duration of infusion, and in part to the use of dextrose solutions near neutrality. Commercially prepared dextrose solutions often have a pH less than 5.0. If the solution is allowed to infiltrate into or beyond the wall of the vein, phlebitis will occur. This is an avoidable complication.

Cyanosis may accompany severe chills and fever during the intravenous treatment of infants. It is doubted whether this is specifically related to amphotericin B, since it has been observed with pyretotherapy with intravenous typhoid vaccine. If this side effect occurs, 100 per cent oxygen should be administered.

Although clonic muscular contractions and convulsions have been observed during severe reactions to intravenous amphotericin therapy, these have been due to improper administration. Uneven and rapid infusion should be avoided.

Hypersensitivity, as to any antibiotic, may occur. It is apparently uncommon, and should be managed as any hypersensitivity reaction to an antibiotic. As a general rule, concomitant corticosteroid administration will be indicated.

Chills and fever may be greatly decreased or abolished by adding approximately 25 mg. (0.25 to 1.0 mg. per kilogram) of hydrocortisone sodium succinate to the infusion fluid. Headache, nausea and anorexia are decreased by corticosteroids, but are not usually abolished. Corticosteroids should not be routinely administered to patients receiving amphotericin intravenously. If reactions are severe, or if maintenance dosage must be reached rapidly, corticosteroids are given. The relatively large initial dose can be reduced gradually after seven to ten days to the level at which mild reactions appear. If at all possible, corticosteroids in any amount should be avoided for patients with coccidioidomycosis. Corticosteriods in the doses recommended have produced no deleterious effect on the course of any of our patients with systemic mycoses.

REFERENCES

Bell, N. H., Andriole, V. T., Sabesin, S. M., and Utz, J. P.: On the Nephrotoxicity of Amphotericin B in Man. *Am. J. Med.*, 33:64, 1962.

Hildick-Smith, G., Blank, H., and Sarkany, I.: *Fungus Diseases and Their Treatment,* Boston, Little, Brown and Co., 1964.

Reynolds, E. S., Tomkeiwicz, Z. M., and Dammin, G. J.: The Renal Lesion Related to Amphotericin B Treatment for Coccidioidomycosis. *Med. Clin. N. Amer.*, 47:1149, 1963.

Seabury, J. H.: Experience with Amphotericin B. *Chemotherapia*, 3:2, 1961.

Seabury, J. H., and Dascomb, H. E.: Experience with Amphotericin B for Treatment of Systemic Mycoses. *Arch. Int. Med.*, 102:960, 1958.

CHAPTER FORTY-EIGHT

Histoplasmosis

AMOS CHRISTIE, M.D.

Pulmonary histoplasmosis is the most prevalent systemic fungous infection. Despite this fact, the disease is still poorly understood by many. Variations in its spectrum are frequently mistaken, overlooked, or misdiagnosed as other disease processes, probably because the wide variety of manifestations caused by parasitization of tissue by *Histoplasma capsulatum* is not sufficiently appreciated by clinicians. Although the scope of this chapter must of necessity emphasize pulmonary histoplasmosis in childhood, it will be necessary to broaden the description of the disease spectrum of human histoplasmosis in order to give the student or the clinician a concept of the pathogenesis as well as the signs and symptoms of this interesting and pleomorphic diease. Its manifestations cut through each specialty and subspecialty of clinical medicine and pediatrics, and it may well be designated as the "great masquerader" of the present.

History

The organism was first described by Darling in Panama in 1906. He observed it in sections of tissue taken at the time of postmortem examination in cases which appeared to be leishmaniasis. Consequently, the organism was thought to be a protozoan. The first case reported in North America was that by Watson and Riley in 1926, but it remained for Demonbrum at Vanderbilt University in 1934 to demonstrate conclusively the fungous origin of this disease by brilliant use of transmission and cultural methods. Until 1945 histoplasmosis was thought to be a systemic fungous disease which was uniformly progressive and fatal. Since that time conclusive evidence has accumulated that there are benign or intermediate forms of the disease as well as the fatal disseminated form. A comprehensive historical review of histoplasmosis has been published by Schwartz and Baum.

General Considerations

Histoplasmosis is caused by the fungus *Histoplasma capsulatum*. This organism grows in two forms according to its environment. Although it is found free in nature in certain soils, particularly in those which have been exposed to avian excreta, it grows in its mycelial form in culture media producing a cottony white mass at room temperature. When properly examined, the tuberculate chlamydospore will be apparent. This is the identifying feature of the fungus. It ap-

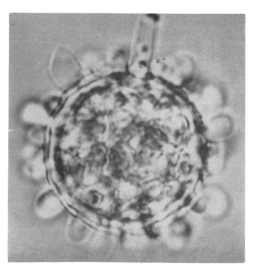

FIGURE 48–1. Tuberculate chlamydospore from a mycelial culture.

pears in the picturesque language of Demonbrum as the "Teutonic war club" (Fig. 1). No other fungi are known to have this feature. Confusion of *Histoplasma capulatum* with any other pathogenic fungi is, therefore, impossible. There are strain differences, however, and the organism produces several antigens: e.g. there is a complement-fixing antigen and a skin test antigen.

In tissue, and when grown on certain forms of enriched culture media at 37°C., the fungus appears as a yeast cell, usually 3 to 5 microns in diameter. In pathologic sections with ordinary stains the yeast cell has a definite border, a capsule and a crescent of deeply stained cytoplasma (Fig. 2) which is the descriptive origin of the term *Histoplasma capsulatum*. *Histoplasma capsulatum* is not a particularly fastidious organism, although it grows slowly on any medium. It has been grown in our laboratory on Sabouraud's dextrose media between wide limits of pH. A more complete medium is that enriched with blood or plasma to which antibiotics have been added. It was originally thought that this was necessary to inhibit the growth of pyogenic organisms so that the rather slow-growing *Histoplasma capsulatum* could emerge. There is now evidence that adequate amounts of antibiotics and

plasma may be necessary for its ideal growth requirements. This, of course, has some therapeutic implications which will be pointed out later.

The fungus not only has been found in the soil, but also has been positively identified in a wide variety of animals. There is no evidence of transmission from animal to man, animal to animal or man to man. Evidence has accumulated that there is probably contamination of the soil with an intermediate saprophytic phase. Infection of man occurs then by inhalation or ingestion, or by both means.

The geographic distribution is interesting. Although histoplasmosis is worldwide, more than half of the recorded disseminated progressive cases have occurred in states that correspond to the area of the Western Appalachian slope and those bordering on the tributaries of the Ohio, Missouri and Mississippi rivers. These represent the endemic areas in this country as evidenced by sensitivity to histoplasmin (Fig. 3). This area has variously been described as avocado- or pear-shaped, the base of which is in Arkansas and Georgia, tapering off along the Western Appalachian slope with the apex in New York State. In addition, endemic foci have been identified in other parts of the country, as far north as Minnesota and

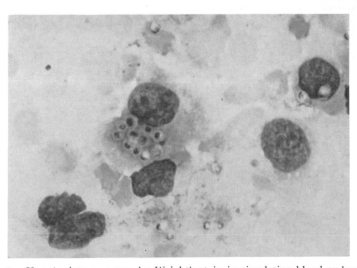

FIGURE 48–2. *H. capsulatum* as seen by Wright's stain in circulating blood or bone marrow.

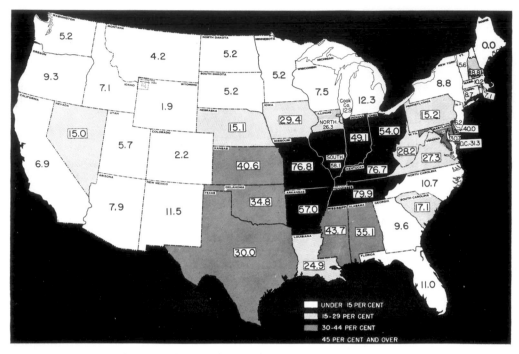

FIGURE 48–3. Prevalence of histoplasmin sensitivity in residents of the United States, by states.

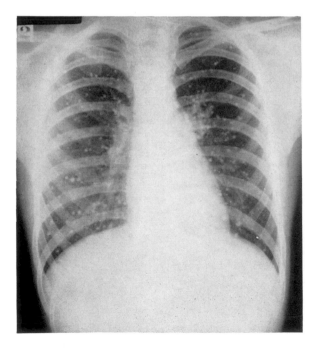

FIGURE 48–4. Healed "miliary tuberculosis" of yesteryear, now well established as healed miliary histoplasmosis. Histoplasmin-positive, tuberculin-negative.

central Pennsylvania. The distribution is more worldwide than is generally appreciated. There are parts of southern Europe, Africa, and Central and South America in which histoplasmin sensitivity is relatively high, and clinical cases have been reported from these regions.

Whenever the prevalence of histoplasmin sensitivity has been demonstrated, calcification in nonreactors to tuberculin has also been shown to be prevalent (Fig. 4).

Pathology

For those who have had an opportunity to study the interesting features of this disease, it is tempting to correlate the pathologic picture with the immunologic maturity of the patient. In the young infant the hallmark of the pathologic picture is the presence of large mononuclear phagocytes which proliferate and contain many conspicuous intracellular parasites. There is little to be seen grossly or microscopically in the way of necrosis or nodular granulomatous formation (Figs. 5, 6).

In later infancy, childhood or adult life, focal lesions occur which are often marked by caseous necrosis, granuloma-tous formation and a paucity of organisms, making their indentification within tissue sections difficult.*

This disease, then, may be characterized pathologically by the formation of granulomatous lesions which may be confused with those of tuberculosis. The characteristic lesion or primary complex is similar. It consists of (1) a primary focus at the site of penetration, (2) lymphangitis from this site to the regional lymph nodes, (3) regional lymphadenitis with inflammation and tendency toward caseation. The yeast cells of the fungus tend to proliferate in the large, mononuclear phagocytic cells of the reticuloendothelial system. They multiply until the mononuclear cells are literally filled with yeast cells. Rupture apparently occurs, and the yeast cells are phagocytized by other large mononuclear cells, thus initiating new cycles. In contradistinction to tuberculosis, this reaction goes on with relatively little inflammatory response in adjacent tissues. Foci tend to become surrounded with giant cells and multinucleated cells, and these foci progress to central caseous necrosis (Fig. 7). In infants with little im-

---

* I am indebted to my colleague, Dr. John Shapiro, for this observation.

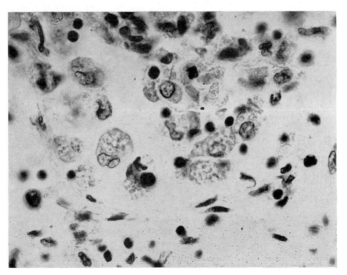

FIGURE 48–5. Large mononuclear phagocytes containing many yeast cells of *Histoplasma capsulatum* (which proliferate). No necrosis.

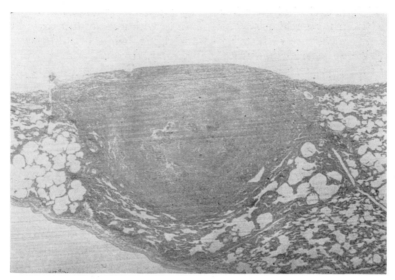

FIGURE 48–6. Proved primary histoplasmosis with granulomatous lesion in lung. Caseous necrosis and calcification present.

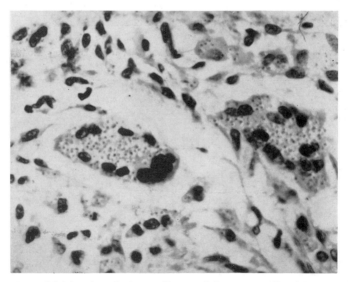

FIGURE 48–7. Multinucleated giant cells containing yeast cells of *H. capsulatum*.

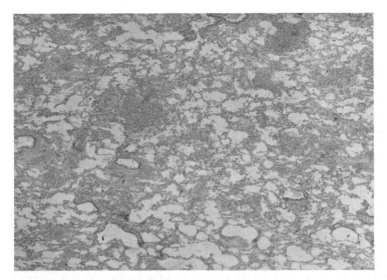

FIGURE 48–8. Interstitial pneumonitis due to histoplasmosis.

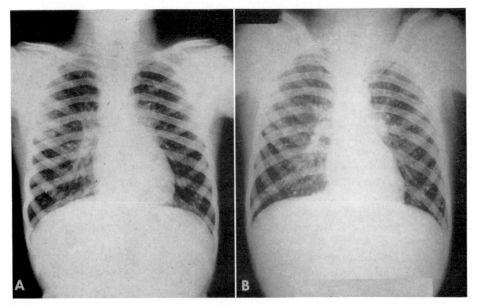

FIGURE 48–9. Multiple primary lesions simulating miliary tuberculosis. Note healing with calcification within 2 years.

munologic maturity or in debilitated adults (depending on the resistance of the host or the virulence of that particular strain of the organism) there is a tendency toward hematogenous spread or progression by postprimary complication. Just as in tuberculosis, spread of the organisms is dependent on tissue resistance of the host, and the dose (immediate or recurrent) of the inoculum. Hypersensitivity now occurs, and histoplasmin sensitivity is established. The time interval from the primary inoculation to this point is usually three to six weeks, similar to that in tuberculosis.

In the postprimary stage the progressive form of the disease may occur. This is characterized by massive enlargement of the liver and spleen, due to pathologic accumulations of proliferative lesions. Pulmonary tissues, including the regional lymph nodes, are similarly involved, and interstitial pneumonitis may be present (Fig. 8). When there is hematogenous spread, roentgenograms of the lungs have much the same soft snowstorm appearance as that seen in miliary tuberculosis (Fig. 9). This may heal with calcification, giving the characteristic "buckshot" x-ray of the chest.

The bone marrow is commonly involved, and with this there is a proliferation of large mononuclear cells filled with the yeast cells. These cells may crowd the normal bone marrow elements and thus produce severe anemia and at times leukopenia and thrombocytopenia. Not infrequently this clinical aspect of histoplasmosis is mistaken for aleukemic leukemia even by experienced clinicians.

In about 50 per cent of the cases there is ulceration of the skin or mucous membranes. Lesions in the oropharynx occur frequently, particularly in adults. Ulcerative lesions have been described in the bowel and colon, and a picture similar to that of tabes mesenterica of tuberculosis is well documented.

Invasion of the adrenal gland with caseous necrosis and adrenal failure produces the signs and symptoms of Addison's disease, another similarity to tuber-

Table 1. *Clinical Forms of Pulmonary Histoplasmosis*

1. Primary
2. Postprimary complications
   a. Intrathoracic
      (1) Miliary, "atypical" pneumonia
      (2) Mediastinal adenopathy
   b. Extrathoracic
      (1) May affect any tissue of the body: e.g. regional adenopathy; meningitis; lytic bone lesions: Addison's disease; eye, skin and mucous membrane ulcerations; myocarditis and endocarditis; ulcerative colitis
   c. Disseminated progressive varieties of histoplasmosis

culosis. This is more commonly found in adults, however, than in children. Involvement of the nervous system is not common, but the disease process can produce signs, symptoms and laboratory findings indistinguishable from those of tuberculous meningitis.

The regional lymph nodes are frequently involved, the cervical, mediastinal or mesenteric being the most common. It is not common, however, to find generalized adenopathy, such as is found in leukemia, and this may be an important differential diagnostic point.

Clinical Manifestations

Table 1 lists the clinical forms of pulmonary histoplasmosis.

Human histoplasmosis, as has been repeatedly pointed out, is a disease of protean nature. It varies with the degree of parasitization. A single primary lesion may be completely asymptomatic and appear only as acquired histoplasmin sensitivity (Fig. 10). On the other hand, infection following inhalation or ingestion of the organisms may commonly produce such symptoms as fever (101° to 103°F.), malaise, and fatigue with desire to rest rather than to play after school, nonproductive cough, weight loss or failure to gain, vomiting, and diarrhea which is occasionally blood-streaked.

The physical examination, particularly

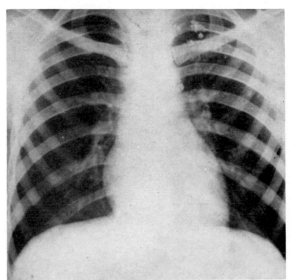

FIGURE 48–10. Healed primary histo-plasmosis. Note berry-like morphology of calcification.

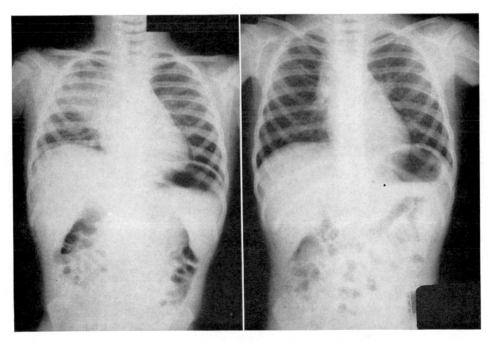

FIGURE 48–11. Primary histoplasmosis with resolution on sulfa therapy in 7 months.

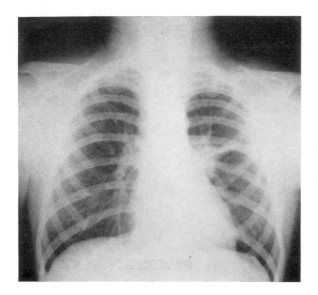

FIGURE 48–12. Primary histoplasmosis. Malaise, cough, low-grade fever of 3 months' duration. Positive histoplasmin and positive histoplasmin complement fixation test results. Note peripheral lesion with mediastinal adenopathy.

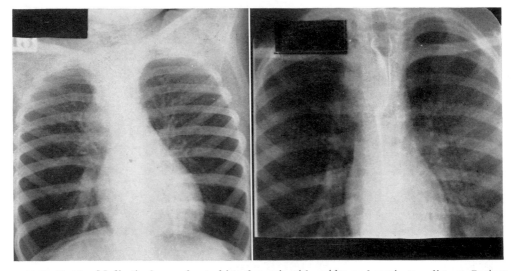

FIGURE 48–13. Mediastinal mass due to histoplasmosis with stridor and respiratory distress. Barium swallow showing narrowing of air passage. Resolution following endobronchial rupture of node (accidental). Histoplasma cultured from bronchial aspiration.

of the chest, may be negative at this time. Careful effort to explain the fatigue and low-grade fever may include skin tests and result in a positive histoplasmin, but negative tuberculin, reaction. Roentgenograms of the chest will then reveal an infiltrative lesion with or without mediastinal adenopathy, suggesting atypical pneumonia or mediastinal malignancy (Figs. 11, 12). A complement fixation test of comparatively low titer (1:4) and a rapid sedimentation rate are good indices of active systemic infection and may become important in judging the prognosis or clinical course of the disease.

Gastric washing, which may be helpful, has been disappointing in the author's considerable experience with histoplasmosis.

Occasionally a mediastinal node is of such size and location as to cause obstruction to venous return. Such instances may require bronchoscopy or exploratory thoracotomy to define the cause and relieve the obstruction (Fig. 13).

If hematogenous dissemination has taken place as the result of overwhelming infection, breakdown of a primary lesion or lowered resistance of the host, the fever rises to higher levels and persists. Hepatomegaly is prominent, and the spleen may enlarge to tremendous proportions (Fig. 14). The pallor, which is due to a normochromic anemia with pancytopenia, may be the presenting clinical manifestation. Experienced house officers will admit these infants with a presumptive diagnosis of aleukemic leukemia. Adenopathy is usually regional instead of generalized as in leukemia, a finding of considerable differential diagnostic importance. As many as 50 per cent of these cases show ulceration of the skin or mucous membranes, and an equal number have evidence of pulmonary infiltration with mediastinal adenopathy.

Purpura is perhaps the commonest cutaneous lesion, and this usually means overwhelming parasitization with crowding out of the normal marrow elements. It is a poor prognostic sign.

To summarize and re-emphasize, the

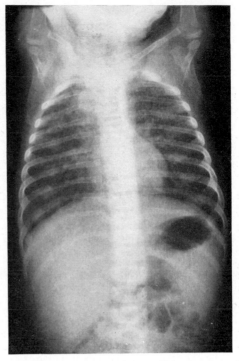

FIGURE 48–14. Postprimary dissemination of pulmonary histoplasmosis. Note fine infiltration with mediastinal adenopathy and hepatosplenomegaly.

clinical manifestations of histoplasmosis are so variable that it is wise and helpful to remember everything known about tuberculosis. The generalized reticuloendotheliosis which has been described accounts for the appearance of the disease in acute, subacute and chronic forms with systematic manifestations of irregular fever, anemia, failure to gain weight or weight loss, hepatosplenomegaly, ulceration of the skin or mucous membranes (particularly of the oronasal pharynx), ulceration of the small intestine, pulmonary infiltration and atypical pneumonia. In the adult, histoplasmosis exhibits another similarity to tuberculosis by involving the adrenal gland and producing classic Addison's disease. We have also observed Histoplasma endocarditis and meningitis, the latter indistinguishable in all its clinical and laboratory manifestations from tuberculous meningitis. There are cases of ulcerative colitis in the

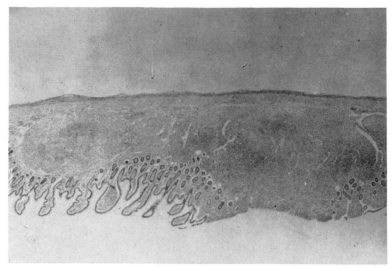

FIGURE 48–15. Ulceration of gastrointestinal mucosa due to histoplasmosis. Note submucosal proliferation suggesting granulomatous enteritis.

Vanderbilt University files which were given the usual University Hospital work-up without avail until the true definitive diagnosis was revealed in the autopsy material (Fig. 15). Pericarditis and myocarditis with endocarditis have been described, and we have seen destructive bone lesions with periosteal new bone formation.

Differential Diagnosis

It has been pointed out that acute disseminated histoplasmosis of a progressive nature must be considered whenever the diagnosis of leukemia is being considered. The absence of generalized adenopathy and of blast forms and the persistence of normal bone marrow elements are helpful. Histoplasmosis adenopathy is inclined to be regional rather than generalized. When histoplasmosis has affected the mesenteric nodes, a picture of tabes mesenterica, tuberculosis, Hodgkin's disease or other malignant lymphomatous diseases must be considered. The differential diagnosis between histoplasmosis and reticuloendothelioses of the Letterer-Siwe type is a most difficult one clinically and histologically save for the finding of yeast cells in the biopsy material or by culture of the organism. Ulcerations of the skin and mucous membranes also suggest tuberculosis, syphilis and epithelioma.

Pulmonary infiltration of histoplasmosis frequently suggests virus or atypical pneumonia or tuberculosis even to the experienced clinician. We have in our files examples of atelectasis resulting from mediastinal gland enlargement due to histoplasmosis and attaining such size as to cause obstruction of the venous return, thereby suggesting a diagnosis of mediastinal malignant lymphoma. When the diagnosis of ulcerative colitis is entertained, it appears wise in endemic areas to obtain cultures and to perform other proper examinations for *Histoplasma capsulatum*. In the presence of organic heart disease with embolic phenomena we have found *Histoplasma capsulatum* in the emboli; the typical picture of infective endocarditis caused by this fungus is well documented.

Prognosis

Histoplasmosis seems to affect most seriously the infant who is immunologically immature and the debilitated older adult who frequently is suffering from concomitant systemic disease. Several factors related to the extent of the inoculation and the virulence of the organism, as well as the resistance of the host, are also operative in determining the prognosis of histoplasmosis.

As in the primary or in the postprimary complications of tuberculosis, an opinion as to prognosis as well as the choice of the therapeutic agent is closely related to a knowledge of the natural course of this disease. In its primary form histoplasmosis is strangely benign, but in its progressive, disseminated form it is almost uniformly fatal unless adequately treated. Nevertheless, particularly in older children, in whom the disease is widely disseminated and appears to be progressive, there have been well documented spontaneous recoveries. In the intermediate forms with ulcerations of the skin and mucous membranes and extensive pulmonary infiltrative disease, patients exhibit few signs and symptoms and usually recover spontaneously or with supportive therapy in a matter of weeks to months.

The difficulty of evaluating a therapeutic agent under these varying conditions is obvious. The duration of the infection and the persistence of skin test sensitivity, as well as the presence of complement-fixing antibodies, are probably related to the degree of infection present. In some instances when the infection is a single minimal primary one, the lesion may heal completely and the patient may lose his sensitivity in a relatively short time. Calcified nodules, when taken from the lungs at autopsy, are seldom if ever associated with the presence of viable organisms. The loss of histoplasmin sensitivity occurs much more often than does loss of tuberculin sensitivity. This is probably related to the absence of viable organisms after healing or to the removal of the subject from reinfection. During childhood and early adult life, however, the opportunity for infection and reinfection is so great that there is a constantly rising level of histoplasmin sensitivity. After thirty years of age there

is a slow decline in histoplasmin sensitivity, suggesting that reinfection does not keep pace with the loss of sensitivity. Little is known about the significance of reinfection, but we have had a number of cases with caseous lesions in the lungs which have broken down and apparently served as a source of generalized dissemination of the infection. This course has been seen particularly in those patients who were receiving corticosteroid therapy.

The question is frequently raised as to whether or not there is danger of a breakdown of the lesions after they have healed to the point of calcification. There are no cases in our files which suggest that such lesions break down and result in hematogenous dissemination of the disease. The most logical explanation for this is the likelihood that the yeast cells are probably all dead or nonviable when calcification occurs, or are incapable of multiplication. As indicated above, the disappearance of signs and symptoms and the gaining of weight are indications of inactivity of the infection. When accompanied by return of the sedimentation rate to normal and the fading out of the complement-fixing antibodies, the infection is considered to be under control or inactivated. In the disseminated form of the disease, decrease in the size of the spleen is a good prognostic sign.

Treatment

Under the conditions described above, the first principle of therapeutics must be exercised. *Primum nole nocere,* which means "to be unwilling to do harm," might be paraphrased as follows: "Try to do some good." A truly effective agent has not been found for the treatment of histoplasmosis. All means of supportive and symptomatic relief should be exercised. Anything which can be done to improve the nutrition or the general hygiene and thus increase the natural resistance of the patient is indicated. Blood transfusion is helpful in improving the general resistance and in correcting the normochromic anemia and

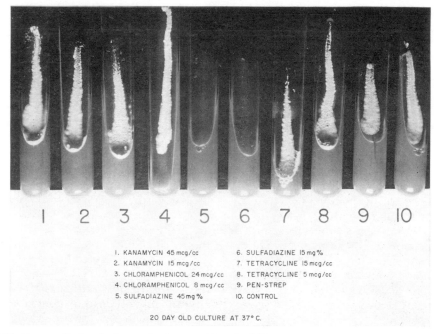

1. KANAMYCIN 45 mcg/cc
2. KANAMYCIN 15 mcg/cc
3. CHLORAMPHENICOL 24 mcg/cc
4. CHLORAMPHENICOL 8 mcg/cc
5. SULFADIAZINE 45 mg %
6. SULFADIAZINE 15 mg %
7. TETRACYCLINE 15 mcg/cc
8. TETRACYCLINE 5 mcg/cc
9. PEN-STREP
10. CONTROL

20 DAY OLD CULTURE AT 37° C.

FIGURE 48–16. Rationale for sulfa therapy. Note inability to grow *H. capsulatum* in presence of 15 mg. of sulfa. (I am indebted to Dr. William Fleet for the preparation of this illustration.)

pancytopenia frequently present. Corticosteroids appear to be contraindicated because of the danger of dissemination of the primary lesion. In-vitro studies reveal that *Histoplasma capsulatum* thrives on antibiotics. It would seem, therefore, that these would be useless, if not contraindicated. In an early observation on biopsy material, we found that growth of the pyogenic organisms could be inhibited by penicillin and streptomycin and that a rather rapid growth of the *Histoplasma capsulatum* occurred in the presence of these antibiotics in the media.

Amphotericin B (Fungizone) has recently come into use in treatment of histoplasmosis, and favorable results have been reported from this institution and elsewhere. In its present form, however, this drug is pyrogenic, producing chills and high fever, is poorly absorbed from the gastrointestinal tract and is nephrotoxic and hepatotoxic. Its use has serious economic repercussions, since the drug should be used only in hospitals under careful observation and the so-called

course of treatment involves prolonged use. It should never be used in the benign forms of the disease, but rather reserved for the progressive disseminated varieties. (See section on amphotericin B in treatment of fungal disease, page 620.)

We have had considerable experience in studying both the natural course of the infection and in treating different forms of histoplasmosis. A triple sulfonamide suspension in a dosage which produces a level of 10 to 15 mg. per 100 ml. in the blood is our antimicrobial of choice in almost all forms of the disease, although evaluation of this or any other therapeutic agent remains a difficult problem. Sulfonamide is well tolerated by patients. The methods of regulating the drug are readily available in most laboratories, including those in private offices (blood serum levels and urinalysis). Less toxic drugs must be developed before a truly effective therapeutic agent can be made available (Fig. 16).

The Present Status of Histoplasmin Sensitivity, Serologic Tests and Other Diagnostic Methods

Histoplasmin is a dilution of a broth culture filtrate. Histoplasmin sensitivity, like old tuberculin sensitivity, is an allergic state induced by infection with *Histoplasma capsulatum*. The test quantitatively and qualitatively has no relation to the state of activity of infection with *Histoplasma capsulatum* and, of course, in this respect is similar to the relation between tuberculosis and tuberculin sensitivity. Sensitivity to histoplasmin appears four to six weeks after infection has begun and may persist for many years after the activity of the infection has disappeared. In disseminated

and progressive infection as many as 50 per cent of the cases will demonstrate no skin test sensitivity. Recent known conversion of histoplasmin sensitivity has the same significance as the acquisition of tuberculin sensitivity and is of considerable clinical importance when one relates it to signs and symptoms associated with unexplained pulmonary pathology or hepatosplenomegaly (Fig. 17).

In our experience the most reliable serologic test is the complement fixation test. Almost invariably, it is strongly positive in postprimary complications of the disease. The presence of complement-fixing antibodies even in low titer, i.e. 1:4, represents an acute phase reaction and is a sign of activity of the disease. The particular antibodies rapidly decrease in titer within a few weeks or

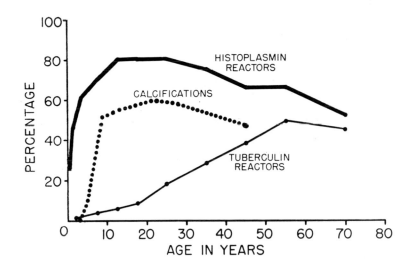

NO. OF CASES		AGE IN YEARS								
HISTOPLASMIN	72,88,205,576	662	338	294	315	243	171	146
TUBERCULIN	323	529	601	289	245	266	210	122	105
X-RAY		2	28	87	238	358	279	70	45

FIGURE 48–17. Pattern of histoplasmin and tuberculin sensitivity by age groups. Note relation of histoplasmin sensitivity to the development of calcification. Note also percentage of persons reacting to histoplasmin and percentage with 2+ or more reaction to 0.1 of old tuberculin and percentage of calcifications, by age group.

months as the infection comes under control or is inactivated by therapy.

Adequate cultural methods of biopsy or other host material will usually reveal *Histoplasma capsulatum* if that is the causative organism.

REFERENCES

Christie, A.: Histoplasmosis and Pulmonary Calcification. *Ann. New York Acad. Sc.,* 50:1283, 1950.

Idem: The Disease Spectrum of Human Histoplasmosis. *Ann. Int. Med.,* 49:544, 1958.

Christie, A., and Peterson, J. C.: Pulmonary Calcification in Negative Reactors to Tuberculin. *Am. J. Pub. Health,* 35:1131, 1945. Also other articles on the same topic.

Darling, S. T.: Protozoan General Infection Producing Pseudotubercles in the Lungs and Focal Necrosis in the Liver, Spleen, and Lymph Nodes. *J.A.M.A.,* 46:1283, 1905.

Idem: Notes on Histoplasmosis: A Fatal Infectious Disease Resembling Kala-Azar Found Among Natives of Tropical America. *Arch. Int. Med.,* 2:107, 1908.

Mayer, R. L., Eisman, P. C., Geftic, S., Konopka, E., and Tanzola, J.: Sulfonamides and Experimental Histoplasmosis. *Antibiotics & Chemotherapy,* 6:215, 1956.

Palmer, C. E.: Nontuberculous Pulmonary Calcification and Sensitivity to Histoplasmin. *Pub. Health Rep.,* 60:513, 1945.

Schwarz, J., and Baum, G.: The History of Histoplasmosis 1906–1956. *New England J. Med.,* 256:253, 1957.

CHAPTER FORTY-NINE

Idiopathic Histiocytosis (Histiocytosis X)

ROBERT H. HIGH, M.D.

The terms "idiopathic histiocytosis" or "histiocytosis X," and many others such as systemic reticuloendotheliosis, histiocytic reticuloendotheliosis, nonlipoid reticuloendotheliosis, nonlipoid histiocytosis, have been used to designate a group of several diseases with varying clinical patterns which have in common proliferation of the histiocytes in the tissues. These diseases, all of unknown origin, include the following in order of decreasing severity of morbidity and mortality: (1) the Letterer-Siwe syndrome, (2) the Hand-Schueller-Christian syndrome, (3) eosinophilic granuloma of bone and (4) histiocytic infiltrations of atypical distribution often involving one organ such as the skin, the lungs, the lymph nodes and others in varying degrees. Although some object to grouping these disturbances together, there seems to be a general consensus that they represent a spectrum of clinical patterns of related processes of unknown causation. These diseases are not malignant, not hereditary, not familial and not infectious in origin. They are not related to the lipoid reticuloendothelioses such as Gaucher's and Niemann-Pick diseases.

Consideration is given to these obscure diseases because all of them except eosinophilic granuloma of the bone can produce pulmonary infiltrations which may cause some of the symptoms and, at times, fatalities. Pulmonary infiltrations are most commonly associated with Letterer-Siwe disease, less commonly with Hand-Schueller-Christian disease, and only occasionally noted in the group designated as "histiocytic infiltrations of atypical distribution." The great variability of the clinical manifestations and pathologic changes in these diseases precludes discussion here. Attention is directed only to the pulmonary component of these disturbances.

Because of the wide variations in the gross and histologic appearances of the lungs, the following descriptions are intended to include, in a general way, only the most important changes. Many details are not mentioned. Histiocytic infiltrations occur in the lungs, chiefly in the interlobular or interalveolar septa or in the perivascular, peribronchial or subpleural tissues. These collections can be of sufficient size to produce nodules in the lungs. Sometimes dilatation of the terminal bronchioles and alveoli develops secondary to the peribronchial infiltrates. This process leads to the development of microcysts which are sometimes the origin of interstitial emphysema, pneumomediastinum or pneumothorax.

In addition to the histiocytic infiltrations, there may also be infiltrations of eosinophils and fibroblasts. Lymphocytes and plasma cells may be present.

The development of pulmonary infiltrations in these diseases is usually a sign of ominous prognostic importance. Extensive pulmonary infiltrates are commonly found in the fatal cases even though the pulmonary involvement was not the cause of death.

The clinical manifestations of the pulmonary histiocytic infiltrations are added to those of the primary problem and may be minor or major, depending upon the extensiveness of the process. Cough and chest pain may be present, and these may be associated with tachypnea, dyspnea and cyanosis. Physical examination seldom reveals the presence of rales or abnormal percussion changes, although evidence of localized or generalized emphysema may be noted. Inspiratory retraction may be present. Rupture of the microcysts can

lead to the development of interstitial emphysema, pneumomediastinum or pneumothorax which produce the changes noted previously (see Pneumothorax p. 487). In general, the abnormalities apparent by physical examination are far less than the extent of the infiltrations demonstrable by roentgenographic examination.

Roentgenographic examination of the chest shows variable findings depending upon the distribution and size of the histiocytic infiltrations. It may be within normal limits or may show evidence of overaeration. When the infiltrations are of sufficient size, generalized hazy densities much like those noted in fulminating miliary tuberculosis are produced (see p. 686). Sometimes discrete nodules are apparent. The roentgenographic abnormalities are not pathognomonic. Examination of other areas, especially the skull and long bones, is indicated when such diffuse densities are noted in the chest roentgenograms.

In this group of diseases, as in most diseases of obscure origin, therapy is largely empiric and supportive and is directed toward the relief of symptoms. Irradiation of the chest may relieve some of the symptoms, and subsequent roentgenographic studies may show some resolution of the infiltrations. The administration of steroid drugs, the alkylating agents or the antimetabolic agents such as aminopterin may retard the progression of the disease, and sometimes recovery, or at least long-term survival, occurs.

The most hopeful therapeutic program at present is the administration of one of the several alkaloid derivatives of the periwinkle plant (*Vinca rosea* Linn). The intravenous administration of vincristine sulfate at weekly intervals for long periods of time seems to be especially beneficial in patients with Letterer-Siwe disease. The paucity of experience with these agents, vincristine and vinblastine, precludes specific recommendation for their use, but the favorable initial experiences with them suggest some value in continuing the appraisal of their effectiveness.

Therapy of the pulmonary aspects of

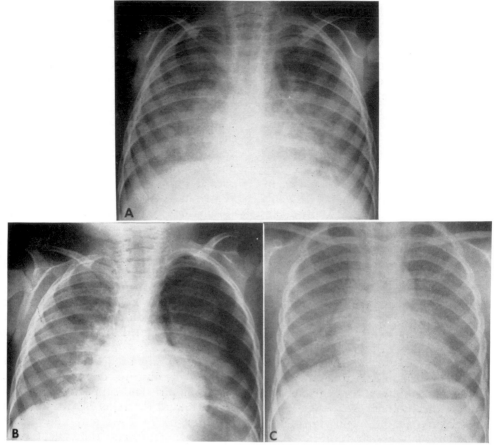

FIGURE 49–1. *A* (5/3/63), Diffuse bilateral pulmonary infiltrates. *B*, Left pneumothorax secondary to rupture of microcysts. *C* (3/12/65), Considerable resolution 22 months later after alternating weekly doses of vincristine and Cytoxan.

the idiopathic histiocytoses is often a minor part of the treatment, especially when the process has a systemic distribution.

It is not possible to state a prognosis for a group of diseases as heterogeneous as those considered here. They are not uniformly fatal. Evaluation of the initial clinical manifestations and of the histologic appearance of tissues may give general indications of the possible outcome. Such appraisals are far from reliable, since some patients with apparently fulminating disease have had the process become quiescent and have survived for long periods. In general terms, the severity of these disturbances in decreasing order of morbidity and mortality is as follows: (1) Letterer-Siwe syndrome, (2) Hand-Schueller-Christian syndrome, (3) eosinophilic granuloma of bone and (4) histiocytic infiltrations of atypical distribution.

REFERENCES

Crocker, A. C.: The Reticuloendothelioses; in S. S. Gellis and B. M. Kagan (Eds.): *Current Pediatric Therapy* 1966-1967. Philadelphia, W. B. Saunders Company, 1966, p. 440.

Holinger, P. H., Slaughter, D. P., and Novak, F. J.: Unusual Tumors Obstructing the Lower Respiratory Tract of Infants and Children. *Tr. Am. Acad. Ophth.,* 54:223, 1950.

CHAPTER FIFTY

Psittacosis (Ornithosis)

ROBERT H. HIGH, M.D.

Psittacosis is an acute infectious disease occurring naturally in many species of birds and transmissible to man. Early reports suggested that the disease was chiefly spread from birds of the psittacine group, such as parrots and parakeets; hence the term "psittacosis." More recent studies have shown that many species of birds, both wild and domesticated, can be infected. These include pigeons, chickens, turkeys, ducks, pheasants, finches and others, and some authors, therefore, prefer to designate the infection as ornithosis. In this chapter the traditional term "psittacosis" will be retained.

The infectious agent is generally regarded as a virus or a group of antigenically related viruses which are included in the psittacosis-lymphogranuloma venereum group of viruses, a group which is intermediate between rickettsiae and viruses. Some doubt that the psittacosis agent is a true virus. Regardless of the eventual resolution of the classification of the organism, it is known that psittacosis can be grown in tissue cultures and on the yolk sac of embryonated eggs. Coccoid-shaped elementary bodies appear to be the causative agent. When grown in tissue culture, inclusion bodies develop in the cells.

In birds the agent has been recovered from nasal secretions, blood, liver, spleen, feces and from feathers presumably contaminated with nasal secretions or feces. Many apparently healthy birds harbor the agent, and birds which have recovered from the infection can continue to shed the agent for long periods. Isolation of the agent from human beings has been made chiefly from secretions from the respiratory tract. The carrier state may persist for long periods of time in human patients who have recovered from psittacosis. The same or a closely related agent has been recovered from other mammalian species.

Man acquires the infection by handling sick or well birds, from inhalation of dust contaminated with fecal droppings or from handling feathers. The portal of entry is the respiratory tract. Since infected human patients shed the agent in their respiratory tract secretions, person-to-person spread is also possible. Indeed, small outbreaks have occurred in hospital personnel caring for patients with psittacosis. Laboratory workers processing live preparations of the agent have likewise become infected. Because of this fact, many laboratories do not attempt direct isolation of the psittacosis agents.

Psittacosis is most common in those caring for birds, such as workers in aviaries, or in those who keep birds as pets. It may also occur in those working with feathers or in those processing domestic fowls for market. Most cases have been noted in adults, but children are not immune, and infections during childhood have been documented.

The actual frequency of psittacosis in this country cannot be stated, since many of the mild cases are not accurately diagnosed and some cases are not reported to the health departments. The United States Public Health Service includes psittacosis among "notifiable diseases of low frequency."

In human beings and monkeys, unlike birds, the disease does not cause widespread visceral involvement, but tends to be localized in the lungs, where a diffuse interstitial pneumonia is produced. Some pleural reaction may occur. The pathologic changes are not pathognomonic for psittacosis, since similar changes occur with other viral infections of the lungs. The liver may show focal necrosis, and the spleen may be enlarged.

The clinical manifestations of psittacosis vary considerably in severity, ranging from a mild influenza-like or "grippelike" illness to severe pneumonia. The manifestations of psittacosis are not sufficiently distinctive to permit a diagnosis on clinical grounds. The diagnosis may be suspected when there is a history of exposure to birds, sick or well, but the diagnosis can be confirmed only by appropriate laboratory studies.

The incubation period varies from several days to two weeks. The onset is usually abrupt with fever, malaise, myalgia, photophobia and chills. Cough may develop as a manifestation of the diffuse pneumonia, but this symptom is often not a prominent one. Epistaxis occurs, and occasionally a rash appears which resembles that seen in typhoid fever. Children may have nonspecific neurologic manifestations such as delirium and convulsions. The fever, in the untreated case, tends to be high during the first week or so and then gradually falls to reach normal by the end of the second or third week of the disease.

Physical examination does not show any characteristic abnormalities. The pulse may be slow despite fever. Examination of the lungs may reveal the signs associated with diffuse pneumonia, but the extent of involvement is usually not in keeping with that noted by roentgenographic examination.

Chest roentgenograms reveal the presence of a diffuse bronchopneumonia or interstitial pneumonitis. The abnormalities are not pathognomonic and are seen in other viral pulmonary infections.

Laboratory studies, other than specific serologic tests, are not helpful in establishing the diagnosis of psittacosis. The diagnosis can be confirmed by specific complement fixation or agglutination tests performed on acute and convalescent-phase serum specimens. The first specimen should be obtained early in the clinical course, and the convalescent one should be obtained during the second or third week of the disease. A rise in titer of four-fold or more is considered diagnostic. As mentioned above, many laboratories do not attempt direct isolation of the agent because of the hazard of infection in the personnel.

The most effective therapy at present is the administration of tetracycline in daily doses of about 50 mg. per kilogram. The duration of treatment should be about two weeks. It is recognized that the infrequent occurrence of this infection makes the appraisal of treatment difficult, and these recommendations are somewhat arbitrary. The remainder of treatment is the application of the usual supportive and symptomatic management of diffuse pneumonia, such as the administration of oxygen, analgesics, parenteral fluids, and the like.

REFERENCES

Berman, S. E.: Ornithosis (Psittacosis); in S. S. Gellis and B. M. Kagan (Eds.): Current Pediatric Therapy 1966-1967. Philadelphia, W. B. Saunders Company, 1966, p. 738.

Dean, D. J., and others: Psittacosis in Man and Birds. Pub. Health Rep., 79:101-106, 1964.

Haig, D. A., and others: Occurrence of Ornithosis in the Wood Pigeon. Nature (London), 200: 381-2, 1963.

Hodes, H. L.: Ornithosis (Psittacosis); in L. E. Holt, Jr., R. McIntosh and H. L. Barnett: Pediatrics. 13th ed. New York, Appleton-Century-Crofts, Inc., 1962, pp. 1155-6.

CHAPTER FIFTY-ONE

Q Fever

ROBERT H. HIGH, M.D.

Q fever is an acute infectious disease caused by infection with *Rickettsia burnetii,* also called *Coxiella burnetii.* The disease was originally described in Australia in 1935, but has subsequently been recognized as having a worldwide distribution. Q fever is not common in this country except in California, where many domesticated animals are infected in certain endemic areas. Q fever has, however, been reported in many other states. Q fever differs from the other major rickettsial infections in several respects: (1) a rash is not present, (2) the primary clinical manifestations are those of pulmonary infection, and (3) it usually is not spread by arthropod vectors.

Q fever occurs as a natural infection in cattle, sheep, goats and many wild animals. Ticks may become infected and can pass the organism to subsequent generations through the ova. Experimental infections have been produced by the bite of ticks, but this mode of spread is not usual for human infections. Ticks may play a significant role in the transmission of Q fever to animals. The rickettsiae are excreted from animals in milk, urine, fetal membranes and discharges, and the rickettsiae are also present in meat from infected animals. The infected animals usually do not appear to be sick.

Man usually acquires Q fever by the inhalation of dust, particles of straw, and the like, contaminated by animal discharges, by contamination with fetal membranes and discharges during the birth of calves or lambs, from contact with infected meat or by the ingestion of infected milk. Commercial pasteurization of milk does not necessarily kill all the rickettsiae. Man-to-man transmission is not likely.

Outbreaks of Q fever have occurred chiefly in slaughter house workers and in the employees of tanneries or processing plants for wool and other animal hair. During World War II, outbreaks occurred in the United States military personnel in Italy. Most of the epidemics were caused by the inhalation of infected dust. The organism is resistant to destruction by drying and can remain viable in dust for long periods.

The epidemiology of Q fever is such that children are not commonly exposed except in rural areas or by drinking infected milk.

The clinical manifestations develop after an incubation period of two to almost four weeks. Studies, chiefly in military personnel, suggest an average incubation period of seventeen to nineteen days. Mild cases may simulate mild influenza and are diagnosed only by serologic studies. The usual manifestations in the typical case include the fairly abrupt onset of fever, malaise and chilliness, and a prominent early complaint is that of severe headache, often frontal, which is worsened by movement of the eyes. A nonproductive cough may develop toward the end of the first week. Chest pain and the production of slightly blood-tinged sputum may occur. Rales and signs of consolidation may be heard when the lungs are examined. A rash does not appear.

The illness tends to have a febrile course for one to two weeks followed by gradual improvement. Convalescence may be moderately prolonged. Complications are rare, and recovery is expected.

Roentgenographic examinations of the chest often show diffuse parenchymal infiltrations which are usually more extensive than is suggested by the findings of

643

the physical examination. Serofibrinous pleurisy is sometimes present. Enlargement of the hilar and mediastinal lymph nodes is not expected. Resolution of the pneumonia is slow, sometimes requiring several weeks before a normal appearance is noted.

The diagnosis may be confirmed by isolation of *R. burnetii* from the blood, urine or sputum during the early stages of the disease, using animal inoculation of guinea pigs, monkeys or mice or by inoculation of embryonated eggs. These methods of isolation are not readily available and offer the possibility of infection of the laboratory personnel. Serologic tests, using acute and convalescent-phase serums, are the most widely recommended studies. Complement-fixing antibody tests and agglutination tests using antigens from *R. burnetii* are available. It should be stressed that the Weil-Felix reaction is not positive in Q fever. Other laboratory findings are not useful in the diagnosis of this disease.

Treatment with tetracycline in daily oral doses of 50 to 100 mg. per kilogram is recommended until the patient has been free of fever for several days. Since tetracycline does not kill the rickettsiae, some recommend two courses of treatment of five days' duration separated by a period of five days without treatment. Improvement is usually rapid, and relapse uncommon. Chloramphenicol is also effective in treating Q fever, but it offers no advantage over tetracycline. Chloramphenicol administration is more hazardous than the program described above. Symptomatic treatment of headache, chest pain and the like may be indicated.

The preventive aspects of Q fever, like those of other rickettsial diseases, are complex and without adequate solution at present. In theory, milk from infected cattle should not be used, but the difficulty in identifying these animals, which do not appear ill, makes such a procedure impractical. Pasteurization of milk from suspected infected herds should be at higher temperatures or for longer periods than usual. Endemic areas should be defined so that patients from them who present the symptoms and findings described above may be diagnosed promptly.

REFERENCES

Gold, E.: Q Fever; in S. S. Gellis and B. M. Kagan (Eds.): *Current Pediatric Therapy* 1966-1967. Philadelphia, W. B. Saunders Company, 1966, pp. 739-40.

Gold, E., and Robbins, F. C.: Q Fever; in W. E. Nelson (Ed.): *Textbook of Pediatrics.* 8th ed. Philadelphia, W. B. Saunders Company, 1964, pp. 611-12.

Luoto, L., and others: Q Fever Vaccination of Human Volunteers. I. The Serologic and Skin-Test Response Following Subcutaneous Injection. *Am. J. Hgy.,* 78:1-15, 1963.

Peterson, J. C.: Q Fever; in L. E. Holt, Jr., R. McIntosh and H. L. Barnett (Eds.): *Pediatrics.* 13th ed. New York, Appleton-Century-Crofts, Inc., 1962, pp. 1166-7.

Wisseman, C. L.: Progress Report on the Development of Q Fever Vaccines. *Mil. Med.,* 129:389-92, 1964.

CHAPTER FIFTY-TWO

Sarcoidosis

EDWIN L. KENDIG, Jr., M.D.

Sarcoidosis seems to be relatively rare among children. In a review of the world literature to February 1953, McGovern and Merritt were able to document only 104 cases in children under fifteen years of age. To these they added nine others, all diagnosed in Washington hospitals.* As far as can be determined, there have been only scattered cases of sarcoidosis in children reported since that time, except for a group of eight cases of rather atypical sarcoidosis reported from Utah and Idaho, an area in which sarcoidosis in adults appears to be extremely rare, eighteen cases reported by Siltzbach and Greenberg, and the seven patients previously reported from the Medical College of Virginia. To date, there have been thirteen cases so diagnosed at the Medical College of Virginia. Niitu has reported sixteen cases of intrathoracic sarcoidosis found in mass chest x-ray surveys among school children in Sendai (Japan), and Mandi noted fourteen such cases among children in Hungary. It is, of course, conceded that there are undoubtedly many other cases of recognized sarcoidosis in children still unreported, but the disease must be considered relatively rare in this age group.†

The criteria for the diagnosis of sarcoidosis were outlined by a subcommittee of the National Research Council in 1948, and redefined in October 1956 as follows:

Sarcoidosis is a systemic disease, or group of diseases, of undetermined etiology and pathogenesis. Histologically it is marked by the presence of epithelioid-cell tubercles, showing little or no necrosis. Varying types of inclusions in giant cells may be present but are not pathognomonic. A similar histological picture may be found in certain other diseases, especially in infectious granulomas and in beryllium poisoning. Clinically, the disease most commonly involves lymph nodes, lungs, skin, eyes, liver, spleen and phalangeal bones. The course is usually chronic and constitutional symptoms vary markedly. More specific symptoms, when present, relate to the tissues and organs involved.

The intracutaneous tuberculin test is frequently negative, but a positive test does not controvert the diagnosis. Hyperglobulinemia and leukopenia are common and hypercalcemia, hypercalciuria, elevated alkaline phosphatase, and eosinophilia are variable but sometimes significant features of sarcoidosis.

The diagnosis of sarcoidosis is based upon the above clinical features associated with a compatible histological picture, provided beryllium poisoning and known infectious processes can be excluded.

Spontaneous clinical recovery, with or without recognizable fibrosis, may result, or sarcoidosis may persist for years with varying functional alterations of the tissues or organs involved, or the disease may follow a progressive course ending fatally.

History

Sarcoidosis was first described in England by Hutchinson in 1875. Contributions clarifying certain clinical and pathologic features were made by Besnier in 1889, Boeck in 1899, and Schaumann in 1917. Heerfordt, and more recently Garland and Thompson and Longcope

---

*The World Group as referred to hereinafter in this text includes the 104 cases documented from the World literature by McGovern and Merritt and the additional nine cases reported by them, a total of 113 cases.

† Siltzbach notes that silent cases are unusual in childhood because children are not included in mass x-ray surveys; it is his feeling that childhood sarcoidosis is more common than is generally realized and that only the advanced cases are diagnosed.

645

and Pierson, have contributed further to the description of the disease.

The use of mass radiography, introduced in many countries in an effort to detect tuberculosis (about the time of World War II), led to a significant advance in the knowledge of sarcoidosis. This method, first used in the Armed Forces and later in the general population, led to the finding of a high incidence of presumptive asymptomatic sarcoidosis.

Age Incidence

Sarcoidosis is encountered more frequently in adults between twenty and forty years of age, but the disease may occur at any age. Although the youngest patient reported, substantiated by biopsy, was a two-month-old infant, most of those cases reported in childhood have occurred in the preadolescent or adolescent age group. Of the patients documented from the World literature by McGovern and Merritt (including their own cases), 75 per cent were between the ages of nine and fifteen years; twelve of the thirteen Medical College of Virginia cases and all of Siltzbach's patients fell into the same age group. It must be noted, however, that one patient in the M.C.V. series had symptoms suggestive of the disease several years before diagnosis was established, and such mild or insidious onset of the disease may cause delay in recognition.

Race

There is a great variation in the racial incidence. In Europe, and particularly in the Scandinavian countries, where the Negro population is low, the disease has been found more often in the white population. In the United States, on the other hand, sarcoidosis occurs more commonly among the Negro race. In three radiographic surveys of the United States Armed Forces, Negroes with sarcoidosis outnumbered white personnel with the disease by a ratio varying from 7:1 to 26:1. Cummings reported the hospitaliza-

tion rate for Negro and white World War II veterans with sarcoidosis to be 40.1 and 3.3 per 100,000, respectively.

Although Siltzbach has noted that the apparent susceptibility of the American Negro is not shared by the Negroes of Central Africa, where the disease is apparently unknown, he also pointed out that cases of sarcoidosis are beginning to be reported in numbers among natives of North and South Africa. He suggests, however, that the latter finding is the result of better facilities now available there for the detection of sarcoidosis.

Among the children for whom the race was stated in the World literature, 34 per cent were Negro, but ten of the thirteen children in the Medical College of Virginia series and twelve of the eighteen in Siltzbach's group were Negroes.

Sex Distribution

It is generally agreed that both sexes appear to be affected with equal frequency, although in the Medical College of Virginia series there were eight females and five males.

Heredity

There appears to be little evidence that heredity is in any way connected with either the incidence of sarcoidosis or predisposition toward it. It is unlikely that such reports as that of three cases among siblings under fifteen years of age are an indication of hereditary involvement.

Geographic Distribution

Sarcoidosis has been observed throughout many parts of the world. Sweden has the highest reported incidence of the disease. In that country the prevalence in the Armed Forces, in the general population and in Stockholm was reported to be above forty per 100,000 population, and one rural county, Jaemtlands, had a rate of 140 per 100,000.

In the United States there have been reports by Michael, Gentry, and Cummings, on the study of the birthplace and residence of persons in the Armed Forces with sarcoidosis, indicating areas with high attack rates of sarcoidosis in in the South Atlantic and Gulf states, with endemic areas in New England and the Midwest.

Etiology and Pathogenesis

Concepts of the cause of sarcoidosis have been reviewed by Jacques and Longcope. Many theories have been advanced, including a causal relation with brucellosis, leprosy, syphilis and infections due to viruses, fungi, protozoa and helminths, and the possibility that sarcoidosis may be a syndrome caused by a number of etiologic agents. Tuberculosis was one of the diseases earlier regarded as a possible causative agent, and this has again been recently championed by Scadding. The similarity of sarcoidosis to berylliosis and to histoplasmosis has been pointed out. Refvem analyzed tissue obtained from patients with sarcoidosis and suggested that calcareous spar found in certain soil types may be a possible etiologic agent; he also demonstrated that particles of quartz and other foreign bodies may provoke localized sarcoid formation. It is interesting to note that organisms resembling unclassified mycobacteria have been isolated with increasing frequency from lesions in patients with sarcoidosis.

Cummings has noted that forest products or even diseases of plant life appear to be related in some way to sarcoidosis, and he has suggested that pine pollen may be involved in the causation.

The discovery of a small area in Virginia where the incidence of sarcoidosis appears to be extremely high (review of 12,000 chest roentgenograms of persons in this area by a tuberculologist of the Virginia State Health Department indicates that the incidence of presumptive asymptomatic sarcoidosis is 500 per 100,-000 population, more than three times greater than the highest previously reported incidence of the disease) has suggested another possible factor. This area is predominantly rural, with pine forests and sandy soil, and the chief crop is peanuts. Among the patients with sarcoidosis no history of contact with any known infectious agent or unusual dietary regimen can be elicited. It is said, however, that practically all those persons in this particular area have worked with peanuts, either in the fields or in factories, and the possibility that in this locality the causative agent is either disseminated from the dust from peanut shells or is activated by it must be considered.

Clinical Manifestations

Lesions may occur in almost any tissue or organ of the body. Since symptoms are due primarily to local tissue infiltration and injury by pressure and displacement by sarcoid lesions, the clinical manifestations depend largely on the organ or system involved.

As noted earlier, sarcoidosis most commonly involves the lungs, lymph nodes, eyes, skin, phalangeal bones, liver and spleen.

LUNGS. Symptoms referable to the chest are usually mild and often consist of a dry, hacking cough, and children are likely to have mild to moderate dyspnea. Gendel, Young and Greiner have classified the pulmonary lesions of sarcoidosis seen on roentgenogram as follows: (1) early bilateral hilar lymph node enlargement, without detectable lung changes; (2) bilateral hilar lymph node enlargement with strandlike infiltration extending from the hilar regions into both lung fields, and small nodular beading and diffuse mottling sometimes occurring along the strands; (3) later, diffuse pulmonary infiltration consisting of patchy coalescent densities; (4) finally, a stage of fibrosis and secondary emphysema with formation of bullae.

The most common roentgenographic finding in children is that of bilateral hilar lymph node enlargement, with or without detectable lung changes (Figs. 1, 2). Cummings noted involvement of the lung and

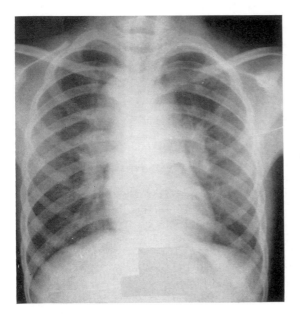

FIGURE 52–1. Bilateral hilar lymph node enlargement. (Courtesy of *New England J. Med.*, 260:962, 1959.)

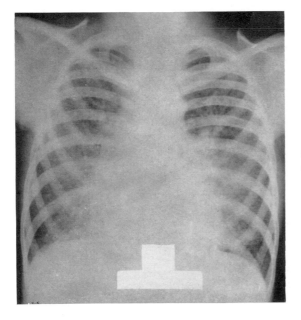

FIGURE 52–2. Bilateral hilar lymph node enlargement and pulmonary infiltration. (Courtesy of *J. Pediat.*, 61:269, 1962.)

hilar lymph nodes in 96 per cent of adult cases, while only sixty-two (55 per cent) of the 113 World cases in children were so affected; nevertheless this 55 per cent constituted the most common finding in that series. Such involvement was noted in all thirteen cases in the Medical College of Virginia group and in sixteen out of eighteen in Siltzbach's series.

LYMPHATICS. Peripheral lymphadenopathy is a common feature of sarcoidosis. The nodes are discrete, painless and freely movable. The typical histologic picture is that of epithelioid cell tubercles, showing little or no necrosis (Fig. 3).

Among the reported World cases in children, there was generalized lymphadenopathy in thirty eight of 113 cases with an additional sixteen cases of isolated or localized lymph node involvement, a total of 48 per cent. Peripheral lymphadenopathy occurred in eight of thirteen Medical College of Virginia cases; thirteen of eighteen cases in Siltzbach's series were so affected.

SKIN. Skin lesions may occur in three different forms (Longcope and Freiman):

(1) small, discrete, slightly elevated nodules; (2) large conglomerate masses, slightly elevated and involving subcutaneous tissues; (3) large flat plaques covering considerable areas of skin over the trunk or extremities.

These lesions may vary in color from waxy, depigmented areas to a reddish blue or violaceous hue. They vary in size from a few millimeters to more than a centimeter in diameter. The lesions are more often seen on the face, but may occur elsewhere. Although Cummings reported the incidence of skin lesions in a series of adults to be only 15 per cent, such lesions may be more common in children. Of the 113 reported World cases, skin lesions were present in fifty seven, but there was involvement of the skin in only three of the thirteen Medical College of Virginia cases and seven of eighteen of Siltzbach's patients.

EYES. The ocular lesions have been described by a number of investigators. Uveitis and iritis constitute the most frequently observed lesions, but keratitis, retinitis, glaucoma, and involvement of

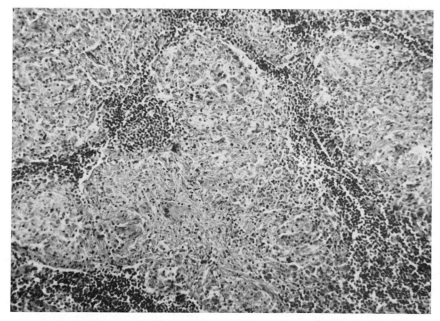

FIGURE 52–3. The architecture of the node is distorted by numerous solid masses of epithelioid cells with occasional giant cells. The masses are surrounded by lymphocytes. No necrosis or caseation is apparent. Lymphoid follicles are almost absent. (Courtesy of *New England J. Med.*, 260:962, 1959.)

the eyelids and lacrimal glands may also occur. Involvement of the eye with resultant partial or total blindness is one of the most feared lesions of sarcoidosis. Although his examination of the World literature suggests that eye lesions in children are not usually severe, McGovern noted one case of partial blindness in his own series. This finding and a survey of the Medical College of Virginia series, in which eye involvement was noted in five of the thirteen cases, appear to refute this conception; such involvement in two patients in the latter group also resulted in partial blindness. Two of Siltzbach's patients suffered blindness in one eye.

UVEOPAROTID FEVER. This syndrome, consisting of ocular disturbances, parotid gland swelling and frequent facial nerve palsy, was first described by Heerfordt in 1909. Uveitis is always present at some time in the course of this syndrome. Usually, low-grade fever, gastrointestinal symptoms and general malaise precede the eye involvement. The World group includes twenty-eight cases (25 per cent), but there were no cases among the Medical College of Virginia group. Siltzbach noted one such patient.

BONES. Osseous lesions, which are usually demonstrable as areas of decreased density and often as "punched out" areas in the metacarpals, metatarsals and distal phalanges, may be either single or multiple. Early changes, not recognizable on roentgenogram, have been revealed by marrow puncture. The incidence of osseous lesions in adults has been variously stated as 2 to 29 per cent; among children there was an incidence of 29 per cent in the World group, 23 per cent (three of thirteen) in the Medical College of Virginia patients and 11 per cent (two of eighteen) in Siltzbach's series. Dunner has suggested that bone lesions may not be as common as was previously suspected.

LIVER. Although hepatic involvement is frequently seen at necropsy, clinical evidence of liver disease is not often apparent. Liver enlargement is the usual finding, and impairment of function is relatively uncommon unless serum protein changes are an indication of liver pathology. In the World series, liver enlargement was noted sixteen times (14 per cent); in the Medical College of Virginia group there were four children with enlarged liver (31 per cent) and Siltzbach noted seven of eighteen patients (39 per cent).

SPLEEN. Although splenic involvement has been demonstrated by needle biopsy, enlargement is practically the only clinical finding. The spleen was palpable in twenty-five of the World cases and in only two of the Medical College of Virginia group; Siltzbach, however, noted splenic enlargement in eight of eighteen cases.

KIDNEY. Kogut and Neumann have reviewed renal involvement in sarcoidosis and reported a case of their own. These authors point out that there have been less than ten reported cases in children; nevertheless this would appear to place the kidney as a not uncommon site of sarcoid involvement in this age group. Renal involvement has been ascribed to one or more of the following processes: (1) sarcoid granulomas infiltrating the renal parenchyma; (2) glomerulitis with basement membrane changes; and (3) hypercalcemia with or without nephrolithiasis and nephrocalcinosis. Abnormal urinary findings may include proteinuria, pyuria, hematuria, granular casts, and calciuria. One of the Medical College of Virginia group had transient hematuria.

HEART. Sarcoid lesions in the myocardium have been found at necropsy in a number of cases. In the 113 World cases there was associated cardiac involvement in six instances; there was no evidence of cardiac involvement in the Medical College of Virginia group. Cardiac changes may be secondary to extensive pulmonary sarcoidosis or may be the result of conduction aberration caused by sarcoid lesions.

NERVOUS SYSTEM. Although central nervous system involvement has been reported in adults, the most commonly noted neurologic involvement in childhood seems to be paralysis of the facial

Table 1. *Comparison of Organs Affected in the World Group and Other Reported Series*

	World Group (113)	Siltzbach (18)	Medical College of Virginia (13)	Mandi (14)	Niitu (16)
Lungs (parenchyma-hilar lymph nodes)	62	16	13	14	16
Peripheral lymphadenopathy	54	13	8	1	0
Skin	57	7	3	0	0
Eyes	55	6	5	0	0
Bones	33	2	3	0	1
Uveoparotid fever	28	1	0	0	0
Spleen	25	8	2	0	0
Liver	16	7	4	0	0

Patients reported by Mandi and Niitu were diagnosed by chest x-ray surveys. One patient in Mandi's series had sarcoid involvement of a tonsil.

nerve. In the 113 World cases there were four instances of facial nerve palsy. Neurologic symptoms apparently result when sarcoid lesions cause local interruption of function.

ENDOCRINE GLANDS. A definite relationship can be demonstrated with the pituitary gland. Diabetes insipidus has been reported in adults, and three of the children in the World group had some evidence of such involvement; none of the Medical College of Virginia group was so involved.

Clinical Picture

The clinical picture of sarcoidosis as reconstructed from the Medical College of Virginia patients is as follows: Ten of the thirteen patients were Negroes, and practically all were in the older age group. Hilar lymph node involvement was always present, the syndrome of uveoparotid fever did not occur, eye lesions were frequently present, and serious eye lesions were noted in two instances.

Laboratory Studies

There are no detailed reports of laboratory findings in the 113 World cases. Among the most frequent significant laboratory changes reported in sarcoidosis are hyperglobulinemia, leukopenia, eosinophilia, hypercalcemia, hypercalciuria

and elevated alkaline phosphatase level.

HYPERGLOBULINEMIA. Salveson was the first to point out that the serum protein concentration may be abnormally high in cases of sarcoidosis. It has since been established that this hyperproteinemia is due to an absolute increase in serum globulin, so that the albumin-globulin ratio is frequently reversed. The Medical College of Virginia series showed hyperglobulinemia in twelve of thirteen cases, and Siltzbach's series showed hyperglobulinemia in ten of seventeen cases.

SERUM CALCIUM. Hypercalcemia occurs in about 20 to 45 per cent of adult patients. Serum calcium concentration above 11 mg. per 100 ml. of serum was noted in two of the ten Medical College of Virginia patients who were tested, and there was hypercalcemia in three of seventeen of Siltzbach's cases.

SERUM ALKALINE PHOSPHATASE. Although Cummings reported the value of serum alkaline phosphatase above 5 Bodansky units in six of twenty adult cases, only one of the nine cases tested at the Medical College of Virginia showed such an increase. Siltzbach's cases showed an elevated alkaline phosphatase in four of eight cases so tested.

LEUKOPENIA. This finding occurred in five of the thirteen Medical College of Virginia patients. In an adult series, leukopenia was found in one fourth of the cases, but was more common among the Negroes.

EOSINOPHILIA. Next to hyperglobulinemia and along with leukopenia, the most consistent laboratory finding among the Medical College of Virginia patients was eosinophilia (above 4 per cent). This occurred in five of thirteen cases, and in three instances there was eosinophilia above 7 per cent. This finding also occurs in adults, although apparently to a lesser degree.

OTHER LABORATORY DATA. Elevation of the erythrocyte sedimentation rate will naturally be expected during the acute phase of the disease. Abnormal urinary findings will be present in those instances in which there is renal involvement; among these may be hematuria, pyuria, proteinuria, granular casts, and hypercalciuria.

Other Diagnostic Procedures

THE KVEIM TEST. This test represents an attempt to elicit a specific skin reaction by the intracutaneous injection of emulsified sarcoid tissue into patients with suspected sarcoidosis. Methods for preparing Kveim suspension have not changed since Williams and Nickerson, Kveim, and Danbolt, first published their work about twenty years ago. Siltzbach has described this method, in which tissue of a sarcoidal lymph node or spleen meeting certain specifications is ground in a mortar with sterile saline solution to make a 10 per cent suspension. The heavier particles are allowed to settle out and are then discarded. The cloudy suspension obtained is then heated to 56°C. for one hour, on two successive days. It is tested for sterility, preservatives are added, and it is then ready for use. The intracutaneous test is performed in the manner of a Mantoux test, with the use of 0.15 to 0.2 ml. per injection. Any nodule which appears at the injection site, no matter how small, is biopsied after twenty-eight days. Although Siltzbach reports a positive Kveim test reaction in sixteen of eighteen patients, scarcity of effective Kveim test

material limits the usefulness of the test at this time.

LYMPH NODE BIOPSY. Biopsy of a lymph node, demonstrating an epithelioid cell tubercle, with little or no necrosis, is an essential in diagnosis. Twelve of the Medical College of Virginia group met this requirement (diagnosis in the other patient was substantiated by lung biopsy).

An enlarged peripheral lymph node is most suitable for biopsy, but if none is present, biopsy of the scalene fat pad is most likely to reveal a lesion compatible with sarcoidosis. Muscle biopsy may also be indicated, and, as noted above, lung biopsy is occasionally helpful.

OTHER TESTS. The tuberculin test, the histoplasmin skin test and the coccidioidin skin test should be performed on each patient with suspected sarcoidosis. Although a positive reaction with one of these antigens does not necessarily controvert the diagnosis, it may be an indication that the infection is merely one which simulates sarcoidosis.

Prognosis

Sones and Israel, in a review of more than 200 adult patients in Philadelphia, have attempted to determine the prognosis of sarcoidosis. They state that sarcoidosis, as observed by them, was neither as benign as indicated in some reports, nor as malignant as in others. Sones and Israel found survival rates, calculated by the life table method, to be 88.8 per cent after five years of observation and 84.8 per cent after ten years, indicating considerable diminution of survival as the result of sarcoidosis.

Treatment

Since the cause of sarcoidosis is unknown, there is no known specific therapy. Corticosteroids and corticotropin are the only agents available at present which can suppress the acute manifestations of sarcoidosis. These agents are used only during the acute and dangerous episodes.

Corticosteroid (or corticotropin) therapy is always indicated in patients with intrinsic ocular disease, with diffuse pulmonary lesions with alveolar-capillary block, with central nervous system lesions, with myocardial involvement, with hypersplenism and with persistent hypercalcemia. Relative indications for corticosteroid therapy include progressive or symptomatic pulmonary lesions, disfiguring cutaneous and lymph node lesions, constitutional symptoms and joint involvement, lesions of the nasal, laryngeal and bronchial mucosa, and persistent facial nerve palsy.

Fresh lesions are apparently more responsive than older ones. Suppressive action is often temporary, but it is beneficial when the unremitting course of such disease will produce loss of organ function. For example, corticosteroids can reduce the level of serum calcium and may thus help prevent nephrocalcinosis and renal insufficiency and possible band keratitis. Whether or not corticosteroids should be utilized in the treatment of those patients whose disease consists only of asymptomatic miliary nodules or bronchopneumonic patches in the lung fields is debatable.

The initial daily dose of prednisone or prednisolone in adults is 20 to 30 mg. and of triamcinolone, 15 to 25 mg. After a few weeks the dose is gradually reduced. In children the dose of prednisone or prednisolone is 1 mg. per kilogram of body weight per day, and of triamcinolone, 0.75 mg. per kilogram of body weight per day, in four divided doses, with gradual reduction as noted above. The course of treatment is usually about six months, but some patients require continuous maintenance therapy. Siltzbach reported the frequent occurrence of temporary relapse following the discontinuation of corticosteroid therapy, but noted that improvement usually follows even if the treatment is not resumed. In the management of ocular sarcoidosis, corticosteroids in the form of either ointment or drops (0.5 to 1 per cent) are utilized in conjunction with the systemic use of these agents. During the course of

such local therapy, the pupils are kept in a state of continuous dilatation by use of an atropine ointment (1 per cent).

Corticosteroid ointment may also be utilized in the treatment of cutaneous lesions, but only in conjunction with systemic therapy, since better results are obtained with the latter.

REFERENCES

Andersen, H.: Sarcoidosis (Boeck) in a Child Treated with Cortisone and ACTH, *Acta paediat.*, 45:343, 1956.

Anderson, J., Dent, C. E., Harper, C, and Philpot, G. R.: Effect of Cortisone on Calcium Metabolism in Sarcoidosis with Hypercalcaemia; Possible Antagonistic Action of Cortisone and Vitamin D. *Lancet*, 2:720, 1954.

Barker, D. H. W.: Benign Lymphogranulomatosis with Apparent Involvement of the Anterior Pituitary. *Brit. J. Dermat.*, 58:70, 1946.

Bauer, H. J., and Gentz, C.: The Results of Mass X-ray Examination in Stockholm City During the Years 1949-1951. *Acta tuberc. Scandinav.*, 29:22, 1953.

Beier, F. R., and Lahey, M. E.: Sarcoidosis Among Children in Utah and Idaho. *J. Pediat.*, 65:350, 1964.

Berger, K. W., and Relman, A. S.: Renal Impairment Due to Sarcoid Infiltration of the Kidney; Report of a Case proved by Renal Biopsies Before and After Treatment with Cortisone. *New England J. Med.*, 252:44, 1955.

Besnier, E.: Lupus pernio de la face, synovitis fongueses (scrofulotuberculeuses) symetriques des extremites superieures. *Ann. Derm. Syph.*, 10:333, 1889.

Block, M.: Sarcoid Diagnosed by Needle Biopsy of the Spleen: Report of a case, *J.A.M.A.*, 149:748, 1952.

Boeck, C.: Multiple Benign Sarkoid of Skin. *J. Cutan. Genito-Urin. Dis.*, 17:543, 1899.

Boman, A.: Diabetes Insipidus vid lymphogranulomatosis benigna. *Nord. Med.*, 47:675, 1952.

Chapman, J. S.: Notes on the Secondary Factors Involved in the Etiology of Sarcoidosis. *Am. Rev. Tuberc.* 71:459, 1955.

Cummings, M. M., and Dunner, E.: Pulmonary Sarcoidosis. *M. Clin. North Amer.*, 43:163, 1959.

Cummings, M. M., and Hudgins, P. C.: Chemical Constituents of Pine Pollen and Their Possible Relationship to Sarcoidosis. *Am. J. M. Sc.*, 236:311, 1958.

Cummings, M. M., Dunner, E., Schmidt, R. H., Jr., and Barnwell, J. B.: Concepts of Epidemiology of Sarcoidosis. *Postgrad. Med.*, 19:437, 1956.

Danbolt, N.: On the Skin Test with Sarcoid-Tissue-Suspension (Kveim's Reaction). *Acta Dermatorener*, 31:184, 1951.

Davidson, C. N., and others: Nephrocalcinosis Associated with Sarcoidosis: A Presentation and Discussion of Seven Cases. *Radiology*, 62:203, 1954.

Deller, D. J., Brodziak, I. A., and Phillips, A. D.: Renal Failure in Hypercalcaemic Sarcoidosis. *Brit. M.J.*, 1:1278, 1959.

Dent, C. E., Flynn, F. V., and Nabarro, J. D. N: Hypercalcaemia and Impairment of Renal Function in Generalized Sarcoidosis. *Brit. M.J.*, 2:808, 1953.

Dressler, M.: Ueber einem Fall von Splenomegalie, durch Sternalpunktion als Boecksche Krankheit verifiziert. *Klin. Wschr.*, 2:1467, 1938.

Dunner, E., Cummings, M. M., Williams, J. H., Jr., Schmidt, R. H., and Barnwell, J. B.: A New Look at Sarcoidosis, a Review of Clinical Records of 160 Patients with a Diagnosis of Sarcoidosis. *South. M.J.*, 50:1141, 1957.

Essellier, A. F., and others: Die zentralnervosen Erscheinungsformen des Morbus Besnier-Boeck-Schaumann. *Schweiz med. Wschr.*, 81:376, 1951.

Fisher, A. M.: In Discussion on A. M. Fisher: Some Clinical and Pathological Features Observed in Sarcoidosis. *Tr. Am. Clin. Climat. A.*, 59:73, 1947.

Garland, H. G., and Thompson, J. G.: Uveoparotid Tuberculosis (Febris Uveoparotid of Heerfordt). *Quart. J. Med.*, 2:157, 1933.

Gendel, B. R., Young, J. M., and Greiner, D. J.: Sarcoidosis: A Review of Twenty-Four Additional Cases. *Am. J. Med.*, 12:205, 1952.

Gentry, J. T., Nitowsky, H. M., and Michael, M., Jr.: Studies on the Epidemiology of Sarcoidosis in the United States; The Relationship to Soil Areas and to Urban-Rural Residence. *J. Clin. Invest.*, 34:1839, 1955.

Gilg, I.: Kliniske undersogelser over Boeck's sarcoid (Sarcoidose): behandling og forlob. *Ugeskr. Laege*, 118:46, 1956.

Gleckler, W. J.: Hypercalcemia and Renal Insufficiency Due to Sarcoidosis: Treatment with Cortisone. *Ann. Int. Med.*, 44:174, 1956.

Heerfordt, C. F.: Ueber eine "Febris uveoparotidea subschronica," an der Glandula Parotis und der Uvea des Auges lokalisiert und haufig mit Paresen cerebrospinaler Nerven kompliaiert. *Arch. Ophthal.*, 70:254, 1909.

Henneman, P. H., Carroll, E. L., and Dempsey, E. F.: The Mechanism Responsible for Hypercalciuria in Sarcoid. *J. Clin. Invest.*, 33:941, 1954.

Henneman, P. H., and others: The Cause of Hypercalciuria in Sarcoid and Its Treatment with Cortisone and Sodium Phytate. *J. Clin. Invest.*, 35:1229, 1956.

Holt, J. F., and Owens, W. I.: The Osseous Lesions of Sarcoidosis. *Radiology*, 53:11, 1949.

Hutchinson, J.: Cases of Mortimer's Malady (Lupus Vulgaris Multiplex Nonulcerans et Non-serpigeneous). *Arch. Surg.* (London), 9:307, 1898.

Israel, H. L., and Sones, M.: Sarcoidosis: Clinical Observations on 160 Cases. A.M.A. *Arch. Int. Med.*, 102:766, 1958.

Jacques, W. E.: Sarcoidosis: A Review and a Proposed Etiologic Concept. *Arch. Path.*, 53:558, 1952.

James, D. G.: Ocular Sarcoidosis, *Am. J. Med.*, 26:331, 1959.

Idem: Quoted in L. E. Siltzbach: The Kveim Test in Sarcoidosis. *Am. J. Med.*, 30:495, 1961 (editorial).

Johnson, J. B., and Jason, R. S.: Sarcoidosis of the Heart: Report of a Case and Review of Literature. *Am. Heart J.*, 27:246, 1944.

Katz, S., Coke, C. P., and Reed, H. R.: Sarcoidosis. *New England J. Med.*, 229:498, 1943.

Kendig, E. L., Jr.: Sarcoidosis in Children. *Am. Rev. Resp. Dis.*, 84:49, 1961.

Idem: Sarcoidosis Among Children, *J. Pediat.*, 61:269, 1962.

Kendig, E. L., Jr., and Wiley, E. J., Jr.: Sarcoidosis in Children. *Postgrad. M. J.*, 37:590, 1961.

Kendig, E. L., Jr., Peacock, R. L., and Ryburn, S.: Sarcoidosis: Report of Three Cases in Siblings Under Fifteen Years of Age. *New England J. Med.*, 260:962, 1959.

Kennedy, A. C.: Boeck's Sarcoid: Report of a Case with Lesions Detected in Material Obtained by Sternal Puncture. *Glasgow M. J.*, 31:10, 1950.

King, D. S.: Sarcoid Disease as Revealed in Chest Roentgenograms. *Am. J. Roentgenol.*, 45:505, 1941.

King, M. J.: Ocular Lesions of Boeck's Sarcoid. *Tr. Am. Ophth. Soc.*, 37:442, 1939.

Klatskin, G., and Gordon, M.: Renal Complications of Sarcoidosis and Their Relationship to Hypercalcemia; With a Report of Two Cases Simulating Hyperparathyroidism. *Am. J. Med.*, 15:484, 1953.

Kogut, M. D., and Neumann, L. I.: Renal Involvement in Boeck's Sarcoidosis. *Pediatrics*, 28:410, 1961.

Kraus, E. J.: Sarcoidosis (Boeck-Besnier-Schaumann Disease) as a Cause of Pituitary Syndrome. *J. Lab. & Clin. Med.*, 28:140, 1942.

Kveim, A.: Preliminary Report on New and Specific Cutaneous Reaction in Boeck's Sarcoid. *Nord. Med.*, 9:169, 1941.

Lindau, A., and Lowegren, A.: Benign Lymphogranulomatosis (Schaumann's Disease) and the Eye. *Acta Med. Scandinav.*, 105:242, 1940.

Longcope, W. T.: Sarcoidosis. *Veterans Admin. Tech. Bull.*, TB-10-73:1015, 1951.

Longcope, W. T., and Fisher, A. M.: Involvement of the Heart in Carcoidosis. *J. Mt. Sinai Hosp.*, 8:784, 1942.

Longcope, W. T., and Freiman, D. G.: A Study

of Sarcoidosis; Based on a Combined Investigation of 160 Cases, Including 30 autopsies, from the Johns Hopkins Hospital and Massachusetts General Hospital. *Medicine,* 31:1, 1952.

Longcope, W. T., and Pierson, J. W.: Boeck's Sarcoid (Sarcoidosis). *Bull. Johns Hopkins Hosp.,* 60:223, 1937.

Mackensen, G.: Veranderungen am Augenhintergrund bei Besnier-Boeck-Schaumannscher Erkrankung. *Klin. Mbl. Augen.,* 121:51, 1952.

Mandi, L.: Thoracic Sarcoidosis in Childhood. *Acta tuberc. Scandinav.,* 45:256, 1964.

Mankiewicz, E.: The Relationship of Sarcoidosis to Anonymous Mycobacteria, *Acta Med. Scandinav.,* Supplement 425:68, 1964.

McCort, J. J., Wood, R. H., Hamilton, J. B., and Erlich, D. E.: Sarcoidosis: Clinical and Roentgenologic Study of 28 Proved Cases. *Arch. Int. Med.,* 80:293, 1947.

McGovern, J. P., and Merritt, D. M.: Sarcoidosis in Childhood. *Advances in Pediatrics,* 8:97, 1956.

McSwiney, R. R., and Mills, I. H.: Hypercalcaemia Due to Sarcoidosis; Treatment with Cortisone. *Lancet,* 2:862, 1956.

Michael, M., Jr., Cole, R., Beeson, P. B., and Olson, B.: Sarcoidosis: Preliminary Report on a Study of 350 Cases with Special Reference to Epidemiology. *Am. Rev. Tuberc.,* 62:403, 1950.

Nagle, R.: Hypercalcemia and Neophrocalcinosis in Sarcoidosis. *J. Mt. Sinai Hosp.,* N.Y., 28:268, 1961.

Niitu, Y., Watanabe, M., Swetake, T., Handia, T., Munakata K., and Shiroishi, K.: Sixteen Cases of Intrathoracic Sarcoidosis Found Among School Children in Sendai in Mass X-ray Surveys of the Chest. *Research Reports of Research Institute for Tuberculosis, Leprosy and Cancer,* 12:99, 1965.

Nitter, L.: Changes in the Chest Roentgenogram in Boeck's Sarcoid of the Lungs. *Acta Radiol.* (suppl. 105), 1, 1953.

Osterberg, G.: Iritis Boeck (Sarkoid of Boeck in Iris). *Brit. J. Ophth.,* 23:145, 1939.

Pautrier, L. M.: Le syndrome de Heerfordt des ophthalmologistes n'est qu'une forme particuliere de la maladie de Besnier-Boeck-Schaumann. *Ann. dermat. et Syph.,* 9:161, 1938.

Idem: *Une nouvelle grande reticulo-endothelioses: La maladie de Besnier-Boeck-Schaumann.* Paris, Masson et Cie, 1940.

Pennell, W. H.: Boeck's Sarcoid with Involvement of the Central Nervous System. *J. Nerv. & Ment. Dis.,* 115:451, 1952.

Phillips, R. W., and Fitzpatrick, D. P.: Steroid Therapy of Hypercalcemia and Renal Insufficiency in Sarcoidosis. *New England J. Med.,* 254:1216, 1956.

Polland, R.: Multipl Benignes Sarkoid bei einem saugling. *Dermz.,* 61:360, 1931.

Refvem, O.: Pathogenesis of Boeck's Disease (Sarcoidosis). *Acta Med. Scandinav.,* 149: (Suppl. 294), 1, 1954.

Reisner, D.: Boeck's Sarcoid and Systemic Sarcoidosis (Besnier-Boeck-Schaumann Disease): Study of 35 Cases. *Am. Rev. Tuberc.,* 49:289, 1944.

Idem: Boeck's Sarcoid and Systemic Sarcoidosis. *Am. Rev. Tuberc.,* 49:437, 1944.

Ricker, W., and Clark, M.: Sarcoidosis: A Clinicopathologic Review of 300 Cases, Including 22 Autopsies. *Am. J. Clin. Path.,* 19:725, 1949.

Riley, E. A.: Boeck's Sarcoid. *Am. Rev. Tuberc.,* 62:231, 1950.

Roos, B.: Cerebral Manifestations of Lymphogranulomatosis Benigna (Schaumann) and Uveoparotid Fever (Heerfordt). *Acta med. Scandinav.,* 104:123, 1940.

Salveson, H. A.: Sarcoid of Boeck, a Disease of Importance to Internal Medicine; Report of Four Cases. *Acta med. Scandinav.,* 86:127, 1935.

Sarcoidosis. *Statistics of Navy Med.,* 13:3, 1957.

Scadding, J. G.: Discussion on Sarcoidosis. *Proc. Roy. Soc. Med.,* 49:799, 1956.

Idem: Mycobacterium Tuberculosis in the Aetiology of Sarcoidosis. *Brit. M. J.,* 2:16, 1960.

Schaumann, J.: Etude sur le lupus pernio et ses rapports avec les sarcoides et la tuberculose. *Ann. dermat. syph.,* 6 (fifth series) : 357, 1916-1917.

Scholz, D. A.: Effect of Steroid Therapy on Hypercalcemia and Renal Insufficiency in Sarcoidosis. *J.A.M.A.,* 169:682, 1959.

Scholz, D. A., and Keating, F. R., Jr.: Renal Insufficiency, Renal Calculi and Nephrocalcinosis in Sarcoidosis. *Am. J. Med.,* 21:75, 1956.

Scholz, D. A., Power, M. H., and Dearing, W. H.: Metabolic Effects of Cortisone in a Case of Sarcoidosis with Hypercalcemia and Renal Insufficiency. *Proc. Staff Meet. Mayo Clin.,* 32:182, 1957.

Siltzbach, L. E.: Effect of Cortisone in Sarcoidosis. *Am. J. Med.,* 12:139, 1952.

Idem: Sarcoidosis: Prevalence and Diagnosis. *Seminar Internat.,* 9:2, 1960.

Idem: The Kveim Test in Sarcoidosis. *Am. J. Med.,* 30:495, 1961 (editorial).

Siltzbach, L. E., and Greenberg, G. M.: To be published.

Sones, M., and Israel, H. L.: Course and Prognosis of Sarcoidosis. *Am. J. Med.,* 29:84, 1960.

Walgren, S.: Pulmonary Sarcoidosis Detected by Photofluorographic Surveys in Sweden, 1950-1957. *Nord. Med.,* 60:1194, 1958.

Walsh, F. B.: Ocular Importance of Sarcoid; Its Relation to Uveoparotid Fever. *Arch. Ophth.,* 21:421, 1939.

Weekly Case Conference: Sarcoidosis. *Clin. Proc. Child. Hosp.,* 12:253, 1956.

Wegelius, C., and Wijkstroem, S.: Mass Radi-
    ography in Sweden. *Nord. Med.*, 60:1191,
    1958.
Williams, R. H., and Nickerson, D. A.: Skin

Reactions in Sarcoid. *Proc. Soc. Exper. Biol.
    & Med.*, 33:403, 1935.
Yesner, R., and Silver, M.: Fatal Myocardial Sar-
    coidosis. *Am. Heart J.*, 41:777, 1951.

CHAPTER FIFTY-THREE

Tuberculosis

EDWIN L. KENDIG, Jr., M.D.

General Considerations

From the beginnings of history, tuberculosis has created a major health problem throughout the civilized world. This disease has been a serious and constant threat, and although great strides toward its eradication have been made in many countries, there are other areas in which it is still largely uncontrolled.

Prior to 1882 there was sharp difference of opinion as to the infectiousness of the disease. In that year, however, Koch announced discovery of the causative agent of tuberculosis, and a more unified and enlightened approach to the problem ensued.

This identification of the tubercle bacillus led subsequently to community action, and finally to organized public health measures aimed at control and eradication of the disease. That these measures, in addition to a far better standard of living, have been effective in the United States, though less so in some parts of the world, is evinced by the sharp drop in mortality from the disease, from 200 per 100,000 population in 1900 to less than fifty per 100,000 in 1940. The advent of the antimicrobial agents, particularly streptomycin in 1944 and isoniazid in 1952, has resulted in an even more precipitate drop, so that mortality from tuberculosis in the United States in 1963 was 4.9 per 100,000 population.

Further evidence of the effectiveness of the campaign against tuberculosis in the United States is the great decrease in the number of persons sensitive to tuberculin. Whereas twenty to thirty years ago the rate of sensitivity among youths of high school or college age was more than 50 per cent, a recent survey of 70,000 Navy recruits of seventeen to twenty-one years of age showed that only 5 per cent were positive reactors.

It is apparent, then, that there has been significant progress toward control of tuberculosis in the United States, but the optimistic feeling that this disease will soon be eradicated which has been engendered by these figures is misleading. The new measure of the seriousness of tuberculosis is the number of new active cases; in 1962 there were 53,315 reported in the United States, a figure which excludes an estimated 10,000 relapses. A report to the Surgeon General by a Task Force on Tuberculosis Control in the United States has indicated that "a realistic measure of the persons now directly affected by tuberculosis is the sum of the 110,000 known active cases on tuberculosis registers, the estimated 250,000 inactive cases whose disease was active less than five years ago, and the 250,000 contacts of newly reported cases: a total of 610,000 persons."

Although it is well known that approx-

Table 1. *New Active Tuberculosis Cases, by Age, Race and Sex, United States, 1962*

Age Groups	Total	White			Nonwhite		
		Total	Male	Female	Total	Male	Female
All ages	53,315	36,012	24,325	11,687	17,303	10,526	6,777
0–4	3,044	1,662	816	846	1,382	655	727
5–14	2,992	1,560	763	797	1,432	658	774
15–24	4,806	2,807	1,409	1,398	1,999	886	1,113
25–44	15,522	9,339	5,805	3,534	6,183	3,646	2,537
45–64	17,182	12,667	9,885	2,782	4,515	3,390	1,125
65 and over	9,769	7,977	5,647	2,330	1,792	1,291	501

This table demonstrates the frequency of tuberculosis in those less than 14 years of age (11 per cent).

From The Future of Tuberculosis Control. A Report to the Surgeon General of the Public Health Service by a Task Force on Tuberculosis Control in the United States, Dec. 1963. (Courtesy of United States Department of Health, Education, and Welfare, Public Health Service, Communicable Disease Center, Atlanta, Georgia.)

imately half of the cases of tuberculosis occurring in the United States in recent years have been in persons over forty-five years of age, few realize that more than 11 per cent of the cases reported in 1962 were in those less than fourteen years of age (Table 1). These are the cases which can be most easily prevented.

Another indication of the high incidence of tuberculosis in infants and young children in certain segments of the population is evident in the results of a ten-year study on BCG vaccine conducted in the Child Chest Clinic at the Medical College of Virginia and involving more than 1800 infants less than six months of age. In this study it was found that 16 per cent of the unvaccinated or control group became infected with tuberculosis, as determined by a positive tuberculin reaction.

That tuberculosis can ever be controlled solely by antimicrobial agents seems extremely doubtful. Certainly this cannot be accomplished with the drugs now available. The present-day approach must still be aimed at early diagnosis, isolation of infected persons, and the judicious use of BCG vaccine and available antituberculosis drugs.

Etiology

In 1882 Koch demonstrated that *Mycobacterium tuberculosis* is the causative agent of tuberculosis in man. This agent is a member of a family (Mycobacteriaceae), the chief characteristic of which is acid fastness, a property which may be defined as resistance to acid discoloration displayed by organisms that have been stained with aniline dyes. Although it is an oversimplification to state that the lipid content is the sole cause of this characteristic of acid fastness, mycolic acid is thought to play a role, perhaps a large one. Lipids also appear to be a factor in the formation of tubercles. Tuberculoproteins, the cause of the hypersensitivity which occurs after infection has taken place, are also important in antibody production.

There is no chemical constituent of the tubercle bacillus which has any demonstrable toxicity for tissues not sensitized to tuberculin.

When stained with an acid-fast stain, and examined under the oil-immersion lens of a microscope, tubercle bacilli appear as slender, bright, refractile red rods, about 4 microns in length and 0.5 micron in width. They are often slightly curved and may be of various sizes and shapes, and may appear to be beaded or segmented (Fig. 1).

Dried tubercle bacilli kept in the dark may survive and remain virulent for many months, but they can be killed by exposure to direct sunlight or ultraviolet rays. In a fluid suspension they are killed

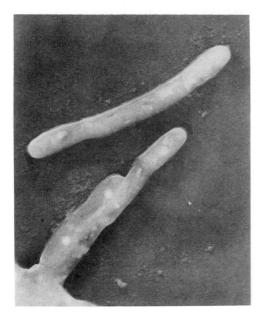

FIGURE 53–1. Virulent tubercle bacilli (H 37 Rv × 38,000). (From NTA Bulletin, June 1961. Courtesy of the National Tuberculosis Association, 1790 Broadway, New York, New York.)

by one minute of boiling or by a temperature of 60°C. (140°F.) within fifteen or twenty minutes. One of the most effective household and hospital disinfectants is 70 per cent isopropyl alcohol.

Epidemiology

Because of the great decrease in mortality and the closure of many sanatoriums, there has been widespread propaganda to the effect that tuberculosis is no longer a serious problem in the United States. This is hardly an accurate estimate of the present status of this disease. As noted above, figures indicating a large reduction in the death rate from tuberculosis do not reflect the seriousness of the problem. The number of newly reported cases is a more accurate measure of the widespread nature of the disease, but even these tell only part of the story.

It should be kept clearly in mind that an adult, adolescent or older child who has active pulmonary tuberculosis has a contagious disease. Spread of the infection is usually accomplished by droplets con-

taining viable tubercle bacilli, and household contacts, particularly children, are extremely susceptible to this danger. In general, those children with nonprogressive primary pulmonary tuberculosis should not be considered contagious.

In recent years there has been a tendency for many physicians to accede to the request of tuberculous adults and attempt to carry out therapy while the patient remains at home. This may be unsatisfactory for several reasons. The patient usually does not receive satisfactory instruction in the ways by which he may lessen the danger of spread of his infection, and even if so instructed, he does not have the advantage of the sanatorium atmosphere which promotes the actual carrying out of these directions. When there are young children in the home, the chance of contact of the child with the patient is great, no matter how much precaution is taken. This may in part account for the high incidence of tuberculous infection in the young age group.

In a study carried out at the Medical College of Virginia, it appears that contact of an infant with a mother who has supposedly inactive tuberculous disease and sputum negative for tubercle bacilli may not be as safe as expected. Twenty of forty-one infants in this category became infected with tuberculosis, and three died with tuberculous meningitis (Table 2). Although contact of the child with other adults in the household may not be as intimate as that with the mother, the risk does not appear inconsequential. It should be noted, however, that there appears to be much less risk in that period during which the tuberculous adult receives adequate antimicrobial therapy.

Among the more common sources of tuberculous disease in the child are the

Table 2. *Infants Born of Tuberculous Mothers with Supposedly Inactive Disease*

Infected	20
Noninfected	21
Total	41

more elderly members of the family, such as grandparents, aunts or uncles, or other older relatives. Baby sitters, household servants, boarders and frequent visitors in the home are often the tuberculosis contact. A one-year-old child in our practice had a positive reaction in a routine tuberculin test. Careful search of family contacts, household servants and frequent visitors to the home was not productive, but six months later the gardener, with whom the little boy often played, announced that he had been to the clinic and found that he had tuberculosis. The possibilities of contact with tuberculosis are numerous, and none should be overlooked.

That epidemic spread may occur in population groups largely unexposed to tuberculosis has been stressed by Mande, who reported twenty-five such epidemics in schools in France. The source case is usually a student or one of the school personnel, more often a teacher.

Predisposing Factors

Most persons who are infected by *Mycobacterium tuberculosis* do not acquire so-called clinical disease. Some persons have a greater resistance than do others, and the resistance of a given person may vary from time to time. Important, too, is the relative virulence of the invading organisms and the number of bacilli in the inoculum.

Chronic illness, malnutrition and chronic fatigue may increase susceptibility to tuberculous disease. A quiescent tuberculous lesion may be activated by nontuberculous infections, such as rubeola and pertussis, by conditions of stress created by surgery, smallpox vaccination, and by corticosteroid therapy. It should be noted, however, that the Medical College of Virginia studies show that rubeola exerts no deleterious effect on either primary tuberculosis or such serious forms of the disease as tuberculous meningitis when the patient is receiving isoniazid therapy at that time. Many studies have also shown that there is no deleterious

effect from corticosteroid therapy when the patient is under treatment with isoniazid.

Heredity

Although the higher incidence of tuberculosis in some families is usually the result of more intimate contact with the disease, Lurie has presented studies with rabbits showing good evidence for the importance of hereditary factors. Congenital infection is rare.

Age, Race and Sex

The mortality rate from tuberculosis is higher during infancy and again at adolescence. It is not so high during the intervening years of childhood. There is a higher death rate from tuberculosis in the United States among nonwhites than among the white population, but differences in racial immunity are not that easily determined. It seems likely that the higher mortality rate among the nonwhite population may be largely the result of social and environmental stress and greater opportunity for infection.

During the latter part of childhood and adolescence, girls have a higher incidence of and mortality from tuberculosis than do boys. Except for the high incidence of disease in older males, there is no such difference between the sexes at other age levels.

Allergy and Immunity

After tuberculous infection there is a two- to ten-week period of incubation. At the close of this period the presence of allergy is manifested by a positive reaction in the tuberculin test. With the appearance of this allergic state there is alteration in the host response to tubercle bacilli, now manifested by exudation and a tendency for the infection to become localized. At some less definite time some immunity also develops. This immunity is a relative one, and the infecting organisms may be so many in number or

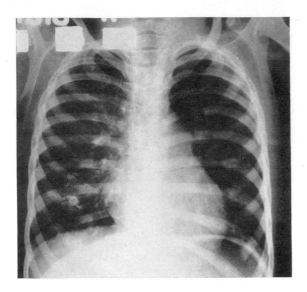

FIGURE 53–2. Multiple calcified primary foci.

Pathogenesis and Pathology

Since the usual mode of tuberculous infection is by inhalation, the primary lesion occurs in the lung parenchyma in more than 95 per cent of the cases. It may, of course, occur elsewhere. In a previously uninfected person there is first an accumulation of polymorphonuclear leukocytes; this is followed by epithelioid cell proliferation, producing the typical tubercle. Giant cells appear, and the whole area is surrounded by lymphocytes.

Almost as soon as infection takes place, tubercle bacilli are carried by histiocytes from the primary focus and travel to the regional lymph nodes. When the primary focus is in the lung parenchyma, the bronchopulmonary glands are usually involved, but an apical focus may drain into the paratracheal lymph nodes.

Hypersensitivity of body tissues to tuberculin does not take place immediately, but makes its appearance only after a period varying from two to ten weeks. During this period the primary focus may grow larger, but does not become encapsulated. When hypersensitivity develops, the perifocal reaction becomes much more prominent and the regional lymph nodes enlarge. The primary focus may become caseous, but with the development of acquired resistance, it usually becomes walled off. This caseous material gradually becomes inspissated and later calcified. The lesion may completely disappear.

Primary foci are usually single, but the occurrence of two or more such lesions is not rare in our experience (Fig. 2). After hypersensitivity has developed, however, the typical primary complex (parenchymal focus and regional gland involvement) does not occur.

Although the usual tendency in primary pulmonary tuberculosis is toward healing, there may be progression of the primary parenchymal focus. The lesion continues to enlarge, the surrounding tissue becomes pneumonic in nature, and the overlying pleura may be thickened. Under these conditions the caseous center may liquefy and empty into one or more of the bronchi, thereby resulting in a residual cavity and one or more new areas of tuberculous pneumonia (cavitating primary).

It is during the stage of caseation, too, that hematogenous dissemination is most likely to occur. This may result in widespread miliary lesions throughout some or all of the viscera or in isolated foci in such parts of the body as the eye, lungs, bones, brain, kidneys, liver or spleen. Although these isolated foci may occur under these conditions, they are more apt to result from the few tubercle bacilli which may reach the blood stream before hypersensitivity develops. This bacillemia may occur either directly or by way of the regional lymph nodes and the thoracic duct.

As a rule, progression of the metastatic lesions occurs as a result of seeding from the blood stream. This may be direct, as in miliary or renal tuberculosis. On the other hand, late progression resulting from a previous hematogenous seeding may occur by continuity. For example, Rich and McCordock have demonstrated that tuberculous meningitis is more likely to result from a tuberculoma contiguous to the meninges.

The involved regional lymph nodes also have a tendency to heal, but less so than does the primary parenchymal focus. Tubercle bacilli may persist for years, even though demonstrable areas of calcification indicate that at least partial healing has occurred.

Because of their location, the hyperemic, edematous hilar lymph nodes may be the cause of considerable pathology, primarily of an obstructive nature. The nodes may encroach on the bronchi, causing occlusion of the lumen with resultant atelectasis of that area of the lung distal to the obstruction. Or, much more often, a caseous node or mass of nodes may become attached to the wall of the bronchus by inflammatory reaction. Infection may progress through the wall and create a fistulous tract. Disease may thus be transmitted through the bronchus to that area of the lung served by that bronchus. Similarly, too, the extrusion of the caseous contents from an affected node into the bronchus may produce complete obstruction, with atelectasis of the distal lung

parenchyma. A lesion thus created is often a combination of atelectasis and pneumonia, however, and not atelectasis alone.

When obstruction of the bronchus is incomplete, a check-valve type of mechanism may result. There may be less hindrance to inspired air than to the exit of respired air, thus resulting in hyperaeration due to the obstruction.

Obstruction of a portion of the wall of a bronchus may lead to a fibrous stricture with resultant partial or complete lack of aeration to that portion of the lung. Tuberculous lymph nodes may also occasionally invade or compress adjacent structures.

Most complications of primary tuberculosis occur during the first year following the onset of the infection. After this time complications are relatively infrequent until the period of adolescence, when pulmonary tuberculosis ("adult or reinfection tuberculosis") becomes a major problem. This occurs twice as often in girls as in boys. Not enough time has yet elapsed so that it can be established whether or not this high incidence of pulmonary tuberculosis in adolescence will follow those cases of primary tuberculosis which have been treated with isoniazid.

It can rarely be determined whether the chronic pulmonary tuberculosis which appears years after primary tuberculosis has healed is the result of activation of the healed primary lesion or the development of a new infection. The presence of an increased resistance toward a new infection which follows the primary infection would seem to favor the endogenous theory.

Diagnosis

THE TUBERCULIN TEST. A positive reaction in the tuberculin test indicates the presence of tuberculous infection, and the test is, therefore, of great aid in the diagnosis of the disease. The degree of activity, if any, or the severity of the disease process cannot be thus determined. There are other limitations of the test,

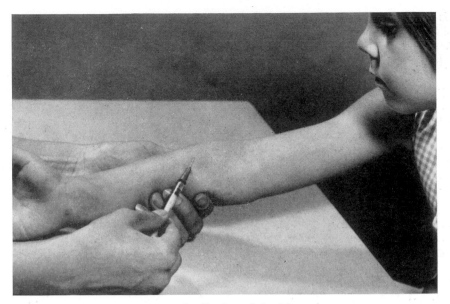

FIGURE 53–3. Application of the Mantoux test.

and these, including the various causes of false-positive and false-negative reactions, will be discussed later.

Tuberculin solution, utilized in skin testing, is available in two forms, OT (Old tuberculin solution) and PPD (purified protein derivative). The former, which has been known since the time of Koch, has some variation of potency in different batches. When kept in a refrigerator, Old tuberculin is satisfactory for skin testing for at least two weeks and probably for a one-month period. It is available as a stable liquid concentrate, and the diluent is a special buffered isotonic fluid available commercially. A dilution of one part concentrated tuberculin to 10,000 parts diluent (1:10,000) supplies approximately 1 international tuberculin unit (TU).

PPD (purified protein derivative) is the protein of the tubercle bacillus which has been precipitated from cultures of the tubercle bacillus on nonprotein medium (Long's medium). Its antigenicity is reduced by heating, and it is filtered free of dead bacilli. The World Health Organization has designated PPD as the international standard tuberculin (PPD-S). PPD is available commercially; it is dispensed in tablet form and is dissolved in a measured amount of diluent before use. When refrigerated and protected from light, PPD-S is said to be satisfactory for skin testing for a six-month period.

The most accurate and reliable method of tuberculin testing is the *Mantoux (intracutaneous) test* (Figs. 3, 4). A measured amount of tuberculin solution of known concentration is injected intracutaneously. For this test, a syringe so graduated that fractional parts of a milliliter may be measured and a short-bevel 26- or 27-gauge needle should be used. Tuberculin is thermostable, and traces of it remain on syringes and glassware after ordinary cleansing methods. A syringe for tuberculin testing should, therefore, not be utilized for other skin tests. A separate needle is used for each patient. If the needle and the syringe are not of the disposable variety, they should be sterilized by autoclaving. If this is not possible, they should be boiled for thirty minutes.

The test must be carefully prepared, and exactly 0.1 ml. of the testing material is injected into the skin on the volar surface of the forearm. Unless a definite wheal follows injection, the test is not sat-

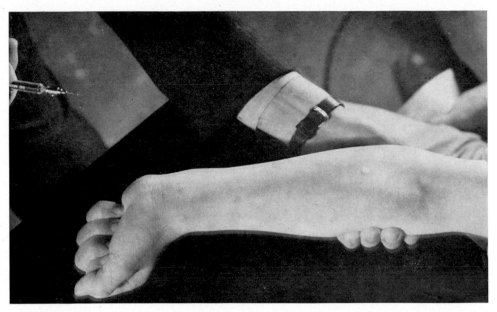

FIGURE 53–4. Demonstration of wheal produced by intracutaneous injection of tuberculin solution (Mantoux test). (Courtesy of the National Tuberculosis Association, 1790 Broadway, New York, New York.)

isfactory and a false-negative reaction may be obtained. This is particularly true if the material is injected subcutaneously.

Either OT or PPD may be utilized in the Mantoux test. In the Child Chest Clinic at the Medical College of Virginia, OT (0.1 mg. or 10 TU) and PPD (0.0001 mg. or 5 TU) have been used concomitantly, and the former has been shown to be only slightly more sensitive. Either, therefore, may be used for routine tuberculin testing.

The test is read forty-eight to seventy-two hours later, and the area of induration should be measured at its greatest transverse diameter. An induration less than 5 mm. in diameter constitutes a negative reaction. If the area of induration measures between 5 and 9 mm. in diameter, the reaction must be considered doubtful, and the test should be repeated with the same dosage of tuberculin. The second test result may be negative, but if it shows the same degree of reaction, an attempt should be made to arrange for simultaneous testing with tuberculin solution (PPD 5 TU) and the antigens of

the atypical (unclassified) mycobacteria. Such tests often result in a small tuberculin reaction (5 to 9 mm. in diameter of induration) and a much larger reaction to one of the antigens of the atypical mycobacteria (15 to 20 mm. in diameter of induration), thereby suggesting that the response to tuberculin is a heterologous reaction. If the tuberculin test, utilizing either OT (0.1 mg.) or PPD (0.0001 mg.), produces an area of induration measuring 10 mm. or more, the result is considered positive (Figs. 5, 6).

A Mantoux test may produce a severe local reaction. There may be much erythema and induration or even vesiculation or ulceration at the site of the injection in persons with a high degree of sensitivity to tuberculin. There may be associated lymphangitis or regional lymphadenopathy. Phlyctenular conjunctivitis is an uncommon complication, and a constitutional reaction with fever is rare.

As noted above, the dosage of tuberculin suggested for routine skin testing and for mass immunization programs is 5 TU. This test presumably detects 99 per cent

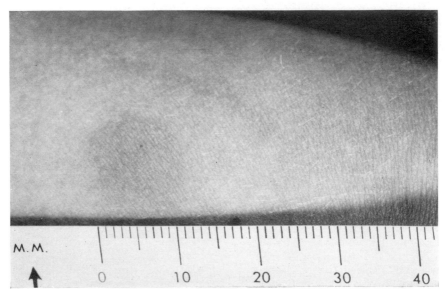

FIGURE 53–5. Positive reaction in the Mantoux test, measuring 10 mm. in diameter of induration.

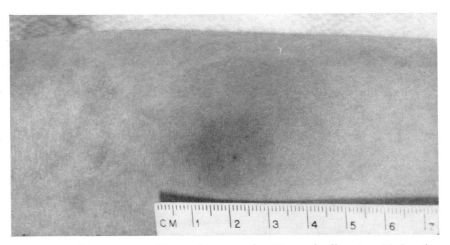

FIGURE 53–6. Mantoux test with reaction measuring 56 mm. in diameter of induration.

of the persons infected with tuberculosis. Nonspecific reactions may occur when the amount of tuberculin is increased beyond 10 TU.

Edwards and Palmer have suggested that the tuberculin reaction measuring between 5 and 9 mm. in diameter of induration is suspect and have pointed out that in certain sections of the United States the number of such reactions is abnormally large. The suggestion has been made that many of these nonspecific reactions may be the result of infection with the so-called unclassified (atypical) mycobacteria. The incidence of these mycobacteria appears to be much greater in some areas of the country than in others. As determined by skin testing, there appears to be a high incidence of infection with atypical mycobacteria among children in Virginia, and it has been shown that not infrequently such infections may, by heterologous reaction, be the cause of a false-positive tuberculin reaction, such as that described above.

Other causes of a false-positive tuberculin reaction are not of great frequency. Hypersensitivity to the phenol, glycerin or bouillon in Old Tuberculin Solution may be productive of redness and induration within the first twenty-four to forty-eight hours after application of the test. If the reading is done forty-eight to seventy-two hours after the test has been performed, the local response produced by such hypersensitivity has practically always disappeared.

It has been our experience that BCG vaccination is usually productive of a tuberculin reaction measuring 5 to 9 mm. in diameter of induration. If a patient who has received BCG vaccine shows a reaction to PPD (0.0001 mg.) measuring 15 mm. or more in diameter of induration, the likelihood of infection with virulent tubercle bacilli must be considered (Fig. 7).

There are a certain number of false-negative tuberculin reactions, also. The most important of these occurs after the time when infection takes place and before allergy sets in, as manifested by a positive tuberculin reaction. It is important to remember that an infant or child who is known to have been exposed to a tuberculous adult must not be adjudged free of infection, as far as that particular contact is concerned, until he has a nega-

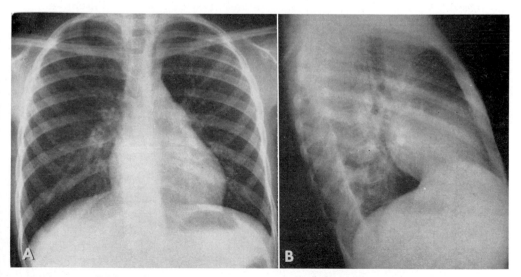

FIGURE 53–7. BCG-vaccinated patient in whom tuberculous infection developed later. Roentgenograms show multiple hilar calcifications. Tuberculin reaction (PPD 0.0001 mg.) measured 12 mm. in diameter of induration 3 years after BCG vaccination. At time of subsequent testing, tuberculin reaction was 52 mm. Roentgenograms taken at that time (*A, B*) indicate presence of healed primary tuberculosis. There had been no evidence of clinical disease.

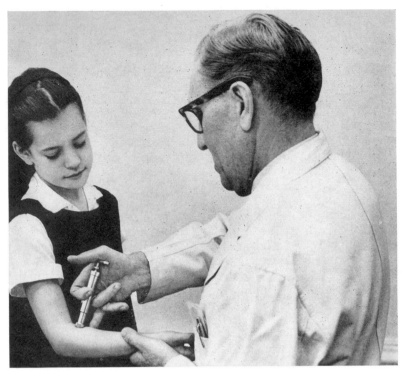

FIGURE 53–8. Application of the Heaf test. (Courtesy of Panray-Parlam Corp., Englewood, N. J.)

tive tuberculin reaction at least ten weeks after contact with the tuberculous person has ceased.

The next most important false-negative reaction may occur in those with overwhelming tuberculous disease, such as an infant moribund with tuberculous meningitis. This does occur, but in our experience is not nearly so frequent as is generally taught.

Certain cases of malnutrition, dehydration and inanition may show a false-negative tuberculin reaction, and the same is true in certain instances of tuberculous bone and joint disease.

During the course of rubeola the tuberculin reaction will be partially or completely depressed, but hypersensitivity again becomes manifest ten days to six weeks later. Tuberculous children vaccinated against measles may have a depressed tuberculin reaction for the same period of time, and those with severe rubella may have a depressed reaction for one to three weeks.

Corticosteroid therapy may be the cause of a false-negative tuberculin reaction, and it is said that antihistaminics also tend to reduce tuberculin sensitivity. Although the latter may be true, our own experience has failed to corroborate the impression that such does occur to any important degree.

Besides the Mantoux test, there are two other important tuberculin tests, the Heaf test and the tuberculin tine test.

The *Heaf test*, devised in England and now utilized to some extent in this country, requires special apparatus for its use. The so-called Heaf gun makes six simultaneous skin punctures 1 mm. deep through a layer of concentrated PPD (100,000 TU per milliliter) (Fig. 8). The test is read three to seven days later, and the presence of four or more papules constitutes a positive reaction (Fig. 9). This apparatus is now available with disposable needle cartridges, and these may be sterilized and used again if so desired (Fig. 10). Anderson and Smith have shown

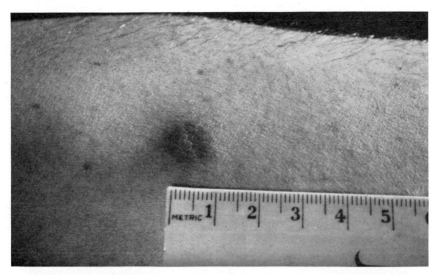

FIGURE 53–9. Strongly positive (4+) reaction in the Heaf test. (Courtesy of Panray-Parlam Corp., Englewood, N. J.)

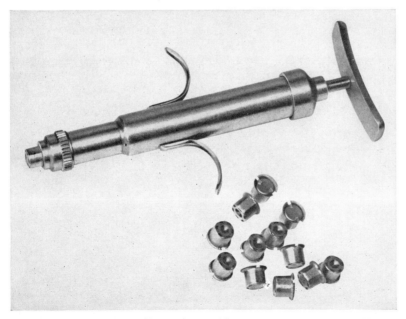

FIGURE 53–10. The Heaf gun with disposable cartridges. (Courtesy of Panray-Parlam Corp., Englewood, N. J.)

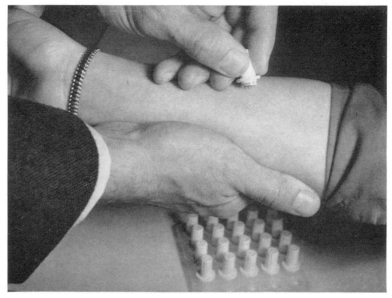

FIGURE 53–11. Application of the tine test. (Courtesy of Lederle Laboratories, A Division of American Cyanamid Co., Pearl River, N. Y.)

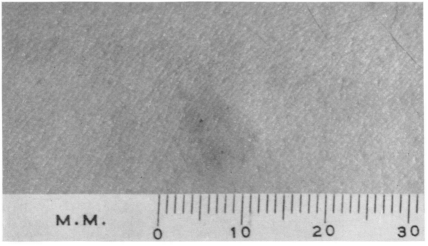

FIGURE 53–12. The tine test. Positive reaction with 4 confluent areas of induration. (Courtesy of Lederle Laboratories, A Division of American Cyanamid Co., Pearl River, N. Y.)

Table 3. *Use of the Routine Tuberculin Test*

Test	Age at Administration
Mantoux (PPD) (0.0001 mg.)	6 to 8 months and
Mantoux (O.T.) (0.1 mg.)	Annually thereafter
Tine	
Heaf	

that results with the Heaf test correlate favorably with the Mantoux test and have found that discrepancies occurred almost entirely among the Heaf "doubtful positives." Our own experience suggests that the Heaf test is so sensitive that a number of false-positive reactions result; a positive reaction should therefore in most instances be corroborated by a Mantoux test.

The *tuberculin tine test* (Rosenthal) is the newest of the tuberculin tests now in use and bids fair to be one of the most useful ones (Fig. 11). The sterilized disposable unit consists of four tines which have been predipped in an Old tuberculin concentrate (four times the standard strength of Old tuberculin). The production of one or more papules measuring 2 mm. or more in diameter constitutes a positive reaction. In a strongly positive reaction a rosette consisting of four confluent areas of induration may result (Fig. 12).

The tuberculin tine test does not have the advantage of quantitative tuberculin testing afforded by the Mantoux test. Nevertheless studies have shown that results obtained in simultaneous tine and Mantoux tests show good correlation. Moreover, the tine test is inexpensive, sterile, disposable and simple to apply. It is also said to be easily interpreted, but in our experience the less extensive reactions (2 to 3 mm. in diameter of induration) do not lend themselves to easy interpretation. Recently Rosenthal has suggested that fusion of at least two papules is necessary for the result to be considered positive. Mild reactions should be corroborated by a Mantoux test.

The *Vollmer patch test* appears to have

outlived its usefulness. The possibilities of technical error are great (unsatisfactory cleansing of the site of application, poor application of the patch, too early or too late removal of the patch, and failure to keep the patch dry), and the accuracy of the test seems suspect, anyway. When utilized simultaneously with a Mantoux test (PPD 5 TU), the patch test failed to detect 6 per cent of the reactions to PPD and produced a reaction in 7 per cent of those who did not react to PPD (Furcolow and Robinson).

A routine tuberculin test should be performed between six and eight months of age, and annually thereafter (Table 3). It is, of course, always indicated when there has been known contact with a tuberculous adult. In the latter instance, if the tuberculin reaction is negative, the test should be repeated eight to ten weeks after the removal of the contact. If the child remains in contact with a tuberculous adult, the tuberculin test should be repeated at three-month intervals.

In the presence of phlyctenular conjunctivitis or erythema nodosum, or if there is a history of intimate exposure to infectious tuberculosis, a lower strength of PPD or Old tuberculin solution or the use of the tine test is indicated. Failure to observe this precaution may lead to worsening of the disease process.

The routine tuberculin test is apparently not utilized to the extent that might be desired. A survey conducted a few years ago among 2500 practicing pediatricians in the United States showed that among 1480 who answered the questionnaire, 821 (55.5 per cent) used the tuberculin test routinely, and, of these, 174 (21 per cent) used the test only after three years of age, too late to be of maximum case-finding value (Table 4).

Table 4. *Utilization of the Routine Tuberculin Test by Pediatricians*

Pediatricians	1480
Use	821*
Do not use	659

*Of 821 using test, 174 used it only after 3 years of age.

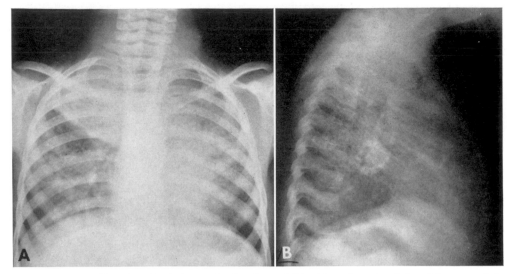

FIGURE 53–13. Negative physical examination in a child with atelectasis of the right upper lobe, cavity in the right lower lobe, and miliary tuberculosis. (Courtesy, A.M.A. *American Journal of Diseases of Children,* 92:558, 1956.)

HISTORY AND PHYSICAL EXAMINATION. History of contact with a tuberculous adult is most important, and should lead immediately to the routine for tuberculin testing outlined above.

The so-called tuberculosis symptom complex consisting of chronic cough, anorexia and failure to gain or even loss of weight may sometimes be helpful in the diagnosis of progressive tuberculous disease, but is of little value in early diagnosis.

Expiratory stridor and bitonal cough, presumably caused by nodal compression of the bronchi, is of rare occurrence, and again is of little value in early diagnosis. Persistent fever of one to two weeks' duration often accompanies the development of primary tuberculosis, and the presence of such fever should arouse suspicion of tuberculosis. Rarely, erythema nodosum may be the first sign of tuberculous disease.

As a rule, the onset of primary tuberculosis is symptomless, and even those with progressive disease present symptoms which are far less prominent than might be expected from the associated disease process. In the Child Chest Clinic of the Medical College of Virginia, review was made of 200 children with tuberculous infection, which ranged from a positive tuberculin reaction without other demonstrable evidence of disease to widespread pulmonary tuberculosis. Not one of these patients exhibited a single symptom or sign which could be associated with any disease process. All were diagnosed by means of a routine tuberculin test or by a tuberculin test performed because of known contact with tuberculosis.

Even in progressive tuberculous disease, symptoms and signs may not be as helpful as might be expected. A three-year-old Negro girl was referred to the Medical College of Virginia Hospital (Dooley) with a diagnosis of pulmonary tuberculosis. There was no history of contact with tuberculosis. The only symptoms were questionable failure to gain weight during the preceding year and a tendency to cough when taking violent exercise. Although physical examination yielded negative results, a chest roentgenogram showed atelectasis of the right upper lobe, a thin-walled cavity in the right lower lobe and miliary tuberculosis (Fig. 13).

Although the clinician should not overlook symptoms and signs which suggest the presence of tuberculosis, it must be stressed that the use of the tuberculin test is by far the most useful diagnostic tool.

ROENTGENOGRAM EXAMINATION. Once the presence of tuberculosis has been established by means of a positive tuberculin reaction, further procedures must be carried out in order to determine the location and the degree of severity of the infection. Since most primary tuberculous infections occur in the lung parenchyma (over 95 per cent), a chest roentgenogram, including both anteroposterior and lateral views, is always indicated and should be taken promptly (Fig. 14).

A primary complex, occurring after conversion of the tuberculin reaction from negative to positive, is more likely to be demonstrable on a roentgenogram in infants and small children. The incidence decreases with age. The primary parenchymal focus is usually small in comparison with the involved lymph nodes, and is more often not demonstrable on a roentgenogram.

Care should be exercised in positioning the patient for a roentgenogram, since relatively minor rotations of the body may result in distortions of the hilar or mediastinal areas. Braids of hair should be pinned up, and all radiopaque objects, such as identification tags or medals, should be removed from the field prior to the roentgenogram.

Most important of all, films should be made on maximal inspiration. During expiration there will be widening of the mediastinum, increase in the transverse diameter of the heart and often suffusion of the lung parenchyma. Figure 15 is an illustration of this. The first film was taken when the child was crying loudly and was in a marked expiratory phase. The second roentgenogram was taken immediately thereafter. The diaphragm should be at least as low as the eighth rib posteriorly, even in the smallest infant.

Care should be taken to avoid unnecessary exposure to radiation, and should always include a protective shield over the lower part of the abdomen.

RECOVERY OF TUBERCLE BACILLI. The diagnosis of tuberculosis is established with certainty by the finding of tubercle bacilli. Careful search for these organisms should always be made.

In infants and children, organisms reaching the pharynx from lung lesions are promptly swallowed. Examination of the gastric contents thus provides a useful way by which the diagnosis of tuberculosis may be proved. Yet the number of bacilli and the frequency of positive cul-

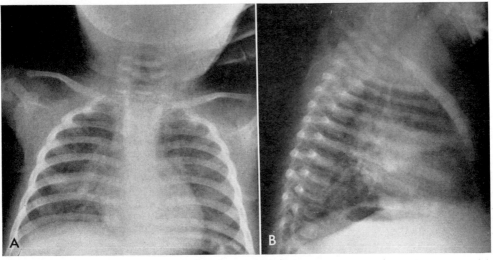

FIGURE 53–14. Roentgenograms showing the value of a lateral view. Extensive infiltration and hilar adenopathy in the lateral view (primary pulmonary tuberculosis). (See also Figure 53-18.)

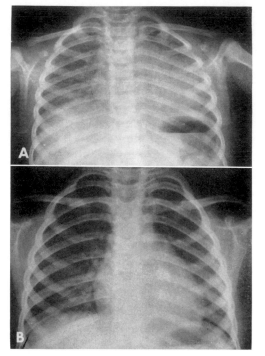

FIGURE 53–15. Films showing the value of proper technique. The first film (*A*) was taken in the expiratory phase, and the second (*B*) in the inspiratory phase. (Same patient a few minutes later.)

tures recovered by gastric lavage is usually small, and it is, therefore, usually recommended that this procedure be carried out each day for three successive days. In the Child Chest Clinic of the Medical College of Virginia, single gastric cultures of children with a positive tuberculin reaction and little or no roentgenographic evidence of disease are productive of tubercle bacilli in only about 6 per cent of the cases. The infrequency of positive gastric cultures lessens the value of this procedure as a diagnostic aid.

Gastric lavage should be performed early in the morning after an overnight fast. The contents of the stomach are aspirated and placed in a sterile container. After this the stomach may be irrigated with 60 ml. of sterile water, and this is aspirated and added to the material in the container. Not all workers believe this second step to be necessary, but if this is done, only sterile water should be used,

since atypical mycobacteria may often be present in tap water. Direct examination of the gastric contents of children with primary pulmonary tuberculosis is of little value, and the material should always be promptly cultured on special media for at least two months. The use of guinea pig inoculation may increase the percentage of cases in which tubercle bacilli are recovered.

Bronchial secretions for both direct examination and culture may be obtained at the time of bronchoscopy. Fluids obtained from the drainage of abscesses, by paracentesis, and especially cerebrospinal fluid, should have direct examination and culture. All cultures should be done immediately. In order to increase the chance of demonstrating the tubercle bacillus, it is recommended that guinea pig inoculation also be done whenever possible, particularly in the examination of the cerebrospinal fluid when tuberculous meningitis is suspected.

BIOPSY. Under satisfactory antimicrobial coverage, biopsy of the pleura and lymph nodes can now be safely performed. Some of the material obtained should be cultured and the rest submitted for histopathologic examination.

BRONCHOSCOPY. Bronchoscopy is indicated in many patients whose roentgenograms show an area of increased density suggestive of segmental obstruction. This procedure should be carried out only under optimum conditions, however. Both the bronchoscopist and the anesthesiologist should be experienced in the management of children, and satisfactory hospital arrangements should be provided.

PULMONARY FUNCTION. Although the majority of children with pulmonary tuberculosis suffer no impairment of lung function, pulmonary function tests may be of help in assessing the possible risks and benefits of surgery.

The Story of Tuberculosis

After tuberculous infection has taken place, there is a two- to ten-week period of incubation during which tubercle bacilli are conveyed from the portal of entry by way of the lymphatics to the regional lymph nodes. The lymph nodes become hyperemic and edematous and may contain areas of caseation. In over 95 per cent of the cases the primary focus is in the lung parenchyma.

At the close of this incubation period, allergy appears, as manifested by a positive tuberculin reaction. At this time, then, the patient has primary pulmonary tuberculosis. There are few, if any, symptoms, and the diagnosis is usually made by means of a routine tuberculin test or by one performed because of known contact with tuberculosis.

Most patients with primary tuberculosis seen at the Medical College of Virginia have a negative chest roentgenogram and no physical evidence of tuberculous disease. The positive reaction in the tuberculin test is the only clue to the presence of tuberculous infection. A smaller number of children have roentgenographic evidence of disease. Most of these have no demonstrable primary parenchymal focus, but the chest roentgenogram shows an area of increased density in the region of the hilus, caused by the edematous lymph nodes. A still smaller group has roentgenographic evidence of a primary parenchymal focus as well as enlarged regional lymph nodes.

In a few cases the primary lesion is not in the lung parenchyma, and physical examination may reveal evidence of tuberculous disease elsewhere.

Primary tuberculosis tends to heal, but the process may become progressive. It may cause progressive destruction at the initial site, or there may be erosion of a bronchus with intrabronchial dissemination and other pulmonary lesions. If there is a massive hematogenous distribution, there will be a widespread formation of tubercles. In any of these instances the patient will usually give some symptomatic evidence of the worsening of the disease process.

Near the close of the incubation period there is often a transient bacillemia. In this way, too, tuberculous foci may be set up throughout the body and remain quiescent for many years. The heaviest distribution of hematogenous seeding is likely to be in the lung, but any of the viscera may be involved. Most of the complications which result later from these foci are not immediately blood-borne. Tuberculous meningitis, for example, is likely to result from the breakdown of a contiguous tuberculoma, previously seeded.

Treatment

Isoniazid and streptomycin have been largely responsible for the drastic reduction in mortality from tuberculosis which has occurred during the past twenty-two years. The present-day approach to the management of this serious disease must include early diagnosis, isolation of infected persons, judicious use of BCG vaccine and the utilization of the available effective antituberculosis drugs.

An optimum therapeutic result can be achieved only when the diagnosis is established early. Since little reliance can be placed on symptoms, a routine tuberculin test is necessary in order to establish the early diagnosis of tuberculosis in childhood. An intradermal tuberculin test (Mantoux), utilizing either PPD (0.0001 mg.) or Old tuberculin solution (0.1 mg.), should be performed on all children between six and eight months of age and annually thereafter. Naturally, such a test is always indicated when there has been known contact with tuberculosis.

PREVENTIVE THERAPY. When the diagnosis has been established, proper therapy for the patient can be promptly instituted and precautions arranged for the prevention of infection of those in contact with the patient. Results from the United States Public Health Service Isoniazid Prophylaxis Study among household contacts suggest that the use of isoniazid may be effective in preventing tuberculous disease in this group.

A group of eighty-three infants born of mothers who had tuberculosis at the time of delivery, shortly beforehand or soon afterward was evaluated in Richmond. The most significant finding was the fact that the removal of the infant or child from the mother was not always enough to prevent later infection in the child. Even though forty-one of the children were isolated from their respective mothers until the mother was sputum-negative, twenty, or almost 50 per cent, became infected with tuberculosis when returned to the home environment, twelve of these during the first two years of life. It is advised that this particular group receive BCG vaccine as soon as practicable.

GENERAL THERAPY. Whenever a child has been found to be tuberculin-positive, removal of the tuberculosis contact must be accomplished as soon as possible. This search entails a chest roentgenogram of all adult contacts, including parents, grandparents, baby sitters, household servants and any others who may have been in contact with the child.

An adequate diet (high protein) and the usual vitamin supplement for a growing child are necessary, but the question of bed rest varies with the type of disease. The child with asymptomatic primary tuberculosis requires no limitation of activity, and even those who are acutely ill should be allowed some activity as soon as possible, since it is recognized that complete bed rest may result in undesirable negative calcium and nitrogen balance.

The child should be protected from intercurrent infection, since not only measles, but also any acute infection, may lower resistance. The tuberculin-positive child who has measles while not then receiving therapy should be given isoniazid for a period of three to four weeks. The tuberculin-positive child who has not had rubeola should be protected against this disease by the use of measles vaccine, but he should receive isoniazid therapy for at least one month when the vaccine is administered. Protection of the child from a source of tuberculous infection in the home is a necessity.

Sharp restriction of activity may be necessary (although today less often and for a shorter time) with certain types of tuberculous disease. Such restriction of activity has psychologic implications which may handicap the child. The child so affected should have a room of his own, comfortable, well lighted, well ventilated and sufficiently accessible that his care can be easily managed. He should be made as self-sufficient as possible and should have a daily schedule of work and play. A Sadler footrest provides additional comfort for the child propped in a sitting position in bed.

The greatest problem is presented by children between two and six years of age. Interest may be promoted for these by picture books, unpainted blocks, housekeeping toys, dolls with numerous changes in costume, crayon color books, clay, simple wooden puzzles, "matching" games, and an occasional grab bag, consisting of a dozen 10-cent toys.

Older children are more easily amused and may find pleasure in reading, drawing or crayon-coloring; weaving, knitting, soap carving and construction sets may also be useful. Carefully selected radio and television programs are entertaining and, indeed, may be helpful for the younger children, too.

Although restlessness and dissatisfaction will occasionally occur in the younger children, the older children, especially those approaching puberty, are the ones most prone to episodes of deep mental depression. These should be carefully watched for, and remedied promptly.

During the convalescent period the older child may find enjoyment in photography or painting, and as soon as possible, arrangements should be made for the school child to keep up with his school work.

Chest x-rays at appropriate intervals are necessary.

ANTIMICROBIAL AGENTS. The three antimicrobial agents of greatest efficacy in the treatment of tuberculosis in childhood are isoniazid (INH), para-aminosalicylic acid (PAS) and streptomycin (SM).

Isoniazid. Isoniazid is the most potent antituberculosis agent yet available. After oral administration of the drug, a plasma concentration twenty to eighty times the usual inhibiting concentration of the drug (0.05 microgram per milliliter) may be attained within a few hours, and effective high concentrations persist for six to eight hours. Isoniazid penetrates the cell membrane and moves freely into the cerebrospinal fluid and into caseous tissue. It is excreted mainly in the urine. The principal side effects of the drug are neurotoxic, manifested as either convulsions or peripheral neuritis, and probably result from competitive inhibition of pyridoxine metabolism. Such side effects have been noted mainly in adults, however, and pyridoxine deficiency does not appear to be a problem in children, although precautions must be exercised during adolescence. Pyridoxine, 25 to 50 mg. daily, should be added to the treatment schedule during this period. Other side effects include gastrointestinal dysfunction and allergic reactions. Rarely, isoniazid may be hepatotoxic.

Dosage of isoniazid is not yet completely established. Isoniazid in the low dosage of 5 mg. per kilogram of body weight is effective in preventing most of the more serious forms of the disease, and has also been effective in the production of a cure in tuberculous meningitis and miliary tuberculosis. Although evidence has been presented that metabolism of isoniazid varies in different patients, by virtue of their different rates of acetylation, studies have indicated that the clinical effectiveness of the drug cannot always be correlated with laboratory results.

The question of adequate dosage may be approached in one of two ways. Since children tolerate isoniazid much better than do adults, the dosage may be increased to 20 or even 30 mg. per kilogram of body weight per day, with a maximum daily dosage of 500 mg. On the other hand, combined therapy with PAS may be utilized. Since para-aminosalicylic acid apparently competes with isoniazid for acetylation in the liver, this competitive effect results in a higher blood level of isoniazid. The present trend in the treatment of tuberculosis is the simultaneous use of isoniazid and para-aminosalicylic acid or another antimicrobial agent (streptomycin). Although triple drug therapy has been shown to have little statistical advantage over treatment by two drugs (if one of the drugs is isoniazid), it is nevertheless preferred by many investigators in the treatment of such serious forms of the disease as tuberculous meningitis and miliary tuberculosis.

Resistance to isoniazid has not yet been of serious clinical significance in children. Often the drug is effective clinically, even though laboratory studies show the organism to be resistant to isoniazid.

Isoniazid is available for oral administration in tablets of 50 mg. and 100 mg., or in a flavored syrup containing 10 mg. per milliliter. A preparation for parenteral administration (intramuscular or intrathecal) is also available.

Streptomycin (SM). Streptomycin was isolated from *Streptomyces griseus* in 1944, and became the first effective antibiotic agent against tuberculosis. The drug inhibits growth of the tubercle bacillus in a concentration of 1.6 micrograms per milliliter. After parenteral administration the drug rapidly appears in the blood stream, reaching a peak value in two hours. It diffuses into the pleural fluid, but does not pass the cerebrospinal fluid barrier to any appreciable extent unless there is inflammation of the meninges. Streptomycin is largely excreted in the urine, with an 80 per cent recovery within twenty-four hours after administration.

The principal toxic effect of streptomycin is involvement of the eighth cranial nerve. Although loss of vestibular function may be permanent, children usually adjust to this defect without symptoms. Involvement of the auditory branch constitutes a real danger, but this effect is much less frequent now than in the days of prolonged streptomycin therapy. Allergic manifestations, such as fever and dermatitis, may occur, and agranulocytosis has been reported.

Although no unusual number of side effects has resulted from the use of a higher dosage of streptomycin in children treated at the Medical College of Virginia, such experience elsewhere seems to indicate use of a lower one. Streptomycin is administered by intramuscular injection in a suggested dosage of 20 to 40 mg. per kilogram of body weight per day, with a maximal daily dosage of 1 Gm. The dosage for small or emaciated children should be at the lower level (20 mg.), except in meningitis or other fulminating forms of tuberculosis. Although a single daily injection of the drug is usually given, the daily dose may be divided into two injections for a small or emaciated patient.

Streptomycin is never used as the sole therapeutic agent because of the rapid development of drug resistance. It is routinely given with at least one other tuberculostatic agent.

Experience at the Medical College of Virginia, as well as elsewhere, has not proved the value of the intrathecal administration of streptomycin, and use of the drug in this manner has been discontinued. Intrathecal administration is still utilized by some investigators, however.

Streptomycin is supplied in crystalline form, usually as a sulfate, in vials containing 1 Gm. and 5 Gm.

Dihydrostreptomycin is a common cause of irreversible damage to the auditory branch of the eighth nerve and is no longer used in the treatment of children.

Para-Aminosalicylic Acid (PAS). Para-aminosalicylic acid has some bacteriostatic activity against the tubercle bacillus, and also acts to delay the emergence of drug resistance to streptomycin. Thus it was of great value when streptomycin was the most effective antimicrobial agent. It also delays bacterial resistance to isoniazid, but such resistance has not yet been of serious clinical significance in children.

As mentioned earlier, the chief value of PAS lies in the fact that it apparently competes with isoniazid for acetylation in the liver, thereby increasing the amount of free isoniazid in the blood.

PAS is administered orally and is readily absorbed. The drug diffuses to some extent into serous surfaces and reaches the cerebrospinal fluid in small amounts. PAS has no intracellular activity. It is rapidly excreted in the urine.

Gastrointestinal disturbances constitute the principal toxicity, but hypokalemia, goitrogenic effect, jaundice and leukopenia may occur. PAS may also be the cause of severe allergic reactions, including dermatoses and an otherwise unexplained fever.

Although children usually have a much better tolerance for all forms of PAS than do adults, many are unable to tolerate the high dosage often recommended. The drug should be prescribed in a dosage of 200 mg. per kilogram of body weight per day in three or four divided doses. When salts of para-aminosalicylic acid (sodium, potassium, calcium) are used, the dose should be correspondingly larger, 250 to 300 mg. per kilogram of body weight per day (maximum daily dose 12 Gm.). PAS is supplied in 0.5-Gm. tablets, as a powder, or as a solution of the sodium salt. The solution is stable for only twenty-four hours, and then only if kept in the dark and refrigerated.

Other Antimicrobial Agents. Although isoniazid, streptomycin and para-aminosalicylic acid are the most useful antimicrobial agents in the therapy of tuberculosis, several other drugs may have limited value: pyrazinamide, viomycin, cycloserine and ethionamide.

Although pyrazinamide has been found to be an effective drug for a short time, its ensuing ineffectiveness cannot be correlated with the emergence of pyrazinamide-resistant tubercle bacilli. There has also been much evidence of hepatic toxicity. The Committee on Therapy of the American Trudeau Society (now The American Thoracic Society) concluded that, when used alone, pyrazinamide had only a limited beneficial effect, and that its serious hepatotoxic action tended to outweigh its therapeutic value. The drug is administered orally in a dosage of 20 to 30 mg. per kilogram of body weight per day (maximum 2 Gm.) in three divided doses. It is supplied in tablets containing 0.5 Gm. of the drug.

Viomycin is another drug derived from a fungus of the streptomyces group. It has tuberculostatic properties which make it available for the treatment of tuberculosis, but it is less potent than streptomycin and is not devoid of toxicity. Such toxic manifestations include depletion of plasma electrolytes, increased blood urea nitrogen level, the appearance of albumin, casts, white and red blood cells in the urine, acoustic nerve damage and the occurrence of urticaria. The drug is rarely used in children, therefore, and is indicated only when other therapy is not effective. It is administered intramuscularly twice weekly in a dosage of 30 mg. per kilogram of body weight and should always be utilized in combination with another antituberculosis agent. It is supplied as a sulfate in vials containing 1 Gm. and 5 Gm.

Cycloserine, also derived from a member of the streptomyces group, is not as effective as isoniazid or streptomycin. It has also shown a number of toxic effects, the tendency toward convulsions being the most important. Cycloserine is given orally in a dosage of 5 to 15 mg. per kilogram of body weight per day in two divided doses (less in renal tuberculosis). Maximum daily dosage is 750 mg. It is supplied in capsules containing 250 mg. of the drug.

A fourth drug, ethionamide, is also available for use in combination with one or more antituberculosis agents when bacterial resistance to isoniazid and streptomycin exists. Dosage for children has not yet been established, but a suggested dose is 10 to 12 mg. per kilogram of body weight per day in two or three divided doses. The maximum daily dose is 750 mg. Ethionamide may be hepatotoxic and is a frequent cause of gastrointestinal dysfunction. The drug is administered orally and is supplied in 250-mg. tablets.

Corticosteroids. Apparently cortisone acts to suppress the usual inflammatory response of the body with impairment of granulation tissue formation, macrophage activity and fibroblastic repair. From the nature of this mechanism it appears likely that cortisone promotes progression of tuberculous disease in the lung. This deleterious effect can be overcome, however, by specific effective antimicrobial treatment. Indications for the use of corticosteroids in specific forms of tuberculosis will be presented under individual headings.

General Principles of Antimicrobial Therapy. Isoniazid is at present the most effective antituberculosis drug known. Not only is it the most effective therapeutic agent, but also it is the only drug which tends to prevent complications of tuberculous disease. Accordingly, it must be included in every therapeutic regimen, unless contraindicated because of the patient's hypersensitivity to the drug or because the causative organism is isoniazid-resistant.

Resistance to isoniazid has not yet been of serious clinical significance in children. As a consequence, the drug can be used alone in the treatment of uncomplicated primary tuberculosis. In progressive primary tuberculosis, isoniazid is used in conjunction with para-aminosalicylic acid. In such severe forms of tuberculosis as miliary tuberculosis and tuberculous meningitis, a triple drug regimen with isoniazid, streptomycin and PAS is utilized.

PRIMARY PULMONARY TUBERCULOSIS

The primary complex is comprised of the primary focus, the involved regional lymph nodes and the lymphatics between them. Primary tuberculosis includes the primary complex and the progression of any of its components.

After tuberculous infection there is a two- to ten-week period of incubation. During this time there is an accumulation of polymorphonuclear leukocytes and then epithelioid cell proliferation, producing a typical tubercle, giant cells make their appearance, and the area is surrounded

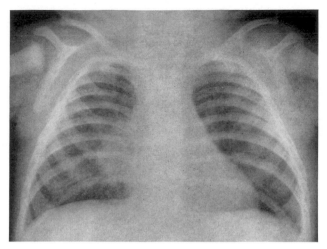

FIGURE 53–16. Primary pulmonary tuberculosis, with enlarged mediastinal lymph nodes, right. (Courtesy of A.M.A. *American Journal of Diseases of Children,* 88:148, 1954.)

by lymphocytes. These organisms are carried by the lymphatics to the regional lymph nodes, and the lymphatics contained in the area between the primary parenchymal focus and the regional lymph nodes constitute the interfocal zone. At the end of the incubation period the presence of allergy is manifested by a positive tuberculin reaction. The patient, who is usually asymptomatic, has primary pulmonary tuberculosis.

Before the body tissues develop hypersensitivity to tuberculin, the primary focus may become larger, but does not become encapsulated. When hypersensitivity develops, the perifocal reaction becomes much more prominent and the regional lymph nodes enlarge. The primary focus may become caseous; however, with the development of acquired resistance, it is usually walled off. The caseous material gradually becomes inspissated and later calcified or may completely disappear. The lesion, of course, may become progressive.

Patients with uncomplicated primary tuberculosis may be divided into four groups: (1) those with a positive reaction to the tuberculin test, with no other demonstrable evidence of disease; (2) those with roentgenographic evidence of mediastinal gland enlargement, but without

evidence of a primary parenchymal focus; (3) those with a demonstrable primary complex; and (4) those with evidence of extrapulmonary tuberculosis.

It has been established that in more than 95 per cent of the cases the initial lesion of primary tuberculosis is in the lung parenchyma. If, therefore, there is a positive tuberculin reaction with no evidence of tuberculous disease elsewhere, it must be assumed that there is a primary focus in the lung parenchyma, too small to be visible on a roentgenogram, with associated regional gland involvement. At the Medical College of Virginia this is the most common form of primary tuberculosis.

Next in frequency is the patient whose chest roentgenogram shows enlarged mediastinal lymph nodes, with no demonstrable primary parenchymal focus (Fig. 16). In such instances, when the disease process has healed, demonstrable calcific deposits will often be present at one or more sites in the lung parenchyma as well as in the hilus (Ghon complex). This calcification in the lung parenchyma is indicative of a healed primary focus which had never been visible on roentgenogram (Fig. 17). Least common is the primary complex with both a demonstrable primary parenchymal focus and

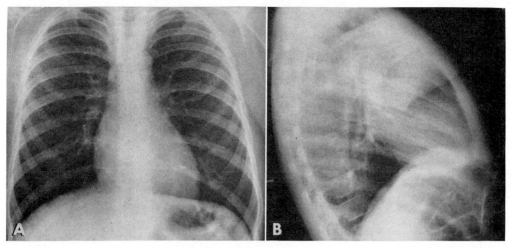

FIGURE 53–17. Calcific densities indicating the presence and location of the healed primary complex (Ghon complex). The primary parenchymal focus was not visible on the roentgenogram taken during the acute phase of the disease.

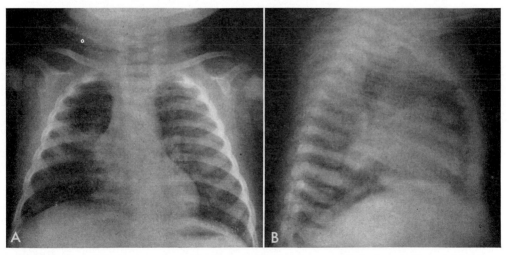

FIGURE 53–18. Primary complex with demonstrable involvement of the interfocal zone (visible on lateral view, *B*).

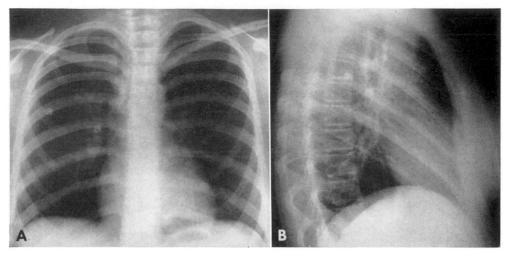

FIGURE 53–19. Calcified primary complex with no evidence of active tuberculous disease.

enlarged hilar lymph nodes. Figure 18 shows a primary complex with demonstrable involvement of the interfocal zone in the lateral view.

Finally, there is a small group of patients who have a positive tuberculin reaction and no roentgenographic evidence of disease, but in whom there is an extrapulmonary tuberculous lesion demonstrable on physical examination, e.g. enlargement of a superficial cervical lymph node.

If the primary complex appears on the roentgenogram at all, it appears at the time of the onset of the disease. It may show progression for one to two months and does not begin to diminish for three to four months. It may remain visible for six to twelve months, or even longer. Resolution of the primary complex is apparently not hastened by antimicrobial therapy.

As far as can be determined, no patient with a primary parenchymal focus without enlarged regional lymph nodes has ever been seen at the Medical College of Virginia. Because of the lymphatic drainage in the mediastinum, a primary focus in the left lung parenchyma is often associated with enlarged lymph nodes on both the left and right sides. In our experience a focus in the right lung has not been the cause of enlarged lymph nodes on the left.

Calcification is more often seen in the regional lymph nodes than in the parenchymal foci, probably because there is early migration of the tubercle bacilli from the parenchymal focus to the regional lymph nodes. The first sign of calcification may appear within six months after the diagnosis of primary tuberculosis in an infant, somewhat later in an older child.

As previously stressed, the diagnosis of primary tuberculosis is practically always accomplished by means of the tuberculin test, either performed routinely or because of the history of contact with a tuberculous adult. Symptoms and signs are rarely of benefit.

Whenever a positive reaction occurs in the tuberculin test, a chest roentgenogram is indicated, and this should include both a posteroanterior and a lateral view.

The prognosis of unhealed primary tuberculosis depends largely on the age of the patient, the duration of infection, and to some degree on the extent of the primary lesion. Whenever calcification is seen on the roentgenogram, it may be assumed that the infection is at least six months old. Thus the presence of calcification is of good prognostic import, but the amount of calcification and the per-

Table 5. *Treatment of Patient with Positive Tuberculin Reaction*

	Drug	Dosage	No. of Daily Doses	Maximum Daily Dosage	Duration of Therapy
< 3 years of age	INH	10–20 mg./kg.	2 or 3	500 mg.	12 months
> 3 years of age	Individualize (see text)				
Recent converter (within 12 months)	INH	10–20 mg./kg.	2 or 3	500 mg.	12 months

sistence of roentgenographic evidence of the primary infection are important, too (Fig. 19).

Treatment

As far as is known, no available antimicrobial agent will eradicate tubercle bacilli. The aim of antimicrobial therapy, therefore, is not only the arrest of the existing tuberculous condition, but also the prevention of the complications of the disease. So far, sufficient evidence is not available for the assumption that antimicrobial therapy is effective in the treatment of primary tuberculosis itself. No drug, other than isoniazid, has shown the ability to prevent the more serious forms of the disease, such as tuberculous meningitis, miliary tuberculosis and Pott's disease.

Whenever a patient less than three years of age has a positive tuberculin reaction, with no physical or roentgenographic evidence of disease, he should be given isoniazid in a dosage of 10 to 20 mg. per kilogram of body weight per day for one year (Table 5). The drug is administered orally in two divided doses at the time of the morning and evening meals. It has been our experience that a crushed tablet in jam, preserves or applesauce constitutes the most practical method of administration, but a flavored syrup is also available. Such a child is not considered infectious, and his activity is not curtailed. Unless complications arise, it is necessary for the patient to be seen by the attending physician only once each month during the period in which he receives medication and annually thereafter. Follow-up roentgenograms, one to three months after diagnosis and again at the completion of one year of therapy, are suggested. Naturally, if there is symptomatic evidence of worsening of the disease process during that period, such a routine must be correspondingly altered. After the first year an annual chest x-ray is indicated. The tuberculous adult is removed from contact with the patient as soon as possible.

The child of any age with roentgenographic evidence of primary pulmonary tuberculosis should be treated in exactly the same manner (Table 6).

Brailey's work indicates that the first year after infection with tuberculosis is the most dangerous period, and it is recommended that any child who converts from a negative to a positive tuberculin reaction within a one-year period be given the same treatment as that outlined above for primary pulmonary tuberculosis. This, of course, accentuates the value of the routine annual tuberculin test (Table 6).

At present it is not nearly so certain that a child over the age of three years with a positive tuberculin reaction and no physical or roentgenographic evidence of tuberculous disease benefits from isoniazid therapy. Such cases must be individualized according to general health, socioeconomic background and the degree of contact with tuberculosis. Until more

Table 6. *Treatment of Asymptomatic Primary Tuberculosis*

	Drug	Daily Dosage	Number of Daily Doses	Maximum Daily Dosage
Isoniazid		10–20 mg./kg.	2 or 3	500 mg.

definite information is available, such a child should have a careful follow-up with routine monthly examinations, an occasional roentgenogram throughout the ensuing year, and an annual chest x-ray thereafter. All children, particularly girls, with a positive tuberculin reaction merit special attention during puberty and adolescence. At present it is our policy to institute a one-year course of isoniazid therapy in those adolescents who for the first time have been demonstrated to have a positive tuberculin reaction. No specific antimicrobial therapy is given during puberty and adolescence to those who have been previously known to be tuberculin-positive.

PROGRESSIVE PRIMARY PULMONARY TUBERCULOSIS

Local progression of the pulmonary component of the primary complex occasionally occurs, but at the Medical College of Virginia it is a rarity. When this does occur, the area of caseation enlarges and then liquefies, and the contents are disseminated into the bronchi, thereby setting up new pulmonary foci of disease. This is a severe form of tuberculosis which occurs much more often in young children, and when it is untreated, the mortality rate is high (above 50 per cent). Symptoms of progressive disease are persistent fever, anorexia, apathy and loss of weight. Physical examination of the chest is most often noncontributory, but there may be moist rales over the diseased area.

Prompt antimicrobial therapy of primary pulmonary tuberculosis is practically always successful in preventing this form of tuberculous disease. When the diagnosis of tuberculosis is not made until the disease has reached this stage, the prognosis is less favorable.

Treatment

Pulmonary progression of primary tuberculosis requires an intense therapeutic approach. Antimicrobial therapy consists of isoniazid, 15 to 20 mg. per kilogram of body weight, with a maximum daily dose of 500 mg., and para-aminosalicylic acid, 200 mg. per kilogram of body weight, with a maximum daily dose of 12 Gm. Isoniazid is given in two daily divided doses and PAS in three or four divided doses. If the child does not respond satisfactorily to this treatment, it will be necessary to add streptomycin, 20 mg. per kilogram of body weight per day, with a maximum daily dose of 1 Gm. Streptomycin is given once each day by the intramuscular route, although for a small or emaciated patient the daily dose may be divided into two injections. Streptomycin therapy is continued for one month after satisfactory clinical response, but isoniazid and PAS therapy should be carried out for at least one year, and sometimes longer (Table 7).

When irreversible damage has occurred, surgical resection of the diseased area of the lung may be necessary.

Table 7. *Treatment of Progressive Primary (Pulmonary) Tuberculosis*

Drug	Daily Dosage	No. of Daily Doses	Maximum Daily Dosage	Duration of Therapy
Isoniazid	15–20 mg./kg.	2 or 3	500 mg.	12 months or longer
PAS	200 mg./kg.	3 or 4	12 Gm.	12 months or longer
If response is unsatisfactory, add streptomycin	20 mg./kg.	1 (2)	1 Gm.	One month after satisfactory clinical response
For endobronchial disease, add prednisone	1 mg./kg.	4	60 mg.	6–12 weeks

TUBERCULOUS PNEUMONIA (HEMATOGENOUS)

Tuberculous pneumonia of hematogenous origin may also occur. This makes its appearance near the close of the incubation period and is usually accompanied by few if any symptoms. On roentgenogram, the lesion itself is indistinguishable from that of a primary parenchymal focus (Fig. 20).

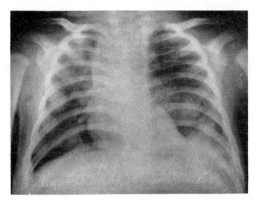

FIGURE 53–20. Roentgenogram of infant whose diagnosis was made at 23 days of age, showing several lesions which may either be primary foci or pneumonia of hematogenous origin (indistinguishable on x-ray film.) (Courtesy of *Amer. Rev. Tuberc.*, 70:161, 1954.)

OBSTRUCTIVE LESIONS OF THE BRONCHI (TUBERCULOUS BRONCHITIS OR LYMPH NODE– BRONCHIAL TUBERCULOSIS)

The regional lymph nodes draining the primary parenchymal focus are tuberculous. They become hyperemic and edematous and may contain areas of caseation. These nodes may be so placed that they impinge upon the wall of a bronchus, causing occlusion of the lumen and atelectasis of that area of the lung distal to the obstruction (extrabronchial or extraluminal tuberculosis).

Much more often, the infected nodes adhere to the adjacent bronchus. This infection may progress no further than the outer wall of the bronchus, but often penetrates to the mucosa. There may be even further progress of the disease process with ulceration of the mucosa and formation of granulation tissue, which may completely obstruct the lumen of the bronchus. Occasionally, too, a tuberculous node penetrates the wall of the bronchus, creating a sinus tract through which caseous material is extruded into the bronchus. When the lumen of the bronchus is thus occluded, there is atelectasis of that area of the lung served by the bronchus (Fig. 22). Under these conditions there

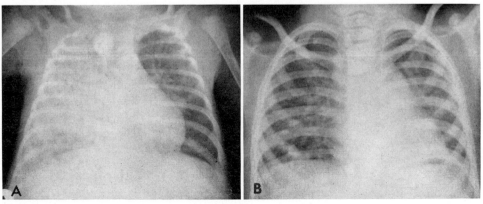

FIGURE 53–21. Roentgenograms of infant whose diagnosis was made at 19 days of age, with widespread pulmonary tuberculosis. Patient recovered from the disease. (Courtesy of *Amer. Rev. Tuberc.*, 61:747, 1950.)

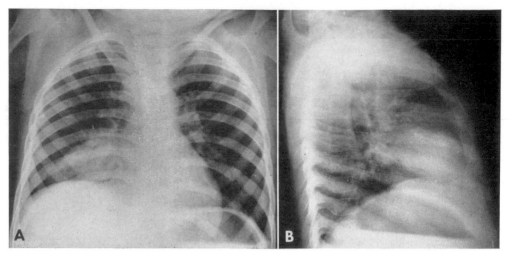

FIGURE 53–22. Atelectasis of the right middle lobe. Convex borders also suggest either early atelectasis or associated pneumonic process.

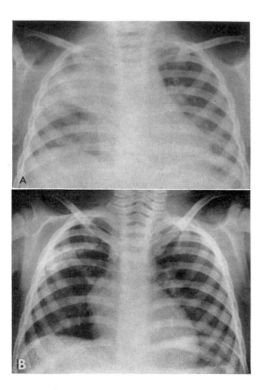

FIGURE 53–23. Roentgenograms illustrating tuberculous pneumonia associated with atelectasis. *B*, shows heavy calcium deposits in lung parenchyma after clearing of atelectasis and pneumonia. (Courtesy of A.M.A. *Journal of Diseases of Children,* 88:148, 1954.)

may also be an associated pneumonia (Fig. 23). Obviously, tuberculous bronchitis must exist whenever this type of tuberculous pneumonia occurs. Tuberculous bronchitis, however, can be present without an accompanying tuberculous pneumonia.

Bronchoscopy is desirable, but should be carried out only if there is available an experienced bronchoscopist and an anesthesiologist, and the hospital is suitably equipped for the study of infants. If the lesion is extraluminal or if there is no obvious obstructive lesion within the lumen, nothing will be accomplished. In due time, however, the edematous nodes will recede, the lumen of the bronchus will again become patent, and that area of the lung which has been atelectatic will usually become reaerated. On the other hand, if the lesion is an endobronchial (intraluminal) one, some of the caseous material can be removed and the patency of the lumen often re-established. Incomplete obstruction of the lumen with a check-valve mechanism, often associated with an intrabronchial polyp, may occur in the same manner and result in hyperaeration (so-called obstructive emphysema) instead of atelectasis (Fig. 24).

Other complications which may occur include the retention of normal secretions, causing edema and congestion of that area of the lung involved and rarely suffocation caused by the extrusion of large masses of caseous material into the bronchus with complete obstruction of the airway.

In our experience atelectasis is seen more often in the right lung, with the middle lobe most often involved and the upper lobe next in frequency.

Treatment

Although the antimicrobial therapy of tuberculous bronchitis is essentially the same as that for other progressive primary tuberculosis, results with this mode of therapy alone have not been satisfactory. For some time there has been a feeling that the use of corticosteroids, in conjunction with antimicrobial therapy, may be of value in such instances. In an excellent double-blind study involving 100 patients, Nemir and her associates have concluded that prednisone as an adjunct to antimicrobial therapy is most successful when given early in the course of lymph node–bronchial disease, i.e. when there is compression of the bronchus as seen by bronchoscopic examination. In her series, when there was a more advanced stage of lymph node–bronchial tuberculosis (evidence of rupture of a caseous lymph node into the bronchus), the difference in results obtained with prednisone and placebo was not conclusive.

The response in those patients treated early in the course of disease may be explained on the basis of the lesion in the lymph node. Since sufficient time has not elapsed for the occurrence of fibrosis, the anti-inflammatory action of prednisone may pave the way for greater penetration of the lymph node by effective antimicrobial agents.

Experience at the Medical College of Virginia, though not as definitive as that

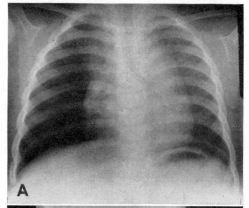

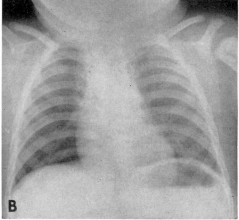

FIGURE 53–24. *A,* Hyperaeration (so-called obstructive emphysema) of right lung. *B,* Nineteen days after the addition of prednisone to the therapeutic regimen (INH and PAS), the roentgenogram showed complete clearing of the process.

contained in Nemir's material, tends to corroborate her results.

Prednisone in a dosage of 1 mg. per kilogram of body weight should be continued for six to twelve weeks.

J.S., a six-month-old Negro female infant, was admitted to a study on the therapy of primary tuberculosis, conducted at the Medical College of Virginia. Chest roentgenogram showed right hilar adenopathy, and the patient was without symptoms. Isoniazid, 15 mg. per kilogram of body weight, was prescribed, and she was seen each month thereafter for follow-up examination. At the time of her visit five months later (eleven months of age) there was a history of anorexia. Physical examination at that time revealed diminished breath sounds and hyperresonance over the entire right side of the chest. Diagnosis of hyperaeration of the right lung (so-called obstructive emphysema) was corroborated by chest roentgenogram. The patient was hospitalized, and bronchoscopy revealed the lumen of the right main bronchus to be almost completely occluded by caseous material. A portion of this material was removed, and para-aminosalicylic acid, 200 mg. per kilogram, and prednisone, 1 mg. per kilogram of body weight, per day, were added to the therapeutic regimen. Within ten days there was clinical improvement, and within three weeks the hyperaeration was no longer apparent on the chest roentgenogram. Prednisone was continued for twelve weeks, with gradual reduction in dosage before the drug was discontinued. Bronchoscopy before discharge from the hospital showed no evidence of disease (Fig. 24).

Mention should be made of the surgical treatment now utilized in England and Wales. In this approach a thoracotomy is performed, the affected node or nodes incised, and the caseous material evacuated. To date this mode of therapy has been rarely used in the United States.

ACUTE MILIARY TUBERCULOSIS

Acute miliary tuberculosis is a generalized hematogenous disease, with multiple tubercle formations and manifestations that are more often pulmonary. It is an early complication of primary tuberculosis and usually occurs within the first six months after the onset of the disease. It is more frequent in infants and young children, but may be seen at any age.

The tubercles, which are of relatively uniform size, result from the lodgment of tubercle bacilli in small capillaries. Necrosis tends to develop in spite of an epithelioid response. The size of the lesions may in part be determined by host resistance. Practically all the organs of the body may be affected, and the lungs are prominently involved.

The onset of miliary tuberculosis is usually acute with high fever, most often remittent. The patient appears acutely ill, but symptoms and signs of respiratory disease may be absent. Enlargement of the spleen, liver or the superficial lymph nodes may be present in about half of the cases. Initially, in rare instances, there are pulmonary manifestations of acute nature.

About one to two weeks after the onset of the disease the mottled lesions, resembling snowflakes, make their appearance on the roentgenogram (Fig. 25). Shortly thereafter fine crepitant rales may be present over the lung fields.

In the untreated cases the mortality

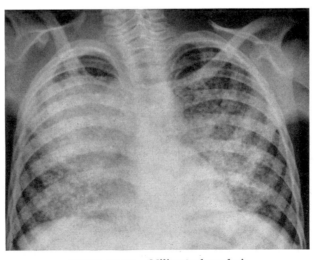

FIGURE 53–25. Miliary tuberculosis.

Table 8. *Treatment of Miliary Tuberculosis*

Drug	Daily Dosage	No. of Daily Doses	Maximum Daily Dosage	Duration of Therapy
INH	20 mg./kg.	2 or 3	500 mg.	12 months or longer
PAS	200 mg./kg.	3 or 4	12 Gm.	12 months or longer
Streptomycin	20–40 mg./kg.	1 (2)	1 Gm.	1 month after satisfactory clinical response
Prednisone	1 mg./kg.	4	60 mg.	Used only during period of extreme dyspnea

rate is almost 100 per cent. Death occurs within four to twelve weeks, usually as the result of tuberculous meningitis. In the successfully treated cases, subsidence of the fever is slow, the temperature usually reaching a normal level in fourteen to twenty-one days after the institution of therapy. Improvement of the lesions on the roentgenogram is usually demonstrable within five to ten weeks, but the lesions do not disappear until later.

Treatment

Therapy consists of a triple drug regimen with isoniazid, 20 mg. per kilogram of body weight per day, para-aminosalicylic acid, 200 mg. per kilogram per day, and streptomycin, 20 to 40 mg. per kilogram per day. Isoniazid and para-aminosalicylic acid are continued for at least one year, but streptomycin is given for one month after satisfactory clinical response. Corticosteroids have been recommended for extreme dyspnea, but are used only for the period necessary to control the dyspnea (Table 8).

Cerebrospinal fluid examinations should be performed at regular intervals in order to make an early diagnosis should meningitis occur. These examinations should be carried out at weekly intervals during the early stages of treatment and less often thereafter.

PLEURISY WITH EFFUSION

Tuberculous pleurisy with effusion is a common early complication of primary pulmonary tuberculosis. It occurs much more often during school age, but is not rare even in young infants. In a group of 303 infants infected with tuberculosis when less than two years of age, reviewed at the Johns Hopkins Hospital, Hardy and Kendig found that 3.3 per cent showed roentgenographic evidence of pleurisy with effusion. Approximately twice as many males as females have this complication.

According to Rich, most of the cases of tuberculous pleurisy with effusion result from extension of the infection from a subpleural focus. Hypersensitivity to tuberculin, too, appears to be a factor (Fig. 26).

The onset is usually acute, with high fever and chest pain, worse on deep inspiration. There may be limitation of respirations on the affected side. Dyspnea and tachycardia may be present when the effusion is massive, and, rarely, there may be bulging of the intercostal spaces.

Fever usually persists for two to three weeks. Although much of the fluid is usually absorbed by the end of this period, some fluid may persist for considerably longer.

Any patient with a serous pleural effusion and a positive reaction in the tuberculin test must be assumed to have tuberculous pleurisy with effusion until proved otherwise. A diagnostic thoracentesis should always be done promptly. No more than 30 ml. of fluid should be withdrawn unless the effusion is so massive that there is respiratory embarrassment. The fluid shows elevation of protein, and

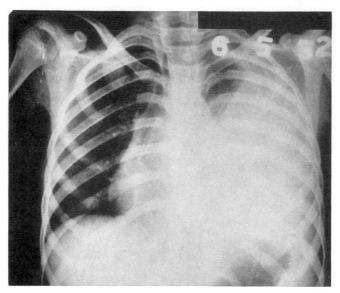

FIGURE 53–26. Tuberculous pleurisy with effusion. (Courtesy of A.M.A. *Journal of Diseases of Children,* 88:148, 1954.)

the cellular content, predominantly lymphocytes except in the very early stages, varies from 200 to 10,000 per cubic millimeter. Culture of the fluid should be done, but the result will be useful only as a corroborative measure.

The prognosis depends on the underlying tuberculous disease.

Spontaneous pneumothorax and caseous pleuritis may occur. Tuberculous empyema is rare now, and no case has been seen at the Medical College of Virginia in recent years.

Scoliosis, presumably due to pleural adhesions, is a not uncommon later result of tuberculous pleurisy with effusion, and contraction of a hemithorax is a rare one.

Treatment

Isoniazid, 15 to 20 mg. per kilogram, and para-aminosalicylic acid, 200 mg. per kilogram of body weight per day, should be given for a twelve-month period (Table 9). Antimicrobial therapy is thus utilized in order to reduce the danger of progressive tuberculous disease and complications such as tuberculous meningitis. There is also evidence that such therapy promotes a reduction in the incidence of later pulmonary tuberculosis. Specific antimicrobial therapy appears to have no direct effect on the pleurisy with effusion.

Although Filler's studies indicate that subsequent pulmonary function is not improved by the use of corticosteroids, it does

Table 9.   *Treatment of Tuberculous Pleurisy with Effusion*

Drug	Daily Dosage	No. of Daily Doses	Maximum Daily Dosage	Duration of Therapy
Isoniazid	15–20 mg./kg.	2 or 3	500 mg.	12 months or longer
PAS	200 mg./kg.	3 or 4	12 Gm.	12 months or longer
Prednisone	1 mg./kg.	4	60 mg.	Until pleurisy with effusion is controlled

appear that they exert an immediately favorable effect on the pleurisy with effusion, promoting a rapid control of fever and the disappearance of the fluid. Moreover, the anti-inflammatory action of the corticosteroids tends to reduce the likelihood of pleural adhesions. The dosage of prednisone is 1 mg. per kilogram of body weight per day in four divided doses. This drug is continued until the effusion is controlled. The dosage is then gradually reduced before discontinuation.

CHRONIC PULMONARY TUBERCULOSIS

Chronic pulmonary tuberculosis occurs as a late involvement in those persons who earlier became infected with tubercle bacilli. The interval between the first infection and chronic pulmonary tuberculosis may be short, but the latter is usually a late complication. In our experience, chronic pulmonary tuberculosis is not common in childhood.

Although it has been established that chronic pulmonary tuberculosis can occur as a result of superinfection (exogenous), the presence of the increased resistance to a second infection which follows the primary infection favors the theory that the majority of the cases of chronic pulmonary tuberculosis in children are endogenous in origin.

The lesion of chronic pulmonary tuberculosis usually appears in the apical or subapical portion of the lung (Fig. 27). Since chronic pulmonary tuberculosis occurs when the tissues have already been sensitized to tuberculin, there is a tendency toward localization of the bacilli and not toward spread by way of the lymphatics. After multiplication of the bacilli has occurred the lesion ulcerates, and the liquefied material is disseminated through the bronchi. The disease, if untreated, will continue to progress, often causing destruction of large areas of lung tissue. At this stage, too, there is occasionally tuberculous enteritis and laryngitis.

Healing occurs by fibrosis and, not nearly so often at this age, by calcification. In addition to the usual closure and obliteration of cavities, there may be re-epithelialization of the bronchocavitary junction, frequently after antimicrobial therapy. This is the so-called open healing (Fig. 28).

The best approach to the early diagno-

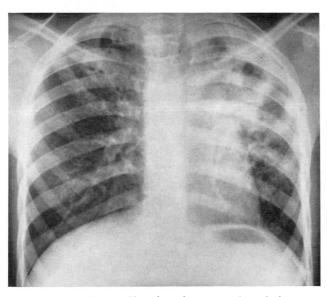

FIGURE 53–27. Chronic pulmonary tuberculosis.

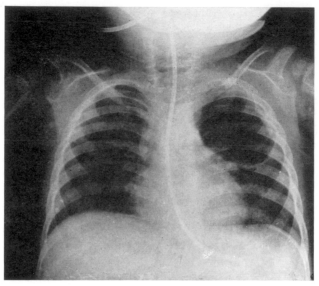

FIGURE 53–28. "Open healing" in a 16-month-old Negro male infant with tuberculous meningitis. Diagnosis corroborated at necropsy. (Courtesy of *American Rev. Tuberc. & Pulmonary Dis.*, 73:99, 1956.)

sis of chronic pulmonary tuberculosis is the routine use of the tuberculin test, between six and eight months of age and annually thereafter. If a child has a positive tuberculin reaction, an annual chest roentgenogram is indicated. In fact, during puberty and early adolescence such a child should have a chest roentgenogram every six months. In girls the year of menarche is an extremely unstable period.

Although symptoms are not a reliable aid to early diagnosis, lassitude, cough, loss of weight, anemia and the suppression of menses are indications for the application of a tuberculin test. If the tuberculin reaction is positive, a chest roentgenogram should be done.

Whenever an older child with a positive tuberculin reaction shows a persistent density on roentgenogram, diagnosis of active tuberculosis should be made unless proved otherwise.

Treatment

Since the lesions of chronic pulmonary tuberculosis in children are extremely unstable, prompt therapy should be instituted. The patient should be hospitalized. If the lesion is a minimal one, prolonged hospitalization may be unnecessary, but the patient will be properly instructed in the necessary measures of hygiene and in his future care. If the lesion is advanced, a longer stay in the hospital will be necessary.

Isoniazid, 10 mg. per kilogram (maximum daily dosage 500 mg.), and para-aminosalicylic acid, 200 mg. per kilogram of body weight (maximum daily dose 12

Table 10. *Treatment of Chronic Pulmonary Tuberculosis*

Drug	Daily Dosage	No. of Daily Doses	Maximum Daily Dosage	Duration of Therapy
INH	10 mg./kg.	2 or 3	500 mg.	2 years after sputum is negative
PAS	200 mg./kg.	3 or 4	12 Gm.	2 years after sputum is negative

Surgical resection may be necessary

Gm.) per day, should be given for two years after the sputum has become negative for tubercle bacilli (Table 10).

If the disease is advanced and there is a great deal of caseation necrosis, surgical resection may be necessary. Pulmonary function studies may be of help in assessing the possible risk and benefits of surgery.

OTHER TUBERCULOUS INVOLVEMENT OF THE RESPIRATORY TRACT

In the past, primary tuberculous infection of the tonsils was not uncommon, but with the advent of the pasteurization of milk and the tuberculin testing of cows such involvement has become a rarity.

That there may be a retropharyngeal abscess accompanying tuberculosis of the cervical vertebrae is well recognized. Nevertheless a tuberculous retropharyngeal abscess arising from caseous lymph nodes in the retropharynx must be rare, and no case has been seen at the Medical College of Virginia in recent years.

There may be tuberculous involvement of the larynx, middle ear, and mastoid and salivary glands.

EXTRAPULMONARY TUBERCULOSIS

Since this is a discussion of respiratory disease in children, little space will be allotted to the extrapulmonary manifestations of tuberculosis. There are several, however, which merit brief discussion.

Tuberculosis of the Superficial Lymph Nodes

Tuberculosis of the superficial lymph nodes does not occur as frequently as in the days before routine tuberculin testing of cows and pasteurization of milk, but the disease is still important.

Involvement of the superficial lymph nodes occurs at the time of the bacillemia

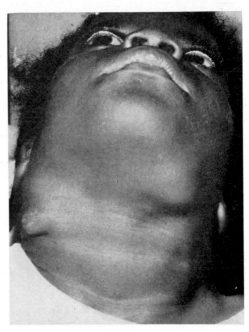

FIGURE 53–29. Multiple areas of suppurative lymphadenitis. (Courtesy of *Journal of Pediatrics,* 47:607, 1955.)

(near the close of the incubation period) when tubercle bacilli are deposited in foci, where they usually remain quiescent unless activated by some trigger mechanism.

There is usually involvement of more than one lymph node. At first there is lymphoid hyperplasia and tubercle formation; later the lesion is that of a chronic granuloma. Caseation and necrosis produce a confluent caseous mass, which, when untreated, will eventuate in a sinus tract. Calcification is often present in a healed tuberculous lymph node.

Since a trigger mechanism is usually required for activation, the disease process more often occurs in the superficial cervical lymph nodes. Here quiescent tubercle bacilli are usually activated by acute tonsillitis or adenoiditis. The bacterial infection is controlled by appropriate antibiotics, but the lymphadenopathy persists, and, indeed, the lymph nodes continue to enlarge. There is usually no associated pain. Later the affected lymph nodes adhere to each other, then to the skin, which

Table 11.   *Treatment of Tuberculosis of the Superficial Lymph Nodes*

1. Excision and	
	INH ...... 15–20 mg./kg. (maximum daily dose 500 mg.) for 12 months
	PAS ...... 200 mg./kg. (maximum daily dose 12 Gm.) for 12 months
or, if excision is not feasible,	
2. Aspiration (when liquefied) and	
	INH ...... 15–20 mg./kg. (maximum daily dose 500 mg.) for 12 months
	PAS ...... 200 mg./kg. (maximum daily dose 12 Gm.) for 12 months

becomes discolored, and the caseous material ruptures into the surrounding tissues. Eventually the caseous material drains externally through a sinus tract (Fig. 29).

Tuberculosis of the superficial lymph nodes may also result from direct lymphatic drainage from an extrapulmonary primary tuberculosis focus. This mode of involvement is uncommon.

Other diseases which must be ruled out as a cause of chronic suppurative lymphadenitis are acute pyogenic infections, coccidioidomycosis, blastomycosis, histoplasmosis, actinomycosis, brucellosis, infectious mononucleosis, leukemia, lymphoma, Hodgkin's disease, cat-scratch fever and infection with the atypical mycobacteria.

Infection with one of the unclassified (atypical) mycobacteria may produce a picture identical to that caused by tuberculous infection. If the positive tuberculin reaction measures less than 10 mm. in diameter, it is probable that infection with one of the unclassified (atypical) mycobacteria exists. Skin testing with both tuberculin solution and the antigens of the atypical mycobacteria may be helpful, too. (See the chapter on Unclassified Mycobacteria, page 701.)

Treatment

Lymphadenitis should be first treated with one of the wide-spectrum antibiotics or with penicillin. Although the former would seem logical, penicillin is usually the most effective agent in the treatment of lymphadenitis of bacterial origin.

If there is a positive tuberculin reaction, and if the lymph nodes measure 2 by 2 cm. or more in diameter, and, in spite of therapy with a wide-spectrum antibiotic or penicillin, are increasing in size, or show early signs of suppuration, prompt excision and the use of isoniazid and para-aminosalicylic acid therapy for a full year are indicated. If the mass of nodes is too great, or if complete liquefaction of the node has already occurred and excision cannot be carried out, the completely liquefied node should be aspirated. It has been suggested that the addition of prednisone in a dosage of 1 mg. per kilogram of body weight per day may be helpful. When used, this drug is continued until healing is effected, but isoniazid and PAS are administered for one year (Table 11). Tonsillectomy is advised only if there are indications for it.

Tuberculous Meningitis

This is the most serious form of tuberculosis. Before the advent of streptomycin it was presumably 100 per cent fatal. At present, with the use of isoniazid, para-aminosalicylic acid and streptomycin, approximately 75 per cent of such patients admitted to the Medical College of Virginia Hospitals recover. Some recover entirely, and others have various degrees of residual involvement. Earlier diagnosis would increase the number with complete recovery and decrease the number and severity of the residua in those who survive.

Tuberculous meningitis is caused by the direct extension of a local contiguous lesion (Rich and McCordock), and is an early complication of tuberculosis. The two principal causes of neurologic sequelae are tuberculous arteritis and obstruction to the flow of the cerebrospinal fluid caused by a thick, gelatinous exudate at the base of the brain.

The clinical course is divided into three stages: (1) the first stage, in which the symptoms are vague and generalized; (2) second, a transitional stage, with early meningeal symptoms and increased intracranial pressure; and (3) third, severe central nervous system involvement, with the patient comatose.

The onset of tuberculous meningitis is usually insidious (although a convulsion may be the first sign), and the symptoms are vague. Apathy, lassitude, anorexia, sometimes irritability, low-grade fever and occasionally vomiting and constipation occur early in the course of the disease.

In the second stage, drowsiness becomes deeper, and there may be convulsions. There is nuchal resistance, often rigidity, and opisthotonos may occur. There may be bulging of the fontanel and ocular paralysis. The patient's condition steadily worsens.

In the final stage the patient lapses into a coma with irregular respirations and high fever. There may be hyperglycemia and glycosuria.

The duration of untreated tuberculous meningitis is approximately three weeks.

Early diagnosis is essential, since the disease, when untreated, is always fatal; even when it is treated it may result in survivors with various neurologic residua.

The *diagnosis* is established by means of the tuberculin test, cerebrospinal fluid findings and a chest roentgenogram. The tuberculin reaction is practically always positive, but may be negative in the last stages of the disease. Most of the patients with tuberculous meningitis have some evidence of primary tuberculosis on the chest roentgenogram. The cerebrospinal fluid is ground glass in appearance and has a cellular content of 10 to 1000 per cubic millimeter. The cells are predominantly polymorphonuclear in the early stages of disease, but lymphocytes are usually more common later. The protein is elevated above 40 mg. per 100 ml., and the sugar is usually decreased. The chlorides are normal in the early stages and frequently below normal later.

Absolute diagnosis can be made only by the isolation of tubercle bacilli from the cerebrospinal fluid. Thus careful direct examination of the fluid should be made. Yet even though direct examination is unsuccessful, treatment should never be deferred until the causative agent has been identified.

Treatment should consist of a triple drug regimen (Table 12): isoniazid in a daily dosage of 20 mg. per kilogram of body weight per day (maximum 500 mg.), PAS in a daily dosage of 200 mg. per kilogram of body weight per day (maximum 12 Gm.), and streptomycin, 20 to 40 mg. per kilogram of body weight per day (maximum 1 Gm.). The first two drugs

Table 12. *Treatment of Tuberculous Meningitis*

Drug	Dosage Daily	No. of Daily Doses	Maximum Dosage Daily	Duration of Therapy
INH	20 mg./kg.	2 or 3	500 mg.	12 months or longer
PAS	200 mg./kg.	3 or 4	12 Gm.	12 months or longer
Streptomycin	20–40 mg./kg.	1 (2)	1 Gm.	1 month after satisfactory clinical response
Prednisone	1 mg./kg.	4	60 mg.	6–12 weeks

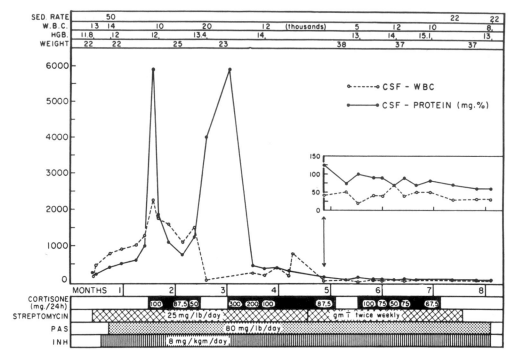

FIGURE 53–30. Diagram depicting precipitous fall of cerebrospinal fluid protein when cortisone therapy was instituted. (Courtesy of *Amer. Rev. Tuberc. & Pulmon. Dis.*, 73:99, 1956.)

are given for at least one year, and streptomycin is given for one month after satisfactory clinical response, as determined by the general condition of the patient, the disappearance of fever and improvement in the cerebrospinal fluid picture.

Antimicrobial agents appear to be reasonably effective in the treatment of tuberculous meningitis if they can reach the organism. The use of prednisone may decrease the likelihood of cerebrospinal fluid obstruction, and, in addition, reduction of the inflammatory process may lessen the danger of irreversible thrombotic phenomena. The use of prednisone after cerebrospinal fluid block has occurred often results in dissolution, as exemplified in the accompanying case report.

Obviously, prevention of such obstruction is more desirable.

CASE REPORT. During the period before the effectiveness of corticosteroid therapy in prevention and dissolution of cerebrospinal fluid obstruction had become recognized, a

two-year-old Negro girl had such a block. Cerebrospinal fluid protein was 5600 mg. per 100 ml. when therapy with cortisone was instituted. After two weeks the cerebrospinal fluid protein was 650 mg. per 100 ml., but as dosage of the drug was decreased and finally discontinued, the cerebrospinal fluid protein gradually rose to 5800 mg. per 100 ml. When it then became apparent that the obstruction could be controlled by cortisone, such therapy was again instituted, and the block rapidly dissolved (Fig. 30).

The promptness of the response to antimicrobial therapy varies considerably. In general, the earlier the diagnosis, the more prompt will be the response. An affected child may lie in a stuporous, semicomatose or even comatose state for months and finally effect an almost complete or even complete recovery.

Tuberculosis of the Bones and Joints

Tuberculosis of the bones and joints usually results from the bacillemia which

Table 13. *Treatment of Tuberculosis of Bones and Joints*

Drug	Daily Dosage	Maximum Daily Dosage	Duration of Therapy
Isoniazid	15–20 mg./kg.	500 mg.	18–24 months
PAS	200 mg./kg.	12 Gm.	18–24 months
Immobilization of involved weight-bearing structures			
Drainage of all superficial and accessible abscesses			

occurs near the close of the incubation period. Clinical disease may occur soon thereafter, or the organism may remain quiescent and reactivate months or even years later. The bones most frequently involved are the head of the femur (hip), the vertebrae and the fingers and toes. The pathologic process usually begins in the metaphysial portions of the epiphyses.

As recommended by the Committee on Respiratory Diseases in Children of the American Thoracic Society, treatment with isoniazid and PAS is carried out for a period of eighteen to twenty-four months. Dosage of these drugs is the same as that mentioned under the therapy of progressive primary tuberculosis. All superficial and accessible abscesses should be drained. Immobilization is not necessary in the nonweight-bearing structures; if, however, weight-bearing structures (vertebrae, hip and others) are involved, whatever means are necessary to prevent weight-bearing are used. For example, the treatment of tuberculosis of the spine (Pott's disease) may vary widely. Some utilize only a hard mattress and the aforementioned drug therapy; others feel that a plaster cast is advisable. Fusion is advised by some orthopedists, and others use fusion only when there appear to be special indications for it (Table 13).

Renal Tuberculosis

Tuberculosis of the kidney is blood-borne in origin, and infection occurs either at the time of the early bacillemia or as part of generalized miliary tuberculosis. Occasionally it may be a late complication.

When the patient does not have associated military tuberculosis and has only a positive tuberculin reaction, the most common finding is a persistent sterile pyuria. There may also be albuminuria, hematuria, dysuria and local renal tenderness. Urine culture or guinea pig inoculation will corroborate the diagnosis, and urograms are indicated in order to determine the area and degree of involvement.

Therapy should be carried out for at least twenty-four months. So-called triple drug therapy with isoniazid, PAS and streptomycin has been advocated for this period, but in those cases in which the urogram shows no abnormality streptomycin may be discontinued after six months. Lattimer has substituted oral cycloserine or ethionamide therapy for streptomycin in the above-noted regimen and gives all three drugs (INH, PAS and one of the other three) for a period of twenty-four months. Dosage of isoniazid is 15 to 20 mg. per kilogram of body weight per day,

Table 14. *Treatment of Renal Tuberculosis*

Drug	Dosage	Maximum Daily Dosage	Duration of Therapy
Isoniazid	15–20 mg./kg./day	500 mg.	2 years
PAS	200 mg./kg./day	12 Gm.	2 years
Streptomycin	20 mg./kg. 3 times	1 Gm.	2 years (6 months in
or	weekly		very mild cases)
Cycloserine	4–5 mg./kg./day	750 mg.	2 years
or			
Ethionamide	10 mg./kg./day	750 mg.	2 years

PAS 200 mg. per kilogram of body weight per day, and streptomycin (when used) 20 mg. per kilogram of body weight three times weekly. The dosage of cycloserine (when used) is 4 to 5 mg. per kilogram, and of ethionamide (when used) 10 mg. per kilogram of body weight per day. (Maximum dosage is indicated in Table 14.) Since there is a possibility that ureteral stricture may appear during therapy, an intravenous pyelogram and ureteral calibration every four months during treatment and annually thereafter for a ten-year period would seem advisable.

Intra-abdominal Tuberculosis

Intra-abdominal tuberculosis has been a rarity on the pediatric service of the Medical College of Virginia in recent years. Tuberculous enteritis may be primary, but is usually secondary to a lesion in the lungs and is nearly always combined with involvement of the mesenteric and retroperitoneal lymph nodes. The main symptoms are tenesmus and chronic diarrhea, with some associated bleeding. There may be fever, abdominal tenderness and distention. There are also debility and anemia. In addition to the antimicrobial therapy routine outlined for progressive primary tuberculosis, the usual general measures for tuberculosis are necessary, and a low residue diet of adequate caloric and vitamin content is also helpful. Therapy is otherwise symptomatic.

When tuberculous enteritis is primary, the principal lesion is in the mesenteric and retroperitoneal lymph nodes. Symptoms are abdominal pain and tenderness. No local treatment is usually required, but rarely excision of enlarged or calcified abdominal lymph nodes may be necessary for the relief of pain.

Tuberculous peritonitis usually results from the rupture of a caseous lesion in a mesenteric lymph node, and also occasionally from an intestinal lesion which has penetrated through the outer coat. The onset is insidious with mild abdominal pain, debilitation and low-grade fever. Later there may be vomiting and abdominal distention.

Tuberculous peritonitis is treated in the same manner as tuberculosis in general, and the addition of corticosteroid therapy may also be helpful. If an exploratory laparotomy is required to establish the diagnosis, it is essential that suitable biopsy material be obtained for tissue section and bacteriologic study. If there is an associated enteritis, a low residue diet provides some symptomatic relief.

Other Extrapulmonary Tuberculosis

There are other less common forms of extrapulmonary tuberculosis. These are tuberculosis of the skin, eye, heart and pericardium, endocrine and exocrine glands, genital tract and fistula in ano. For consideration of these entities the reader is referred to those publications which deal with tuberculosis in its entirety.

THE PREVENTION OF TUBERCULOSIS

There are two accepted methods which have been demonstrated to be reasonably effective in preventing tuberculous infection: isolation of those adults with infectious tuberculosis, and the use of BCG vaccine.

Results from the United States Public Health Service Isoniazid Prophylaxis study among household contacts of tuberculous patients suggest a third method of control. Results of this study indicate a beneficial effect from the administration of isoniazid to household contacts of tuberculous patients. Families of patients with active tuberculosis who received isoniazid in a dosage of 5 mg. per kilogram of body weight per day for a one-year period showed an 80 per cent reduction in the incidence of tuberculosis during the year in which isoniazid was administered and a 50 per cent reduction for the five years during which they have been observed since the drug was stopped. This finding appears to introduce an important new method of tuberculosis control.

BCG vaccine has been conclusively shown to increase resistance to exogenous tuberculous infection, and is mainly of use in this country in those children living in a home in which there is an adult with infectious tuberculous disease, or one with potentially infectious disease, such as a mother who has been discharged from a sanatorium with apparently arrested tuberculosis. It is also useful in those population groups in which there is a high incidence of tuberculous infection. BCG vaccination may be effected by the multiple puncture technique or by the intracutaneous route. One of the main disadvantages of BCG vaccination is said to be the positive tuberculin reaction which results. It has been our experience that the resultant positive tuberculin reaction nearly always measures 5 to 9 mm. and rarely above 12 to 14 mm. in diameter of induration. If the reaction is 15 mm. or more in diameter of induration, the physician can be reasonably sure that there has been

infection with virulent tubercle bacilli, and further investigation is indicated.

In order to be eligible for BCG vaccination, the patient must have a negative tuberculin reaction (PPD 0.0001 mg. or OT 0.1 mg.) and a negative chest roentgenogram within the previous two weeks. Eight to twelve weeks after vaccination the same procedures should be carried out. This time the tuberculin reaction should be positive, and if this is not the case, the vaccination is repeated.

The multiple puncture disk method, as described by Rosenthal, is the preferable procedure. The vaccination is performed over the deltoid region, and the area should be cleansed with acetone and allowed to dry thoroughly. There should be no constriction of the arm. Three drops of BCG vaccine are placed on the skin of the deltoid area, using a syringe and a 22-gauge needle. The disk is picked up by a sterile magnet-type holder (Fig. 31), allowing the wide margin of the disk to extend beyond the magnet and away from the operator. The operator holds the disk at a 30-degree angle and distributes the vaccine over an area about 2.5 cm. square,

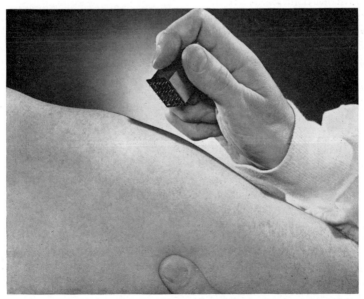

FIGURE 53–31. Multiple puncture disk and magnet-type of holder held in position before depressing for BCG vaccination. (Courtesy of S. R. Rosenthal, Research Foundation, 70 W. Hubbard Street, Chicago, Ill.)

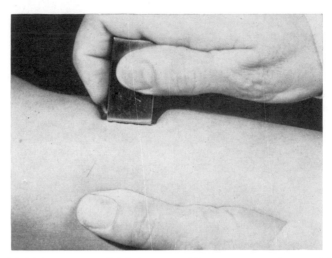

FIGURE 53–32. Multiple puncture disk being pressed in outer aspect of arm. Disk is pressed downward through drop of BCG vaccine. (Courtesy of S. R. Rosenthal, Research Foundation, 70 W. Hubbard Street, Chicago, Ill.)

tapping with the wide margin of the disk. The points of the disk are dipped into the vaccine, rotating the disk slightly, so that all points become moistened with BCG vaccine. The disk is placed in the center of the vaccine site, with the long axis of the holder at a right angle to the arm, and the magnet is moved to the center of the disk. This will avoid bending of the disk. The arm under the vaccine site is grasped with the operator's other hand, thereby tensing the skin over the vaccination area. With the butt or the magnet in the curve of the index finger, downward pressure is applied so that the points of the disk are well buried in the skin (Fig. 32). Enough pressure is applied so that penetration of the points is readily felt by the hand. With pressure still exerted as above, the disk is rocked forward and backward and from side to side twice. The grasp underneath the arm is then released. The operator slides the magnet toward himself and off the disk, maintaining a slight downward pressure. After a successful procedure the disk remains flat on the arm, with the points still in the skin. If the points are on top of the skin, the procedure must be repeated. The disk is again picked up with the magnet, allowing the wide margin to extend beyond the mag-

net. By utilizing the wide margin of the disk, the vaccine is gently tapped so that each perforation of the skin is covered with vaccine. If too much pressure is exerted, the vaccine will be pressed out of the perforations. The vaccine is allowed

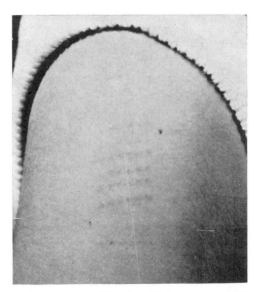

FIGURE 53–33. Size of multiple puncture BCG vaccination, 13 days after vaccination (actual photograph). (Courtesy of S. R. Rosenthal, Research Foundation, 70 W. Hubbard Street, Chicago, Ill.)

to dry on the arm without a dressing. The vaccinated area should not be washed for twenty-four hours (Fig. 33).

Infants and children from tuberculous households (and all adults) should receive the two-site method of BCG vaccination. This procedure differs from the foregoing only in that a larger area of the deltoid region is cleansed and utilized with one vaccination site in the upper portion and a second in the lower one.

Materials for use in BCG vaccination may be obtained from the Research Foundation, 70 West Hubbard Street, Chicago, Illinois 60610. BCG vaccine is also commercially available from the Eli Lilly Company, 740 South Alabama Street, Indianapolis 6, Indiana.

REFERENCES

Adams, W. C.: Variations in the Endurance of Positive Mantoux Reactions in Primary Childhood Tuberculosis. *Am. Rev. Resp. Dis.*, 81:955, 1960.

Anderson, S. R., and Smith, M. H. D.: The Heaf Multiple Puncture Tuberculin Test. *Am. J. Dis. Child.*, 99:764, 1960.

Aronson, J. D.: BCG Vaccination Among American Indians. *Am. Rev. Tuberc.*, 57:96, 1948.

Aspin, J., and O'Hara, H.: Steroid-Treated Tuberculous Pleural Effusion. *Brit. J. Tuberc.*, 52:81, 1958.

Auerbach, O.: The Progressive Primary Complex. *Am. Rev. Tuberc.*, 37:346, 1938.

Barclay, W., Ebert, R. H., and Koch-Weser, D.: Mode of Action of Isoniazid. *Am. Rev. Tuberc.*, 67:490, 1953; 70:784, 1954.

Bentley, F. J., Grzybowski, S., and Benjamin, B: *Tuberculosis in Childhood and Adolescence: With Special Reference to the Pulmonary Form of the Disease.* London, The National Association for the Prevention of Tuberculosis, 1954.

Brailey, M. E.: Prognosis in White and Colored Tuberculous Children According to Initial Chest X-Ray Findings. *Am. J. Pub. Health*, 33:343, 1944.

Committee on Control of Infectious Diseases. Chicago, American Academy of Pediatrics, 1961.

Committee on Therapy, American Trudeau Society: A Statement on Pyrazinamide. *Am. Rev. Tuberc.*, 75:1012, 1957.

Dahlström, G. and Difs, H.: Efficacy of BCG Vaccination; Study on Vaccinated and Tuberculin Negative Non-vaccinated Con-

scripts. *Acta Tuberc. Scandinav.*, Suppl. 27, 1951.

Débre, R. and Brissaud, H. E.: *Méningite tuberculeuse et tuberculose miliare de l'enfant; Leur traitement.* Paris, Masson et Cie, 1953.

Débre, R., and Papp, K.: About the Tuberculin Skin Test During the Course of Measles and Rubella. *Compt. rend. Soc. de biol.*, 95:29, 1926.

Edwards, L. B., Edwards, P. Q., and Palmer, C. E.: Sources of Tuberculin Sensitivity in Human Populations. *Acta Tuberc. Scandinav.*, Suppl. 47, 1959.

Edwards, L. B., Palmer, C. E., Affronti, L. F., Hopwood, L., and Edwards, P. Q.: Epidemiologic Studies of Tuberculin Sensitivity. II. Response to Experimental Infection with Mycobacteria Isolated from Human Sources. *Am. J. Hyg.* 71:218, 1960.

Edwards, P. Q., and Edwards, L. B.: Story of the Tuberculin Test from an Epidemiologic Viewpoint. *Am. Rev. Resp. Dis.*, 81 (part 2): 1, 1960.

Elmendorf, D. F., Jr., Cauthorn, W. W., Muschenheim, C., and McDermott, W.: The Absorption, Distribution, Excretion and Short Term Toxicity of Isoniazid (Nydrazid) in Man. *Am. Rev. Tuberc.*, 65:429, 1952.

Ferebee, S. H., and Mount, R. W.: Prophylactic Effect of Isoniazid on Primary Tuberculosis in Children, a Preliminary Report: United States Public Health Service Tuberculosis Prophylaxis Trial. *Am. Rev. Tuberc.*, 76: 942, 1957.

Filler, J., and Porter, M.: Physiologic Studies of the Sequelae of Tuberculous Pleural Effusion in Children Treated with Antimicrobial Drugs and Prednisone. *Am. Rev. Resp. Dis.*, 88:181, 1963.

Furcolow, M. L., and Robinson, E. L.: Quantitative Studies of the Tuberculin Reaction. II. The Efficiency of a Quantitative Patch Test in Detecting Reactors to Low Doses of Tuberculin. *Pub. Health Rep.*, 56:2405, 1941.

The Future of Tuberculosis Control: A Report to the Surgeon General of the Public Health Service by a Task Force on Tuberculosis Control, United States Dept. of Health, Education, and Welfare, Public Health Service, Communicable Disease Center, Atlanta, Georgia, 1963.

Gerbeaux, J., Baculard, Jr., and Beaucher, A.: Prevention of Bronchial Sequelae in a Primary Tuberculous Lymph Node by Hormonal Treatment. *Presse méd.*, 67:1285, 1959.

Ghon, A., and Kudlich, H.: Die Eintrittspforten der Infektion vom Standpunkte der pathologischen Anatomie; in S. Engel and C. Pirquet: *Handbuch der Kindertuberkulose.* Stuttgart, Georg Thieme Verlag, 1930, Vol. 1.

Hardy, J. B., and Kendig, E. L., Jr.: Tuberculous Pleurisy with Effusion in Infancy. *J. Pediat.*, 26:138, 1945.

Heimbeck, J.: Vaccination sous-cutanée et cutanée au B.C.G., 1926-1948. *Semaine Hôp. Paris,* 25:771, 1949.

Jacobs, J.: A Concept of Pulmonary Tuberculosis in Childhood. *Brit. J. Clin. Prac.,* 12:778, 1958.

Johnson, J. R., and Davey, W. N.: Cortisone, Corticotropin and Antimicrobial Therapy in Tuberculosis in Animals and Man. *Amer. Rev. Tuberc.,* 70:623, 1954.

Johnson, W. J.: Biological Acetylation of Isoniazid. *Nature,* 174:744, 1954.

Johnston, J. A.: *Nutritional Studies in Adolescent Girls and Their Relation to Tuberculosis.* Springfield, Ill., Charles C Thomas, 1953.

Kendig, E. L., Jr.: The Effect of Antihistaminic Drugs on the Tuberculin Patch Test. *J. Pediat.,* 35:750, 1949.

Idem: The Routine Tuberculin Test—A Neglected Pediatric Procedure. *J. Pediat.,* 40: 813, 1952.

Idem: Tuberculosis in the Very Young. *Amer. Rev. Tuberc.,* 70:161, 1954.

Idem: Incidence of Tuberculous Infection in Infancy. *Am. Rev. Tuberc.,* 74:149, 1956.

Idem: Early Diagnosis of Tuberculosis in Childhood. A.M.A. *J. Dis. Child.,* 92:558, 1956.

Idem: BCG Vaccination in Virginia. *J. Pediat.,* 51:54, 1957.

Idem: Prognosis of Infants Born of Tuberculous Mothers. *Pediatrics,* 26:97, 1960

Idem: Unclassified Mycobacteria in Children: Correlation of Skin Tests and Gastric Cultures. *Am. J. Dis. Child.,* 101:749, 1961.

Idem: Unclassified Mycobacteria as a Causative Agent in the Positive Tuberculin Reaction. *Pediatrics,* 30:221, 1962.

Idem: Unclassified Mycobacteria: Incidence of Infection and Cause of a False Positive Tuberculin Reaction. *New England J. Med.,* 268:1001, 1963.

Kendig, E. L., Jr., and Burch, C. D.: Short-Term Antimicrobial Therapy of Tuberculous Meningitis. *Am. Rev. Resp. Dis.,* 82:672, 1960.

Kendig, E. L., Jr., and Hudgens, R. O.: The Effect of Rubeola on Tuberculosis Under Antimicrobial Therapy. I. Primary Tuberculosis Treated with Isoniazid. II. Tuberculous Meningitis Treated with Isoniazid, Streptomycin and Para-aminosalicylic Acid. *Pediatrics,* 24:616, 619, 1959.

Kendig, E. L., Jr., and Johnston, W. B.: Short-Term Antimicrobial Therapy of Tuberculous Meningitis. *New England J. Med.,* 258: 928, 1958.

Kendig, E. L., Jr., and Rogers, W. L.: Tuberculosis in the Neonatal Period. *Amer. Rev. Tuberc.,* 77:418, 1958.

Kendig, E. L., Jr., and Wiley, T. M.: The Treatment of Tuberculosis of the Super-

ficial Cervical Lymph Nodes in Children. *J. Pediat.,* 47:607, 1955.

Kendig, E. L., Jr., Choy, S. H., and Johnson, W. H.: Observations on the Effect of Cortisone in the Treatment of Tuberculous Meningitis. *Am. Rev. Tuberc.,* 73:99, 1956.

Kendig, E. L., Jr., Trevathan, G. E., and Ownby, R. J.: Isoniazid in Treatment of Tuberculosis in Childhood. A.M.A. *J. Dis. Child.,* 88:148, 1954.

Lanier, V. S., Russell, W. F., Jr., Heaton, A., and Robinson, A.: Concentrations of Active Isoniazid in Serum and Cerebrospinal Fluid of Patients with Tuberculosis Treated with Isoniazid. *Pediatrics,* 21:910, 1958.

Lattimer, J. K.: Kidney Tuberculosis in Children. *Pediat. Clin. N. Amer.,* 2:793, 1955.

Leunda, J. J., Panizza Blanco, A., and Raggio, O. V.: The Tuberculous Infection and the Measles Infection. *Arch. Ped. Uruguay,* 14: 502, 1943.

Lincoln, E. M., and Sewell, E. M.: *Tuberculosis in Children.* New York, McGraw-Hill Book Company, Inc., 1963.

Lincoln, E. M., Davies, P. A., and Bovornkitti, S.: Tuberculous Pleurisy with Effusion in Children: A Study of 202 Children, with Particular Reference to Prognosis. *Am. Rev. Tuberc.,* 77:271, 1958.

Long, E. R.: *The Chemistry and Chemotherapy of Tuberculosis.* 3rd ed. Baltimore, Williams & Wilkins Company, 1958.

Lorriman, G., and Bentley, F. J.: The Incidence of Segmental Lesions in Primary Tuberculosis: With Special Reference to the Effect of Chemotherapy. *Am. Rev. Tuberc.,* 79: 756, 1959.

Lurie, M. B., Zappasodi, P., and Tickner, C.: On the Nature of Genetic Resistance to Tuberculosis in the Light of the Host-Parasite Relationship in Natively Resistant and Susceptible Rabbits. *Am. Rev. Tuberc.,* 72:297, 1955.

Mande, R., Herrault, A., Loubry, P., and Bouchet, C.: Les epidémies scolaires de tuberculose. *Semaine Hôp. Paris,* 34:1837, 1958.

McDermott, W., and others: Pyrazinamide-Isoniazid in Tuberculosis. *Am. Rev. Tuberc.,* 69:319, 1954.

Morales, S. M., and Lincoln, E. M.: The Effect of Isoniazid Therapy on Pyridoxine Metabolism in Children. *Amer. Rev. Tuberc.,* 75:594, 1957.

Nemir, R. L., Cardona, J., Lacoius, A., and David, M.: Prednisone Therapy as an Adjunct in the Treatment of Lymph Node-Bronchial Tuberculosis in Childhood. *Am. Rev. Resp. Dis.,* 88:189, 1963.

Palmer, C. E., and Edwards, L. B.: Geographic Variations in the Prevalence of Sensitivity to Tuberculin (PPD-S) and to the Battey Antigen (PPD-B) Throughout the United

States. *Bull. Int. Union Against Tuberculosis,* 32:373, 1962.

Renzetti, A. D., Wright, K. W., Edling, J. H., and Bunn, P.: Clinical, Bacteriologic and Pharmacologic Observations upon Cycloserine. *Am. Rev. Tuberc.,* 74:128, 1956.

Rich, A. R.: *The Pathogenesis of Tuberculosis.* 2nd ed. Springfield, Ill., Charles C Thomas, 1951.

Robinson, A., Meyer, M., and Middlebrook, G.: Tuberculin Hypersensitivity in Tuberculous Infants Treated with Isoniazid. *New England J. Med.,* 252:983, 1955.

Rosenthal, S. R.: *BCG Vaccination Against Tuberculosis.* Boston, Little, Brown & Co., 1957.

Idem: The Disk-Tine Tuberculin Test (Dried Tuberculin-Disposable Unit). *J.A.M.A.,* 177:452, 1961.

Rosenthal, S. R., Nikurs, L., Yordy, E., Hoder, B., and Thorne, M.: Tuberculin Tine and Mantoux Tests. *Pediatrics,* 30:385, 1965.

Schwartz, W. S., and Moyer, R. E.: The Chemotherapy of Pulmonary Tuberculosis with Pyrazinamide Used Alone and in Conjunction with Streptomycin, Para-aminosalicylic Acid or Isoniazid. *Am. Rev. Tuberc.,* 70:413, 1954.

Starr, S., and Berkovich, S.: Effects of Measles, Vaccine Measles on the Tuberculin Test. Gamma Globulin Modified Measles and *New England J. Med.,* 270:386 1964.

Storey, P. B., and McLean, R. L.: Some Considerations of Cycloserine Toxicity. *Am. Rev. Tuberc.,* 75:514, 1956.

Ström, L.: Vaccination Against Tuberculosis. *Am. Rev. Tuberc.,* 74:28, 1956.

Viomycin. *Am. Rev. Tuberc.,* 63:1, 1951.

Wallgren, A.: Pulmonary Tuberculosis: Relation of Childhood Infection to the Disease in Adults. *Lancet,* 1:417, 1938.

Idem: Pulmonary Tuberculosis in Children; in J. A. Miller and A. Wallgren: *Pulmonary Tuberculosis in Adults and Children.* New York, Thomas Nelson and Sons, 1939.

Idem: The Time Table of Tuberculosis. *Tubercle,* 29:245, 1948.

Wasz-Höckert, O.: Variola Vaccination as an Activator of Tuberculous Infection. *Ann. Med. Exper. et Biol., Fenniae,* 32:26, 1954.

Zumstein, P.: Des effets secondaires de l'acide para-aminosalicylique (PAS). *Praxis,* 45:48, 1956.

CHAPTER FIFTY-FOUR

Infections with the Unclassified Mycobacteria

EDWIN L. KENDIG, Jr., M.D.

In recent years it has been established by examination of resected pulmonary lesions and suppurative lymph nodes that human disease can be caused by mycobacteria previously considered to be harmless. These pathogenic organisms are called unclassified (anonymous, atypical) mycobacteria.

General Characteristics of Mycobacteria

Many types of mycobacteria have been isolated from water, vegetable matter and soil; occasionally pathogens have been found in swimming pools and in sewage. In general, the unclassified mycobacteria are nonpathogenic for guinea pigs, although many can produce disease in mice. They are much less susceptible to therapy with isoniazid and the other antituberculosis chemotherapeutic agents.

It is not yet completely settled whether or not these organisms may be mutations of *M. tuberculosis* treated with antituberculosis drugs, but the fact that many acid-fast organisms exist in nature, and existed for many years before the advent of the antituberculosis chemotherapeutic agents, indicates that this is, at best, not the entire answer.

Classification of Mycobacteria

The most important consideration from a clinical point of view is the differentia-tion of the human tubercle bacillus from the unclassified mycobacteria. Although additional subclassification of these organisms is, therefore, not essential, it may be helpful. The most useful classification to date is that suggested by Runyon and based on the cultural characteristics of the organisms (Table 1). *Group I (the*

Table 1. *Differential Characteristics of Some Mycobacteria*

Group I Photochromogens (M. kansasii, M. luciflavum)	Group II Scotochromogens	Group III Nonphotochromogens (Battey bacillus)	Group IV Rapid Growers
Appearance of colonies			
These are characterized by a yellow color, often a bright lemon-yellow pigment which appears only on exposure to light. Exposure for a few minutes may suffice, but several hours are required for maximum pigment production. Exposure to light followed by further incubation will reveal this pigment. When grown in total darkness, they show only slight creamy color	These organisms produce pigment in darkness as well as in light and usually produce an orange-yellow pigment	Colony form is smooth, often glossy, with a moist appearance, a white or off-white appearance or dull creamy tint. No pigment is produced on exposure to light	These organisms are a mixed group not well characterized by colony type
Appearance of growth in liquid media			
These suspend in liquid and are reported to show a swirling pattern	These suspend easily, like many other organisms	Suspension is easy, and uniform ground-glass appearance is characteristic	
Rate of growth			
Grow more rapidly than tubercle bacilli, reaching good maturity in about 2 weeks	Ordinarily are well matured in 1 or 2 weeks	Mature well in 1 to 2 weeks	Are able to produce well formed colonies in 2 to 4 days
Sensitivity to isoniazid			
Only slightly sensitive; often highly resistant	Usually resistant	Usually highly resistant	
Morphology in smears			
Longer, thicker and straighter than tubercle bacilli; often large granules are seen	Long, thick and often granular	Very variable, pleomorphic, some organisms being almost spherical, others more bacillary in appearance and often containing heavy granules	
Cording			
Cording is less pronounced and loose in nature	No cording	No cording	

Adapted from Hinshaw and Garland: *Diseases of the Chest.*

photochromogens, M. kansasii, M. luci-flavum, yellow bacillus). These organisms grow creamy white in the dark, but become bright yellow to orange when exposed to the light. Growth is more rapid than that of tubercle bacilli, reaching good maturity in about two weeks. *Group II (the scotochromogens, orange bacillus).* These mycobacteria produce pigment in the darkness as well as in the light and are orange to brick-red in color. They mature in one to two weeks. *Group III (the nonphotochromogens, Battey bacillus).* No pigment is produced either in the dark or when exposed to light. There is good maturity in one to two weeks. *Group IV (rapid growers).* The chief characteristic of this heterogeneous group is the rapid rate of growth. They are able to produce well formed colonies in two to four days.

Incidence and Epidemiology

In the United States, disease caused by the unclassified mycobacteria is seen more frequently in the southern states, particularly those bordering the Gulf of Mexico. Edwards and Palmer have noted a high incidence of infection without clinical symptoms in persons living in the southeastern states, and studies in Richmond have corroborated this observation. In this warm, moist climate it has been suggested that infection may be acquired from the soil or from vegetation. Person-to-person transmission has not been demonstrated. It is interesting also to note that organisms resembling unclassified mycobacteria have been isolated with increasing frequency from lesions in patients with sarcoidosis.

Pathology

In the light of present knowledge, the pathology appears similar to that of tuberculosis, and only a few minor differences have been noted. In children particularly, there seems to be a greater tendency toward lymph node involvement than in tuberculosis. Such involvement of the hilar lymph nodes may also account

for the higher incidence of endobronchial involvement.

Necrosis occurs relatively early in those infected with the unclassified mycobacteria, and there is a tendency more toward liquefaction than to semisolid caseation. The inflammatory reaction is generally more nonspecific than granulomatous.

For all practical purposes, however, the lesions of tuberculosis and those caused by the unclassified mycobacteria are indistinguishable.

Clinical Disease

Chronic suppurative lymphadenitis is the usual form of the disease as it occurs in children. Photochromogens, scotochromogens or the Battey bacillus may be the causative agent, and all three have on occasion been demonstrated at the Medical College of Virginia. The superficial cervical lymph nodes are more often involved, and Chapman has cultured identical organisms from the adenoids, tonsils

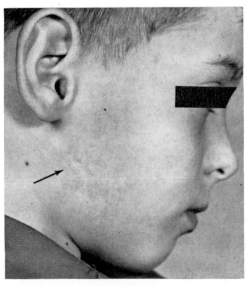

FIGURE 54–1. Chronic suppurative lymphadenitis usually involves a node or node group at the angle of the mandible. The healed lesion depicted here was caused by a scotochromogen. This mass of nodes liquefied before excision could be carried out, and aspirations were substituted. The patient fell from a bicycle, the mass ruptured, and healing ensued.

and the affected lymph nodes. The cervical lesion is usually unilateral and more often involves a node or node group at the angle of the mandible (Fig. 1). Involvement of the superficial cervical lymph nodes usually follows one or more acute attacks of tonsillitis or adenoiditis, and when the disease involves a lymph node elsewhere, there is usually some evidence of an associated skin lesion.

The development of the lesion in the lymph nodes seems to be more rapid than that noted in tuberculosis, and fluctuation occurs early. Liquefaction is often complete by the time surgery is instituted.

The pulmonary form of the disease, rarely seen in children, resembles tuberculosis. Symptoms are relatively nonspecific and include malaise, low-grade fever, mild cough, rhinorrhea, generalized aching and occasionally small hemoptyses. The lesion in the lung tends to remain localized and to undergo cavitation (with thin walls) and heavy fibrosis. Bronchogenic dissemination is rare. The diagnosis should be suspected if the patient does not make a satisfactory response to antituberculosis chemotherapy and is established by repeated isolation of the organism from the sputum, pus or tissue.

Another form of disease is the so-called swimming pool granuloma, of which the causative agent is *M. balnei*. This organism usually grows along the side of the pool, and lesions occur when the swimmer suffers abrasions of the skin when entering or leaving the pool. The lesions are chronic and ulcerative.

Other reported variations of disease caused by the unclassified mycobacteria include lesions of the bone and generalized systemic involvement.

Sensitivity to Tuberculin

In children the most important problem posed by infection with the unclassified mycobacteria is that of the heterologous reaction produced on tuberculin testing, the so-called false-positive tuberculin reaction. This was first demonstrated by Edwards and Palmer, who suggested that the tuberculin reaction measuring less than 10 mm. in diameter of induration is suspect. At the Medical College of Virginia there have been three corroborative studies. Whenever there is a positive tuberculin reaction measuring 5 to 9 mm. in diameter of induration, the tuberculin test should be repeated. If the same result occurs, concomitant skin testing with tuberculin solution and the antigens of the more common unclassified mycobacteria is indicated. Such testing often results in a small tuberculin reaction (5 to 9 mm. in diameter of induration) and a much larger reaction to one of the antigens of the unclassified mycobacteria (15 to 20 mm. in diameter of induration), thereby suggesting that the response is a heterologous reaction.

Since the value of such testing lies in the differentiation between infection caused by *M. tuberculosis* and that caused by the unclassified mycobacteria, the fact that the antigens of the unclassified mycobacteria are apparently not sufficiently specific to distinguish between the Timpe-Runyon groups is not of foremost importance.

If the results obtained on concomitant skin testing do not clearly differentiate between tuberculosis and infection with the unclassified mycobacteria, repeat skin testing two or three months later is often helpful.

Treatment

Most of the unclassified mycobacteria are relatively resistant to the antituberculosis chemotherapeutic agents, and only a few are sensitive. Streptomycin is more likely to be an effective drug than is isoniazid, but both, along with para-aminosalicylic acid, should be given until sensitivity studies have been completed. Recently, ethionamide has been recommended, too.

Isoniazid should be given orally in a dosage of 20 mg. per kilogram of body weight per day in two divided doses (maximum daily dose 500 mg.), and para-aminosalicylic acid in a dosage of 200 mg.

per kilogram of body weight per day in three or four divided doses (maximum daily dose 12 Gm.). If the organism is even partially sensitive, medication should be continued for one year. Streptomycin in a single intramuscular daily dose of 20 to 40 mg. per kilogram of body weight (maximum daily dose 1 Gm.) is continued until clinical improvement is noted, and the drug may then be administered three times each week. The duration of treatment with this drug will depend upon the course of the disease, but if such treatment is prolonged, the patient should be carefully watched for possible damage to the eighth cranial nerve.

Prompt excision of suppurative lymph nodes is the most important part of the therapeutic approach. As noted earlier, there is a tendency toward early and complete liquefaction of the affected lymph nodes, and these nodes should be completely removed as soon as possible. In those children with pulmonary disease who have localized lesions which have not responded to chemotherapy and are in satisfactory general condition, pulmonary resection is the treatment of choice. They should continue to receive the same antimicrobial therapy as that outlined above.

Skin lesions caused by *M. balnei* should be excised and the patient given the same antimicrobial therapy.

Those patients with clinical disease caused by the unclassified mycobacteria should not be treated in a tuberculosis sanatorium.

REFERENCES

Bates, R. D., and Chapman, J. S.: Tuberculin Test: Some Inherent Limitations. *Texas State J. Med.*, 60:517, 1964.

Bialkin, G., Pollak, A., and Weil, A. J.: Pulmonary Infection with Mycobacterium Kansasii. *Am. J. Dis. Child.*, 101:739, 1961.

Black, B. G., and Chapman, J. S.: Cervical Adenitis in Children Due to Human and Unclassified Mycobacteria. *Pediatrics*, 33:887, 1964.

Chapman, J. S.: The Anonymous Mycobacteria in Human Disease. Springfield, Ill., Charles C Thomas, 1960.

Chapman, J. S., and Guy, L. R.: Scrofula Caused by Atypical Mycobacteria. *Pediatrics*, 23:323, 1959.

Cuttino, J. T., and McCabe, A.: Pure Granulomatous Nocardiosis: A New Fungus Disease Distinguished by Intracellular Parasitism. *Am. J. Path.*, 25:1, 1949.

Davis, S. D., and Comstock, G. W.: Mycobacterial Cervical Adenitis in Children. *J. Pediat.*, 58:771, 1961.

Edwards, L. B., and Palmer, C. E.: Isolation of "Atypical" Mycobacteria from Healthy Persons. *Am. Rev. Resp. Dis.*, 80:747, 1959.

Edwards, L. B., Edwards, P. Q., and Palmer, C. E.: Sources of Tuberculin Sensitivity in Human Populations. *Acta Tuberc. Scandinav.*, 47 (Suppl): 77, 1959.

Edwards, L. B., and others: Epidemiologic Studies of Tuberculin Sensitivity. II. Response to Experimental Infection with Mycobacteria Isolated from Human Sources. *Am. J. Hyg.*, 71:218, 1960.

Edwards, P. Q., and Edwards, L. B.: Story of the Tuberculin Test. *Am. Rev. Resp. Dis.*, 81: (part 2): 1, 1960.

Guy, L. R., and Chapman, J. S.: Susceptibility in Vitro of Unclassified Mycobacteria to Commonly Used Antimicrobials. *Am. Rev. Resp. Dis.* 84:746, 1961.

Hsu, K. H. K.: Nontuberculous Mycobacterial Infections in Children: Preliminary Clinical and Epidemiologic Study. *J. Pediat.*, 60:705, 1962.

Jenkins, D. E., and others: The Clinical Problem of Infection with Atypical Acid-Fast Bacilli. *Tr. Am. Clinical & Climatological Assoc.*, 71:21, 1959.

Kendig, E. L., Jr.: Unclassified Mycobacteria in Children: Correlation of Skin Tests and Gastric Cultures. *Am. J. Dis. Child.*, 101:749, 1961.

Idem: Unclassified Mycobacteria as a Causative Agent in the Positive Tuberculin Reaction. *Pediatrics*, 30:221, 1962.

Idem: Unclassified Mycobacteria: Incidence of Infection and Cause of a False-Positive Tuberculin Reaction. *New England J. Med.*, 268:1001, 1963.

Krieger, I., Hahne, O. H., and Whitten, C. F.: Atypical Mycobacteria as a Probable Cause of Chronic Bone Disease. *J. Pediat.*, 65:340, 1964.

Lunn, H. F.: Mycobacterial Lesions in Bone. *East African Med.*, 40:113, 1963.

Mankiewicz, E.: The Relationship of Sarcoidosis to Anonymous Mycobacteria. *Acta Med. Scandinav.*, Supplement No. 62:403, 1964.

Millman, W. J., and Barness, L. A.: Unclassified Mycobacteria: Cause of Nonspecific Tuberculin Reactions. *Am. J. Dis. Child.*, 104:21, 1962.

Mollohan, C. S., and Romer, M. S.: Public Health Significance of Swimming Pool Granuloma. *Am. J. Pub. Health*, 51:883, 1961.

Prissick, F. H., and Masson, A. M.: Cervical Lymphadenitis in Children Caused by Chromogenic Mycobacteria. *Canad. M.A.J.*, 75:798, 1956.

Runyon, E. H.: Anonymous Mycobacteria in Pulmonary Disease. *Med Clin. N. Amer.*, 43:273, 1959.

Schaefer, W. B., and Davis, C. L.: Bacteriologic and Histopathologic Study of Skin Granuloma Due to Mycobacterium Balnei. *Am. Rev. Resp. Dis.*, 84:837, 1961.

Tarshis, M. S.: The Impact of Chemotherapy on the Tubercle Bacillus and Its Significance. *Dis. of Chest*, 41:471, 1962.

Timpe, A., and Runyon, E. H.: Relationship of "Atypical" Acid-Fast Bacteria to Human Disease: Preliminary Report. *J. Lab. & Clin. Med.*, 44:202, 1954.

Van der Hoeven, L. H., Rutten, F. J., and Van der Sar, A.: An Unusual Acid-Fast Bacillus Causing Systemic Disease and Death in a Child, with Special Reference to Disseminated Osteomyelitis and Intracellular Parasitism. *Am. J. Clin. Path.*, 29:433, 1958.

Weed, L. A., McDonald, J. R., and Needham, G. M.: The Isolation of Saprophytic Acid-Fast Bacilli from Lesions of Caseous Granulomas. *Proc. Staff Meet., Mayo Clin.*, 31: 246, 1956.

Weed, L. A., Karlson, A. G., Ivirs, J. C., and Miller, R. H.: Recurring Migratory Osteomyelitis Associated with Saprophytic Acid-Fast Bacilli. *Proc. Staff Meet., Mayo Clin.*, 31:238, 1956.

Yakovac, W. C., Baker, R., Sweigert, C., and Hope, J. W.: Fatal Disseminated Osteomyelitis Due to an Anonymous Mycobacterium. *J. Pediat.*, 59:909, 1961.

CHAPTER FIFTY-FIVE

Tularemia

WILLIAM A. HOWARD, M.D.

Tularemia is primarily a septicemic disease of rodents, which may be transmitted to man by the handling of infected material or by the bite of certain insect vectors. The disease was first described in ground squirrels in Tulare County, California, in 1912 by McCoy of the United States Public Health Service, and the first human case was described by Wherry in 1914.

Incidence

Tularemia probably has worldwide distribution and is found in all those parts of the United States and Canada where rodents and small game abound. The disease apparently occurs regularly in Europe and the USSR. Individual cases are not common, and at present the greatest incidence is found in laboratory workers handling the infectious agent.

Etiology

The disease is caused by *Pasteurella tularensis (Bacterium tularense)*, a small nonmotile, gram-negative, coccoid bacillus, 0.3 to 0.7 micron in length. The organism is readily destroyed by heating at 56°C. for ten minutes, and by most disinfectants, including one part per million of chlorine in drinking water. This probably accounts for the rarity of the gastrointestinal, oropharyngeal and glandular varieties of the disease in the United States, since potentially infected foods are nearly always cooked before being eaten, and chlorination of water is the rule.

Pathogenesis

Although tularemia is usually found in rodents, including the rabbit and the hare, the organism may infect the deer, fox, coyote, woodchuck, sheep, skunk, squirrel, opossum, water rat, cat, dog and many other animals. Birds and quail may also harbor *P. tularensis*. The disease is transmitted from animal to animal by several species of ticks of the family Ixodidae, including the rabbit tick (*Haemaphysalis leporis-palustris*), the brown dog tick (*Rhipicephalus sanguineus*), Ixodes and Amblyomma.

Transmission from animal to man may also be mediated by members of the family Ixodidae, most commonly the American dog tick (*Dermacentor variabilis*), the Rocky Mountain wood tick (*D. andersoni*), the Pacific coast tick (*D. occidentalis*) and the southern lone star tick (*Amblyomma americanum*). In the tick the infection is perpetuated by congenital transmission through the egg, and the organism is present in both the gut and hemocele. The deer fly (*Chrysops discalis*) transmits tularemia in the northwestern United States, and it is probable that other tabanid flies are responsible for the spread of the disease in the USSR. In Russia the common mosquitoes, *Aedes aegypti* and *Culex apicalis*, have been implicated as vectors. To date mosquito

transmission has not been reported in this country, but with the recognized mosquito population of the United States this remains a distinct possibility. *Pasteurella tularensis* has survived for fifty days in *Anopheles maculipennis*. Squirrel and rabbit fleas may also be vectors in occasional instances.

Naturally acquired infection is almost always obtained by the handling of infected small game, primarily rabbits. Rarely it may be caused by the bite of an infected tick or by the crushing of a tick on the skin. The organism seems able to penetrate the unbroken skin, and a remarkably small number of bacteria (ten to fifty) are regularly capable of causing the infection in the experimental subject. Man-to-man transmission has not been recorded, but laboratory infections are common.

Recent evidence indicates that host resistance in acquired immunity to tularemia may be dependent primarily on the development of phagocytic cells which have a greatly increased intracellular destructive capacity. Humoral factors (circulating antibody) appear to be of secondary importance.

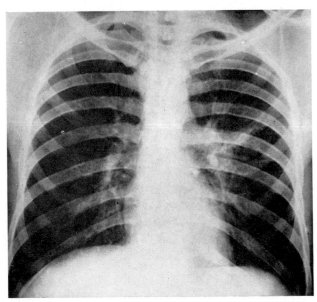

FIGURE 55–1. Tularemia. (Courtesy of Walter T. Hughes, M.D., University of Louisville School of Medicine, Louisville, Kentucky.)

Clinical Manifestations

Tularemia is usually more prevalent during the fall and winter months, coincident with the hunting season. The incubation period of the disease is nearly always less than two weeks, and usually less than one week. Depending on the portal of entry and the mode of infection, six clinical types are described: (1) ulceroglandular (most common), (2) oculoglandular, (3) oropharyngeal, (4) pulmonic, (5) glandular, and (6) intestinal (typhoidal).

There obviously may be some overlapping, and some reports indicate that a high percentage of patients, regardless of the type of clinical picture, will have x-ray evidence of lung involvement.

In naturally occurring infections, mostly from handling infected animals, approximately 90 per cent are of the ulceroglandular type, while laboratory infections are almost always of the pneumonic variety. In natural infections the onset is abrupt with chills, fever as high as 105 or 106°F., headache and vomiting. Evidence of the portal of entry may not be present for the first twenty-four hours, though regional lymphadenopathy may be evident. The initiating lesion begins as a localized inflammatory area, 2 to 3 cm. in diameter, with a central papule. The lesion progresses to central necrosis with abscess formation and ulceration. The regional lymph nodes become enlarged, firm, reddened and tender, and may undergo abscess formation, requiring surgical drainage. Other systemic symptoms include generalized muscular aches and pains, prostration, sweating and somnolence. Skin rashes may be present and vary from macules and papules to petechiae. Hepatosplenomegaly may be observed. Variations occur, depending upon the portal of entry, and ulcers may be found on the tonsils, pharynx or conjunctiva. Corneal ulcers have also been reported.

Many patients have evidence of pulmonary involvement both clinically and by x-ray, often with an associated hilar adenopathy. In obscure pulmonary lesions, one should consider tularemia, since the portal of entry may not be obvious, and primary lesions may not be found. Infection acquired by laboratory workers is nearly always of the pulmonic variety, and respiratory symptoms include dry cough, sore throat, substernal discomfort and pleuritic pain. Physical signs may include those of bronchopneumonia. X-ray findings may be indicative of patchy bronchopneumonia, pleural effusion, peribronchial thickening and nodular infiltration. Residual changes include fibrosis and an apparent increase in calcification.

The oropharyngeal type usually results from the ingestion of contaminated food or water and may involve more than one member of the family, since there is a common source of infection. This form produces the characteristic ulcerations in the mouth, throat or tonsils, with cervical adenitis and occasionally exudate or pseudomembrane on the tonsils.

Eye involvement causes lacrimation, photophobia, itching and swelling of the eyelids, and enlargement of the preauricular lymph nodes. Rarely corneal ulcers may cause permanent impairment of vision.

Diagnosis

The presence of tularemia usually may be suspected when the patient gives a history of contact with some sort of small wild animal, usually a rabbit. This, combined with the classic appearance of the ulceroglandular form of the disease, may suggest the proper diagnosis. The leukocyte count may be as high as 14,000 to 16,000 per cubic milliliter at the onset, and the erythrocyte sedimentation rate and C-reactive protein level are usually slightly elevated. Laboratory confirmation may be obtained by the isolation of the causative agent from material from ulcers or buboes cultured on glucose-cystine blood agar. Animal inoculation is also an effective way of establishing the diagnosis. Unfortunately, both methods carry a high degree of risk to laboratory personnel, and are not normally recommended. Blood drawn early in the disease and three to four weeks after onset may be used for comparative complement fixation, hemagglutination inhibition and antibody neutralizing studies. Agglutination titers of 1:80 are considered diagnostic, but a definite rise in titer in the convalescent blood is more conclusive. The intradermal skin test (Foshay) is felt by some to be specific and diagnostic. It is of the delayed type, indicating that cellular factors may play a prominent part in host resistance; it generally becomes positive after the first week of the disease.

Differential diagnosis includes atypical pneumonia, influenza, tuberculosis, psittacosis, histoplasmosis, the typhoid group of diseases, brucellosis, sepsis, anthrax, rat-bite fever and relapsing fever.

Pathology

In addition to the local lesion, pathologic findings include enlarged regional lymph nodes which contain focal lesions with central suppurative necrosis, characteristically bordered by a granulomatous infiltrate consisting of epithelioid cells and multinucleated giant cells of the foreign body type. In addition, there are focal necrotic lesions in various organs throughout the body, especially the liver, spleen, kidneys, lungs and bone marrow. Polymorphonuclear leukocytes are plentiful in the center of these lesions, while in older lesions evidence of fibrosis is usually present.

Complications

Involvement of the respiratory tract occurs most commonly and includes bronchopneumonia, chronic bronchitis, and pleural effusion. Encephalitis and meningitis have been reported, and painful arthritis may occur. Other rare complications include thrombophlebitis, osteomyelitis, peritonitis and pericarditis.

Prevention

Tularemia is most effectively prevented by the avoidance of contact with infected wild game and with various insect vectors. One should reject for use and destroy by burying or burning any game with evidence of liver involvement such as abscesses or spots. Vaccine prophylaxis has been used in laboratory workers, but is rarely indicated for children. The killed vaccine does not appear to prevent local infection, but may prevent the resulting systemic infection or may modify the severity of the disease. The viable attenuated vaccine recently in use appears to offer protection against respiratory challenge in experimental subjects, and appears to be the material of choice. In spite of the routine use of vaccines in laboratory workers, there are now over 200 cases of tularemia recorded in this group.

Treatment

Streptomycin is the most effective drug in the treatment of tularemia. It is bactericidal at concentrations of 1.9 micrograms per milliliter; if the strain is resistant to the drug, it will remain resistant regardless of concentration. Dosage in children should be 20 to 40 mg. per kilogram per day in divided doses, the total dosage not to exceed 1 Gm. daily. Treatment is continued for seven to ten days; relapses have not been observed with this plan of therapy. The later in the course of the disease that streptomycin is started, the slower will be the response.

The tetracyclines are also effective drugs in the treatment. Because they are bacteriostatic, relapses are common if they are begun too early in the course of the disease, before host immune response has been initiated. Relapses respond promptly, however, to a second course of the drug. Tetracyclines are used in a dosage of 20 to 40 mg. per kilogram per day in divided doses orally, or 12 to 20 mg. per kilogram per day intramuscularly or intravenously for at least ten days.

Chloramphenicol in dosage of 50 to 100 mg. per kilogram per day orally or intramuscularly may be used when the other drugs are for any reason contraindicated.

For the individual case, general supportive measures are used for fever and pain, including the use of acetylsalicylic acid, analgesics and sedatives. Local treatment is largely symptomatic, with emphasis on the maintenance of cleanliness. Surgical intervention with the drainage of suppurative processes may be necessary, but may be accompanied by systemic reactions. Isolation is generally not considered necessary, although exudates and dressings should be handled with rubber gloves.

Untreated, the majority of patients will recover in six to eight weeks, but with a rather protracted convalescence. Suitable antibiotic therapy greatly shortens both the duration and severity of the infectious process.

REFERENCES

Archer, V. W., Blackford, S. D., and Wissler, J. E.: Pulmonary Manifestations in Human Tularemia. *J.A.M.A.*, 104:895, 1935.

Burroughs, A. L., Holdenried, R., Longanecker, D. B., and Meyer, K. F.: A Field Study of Latent Tularemia in Rodents with a List of All Known Naturally Infected Vertebrates. *J. Infect. Dis.*, 76:115, 1945.

Faust, E. C., and Russell, P. F.: Tularemia; in *Clinical Parasitology*. 7th ed. Philadelphia, Lea & Febiger, 1964, p. 762.

Gould, S. E., Hinerman, D. L., Batsakis, J. G., and Beamer, P. R.: Diagnostic Patterns in Diseases of the Reticulo-endothelial System. Tularemia. *Am. J. Clin. Path.*, 41:419, 1964.

Hughes, W. T.: Tularemia in Children. *J. Pediat.*, 62:495, 1963.

Hughes, W. T., and Etteldorf, J. N.: Tularemia; in S. S. Gellis and B. M. Kagan (Eds.): *Current Pediatric Therapy* 1966-1967. Philadelphia, W. B. Saunders Company, 1966.

Ljung, O.: Intradermal and Agglutination Tests in Tularemia. *Acta Med. Scand.*, 160:149, 1958.

Idem: The Intradermal Test in Tularemia. *Acta Med. Scand.*, 160:135, 1958.

Overholt, E. L., Tigertt, W. D., Kadull, P. J., and Ward, M. K.: An Analysis of Forty-Two Cases of Laboratory Acquired Tularemia. *Am. J. Med.*, 30:785, 1961.

Parker, R. T., Lister, L. M., Bauer, R. E., Hall, H. E., and Woodward, T. E.: Use of Chloramphenicol in Experimental and Human Tularemia. *J.A.M.A.*, 143:7, 1950.

Saslaw, S., Eigelsbach, H. T., Wilson, H. E., Prior, J. A., and Carhart, S.: Tularemia Vaccine Study. I. Intracutaneous Challenge. *Arch. Int. Med.*, 107:689, 1961.

CHAPTER FIFTY-SIX

Varicella Pneumonia

ROSA LEE NEMIR, M.D.

Varicella, a highly contagious viral disease of childhood, has taken on new interest and importance in recent years. Since the early detailed reports of fatalities from pneumonia in congenital varicella and in adults following varicella infection, the literature has been filled with accounts of chickenpox pneumonia and descriptions of disseminated varicella occurring at all ages, with some fatalities.

The virus of varicella has been fully described, and it can be isolated readily from "pox" lesions. Its similarity to the virus of herpes zoster, however, is so great that exact differentiation between the two cannot be made either by growth and cultural methods or by cytopathology from infected tissue, although clinical differentiation is usually not too difficult. The virus of *variola*, on the other hand, can be distinguished from varicella by both its cytology and its pathologic lesions. The clinical manifestations produced by each of these two viruses differ also—an interesting point, especially since the name "varicella" is the diminutive of variola.

Pathology

The lungs are congested, and the alveoli are filled with protein-rich edema fluid. Occasionally, hemorrhagic areas are described. The outstanding microscopic findings in the lungs are the cellular exudate in which large mononuclear cells predominate, proliferation of septal cells to form a prominent alveolar lining, alveolar necrosis, and vascular damage. Evidence for viral infection is supported by the frequency of type A inclusion bodies and the absence or rarity of bacteria on staining. The many patchy lobular lesions radiating out from the hilus into all lobes of the lung may show coalescence.

In uncomplicated varicella there is no mediastinal or hilar adenopathy, a helpful point in differentiation from tuberculosis.

Disseminated nodular lesions of varying sizes are found in many organs of the body in addition to the skin: namely, in the liver, lung, spleen, adrenal glands, gastrointestinal tract, renal pelvis, bladder and pancreas. The central portion of these lesions shows necrosis. Vesicular lesions may be seen on the surface of the pleura. Grayson and others have described effusion in both pleural and pericardial cavities observed at autopsy and in x-ray films.

Oppenheimer, in her report on the pathology of congenital varicella, added to these observations the description of foci of necrosis containing intranuclear inclusion bodies in the thymus and lesions on the placenta.

Epidemiology

This highly contagious disease spreads by droplet infection from contact, with a usual incubation period of fourteen to

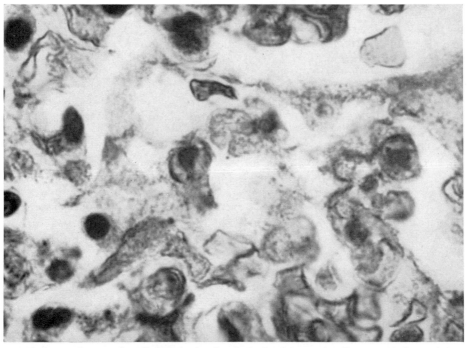

FIGURE 56–1. Intranuclear inclusions in sloughed alveolar septal cells, × 1200, in an infant.

sixteen days and varying from seven to twenty days. Infection by way of the maternal blood stream to the fetus also occurs. The infant may be born prematurely because of the varicella infection. Both the mother and the newborn may show the lesions of chickenpox varying in severity from a mild to a rapidly fulminating course ending in death and usually involving the lung. Fish recently described four such instances which were fatal for both mother and infant. There is no evidence at present that pregnancy increases susceptibility to varicella.

Although varicella is primarily a disease of childhood, it may occur at any age. When it develops in adults, the infection may produce pulmonary complications ranging from mild to serious; therefore recognition of the susceptibility of adults is important. An infected child should be isolated promptly, and adults with no previous history of varicella infection—especially pregnant women and any patient under corticosteroid therapy—should be protected from exposure.

Occasionally the history of the spreading of varicella to contacts is helpful in differentiating variola from acute fulminating hemorrhagic varicella. Fitz and Meiklejohn found it necessary to vaccinate seventy contacts of one such patient whose diagnosis was later clarified when variola antibodies failed to develop.

Although one attack of varicella is believed to confer lifelong immunity, Shee and Fehrsen have described the recurrence of varicella one month after the first attack in a nine-year-old boy. Reactivation of dormant varicella virus in the tissues was believed to be related to cortisone treatment that was given immediately after the first crop of chickenpox lesions to control giant urticaria thought to have been induced by penicillin.

Incidence

It is difficult to give a statistical analysis of the frequency of pneumonia in patients with varicella, a frequent and mild contagious disease of childhood usually not requiring hospitalization. A recent publication by Bastin and others covering a period from January 1960 to June 1962 reported only three cases of pneumonia among 2225 children and 143 adults.

At Bellevue Hospital (on the Infectious Disease Ward) for the period from November 1963 to November 28, 1964, ninety-eight patients with varicella were observed; there were two with pulmonary complications, one with varicella pneumonia (an adult) and one with bronchiolitis.

Congenital varicella is rare, and only eighteen cases have been reported. Ehrlich and others pointed out that congenital varicella developing between the fifth and tenth days after birth appears to be more severe than chickenpox which develops earlier. Transplacental antibodies may ameliorate the infection in the latter instance. In their review of the literature they found a mortality rate of almost 25 per cent (four deaths in the group of seventeen infants).

Clinical Features

Pneumonia as a complication of varicella may be viral (varicella virus) or bacterial in origin. Typically, the viral pneumonia parallels the rash, whereas the bacterial pneumonia usually occurs later in the course of the disease with recrudescence of fever and the development of respiratory signs. The diagnosis of bacterial pneumonia may be established by obtaining pathogens from cultures of the nasopharynx or blood, by finding foci of bacterial infection, by laboratory aids such as the white blood cell count and sedimentation rate, and by x-ray examination of the lungs. There is no uniform roentgenographic picture in bacterial infection, in contrast to varicella viral pneumonia. The symptoms and signs of bacterial pneumonia vary with the organisms responsible; hemolytic *Staphylococcus aureus, Hemophilus influenzae*, beta hemolytic streptococcus and pneumococcus are the predominant bacteria involved.

The earliest large study, made by Bul-

Iowa and Wishik of 2342 patients, reported a very small incidence (5.2 per cent) of complications of any sort with varicella; only 0.5 per cent were diagnosed as pneumonia, and these were associated with secondary bacterial infection.

In a 1961 study Weinstein and Meade reported on 453 patients with chickenpox during the period between 1944 and 1955. They described forty-one cases with disease of the respiratory tract, twenty of them in children under seven and twenty-one in adults over nineteen years of age. The bacterial respiratory complications described by these authors were found only in children. Pneumonia or tracheobronchitis, presumably due to bacterial infection, occurred in fifteen of the two hundred twenty-two children with varicella, all under seven years. In eleven patients pathogenic organisms were reported, *Hemophilus influenzae* in six cases, beta hemolytic streptococcus in four cases, and pneumococcus in one case. None of the children in this study was thought to have viral pneumonia.

Pneumonia as a complication of the varicella infection occurs in the first few days of the disease and appears to be much more frequent among adults than among children. Pulmonary and respiratory tract complications do occur in children, however, not only as congenital varicella in full-term infants and prematures, but also in older children, some of whom fail to survive. In some of these, autopsy reports have verified the clinical diagnosis.

The first signs of pulmonary involvement by the varicella virus appear between the second and fifth days. They include cough, increasing in severity, some dypsnea, and occasionally fever and cyanosis. These signs may progress rapidly to fatal termination within a few days after onset, but usually they disappear after five to seven days. Approximately one fourth of the patients complain of chest pain. In adults, especially, blood-streaked sticky sputum and hemoptysis may be a disturbing feature. The physical findings in the lungs depend in part on the degree of coalescence of the patchy nodular areas. When the latter occurs, some dullness and diminished breath sounds may be heard. The most common findings are wheezes, rhonchi, and scattered, fine or moist rales. The paucity of physical findings in the lungs as compared to the extent of pathology noted in the x-ray film is well known. In rare instances a pleural friction rub may be present. Varicella lesions on the pleura and pleural effusion described pathologically may well account for the occasional physical findings of pleurisy. Krugman, Goodrich and Ward described massive pleural effusion, which cleared in one week in one patient. The pleural fluid was bacteria-free. The majority of patients have minimal lung involvement, and, in general, the pulmonary infection is more frequently diagnosed by roentgenogram than by physical findings. The severity of the pneumonia parallels the progression of the skin lesions, which in some instances may be confluent and hemorrhagic. Mermelstein and Freireich have noted that all patients requiring oxygen had widespread rash. It has been emphasized repeatedly that pulmonary complications of varicella are more frequent than the clinicians may suspect from physical examination of the lung alone; x-ray examination of the lungs may show extensive pathology even though the physical examination gives negative results.

The range of severity is indicated in a study made by Weinstein and Meade. They classified pulmonary complications into three groups. In type I, viral respiratory involvement concerned patients whose respiratory disease was mild and subsided rapidly without treatment; most of these patients were children, and many had laryngotracheobronchitis. Type II included more severely ill patients who had an extensive rash and distressing cough. Almost all of those in this group had fever ranging from 102° to 105°F. Auscultation of the lungs gave normal results, and the patients recovered without specific treatment. The x-ray findings in the lungs varied from extensive interstitial infiltration to minimal lung changes, e.g. peribronchial thickening with occasional hilar enlargement. Type III included patients whose main complaint was respiratory distress and who were severely ill with definite primary varicella pneumonia and extensive skin rash, often suggesting variola, and whose illness lasted for a period ranging from one day to two weeks. In all these, the authors reported typical x-ray findings of numerous, soft, rounded infiltrates scattered throughout the lungs, and hilar lymphadenopathy. Treatment of some patients with various antibiotics (including tetracyclines) had no apparent effect on the course of the disease as compared with the untreated cases.

Diagnosis and Laboratory Aids

The clinical diagnosis of varicella with its typical location and progression of skin lesions is usually relatively simple. Variola must be considered in acute fulminating cases. Laboratory aids such as isolation of type A inclusion bodies from the sputum of patients with varicella pneumonia as described by Williams and Capers may be used when indicated. The cultural and basic differences of variola and varicella viruses may be pursued if ultimate confirmatory evidence is desired. The varicella virus may be cultured from the vesicles of chickenpox. Complement-fixing antibodies to varicella virus appear rapidly, beginning on the fourth day, and neutralizing antibodies on the tenth day.

The differentiation of herpes zoster from varicella is much more difficult. These two viruses cannot be differentiated by means of tissue culture or microscopy studies. The discovery of contact cases of varicella may be helpful, although contact of a patient with one of these two diseases may trigger the appearance of the other. Pek and Gikas have reported a fatal herpes zoster pneumonia occurring in a patient with Hodgkin's disease. The clinical and pathologic picture was indistinguishable from varicella pneumonia.

In uncomplicated chickenpox pneumonia, the white blood cell count is normal, the cold agglutinin and streptococcus MG titers are negative, the bacterial cultures of the nose and throat are negative or show normal flora, blood cultures are negative, and blood clotting time, even in hemorrhagic cases, is normal.

The most helpful diagnostic aid is the roentgenogram of the lungs. The typical widespread, nodular soft densities of varying sizes in all five lobes of the lungs, usually more prominent in the bases and in the hilar regions, are characteristic, but not pathognomonic. A long list of diseases, notably among them tuberculosis and sarcoidosis, have been considered in the differential diagnosis by Felson and Buechner. In varicella pneumonia there are increased bronchovascular markings and increased prominence of root shadows. We have never seen enlargement of the superior mediastinum in these patients as is often present in childhood tuberculosis with miliary or bronchogenic spread (see the chapter on tuberculosis, p. 656). The knowledge of a previously normal chest x-ray and the early and rapid, although partial, regression paralleling the course of the skin lesion is a diagnostic feature of varicella infection. The lobular infiltrate clears quickly; increased bronchovascular markings persist longer. Endress and Schnell in their study of clearing in the chest x-ray have indicated that the x-ray picture is usually normal within six weeks, although complete return to normal may require months. Saslaw, Prior and Wiseman described a patient in whom residual findings in x-ray films of the lungs remained two months.

Pulmonary function studies by Bocles, Ehrenkranz and Marks in ten adult patients with varicella pneumonia disclosed a significant diffusion defect, with abnormal alveolar capillary exchange persisting long after clinical recovery and x-ray clearing. Similar observations were not found in a control group of eight varicella patients without pneumonia.

FIGURE 56–2. Typical varicella pneumonia. *A,* Roentgenogram of the lungs on the day of admission of a 20-year-old male showing diffuse mottling bilaterally. Note the normal mediastinum.

This patient was admitted for a sore throat, cough and pain in the chest for 24 hours. Difficulty in breathing and swallowing was present for 12 hours. Extensive vesicular rash characteristic of varicella developed during the previous 5 days. The body on admission was covered with macular, pustular and crusted lesions; there were vesicles on the hard palate and tonsils, the temperature was 102° F., respirations were slow (20 per minute) and comfortable, and the white blood cell count was normal. No pathogens were found in the nose and throat cultures. Tine test was positive.

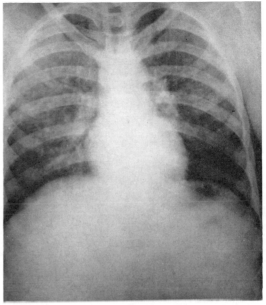

A

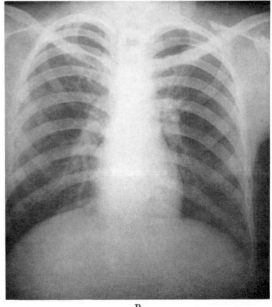

B, Five days later the mottlings in the lungs have cleared. The patient was afebrile and symptom-free within 36 hours with symptomatic treatment only. Although the tine test was positive, the rapid clearing eliminates the diagnosis of miliary tuberculosis. The first x-ray picture of the lung (*A*) appearing at the height of the rash and the prompt clearing are characteristic of varicella pneumonia.

B

Complications

As previously mentioned, pleurisy with effusion may be found in patients with varicella pneumonia. Claudy described at autopsy the typical varicella "pock" lesions on the surface of the pleura of an infant. A pathologic report of pericarditis in a child with rheumatic fever dying from varicella has been noted. Clinically, pericarditis has been reported in adults. Mandelbaum and Terk, in describing pericarditis in an adult who recovered in eight days, noted that it was proved only by electrocardiographic changes. This case indicates that pericarditis may occur without serious consequences and suggests that it may be diagnosed more often if electrocardiograms are made more frequently in these patients.

Other complications reported in patients with varicella pneumonia have been heart failure with shock, orchitis, nephritis, encephalitis, Waterhouse-Friederichsen syndrome, conjunctivitis and iritis, and laryngitis (one case reported as croup). All these and other reports testify to the diffuse spread of the varicella virus at the time of the lung infection.

From New Zealand, a country which has not reported histoplasmin infections, Mackay and Cairney described calcification of the lung following varicella in seven adult patients. Their theory that this calcification was etiologically related to varicella (tuberculosis was ruled out) was supported by the pathologic finding in one adult with carcinoma of the lung who required pneumonectomy shortly after varicella. Caseation was found in the central area of the calcified lesion.

Treatment

There is no specific treatment for varicella pneumonia. Attention to electrolyte and fluid balance is essential. Oxygen for cyanosis is certainly indicated, usually in a humidified atmosphere. Artificial respiration together with nasal administration of oxygen has been described as a lifesaving measure in a desperately ill young man. Fortunately, therapy of this extreme nature is rarely required. There is no evidence that antibiotic therapy is useful except for secondary bacterial infection. (See Chapter 21 for the treatment of bacterial pneumonia.)

The several papers in which the use of corticosteroids in the treatment of varicella pneumonia is reported suggest that these hormones may be harmful unless they are necessary for the therapy of concomitant disease such as definite adrenal insufficiency. There have been some instances in which corticosteroids were used without untoward results. Helmly and Smith described the recovery of an adult with pericarditis following treatment with prednisolone. The reactivation of the varicella virus, however, as described earlier, is always a possibility. In our own experience on the Children's Chest Service, Bellevue Hospital, corticosteroid therapy is avoided during periods of known exposure to varicella on the ward or elsewhere. In one instance, however, a child acquired varicella twelve days after the termination of a six-weeks period of prednisone therapy for tuberculous lymph node-bronchial disease. The patient had a mild uneventful course of chickenpox and recovered without untoward effect. The best approach, however, is the avoidance of the use of corticosteroids and the reduction of the dosage of patients on such medication to half the current dosage, aiming at a maximum of 50 mg. a day.

There is no effective prophylactic measure; neither convalescent serum nor gamma globulin has been shown to prevent infection. Ross, in a recent study of household contacts, found that the disease was modified by the administration of gamma globulin. He has recommended its use for high-risk, susceptible patients, suggesting an intramuscular dosage of 0.2 to 0.3 ml. per pound of body weight. Trimble also reported attenuation of varicella in two hospital interns by the use of gamma globulin. Both Trimble and Ehrlich have recommended that gamma globulin be used when infants are exposed to varicella in the immediate perinatal period. Debilitated children, those with chronic disease, children on corticosteroid therapy, and premature and newborn infants are most vulnerable to the development of disseminated varicella with pulmonary complication. Because some of these children do not survive, this group of patients may be benefited by the possible protection obtained from gamma globulin until some other more effective preventive treatment is found.

Most important is the realization that chickenpox, long treated lightly as an unimportant disease of childhood, can be a serious and fatal infection in an adult, who may quickly suffer pneumonia. In adults, varicella pneumonia is a serious infection with a number of fatalities. Recently with greater recognition of these complications by means of lung x-rays, reports of complete recovery and no fatalities are increasing. The incidence of varicella pneumonia in children is much lower than in adults. DiMase and others, in a survey of the accumulated literature, found that 90 per cent of the pneumonia reported is in adults. Successful isolation of previously noninfected adults from the child with chickenpox, though difficult, may save lives and, in the case of pregnant women, prevent premature births and possible congenital varicella.

REFERENCES

Almeida, J. D., Howatson, A. F., and Williams, M. G.: Morphology of Varicella (Chickenpox) Virus. *Virology,* 16:353, 1962.

Andrews, C. H., and others: Virus Infecting Vertebrates: Present Knowledge and Ignorance. *Virology,* 15:52, 1961.

Baroody, N. B., Jr., Baroody, W. G., Jr., and Cakell, B. B.: Varicella Pneumonia in Pregnancy; Report of Case Treated with Corticosteroids. *Am. Pract.,* 12:739, 1961.

Bastin, R., Binard, C., and Phav-Sany: Les manifestations pulmonaires au cours de la varicelle. *Presse Méd.,* 71:1873, 1963.

Bereston, E. S., and Robinson, R. C.: Herpes Zoster and Varicella in Identical Twins. *Arch. Dermatol.,* 83:503, 1961.

Bocles, J. S., Ehrenkranz, N. J., and Marks, A.: Abnormalities of Respiratory Function in

Varicella Pneumonia. *Ann Int. Med.,* 60:183, 1964.

Buechner, H. A.: The Differential Diagnosis of Miliary Diseases of the Lungs. *Med. Clin. N. Amer.,* 43:89, 1959.

Bullowa, J. G. M., and Wishik, S. M.: Complications of Varicella, I. Their Occurrence Among 2,534 Patients. *Am. J. Dis. Child.,* 49:923, 1935.

Bunn, P. A., and Hammond, J. D.: Chickenpox Complicated by Severe Pneumonia Treated with Aureomycin. *New York J. Med.,* 50:-1485, 1950.

Cheatham, W. J., Weller, T. H., Dolan, T. F., Jr., and Dower, J. C.: Varicella; Report of 2 Fatal Cases with Necropsy, Virus Isolation, and Serologic Studies. *Am. J. Path.,* 32:1015, 1956.

Claudy, W. D.: Pneumonia Associated with Varicella; Review of Literature and Report of Fatal Case with Autopsy. *Arch. Int. Med.,* 80:185, 1947.

DiMase, J. D., Groover, R., and Allen, J. E.: Artificial Respiration in the Therapy of Primary Varicella Pneumonia. *New Eng. J. Med.,* 261:553, 1959.

Downie, A. W.: Chickenpox and Zoster. *Brit. M. Bull.,* 15:197, 1959.

Drips, R. C.: Varicella in a Term Pregnancy Complicated by Postpartum Varicella Pneumonia and Varicella in the Newborn Infant. *Obstet. & Gynec.,* 22:771, 1963.

Editorial: Chickenpox and Pregnancy. *J.A.M.A.,* 173:1030, 1960.

Ehrlich, R. M., Turner, J. A., and Clarke, M.: Neonatal Varicella; A Case Report with Isolation of the Virus. *J. Pediat.,* 53:139, 1958.

Eisenbud, M.: Chickenpox with Visceral Involvement. *Am. J. Med.,* 12:740, 1952.

Endress, Z. F., and Schnell, F. R.: Varicella Pneumonitis. *Radiology,* 66:723, 1956.

Esswein, J. G., and DiDomenico, V. P.: Hemorrhagic Varicella Pneumonia. *Ann. Int. Med.,* 53:607, 1960.

Farrell, G. F., and Banshoff, A. M., Jr.: Primary Varicella Pneumonia, *W. Va. Med. J.,* 60:204, 1964.

Felson, B.: Acute Miliary Diseases of the Lung. *Radiology,* 59:32, 1952.

Fish, S. A.: Maternal Death Due to Disseminated Varicella. *J.A.M.A.,* 173:978, 1960.

Fitz, R. H., and Meiklejohn, G.: Varicella Pneumonia in Adults. *Am. J. Med. Sc.,* 232:489, 1956.

Frank, L.: Varicella Pneumonitis; Report of Case with Autopsy Observations. *Arch. Path.,* 50:450, 1950.

Gable, J. J., Jr.: Primary Chickenpox (Varicella) Pneumonia; Report of Two Cases Seen in the Private Practice of Internal Medicine. *Ann. Int. Med.,* 51:583, 1959.

Good, R. A., Vernier, R. L., and Smith, R. T.: Serious Untoward Reactions to Therapy with

Cortisone and Adrenocorticotropin in Pediatric Practice. *Pediatrics*, 19:272, 1957.

Grayson, C. E., and Bradley, E. J.: Disseminated Chickenpox (Pneumonia and Nephritis). *J.A.M.A.*, 134:1237, 1947.

Haggerty, R. J., and Eley, R. C.: Letters to the Editors: Varicella and Cortisone. *Pediatrics*, 18:160, 1956.

Helmly, R. B., Smith, J. O., Jr., and Eisen, B.: Chickenpox with Pneumonia and Pericarditis. *J.A.M.A.*, 186:870, 1963.

Johnson, H. N.: Visceral Lesions Associated with Varicella. *Arch. Path.*, 30:292, 1940.

Krugman, S., and Ward, R.: *Infectious Diseases of Children*, 3rd ed. St. Louis, C. V. Mosby Company, 1964.

Krugman, S., Goodrich, C. H., and Ward, R.: Primary Varicella Pneumonia, *New England J. Med.*, 257:843, 1957.

Lucchesi, P. F., LaBoccetta, A. C., and Peale, A. R.: Varicella Neonatorum. *Am. J. Dis. Child.*, 73:44, 1947.

MacKay, J. B., and Cairney, P.: Pulmonary Calcification Following Varicella, *New Zealand Med. J.*, 59:453, 1960.

Mandelbaum, T., and Terk, B. H.: Pericarditis in Association with Chickenpox. *J.A.M.A.*, 170:191, 1959.

Mermelstein, R. H., and Freireich, A. W.: Varicella Pneumonia. *Ann. Int. Med.*, 55:456, 1961.

Michel, J. C., Coleman, D. H., and Kirby, W. M. M.: Pneumonia Associated with Chickenpox; Report of a Patient Treated with Aureomycin. *Am. Pract. & Digest Treat.*, 2:57, 1951.

Montgomery, R. R., and Olafsson, M.: Waterhouse-Friderichsen Syndrome in Varicella. *Ann. Int. Med.*, 53:576, 1960.

Nelson, W. E. (Ed.): *Textbook of Pediatrics*. 8th ed. Philadelphia, W. B. Saunders Company, 1964.

Nemir, R. L., Cardona, J., Lacouis, A., and David, M.: Prednisone Therapy as an Adjunct in the Treatment of Lymph Node-Bronchial Tuberculosis in Childhood. *Am. Rev. Resp. Dis.*, 88:189, 1963.

O'Neil, R. R.: Congenital Varicella. *Am. J. Dis. Child.*, 104:391, 1962.

Oppenheimer, E. H.: Congenital Chickenpox with Disseminated Visceral Lesions. *Bull. Johns Hopkins Hosp.*, 74:240, 1944.

Pek, S., and Gikas, P. W.: Pneumonia Due to Herpes Zoster. Report of a Case and Review of the Literature. *Ann. Int. Med.*, 62:350, 1965.

Rake, G., Blank, H., Coriell, L. L., Nagler, F. P. O., and Scott, T. F. McN.: Relationship of Varicella and Herpes Zoster: Electron Microscopic Studies. *J. Bact.*, 56:293, 1948.

Rausch, L. E., Grable, T. J., and Musser, J. H.: Atypical Pneumonia Complicating Severe

Varicella in an Adult. *New Orleans M. & S. J.*, 96:271, 1943.

Reich, J. S., and Baumal, A.: Herpes Zoster and Varicella Occurring in Siblings Following Contact with Chickenpox. *J. Mount Sinai Hosp. N.Y.*, 28:473, 1961.

Rosecan, M., Baumgarten, W., Jr., and Charles, B. H.: Varicella Pneumonia with Shock and Heart Failure. *Ann. Int. Med.*, 38:830, 1953.

Ross, A. H.: Modification of Chickenpox in Family Contacts by Administration of Gamma Globulin. *New England J. Med.*, 267:369, 1962.

Saslaw, S., Prior, J. A., and Wiseman, B. K.: Varicella Pneumonia, *Arch. Int. Med.*, 91:35, 1953.

Schleussing, H.: Nekrosen im Leber, Milz, und Nebennieren bei nicht vereiterten Varicellen. *Verhandl. d. deutsch. path. Gesellsch.*, 22:228, 1927.

Shee, J. C., and Fehrsen, P.: Reactivation of Varicella Virus by Cortisone Therapy. *Brit. M. J.*, 2:82, 1953.

Southard, M. E.: Roentgen Findings in Chickenpox Pneumonia; Review of Literature; Report of 5 Cases. *Am. J. Roentgenol.*, 76:533, 1956.

Strachman, J.: Uveitis Associated with Chickenpox. *J. Pediat.*, 46:327, 1955.

Tan, D. Y. M., Kaufman, S. A., and Levene, G.: Primary Chickenpox Pneumonia. *Am. J. Roentgenol.*, 76:527, 1956.

Taylor-Robinson, D.: Herpes Zoster Occurring in a Patient with Chickenpox. *Brit. M.J.*, 5187:1713, 1960.

Thompson, C. A., and Cantrell, F. P.: Chickenpox Pneumonia Treated with Prednisolone—A Case Report. *Ann. Int. Med.*, 49:1239, 1958.

Trimble, G. X.: Attenuation of Chickenpox with Gamma Globulin. *Canad. M.A.J.*, 77:698, 1957.

Waddington, H. K.: Congenital Chickenpox; Report of a Case in Twins. *Obstet. & Gynec.*, 7:319, 1956.

Waring, J. J., Neubuerger, K. T., and Geever, E. F.: Severe Forms of Chickenpox in Adults with Autopsy Observation in Case with Associated Pneumonia and Encephalitis. *Arch. Int. Med.*, 69:384, 1942.

Weinstein, L., and Meade, R. H.: Respiratory Manifestations of Chickenpox. *Arch. Int. Med.*, 98:91, 1956.

Weller, T. H.: Observations on the Behavior of Certain Viruses That Produce Nuclear Inclusion Bodies in Man. *The Harvey Lectures*, 1956-1957, New York, Academic Press, Inc., pp. 228-54.

Weller, T. H., and Stoddard, M. B.: Intranuclear Inclusion Bodies in Cultures of Human Tissue Inoculated with Varicella Vesicle Fluid. *J. Immunol.*, 68:311, 1952.

Weller, T. H., Witton, H. M., and Bell, E. J.:

Etiologic Agents of Varicella and Herpes Zoster. *J. Exper. Med.*, 108:869, 1958.

Wesselhoeft, C., and Pearson, C. M.: Orchitis in the Course of Severe Chickenpox with Pneumonitis, Followed by Testicular Atro-

phy. *New England J. Med.*, 242:651, 1950.

Williams, B., and Capers, T. H.: The Demonstration of Intranuclear Inclusion Bodies in Sputum from a Patient with Varicella Pneumonia. *Am. J. Med.*, 27:836, 1959.

CHAPTER FIFTY-SEVEN

Measles Pneumonia

ROSA LEE NEMIR, M.D.

Measles, the most common contagious exanthematous disease of childhood, known since ancient times, should soon be rare now that there are available preventive vaccines which, it is hoped, will confer lifelong immunity. These successes with vaccines, both live attenuated and killed, have been possible because of the isolation of measles virus in tissue culture by Enders and co-workers and shortly afterwards by Cohen and others.

Measles pneumonia caused by the measles virus alone may occur early in the disease. More commonly, pneumonia may occur later, after the fading of the rash, when it is associated with secondary bacterial invaders. The most frequent complications of measles are otitis media, pneumonia and encephalitis. Bronchitis, laryngotracheitis and even bronchiolitis may be manifestations of a severe attack of measles. The acute inflammatory process throughout the bronchial tree may produce special symptoms of laryngeal obstruction resulting in the clinical and alarming picture of croup. Tracheolaryngitis is a part of the measles infection; therefore, accurately speaking, clinical "croup" in measles represents tracheolaryngitis of increased severity. Laryngitis was the most common "complication" (147 instances) reported in 1960-61 in 287 patients with measles in Chile. Laryngitis,

sometimes severe, is still common today. The ensuing discussion is confined to measles pneumonia.

Pathology

All epithelial cells of the respiratory tract from the nasal mucosa to the bronchioles are inflamed. Hyperplasia of the lymphoid tissue is found. There is an interstitial pneumonia with peribronchial infiltration by mononuclear cells. Two types of giant cells are found: large multinucleated syncytial cells containing inclusion bodies, and the Warthin-Finkeldey cell, found in the lymph nodes and the reticuloendothelial system, probably formed by the clumping and fusion of lymphoid cells and rarely showing inclusion bodies. The first, the epithelial multinucleated cell, has been described in "giant cell" pneumonia (see the chapter on Giant Cell Pneumonia, p. 301); the second giant cell is pathognomonic for measles. These Warthin-Finkeldey cells were first described in the tonsils and appendix; subsequently they have been found in lymph nodes throughout the respiratory and gastrointestinal tracts, and in the spleen, thymus and bone marrow. Recognition of the multinucleated epithelial giant cells in pathologic sections is credited to the careful descriptions of Denton.

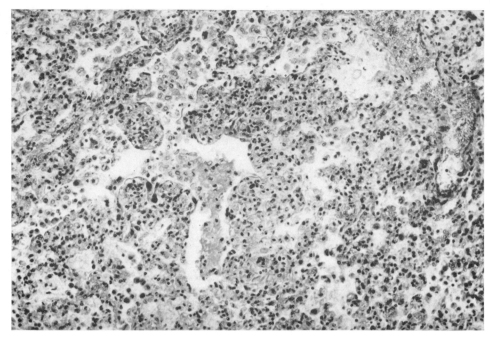

FIGURE 57–1. Measles pneumonia. Section of lung showing extensive interstitial inflammation. Desquamated bronchial epithelium, giant cells and mononuclear cells in alveoli and ducts. H. & E., × 150. (Courtesy of Dr. Renata Dische, Department of Pediatric Pathology, New York University School of Medicine.)

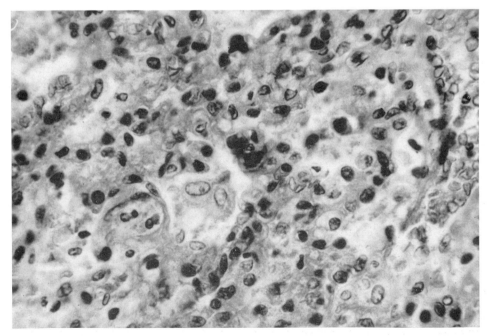

FIGURE 57–2. Measles pneumonia. Alveolar septa infiltrated by mononuclear cells. H. & E., × 500. (Courtesy of Dr. Renata Dische, Department of Pediatric Pathology, New York University School of Medicine.)

The first description in tissues of the tongue was made by Semsbroth.

The alveoli may become filled with the syncytial giant cells, and these, together with desquamated, degenerative cells, may line the alveolar wall in a manner similar to a hyaline membrane. In some instances, obstructions to bronchioles may occur, resulting in emphysematous bullae.

Pathogenesis

By both experimental and epidemiologic evidence, measles is a respiratory disease, beginning with infection in the upper respiratory tract and in the conjunctivae. The infectious droplets from the nasopharyngeal secretions of an acute case lodge on the respiratory epithelium of the new host. The progress of infection thereafter has been ably described by Grist. As Anderson and Goldberger showed experimentally, the virus invades the blood stream, producing a viremia. As the virus progresses to the reticuloendothelial system, generalized lymphadenopathy develops. This first viremia was demonstrated by Enders and others by inoculating monkeys with measles virus from tissue culture. They recovered the virus from the blood within five to seven days after inoculation. Using blood from patients with measles to inoculate monkeys, Sergiev and co-workers recovered the virus as early as the third day. There is a short period of decrease in virus titer in the blood after inoculation, followed by a demonstrable viremia (the second viremia) starting six to eleven days before the appearance of the rash, and persisting for a day or two after the appearance of the rash. The prodromal signs of measles— fever, coryza and conjunctivitis—usually occur ten to twelve days after the initial infection and during this second viremia. Measles virus may be cultured from the respiratory tract during the early prodromal period of respiratory infection. Early infection of the epithelial cells of the respiratory tract and the lymphatic nodes, including those in the hilar and mediastinal areas, has been demonstrated

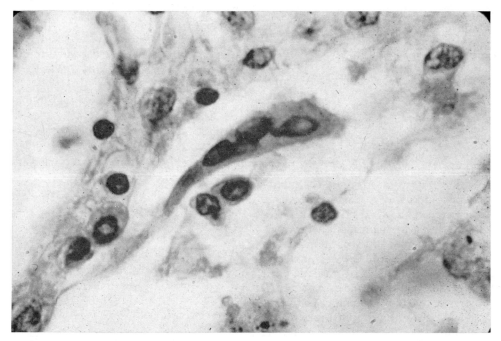

FIGURE 57–3. Measles pneumonia. Giant cell lining alveolus. H. & E., $\times$ 1500. (Courtesy of Dr. Renata Dische, Department of Pediatric Pathology, New York University School of Medicine.)

by experimental measles in monkeys. Sherman and Ruckle isolated interstitial pneumonia virus from the lung, as well as other tissues, of a patient dying during the prodromal stage of the disease.

By applying these observations clinically, tracheobronchitis is usually found at this time, and pneumonia occasionally. X-ray films taken during the first days of the rash show increased hilar markings which correlate with the peribronchial infiltration present in the first few days of the posteruptive stage of measles.

During the eruptive stage of measles the inflamed epithelial lining of the respiratory tract with its disturbed physiology is ripe for secondary bacterial infection and the consequent development of bacterial complications. Accumulated bronchial secretions, desquamated giant cells and epithelial cells often fill the lumen of the bronchi and produce obstruction of the bronchial tree, thus promoting areas of atelectasis, areas of emphysema, and the growth of bacterial pathogens in pulmonary tissues, resulting in superimposed bacterial pneumonia.

Incidence

The frequency of *pulmonary complications* varies from epidemic to epidemic and from country to country. A recent study in England utilized questionnaires sent to all physicians to cover the period from January 1 to April 30, 1963. The 53,000 replies (95 per cent) indicated that 38 per 1000 had respiratory tract disease: namely, pneumonia, severe bronchitis, bronchiolitis and croup, most commonly in infants and children under five years. There were six known deaths from pneumonia and one from bronchiolitis.

In a longitudinal study of 400 children in an African village in Nigeria, and the analysis of 1232 additional patients with measles, Morley found that bronchopneumonia was the most common complication. Many of these children were treated on an ambulatory basis, but 45 per cent of those requiring admission to the hospital and 54 per cent of the fatalities had bronchopneumonia. These observations may well relate to the extensive and frequent malnutrition in the Nigerian children, predisposing them to pulmonary complications. Morley found that over half of the children had contracted the disease before two years of age. Christensen and others, reporting on the measles epidemic in southern Greenland in 1951, noted that half of the pulmonary complications developed early in the course of disease, in direct connection with the rash, and during the prodromal period; the other half developed late in the disease. In the United States both the incidence of severe measles with complications and the mortality have decreased in recent years. Several factors, including the widespread use of antibiotics, are responsible for this decline. Cooch reviewed the incidence in the United States during the two World Wars and cited a declining rate since 1957, emphasizing especially the decrease in secondary infections associated with the hemolytic streptococcus. Fatalities from measles pneumonia largely occur late in the course of the disease and are due to secondary bacterial infection. Top has stated that 90 per cent of the deaths in patients with measles are attributable to pneumonia, and suggested that most of these are associated with bacterial infections.

Babbott and Gordon pointed out that the changing picture of measles in the United States may be seen in the Army experience during the two World Wars. They suggested at the time (1954) that antibiotic therapy might be an effective tool in the treatment of the bacterial complications that are the usual cause of fatality in patients with measles.

At Bellevue Hospital on the infectious disease ward where only the acutely ill patients are admitted, there were 167 patients ill with measles between November 1, 1963, and November 30, 1964. Pulmonary complications were responsible for 26 per cent of these admissions; twenty-nine of these patients had pneumonia, sixteen had croup, and three had bronchiolitis.

Respiratory Symptoms and Signs

Inflammation of the conjunctivae and mucous membrane of the nasopharynx may occur even at the time of the initial invasion of the virus, with mild transient respiratory symptoms and the horizontal red lines in the conjunctivae described by Papp. In general, however, the first signs of measles infection occur later, during the prodromal period, after an average incubation period of ten to twelve days. These signs include profuse mucoserous nasal discharge, sneezing, excessive tearing and photophobia, a mild irritating cough, Koplik spots and some fever. As the rash develops, the fever mounts and the inflammation in the tracheobronchial tree progresses. Cough increases and often develops a "barking" quality. Transient musical and occasional moist rales and rhonchi may be heard in the lungs.

Most patients recover within a few days, although there may be a mild cough that lingers for a while. In some patients a recrudescence of the disease or an increasing severity of the initial symptoms is noted with increase in the fever. These patients must be examined carefully for evidence of complications, encephalitis, otitis media, lymphadenitis, sinusitis and pulmonary disease—either bronchitis, tracheobronchitis, bronchiolitis or pneumonia. Excessive mucoid and mucopurulent secretions may be found in the posterior pharyngeal spaces. A hoarse voice or barking cough may call attention to increased infection in the larynx. Physical findings suggesting obstruction of bronchi, either partial or complete, may be obtained. Hyperresonance and decreased breath sounds suggest emphysematous areas and large bullae. These areas may clear quickly if they are due to endobronchial obstruction from mucoid secretions and desquamated epithelial material, or they may remain longer if they are also associated with bronchopneumonia and peribronchial inflammation. Similarly, complete obstruction with segmental collapse may clear readily or remain longer, depending on the underlying pathology.

Bacterial pneumonia during the course of measles may be detected not only by means of laboratory aids described above, but also by clinical observations of the patients. An increase in respiratory distress, and areas of consolidation, for example, found in examination of the lungs, suggest the presence of bacterial pneumonia in measles.

Diagnosis

When pneumonia occurs during the typical clinical picture of measles, there is usually no difficulty in making the diagnosis. In most instances when the diagnosis of measles is not clear, laboratory and immunologic aids may be helpful.

Antibody formation in measles can be measured by the technique as described by Enders, and others. The complement-fixing antibodies appear within two to three days, and neutralizing antibodies appear as the rash begins to subside, often as early as the fourth day after the appearance of the rash.

The measles epidemic in Greenland in 1951, a virgin area for measles infection, furnished a unique opportunity for the study of antibody titers. Bech showed that one third of seventy-one patients had complement-fixing antibodies on the first day after the onset of the exanthem. Within a short time the titers reached high levels; on the second postexanthematous day the majority had titers of 1:32 to 1:512.

The usual antibody response, however, may be suppressed in patients who are debilitated or have long-standing disease, notably leukemia. Determination of antibody titer may differentiate the immune person from the nonimmune. Bech showed a more rapid rise in antibody level in immune persons after exposure to measles.

Krugman and his co-workers have reported extensive studies of the immunity to measles in a longitudinal study of well infants during the first year of life, in

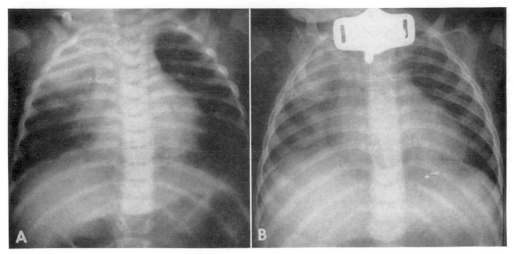

FIGURE 57–4. *A,* X-ray of chest, taken on admission 3 days after onset of measles rash, showing homogeneous density in the right upper lobe and some prominence of the right root. *B,* Three days after admission and 2 days after tracheostomy. Respiratory distress was relieved, although the right upper lobe pulmonary shadow remains.

patients with measles, in persons receiving various vaccines, and cross-sectional sampling of various populations of peoples. Complement-fixing, hemagglutination-inhibition and neutralizing antibody tests were used. The infant at birth receives transplacental antibodies which disappear usually by five months of age. Tompkins and Macaulay have showed that smears from nasal secretions during the prodromal period (forty-eight hours before the rash) contain giant multinucleated epithelial cells with typical inclusion bodies. These cells may continue in the secretions for several days.

Fluorescent antibody technique may enable us to make an early presumptive diagnosis. It may be helpful when the disease is atypical, in experimental work, or when a retrospective or necropsy diagnosis of the origin is to be made, or in the clarification of the agent of giant cell pneumonia.

Measles pneumonia of viral origin alone occurs early in the course of the disease. Later bacterial infection may produce symptoms of pulmonary disease. Certain tests are diagnostically helpful, such as blood cell counts, bacterial cultures, associated tests, and x-ray studies. For example, the white blood cell count shifts from the usual leukopenia with slight lymphocytosis at the onset of disease to a leukocytosis with polymorphonuclear increase as secondary bacterial infections occur. The most common bacterial invader of the respiratory tract is the hemolytic streptococcus, the frequent culprit during the epidemic among military personnel in World War I. Top has listed hemolytic streptococcus, pneumococcus and *Haemophilus influenzae* as the organisms most often cultured in patients with measles pneumonia. The staphylococcus and the organisms listed above were reported as etiologic agents by Weinstein and Franklin in their study of 163 children with measles, 25 per cent of whom had pneumonia.

An x-ray film of the chest is essential in the diagnosis of pulmonary complications in measles. Since the tracheobronchial tree and bronchopulmonary lymph nodes are always infected in measles, it is logical to assume that the chest x-ray will show some evidence of this involvement. When x-ray films were taken routinely in those patients with measles seen by Kohn and Koiransky, one fourth were found to show minimal hilar adenopathy in the pre-

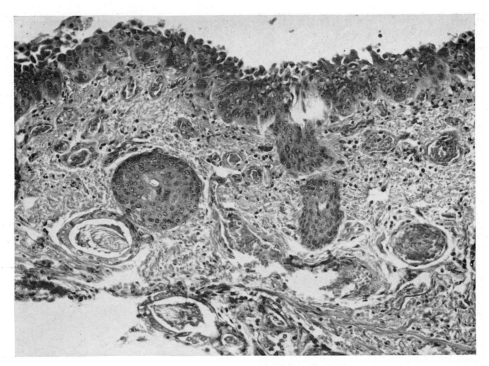

FIGURE 57–5. Measles tracheitis. × 150.

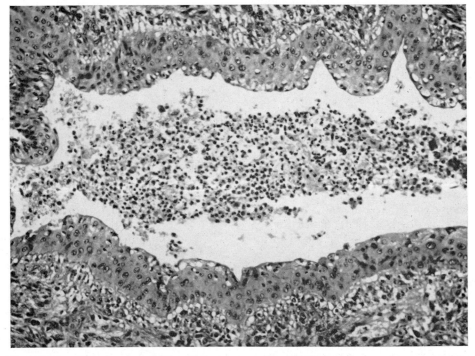

FIGURE 57–6. Extensive bronchitis and squamous cell metaplasia seen in autopsy material of a patient dying of measles pneumonia. × 150.

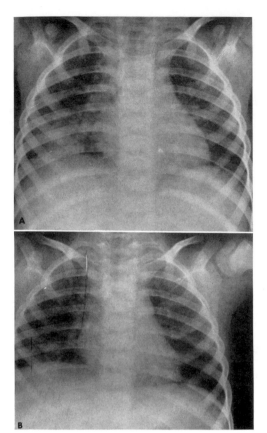

FIGURE 57–7. *A,* Four days after admission pulmonary infiltration is seen in the right base above the diaphragm. There are also mottled soft lesions of irregular size in the right lung near the hilus and in the left upper lobe. *B,* There is complete clearing of the lungs 6 days later.

eruptive stage. In their subsequent studies, lateral views of the chest were taken, and enlargement of the hilar nodes was visualized in almost all the seventy-three children studied. Most of these patients were very young.

Our experience on the Pediatric Service at Bellevue Hospital is that the majority of chest x-rays show a picture commonly seen in viral pneumonia. There are increased bronchovascular markings radiating out from the hilar areas, especially into the lower lobes, and enlargement of the bronchopulmonary nodes in the hilar areas. These radiographic findings may persist several weeks after recovery from measles. Rarely, pronounced enlargement

in the superior mediastinum is seen, similar to that in childhood tuberculosis.

When bronchopneumonia becomes established, the areas of increased density may coalesce. Patchy areas of atelectasis may appear and disappear; emphysematous blebs may also be a complication. These findings are not specific for measles and are found in common with other viral bronchopneumonias. Occasionally segmental collapse occurs, but usually clears as the infection subsides.

The radiologic lung changes of 897 cases from Manchester, England, seen from January 1948 to June 1955 were categorized by Fawcitt and Parry. They described atelectasis, consolidation, hilar glandular enlargement, bronchopneumonia, and an infiltration such as is commonly seen in viral interstitial pneumonia, consisting of a "loss of translucency of the lung fields . . . not amounting to bronchopneumonia, or lobar consolidation." The authors did not distinguish between pneumonia of viral origin alone and that associated with bacterial infection; however, it is noteworthy that hilar glandular enlargement was present in 63 per cent and lung infiltrations in 21.3 per cent, both observations being the anticipated findings for viral measles pulmonary infection.

At present, with antibiotics readily available, the majority of pulmonary lesions are due to measles virus alone. X-ray evidence of superimposed bacterial pulmonary infection will vary, depending on the type of invading organism.

A word of caution needs to be given with reference to a persisting pulmonary shadow and a clinical picture of possible bacterial pneumonia in the face of negative bacterial cultures. Tuberculosis cannot be ruled out because the tuberculin skin reaction obtained around the time of the measles infection is usually negative. We recommend repeated tests for a period of four to six weeks after the onset of measles for accurate diagnosis. (See ensuing section on tuberculin testing in measles.)

DIAGNOSIS OF MEASLES PNEUMONIA

WITHOUT RASH. The verification of such an entity was made by Enders and his co-workers when they cultured measles virus from three children dying of "giant cell" pneumonia. All of them were ill with other serious conditions, mucoviscidosis, leukemia and Letterer-Siwe disease. A 1959 report in a twelve-month-old infant added another instance of pulmonary disease without rash, diagnosed as measles at autopsy. This baby had been exposed to measles shortly before the fatal illness. Immunologic studies and nasal secretion smears for giant epithelial cells described above may be of diagnostic value in such instances.

The question of the relation of measles to distemper virus infections and especially to giant cell pneumonia (Hecht's disease) is provocative. The histopathologic similarity described by Pinkerton and others initiated many subsequent articles and studies, and Janigan concluded that the measles virus is a specific etiologic agent in giant cell pneumonia. A full discussion of giant cell pneumonia is given in Chapter 23 (p. 301).

Complications

Obstructive lesions in the diseased lower respiratory tract may lead to *mediastinal emphysema,* although this is not a common complication. There were three in the 897 patients studied by Fawcitt and Parry, and occasional other references are found in the literature.

The mechanism for the development of mediastinal emphysema has been described by Macklin and Macklin. Rupture of diseased alveoli with blebs and the coalescence of adjacent blebs into large bullae form the framework for pulmonary interstitial emphysema. The trapped air follows the path of least resistance and proceeds along the sheaths of blood vessels and adjacent bronchi either toward the mediastinum and along the structures upward to the mediastinum and around the heart, the usual route, or peripherally to the pleura, producing a pneumothorax.

Atelectasis in single or multiple lobes of the lungs occurs in patients of all ages with measles, although less frequently than in patients with pertussis. Fawcitt and Parry obtained x-ray evidence of atelectasis in 28.4 per cent of the patients in their series, practically all of whom were over one year of age. If atelectasis persists for a time and secondary bacterial infection occurs, bronchiectasis may be the ultimate outcome (see Chap. 28, p. 315). A patient with long-standing atelectasis should be considered a potential candidate for bronchiectasis. If clinical signs and impairment of health corroborate the suspicion of lung damage, bronchograms should be obtained.

With the possible exception of staphylococcal infections, *empyema* is a rare complication today when broad-spectrum antibiotic therapy is available. Certainly this is our experience on the Children's Service, Bellevue Hospital, in recent years. In contrast, in the 1937 pathologic study by Degen of 100 total cases of measles, empyema was described in 13 per cent and pleurisy in 27 per cent. In this same study, four patients were described with exudative pericarditis.

The deleterious effect of measles on tuberculosis has been common knowledge, especially to those responsible for children with tuberculosis. There have been many instances on our Children's Tuberculosis Ward at Bellevue Hospital of tuberculous meningitis, bronchogenic spread of tuberculosis, and miliary tuberculosis following measles. Recognizing the possible flare-up of tuberculosis precipitated by measles, we have stressed the importance of isoniazid therapy "to cover" this period of greater susceptibility. We have arbitrarily suggested a three-week period of therapy for children known to be positive tuberculin reactors who are not receiving therapy. (For further details see page 674.)

A most instructive documentation of the effect of measles on tuberculosis was made during the Greenland epidemic in 1951 by Bech. Of 352 patients x-rayed one month prior to the epidemic and found negative, nineteen showed pulmonary infiltration on re-examination three

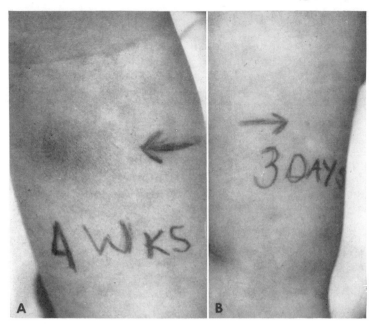

FIGURE 57–8. Tuberculin test on a patient with tuberculosis admitted to the hospital for measles. *A*, The pigmented areas resulting from an intermediate PPD given 4 weeks before onset of measles. *B*, Negative result to similar tuberculin test 3 days after onset of measles. The positive tuberculin reaction returned 17 days after the measles rash.

months later. Acid-fast bacilli were found in the sputum of thirteen of these.

A second effect of measles on tuberculosis is the suppression of tuberculin sensitivity as measured by the tuberculin reaction. Clinically, we are quite familiar with this phenomenon. Helms and Helms in the well documented Greenland epidemic demonstrated a suppression of tuberculin reaction to 5 tuberculin units given on the first or second day of the rash, with sensitivity returning gradually and irregularly, from one week to one month afterwards. A carefully designed study on the effects of measles and measles vaccine on the tuberculin test was made by Starr and Berkovich. A negative reaction to the tuberculin test was almost uniform in patients with regular and gamma-globulin-modified measles during the first four days of the rash. Considerable variation in time occurs in the return of tuberculin sensitivity, ranging from ten days to five weeks, with an average of eighteen days after the onset of the rash.

Treatment

Symptomatic care of patients with measles should be carefully supervised; whenever complications arise, close observation and appropriate specific therapy must be provided. Bendz and Engstrom, for example, reported the risk of asphyxiation in measles encephalitis. Cough may require medication, but we are cautious in the use of codeine mixtures for infants under one year. Humidified atmosphere is helpful for tracheitis. Patients with signs of obstructive laryngotracheitis should be observed closely, preferably in a hospital, where tracheostomy may be done if the symptoms of increased respiratory distress and restlessness suggest impending serious obstruction.

There is no specific treatment for measles interstitial pneumonia. Humidity and oxygen therapy are used as indicated for anoxia. Antibiotic therapy as a preventive measure was studied by Karelitz and his co-workers, and by Weinstein without demonstrating success; in fact, Weinstein suggested there was possible harm by promoting superimposed infection. Nevertheless our experience at Bellevue Hospital leads us to suggest that though antibiotics should not be given routinely to prevent complications, they should be given to high-risk patients, such as very young patients with severe measles. For such special cases Krugman and Ward have recommended penicillin, tetracycline or one of the sulfones. Karelitz has also advised prophylactic chemotherapy for patients under three years of age and for debilitated patients. Bacterial cultures in the severely ill patient should be taken early in the course of disease as a guide to therapy in the event of complications.

The treatment of bacterial pneumonia is described in Chapter 21 (p. 283). Careful and repeated cultures of the nasopharynx and blood help to determine the choice of therapeutic agents.

Prevention

Nonimmune persons known to have been exposed within a period of four days should be protected with gamma globulin.

The steady progression toward the perfection of a vaccine for the prevention of measles suggests the possibility that in the United States measles pneumonia may soon be of historic interest only.

REFERENCES

Adams, J. M., and Imagawa, D. T.: The Relationship of Canine Distemper to Human Respiratory Disease. *Pediat. Clin. N. Amer.*, 4:193, 1957.

Idem: Immunological Relationship Between Measles and Distemper Viruses. *Proc. Soc. Exper. Biol. & Med.*, 96:240, 1957.

Anderson, J. F., and Goldberger, J.: The Period of Infectivity of the Blood in Measles. *J.A.M.A.*, 57:113, 1911.

Babbott, F. L., Jr., and Gordon, J. E.: Modern Measles. *Am. J. Med. Sc.*, 228:331, 1954.

Bech, V.: Studies on the Development of Complement Fixing Antibodies in Measles Patients. *J. Immunology*, 83:267, 1959.

Idem: Measles Epidemics in Greenland. *Amer. J. Dis. Child.*, 103:252, 1962.

Bendz, P., and Engström, C. G.: Risk of Death from Asphyxiation in Measles Encephalitis. *Am. J. Dis. Child.*, 86:772, 1953.

Blake, F. G., and Trask, J. D., Jr.: Studies on Measles. II. Symptomatology and Pathology in Monkeys Experimentally Infected. *J. Exp. Med.*, 33:413, 1921.

Carlstrom, G.: Neutralization of Canine Distemper Virus by Serum of Patients Convalescent from Measles. *Lancet*, 273:344, 1957.

Idem: Relation of Measles to Other Viruses. *Am. J. Dis. Child.*, 103:287, 1962.

Cheatham, W. J.: A Comparison of *in Vitro* and *in Vivo* Characteristics as Related to the Pathogenesis of Measles, Varicella, and Herpes Zoster. *Ann. New York Acad. Sc.*, 81:6, 1959.

Christensen, P. E., and others: An Epidemic of Measles in Southern Greenland, 1951. *Acta Med. Scand.*, 144:430, 1952-53.

Cohen, S. M., Gordon, I., Rapp, F., Macaulay, J. C., and Buckley, S. M.: Fluorescent Antibody and Complement Fixation Tests of Agents Isolated in Tissue Culture from Measles Patients. *Proc. Soc. Exper. Biol. & Med.*, 90:118, 1955.

Cooch, J. W.: Measles in U. S. Army Recruits. *Am. J. Dis. Child.*, 103:264, 1962.

Corkett, E. U.: The Visceral Lesions in Measles. *Am. J. Path.*, 21:905, 1945.

De Carlo, J., Jr., and Startzman, H. H., Jr.: The Roentgen Study of the Chest in Measles. *Radiol.*, 63:849, 1954.

Degen, J. A.: Visceral Pathology in Measles; A Clinicopathologic Study of 100 Fatal Cases. *Am. J. M. Sc.*, 194:104, 1937.

Denton, J.: The Pathology of Fatal Measles. *Am. J. M. Sc.*, 169:531, 1925.

Enders, J. F.: Development of Attenuated Measles-Virus Vaccines. *Am. J. Dis. Child.*, 103:335, 1962.

Enders, J. F., and Peebles, T. C.: Propagation in Tissue Cultures of Cytopathogenic Agents from Patients with Measles. *Proc. Soc. Exper. Biol. & Med.*, 86:277, 1954.

Enders, J. F., Katz, S. L., and Medearis, D. N.: Recent Advances in Knowledge of the Measles Virus; in *Perspective in Virology*. New York, John Wiley & Sons, Inc., 1959, Vol. I, pp. 103-20.

Enders, J. F., McCarthy, K., Mitus, A., and Cheatham, W. J.: Isolation of Measles Virus at Autopsy in Cases of Giant-Cell Pneumonia Without Rash. *New England J. Med.*, 261:-875, 1959.

Enders, J. F., and others: Measles Virus: A Summary of Experiments Concerned with Isolation, Properties, and Behavior. *Am. J. Pub. Health*, 47:275, 1957.

Fawcitt, J., and Parry, H. E.: Lung Changes in Pertussis and Measles in Childhood. A Review of 1894 Cases with a Follow-up Study of the Pulmonary Complications. *Brit. J. Radiol.*, 30:76, 1957.

Feyrter, F.: Ueber die Histopathologie der Masern des Menschen. *Wien. Zschr. f. inn. Med. u. ihre grenzgebiete*, 28:Suppl. 1-39, 1947.

Finkeldey, W.: Ueber Riesenzellbefunde in den Gaumenmandeln, zugleich ein Beitrag zur Histopathologie der Mandelveranderungen im Maserninkubationsstadium. *Virchows Arch. f. path. Anat.*, 281:323, 1931.

Grist, N. R.: The Pathogenesis of Measles: Review of the Literature and Discussion of the Problem. *Glasgow Med. J.*, 31:431, 1950.

Helms, S., and Helms, P.: Tuberculin Sensitivity During Measles. *Acta Tuber. Scand.*, 35:166, 1958.

Hers, J. F.: Fluorescent Antibody Techniques in Respiratory Viral Diseases. *Amer. Rev. Resp. Dis.*, 88:316, 1963.

Hilleman, M. R., and others: Enders' Live Measles-Virus Vaccine with Human Immune Globulin. II. Evaluation of Efficacy. *Am. J. Dis. Child.*, 103:372, 1962.

International Conference on Measles Immunization. Session I-VI. *Am. J. Dis. Child.*, 103:- 219, 1962.

Janigan, D. T.: Giant Cell Pneumonia and Measles: An Analytical Review. *Canad. M.A.J.*, 85:741, 1961.

Jones, O. R.: Measles: A Case of Emphysema Correspondence. *Am. Rev. Resp. Dis.*, 87:597, 1963.

Karelitz, S.: in L. E. Holt, Jr., R. McIntosh, and H. L. Barnett: *Pediatrics*. 13th ed. New York, Appleton-Century-Crofts, Inc., 1964.

Karelitz, S., King, H., Curtis, B., and Wechsel, M.: Use of Aureomycin and Penicillin in the Treatment of Rubeola in the Pre-Eruptive and Early Eruptive Phase. *Pediatrics*, 7:193, 1951.

Karelitz, S., and others: Inactivated Measles Virus Vaccine. Subsequent Challenge with Attenuated Live Virus Vaccine. *J.A.M.A.*, 184:673, 1963.

Koffler, D.: Giant Cell Pneumonia. *Arch. Path.*, 78:267, 1964.

Kohn, J. L., and Koiransky, H.: Roentgenographic Reexamination of the Chests of Children from Six to Ten Months After Measles. *Am. J. Dis. Child.*, 41:500, 1931.

Idem: Relation of Measles and Tuberculosis in Young Children. A Clinical and Roentgenographic Study. *Am. J. Dis. Child.*, 44:1187, 1932.

Idem: Further Roentgenographic Studies of the Chests of Children During Measles. *Am. J. Dis. Child.*, 46:40, 1933.

Krugman, S., and Ward, R.: *Infectious Diseases of Children*. 3rd ed. St. Louis, C. V. Mosby Company, 1964.

Krugman, S., Giles, J. P., Friedman, H., and

Stone, S.: Studies on Immunity to Measles. *J. Pediat.*, 66:471, 1965.

Krugman, S., Giles, J. P., Jacobs, A. M., and Friedman, H.: Studies with Live Attenuated Measles-Virus Vaccine. *Am. J. Dis. Child.*, 103:353, 1962.

McCarthy, K.: Measles. *Brit. Med. Bull.*, 15:201, 1959.

McConnell, E. M.: Giant Cell Pneumonia in an Adult. *Brit. Med. J.*, 2:288, 1961.

McCrumb, F. R., Jr., and others: Studies with Live Attenuated Measles-Virus Vaccine. *Am. J. Dis. Child.*, 101:689, 1961.

Macklin, M. T., and Macklin, C. C.: Malignant Interstitial Emphysema of the Lungs and Mediastinum as an Important Occult Complication in Many Respiratory Diseases and Other Conditions: An Interpretation of the Clinical Literature in the Light of Laboratory Experience. *Med.*, 23:281, 1944.

Massey, A., and Oldershaw, W. L.: Surgical Emphysema as a Complication of Measles. *Brit. Med. J.*, 1:61, 1933.

Miller, D. L.: Frequency of Complications of Measles, 1963. *Brit. Med. J.*, 2:75, 1964.

Mitus, A., Enders., J. F., Craig, J. M., and Holloway, A.: Persistence of Measles Virus and Depression of Antibody Formation in Patients with Giant-Cell Pneumonia After Measles. *New England J. Med.*, 261:882, 1959.

Morley, D. C.: Measles in Nigeria. *Am. J. Dis. Child.*, 103:230, 1962.

Namiki, H.: Giant Cell Pneumonia. *J. Okla. M. A.*, 52:311, 1959.

Panum, P. L.: Observations During the Epidemic of Measles on the Faroe Islands in the Year 1846. Translated by Mrs. A. S. Hatcher, United States Public Health Service. *Medical Classics*, 3:829, 1939.

Papp, K.: Experiences prouvant que la voie d'infection de la rougeole est la contamination de la muqueuse conjonctivale. *Revue Immunol.*, 20:27, 1956.

Pinkerton, H., Smiley, W. L., and Anderson, W. A. D.: Giant Cell Pneumonia with Inclusion; A Lesion Common to Hecht's Disease, Distemper and Measles. *Am. J. Path.*, 21:1, 1945.

Rauh, L. W., and Schmidt, R.: Measles Immunization with Killed Virus Vaccine. *Am. J. Dis. Child.*, 109:232, 1965.

Ristori, C., Boccardo, H., Borgono, J. M., and Armijo, R.: Medical Importance of Measles in Chile. *Am. J. Dis. Child.*, 103:236, 1962.

Robbins, F. C.: Measles: Clinical Features. *Am. J. Dis. Child.*, 103:266, 1962.

Ruckle, G., and Rogers, K. D.: Studies with Measles Virus. II. Isolation of Virus and Immunologic Studies in Persons Who Have Had the Natural Disease. *J. Immun.*, 78:341, 1957.

Semsbroth, K. H.: Multinucleate Epithelial Giant Cells with Inclusion Bodies with Prodromal

Measles: Report of an Autopsy. *Arch. Path.*, 28:386, 1939.

Sergiev, P. G., Ryazantseva, N. E., and Shroit, I. G.: The Dynamics of Pathological Processes in Experimental Measles in Monkeys. *Acta Virol.*, 4:265, 1960.

Sherman, F. E., and Ruckle, G.: In Vivo and in Vitro Cellular Changes Specific for Measles. *Arch. Path.*, 65:587, 1959.

Soto, P. J., and Deauville, G. A.: Spontaneous Simian Giant-Cell Pneumonia with Coexistent B Virus Infection. *Am. J. Vet. Research*, 25:793, 1964.

Starr, S., and Berkovich, S.: Effects of Measles, Gamma-Globulin-Modified Measles, and Vaccine Measles on Tuberculin Test. *New England J. Med.*, 270:386, 1964.

Stokes, J., Jr., Maris, E. P., and Gellis, S. S.: Chemical, Clinical, and Immunological Studies in the Products of Human Plasma Fractionation. XI. The Use of Concentrated Normal Human Serum Gamma Globulin (Human Immune Serum Globulin) in the Prophylaxis and Treatment of Measles. *J. Clin. Invest.*, 23:531, 1944.

Tompkins, V., and Macaulay, J. C.: A Characteristic Cell in Nasal Secretions During Prodromal Measles. *J.A.M.A.*, 157:711, 1955.

Top, F. H.: *Communicable and Infectious Diseases.* 5th ed. St. Louis, C. V. Mosby Company, 1964, pp. 431-42.

Warthin, A. S.: Occurrence of Numerous Large Giant Cells in the Tonsils and Pharyngeal Mucosa in the Prodromal Stage of Measles. Report of Four Cases. *Arch. Path.*, 11:864, 1931.

Weinstein, L.: Failure of Chemotherapy to Prevent the Bacterial Complications of Measles. *New England J. Med.*, 253:679, 1955.

Weinstein, L., and Franklin, W.: The Pneumonia of Measles. *Am. J. M. Sc.*, 217:314, 1949.

CHAPTER FIFTY-EIGHT

Pertussis Pneumonia

ROSA LEE NEMIR, M.D.

Pneumonia due to *Bordetella pertussis*, formerly called *Haemophilus pertussis*, usually occurs during the paroxysmal stage of the disease. Pertussis may cause interstitial pneumonia, or in association with secondary bacterial invaders may produce bronchopneumonia.

Incidence

The frequency and severity of pertussis have diminished greatly in recent years. The mortality rate in the United States declined from two per 100,000 population in 1945 to 0.5 in 1960, and the morbidity from 849,140 in 1945 to one sixth this figure (146,989) in 1960. Unfortunately, 10 per cent of these infections occur during the first year of life, a time when the mortality rate is highest and pneumonia is most likely to develop.

Most of the studies on this disease were made at a time when pertussis was more prevalent and more severe. Indeed, the National Health Survey in 1963-64 no longer lists pertussis separately, but includes it in the category of "common childhood disease." This decline in prevalence and severity began before 1940, when pertussis vaccine immunization was introduced, but accelerated rapidly in the years that followed.

The incidence of pneumonia as a complication of pertussis is not usually indicated in large statistical or official records. In addition, there is a paucity of literature in recent years on pulmonary complications of pertussis even though pneumonia is the most frequent complication, excluding otitis media, and the most common cause of death.

In 1964 Jernelius reported fifty-eight cases of bronchopneumonia or atelectasis among 602 pertussis patients observed between the years 1951 and 1953 in the Stockholm Hospital for Infectious Diseases. This 10 per cent incidence corresponds to the rate reported from England in 1947 by Oswald. In Glasgow, in 1946-47, Lees reported a 20 per cent incidence of bronchopneumonia in 150 patients. Before the advent of antibiotics, pneumonia produced by secondary bacterial invaders was probably more frequent.

Pathology

In pertussis the entire mucosal lining of the respiratory tract is congested, edematous, and infiltrated with cells. Characteristic lesions consist of necrosis of basilar midzonal portions of bronchial epithelium with clumps of organisms in the cilia of the bronchial and tracheal epithelium (Mallory and Horner). The presence of pneumonia is indicated both by polymorphonuclear leukocytic infiltration of the bronchial walls and by the peribronchial collar of mononuclear cells. The alveolar walls are thickened and are also infiltrated by mononuclear cells. Viscous mucus, so characteristic of pertussis, may fill the bronchi or bronchioles. Atelectasis is common, and emphysema occurs often. Early in the disease edema and hemorrhage may be found in the parenchyma. Terminal pneumonia may be produced by *Bord. pertussis* alone or in combination with secondary bacterial invaders, the latter accounting for pus, cellular debris and mucus within the alveolus. Rich, in his discussion of the pathology, described the interstitial pneumonia in pertussis as similar to that of influenza and other viral infections.

There has been considerable difference of opinion as to the presence of enlarged tracheal and bronchial lymph nodes. Certainly such enlargement, if present, is not impressive clinically or in the roentgeno-

grams and does not approach that seen in primary tuberculosis. In a roentgenographic study using lateral and posteroanterior views, Kohn and others noted enlarged glands in only five of 154 cases, thus confirming their postmortem findings.

Pathogenesis

Inflammation of the mucosal lining of the trachea and bronchi is an essential part of the disease. The thick, tenacious mucus is not easily expelled, and its stagnation or presence in the bronchi produces obstruction resulting in atelectasis or emphysema. The paroxysmal cough is associated with peribronchial mononuclear infiltration. Cyanosis often occurs after a long bout of coughing and is associated with obstruction to the airways by mucus, spasm and congestion. Any secondary bacterial or viral invaders will alter the clinical picture.

Clinical Features

Pneumonia develops during the paroxysmal stage. When there is a sudden reappearance of fever in pertussis, pulmonary complication must always be considered. Rales are found early, followed by dullness and bronchial breathing. The cough often becomes less paroxysmal, the respiratory rate increases out of proportion to the temperature elevation, and dyspnea becomes apparent. If sufficient pulmonary tissue is involved, cyanosis alternating with pallor may be observed, and occasionally apnea is noted, especially post-tussic. The disease is more severe and the mortality rate is higher in young infants under one year of age. Fawcett and Parry reviewed 1163 children under fifteen years of age showing pulmonary complications of pertussis between the years 1948 and 1955. Thirty per cent of these were under one year of age.

Scattered areas of emphysema are regularly a part of the pathology of pertussis and may alter the physical findings associated with areas of collapse or consolidation. Emphysematous blebs may coalesce and rupture, peripherally to produce pneumothorax or centrally to cause mediastinal emphysema. The latter may be discovered by crepitus in the tissues of the neck and chest if the air escapes from the mediastinum along the great vessels. The physical findings of hyperresonance, the possible shift of mediastinal structures, the increased respiratory distress and finally the chest x-ray confirm the diagnosis.

Restlessness and irritability are associated with anoxia. Fatigue from bouts of coughing and loss of weight associated with vomiting are also observed.

Diagnosis

Aids to diagnosis consist of blood cell counts, immunologic tests, and roentgen examination of the lungs. A clinical history of exposure to pertussis, of infection in a sibling, and the lack of pertussis immunization all lend support to the diagnosis of pertussis as a cause of the presenting pulmonary disease. The white blood cell count is particularly high (as much as 100,000 per cubic millimeter) with a decided lymphocytosis (all normal cells). Immunization does not always prevent pertussis, but it does prevent a severe infection, and pneumonia is less likely to develop.

Antibodies produced by *Bord. pertussis* infection include humoral antibodies, agglutinins and antihemagglutinins, complement-fixing and mouse protection antibodies, and opsonocytophagic antibodies; the last appear in the third week of disease. A positive intradermal reaction to the injection of agglutinogen in the convalescent stage of pertussis may be valuable in detecting sensitivity to the disease, thereby casting doubt on the diagnosis.

Accurate diagnosis can best be made by bacterial cultures on appropriate Bordet-Gengou media, using the customary cough plate. *Bordetella pertussis* is easily cultured from the nasopharynx in the early stage of the disease, and it is possible to culture the organisms in untreated cases as late as the sixth week of disease. Felton obtained 74.4 per cent positive cultures from 239 children.

Roentgen Diagnosis

The majority of patients show some changes in the chest roentgenogram during pertussis infection. The extent of pulmonary lesions seen on chest x-ray is directly related to the severity of the disease.

Patients with mild illness may show only some decrease in radiotranslucency of the lung fields and increased bronchopulmonary markings. As pneumonia becomes clinically apparent, these infiltrations along the larger bronchi increase and produce a picture of interstitial pneumonia. Occasional emphysematous areas and small scattered areas of increased density may be found in the lung parenchyma. Some of these clear quickly and may represent patchy areas of alveolar collapse; others may represent alveolar infiltration due to *Bord. pertussis* or intercurrent bacterial infection. An associated

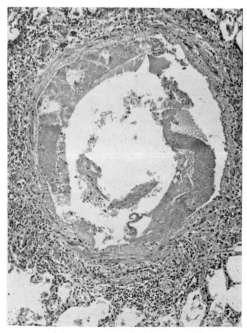

FIGURE 58–1. Necrotizing bronchitis. × 100.

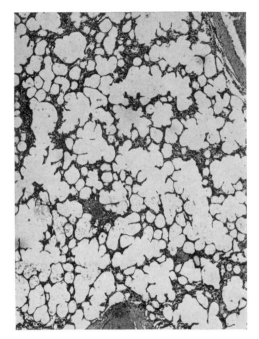

FIGURE 58–2. Emphysema. $\times$ 30.

febrile illness is usually present in the latter instance. Lobar consolidation is rarely seen and is most often a combination of pertussis and other bacterial infection. Rarely mediastinal emphysema with infiltration of air pockets into the subcutaneous tissue of the neck and chest as well as the mediastinum may be present. Pneumothorax is also rare.

Segmental collapse is more frequent in the older child than in the infant; it also occurs more often in severe cases. The segments affected are usually the lower lobes, frequently the right middle, and rarely the upper lobes. Occasionally, bilateral segmental collapse is encountered. The left lower lobe is affected somewhat more frequently than the right, apparently because of the sharper angulation of the left main bronchus and its proximity to the arch of the aorta and the pulmonary artery. James and others found collapse of the right middle lobe most common, and Kohn and co-workers reported similar findings.

In general, the segment or segments re-expand as the patient improves, usually within a few weeks. The age of the pa-tient is also a factor in the speed of expansion; infants reaerate rather quickly. Persistent collapse is uncommon in infants and in young children below the age of five years. Today, long-standing collapsed segments are much less frequent, but it is important to recognize such complications when they occur. Prolonged periods of collapse may be associated with the development of bronchiectasis.

In establishing the diagnosis of collapse by roentgenography both posteroanterior and lateral films are needed. The collapsed segment or lobe is visualized as a dense shadow, frequently smaller than the normal lobe; however, very early, after obstruction, the lobe may be swollen and larger than normal with distorted convex fissure lines.

Differential Diagnosis

Pertussis in its typical form is easily identified. Difficulty may arise when the disease is modified by the partial protection of an old immunization. In the very young infant a whoop usually is not present in pertussis; a paroxysmal cough in such a patient should arouse suspicion. Pertussis is simulated almost exactly, but to a milder degree, by *Bord. parapertussis*. Although it is customary to think of parapertussis as a mild disease, fatal pneumonia due to *Bord. parapertussis* was described in two children by Zuelzer and Wheeler.

The cough attributed to pertussis may be observed in patients infected with another member of the Bordetella group, *Bord. bronchiseptica*, and occasionally in cases of *Haemophilus influenzae*. Hoarseness is characteristic of *H. influenzae* infections, not of pertussis. Di Sant'Agnese calls attention to the similarity of the pertussis cough to the paroxysms of patients with cystic fibrosis of the pancreas, a disease with frequent protean pulmonary complications.

Some patients with extensive bronchopneumonia and interstitial pneumonia unassociated with *Bord. pertussis* may also have paroxysmal, spasmodic cough without whoop or vomiting. These patients usually have extensive physical findings in the lungs consisting of many scattered rales and suffer from much respiratory difficulty. These patients continue to be quite ill between the bouts of coughing, with rapid and often shallow respirations. A pertussoid eosinophilic pneumonia with a pertussis-like cough (see p. 737) has been described in very young infants. A similar syndrome associated with adenovirus type 12 was reported in 1964 by Olson and co-workers. Laboratory studies and a careful history of onset and progression of signs and symptoms should clarify the diagnosis.

Occasionally patients with enlarged tuberculous bronchopulmonary glands have a paroxysmal spasmodic cough similar to that noted in pertussis; there may also be an associated collapse of a segment of the lung. In this instance pressure by enlarged lymph nodes causes the obstruction; in pertussis, obstruction results from the thick mucus within the bronchus. The presence of a whoop in pertussis and a barking metallic cough in tuberculosis

may aid in diagnosis. Cyanosis, rather than suffusion of the face, is more commonly associated with the paroxysmal coughing of the tuberculous child, and vomiting is rare. Cough plates, the white blood cell count and lymphocytosis, tuberculin tests, pertussis antibody studies and the chest roentgenogram are helpful aids. Enlarged mediastinal nodes are rare in pertussis. Physical findings in the chest of a child with tuberculosis are often negative except for a localized wheeze at the site of obstruction.

Complications

Collapse occurs so frequently in pertussis, with or without pneumonia, that it is perhaps improper to consider it under the category of complication. Indeed, pertussis, until the past decade, was the most frequent cause of pulmonary collapse in children. This was statistically demonstrated by James and others who found collapse caused by pertussis in 18.9 per cent of 854 consecutive cases seen from 1945 to 1952. In a few of these children

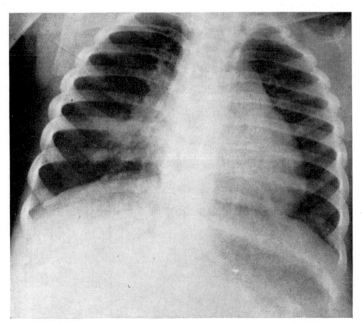

FIGURE 58–3. Roentgenogram of chest showing increased bronchovascular markings and pulmonary density obscuring the right heart border.

the collapse persisted several months despite bronchoscopy. In an analysis of 150 consecutive cases of pertussis (1946-47) 43 per cent were found to have collapse, although the atelectatic areas were small and of short duration. In our own experience on the Infectious Disease Ward, Bellevue Hospital, collapse is common when pertussis is severe; however, it is short-lived.

Bronchiectasis is a late complication of pertussis pneumonia, and is apt to follow atelectasis. Nicholson states that failure to re-expand after nine months produces irreversible damage to the bronchi. Although all observers agree that long-standing collapse leads to bronchiectasis, they differ as to the exact length of time required.

Biering made follow-up observations on sixty-two children seen in the Blegdam Hospital nine years previously and found only one with bronchiectasis. The rarity of this complication is certainly in line with our experience in recent years. We have not observed symptoms suggesting bronchiectasis, but a long-term follow-up study has not been made.

Pulmonary function studies of forty-nine children with pertussis complicated by bronchopneumonia or atelectasis were made by Jernelius seven to ten years later. Significantly lower static lung volumes than the predicted normal values were found. The maximum breathing capacity and the intrapulmonary gas mixing showed normal values.

Because of the constant coughing with increased intrapulmonary pressure and the intense venous congestion with each paroxysm, pertussis may conceivably reactivate or spread pulmonary tuberculous foci. In our experience this is rare today.

Treatment

Tetracycline and chloramphenicol are almost equally effective, but because of the possible toxicity of the latter, tetracycline is preferred. The usual dosage is 10 mg. per pound of body weight per twenty-four hours. For the very young infant, and the seriously ill patient, hyperimmune pertussis gamma globulin intramuscularly in dosage of 1.25 to 2.5 ml. per pound of body weight per twenty-four hours is recommended; this is repeated every other day for a total of three injections. Oxygen (40 per cent) with increased humidity (40 to 50 per cent) is indicated; this adds to the patient's comfort and decreases symptoms. Care must be used in the selection of medication for cough. Sedatives depressing the respiratory center are to be avoided.

When intercurrent bacterial infections are suspected, an antibiotic selected by the clinician in accordance with his best judgment may be used until bacterial cultures and other aids to diagnosis clarify the etiologic pathogen.

Good nursing care is of paramount importance because of the danger of asphyxia during bouts of coughing, when the bronchi are filled with tenacious mucus, and because of the possibility of aspiration following vomiting. Gentle suction, performed promptly, relieves the airways. Infants, especially, require the most careful watching because of vomiting in the prone position, with its danger of aspiration of vomitus, and because of discomfort, cyanosis from coughing, and emotional fatigue and distress. Refeeding after vomiting may be effective in maintaining nutrition, and attention must be given to providing adequate fluid intake.

Prognosis

Pneumonia is the common cause of death from pertussis and is an especially serious complication during infancy. The present low incidence of severe pertussis, with great decline in fatality and, therefore, in pneumonia associated with pertussis, can be attributed, in large measure, to the widespread use of prophylactic vaccine and to improved methods of treatment. Krugman and Ward have listed other factors, including greater host resistance, possible decreased virulence of the infecting agent, and environmental factors that affect either host resistance or activity of the infecting agent. With continuing vigilance in the preventive immunization program and with continuing research in the field of vaccine production and related problem areas, pertussis and the pneumonia it causes should rapidly disappear.

REFERENCES

Biering, A.: Childhood Pneumonia, Including Pertussis Pneumonia and Bronchiectasis. A Follow-up Study of 151 Patients. *Acta Pediat.*, 45:348, 1956.

Botsztejn, A. von: Die pertussoïde, eosinophile Pneumonie des Säuglings. *Ann. Paed.* (Basel), 157:28, 1941.

Fawcitt, J., and Parry, H. E.: Lung Changes in Pertussis and Measles in Childhood. A Review of 1894 Cases with a Follow-up Study of the Pulmonary Complications. *Brit. J. Radiol.*, 39:76, 1957.

Felton, H. M.: Pertussis: Current Status of Prevention and Treatment. *Pediat. Clin. N. Amer.*, 5:271, 1957.

Felton, H. M., and Flosdorf, E. W.: The Detection of Susceptibility to Whooping Cough. I. Institutional Experience with the Pertussis Agglutinogen as Skin Test Reagent. *J. Pediat.*, 29:677, 1946.

Gallavan, M., and Goodpasture, E. W.: Infection of Chick Embryos with H. Pertussis Reproducing Pulmonary Lesions of Whooping Cough. *Am. J. Path.* 13:927, 1937.

James, U., Brimblecombe, F. S. W., and Wells, J. W. The Natural History of Pulmonary Collapse in Childhood. *Quart. J. Med.*, No. 97, p. 121, 1956.

Jernelius, H.: Pertussis with Pulmonary Complications—A Follow-up Study. *Acta Paediat.*, 53:247, 1965.

Kohn, J. L., Schwartz, I., Greenbaum, J., and Daly, M. M. I.: Roentgenograms of the Chest Taken During Pertussis. *Am. J. Dis. Child.*, 67:463, 1944.

Krugman, S., and Ward, R.: *Infectious Diseases of Children.* 3rd ed. St. Louis, C. V. Mosby Company, 1964, pp. 371-73.

Lees, A. W.: Atelectasis and Bronchiectasis in Pertussis. *Brit. M.J.*, 2:1138, 1950.

Mallory, F. B., and Horner, A. A.: The Histological Lesion in the Respiratory Tract. *J. Mod. Research*, 27:115, 1912-1913.

Nicholson, D. P.: Pulmonary Collapse in Pertussis. *Arch. Dis. Childhood*, 24:29, 1949.

Olson, L. C., Miller, G., and Hanshaw, J. B.: Acute Infectious Lymphocytosis Presenting as a Pertussis-like Illness: Its Association with Adenovirus Type 12. *Lancet*, 1:200, 1964.

Oswald, N. C.: Collapse of the Lower Lobes of the Lungs in Children. *Proc. Roy. Soc. Med.*, 40:736, 1949.

Rich, A. R.: The Etiology and Pathogenesis of Whooping Cough. *Bull. Johns Hopkins Hosp.*, 51:346, 1932.

Sant'Agnese, P. A. di: The Pulmonary Manifestations of Fibrocystic Disease of the Pancreas. *Dis. Chest*, 27:654, 1955.

Zuelzer, W. W., and Wheeler, W. E.: Parapertussis Pneumonia. A Report of 2 Fatal Cases. *J. Pediat.*, 29:493, 1946.

CHAPTER FIFTY-NINE

Pertussoid Eosinophilic Pneumonia

ROSA LEE NEMIR, M.D.

Pertussoid eosinophilic pneumonia is a term first used by Botsztejn in 1941 to describe a subacute, benign illness characterized by a pertussis-like cough associated with lymphocytosis and eosinophilia; the syndrome occurred in very young infants. Since this first report there has been a publication by Biro from the same hospital in Zurich. The syndrome of acute lymphocytosis with eosinophilia described by Smith the same year, also a disease of unknown origin, did not include a pertussoid-like cough; in fact, there were minimal and insignificant signs of respiratory infection.

Clinical Features

The patients so far described vary in age from three weeks to four months.

Bouts of coughing spells associated with dyspnea, but usually with minimal temperature elevation, are the chief symptoms. The patients are only moderately ill, and all reported patients have recovered. The physical findings in the lungs vary from negative findings and occasional rales to signs indicating bronchopneumonia.

The distinguishing feature of the syndrome is the absolute and relative lymphocytosis and eosinophilia. These blood changes parallel the pneumonia, which subsides slowly, often persisting several weeks and varying from three to eight weeks.

The roentgenograms uniformly show increased bronchovascular markings bilaterally radiating out from the hili and filling the inner half of the lung fields and obscuring the heart borders. In the original description pleurisy was diagnosed from the visualization of the horizontal fissures in the roentgenogram of the lungs. Biro proposed a new title for this syndrome, *interstitial pertussoid eosinophilic pneumonia,* because the roentgenograms of the lungs were characteristic of an interstitial pneumonia, which is produced by many agents with or without eosinophilia.

Course

The disease runs a subacute course after the initial few days of severe dyspnea and cough. The symptoms disappear before the roentgenograms of the lungs become normal. It requires three to eight weeks before the x-ray films show final resolution of the pneumonia. The absolute eosinophilia is highest early in the disease, within the first week to ten days, and is usually normal within a month. Leukocytosis is rarely above 18,000, although an occasional count of 22,000 to 28,000 cells has been reported.

Treatment and Prognosis

All the patients so far reported have recovered despite their prematurity, small size, and the severity of the dyspnea at onset. Treatment is nonspecific, supportive and symptomatic, directed toward relief of the cough and the respiratory symptoms. Biro in 1960 varied his treatment from purely symptomatic to the use of penicillin, streptomycin, and broad-spectrum antibiotics, singly or in combination. There appeared to be no difference in the response to the various therapeutic regimens in this group of twelve patients.

Comment

The causation of the syndrome described by Botsztejn and elaborated by Biro is unknown. A subsequent report of a similar syndrome has been described and an etiologic agent discovered. In 1964 Olson and others reported a similar illness in a family of nine which they called acute lymphocytosis with eosinophilia and presenting as a pertussis-like illness. In all these patients *Bord. pertussis* could not be cultured on Bordet-Gengou media. They did isolate *adenovirus type 12* from throat swabs of these children and showed in all members of the family a marked and significant complement-fixing antibody rise persisting for months.

REFERENCES

Biro, Z.: Twelve More Cases of Interstitial Pertussoid Eosinophilic Pneumonia in Infants. *Helvet. paed. Acta,* 15:135, 1960.

Botsztejn, A. von: Die pertussoïde, eosinophile Pneumonie des Säuglings. *Ann. Paed.* (Basel), 157:28, 1941.

Olson, L. C., Miller, G., and Hanshaw, J. B.: Acute Infectious Lymphocytosis Presenting as a Pertussis-like Illness: Its Association with Adenovirus Type 12. *Lancet,* 1:200, 1964.

Smith, C. H.: Infectious Lymphocytosis. *Am. J. Dis. Child.,* 62:231, 1941.

CHAPTER SIXTY

Rheumatic Pneumonia

ROSA LEE NEMIR, M.D.

Rheumatic fever, the center of much attention and study some decades ago, has been steadily receding into the background as a frequent cause of childhood disease. The therapeutic use of the sulfones and antibiotics, particularly penicillin, against the group A streptococcus, which is generally accepted as the underlying etiologic agent in rheumatic fever, has been largely responsible for this change. Rheumatic pneumonia, the pulmonary manifestation of the infection, therefore, is also less frequently diagnosed. This does not, however, mean that either rheumatic fever or rheumatic pneumonia has been entirely conquered. Unrecognized, subacute attacks of infection still occur, and there is evidence that rheumatic pneumonitis may precede recognized rheumatic carditis or arthritis. Such pulmonary infections are most likely to receive various nonrheumatic diagnoses without challenge. This is particularly true because there is no pathognomonic sign or test for rheumatic pneumonia, and more especially because the pneumonia, like the rheumatic fever itself, follows the streptococcal infection after a short latent period.

The frequency of rheumatic pneumonia is difficult to determine; for a long time there has been much discussion as to its actual existence. Now sufficient carefully documented pathologic material has accumulated to substantiate the diagnosis of rheumatic pneumonia, thus implicating the lung as one of the organ systems affected in the total rheumatic disease pattern. In the opinion of Scott and others, the lung is commonly involved in varying degrees. Reporting an analysis of eighty-seven children (three to sixteen years of age) who died during the acute active rheumatic infection, between 1919 and 1954, these writers found fifty-four cases of rheumatic pneumonia, an over-all incidence of 62 per cent. Over a third of these (39 per cent) had only slight pulmonary involvement; half (54 per cent) showed moderate rheumatic pulmonary disease. On the other hand, Griffith and others in 1946 reported an 11.3 per cent incidence of rheumatic pneumonia based on the autopsy analysis of 119 fatal cases from the 1046 patients in the United States Naval Hospital. The experience of Neubuerger and others with postmortem material is similar; they found an incidence of 12.7 per cent among sixty-three patients, some with quiescent and others with active rheumatic disease. Brown and others accumulated from the literature references as to the frequency of pneumonia and pleurisy from 1844 to 1954.

They reported a frequency range from 27.8 per cent to less than 1 per cent. These figures are based in part on clinical impressions, and serve best to indicate the difficulty in diagnosis and the long-standing attempts to clarify the relation of the pulmonary findings to the rheumatic infection.

Pathologic Features

The first histologic description of rheumatic pneumonia was made in 1928 by Naish. In gross appearance the lung is characteristically larger than normal, with dark red areas due to hemorrhage (unilateral and bilateral) scattered in various parts of the lung, usually hilar or peripheral. The lungs are elastic and resilient on palpation with a consistency comparable to India rubber (Hadfield). Microscopically, the following features are found: alveolar hemorrhage, necrosis of alveolar walls, and arteriolitis and vasculitis with occasional thrombosis in alveolar capillaries, hyaline membrane lining of alveoli and alveolar ducts and alveolar proliferation of mononuclear fibroblast cells, sometimes called Masson bodies. The pleura may show fibrinous exudate, usually without effusion. None of these lesions is pathognomonic.

Many pathologists have contributed to the present understanding of the pulmonary findings in rheumatic pneumonitis. Scott feels that the most satisfactory criterion for diagnosis is the focal mononuclear, fibrinous intra-alveolar or intraductal exudate containing protein-rich fluid. Lustock and Kuzma have called attention to unusual bronchiolar changes in which the epithelial cells are desquamated, often stripped completely from the bronchi, and also to the presence of eosinophilic granular necrosis of the lamina. This destruction of the bronchial wall and mucosa was also described by Frazer. Von Glahn and Pappenheimer reported the presence of arteriolitis in the smaller pulmonary arterial vessels. The cellular tissue mass filling the alveoli and alveolar ducts described by Masson was

given the name "Masson bodies" by Neuburger and his associates, and though there is a difference of opinion in this regard, it is possible that "Masson bodies" are the equivalent of a modified form of Aschoff nodules.

The best explanation for the lung changes is that proposed by Rich and Gregory; these workers feel that the lung changes result from a sensitivity phenomenon secondary to arteriolar damage. They were able to reproduce in animals pathologic lesions of the heart identical with those seen in patients with rheumatic pneumonitis. Rich and Gregory also pointed out the pathologic similarity of rheumatic pneumonia to other hypersensitivity, such as that to sulfathiazole. Van Wijk, Mossberger and Jensen have all attributed the pneumonia to an allergic basis. It appears likely, then, that there is capillary endothelial injury, and the hyaline membrane, a predominant feature of rheumatic pneumonia, can best be explained on the basis of capillary injury with the seepage of fibrinogen into the alveoli, where it is converted to fibrin.

With the acceptance of Group A streptococci as the etiologic agent of rheumatic fever, the development of pneumonia as an allergic reaction to this organism seems the most attractive explanation for the pathology, especially for the alveolar exudative membrane, the reputed severity of the lung manifestations, and for the transitory, rapidly changing x-ray findings in which the pulmonary lesions appear to move from one area of the lung to another, not unlike the clinical picture of Loeffler's pneumonia. Even the transient development of pleural fluid is compatible with this theory.

Clinical Features

With the foregoing descriptions of the pulmonary pathology in mind, especially the asphyxiating hyaline membrane and the hemorrhagic alveolar exudate, the predominant symptoms of dyspnea, tachypnea, tachycardia (usually out of proportion to the general appearance of illness and to the amount of fever), persistent cough and blood-streaked sputum are readily understandable. Chest pain and restlessness are frequent, and cyanosis may develop. The presence, degree and duration of fever are variable. It is usually intermittent and irregular, ranging from 101° to 105°F., gradually tapering off to normal. The onset of pneumonia may be mild, simulating an upper respiratory tract infection, or it may appear as a sudden acute attack of dyspnea. The latter is particularly evident if there is a concurrent acute carditis. Other symptoms and signs referable to rheumatic infection elsewhere in the body may be present if carditis or arthritis is also manifest, e.g. arthralgia, swelling of joints, gallop rhythm, heart murmur, skin manifestations or, rarely, chorea.

At one time, on the Children's Rheumatic Fever Service at Bellevue Hospital, the diagnosis of rheumatic pneumonia was withheld unless there was also other evidence of active rheumatic infection, especially carditis. Today there is evidence that rheumatic pneumonia may precede other forms of rheumatic infection. This argument has been presented by Rubin and Rubin and documented by Jensen and others.

Griffith has produced evidence that rheumatic pneumonia is more apt to develop in conjunction with acute rheumatic fever, and Seldin found that pneumonia may occur at any time from four days to twelve months after the onset of rheumatic fever. On the basis of Griffith's observations, the following classification of rheumatic pneumonitis is offered: (1) primary acute pneumonitis, often the presenting manifestation of rheumatic fever; (2) secondary acute pneumonitis occurring during the course of rheumatic fever, often the polycyclic type; and (3) subclinical pneumonitis, when the pulmonary infection may be overlooked entirely. There are few symptoms or signs. The diagnosis is dependent on the study and interpretation of the pulmonary findings in the roentgenograms. Evidence of streptococcal group A infection helps to establish the diagnosis of rheumatic pneumonitis.

A summary of the dominant symptoms of rheumatic pneumonitis (dyspnea, tachypnea, cough with sputum which is occasionally blood-streaked and usually bacteria-free, and chest pain) clearly indicates the importance of a careful assembling of diagnostic data for rheumatic pneumonitis by physical examination, laboratory tests, and certainly by a study of the chest roentgenograms. Often the x-ray films, supplemented by appropriate laboratory tests or history of previous streptococcal infection, give support to the diagnosis.

Physical examination of such a patient may reveal a sick child whose pulmonary symptoms are greater than the demonstrable lung findings. There is often a paucity of the latter. Debré and others have pointed out that pulmonary lesions may exist in the absence of clinical signs. Early there may be dullness and diminished breath sounds, progressing to flatness and bronchial breathing, depending on the extent of the lung involvement and amount of pleural reaction. Occasional fine or moist rales, usually transitory, are heard, and a friction rub, pleural or pericardial, is common. Pleurisy, although short-lived and transient, is common and may or may not be associated with pleural effusion. If the effusion is present, displacement of the heart and mediastinum may or may not occur. Associated findings of active carditis such as gallop rhythm, newly developed murmurs, muffled heart sounds, and pericardial friction rub may be heard.

Laboratory Findings

The leukocyte count is high, the erythrocyte sedimentation rate is increased, and there is a moderate anemia just as in active rheumatic fever. Bacteriologic study of the blood, nose and throat usually gives negative results. Tests for the reaction to a recent streptococcal infection should always be made, especially the antistreptolysin O titer (and when possible, other tests for streptococcal antibodies such as antihyaluronidase titers); these are helpful diagnostically and also as a measure of successful response to therapy. Electrocardiographic studies made at frequent intervals are important in relating and finding evidence of an active carditis. Although pleural effusion may be suspected from the x-ray of the chest, a pleural tap may be unsuccessful. The fluid, when found, is sterile and often sanguineous.

The roentgenogram of the lung shows the rapid appearance and disappearance of hazy-edged densities in the periphery or the central portion of the lungs, usually in the left midlung and the right upper lobe, although there are often bilateral shadows. Pleurisy, when present, is commonly transitory. The x-ray shadows may vary from increased bronchovascular markings to a large homogeneous segmental density and may even include small, soft, mottled shadows resembling miliary tuberculosis. Lobar shadows are rare and are usually transitory. The apices and bases of the lungs are relatively clear. The size of the heart should be carefully observed on each roentgenogram. It frequently shows an enlarging cardiac silhouette and occasionally exhibits the presence of pericarditis.

Differential Diagnosis

Since there is no pathognomonic sign of rheumatic pneumonitis and since rheumatic fever patients with quiescent or active infection are subject to intercurrent infections, it is easy to understand why a differential diagnosis is difficult. Nevertheless antemortem diagnosis can be established if careful attention is given to the possibility. The list of disease processes simulating rheumatic pneumonitis is long; only the more important ones will be listed. Foremost among them are viral pneumonitis, congestive heart failure, bacterial pneumonia, tuberculosis, azotemic pneumonia and Loeffler's pneumonia (reacting to antigens other than to the streptococcus).

The greatest difficulty in diagnosing

rheumatic pneumonitis lies in distinguishing between viral pneumonitis on the one hand and pulmonary edema on the other, especially in patients severely ill with carditis. With improved diagnostic techniques these forms of pneumonopathy, as well as bacterial and other infections, may be more readily differentiated now than two decades ago. There are new, refined methods not only for bacteriologic cultures of group A streptococci and other organisms, available even for office practice, but also for the identification of respiratory viral infections, whether by tissue culture techniques or by immunologic methods such as complement-fixing antibody tests or viral neutralization tests.

Feinstein and Spagnuola, in their review of material from Irvington House (chiefly a convalescent home for cardiac patients and for later stages of acute illness at Irvington on the Hudson), did not see rheumatic pneumonitis. They described two types of pulmonary pathology: (1) viral pneumonitis and (2) congestive heart failure. This selected population would be more likely to have congestive heart failure and less likely to have recent or fresh rheumatic infection. Presumably almost all these patients were under continuous antistreptococcal prophylaxis therapy, and one would not expect appreciable streptococcal infection to develop. Thus rheumatic pneumonitis associated with active or recent infection most likely would not be seen in this group.

Figure 1 is an example of rheumatic pneumonitis as the presenting symptom of rheumatic involvement in a patient. For such a person, prophylactic penicillin therapy is a wise choice, since the prevention of serious rheumatic cardiac damage can thereby be prevented. The opportunity to prevent recurrent rheumatic illness should not be overlooked.

Subacute and unrecognized streptococcal infections still occur. It is in these patients that the physician must be most alert to the possibility of rheumatic infection when the proper respiratory symptoms present themselves. Rabinowitz, as early as 1926, suggested that rheumatic

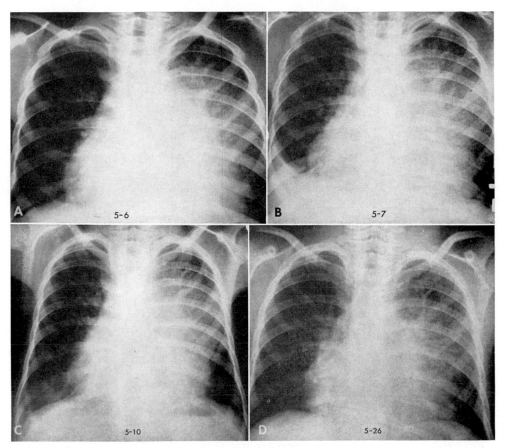

FIGURE 60–1. *A,* Roentgenogram of chest taken 24 hours after onset of symptoms shows a fuzzy-edged, homogeneous nonsegmental shadow in the middle third of the lung. The cardiac silhouette seems enlarged to right and left. Trachea is in the midline. In the original film a fine, pleural line may be seen extending bilaterally from costophrenic angle upward 2 interspaces. *B,* The left pulmonary shadow is unchanged. The right costophrenic angle is obliterated by a small triangular shadow consistent with pleural fluid. The cardiac shadow is somewhat larger bilaterally; this may be due to pericardial fluid. *C,* Almost complete clearing at the right base on the third day. No tap was done. Note obliteration of right costophrenic angle and a fine oblique fissure line above diaphragm extending to right heart border in the cardiohepatic angle. *D,* The right diaphragm and costophrenic angle are clear. The pulmonary shadow in left midlung shows some clearing at the periphery, 20 days after onset of symptoms. The cardiac silhouette seems smaller. The left border especially is obscured by fuzzy, mottled pulmonary infiltrate and increased bronchovascular shadows.

Table 1. *Differential Diagnosis of Rheumatic Pneumonia, Acute Pulmonary Edema,* Bacterial Pneumonia and Viral or Primary Atypical Pneumonia*

		Bacterial Pneumonia	Viral or PAP Pneumonia	Rheumatic Pneumonia	Pulmonary Edema
PHYSICAL FINDINGS	Clinical history	U.R.I., immediately preceding infection	Insidious onset usually with respiratory symptoms	Preceding beta H. strep. infection; often previous rheumatic fever	Usually previous rheumatic fever and often associated carditis
	Predominant presenting symptom	High fever, occasionally hacking cough	Frequent cough	Respiratory distress	Respiratory distress (with edema peripherally and liver enlargment)
	Lungs	Segmental, constant over the area, corresponding to x-ray lesions; rales follow signs of consolidation	Nonsegmental, variable, inconstant signs. Rales predominate and precede signs of consolidation when present	Nonsegmental, fleeting minimal findings, dull and diminished to bronchial B.S., few rales	Nonsegmental, bilateral findings at bases, rales, pleural fluid ± fluid elsewhere, edema, ascites
	Pleurisy ± fluid	Positive with fluid; tap often productive and culture positive	Rarely occurs; when present, cultures are sterile	Frequent, migratory and bilateral as fibrinous pleurisy ± fluid, transient and sterile	Common with fluid
	Heart	Normal (tachycardia)	Normal	Usually active carditis, occasionally pericarditis; often enlarged heart	Not necessarily active carditis; enlarged always
X-RAY CHEST	Location and type of lesions	Segmental, homogeneous, dense shadow, develops early	Nonsegmental, lesions scattered, often bilateral, different degrees of density and extent	Nonsegmental, migratory, fleeting, soft hazy shadows from hilus, often bilateral	Nonsegmental, dense, diffuse, extensive shadows usually bilateral from hilus
	Pleurisy	Fibrinous moderately frequent Effusion occasionally	Fibrinous and interlobar Rare otherwise	Frequent, fleeting ± pericarditis	Pleural fluid frequent
	Heart	Normal	Normal	Sometimes enlarged at beginning, may increase in size	Abnormal always, frequently large
	Duration of pulmonary shadow	Resolves shortly (few days) after effective antibiotic therapy	Slowly resolving, unrelated to therapy	Short time clearing unrelated to any therapy	Often responsive to diuretics and cardiac therapy Watch heart shadow
	Relation to pulmonary edema	Corresponds	Scattered, transient, often not found over x-ray shadow	Corresponds	Corresponds

* In patients with rheumatic heart disease.

pneumonia may occur in patients with subacute infection before carditis is clearly diagnosed.

Some of the salient features in the diseases most commonly requiring differentiation are given in Table 1. Additional aids from the laboratory include blood cultures, bacteriologic cultures from the nose and throat, cold agglutinin tests, antistreptolysin O titers, and electrocardiograms. All of these may aid in clarifying the diagnosis.

Additional observations of diagnostic value from a clinical standpoint are the frequency of pleuritic pain, the unusual degree of dyspnea, and the presence of blood-tinged sputum (when, indeed, sputum is available).

There may be other evidences of rheumatic fever, including skin manifestations such as erythema nodosum, erythema mar-ginatum and an undifferentiated rash (also possibly erythema marginatum). Chorea is rarely reported with rheumatic pneumonitis.

Therapeutic trial and response are often revealing. Patients with pulmonary edema may show prompt response to the use of digitalis, diuretics, oxygen and other supportive measures; this response is not seen in uncomplicated rheumatic pneumonitis.

Treatment

Supportive therapy should be given for the respiratory distress, for the chest pain and for the restlessness so frequently seen. Oxygen is usually required. Digitalis should be given as indicated.

Various therapeutic agents such as salicylates, sulfonamides (which were actu-

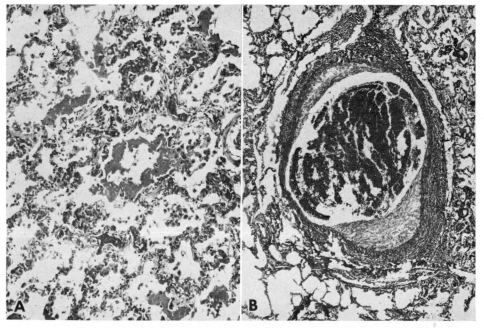

FIGURE 60–2. A 4-year-old girl was admitted to the rheumatic fever ward in Bellevue Hospital in January 1947 with acute arthritis and active carditis. She was digitalized and treated with salicylates and improved thereafter. Three months later fever, substernal pain and pericarditis developed. Rales were also heard in the chest. She was in acute respiratory distress and died 4 months after admission. The final diagnosis was rheumatic myocarditis, endocarditis of the tricuspid and mitral valves, and hypertrophy and dilatation of the heart with organizing fibrinous pericarditis. The lungs showed some pathologic features described in rheumatic pneumonia. *A,* Hyaline membranes and congestion. × 150. *B,* Arterial thrombus, organized. × 30.

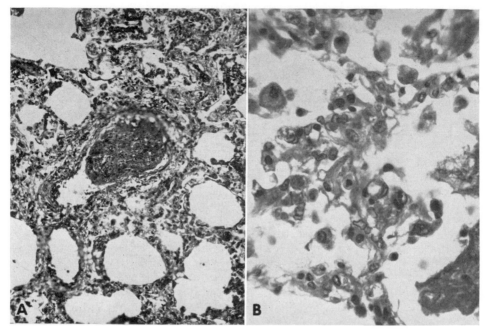

FIGURE 60–3. A 15-year-old Puerto Rican girl who died within 12 days after admission to Bellevue Hospital in 1947. Her clinical diagnosis was active rheumatic heart disease with enlarged heart, mitral stenosis and insufficiency and bronchopneumonia. At autopsy she was found to have rheumatic myocarditis; endocarditis of the mitral, aortic and tricuspid valves; rheumatic pericarditis and arteritis. In the lungs there was congestion, pulmonary embolism and rheumatic pneumonia with hyaline membranes. *A,* Pulmonary thromboembolus, acute. × 150. *B,* Exudate of mononuclear cells. × 500.

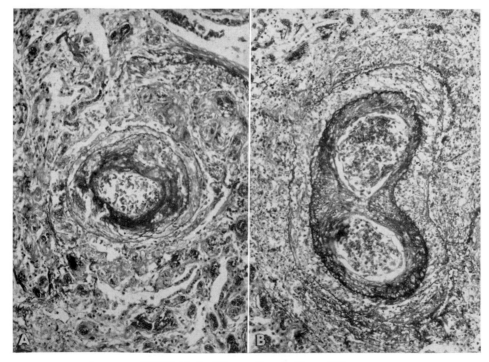

FIGURE 60–4. Rheumatic arteritis. × 100.

ally harmful) and B-dimethyl-amino-ethyl-benzhydryl ether (benadryl) have been used without success.

There is evidence that corticosteroid therapy may be helpful.

Prognosis

There is fairly uniform opinion that rheumatic pneumonitis has a grave prognosis. One must be constantly alert to the possibility of widespread pulmonary involvement; it appears that this finding has prognostic significance, especially in the initial attack. For those who survive, pulmonary damage may occur later in the form of chronic interstitial fibrosis.

It is probably safe to predict that the prophylactic therapy of streptococcal infections not only will diminish the recurrence of rheumatic fever itself, but also will help to decrease the incidence of the protean manifestations, including rheumatic pneumonitis. Prompt and early use of penicillin in the treatment of acute rheumatic fever will eliminate foci of streptococci and thereby lessen its antigenic elaboration. The use of corticosteroids during the acute phase is also helpful, to a greater degree than salicylates, in diminishing inflammation in acute rheumatic processes. Early diagnosis of rheumatic fever must be made in time for the prophylaxis of complications to be effective. In some instances, however, when the first rheumatic manifestation is the occurrence of pulmonary signs and symptoms instead of the classic joint and cardiac ones, arriving at the correct diagnosis may be virtually impossible in the absence of cardiac manifestations or other signs pointing to its rheumatic origin.

REFERENCES

Brown, G., Goldring, D., and Behrer, M. R.: Rheumatic Pneumonia. *J. Pediat.*, 52:598, 1958.

Chancey, R. L.: Intravenous Use of ACTH in Rheumatic Pneumonitis. *U.S. Armed Forces M.J.*, 4:1129, 1953.

Daugherty, S. C., and Schmidt, W. C.: Current Considerations Regarding the Prevention of Primary and Recurrent Rheumatic Fever. *M. Clin. N. Amer.*, 47:1301, 1963.

Debré, R., Marie, J., Bernard, J., and Normand, E.: Pneumonie rhumatismale. *Presse méd.*, 45:273, 1937.

Epstein, E. Z., and Greenspan, E. B.: Rheumatic Pneumonia. *Arch. Int. Med.*, 68:1074, 1941.

Feinstein, A. R., and Spagnuola, M.: The Clinical Patterns of Acute Rheumatic Fever: A Re-Appraisal. *Medicine*, 41:279, 1962.

Fraser, A. D.: The Aschoff Nodule in Rheumatic Pneumonia. *Lancet*, 1:70, 1930.

Geever, E. F., Neubuerger, K. T., and Rutledge, E. K.: Atypical Pulmonary Inflammatory Reactions. *Dis. Chest*, 19:325, 1951.

Glahn, W. C. von, and Pappenheimer, A. M.: Specific Lesions of Peripheral Blood Vessels in Rheumatism. *Am. J. Path.*, 2:235, 1926.

Goldring, D., Behrer, M. R., Brown, G., and Elliott, G.: Rheumatic Fever: Report on the Clinical and Laboratory Findings in Twenty-Three Patients. *J. Pediat.*, 53:547, 1958.

Goldring, D., Behrer, M. R., Thomas, W., Elliott, G., and Brown, G.: Rheumatic Pneumonia in Children. *Postgrad. Med.*, 26:739, 1959.

Gouley, B. A.: Acute and Subacute Pulmonary Involvement in Rheumatic Fever, with Notes on the Complication of Basal Pulmonary Collapse. *Ann. Int. Med.*, 11:626, 1937.

Gouley, B. A., and Eiman, J.: The Pathology of Rheumatic Pneumonia, *Am. J.M. Sc.*, 183:359, 1932.

Griffith, G. C., Phillips, A. W., and Asher, C.: Pneumonitis Occurring in Rheumatic Fever. *Am. J.M. Sc.*, 212:22, 1946.

Hadfield, G.: The Rheumatic Lung. *Lancet*, 2:710, 1938.

Harris, S., and Harris, T. N.: Serologic Response to Streptococcal Hemolysin and Hyaluronidase in Streptococcal and Rheumatic Infection. *J. Clin. Invest.*, 29:351, 1950.

Harris, T. N., Friedman, S., Needleman, H. L., and Saltzman, H. A.: Therapeutic Effects of ACTH and Cortisone in Rheumatic Fever: Cardiologic Observations in a Controlled Series of 100 Cases. *Pediatrics*, 17:11, 1956.

Harris, T. N., Needleman, H. L., Harris, S., and Friedman, S.: Antistreptolysin and Streptococcal Antihyaluronidase Titers in Sera of Hormone-Treated and Control Patients with Acute Rheumatic Fever. *Pediatrics*, 17:29, 1956.

Herbut, P. A., and Manges, W. E.: The "Masson Body" in Rheumatic Pneumonia. *Am. J. Path.*, 21:741, 1945.

Honma, M.: A Case of Rheumatic Pneumonitis. *J. Therapy* (Tokyo), 45:1169, 1963.

Jensen, C. R.: Non-suppurative Post-streptococcal (Rheumatic) Pneumonia. *Arch. Int. Med.*, 77:237, 1946.

Levy, H. B., Coffey, J. D., and Anderson, C. E., Jr.: Rheumatic Pneumonitis in Childhood. *Pediatrics,* 2:688, 1948.

Lustock, M. J., and Kuzma, J. F.: Rheumatic Fever Pneumonitis: A Clinical and Pathological Study of 35 Cases. *Ann. Int. Med.,* 44:337, 1956.

Markowitz, M., and Kuttner, A. G.: *Rheumatic Fever: Diagnosis, Management, and Prevention.* Philadelphia, W. B. Saunders Company, 1965, pp. 1-19, 26-32.

Massell, B. F., Fyler, D. C., and Roy, S. B.: Clinical Picture of Rheumatic Fever: Diagnosis, Immediate Prognosis, Course and Therapeutic Implications. *Am. J. Cardiol.,* 1:436, 1958.

Masson, P., Riopelle, J. L., and Martin, P.: Poumon rhumatismal. *Ann. Anat. Path. Med. Chir.,* 14:359, 1937.

Mossberger, J. I.: Rheumatic Pneumonia: Report of Two Cases. *J. Pediat.,* 30:113, 1947.

Muirhead, E. E., and Haley, A. E.: Rheumatic Pneumonitis: A Case of Widespread Chronic (Proliferative) Type with Acute (Exudative) Foci. *Arch. Int. Med.,* 80:328, 1947.

Myers, W. K., and Ferris, E. B., Jr.: Pleurisy in Rheumatic Fever. *Arch. Int. Med.,* 52:325, 1933.

Naish, A. E.: The Rheumatic Lung. *Lancet.* 2:10, 1928.

Neubuerger, K. T., Geever, E. F., and Rutledge, E. K.: Rheumatic Pneumonia. *Arch. Path.,* 37:1, 1944.

Nittono, F., and Hoshiyama, J.: Necropsy Findings in Rheumatic Pneumonia. *Jap. J.M. Sc. V. Path.,* 5:315, 1940.

Paul, J. R.: Pleural and Pulmonary Lesions in Rheumatic Fever. *Medicine,* 7:383, 1928.

Rabinowitz, M. A.: Rheumatic Pneumonia. *J.A.M.A.,* 87:142, 1926.

Reimann, H. A.: *Pneumonia.* Springfield, Ill., Charles C Thomas, 1954, p. 145.

Rich, A. R., and Gregory, J. E.: Experimental Evidence That Lesions with the Basic Characteristics of Rheumatic Carditis Can Result from Anaphylactic Hypersensitivity. *Bull. Johns Hopkins Hosp.,* 73:239, 1943.

Idem: On the Anaphylactic Nature of Rheumatic Pneumonitis. *Bull. Johns Hopkins Hosp.,* 73:465, 1943.

Idem: Further Experimental Cardiac Lesions of the Rheumatic Type Produced by Anaphylactic Hypersensitivity. *Bull. Johns Hopkins Hosp.,* 75:115, 1944.

Rubin, E. H., and Rubin, M.: Rheumatic Fever Pneumonia; in *Thoracic Diseases.* Philadelphia, W. B. Saunders Company, 1961, pp. 770-71.

Scott, R. F., Thomas, W. A., and Kissane, J. M.: Rheumatic Pneumonitis: Pathologic Features. *J. Pediat.,* 54:60, 1959.

Seldin, D. W., Kaplan, H. S., and Bunting, H.: Rheumatic Pneumonia. *Ann. Int. Med.,* 26: 496, 1947.

Shopfner, C. E., and Seife, M.: Rheumatic Carditis and Hemorrhagic Pneumonitis Treated with ACTH. *U.S. Armed Forces M.J.,* 3:819, 1952.

Smith, J. C.: Clinicopathologic Conference: Rheumatic Pneumonitis. *Am. J. Clin. Path.,* 20:783, 1950.

Swift, H. F., Moen, J. K., and Hirst, G. K.: Action of Sulfanilamide in Rheumatic Fever. *J.A.M.A.,* 110:426, 1938.

Tragerman, L. J.: Rheumatic Pneumonia. *Arch. Path.,* 22:566, 1936.

Tudor, R. B., and Kling, R. R.: Rheumatic Pneumonia. *Minnesota Med.,* 34:437, 441, 1951.

Van Wijk, E.: Rheumatic Pneumonia. *Acta paediat.,* 35:108, 1948.

Von Glahn, W. C., and Pappenheimer, A. M.: Specific Lesions of Peripheral Blood Vessels in Rheumatism. *Am. J. Path.,* 2:235, 1926.

Wilson, M. G., Lim, W. N., and Birch, A. M.: Decline of Rheumatic Fever: Recurrence Rates of Rheumatic Fever Among 782 Children for Twenty-One Consecutive Calendar Years (1936-1956). *J. Chron. Dis.,* 7:183, 1958.

CHAPTER SIXTY-ONE

Salmonella Pneumonia

ROSA LEE NEMIR, M.D.

Although typhoid bacilli were isolated from the sputum in 1884, the pulmonary manifestations of salmonella infections have received little attention. Salmon and Smith published the first reports of salmonella infections in 1886, and as early as 1895 Osler described pulmonary lesions in typhoid fever. Jehle again called attention to the presence of typhoid bacilli in the sputum of fifteen patients in 1902. Shortly thereafter reports of various types of lung pathology due to infections with the typhoid bacillus appeared, and recognition of a similar pulmonary disease produced by the paratyphoid organism followed.

Etiology

Data have been collected and classifications of the ever-increasing Salmonella groups have been drawn up in this country and elsewhere. In 1961 Huckstept reported the existence of approximately 700 types. Among the most frequently encountered types in this country are *S. typhimurium, Montevideo, Newport, Oranienburg, Paratyphi B,* and *Bareilly.* Of these, *S. choleraesuis* (paratyphoid group C_1), previously called *S. suipestifer,* is the type most often associated with pulmonary complications. *S. typhimurium* is the organism most commonly responsible for infection, but pulmonary complications with this organism are less common; however, it has been cultured from the pleural fluid in an appreciable number of cases.

Pathology and Pathogenesis

In an early textbook of pathology Mac-Callum states that "lobar and lobular pneumonia may accompany typhoid fever, the former rarely, the latter as a common terminal affection. Lobar pneumonia caused by *B. typhosus* has a peculiarly hemorrhagic character. . . . In the bronchopneumonia the typhoid bacillus may cause the lesions and appear in the sputum . . . . In the pharynx and larynx there is sometimes an extensive diphtheritic and haemorrhagic inflammation in the late stage of disease." Today the last-named lesion is exceedingly rare, and other pulmonary manifestations such as pulmonary thrombi, lung abscess, pleurisy and empyema, have been added to the list.

The etiologic relation of Salmonella to pulmonary lesions has been demonstrated by culture of the bacilli from sputum, from bronchial secretions, from pus from abscess, and from pleural fluid. *S. choleraesuis* is most often identified with sepsis and lung pathology.

The organisms usually enter the body through the mouth by the ingestion of contaminated food or water, rarely through the handling of contaminated toys or other objects. An unusual epidemic in a newborn nursery was traced to the contamination of resuscitators and suction machines. The trap water fluid was found to harbor *S. Montevideo* and *S. Bareilly* in each of two epidemics, and it was thought that the infection was disseminated in the nursery by the inhalation of contaminated air.

Bronchitis is the most common pulmonary manifestation, especially in *S. typhi* infections. Bronchopneumonia and pulmonary congestion are next in frequency. Lobar pneumonia due to the Salmonella agent alone may also occur, and Bullowa first reported lobar pneumonia due to *S. suipestifer* (now called *S. choleraesuis*) in an adult; the organism was isolated on culture of the blood and sputum, and by postmortem lung puncture.

The pathogenesis may be described as follows: Lesions may begin in the mucous membranes of the bronchopulmonary tree, producing tracheobronchitis, bronchitis or subsequently bronchopneumonia. The parenchyma may be infected by way of the blood stream, producing separate areas of inflammatory reaction which, by necrosis and excavation, result in abscess formation. Pulmonary thrombi may be produced, resulting in pulmonary infarction. The bones, particularly the ribs and the cartilages, are often the target of focal salmonella infections; pleurisy and empyema may result from the spread of infection from these foci into the pleura. One such case of empyema and bronchopleural fistula has been reported in an adult eleven years after a gunshot wound in the chest. Empyema and, rarely, bronchopleural fistula may result from the rupture of a pulmonary abscess into the pleura. Some of these pulmonary manifestations, such as abscess or empyema, are late complications of salmonella infection. In patients with empyema, subsequent pneumonitis may occur.

Pleural fluid varies from purulent to serofibrinous or hemorrhagic, the latter two being more frequent, and salmonellae are often cultured from these fluids.

Incidence

The chief pulmonary manifestations of salmonella infection, especially *S. typhi,* are bronchitis and secondary bronchopneumonia. Pneumonia and the more serious manifestations of lung disease have always been uncommon, and since the advent of the antibiotics have decreased still further. In an analysis of ninety-five cases of bacteriologically proved salmonellosis (forty-five children), Eisenberg and associates did not find a single instance of abscess, pneumonia or other localizing bacterial infection among the children.

The rarity of salmonella pulmonary complications in fatal cases may be further judged by the fact that there has not been such a case since 1947 at Bellevue Hospital, a large municipal hospital in New York City. The author obtained similar information from pathologists in Chicago, St. Louis and Richmond, Virginia. One fatality was reported by Szanton in an epidemic of *Salmonella Oranienburg* in a newborn nursery in 1957. An infant 144 days old died on arrival at the hospital, and necropsy revealed bronchitis and bronchiolitis.

From other countries where salmonella infection is more frequent, the incidence of pulmonary infection and mortality is also low. Rowland, in 1961, reporting his experience in Iran with 191 children with typhoid fever treated with chloramphenicol, reported no instances of pneumonia. In 1948 Kao, reporting from China, described two deaths from typhoid fever and bronchopneumonia among 126 cases of sulfadiazine-treated children.

Clinical Features

The clinical pattern of salmonella infection has been categorized as follows: (1) gastroenteritis, the most common; (2) typhoid-like or septic syndrome; (3) focal manifestations; and (4) the carrier state involving apparently healthy persons who harbor the infection and may serve as a reservoir.

Bronchitis or tracheobronchitis may occur during any one of the first types of involvement. Nelson and Pijper, in a series of 876 patients with salmonella infections in Pretoria, South Africa, and Goulder and others in this country, list the presence of bronchitis in 30 per cent of the patients. Both series include children. Our own early experience on the Children's Medical Service, Bellevue Hospital, is similar; however, today there is a decreased incidence of *S. typhi* infections, and such pulmonary complications are less frequent.

Cough, usually resulting from a simple tracheitis or tracheobronchitis, is one of the most frequent symptoms. The accompanying signs and symptoms include fever, varying in degree, abdominal pain or tenderness, headache, drowsiness or irritability, and occasionally mild chest pain aggravated by coughing. When rales appear, the diagnosis of bronchitis is assured. Diarrhea may not be present; indeed, in S. *typhi* infections in children constipation is more frequent. Hepatomegaly and splenomegaly are often present.

The pulmonary complications of bronchopneumonia, "lobar" pneumonia, abscess formation and pleural infections usually occur after the first week of infection. They may appear during the period of acute infection, especially with bronchopneumonia and disseminated pneumonia, and are often associated with septicemia. Bronchopneumonia usually follows shortly after the appearance of the early symptoms of salmonella infection. There may be a new elevation in temperature following defervescence or absence of fever, increasing cough, and the occurrence of chest pain following cough; physical findings include scattered transient rales and some patchy areas of altered breath sounds. The physical findings are not characteristic and differ from other pulmonary infections in only one way; the sputum frequently is hemorrhagic or blood-streaked. There have been few descriptions of abscess formation or pleural complications in children. Focal manifestations of salmonella infection occur late in the course of the disease, sometimes years afterwards, and may include lung abscess or pleurisy and empyema.

Diagnosis

In order to establish the diagnosis of salmonella infection, cultures should be made from the stools, urine and blood, and to clarify the origin of pulmonary complications, cultures from the sputum, pleural fluid and bronchial aspirations should be included. Occasionally cultures of the cerebrospinal fluid are made. Diarrhea must not be the only indication for

suspicion. A successful isolation of Salmonella is more likely during the first week of illness. Agglutination reactions to both O and H antigens, suitably grouped, furnish valuable evidence and were positive in more than 90 per cent of the 876 cases observed by Nelson and Pijper. Serums for groups C and E Salmonella should be included in the diagnostic antigens, since group C, especially S. *choleraesuis,* is the most frequently involved agent in pulmonary complications.

Other laboratory aids, such as blood cell counts, are of little aid in diagnosis. Leukopenia may be present, but the white blood cell count may vary, with elevations as high as 22,000 per cubic millimeter.

The findings noted in the x-ray of the chest in salmonella infections vary with the underlying pathology. Increased broncovascular markings may be seen in bronchopneumonia. When bacteremia is present and the parenchyma is infected by dissemination, mottled areas of infiltrate resembling miliary tuberculosis have been described. In patients with known salmonella septicemia, examination of the chest x-ray for focal involvement of the bony structures, especially ribs, may be rewarding. These lesions may be forerunners of pleural infection.

Certain diseases predispose the patient to infection by Salmonella. Bennett and Hook have given an excellent discussion of host factors and of the disease and nutritional status predisposing the patient to such infections. Among the more frequent are malaria, relapsing fever, bartonellosis, viral hepatitis, sickle cell anemia and postoperative complications. Such patients merit diagnostic tests for salmonellae when evidence of infection appears and when unexplained chest pathology is found.

Treatment

Treatment for pulmonary manifestations is the same as for other salmonella infections, with respiratory symptoms treated as indicated. Chloramphenicol is the drug of choice and is effective against virtually all strains of Salmonella. In the case of purulent complications, empyema or lung abscess, it is important to test the sensitivity of the organism isolated by culture. The emergence of drug-resistant strains during therapy is unusual, although it has been produced experimentally. Usually there is a prompt clinical response within a few days, an average of four days in children. When *Salmonella choleraesuis* is cultured, it is desirable to continue treatment longer than usual because of the high invasiveness and fatality rate, including those resulting from pulmonary infections. Balkin has suggested that short periods of therapy may be responsible for the later appearance of pulmonary complications.

Corticosteroid therapy should be reserved for the very toxic patient; then it may be used in conjunction with antibiotics. A controlled study by Rowland, in which one half of the patients received prednisoline, indicated that the addition of a corticosteroid affected neither the incidence of complications nor the relapse rate.

The management of lung abscess, pleural effusion or empyema is much the same as when these complications are produced by other organisms. These serious complications require longer therapy, but in time usually respond to medical treatment. Adequate medical therapy should always precede any decision as to the necessity for surgical intervention.

The Carrier State

Thomson, in a study of pathogenic bacilli in feces, has pointed out that infants and young children, as well as adults, can act as symptomless carriers, excreting large numbers of pathogens.

Jones and Pantin, studying an outbreak of *S. paratyphoid* B in a maternity home where adults and child contacts became infected, found that infants remained carriers longer than older children or adults. Three infants were still excreting *S. paratyphoid* B nine months after infection. Chloromycetin was valu-

able in combating symptoms, but had no effect on the carrier state.

Bille and others reported one case of an infant infected at birth from the maternal amniotic fluid. The newborn did not become ill, but at ten weeks of age, long after its mother had become negative, the infant was still excreting *S. Newport*.

Prognosis

There are several factors which determine the prognosis in salmonella infections. These include the speed and accuracy of diagnosis, appropriate selection of therapeutic agents, the general health and age of the patient, the extent or massiveness of bacterial invasion, and the type of Salmonella organism. That age is a factor is shown by the figures computed by Saphra from 174 fatalities; in infants the mortality rate was 5.8 per cent; the rate was 2 per cent in those from ages one to fifty years; and for patients past fifty years of age the mortality rate was 15 per cent.

Saphra and Winters also found that the fatality rate of *S. choleraesuis* infections was 21.3 per cent as compared to 5.3 per cent for the total group (174 cases). Twenty patients, who failed to survive, had pneumonia or pleurisy (*S. choleraesuis*, cultured from seven cases). In the report by MacCready and others, of thirty-seven fatalities (1.4 per cent) among 2605, *S. choleraesuis* was responsible for five (16 per cent) deaths in thirty-one patients. The high invasiveness of *S. choleraesuis* was suggested by the observations of these authors that ten of the thirty-one bacterial isolations came from the blood stream.

In summary, it appears that pulmonary manifestations other than bronchitis are rare in salmonella infections and that, in general, the prognosis is good. It must be pointed out that with the exception of *S. typhi* infections, salmonella diseases appear to be increasing in incidence. There was a sevenfold rise in the series reported by MacCready and others between 1950 and 1956 in Massachusetts. This indicates a need for increased alertness, not only for the initial salmonella infections, but also for their possible complications.

REFERENCES

Abram, J. H.: Paratyphoid Infections of the Pleura. *Lancet,* 2:283, 1919.

Balkin, S. S.: Bronchopneumonia, Empyema, Pneumothorax and Bacteremia Due to Salmonella (Var. Kunzendorf) Treated with Chloramphenicol. *Am. J. Med.,* 21:974, 1956.

Basch, S.: Report of a Case of Typhoid Fever Complicated by a Pure Typhoid Pneumonia and Pulmonary Abscess. *Med. Rec.,* 87:539, 1915.

Bennett, I. L., Jr., and Hook, E. W.: Infectious Diseases (Some Aspects of Salmonellosis). *Am. Rev. Med.,* 10:1, 1959.

Bille, B., Mellbin, T., and Nordbring, F.: An Extensive Outbreak of Gastroenteritis Caused by Salmonella Newport I. Some Observations on 745 Known Cases. *Acta Med. Scand.,* 175:557, 1964.

Bokra, S. T.: Chronic Empyema Due to Salmonella Oranienburg Complication of Old Chest Wound. *Canad. M.A.J.,* 78:599, 1958.

Bornstein, S., and Schwarz, H.: Salmonella Infection in Infants and Children. *Am. J.M. Sc.,* 204:546, 1942.

Bullowa, J. G. M.: Bacillus Suipestifer (Hog Cholera) Infection of the Lung. *M. Clin. N. Amer.,* 12:691, 1928.

Cohen, L., Fink, H., and Gray, I.: Salmonella Suipestifer Bacteremia with Pericarditis, Pneumonitis and Pleural Effusion (Report of a Case). *J.A.M.A.,* 107:331, 1936.

Eisenberg, G. M., Palazzolo, A. J., and Flippin, H. F.: Clinical and Microbiologic Aspects of Salmonellosis. A Study of Ninety-Five Cases in Adults and Children. *New England J. Med.,* 253:90, 1955.

Finley, F. G.: Typhoid Pleurisy. *Canad. M.A.J.,* 2:764, 1912.

Goulder, N. E., Kingsland, M. F., and Janeway, C. A.: Suipestifer Infection in Boston. Report of 11 Cases with Autopsy Findings in Case of Bacterial Endocarditis Due to This Organism and Study of Agglutination Reactions in This Infection. *New England J. Med.,* 226:127, 1942.

Hahne, O. H.: Lung Abscess Due to Salmonella Typhi. *Am. Rev. Resp. Dis.,* 89:566, 1964.

Harvey, A. M.: Salmonella Suipestifer Infection in Human Beings. *Arch. Int. Med.,* 59:118, 1937.

Harvill, T. H.: Typhoid Pulmonary Abscess. *J.A.M.A.,* 119:494, 1942.

Huckstept, R. L.: *Typhoid Fever and Other Salmonella Infections.* Edinburgh, E. and S. Livingstone, Ltd., 1962, p. 282.

Jameson, H. P., and Signy, A.: A Case of Paratyphoid B Infection with Purpura and Spe-

cific Bronchopneumonia. *Arch. Dis. Childhood,* 34:238, 1928-9.

Jehle, L.: Ueber den Nachweis von Typhusbacillen in Sputum der Typhenkranker. *Wien. klin. Wchnschr.,* 25:232, 1902.

Jones, D. M., and Pantin, C. G.: Neonatal Diarrhea Due to Salmonella. *J. Clin. Path.,* 9:128, 1956.

Kao, Yung-En: A Study of Typhoid Fever in Children in Kweichow. *Chinese Med. J.,* 66: 391, 1948.

Kuncaitis, J., and Okutan, A.: Empyema Due to Salmonella Typhimurium. *Am. Rev. Resp. Dis.,* 83:741, 1961.

Kuttner, A. G., and Zepp, H. D.: Salmonella Suipestifer Infections in Man. *J.A.M.A.,* 101: 269, 1933.

Layles, A. M.: Human Infection with Salmonella Choleraesuis. *Brit. M.J.,* 1:1284, 1957.

MacCallum, A. G.: *A Textbook of Pathology.* 3rd ed. Philadelphia, W. B. Saunders Company, 1925, p. 613.

MacCready, R. A., Reardon, J. P., and Saphra, I.: Salmonellosis in Massachusetts. A Sixteen Year Experience. *New England J. Med.,* 256: 1121, 1957.

McLean, I. W., Jr., Schwab, J. L., Hillegas, A. B., and Schlingman, A. S.: Susceptibility of Micro-Organisms to Chloramphenicol (Chloromycetin). *J. Clin. Invest.,* 28:953, 1949.

Minet, J.: Congestions pulmonaires à bacilles paratyphiques. *Bull. Acad. de Méd.,* 35:196, 1916.

Minor, G. R., and White, M. L., Jr.: Some Unusual Thoracic Complications of Typhoid and Salmonella Infections. *Ann. Int. Med.,* 24:27, 1946.

Nelson, H., and Pijper, A.: Typhoid and Paratyphoid Fevers; in H. S. Banks (Ed.): *Modern Practices in Infectious Fevers.* New York. Paul B. Hoeber, Inc., 1951, pp. 349-75.

Osler, W.: Typhoid Fever. II. Special Features, Symptoms and Complications. *Johns Hopkins Hosp. Rec.,* 5:283, 1895.

Robinson, C. C.: The Role of the Typhoid Bacillus in the Pulmonary Complications of Typhoid Fever. *J. Infect. Dis.,* 2:498, 1905.

Roque and Bancel: *Lyon méd.,* 100:578, 1903.

Rowland, H. A.: The Treatment of Typhoid Fever. *J. Trop. Med. & Hyg.,* 64:101, 1961.

Idem: The Complications of Typhoid Fever. *J. Trop. Med. & Hyg.,* 64:142, 1961.

Rubenstein, A. D., and Fowler, R. N.: Salmonellosis of the Newborn with Transmission by Delivery Room Resuscitators. *Am. J. Pub. Health,* 45:1109, 1955.

Sachs, J., and Antine, W.: Salmonella Infection in Man. A Report of Five Cases with Autopsies in Two Cases and a Review of the Clinical Aspects. *Am. J.M. Sc.,* 208:633, 1944.

Sahli: *Mitt. a. klin. u. med. Inst. d. Schweiz.,* 1:749, 1894.

Salmon, D. E., and Smith, T.: Investigations in Swine Plague. Annual Report, Bureau Animal Ind., U.S. Department of Agriculture, 1886.

Saphra, I.: Fatalities in Salmonella Infections. *Am. J.M. Sc.,* 220:74, 1950.

Saphra, I., and Wassermann, M.: Salmonella Choleraesuis: Clinical and Epidemiological Evaluation of 329 Infections Identified Between 1940 and 1954 in New York Salmonella Center. *Am. J.M. Sc.,* 228:525, 1954.

Saphra, I., and Winter, J. W.: Clinical Manifestations of Salmonellosis in Man. An Evaluation of 779 Human New Infections Identified at the New York Salmonella Center. *New England J. Med.,* 256:1128, 1957.

Stuart, B. M., and Pullen, R. L.: Typhoid: Clinical Analysis of Three Hundred and Sixty Cases. *Arch. Int. Med.,* 78:629, 1946.

Szanton, V. L.: Epidemic Salmonellosis. A 30-Month Study of 80 Cases of Salmonella Oranienburg Infection. *Pediatrics,* 20:794, 1957.

Thomson, S.: The Number of Pathogenic Bacilli in Faeces in Intestinal Diseases. *J. Hyg.,* 53:217, 1955.

Weiss, W., Eisenberg, G. M., and Flippin, H. F.: Salmonella Pleuropulmonary Disease. *Am. J.M. Sc.,* 233:487, 1957.

CHAPTER SIXTY-TWO

Visceral Larva Migrans

WILLIAM A. HOWARD, M.D.

Visceral larva migrans is the term applied to a clinical syndrome consisting of eosinophilia, hepatomegaly and pneumonitis which results from the invasion of human viscera by nematode larvae normally parasitic to lower animals. Although aberrant human ascarid and hookworm larvae may occasionally produce the disease, the most common cause appears to be the dog ascarid, *Toxocara canis,* and possibly the cat ascarid, *T. cati.* The disease is widespread and apparently may occur anywhere that infected dogs are present, cases being reported from North and South America, England and Europe.

Etiology

The etiologic agent, *Toxocara canis* (and possibly *T. cati*), is a common parasite of dogs, but is only accidentally infective to man, who is an unnatural host. *T. canis* in dogs produces lesions and symptoms similar to those of *Ascaris lumbricoides* infection in man, to which it is related, since both are members of the family Ascarididae. The adult male Toxocara is approximately 4 to 6 cm. long, while the female may be 10 cm. or more in length. The ova of this parasite measure 75 by 85 microns, and are passed unembryonated into the soil in the feces of the infected animal. Although the dog and the cat are the most likely sources of human infection, it is possible that the fox is a natural host. True intestinal infection with adult worms in man has not been substantiated.

Pathogenesis

The unembryonated ova of *T. canis* are passed onto the soil and under suitable conditions of temperature and humidity become embryonated and infective for the accidental and unnatural human host, usually a small child with pica who is a dirt-eater. The ingested, embryonated eggs pass through the stomach, and their larvae hatch in the upper levels of the small intestine. The freed larvae penetrate the intestinal wall and migrate through blood and lymph channels to the liver, lungs, brain and other organs. In these areas the larvae are attacked by a host cell reaction of granulomatous nature, which effectively blocks their further migration. In the unnatural host the larvae do not grow or moult, but may remain alive for a period up to one year. Since the larvae cannot complete their migration through the lungs to the tracheobronchial tree, there is no opportunity for *T. canis* to mature in the human intestine.

The immune response to such helminthic infections is caused primarily by and operates against larval migration stages in tissues. Lesions produced by various nematode larvae in tissues of immune hosts are strikingly similar in different hosts and in different tissues, all resembling the eosinophilic granuloma. The tissue reaction, including the peripheral eosinophilia, is proportional in both intensity and promptness to the immune state and the unnatural degree of the host.

Clinical Manifestations

Clinical symptomatology is derived primarily from the number and location of the granulomatous lesions and from the allergic response of the human host to the presence of the nematode larvae. Visceral larva migrans occurs primarily in the young child under the age of four or five years who has a history of pica and dirt-eating and has ample opportunity for contact with dogs. The usual early signs and symptoms include mild anorexia, failure to gain weight, low-grade fever, anemia, eosinophilia and hepatomegaly of varying degree. There may be evidence of bronchitis, pneumonitis or asthma. More severe involvment may produce gross liver enlargement, abdominal pain, pains in muscles and joints, weight loss, high intermittent fever, severe pulmonary involvement, and various neurologic disturbances. The eye may be involved with iritis, choroiditis and ocular hemorrhage.

Relative eosinophilia is usually pronounced, ranging from 50 to 90 per cent,

but unless above 30 per cent, the diagnosis may be questionable. Leukocytosis is common and may be extreme, above 100,000 cells per cubic millimeter.

Hepatomegaly is an almost constant finding, since this is the first organ invaded and is usually most heavily involved; this finding is absent in only the mildest infections. Fever, regardless of degree, may be associated with profuse sweating.

Pulmonic involvement is manifested clinically as bronchitis, pneumonitis or asthma in approximately 20 per cent of the cases, but pulmonary infiltrates are found in as many as 50 per cent of those patients who have chest x-rays. These lesions may represent actual migration of larvae, since studies in fatal cases have shown larval granulomatoses in the lungs as well as in other tissues. An occasional patient may show severe pulmonary involvement with widespread pneumonia, high fever and x-ray findings similar to those seen in miliary tuberculosis.

Neurologic disturbances are reported in severe cases. The author has observed a young Negro boy with epilepsy in whom a presumptive diagnosis of visceral larva migrans was made on the basis of a history of pica and dirt-eating, close association with dogs, and a 56 per cent blood eosinophilia. Encephalitis has also been reported as occurring in *T. canis* infection.

Other laboratory findings in visceral larva migrans include hyperglobulinemia, primarily an increase in the $gamma_2$ (IgG) fraction of gamma globulin, with normal levels of serum albumin, elevated erythrocyte sedimentation rate and albuminuria. Most liver function tests have been reported as normal or equivocal, with the exception of the cephalin flocculation test, which may be elevated. Transaminase levels have not been recorded.

Complications

Eye involvement, occurring without the usual findings of eosinophilia and hepatomegaly, may prove serious. There may be iritis, choroiditis, retinal detachment, fibrous tumors and keratitis. In some instances the appearance of the eye may be suspicious of retinoblastoma, and occasionally diagnosis can be made only after removal of the eye.

Pica is associated not only with visceral larva migrans, but also with lead poisoning, and the finding of refractory anemia, eosinophilia and abdominal pain may be part of either picture. Cases are reported in which both conditions have existed simultaneously, with disastrous results.

Course and Prognosis

Jung divides the clinical course of visceral larva migrans into three stages. During stage I, usually lasting several weeks, there is increasing eosinophilia, low-grade fever, and episodes of bronchitis, pneumonia and asthma. Stage II, lasting approximately one month, encompasses the cardinal signs of eosinophilia, heptomegaly, pulmonary involvement, hyperglobulinemia and intermittent high fever. This is followed by stage III, the period of recovery, which may last as long as one to two years, although eventual return to normal may be expected. A few patients die, either because of a massive involvement or because of a severe hypersensitivity reaction to the parasite.

Diagnosis

The diagnosis of visceral larva migrans is based upon the clinical history of pica, dirt-eating and adequate exposure to dogs, plus the clinical findings of chronic sustained eosinophilia, hepatomegaly and hypergammaglobulinemia. Additional findings may be referable to other organs involved, including the lung, brain and eye. Search has been made for suitable diagnostic techniques, but at present the only adequate accurate diagnosis is established by biopsy of a lesion, usually in the liver, and the finding of the typical nematode larva in an eosinophilic granuloma. The hemagglutination reaction and skin tests have been used and may give suggestive but not conclusive findings.

Differential diagnosis should include the visceral lesions which may be produced by a number of other nematode worms, including *Ascaris lumbricoides, Ancylostoma braziliense, Ancylostoma caninum, Strongyloides stercoralis,* as well as immature stages of certain spiruroid nematodes and filarial worms. Invasion of the liver by *Fasciola hepatica,* a nematode worm, or *Capillaria hepatica,* a trematode, might also be included. It is apparent that *Toxocara canis* may be one cause of the picture of Loeffler's syndrome of transient pulmonary infiltrations and eosinophilia, but other causes may mimic the picture. Also to be considered in the diagnosis are trichinosis, hepatitis, leukemia, familial eosinophilia, tropical eosinophilia, tuberculosis, asthma, lead poisoning, and the leukemoid reaction occurring in certain severe bacterial pneumonias.

Treatment

No satisfactory treatment for visceral larva migrans is recognized at present. Diethylcarbamazine (Hetrazan) in doses of 10 to 30 mg. per kilogram per day for fourteen days has been suggested, but has proved disappointing. More recently a new drug, thiabendazole, successfully used in cutaneous larva migrans (creeping eruption), in dosage of 25 to 100 mg. per kilogram per day has been used for the visceral form, but results so far are equivocal. Corticosteroids in adequate dosage may be lifesaving for patients who are highly sensitive to the larval nematode, especially those with severe pneumonitis. Otherwise treatment is primarily symptomatic and supportive, with stress on correction of the anemia.

REFERENCES

Beaver, P. C., Snyder, C. H., Carrera, G. M., Dent, J. H., and Lafferty, J. W.: Chronic Eosinophilia Due to Visceral Larva Migrans. *Pediatrics,* 9:7, 1952.
Brain, Lord, and Allen, B.: Encephalitis Due to

Infection with Toxocara Canis. Report of a Suspected Case. *Lancet*, 1:1355, 1964.

Chandra, R. K.: Visceral Larva Migrans. *Indian J. Pediat.*, 30:388, 1963.

Faust, E. C., and Russell, P. F.: *Clinical Parasitology. Philadelphia*, Lea & Febiger, 1964.

Friedman, S., and Hervade, A. R.: Severe Myocarditis with Recovery in a Child with Visceral Larva Migrans. *J. Pediat.*, 56:91, 1960.

Galvin, T. J.: Experimental Toxocara Canis Infections in Chickens and Pigeons. *J. Parasit.*, 50:124, 1964.

Karpinski, F. E., Jr., Everts-Saurez, E. Z., and Sawitz, W. G.: Larval Granulomatosis (Visceral Larva Migrans). *Am. J. Dis. Child.*, 92:34, 1956.

Smith, M. H. D., and Beaver, P. C.: Persistence and Distribution of Toxocara Larvae in the Tissues of Children and Mice. *Pediatrics*, 12:491, 1953.

Snyder, C. H.: Visceral Larva Migrans. *Pediatrics*, 28:85, 1961.

Vinke, B.: Application of Haemagglutination Test for Visceral Larva Migrans in Adult. *Trop. & Geog. Med.*, 16:43, 1964.

Woodruff, A. W., and Thacher, C. K. M.: Infections with Animal Helminths. *Brit. M.J.*, 1:1001, 1964.

CHAPTER SIXTY-THREE

Loeffler's Syndrome

WILLIAM A. HOWARD, M.D.

In 1932 Loeffler described a group of patients whose chest x-rays showed shadows of variable structures and fleeting density, accompanied by a moderate eosinophilia (10 to 20 per cent) and mild systemic symptoms. This combination of symptoms was generally called Loeffler's syndrome and was presumed to be benign and of short duration, usually a matter of a few weeks. Although no etiologic agent was established, infection with *Ascaris lumbricoides* was known to be present in some of Loeffler's cases. A year later Weingarten reported the same pulmonary and blood findings in cases of tropical eosinophilia from India. Since that time a number of other similar clinical pictures have been described, and the many variants are now often grouped together under the term "eosinophilic pneumonopathy."

Classification

Crofton and his associates proposed the following classification of this heterogeneous group, though it obviously goes far beyond Loeffler's original concept:

GROUP I. SIMPLE PULMONARY INVOLVEMENT WITH EOSINOPHILIA, OR LOEFFLER'S SYNDROME. This group is limited to those cases in which pulmonary infiltration persists for no more than one month, with mild or absent systemic symptoms.

GROUP II. PROLONGED PULMONARY EOSINOPHILIA. Here the duration is two to six months with definite symptomatology and occasional recurrences, but with ultimate recovery.

GROUP III. TROPICAL EOSINOPHILIA (WEINGARTEN'S SYNDROME). The cause of this syndrome is unknown, but it may be associated with filarial or other parasitic infections; improvement often follows treatment with arsenicals. The eosinophilia is pronounced, and, when untreated, the disease runs a benign but prolonged course.

GROUP IV. PULMONARY EOSINOPHILIA WITH ASTHMA. This is an attempt to place asthmatics in the group of eosino-

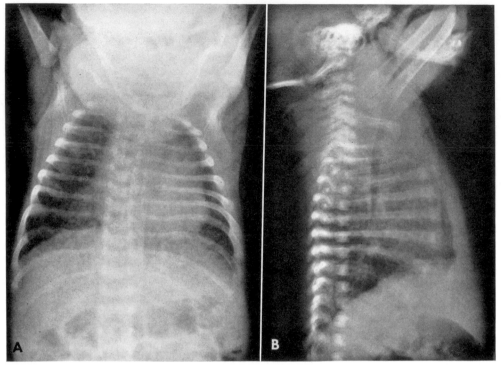

FIGURE 63–1. Loeffler's syndrome. Increased density at the right lung base. (Courtesy of John Kirkpatrick, M.D., St. Christopher's Hospital for Children and Temple University School of Medicine, Philadelphia.)

philic pneumonopathies whenever they have pulmonary infiltrates which may be shifting in nature.

GROUP V. POLYARTERITIS NODOSA. These patients usually are severely ill, with an asthmatic component and a poor prognosis.

Etiology and Pathogenesis

In many cases of Loeffler's syndrome no specific etiologic agent can be demonstrated. When a specific cause has been found, it most often appears to be infection with parasitic nematodes, usually Ascaris or Toxocara, although amebiasis, trichinosis and filiarial infections may give a similar picture. It may be difficult to determine the presence of a nematode worm in the patient, since in the case of Ascaris the pulmonary phase may occur some days or weeks before ova from adult worms will be found in the stool.

The larval forms of Toxocara become encysted in the tissue, including the lungs, and never reach the intestinal tract to develop into mature worms passing diagnostic ova, such as occurs in the dog.

A number of cases of Loeffler's syndrome caused by a variety of drugs and chemicals have now been reported. The list includes nitrofurantoin, para-aminosalicylic acid, hydralazine, mecamylamine, penicillin, imipramine, mephenesin and chlorpropamide, and the list will probably lengthen.

The eosinophilia and pulmonary findings are generally considered to be the result of a hypersensitivity reaction to the etiologic agent, and the syndrome occurs most commonly in persons with a personal or family history of allergy.

Clinical Manifestations

In general the symptoms are very mild or absent, even in the presence of fairly large pulmonary lesions. There may be a

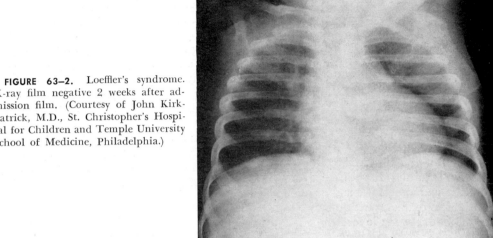

FIGURE 63–2. Loeffler's syndrome. X-ray film negative 2 weeks after admission film. (Courtesy of John Kirkpatrick, M.D., St. Christopher's Hospital for Children and Temple University School of Medicine, Philadelphia.)

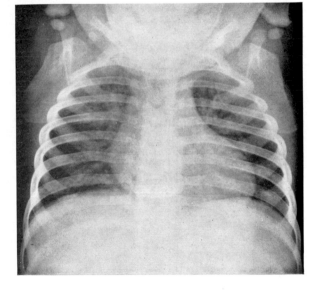

FIGURE 63–3. Loeffler's syndrome. Film one month after Figure 2, showing area of infiltration at the right lung base. (Courtesy of John Kirkpatrick, M.D., St. Christopher's Hospital for Children and Temple University School of Medicine, Philadelphia.)

cough or wheeze, and occasionally scattered rales may be heard. On the roentgenogram the pulmonary lesions are usually simple infiltrations, pneumonic or occasionally atelectatic, somewhat similar in appearance to those caused by tuberculosis. In other instances the x-ray findings may resemble bronchopneumonia or a viral pneumonitis. Within a few days these lesions begin to clear, but new involvement appears in other areas.

There may be a moderate leukocytosis, and eosinophils range from 10 to 50 per cent. When toxocara infection is the underlying cause, hepatomegaly is usually present.

Pathology

In the rare case observed at autopsy the principal findings have been irregular bronchopneumonic foci, and small areas of alveolar exudate with many eosinophils. Giant cells of the foreign body type, such as are seen in visceral larva migrans, may also be seen. Vascular damage is rare.

Diagnosis

Diagnosis is dependent upon x-ray evidence of transient and migratory pulmonary infiltrations with eosinophilia and only mild systemic manifestations. A consideration of possible etiologic agents should include a careful history of recent drug ingestion and a careful search for parasites. Among those responsible besides Ascaris and Toxocara are included the hookworms, strongyloides infection and trichinosis. A careful search should be made for tubercle bacilli in the sputum, and a tuberculin test result which remains

negative will be helpful in differentiation. The possibility of polyarteritis should be kept in mind. Skin tests to Ascaris antigen may occasionally be helpful in diagnosis.

Treatment

Typically, Loeffler's syndrome is self-limited, and treatment may not be necessary. If pulmonary lesions are bothersome or cough or wheeze is significant, rapid resolution of the pulmonary process can be produced by administration of a suitable corticosteroid preparation. These should be used only when the presence of tuberculosis has been excluded. If worm infestations are present, these should be treated appropriately. Such therapy, however, will have no effect on the pulmonary phase of the disease.

REFERENCES

Bell, R. J. M.: Pulmonary Infiltrations with Eosinophilia Caused by Chlorpropamide. *Lancet,* 1:1249, 1964.

Crofton, J. W., Livingston, J. L., Oswald, N. C., and Roberts, A. T. M.: Pulmonary Eosinophilia. *Thorax,* 7:1, 1952.

Incaprera, F. P.: Pulmonary Eosinophilia. *Am. Rev. Resp. Dis.,* 84:730, 1961.

Loeffler, W.: Zur Differential-Diagnose der Lungeninfiltrierungen. II. Ueber fluchtige Succedan-Infiltrate (mit Eosinophilie). *Beitr. z. Klini. Tuberk.,* 79:368, 1932.

Mark: L.: Loeffler's Syndrome. *Dis. Chest.,* 25: 128, 1954.

Scheer, E. H.: Loeffler's Syndrome. *Arch. Pediat.,* 68:407, 1951.

Wilson, I. C., Gambill, J. M., and Sandifer, M. G.: Loeffler's Syndrome Occurring During Imipramine Therapy. *Am. J. Psychiatry,* 119: 892, 1963.

CHAPTER SIXTY-FOUR

Viral Etiology of Respiratory Illness

VINCENT V. HAMPARIAN, Ph.D.,
and HENRY G. CRAMBLETT, M.D.

The application of modern cell culture methodology to the study of viruses launched the field of virology into an era of intense activity with the consequent rapid accumulation of an overwhelming body of new knowledge. In the decade 1953 to 1963 approximately 150 new viruses were recovered from human patients, an average of fifteen viruses per year. Most of these agents are either proved or probable causes of respiratory illness. This chapter will endeavor to present exemplary methods for the laboratory diagnosis of viral respiratory disease and to summarize the salient aspects of the clinical picture produced by viruses infecting the respiratory tract of man. The mycoplasma, rickettsiae and members of the psittacosis–lymphogranuloma venereum–trachoma group of agents are not true viruses and are considered elsewhere in this volume. Table 1 shows the vi-

Table 1. *Viruses Affecting the Respiratory Tract of Man*

Virus Designation	Number of Known Serotypes
I. Picornaviruses	
A. Enteroviruses	
1. Poliovirus	3
2. Coxsackie A	23
3. Coxsackie B	6
4. ECHO	29
B. Rhinoviruses	At least 53 types
II. Adenoviruses	28
III. Myxoviruses	
A. Influenza	
1. Influenza A	3 subtypes
Influenza B	3 subtypes
Influenza C	1
B. Parainfluenza	4
C. Respiratory syncytial	1
D. Rubeola	1
E. Rubella	1
IV. Reoviruses	3
V. Miscellaneous	
A. Lymphocytic choriomeningitis	1
B. Infectious mononucleosis	1 ? (presumed viral)
C. Varicella	1
D. Variola	1
E. Cytomegalovirus	1

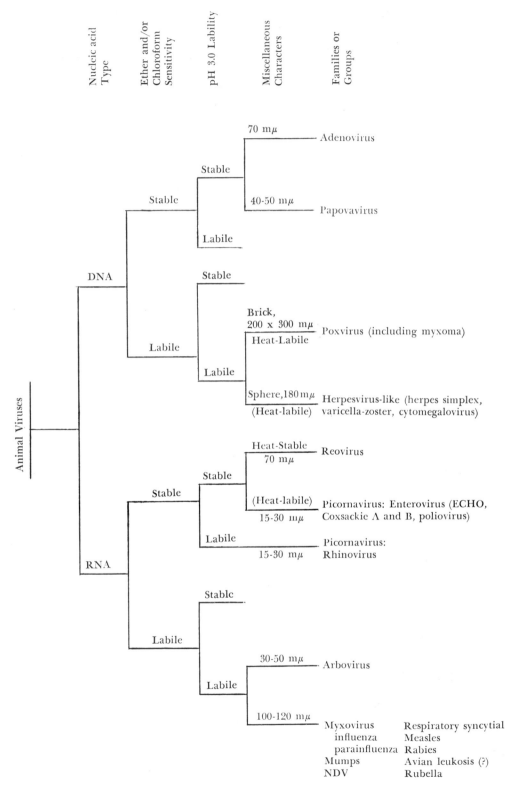

FIGURE 64–1. A practical classification of viruses. (From Hamparian et al.)

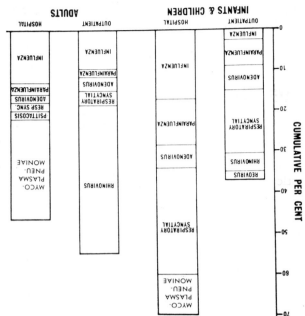

FIGURE 64–2. Interpretive estimate of relative importance of nonbacterial respiratory disease agents according to age and case selection. (Adapted from Hilleman et al.)

ruses or groups of viruses known to be associated with respiratory tract illness in man. Figure 1 presents a practical classification of viruses based upon presently recognized chemical and physical properties. Figure 2 presents an over-all interpretive estimate of the relative importance of nonbacterial respiratory disease agents, according to age and case selection.

Laboratory Diagnosis: General Considerations

For viral diagnostic procedures, it is axiomatic that acute-phase serum samples and materials for virus recovery attempts be obtained as early in the course of the illness as possible. Convalescent-phase serum specimens should be taken three to four weeks after the onset of the illness. In general, serologic procedures alone are not practical for diagnostic purposes. The great number of known respiratory viruses, the difficulties and expense of preparing potent specific antigens and, in many cases, the undependable specificity of the antibody response all serve to pre-

clude the routine use of serologic procedures for laboratory diagnosis. Serology is most useful after the recovery of a virus from a patient. The presence of a fourfold or greater increase in neutralizing antibody titer with paired patient's serums for a particular virus provides added assurance that the virus caused an infection in the patient. In addition, serologic procedures are often of particular value for obtaining sero-epidemiologic data on individual viruses or on a single group of viruses.

For laboratory diagnosis, viral isolation procedures are preferable because they yield specific answers and, although expensive, are suitable for routine application on a large scale. Ideally, clinical specimens such as throat washings should be collected in a menstruum rich in protein and should arrive in the laboratory with minimal delay. Specimens should be kept in wet ice during transportation over short distances or frozen in dry ice if time in transit is longer than twenty-four hours. Information such as the kind of specimen, the clinical diagnosis and the date of the onset of the illness should be forwarded with the specimen.

Although the recovery and the identification of viruses are slow and laborious, and no specific therapeutic drugs are available for most viral diseases, the diagnostic laboratory performs a vital function by keeping under constant surveillance the prevalence of viruses within a given population. Such knowledge is not only helpful to the physician in establishing diagnoses, but will also provide the necessary epidemiologic data to help determine which viruses are worthy candidates for inclusion in vaccines or for attempts at other methods of control.

PICORNAVIRUSES

General Properties

The picornaviruses (pico, very small; RNA, ribonucleic acid) are one of the largest, if not the largest, single group of viruses known. They contain a ribonucleic acid core (RNA) and range in size from 15 to 30 microns in diameter. The few types adequately studied by electron microscopy have been found to have cubic icosahedral symmetry. These viruses do not have an outer envelope and are not susceptible to lipid solvents. As can be seen in Table 1, the picornaviruses are divided into two major subgroups—the enteroviruses and the rhinoviruses.

Biologically, these subgroups differ in that the enteroviruses primarily inhabit the gastrointestinal tract and are most commonly isolated from the feces of the infected person. The enteroviruses are capable of causing a spectrum of illness ranging from common colds to aseptic meningitis. They do not appear to be associated with lower respiratory tract illness. Rhinoviruses, on the other hand, are rarely if ever found in the feces and to date have been found associated only with respiratory tract illness. In the laboratory these two subgroups can be differentiated easily on the basis of stability at pH 3.0.

Rhinoviruses are extremely labile under these conditions, while the enteroviruses are unaffected. The lability of rhinoviruses at acid pH might explain their absence from the alimentary tract.

Enteroviruses

Clinical Aspects

The enteroviruses cause a wide spectrum of illnesses, including aseptic meningitis with or without paralysis, pleurodynia, exanthems, gastroenteritis, myocarditis and pericarditis, in which the respiratory tract is not involved or is involved only to a minor degree. Only the diseases in which there is major involvement of the respiratory tract will be discussed in this section.

As with most viruses, the enteroviruses rarely cause clinically distinguishable respiratory disease. Rhinitis, tonsillitis, pharyngitis and croup due to various enteroviruses have been reported. These syndromes, however, do not differ sufficiently from those due to other viruses to permit the clinician to make an etiologic diagnosis on clinical grounds alone.

Herpangina caused by Coxsackie group A viruses types 2, 4, 5, 6, 8 and 10 is a disease in which the clinical diagnosis can be made with some certainty. The disease occurs most commonly between the ages of one and four years. There is usually fever, irritability and occasionally vomiting and diarrhea with associated abdominal pain. The lesions characteristic of the disease begin as papules which progress to fragile vesicles which are easily broken, leaving behind small ulcers surrounded by inflammatory areolae. The lesions are characteristically located on the soft palate, uvula and tonsillar fauces. This is in contradistinction to the lesions caused by the herpes simplex virus which are located in the anterior portion of the oral cavity. There is no specific therapy. An individual child may have recurrent episodes of herpangina due to different serotypes of

Coxsackie group A viruses, since immunity is type-specific.

Laboratory Diagnosis

On a routine basis, enteroviruses are best isolated by the inoculation of clinical specimens such as washings from rectal swabs and throat swabs into monkey renal cell cultures. All known enteroviruses with the exception of most of the Coxsackie A group can be recovered in such cell cultures. Most Coxsackie A viruses do not propagate in cell cultures, but can be isolated by the inoculation of newborn mice. The isolation, standardization and identification of Coxsackie A viruses using mice is so time-consuming and laborious that few laboratories use this procedure. Usually, Coxsackie A viruses can be presumptively identified by the type of pathology produced in infant mice. These agents primarily involve the skeletal muscles and result in a flaccid type of paralysis. Since herpangina is the usual clinical finding in human patients infected by these agents and since no other viruses have been found to cause this syndrome, the cause can be determined with reasonable certainty on a clinical basis.

To the experienced person the type of cytopathology produced by a virus in cultured cells provides an important clue to the identity of the agent. The cytopathic effects (CPE) produced by Picornaviruses are typical, and if the agent recovered is stable at pH 3.0, this is good presumptive evidence that the virus is an enterovirus. For specific identification, the virus can be tested against immune serum pools utilizing the "intersecting serum scheme" in which each type-specific serum is present in two pools. The unknown virus is presumptively identified when it is neutralized by pools sharing identical antiserums. An additional aid in simplifying the identification of an unknown enterovirus is the ability of a large number of such viruses to agglutinate type O human erythrocytes. If demonstrable, this property can provide a clue to the identity of the virus, thus reducing the amount of serologic testing necessary. Hemagglutinating enteroviruses include ECHO virus types 3, 6, 7, 11-13, 19-21, 25, 29, 30; Coxsackie virus types B_1, B_3, B_5, B_6, A_7, A_{20}, A_{21} and A_{24}.

Rhinoviruses

Clinical Aspects

More data are available at present concerning clinical illnesses resulting from rhinovirus infections in adults than in children. These viruses have been shown to be responsible for approximately 30 per cent of the upper respiratory tract illnesses in adults. For the most part the predominant signs and symptoms have included rhinorrhea, coryza, and minimal soreness or "scratchiness" of the throat, usually without fever. In children, rhinovirus infections appear to result in lower almost as commonly as upper respiratory tract illnesses. Further, upper respiratory tract illness in children is frequently accompanied by fever. Croup, bronchitis, pneumonia and bronchiolitis have been observed in children from whom rhinoviruses have been recovered. Data are not available at present to determine the relative importance of the various serotypes as causes of respiratory disease in children. Present data indicate that rhinoviruses do not account for more than 5 per cent of the respiratory diseases in infants and children.

Laboratory Diagnosis: General Considerations

The initial virus in this group to be isolated and described in detail was the 2060 virus, also known as the ECHO 28 virus. Although the 2060 virus was isolated in monkey kidney cell cultures, success in the isolation of a number of agents from common colds in adults was accomplished by using cell cultures derived from human tissues. The early laboratory methods necessary to propagate these agents were different from those routinely used for other viruses. A unique property of these agents is the necessity to roll inoculated cell cultures at 33 °C. during the virus isolation procedure. The cell culture system consisted of primary human fetal kidney cultures maintained on a relatively low pH medium. Human fetal tissues are not routinely available and do not have the desirable quality of uniformity of susceptibility to viruses.

The first significant technologic advance for simplifying the work with these agents was provided by the development of diploid cell strains from human fetal tissue. Such cells can be made available in quantity, maintain a normal karyotype throughout their useful life span and do not have the properties of "malignant" cells. Human diploid cell strains are highly sensitive to rhinoviruses, which produce a distinct and easily recognizable cytopathology in such cell cultures. Although other Picornaviruses produce a similar cytopathic effect, the rhinoviruses are easily distinguished by their property of lability at pH 3.0.

At present specific identification of rhinoviruses is not feasible for the ordinary virus laboratory. It seems likely that a multiplicity of serotypes are present in the population at any one time. The great diversity and the rapid turnover of serotypes in a given geographic area suggest that the total number of antigenic types may be very large. In the relatively short time period in which these agents have been recognized as a distinct group, fifty-three serotypes have been described, and there is a constantly increasing number of isolates in laboratories around the world still waiting to be recognized. At present typing serums are not available from commercial or private sources, and isolates must be stored for identification at some future date unless the individual laboratory is willing to expend the time, labor and expense in preparing suitable antiserums.

ADENOVIRUSES

General Properties

The adenoviruses are composed of a DNA core enclosed in a protein shell of about 70 microns in diameter. No outer envelope has been demonstrated. These agents are not affected by lipid solvents or by exposure to pH 3.0. All the human adenoviruses share a common complement-fixing antigen. With the exception of types 12 and 18, all human types agglutinate rat or monkey erythrocytes. These agents propagate and mature within the nucleus of the infected cell, producing type B intranuclear inclusions and a characteristic cytopathic effect. A recently discovered property of certain members of this group is the ability to induce the formation of malignant tumors when inoculated into newborn hamsters. This is the first recognized example of tumor induction in animals by human viruses.

Clinical Aspects

The adenoviruses are responsible for approximately 5 per cent of all respiratory disease in infants and children. They may infect any portion of the respiratory tract and hence cause a wide spectrum of disease ranging from rhinitis to bronchiolitis. Adenovirus types 3, 4 and 7 are the most frequent serotypes causing respiratory disease. Types 1, 2 and 5 are less common causes of disease and apparently cause illness only in infants and younger children.

Pharyngoconjunctival fever is the only clinically distinguishable syndrome caused by the adenoviruses. Most patients with this disease are infected with adenovirus types 3 and 7, with occasional cases due to types 4 and 14. The signs and symptoms of pharyngoconjunctival fever include erythema and injection of the palpebral and bulbar conjunctivae (unilateral or bilateral) and erythema of the tonsils and pharynx, occasionally accompanied by exudate, coryza and fever. As the child recovers, there may be enlargement and tenderness of the posterior cervical and preauricular lymph nodes. Pharyngoconjunctival fever is clinically similar to prodromal measles prior to the appearance of Koplik spots and the exanthem.

The other respiratory diseases due to the adenoviruses are not clinically distinguishable. Nevertheless the presence of conjunctivitis associated with respiratory disease is suggestive of an adenovirus infection.

Adenovirus types 1, 2, 3 and 7 have been recovered by postmortem examination of lung tissue of children with primary viral pneumonia. Adenovirus pneumonia, however, is not clinically different from pneumonia due to other viruses.

Laboratory Aspects

Most laboratories utilize stable cell lines such as HeLa, KB and Hep-2 for the isolation of adenoviruses from throat or rectal specimens. For the optimum recovery of adenoviruses, cell cultures of primary human fetal kidney tissue also should be used. Such cultures can be maintained for long periods of time and are particularly useful for certain slow-growing adenoviruses. Identification of an isolate such as an adenovirus is relatively easy. These agents produce a characteristic cytopathic effect in cell cultures. In addition, all the known human adenoviruses produce a group-specific complement-fixing (C.F.) antigen which is best demonstrated by the use of a specific, standardized animal antiserum. When utilizing the complement fixation reaction for the identification of viruses, a negative test result should be interpreted with caution, since it may be due to an inadequate complement-fixing antigen content in the preparation used.

Specific identification of adenoviruses can be accomplished by use of type-specific antiserums in neutralization or hemagglutination-inhibition tests. The hemagglutination-inhibition test is particularly helpful, since the type of red cell agglutinated and the pattern of agglutination obtained place the virus in a subgroup, substantially reducing the number of antiserums needed for final identification. Knowledge of adenovirus types most likely to be encountered in a given clinical situation is also helpful in the rapid identification of isolates.

MYXOVIRUSES

General Properties

The myxoviruses contain a ribonucleoprotein core enclosed in an outer envelope and range in particle size from 80 to 250 millimicrons. These agents contain essential lipid and are inactivated by lipid solvents. Myxoviruses are also inactivated at pH 3.0. Most of the human myxoviruses agglutinate erythrocytes by attachment to mucoprotein receptor sites on red blood cells. This is due to an enzyme reaction, and once the substrate is destroyed, the virus elutes from the red blood cell. Most myxoviruses cause a phenomenon termed hemadsorption in which erythrocytes are adsorbed to cells in infected cultures, a phenomenon used extensively for demonstrating the presence of virus in infected cells.

The two primary subgroups of myxoviruses which are important in the causation of human respiratory illness are the influenza and parainfluenza viruses. Although these subgroups share many common properties, they have certain distinguishing characteristics. The influenza viruses are smaller, 80 to 120 millimicrons, as opposed to a size of 150 to 250 millimicrons for the parainfluenza viruses. The parainfluenza viruses can hemolyze certain kinds of erythrocytes and have common antigens not related to the common antigens shared by the influenza viruses. The parainfluenza viruses appear to be relatively stable antigenically, while the influenza viruses, particularly type A, are notorious for the instability of their antigenic composition. For example, it appears likely that in the last seventy years approximately five major and many minor changes have occurred in the influenza A virus, while only two demonstrable antigenic shifts have occurred in influenza B virus since its original isolation in 1940. No changes have occurred in the antigenic structure of influenza C virus. In contrast to the influenza A and B viruses and up to the present time, there is no evidence that any important antigenic changes have occurred in the members of the parainfluenza group of viruses.

Clinical Aspects

Illnesses due to influenza types A, B and C are similar. Most pandemics and epidemics of influenza are due to strains of type A virus, while type B virus is usually endemic or epidemic. Type C influenza virus causes only sporadic cases of disease.

In children the most common symptoms of influenza are headache, cough, sore throat and nasal discharge or obstruction. Other symptoms include pain, lacrimation, vomiting, abdominal pain and weakness or dizziness. On physical examination, fever is usually present with an impressive absence of physical findings. There may be mild to moderate erythema of the pharynx and erythema of the conjunctivae, and coarse rhonchi may be present.

Laboratory Aspects

The classic technique for the isolation of influenza viruses has been the inoculation of throat specimens into the amniotic cavity of the ten-day-old embryonated chicken egg. The presence of the virus in amniotic fluid is detected by hemagglutination, and the exact identity can be established by the use of specific inhibitor-free antiserums in hemagglutination-inhibition tests. Primary monkey kidney cell cultures also appear to be useful for the recovery of influenza viruses from clinical materials. Furthermore, the influenza viruses, like other myxoviruses, are capable of causing hemadsorption in infected cell cultures.

During recognized epidemics the complement fixation test can be used to great advantage for diagnostic purposes. Strain-specific complement-fixing antigens for contemporary influenza viruses can be prepared in the laboratory or obtained commercially. When serums collected from patients during the acute and convalescent phases of illness are available, serologic tests incorporating these antigens can be utilized to demonstrate strain-specific antibody increases with a minimum of labor and cost. An additional advantage of this technique is that nonspecific inhibitors present in most serums do not affect the outcome of the test.

Parainfluenza Viruses

Clinical Aspects

The parainfluenza viruses have been recovered from children with syndromes varying from mild rhinitis to severe bronchiolitis. In general, infections with types 1 and 3 viruses are more common than those with type 2. The significance of type 4 virus in the causation of respiratory illness is uncertain at present. Collectively, parainfluenza viruses types 1, 2 and 3 are the most important agents etiologically associated with croup. In contrast to types 1 and 3 viruses, which cause a diverse number of respiratory illnesses, type 2 virus is usually associated only with croup.

Laboratory Aspects

Serologic procedures such as the complement fixation and hemagglutination-inhibition tests are useful, but suffer from the lack of specificity of the antibody response. Heterotypic antibody responses in human subjects following parainfluenza virus infections are not uncommon, and in the absence of virus isolation studies, serologic results are difficult to interpret precisely; however, they can be utilized to delegate causation to the parainfluenza virus group.

The development of the hemadsorption technique has simplified the virus isolation and identification methodology for the parainfluenza viruses. Primary monkey renal cell cultures appear to be the most sensitive system for the recovery of these agents from clinical materials. The cytopathic effects produced by these agents on initial inoculation into such cultures are subtle at best, making the hemadsorption phenomenon basic to the early and certain recognition of these agents in infected cell cultures. The specific identification of a hemadsorbing agent is carried out by use of type-specific antiserums in neutralization tests. The number of known hemadsorbing viruses recoverable in monkey renal cell culture from human sources is at present relatively small, and antiserums are needed for only seven or eight viruses. It is worthy of note that some lots of monkey kidney cell cultures harbor endogenous simian viruses capable of causing cytopathic effects or the hemadsorption phenomenon. The isolation of "new" viruses in such cell cultures or even in nonsimian cell culture systems must be interpreted with caution, especially if monkey kidney cell cultures are used routinely in the laboratory.

Respiratory Syncytial Virus

General Properties

The presently recognized biological and physical properties of the respiratory syncytial (R.S.) agent appear to resemble closely those of the known myxoviruses. It is of medium size and contains an RNA core. It is inactivated by lipid solvents and is extremely labile at pH 3.0. In sharp contrast to the myxoviruses, however, it lacks the ability to agglutinate erythrocytes or to cause hemadsorption. The respiratory syncytial virus generally is classified with the myxoviruses.

Clinical Aspects

The respiratory syncytial virus is the most important single virus causing respiratory disease in infants and children so far recovered. It is estimated that as many as 15 per cent of the cases of respiratory disease seen in outpatients and as many as 25 per cent of the cases of respiratory disease in hospitalized children are due to the respiratory syncytial virus.

Bronchiolitis is the most severe respiratory illness caused by this virus. The virus is responsible for over 50 per cent of the cases of this syndrome. It may also cause pneumonia, bronchitis, croup and rhinitis. The less severe upper respiratory tract illnesses are often the clinical expression of reinfections with the virus.

Laboratory Aspects

This agent is particularly susceptible to inactivation, a factor which emphasizes the importance of the careful collection and handling of clinical specimens. Stable cell line cultures such as HeLa, KB and Hep-2 are highly sensitive to respiratory syncytial virus, although recent reports indicate that some strains propagate best in monkey kidney cell cultures. The cytopathology is characteristically lytic in nature with the formation of syncytia, cell rounding and swelling. Absence of hemadsorption concomitant with this kind of cytopathic effect suggests the presence of respiratory syncytial virus. Specific identity can be established by the neutralization technique using specific animal antiserum. Since the virus produces a potent complement-fixing antigen, some laboratories prefer to use the complement fixation test for the purpose of viral identification.

COMMENT

Although a number of viruses, including rubeola, rubella, varicella, variola, cytomegalovirus and lymphocytic choriomeningitis viruses, are capable of causing symptoms of acute respiratory disease, their primary manifestations are not usually in the respiratory tract, and for this reason they will not be discussed here. (See chapters on Measles Pneumonia, Varicella Pneumonia and Cytomegalic Inclusion Disease.) The reoviruses also are omitted from discussion, since there is no definite proof that they play a significant role in the origin of human respiratory disease. Moreover, the existing evidence is merely suggestive, and final judgment must await the results of future investigations.

It must be emphasized that the methodology for laboratory diagnosis of virus infections varies considerably from laboratory to laboratory. The techniques utilized are often governed by the special interests, experience and background of the laboratory personnel. These differences are not vital as long as the laboratory adequately performs the task for which it exists.

Hopefully, the techniques described above will be improved in the future and replaced by more rapid and accurate means for laboratory diagnosis of viral infections. Among others, methods presently being explored in a number of laboratories with varying degrees of success include the use of fluorescent antibody techniques and the direct application of electron microscopy to clinical materials.

REFERENCES

Conference on Newer Respiratory Disease Viruses. *Am. Rev. Resp. Dis.*, 88: September 1963, part 2 of two parts, number 3.

Gwaltney, J. M., and Jordan, W. S., Jr.: The Present Status of Respiratory Viruses. *Med. Clin. N. Amer.*, 47:1155, 1963.

Hamparian, V. V., Hilleman, M. R., and Ketler, A.: Contributions to Characterization and Classification of Animal Viruses. *Proc. Soc. Exper. Biol. & Med.*, 112:1040-50, 1963.

Hilleman, M. R., Hamparian, V. V., Ketler, A., Reilly, C. M., McClelland, L., Cornfeld, D., and Stokes, J., Jr.: Acute Respiratory Illnesses Among Children and Adults. Field Study of Contemporary Importance of Several Viruses and Appraisal of the Literature. *J.A.M.A.*, 180-445-53, 1962.

Hsiung, G. D., Pinheiro, F., and Gabrielson, M. O.: The Virus Diagnostic Laboratory: Functions and Problems Based on Three Years' Experience. *Yale J. Biol. & Med.*, 36: 104-23, 1963.

Lennette, E. H., and Schmidt, N. J. (Eds.): *Diagnostic Procedures for Viral and Rickettsial Diseases.* 3rd ed. New York, American Public Health Association, 1964.

Schmidt, N. J.: Trends in the Laboratory Diagnosis of Viral Infections. *Postgrad. Med.*, 35:488-95, 1964.

Wulff, H., Kidd, P., and Wenner, H. A.: Etiology of Respiratory Infections. Further Studies During Infancy and Childhood. *Pediatrics*, 33:30-44, 1964.

CHAPTER SIXTY-FIVE

Collagen Diseases (Dermatomyositis, Diffuse Scleroderma [Progressive Systemic Sclerosis], Disseminated Lupus Erythematosus [SLE] and Periarteritis Nodosa [Polyarteritis Nodosa])

WILLIAM CURTIS ADAMS, M.D.

Dermatomyositis, diffuse scleroderma, disseminated lupus erythematosus and periarteritis nodosa are regarded today as specific entities. Overlapping clinical and immunochemical findings in these diseases and with rheumatic fever, rheumatoid arthritis, thrombotic thrombocytopenic purpura and anaphylactoid purpura have led to their common grouping as the collagen or connective tissue or mesenchymal diseases. Future developments, perhaps most likely in the field of immunoserology, may alter such groupings.

As the origin and pathogenesis of dermatomyositis, diffuse scleroderma, disseminated lupus erythematosus and periarteritis nodosa are clarified, the therapy of the individual entity and its pulmonary complications may well become primarily prophylactic. The theoretical elimination of rheumatic fever by early recognition and control of streptococcal infections is cited by way of illustration. Presently we are limited to the recognition of these four diagnostic possibilities from clinical findings, i.e. skin involvement, muscle pain, arthritis, fever, and cardiac, visceral and pulmonary involvement. Alteration of the hemoglobin, white blood cell count, platelet count, serum protein fractions, demonstration of the L.E. cell phenomenon and carefully selected skin, muscle, renal and lung biopsies may provide important substantiating information.

For practical purposes, the pulmonary manifestations are so similar for all four of these entities that they will be arbitrarily discussed as a group. (Figures 1 through 4 illustrate the variety of pulmonary involvement found in these conditions.) Although the occurrence of primary involvement is questioned by some, various pulmonary findings have been reported. These range from miliary involvement in dermatomyositis to pleural effusion in systemic lupus erythematosus. The very nature of these entities predisposes to altered pulmonary function, vascular change, aspiration, mediastinitis from esophageal perforation, cardiac failure and a natural potentiation for super-

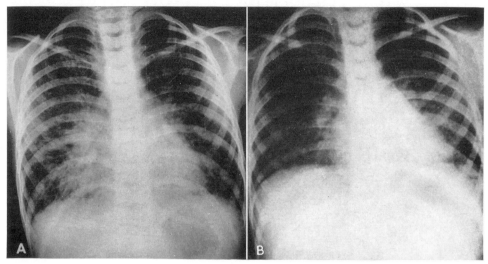

FIGURE 65–1. *A,* Dermatomyositis presenting with pulmonary manifestations resembling miliary tuberculosis. Five year-old white boy with clinical and associated features consistent with a diagnosis of acute dermatomyositis. *B,* Same patient showing clearing of lesion 6 days after film taken on admission. During the interval the child received steroid therapy without antituberculous therapy. (From Dubowitz and Dubowitz: *Arch. Dis. Childhood,* 39:294, 1964.)

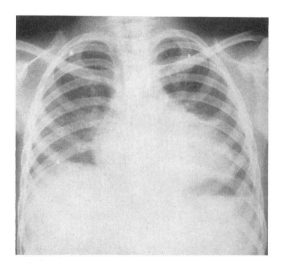

FIGURE 65–2. Disseminated lupus erythematosus. A 10-year-old Negro girl with arthritis, fever and shortness of breath. Clinical course and laboratory findings were consistent with the diagnosis. Illustration shows cardiac enlargement and secondary pulmonary findings despite antimicrobial, steroid and digitalis therapy. Respiratory symptoms were a definite part of this child's illness. (Supplied by the kindness of M. Q. Jenkins, M.D., and J. R. Paul, Jr., M.D., Department of Pediatrics, Medical College of South Carolina)

imposed infection. In addition, the naturally increased susceptibility to infection is further increased and masked by present-day modalities of therapy (corticosteroids and other immunosuppressant agents).

The fact remains that whether primary or secondary, varied and nonspecific pulmonary involvement does occur and contributes significantly to the morbidity and mortality of these cases. Rose reports that at least one third of the cases of periarteritis have major pulmonary disease antedating the establishment of the diagnosis. All of these, with the exception of progressive systemic sclerosis, have been reported throughout childhood, and progressive systemic sclerosis makes its appearance with puberty.

Interpretation of the pulmonary findings is further complicated by the frequency of cardiac involvement and renal failure. Unfortunately, the roentgenographic examination of the chest usually does not provide an indication of the causation of the lung pathology.

Prophylaxis

If pulmonary manifestations are not present when either dermatomyositis, dis-

seminated lupus erythematosus, diffuse scleroderma or periarteritis nodosa is diagnosed, the likelihood of later occurrence is high. The best prophylactic measures cannot ensure against such pulmonary involvement, but every attempt at prevention should be made.

1. Each patient should be provided maximum protection from preventable diseases, e.g. measles, pertussis, diptheria, poliomyelitis.

2. Immunologic deficiencies should be corrected, e.g. agammaglobulinemia when present.

3. Therapy of specific superimposed infectious diseases should be designed to include prevention of expected complications, e.g. penicillin for streptococcal infections to prevent rheumatic fever or isonicotinic acid hydrazide for active primary tuberculosis to prevent postprimary complications. (See the chapter on Tuberculosis, page 656.)

4. Suspected etiologic agents should be eliminated, e.g. avoidance of a drug or drugs suspected of being the cause of systemic lupus erythematosus.

5. A carefully planned physiotherapy program to provide maximum pulmonary function and to teach the patient the essentials of postural drainage and respira-

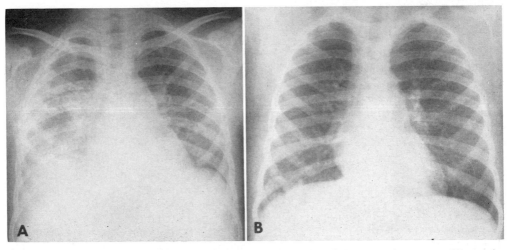

FIGURE 65–3. *A,* Twelve-year-old Negro boy with disseminated lupus erythematosus. Illustration shows nonspecific pulmonary findings during acute exacerbation. *B,* Same patient 10½ months after acute phase seen in *A.* Persistent findings in right lower lobe are striking. (From Dubowitz and Dubowitz: *Arch. Dis. Childhood,* 39:294, 1964.)

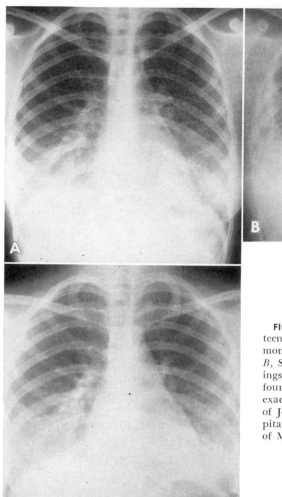

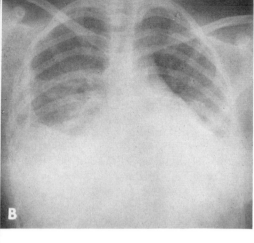

FIGURE 65–4. *A*, Periarteritis nodosa. Thirteen-year-old Negro girl with nonspecific pulmonary findings preceding acute exacerbation. *B*, Same patient 2 weeks later. Nonspecific findings of effusion and cardiac enlargement are found. *C*, Four months after treatment of acute exacerbation depicted in *A*, *B* and *C*. (Courtesy of John Kirkpatrick, M.D., St. Christopher's Hospital for Children and Temple University School of Medicine, Philadelphia.)

tory control before they are needed for active therapy should be instituted. Many of the related symptoms of each of these four syndromes require physiotherapy, e.g. arthritis and muscle pain, but the use of physiotherapy to prevent or treat potential pulmonary complications is often overlooked.

Inspiration is basically an active muscular activity, and expiration results from the relaxation of the inspiratory muscles coupled with the elastic lung tissue reaction to the stretching of inspiration. The diaphragm and the external intercostal muscles are the main muscles of inspiration producing chest expansion antero-

posteriorly, transversely and vertically. Restrictions of chest motion by the muscular, skin or pulmonary involvement of one of these syndromes will understandably lead to pulmonary complications; hence the need for maintaining maximum possible function.

The removal of secretions within the lung is accomplished by the ciliary movement of the epithelial cells coupled with the constant change of the bronchi, which widen and lengthen with inspiration and narrow and shorten with expiration. The cough is used to augment the cleaning of the bronchi and trachea. Correct coughing does not always occur naturally. Demonstration of the basic tussive mechanism in anticipation of need can be helpful. Since sufficient air must be peripheral to the material to be expressed, a slow inspiration permitting alveolar filling is essential. If this action is rapid, secretions may be driven deeper into the bronchus. A sudden cessation of inspiration and glottic relaxation timed with the contraction of the abdominal, serratus anterior, latissimus dorsi and other muscles causes a rush of air through a narrowing bronchus, giving sufficient pressure to move mucus into larger air passages for expectoration. With muscle fatigue, thickening of mucus, prolonged expiration, and so on, cough efficiency may be reduced. In every case positioning of the patient to permit postural drainage of each lung segment separately, maximum use of the local muscular effort and possibly frappage may be valuable adjuncts toward the maintenance or restoration of pulmonary function. (See the chapter on Diagnostic and Therapeutic Procedures, page 80.)

The positioning for postural drainage does have special problems with babies and small children. Firm mummification with a blanket and careful positioning on the lap of a therapist make it easy to place a child in any needed position and to provide the greatest security for the child. In addition, most children are carefully taught at home and at school that they must not spit. This training must be overcome to provide a good pulmonary toilet.

6. Since aspiration becomes a serious threat in each of these conditions, proper eating techniques emphasizing small size of bolus, care in deglutination and avoidance of distractions while swallowing should be emphasized as the disease progresses.

Treatment

Once pulmonary involvement is associated with any of these collagen diseases, active therapy must be instituted.

1. The patient's history of exposure to infectious disease must be carefully considered along with bacteriologic and viral cultures and serologic control, and clinical and roentgenographic findings.

2. Regardless of the cause of the pulmonary involvement, appropriate effort to improve pulmonary function should be made. The aspects of physiotherapy and postural drainage discussed under Prophylaxis will be brought into play now as part of active therapy.

3. Intermittent or continuous surgical drainage of fluid collections may be in order.

4. The individual patient will require respiratory support carefully selected to meet his needs. Such support will vary from increased humidification or oxygenation in the inspired air to the provision of a complete mechanical substitute for the breathing process. When the latter extreme becomes necessary, the selection will depend upon the availability of equipment and the experience of the physician and nursing personnel. Intermittent positive-pressure breathing, with or without wetting agents, as well as complete positive- or negative-pressure breathing replacement, may be considered. Today such equipment will provide variability in both the duration and the pressure involved in the inspiratory effort, in the duration of the respiratory lag period and in the amount of patient effort needed to initiate respiratory movements.

5. When tracheostomy or endotracheal intubation is required as a part of the therapy, careful tracheal toilet must be observed to reduce the morbidity of the procedure. Detailed attention must be paid to the amount of suctioning pressure, the cycling and duration of the suctioning attempt, the cleanliness of equipment, and so forth. The basic principles include clean technique, suctioning during the expiratory phase, and the avoidance of trauma. These same basic principles must be applied to the suctioning of the entire respiratory tree.

6. If aspiration secondary to palatorespiratory involvement is a problem, nasogastric or gastrostomy tube feedings

should be considered. The advantages of gastrostomy feedings for the critically ill patient or for the patient with long-term debilitating disease are often overlooked today. Either method, when appropriate, affords an opportunity for nutritional support not possible with parenteral feeding.

If superimposed infection is not ruled out, appropriate antimicrobial agents should be administered. The therapy may be altered when culture and serologic results become available.

7. Every effort must be made to provide maximal cardiac and renal function, to prevent the development of contractures or pressure sores, and to provide optimum evacuation of bowel and bladder without increasing dangers of infection, perforation, and the like. The selection of appropriate medical therapeutic aids ranging from aspirin to the immunosuppressive drugs such as the corticosteroids should be based upon the symptomatology of the individual patient. The argument as to the immunosuppressive agents will continue, but such therapy must be given serious consideration in every case.

Basically, all the modalities of therapy must be carefully tailored to the individual patient in an attempt to maintain maximum comfort and as normal physiologic function as is possible without inducing complications.

REFERENCES

General

Talbot, S. H.: The Nonrheumatoid Connective Tissue Disorders. A.M.A. *Arch. Int. Med.,* 100:535, 1957.

Thacker, E. W.: *Postural Drainage and Respiratory Control.* 2nd ed. London, Lloyd-Luke (Medical Books), Ltd., 1963.

Venters, H. D., Jr., and Good, R. A.: Current Concepts of the Pathogenesis of the So-Called Collagen Diseases. *Pediat. Clin. N. Amer.,* 10:1017, 1963.

Wedgwood, R. J.: Diseases of Mesenchymal Origin; in W. E. Nelson, (Ed.): *Textbook of Pediatrics.* 8th ed. Philadelphia, W. B. Saunders Company, 1964.

Wolf, J. K.: Primary Acquired Agammaglobinemia with Family History of Collagen Diseases and Hematologic Disorders. *New England J. Med.,* 266:473, 1962.

Dermatomyositis

Bitnum, S., Daeschner, C. W., Jr., Traves, L. B., Dodge, W. S., and Hopps, H. C.: Dermatomyositis. *J. Pediat.,* 64:101, 1964.

Carlisle, J. W., and Good, R. A.: Dermatomyositis in Childhood. *Jour. Lancet,* 79:266, 1959.

Cook, C. D., Rosen, F. S., and Banker, B. Q.: Dermatomyositis and Focal Scleroderma. *Pediat. Clin. N. Amer.,* 10:979, 1963.

Dubowitz, L. M. S., and Dubowitz, V.: Acute Dermatomyositis Presenting with Pulmonary Manifestations. *Arch. Dis. Childhood,* 39:293, 1964.

Farber, S., and Vawter, G. F.: Clinical Pathological Conference (Dermatomyositis). *J. Pediat.,* 57:784, 1960.

Pearson, C. M.: Rheumatic Manifestations of Polymyositis and Dermatomyositis. *Arth. & Rheum.,* 2:127, 1959.

Roberts, H. N., and Brunsting, L. A.: Dermatomyositis in Children; A Summary of 40 Cases. *Postgrad. Med.,* 16:396, 1954.

Williams, R. C., Jr.: Dermatomyositis and Malignancy: A Review of the Literature. *Ann. Int. Med.,* 50:1174, 1959.

Polyarteritis

Dodge, W. S., Travis, L. B., and Daeschner, C. W., Jr.: Anaphylactoid Purpura, Polyarteritis and Purpura Fulminans. *Pediat. Clin. N. Amer.,* 10:879, 1963.

Fager, D. B., Bigler, J. A., and Simonds, J. P.: Polyarteritis Nodosa in Infancy and Childhood. *J. Pediat.,* 39:65, 1951.

Farber, S., and Craig, J. N.: Clinical Pathological Conference (Polyarteritis). *J. Pediat.,* 56:120, 1960.

Miller, H. G., and Daby, R.: Clinical Aspects of Polyarteritis Nodosa. *Quart. J. Med.,* 15:255, 1946.

Mundy, W. L., Walker, W. G., Jr., Bickerman, H. A., and Beck, G. J.: Periarteritis Nodosa, Report of a Case Treated with ACTH and Cortisone. *Am. J. Med.,* 11:630, 1951.

Rich, A. R., and Gregory, J. E.: Experimental Demonstration that Periarteritis Nodosa Is a Manifestation of Hypersensitivity. *Bull. Johns Hopkins Hosp.,* 72:65, 1943.

Rose, G. A., and Spencer, H.: Polyarteritis Nodosa. *Quart. J. Med.,* 26:43, 1957.

Scleroderma

Bloch, K. J., and Bunim, J. J.: Sjogren's Syndrome and Its Relation to Connective Tissue Diseases. *J. Chron. Dis.,* 16:915, 1963.

Castleman, B., and Kibbee, B. W.: Clinical Pathological Conference (Scleroderma). *New England J. Med.,* 262:981, 1960.

Chazen, E. M., Cook, C. D., and Cohen, J.: Focal Scleroderma. *J. Pediat.,* 60:385, 1962.

Greenberg, L. M., Geppert, C., Worthin, H. G., and Good, A.: Scleroderma "Adultorum" in Children. *Pediatrics*, 32:1044, 1963.

Opie, L. H.: The Pulmonary Manifestations of Generalized Scleroderma (Progressive Systemic Sclerosis). *Arch. Dis. Childhood*, 28:665, 1955.

Rodnan, G. P.: A Review of Recent Observations and Current Theories on the Etiology and Pathogenesis of Progressive Systemic Sclerosis (Diffuse Scleroderma). *J. Chron. Dis.*, 16:929, 1963.

Shuford, W. H., Seaman, W. B., and Goldman, A.: Pulmonary Manifestations of Scleroderma. A.M.A. *Arch. Int. Med.*, 92:85, 1953.

Zarafonitis, C. J. D.: Treatment of Scleroderma. *Ann. Int. Med.*, 50:343, 1959.

Systemic Lupus Erythematosus

Domz, C. A., McNamara, O. H., and Holzapfel, N. F.: Tetracycline Provocation in Lupus Erythematosus. *Ann. Int. Med.*, 50:1217, 1959.

Harvey, A. McG., Schulman, L. E., Tumulty, P. A., Conely, C. L., and Schoenrich, E. H.: Systemic Lupus Erythematosus: Review of the Literature and Clinical Analysis of 138 Cases. *Medicine*, 33:291, 1954.

Holman, H.: Systemic Lupus Erythematosus. *J. Pediat.*, 56:109, 1960.

Nice, C. N., Jr.: Congenital Disseminated Lupus Erythematosus. *Am. J. Roent.*, 88:585, 1962.

Peterson, R. D. A., Vernier, R. L., and Good, R. A.: Lupus Erythematosus. *Pediat. Clin. N. Amer.*, 10:941, 1963.

CHAPTER SIXTY-SIX

Familial Dysautonomia

EDWIN L. KENDIG, JR., M.D.

Familial dysautonomia is a rare, heritable disorder found mostly in Jewish children. The diagnosis is a clinical one in which the symptoms and signs are primarily referable to the nervous system; although disseminated lesions in the reticular formation of the brain stem have been described, no satisfactory pathologic basis has been established.

The constant features of the syndrome are defective lacrimation and corneal sensory impairment, often resulting in ulcers of the cornea; erythematous blotching of the skin and excessive perspiration; drooling, excessive salivation and lessened ability to swallow; emotional instability; hyporeflexia or areflexia, hypotonia, poor motor coordination and relative indifference to pain.

The children are small and may be mentally retarded. Frequently there is intermittent hypertension, and postural hypotension may occur. Urinary frequency occurs in a large number of the cases.

Lingual fungiform papillae may be absent or decreased in number. Impaired temperature regulation and feeding problems may be present during infancy.

Several of the altered responses in these children may be used to support the clinical diagnosis of familial dysautonomia, although none is itself diagnostic. Smith and co-workers have suggested four as test possibilities: (1) reduced skin reactivity to intradermally injected 1:1000 histamine phosphate solution; (2) pupillary supersensitivity to 2.5 per cent methacholine (Mecholyl) instilled into the eye; (3) exaggerated parasympathetic responses to intravenously administered methacholine; and (4) decreased taste perception and discrimination.

Riley noted that frequent pulmonary infection is an almost constant feature in this syndrome. The recurrent pulmonary lesions are probably the result of a defective swallowing mechanism with associated aspiration. Roentgenograms may re-

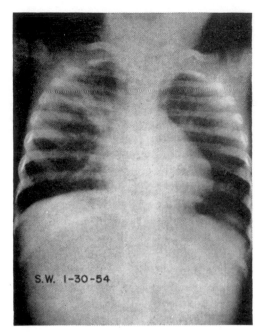

FIGURE 66–1. Fine bilateral interstitial infiltrations with diffuse emphysema, depressed diaphragms and atelectasis of the upper lobe of the right lung. (R. E. Moloshok and J. E. Moseley: *Pediatrics,* 17:327, 1956.)

veal varying combinations of infiltration, atelectasis and emphysema, the findings closely resembling those seen in fibrocystic pulmonary disease.

Because of their inability to respond normally to an atmosphere with increased carbon dioxide concentration or low oxygen concentration, these children should be protected from high altitudes and warned against underwater swimming.

The prognosis is poor; some children attain adult life.

Treatment of the syndrome is supportive and symptomatic (see p. 51) and should include protection of the cornea. Since the pulmonary lesions so closely resemble those of fibrocystic disease, therapy for this important manifestation of the disease is essentially the same as that for pulmonary fibrocystic disease, and the reader is referred to that discussion (p. 557).

REFERENCES

Moloshok, R. E., and Moseley, J. E.: Familial Dysautonomia: Pulmonary Manifestations. *Pediatrics,* 17:327, 1956.

Moloshok, R. E., and Reuben, R. N.: Familial Autonomic Dysfunction. *J. Mt. Sinai Hosp.,* 21:137, 1954.

Riley, C. M.: Familial Autonomic Dysfunction. *J.A.M.A.,* 149:1532, 1952.

Riley, C. M., Freedman, A. M., and Langford, W. S.: Further Observations on Familial Dysautonomia. *Pediatrics,* 14:475, 1954.

Riley, C. M., Day, R. L., Greeley, D. McL., and Langford, W. S.: Central Autonomic Dysfunction with Defective Lacrimation. *Pediatrics,* 3:468, 1949.

Riley, C. M., and Moore, R. H.: Familial Dysautonomia and Related Disorders. *Pediatrics,* 37:435, 1966.

Smith, A. A., and Dancis, J.: Response to Intradermal Histamine in Familial Dysautonomia —A Diagnostic Test. *J. Pediat.,* 63:889, 1963.

Smith, A. A., Hirsch, J. I., and Dancis, J.: Responses to Infused Methacholine in Familial Dysautonomia. *Pediatrics,* 36:225, 1965.

Smith, A. A., Taylor, T., and Wortis, S. B.: Abnormal Catecholamine Metabolism in Familial Dysautonomia. *New England J. Med.,* 268:705, 1963.

SECTION XI

Disorders of the Respiratory Tract Due to Trauma

CHAPTER SIXTY-SEVEN

Disorders of the Respiratory Tract Due to Trauma

ARNOLD M. SALZBERG, M.D.

The incidence of thoracic trauma in the infant and the child is exceedingly low and is usually confined to automobile accidents, the battered child syndrome, and falls from a considerable height. Stab and bullet wounds are rare. Nevertheless the complete spectrum of chest trauma has been recorded and includes pneumothorax, hemothorax, destruction of the integrity of the chest wall and diaphragm, thoracic visceral damage, and combined thoracoabdominal injuries (Fig. 1).

As in the adult, the significance of thoracic trauma parallels the pulmonary, cardiac and systemic dysfunction which follows, and in the pediatric age group, because of chest wall resiliency, physiologic aberrations can occur with trauma that does not fracture or penetrate. The interruption of satisfactory respiration and circulation secondary to chest injury is frequently complicated by blood loss and hypotension, and all three factors must be quickly reversed for survival. Shock from hemorrhage can usually be managed by intelligent, arithmetic replacement which is monitored by serial blood pressures, hematocrit, central venous pressure and, if necessary, blood volume determinations. Restoration of the normal cardiopulmonary function fundamentally depends on a clear airway, intact chest and diaphragm and unrestricted heart-lung dynamics. This, in most instances, can be accomplished by maneuvers other than thoracotomy.

STERNAL FRACTURES

Fractures of the sternum in infancy and childhood follow high compression crush injuries, and are usually associated with other thoracic and orthopedic problems elsewhere.

On physical examination there is local tenderness, ecchymosis and sometimes a peculiar concavity or paradoxical respiratory movement, but usually the sternal segments are well aligned without too much displacement. Dyspnea, cyanosis, tachycardia and hypotension may be evidence of an underlying contused heart.

Cardiac tamponade and acute traumatic myocardial damage must be ruled out by various studies, including serial electrocardiograms. If the bony deformity is minimal, injection of a local anesthetic and appropriate posture will suffice. Markedly displaced fragments are reduced under general anesthesia by the closed or open technique in order to prevent a traumatic pectus excavatum. Violent paradoxical respirations can be controlled by strapping, sand bags, operative fixation or assisted mechanical respiration.

FRACTURED RIBS

Rib fractures are unusual in pediatrics because of the extreme flexibility of the osseous and cartilaginous framework of the thorax. Crush and direct blow injuries are the usual etiologic factors. In

781

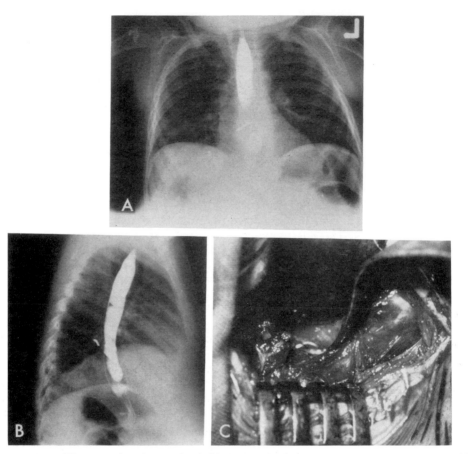

FIGURE 67–1. The posterior chest wall of this 8-year-old boy was penetrated by an object which was apparently accelerated by a power mower operating 8 feet away. *A, B,* Posteroanterior and lateral chest films with barium in the esophagus demonstrate an opaque foreign body in the posterior mediastinum. *C,* Through an extrapleural approach a curved nail, seen just below the stump of the resected rib, and lying on the aorta, was removed from the posterior mediastinum.

addition, manual compression of the lateral chest wall, rickets and osteogenesis imperfecta have been incriminated. Multiple fractures of the middle ribs can be seen in the battered child syndrome (Fig. 2). The upper ribs are protected by the scapula and related muscles, and the lower ones are quite resilient.

Violence to the chest wall may produce pulmonary and cardiac lacerations and contusions, and a variety of pneumothoraces or hemothorax. Critical respiratory distress may also follow multiple anterior rib fractures, in which the integrity of the thoracic cage is destroyed and the involved chest becomes flail. This unsupported area of chest wall moves inward with inspiration and outward with expiration, and these paradoxical respiratory excursions inexorably lead to dyspnea. The explosive expiration of coughing is dissipated and made ineffectual by the paradoxical movement and intercostal pain. In effect, the ideal preparation for the wet lung syndrome, airway obstruction, atelectasis and pneumonia has been established.

The clinical picture includes local pain which is aggravated by motion. Tenderness is elicited by pressure, applied directly over the fracture, or elsewhere on the same rib. The fracture site may be edematous and ecchymotic. These minimal findings with simple, restricted fractures can be expanded to the severest form of ventilatory distress with a flail chest and lung injury.

Chest x-rays demonstrate the extent and displacement of the fractures and underlying visceral damage.

Treatment of the uncomplicated fracture involves control of pain in order to permit unrestricted respiration. Mild sedation, strapping, and intercostal nerve block with short- and long-acting local anesthetics all have a place. Displacement requires no therapy. With severe fractures, the alleviation of pain and restoration of cough are important and can be provided by nerve blocks. Thoracentesis and insertion of intercostal tubes should be done promptly for pneumothorax and hemothorax, and shock should be managed by appropriate replacement therapy and oxygen.

Paradoxical respiratory excursions with flail chest must be brought under prompt control to help prevent the wet lung syndrome, which may be the morbid pulmonary complication. Strapping over a bol-

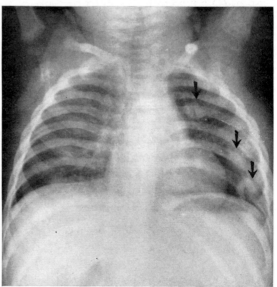

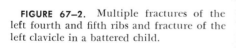
FIGURE 67–2. Multiple fractures of the left fourth and fifth ribs and fracture of the left clavicle in a battered child.

ster may provide some rigidity; if this fails, immobilization by towel clips or nonabsorbable sutures may be tried. Recently intermittent positive-pressure respiration has been used for the paradox and respiratory insufficiency. In spite of vigorous therapy, secretions cannot be avoided and are attacked by tracheal catheterization and bronchoscopy. Tracheostomy, then, becomes useful in providing an avenue for the control of profuse secretions, diminishing the dead space and bypassing an obstructed airway. Mechanical respiration can be applied and maintained through the tracheostomy for several weeks.

During the first year of life tracheostomy is a morbid operation and should be avoided, if possible. Secretions may be difficult to aspirate, and the small tracheostomy tube becomes easily plugged; distal infection, often with staphylococci, is poorly handled, and withdrawal of the tracheostomy tube, at times, is a precarious and unpredictable adventure. Nevertheless, even in this age group, and certainly later, tracheostomy can be mandatory and lifesaving in specific instances of chest trauma.

The decision for tracheostomy in cases of chest injury can often be made on the basis of (1) a mechanically obstructed airway which cannot be managed more conservatively, (2) flail chest. The unstable, paradoxing chest wall can be controlled for long periods of time by assisted positive-pressure respirations through a short, cuffed laryngectomy tube.

Often, however, the decision for tracheostomy is first broached in the presence of minimal dyspnea. In this situation use of blood alveolar gas studies can augment the clinical impression and intercept clinical respiratory failure. Serial measurements of arterial carbon dioxide tension are a satisfactory chemical guide to imminent ventilatory distress and the need for and efficiency of assisted or controlled mechanical respiration, since normal values rule out the presence of anoxia.

TRAUMATIC PNEUMOTHORAX

Traumatic tension and open pneumothorax are rare in infants and children, in whom a very mobile mediastinum would compound the usual cardiorespiratory distress. Both types of injuries are formidable and require specific maneuvers to reverse a malignant chain of events.

The creation of a tension pneumothorax in which intrapleural pressures approach or exceed atmospheric pressures requires a valvular mechanism through which air entering the pleura exceeds the amount escaping. The positive intrapleural pressure is dissipated by a mediastinal shift, which compresses the opposite lung in the presence of ipsilateral pulmonary collapse, and angulates the great vessels entering and leaving the heart. Intrapleural tension can be increased by traumatic hemothorax, and respiratory exchange and cardiac output are critically diminished by this form of mediastinal tamponade.

The etiologic possibilities, in addition to chest wall and lung trauma, include rupture of the esophagus, a pulmonary cyst, and an emphysematous lobe and postoperative bronchial fistula. These latter sources of tension pneumothorax almost always require thoracotomy for control.

The clinical findings may include external evidence of a wound, tachypnea, dyspnea, cyanosis with hyperresonance, absent or transmitted breath sounds and dislocation of the trachea and apical cardiac impulse. The hemithoraces may be asymmetrical, with the involved side larger.

A confirmatory x-ray film is comforting, but often cannot be afforded in this thoracic emergency. Needle aspiration is indicated for tension or a pneumothorax exceeding 25 per cent. Prompt relief and pulmonary expansion can be anticipated if the source of the intrapleural air has been controlled. Obviously, a traumatic valvular defect in the chest wall can be occluded. If the pulmonary air leak persists or recurs, the possibility of further tension pneumothorax is circumvented by the insertion of one or more intercostal tubes connected to underwater drainage with mild suction. Most instances of traumatic tension pneumothorax will require tube drainage for permanent decompression, although the needle is indispensable for its emergency management. Stubborn bronchopleural fistulas which continue to remain widely patent in spite of adequate intercostal tube deflation may require operative closure.

An open, sucking pneumothorax is a second, equally urgent thoracic emergency in which atmospheric air has direct, unimpeded entrance into and exit from a relatively free pleural space. This is almost invariably accomplished through a good-sized, traumatic hole in the chest wall. Ingress of air during inspiration and egress during expiration produce an extreme degree of paradoxical respiration and mediastinal flutter which is partially regulated by the size of the chest wall defect in comparison to the circumference of the trachea. If a considerable segment of chest wall is absent, more air is exchanged at this site than through the trachea, since pressures are similar. Inspiration collapses the ipsilateral lung and drives its alveolar air into the opposite side. During expiration the air returns across the carina. In addition, the mediastinum becomes a wildly swinging pendulum compressing uninjured lung on inspiration and lung on the injured side during expiration. Obviously, under these circumstances little effective ventilation is taking place because of the tremendous increase in the pulmonary dead space and decreased tidal exchange. A totally ineffective cough completes the clinical picture.

The diagnosis is readily made by inspection of the thoracic wound and the peculiar sound of air going in and coming out of the chest.

The emergency management of this critical situation demands prompt occlusion of the chest wall defect by bulky sterile dressings and measures to prevent conversion of this open pneumothorax into an equally aggravating tension pneumothorax which can occur if the underlying lung has been traumatized. In this regard, Haynes has emphasized the importance of simultaneous pleural decompression through the original wound by closed intercostal tube drainage. After systemic stabilization more formal surgical débridement, reconstruction and closure can be done in the operating room.

HEMOTHORAX

Blood in the pleural cavity is perhaps the commonest sequela of thoracic trauma, regardless of type. The source of the bleeding is either systemic (high pressure) from the chest wall, or pulmonary (low pressure). Hemorrhage from pulmonary vessels is usually self-limiting unless major tributaries have been transected.

Intrapleural blood eventually clots and becomes organized fibrous tissue. Prior to this, pulmonary compression and mediastinal displacement, with reduced vital capacity and atrial filling, can occur. With the development of a fibrothorax, the changes in cardiorespiratory dynamics become chronic as the lung becomes incarcerated and the chest wall immobilized. Finally, empyema from secondary contamination is always a threat in the presence of a pleural space filled with blood.

The acute findings are those of blood loss compounded by respiratory distress and perhaps hemoptysis. The trachea and apical cardiac impulse are dislocated, the percussion note is flat, and the breath sounds are indistinct. The actual diagnosis is confirmed by thoracentesis after adequate x-ray studies, if time allows.

It has been established that aspiration of a hemothorax and expansion of the underlying lung do not instigate additional bleeding. Accordingly, the local management of hemothorax is prompt and total evacuation without air replacement. The dead space is abolished, and without it empyema cannot occur.

clotting is circumvented, and pulmonary function restored by pulmonary expansion. Further extensive bleeding must be controlled by operation. Obviously, systemic resuscitation has not been overlooked.

In spite of vigorous initial therapy, clotting, loculation and infection may supervene. Enzymatic pleural débridement should be attempted, but is often disappointing. Many of these patients eventually come to decortication.

TRACHEOBRONCHIAL TRAUMA

Rupture of the trachea or bronchus in the infant and the child is usually preceded by a severe compression injury of the chest or sharp blow to the anterior part of the neck. This discontinuity of a major airway is characterized by intrathoracic tension phenomena; later, stricture at the site of rupture leads to loss of lung function by sepsis and atelectasis.

Violently progressive interstitial emphysema, pneumomediastinum, tension pneumothorax and hemoptysis are fairly specific. Upper rib fractures usually occur on the involved side, but certainly are not constant in children with partial tracheal or bronchial transection.

Conventional chest roentgenograms and the air tracheobronchogram can suggest the diagnosis in the presence of a compatible clinical picture, but bronchoscopic demonstration of the rupture is usually necessary. The diagnosis may not be suspected during the acute phase of smaller transections of major or minor bronchi, but becomes obvious when late stricture with distal atelectasis and chronic pneumonitis is related retrospectively with a history of fairly severe chest trauma.

The initial management of bronchial rupture is concerned with the maintenance of a patent airway and decompression of the pleura and mediastinum by one or more intercostal tubes connected to closed drainage. Confirmatory endoscopy and elective bronchoplasty within several months is followed by little or no

loss of pulmonary function distal to the narrowed segment (Weisel and Jake; Mahaffey). Emergency bronchoscopy and repair of the defect are done if the air leak and intrathoracic tension cannot be otherwise controlled.

Severe lacerations of the trachea can be immeasurably helped by bypassing the glottis with a tracheostomy during the acute phase while preparing the patient for emergency tracheal repair. Smaller tears may heal spontaneously with tracheostomy alone; others will result in stricture and require later tracheorrhaphy.

PULMONARY COMPRESSION INJURY

Explosive blasts compress flexible ribs, the sternum and cartilages against the lungs with sudden, violent increase in intra-alveolar pressure. Alveolar disruption, interstitial emphysema and pneumothorax may follow if the glottis is closed when the compression occurs. Distribution of this force to the great, valveless veins of the mediastinum leads to venous distention, extravasation of blood and purplish edema of the head, neck and upper extremities. The pulmonary contusion is represented pathologically by edema, hemorrhage and atelectasis.

Clinically, there may be dyspnea, cough, chest pain and hemoptysis. The face and the neck can be grotesquely swollen with crepitus and submucous and subconjunctival hemorrhage (Fig. 3). There need not be evidence of external trauma or fractured ribs in a child, and, accordingly, the indication for chest x-ray is merely the possible history of a blast, acceleration (fall) or deceleration (automobile) injury. Unilateral or bilateral pulmonary hematoma, hemothorax, pneumothorax and pneumomediastinum can be seen.

With mild injuries the subcutaneous emphysema and purplish hue gradually and spontaneously disappear over several days. Patients with more serious blast injuries are treated initially for anoxia and

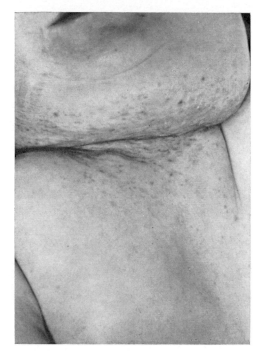

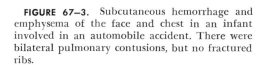

FIGURE 67–3. Subcutaneous hemorrhage and emphysema of the face and chest in an infant involved in an automobile accident. There were bilateral pulmonary contusions, but no fractured ribs.

hypotension, and attention is then directed toward the wet lung, atelectasis and pleural complications. Rapid progression of the mediastinal and subcutaneous emphysema would implicate a serious disruption of the trachea, bronchi or lungs and perhaps require thoracotomy.

POST-TRAUMATIC ATELECTASIS (WET LUNG)

With pulmonary contusion from any source, production of tracheobronchial secretions is stimulated, but elimination is impeded by airway obstruction, pain, and depression of cough. The addition of hemorrhage to these accumulated secretions produces atelectasis in the damaged lung and inevitable infection—a syndrome aptly called "wet lung."

The clinical findings are dyspnea and cyanosis, an incessant, unremunerative little cough with wheezing and audible rattling, and gross rhonchi and rales. Chest x-rays show varying degrees of unilateral and bilateral atelectasis.

The syndrome demands vigorous treatment to avoid morbidity and mortality. This should be started, in a preventive sense, in all instances of chest trauma, by frequent changes of position, insistence on coughing, small amounts of depressant drugs, oxygen, humidification and antibiotics. If a child with chest trauma will not cough, tracheal catheterization, popularized by Haight, should be started prior to early signs of the wet lung syndrome. Failure at this step should be followed in quick succession by bronchoscopy and even tracheostomy if endoscopic aspiration is required too frequently. Spencer has recently emphasized the advantages of endoscopy through the tracheal stoma.

CARDIAC TRAUMA

Cardiac wounds should be suspected after penetration of any part of the chest, lower part of the neck or upper part of the abdomen. The possibility of heart injury also exists in the presence of blunt trauma to the anterior or left hemithorax with laceration by fractured sternum or ribs or severe compression between sternum and vertebral column. Blood loss with perforation varies between exsanguination internally or externally, to minimal bleeding with or without acute cardiac tamponade. Tamponade usually follows trauma to the myocardium in the presence of intact pleura bilaterally. The hemopericardium cannot decompress into the pleura or externally, since the pericardial wound is dislocated from the soft tissue wound of entrance by the pericardial blood. This increased intrapericardial pressure constricts the heart and great veins, and the venous return and cardiac output are critically impaired.

The physical findings with acute tamponade are often classic. The veins of the neck and upper extremity may be distended. The heart sounds are distant and perhaps inaudible. The systolic pressure is depressed, the pulse pressure is narrow, and the pulse rate relatively slow in spite of the lowered blood pressure.

The venous pressure is the most valuable laboratory determination and will be elevated. Fluoroscopy demonstrates an inactive cardiac silhouette whose margins may not be widened.

With this picture, in addition to systemic resuscitation, emergency aspiration of the pericardial sac through a left costoxiphoid approach should be performed while the operating suite is being prepared. Aspiration of small amounts of blood can restore cardiopulmonary dynamics. If bleeding and tamponade recur promptly, thoracotomy is indicated.

Nonpenetrating trauma can produce varying degrees of myocardial contusions ranging from a small area of edema to a ruptured chamber. The chest pain and tachycardia may be difficult to evaluate without evidence of cardiac failure. Immediate and serial electrocardiograms are essential for the emergency and late diagnosis of myocardial damage secondary to trauma.

The treatment can follow the standard regimen for coronary occlusion with the exclusion of anticoagulants, and complete rehabilitation can be anticipated. Late complications include chronic constrictive pericarditis, congestive heart failure and ventricular aneurysm.

INJURIES TO THE ESOPHAGUS

Perforation of the esophagus in the pediatric age group can begin in the delivery room from extreme positive-pressure resuscitation or aspiration with a stiff catheter. Later in infancy and childhood, rupture can follow ingestion of lye or a solid foreign body, esophagoscopy, and dilatation without a guiding string. Spontaneous rupture proximal to an esophageal web has been described. Stab and gunshot wounds, as in the adult, can perforate the esophagus.

Clinically, hyperthermia, hypotension, and chest and neck pain mirror the mediastinitis. Pneumomediastinum, tension pneumothorax, subcutaneous emphysema and hematemesis can be seen.

Plain chest x-rays followed by a contrast esophagogram and thoracentesis may demonstrate the tension sequelae, esophageal defect, and perhaps high acid fluid.

The tension pneumothorax must be quickly decompressed and followed promptly by closure of the esophageal defect, mediastinal drainage and massive antibiotics.

THORACOABDOMINAL INJURIES

In the infant and the child combined injury to the thorax and abdomen, including ruptured diaphragm, is usually preceded by a violent traffic accident or other forms of sudden, jolting impact. Splenic and hepatic lacerations commonly occur with minimal external evidence of injury and need not be associated with fractured ribs or soft tissue mutilation.

Clinically, upper abdominal tenderness, rigidity and rebound tenderness almost uniformly accompany lower chest trauma and are explained by the abdominal distribution of the intercostal nerves. Therefore peritoneal irritation, of itself, is not conclusive evidence of a combined or abdominal injury. Careful, repeated examinations correlated with laboratory data are necessary for the diagnosis of intra-abdominal perforation or hemorrhage in the presence of chest trauma. Needle aspiration of the peritoneum may have a place and perhaps should be used more often.

A ruptured diaphragm can occur with an extensive soft tissue injury, and there may be chest pain, dyspnea and hypotension. On inspection the involved chest wall lags during inspiration, and percussion can be dull or hyperresonant. Chest x-rays may show fractured ribs and a mediastinal shift to the right, since in 90 per cent of the cases the posterolateral left leaf of the diaphragm is torn in a radial manner. At times a pneumoperitoneum is seen.

The preliminary management of combined chest-abdominal injuries must provide an adequate airway and circulation, and gastric decompression. Intra-abdominal hemorrhage and perforation with thoracic and abdominal soiling is an obvious indication for immediate exploration. Ideally, a ruptured diaphragm should be repaired within seventy-two hours after the injury, after systemic stabilization.

REFERENCES

Chest Trauma

Avery, E. E., Morch, E. T., and Benson, D. W.: Critically Crushed Chests. *J. Thorac. Surg.,* 32:291, 1956.

Berry, F. B.: Chest Injuries. *Surg., Gynec. & Obst.,* 70:413, 1940.

Betts, R. H.: Thoraco-abdominal Injuries: Report of Twenty-Nine Operated Cases. *Ann. Surg.,* 122:793, 1945.

Blades, B., and Salzberg, A. M.: The Importance of Tracheostomy in Acute Ventilatory Distress. *Milt. Surg.,* 114:184, 1954.

Burke, J., and Jacobs, T. T.: Penetrating Wounds of the Chest. *Ann. Surg.,* 123:363, 1946.

Burke, J. F.: Early Diagnosis of Traumatic Rupture of Bronchus. *J.A.M.A.,* 181:682, 1962.

Carter, B. N., and Guiseffi, J.: Tracheostomy—A Useful Procedure in Thoracic Surgery, with Particular Reference to Its Employment in Crushing Injuries of the Thorax. *J. Thorac. Surg.,* 21:495, 1951.

Carter, R., Wareham, E. E., and Brewer, L. A., III: Rupture of the Bronchus Following Closed Chest Trauma. *Am. J. Surg.,* 104:177, 1962.

Childress, M. E., and Grimes, O. F.: Immediate and Remote Sequelae in Traumatic Diaphragmatic Hernia. *Surg. Gynec. & Obst.,* November 1961, p. 573.

DeBakey, M. E. (Ed.): *The Year Book of General Surgery* (1963-1964 Year Book Series). Chicago, Year Book Medical Publishers, Inc., p. 186.

Edwards, H. C.: *Surgical Emergencies in Children.* Baltimore, William Wood and Company, 1936, p. 213.

Flavell, G.: *An Introduction to Chest Surgery.* London, Oxford University Press, 1957, pp. 67, 68, 70, 71.

Fraser, J.: *Surgery of Childhood.* New York, William Wood and Company, 1926, Vol. II, p. 675.

Fryfogle, J. D.: Discussion of paper by R. L. Anderson: Rupture of the Esophagus. *J. Thorac. Surg.,* 24:369, 1952.

Graivier, L., and Freeark, R. J.: Traumatic Diaphragmatic Hernia. *Arch. Surg.,* 86:33, 1963.

Haight, C.: Intratracheal Suction in the Management of Postoperative Pulmonary Complications. *Ann. Surg.,* 107:218, 1938.

Haynes, B. W., Jr.: Dangers of Emergency Occlusive Dressing in Sucking Wounds of the Chest. *J.A.M.A.,* 150:1404, 1952.

Howell, J. F., Crawford, E. S., and Jordan, G. L.: Flail Chest: Analysis of 100 Patients. *Am. J. Surg.,* 106:628, 1963.

Johnson, J.: Battle Wounds of the Thoracic Cavity. *Ann. Surg.,* 123:321, 1946.

Keshishian, J. M., and Cox, P. A.: Diagnosis and Management of Strangulated Diaphragmatic Hernias. *Surg., Gynec. & Obst.,* 115:626, 1962.

Lindskog, G. E.: Some Historical Aspects of Thoracic Trauma. *J. Thorac. Cardiov. Surg.,* 42:1, 1961.

Lindskog, G. E., Liebow, A. A., and Glenn, W. W. L.: *Thoracic and Cardiovascular Surgery, with Related Pathology.* New York, Appleton-Century-Crofts, Inc., 1962, pp. 3, 6, 13, 16, 17, 19, 22, 25.

Lucido J. L., and Wall, C. A.: Rupture of Diaphragm Due to Blunt Trauma. *Arch. Surg.,* 86:989, 1963.

Mahaffey, D. E., and others: Traumatic Rupture of the Left Main Bronchus Successfully Repaired Eleven Years After Injury. *J. Thorac. Surg.,* 32:312, 1956.

Maloney, J. V., Jr., and McDonald, L.: Treatment of Trauma to Thorax. *Am. J. Surg.,* 105:484, 1963.

Nealon, T. F.: Trauma to the Chest; in J. H. Gibbon (Ed.): *Surgery of the Chest.* Philadelphia, W. B. Saunders Company, 1962, pp. 177, 183.

Paulson, D. L.: Traumatic Bronchial Rupture

with Plastic Repair. *J. Thorac. Surg.*, 22:636, 1951.

Perry, J. F., and Galway, C. F.: Chest Injury Due to Blunt Trauma. *J. Thorac. Cardiov. Surg.*, 49:684, 1965.

Pilcher, R. S.: Trachea, Bronchi, Lungs and Pleura; in J. J. M. Brown (Ed.): *Surgery of Childhood*. Baltimore, Williams & Wilkins Company, 1963, pp. 659, 660, 661, 664.

Ransdell, H. T., and others: Treatment of Flail Chest Injuries with a Piston Respirator. *Am. J. Surg.*, 104:22, 1962.

Richardson, W. R.: Thoracic Emergencies in the Newborn Infant. *Am. J. Surg.*, 105:524, 1963.

Said, S.: Personal communication.

Schwartz, A., and Borman, J. B.: Contusion of the Lung in Childhood. *Arch. Dis. Childhood,* 36:557, 1961.

Segal, S.: Endobronchial Pressure as an Aid to Tracheobronchial Aspiration. *Pediatrics,* 35: 305, 1965.

Shaw, R. R., Paulson, D. L., and Kee, J. L., Jr.: Traumatic Tracheal Rupture. *J. Thorac. Cardiov. Surg.*, 42:281, 1961.

Spencer, F. C.: Treatment of Chest Injuries. *Curr. Probl. Surg.*, January 1964.

Strug, L. H., and others: Severe Crushing In-

juries of the Chest. *J. Thorac. Cardiov. Surg.*, 39:166, 1960.

Swenson, O.: *Pediatric Surgery*. 2nd ed. New York, Appleton-Century-Crofts, Inc., 1962, p. 150.

Taylor, S. F.: *Recent Advances in Surgery*. Boston, Little, Brown and Company, 1946, p. 143.

Warden, H. D., and Mucha, S. J.: Esophageal Perforation Due to Trauma in the Newborn. *Arch. Surg.*, 83:813, 1961.

Webb, W. R.: Chest Injuries. *J. Louisiana Med. Soc.*, 116:1, 1964.

Weisel, W., and Jake, R. J.: Anastomosis of Right Bronchus to Trachea 46 Days Following Complete Bronchial Rupture from External Injury. *Ann. Surg.*, 137:220, 1953.

White, M., and Dennison, W. M.: *Surgery in Infancy and Childhood, a Handbook for Medical Students and General Practitioners*. Edinburgh, E. & S. Livingstone, Ltd., 1958, p. 292.

White, P. D., and Glenby, B. S.; in L. Brahdy and S. Kahn; *Trauma and Disease*. Philadelphia, Lea & Febiger, 1937.

Zollinger, R. W., Creedon, P. J., and Sanguily, J.: Trauma in Children in a General Hospital. *Am. J. Surg.*, 104:855, 1962.

Index